W9-BOE-178

Personal Fitness Training
Theory & Practice

by

Mary Yoke, MA

Editor

Laura A. Gladwin, MS

Published by
Aerobics and Fitness Association of America
15250 Ventura Blvd., Suite #200
Sherman Oaks, California 91403-3297
(818) 905-0040 FAX (818) 990-5468
www.afaa.com
contactafaa@afaa.com

AFAA certification exams are accredited by Vital Research.
AFAA is a National Board of Fitness Examiners (NBFE) Affiliate.
AFAA also applied for an additional accreditation through an organization recognized by the Council for Higher Education Accreditation (CHEA) and the U.S. Dept. of Education, meeting IHRSA's 2005 recommendation on accreditation for fitness certification organizations.

AFAA and logo, Aerobics and Fitness Association of America, AFP Fitness Practitioner, Fitness Triage, Fitness Gets Personal, Mat Science, American Fitness, FitMarkers, Fitness Management for Life are registered trademarks of Aerobics and Fitness Association of America. The Sunrise Yoga Format and AFAA 5 Questions are trademarks of Aerobics and Fitness Association of America. Other marks referenced in this book may be trademarks or registered trademarks of other companies, and are used only for informational purposes and to the owner's benefit, without intent to infringe.

 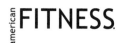 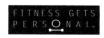 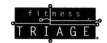

ISBN 0-9777102-0-3

Printed in the United States of America
10 9 8 7 6 5 4 3

First Edition, 2006, revised 2007

Acknowledgements

The editor wishes to acknowledge the guidance and talents of the following people in the creation of this book.

AFAA President: Linda D. Pfeffer, RN

AFAA Board of Certification and Training: Laura A. Gladwin, MS, Chair, Nancy Gillette, MA, Meg Jordan, PhD, RN, Kathy Stevens, MA

Editorial Production

Managing Editor: Julie van Roden

Graphic Design/Production: Laura Carrington

Illustrations: Laura Carrington, Michael Aniel

Editorial Support: Marcia Ditmyer, Dena Feingold, Lauri Reimer

Photographers: Chuck Zlotnick, Tom Ivicevic

Photo Shoot Coordinators: Lauri Reimer and Kathy Stevens

Models: Ryan Baylor, Steve Ford, Shilo Nelson, Lauri Reimer, Kathy Stevens

Acknowledgements from the Author

I am grateful for the opportunity to have written *Personal Fitness Training: Theory & Practice*. I thank Linda D. Pfeffer, RN, President of AFAA, for without her vision and support this project would not have been possible. I owe a debt of thanks to Laura Gladwin, my tireless supporter and friend, who took on the daunting task of editing, and re-editing, this book. The support from the AFAA office, and most especially from Lauri Reimer and Tere Filer, has been extremely valuable. On a personal level, I continue to be grateful for my parents, James and Margaret Yoke, who provide me with such love, support, and inspiration. And I am very thankful for my two wonderful sons, Nathaniel and Zachary, who have been so understanding, helpful, and loving to me.

I would also like to thank the following contributors for the use of selected material from their chapters in AFAA's *Fitness: Theory & Practice* (4th ed., 2002): William C. Beam, PhD (Chapter 2), Sharon Cheng, MS, PT (Chapter 5), Patti Mantia, EdD (Chapter 6), Judith Gantz, MA, CMA (Chapter 9), Tracy Gordner-Cherry, RD, CDE, CDN (Chapter 23), Lawrence Biscontini, MA, NC, CPT (Chapter 32), David L. Herbert, JD (Chapter 33), and Diana McNab, MEd (Chapter 47).

About the Author

Mary Yoke has a master's degree in exercise physiology, two degrees in music, and has obtained certifications from such organizations as ACSM, AFAA, ACE, NASM, NBFE, Pilates Method Alliance, Stott, Physical-Mind, Yogafit, and Johnny G. Spinning. She is an adjunct professor at Adelphi University in New York where she has authored numerous group exercise research studies and teaches a graduate course in functional anatomy and exercise leadership. She continues to teach a variety of group exercise classes and trains approximately 16 clients per week on both traditional weight-room equipment and on Pilates apparatus. She is in demand as a presenter and is known as the "trainer's trainer" as she travels internationally and throughout the country leading workshops for fitness professionals. Additionally, she presents popular seminars on health and wellness to the general public. She has frequently served as a fitness video consultant and reviewer (for *SHAPE*, *Consumer Reports*, and *Good Housekeeping*), and has served as an expert witness in lawsuits involving injuries related to fitness videos. Mary has worked in the areas of cardiac rehabilitation, physical therapy, and corporate fitness and health promotion, served on the advisory board for ACSM's *Health & Fitness Journal,* and served 6 years on ACSM's credentialing committee. She is on AFAA's adjunct board and is a master trainer for AFAA. In addition to *Personal Fitness Training: Theory & Practice* (2006), Mary has written three other books: *A Guide to Personal Fitness Training* (1996, 2001), *Functional Exercise Progressions* (2004), and *Methods of Group Exercise Leadership* (2005), and has been featured in six educational videos.

About the Editor

Laura A. Gladwin, MS

Former Director, You're in Charge!sm health promotions, Preferred Care/MVP Health Plan, Rochester, New York; AFAA's Director of Education; chair, AFAA board of certification and training; Master AFAA Fitness Practitioner (MAFP); editor, AFAA's *A Guide to Personal Fitness Training, Fitness: Theory & Practice* (3rd and 4th eds.), and *Fitness Gets Personal* series; fitness consultant and contributing author, *American Fitness* magazine; author of published articles in peer reviewed journals in the areas of health care and exercise science; member, board of directors, Center for the Study of Aging; member, National Coalition for Developing Curriculum Standards for Senior Fitness Specialists; faculty member, St. John Fisher/Lifespan Gerontology Certificate Program; presenter for such groups as ACSM, AAPHERD, AFAA, World Congress on Physical Activity and Aging, and Marketing Strategies for Medicare Advantage Health Plans; more than 30 years of experience in the fitness industry.

AFAA's Notice

PLEASE READ BEFORE USING AFAA PROGRAMS AND MATERIALS

The programs and materials offered by the Aerobics and Fitness Association of America (AFAA) are intended to provide general educational information to you in your efforts to obtain certification and in working with your clients to reach definable goals. "You," as used here, includes, but is not limited to, fitness trainers and other fitness professionals of all kinds, fitness trainer candidates and other professional fitness candidates of all kinds, providers of continuing education services, AFAA educational contractors, and all other readers and users of the programs and materials offered by AFAA.

The programs and materials of AFAA are intended to provide what is believed to be accurate information. However, please note the following important cautions before making use of AFAA programs and materials.

- To the best of the knowledge of the authors, publishers, and presenters of AFAA programs and materials, the contents of such programs and materials were accurate as of the date of publication and/or presentation. However, you are strongly encouraged to keep yourself informed of new developments in the field to make sure that the contents are still accurate when you consult the programs and materials.

- AFAA programs and materials are made available with the understanding that the authors, publishers and presenters are not engaged in rendering legal, medical, or other professional services by reason of their authorship, publication or presentation of such programs and materials. You are strongly encouraged to consult an appropriate legal, medical, or other expert if you are seeking such advice or assistance. This is an especially important precaution in the field of fitness and exercise, personal fitness training, and fitness practice.

- AFAA programs and materials are made available without warranties or guarantees of any kind, express or implied, all of which are disclaimed. By way of example only, and without limiting the general disclaimer given above, the authors, publishers and presenters of AFAA programs and materials cannot and do not promise or guarantee that the contents of such programs and materials are appropriate for every reader or user, or that use of such programs and materials will result in certification or in obtaining employment; or that, if you are certified, you will be able to obtain third-party insurance payments for any services that you may render to your clients.

- You acknowledge that all of the above-referenced authors, publishers and presenters are independent contractors whom AFAA has engaged for their respective purposes, and that consistent with their independent contractor status, AFAA neither has nor had any right of control over the manner or methods by which they provide their services, and is not legally responsible for their acts or omissions while performing services in their respective capacities.

- The laws that define the practice of medicine or other health care fields reserved for those who are licensed to provide such services vary from state to state and according to specific circumstances. In some states, and under some circumstances, the rendering of services may be actually or potentially in violation of law. For that reason, you are cautioned to obtain specific professional advice about the laws and regulations that may apply to you in a particular locality.

- The documents, forms, and other content found in AFAA programs and materials are offered as illustrative examples only. No such documents, forms, graphs, or other content should be used or adapted for use in violation of copyright or other applicable law. Since the use of these documents, forms, and other content may have legal implications, you are strongly cautioned to consult a qualified attorney before using or adapting them.

- AFAA programs and materials are not intended to establish or define any specific professional standards that apply to all fitness trainers or other fitness professionals and their clients in all circumstances or to limit the exercise of your independent professional judgment as to what is in the best interest of any particular client. The standard of care that you must observe may change from time to time or vary from place to place, and you are strongly cautioned to familiarize yourself with the standard of care that applies to you.

- All of these cautions apply to you regardless of your location. However, since AFAA programs and materials were prepared for use in the United States, special care should be taken if you are outside the U.S. to make sure you are familiar with the laws and regulations that apply in your country and locality.

- Participation in AFAA programs, use of AFAA materials, and/or any certification of a fitness trainer or other fitness professional that may result do not qualify you to approve, endorse or recommend dietary supplements or other ingestibles, ergogenic aids, or any other products or services that claim to enhance physical performance or appearance, nor does AFAA itself issue any such approvals, endorsements or recommendations. AFAA disclaims any responsibility or liability for any claim resulting from any such approvals, endorsements or recommendations that you may offer.

- By participating in and/or using programs and materials offered by AFAA, and as condition for providing and presenting such materials and programs to you, you are acknowledging and agreeing that (a) you are solely responsible for all aspects of the conduct of your business and practice as a fitness trainer or other fitness professional; (b) you are not sponsored or endorsed by or otherwise affiliated with AFAA by reason of any certification that AFAA may issue to you; (c) AFAA is not responsible or liable in any manner whatsoever for claims or liabilities arising from the conduct of your business; (d) AFAA disclaims any liability, loss or damages that may result from the conduct of your business or practice, and/or your use of such programs and materials, and/or the information, advice and techniques embodied in such programs and materials; and (e) AFAA does not assume any responsibility, obligation, or duty toward you or any client or person to whom any service or product is rendered or provided by you or otherwise.

Part of the foregoing was adapted from a Declaration of Principles of the American Bar Association and a Committee of Publishers and Associations

Table of Contents

Reviewers

Gina Blunt, MA

Assistant director, campus recreation, University of Tennessee Health Science Center, Memphis, TN, with a master's in exercise physiology; currently working toward a PhD in exercise science with an emphasis in exercise behavior; AFAA primary and personal fitness trainer specialist.

Marcia Mastracci Ditmyer, PhD, MBA, MS, CHES

Statistician, department of health and nutrition sciences and school of dental medicine, University of Nevada, Las Vegas, with a doctorate in public health and a master's of science in health education; program director for the master's of public health program, California College for Health Sciences; over 20 years in the fitness industry; author of published articles in peer-reviewed journals in the areas of public health, nutrition, and diabetes.

Tere Filer, MS, MPH

Owner, Action Plus Consulting Services, Los Angeles, CA, providing health education seminars, coordinating and implementing wellness programs, special events, and health fairs at the worksite, and conducting risk appraisals and follow-up counseling for employees; over 25 years in the fitness industry, with master's degrees in both nutritional sciences and public health; AFAA international presenter; certified with AFAA, ACSM, and ACE in personal fitness training; ACSM certified health fitness instructor.

Nancy Gillette, MA

Physical educator with two California state K-12 teaching credentials and a master's degree in adapted physical education; certified Master AFAA Fitness Practitioner (MAFP); AFAA master specialist; national master trainer for Nordic Walking and Flow Motion; senior fitness specialist; member, AFAA board of certification and training since 1984; lecturer, author, workshop leader, personal trainer, and career mentor.

David L. Herbert, JD

Senior partner, Herbert & Benson, Attorneys At Law, Canton, Ohio; co-editor of *The Exercise Standards and Malpractice Reporter, The Sports Medicine Standards of Malpractice Reporter,* and *The Sports Parks and Recreations Law Reporter;* author of over a dozen books, numerous book chapters, and over 500 articles on various legal and risk management issues associated with health and fitness facilities, personal fitness training, sports medicine, and sports and recreation; frequent speaker before such groups as AFAA, ACSM, ACE, NSCA, as well as other organizations.

Patti Mantia, EdD

Faculty chair and professor, department of health, fitness, and nutrition, Holyoke Community College, Holyoke, MA, with a doctorate in curriculum and teaching human movement; owner, The Fitness Firm, Mansfield, MA, providing education and training for fitness professionals; AFAA master certification specialist.

Dorette M. Nysewander, MS, AFP, NBFE

Director of business development, MediFit Corporate Services, Inc., Florham Park, NJ; AFAA master consultant and certification specialist; member, AFAA Fitness Practitioner (AFP) board; fellow of the National Board of Fitness Examiners (NBFE); contributor to AFAA's *American Fitness* magazine and AFAA training manuals; industry leadership and experience in the academic, military, and corporate sectors.

Yusuf (J.P.) Saleeby, MD

Co-director, emergency department, Liberty Regional Medical Center, Hinesville, GA; adjunct professor, school of allied health, Georgia Southern University, Statesboro, GA; author of *Wonder Herbs: A Guide To Three Adaptogens;* frequent lecturer on topics concerning integrative medicine; medical/health writer for numerous regional and national journals; president, Vita Sanus Nutraceuticals; competitive Olympic-style weight lifter.

Jan Schroeder, PhD

Associate professor of kinesiology, California State University, Long Beach; senior exercise physiologist for IDEA Health and Fitness Association; member, ACSM Fit Society board; active member of eight professional and academic associations; author of 11 peer-reviewed journal articles and 5 peer-reviewed manuals and book chapters; has delivered over 30 research presentations at the regional, national, and international level.

Kathy Stevens, MA

Master's degree in kinesiology; member, AFAA board of certification and training; certified Master AFAA Fitness Practitioner (MAFP); group and personal trainer; certified National Academy of Sports Medicine (NASM) group trainer; Reebok master trainer, program development manager, and international presenter.

Gregory L. Welch, MS

Exercise physiologist and owner of SpeciFit, An Agency of Wellness, Seal Beach, CA; over 20 years in the fitness industry with a focus on the special needs population; author and lecturer; creator, SpeciFit Foundation, designed to further wellness concepts for adolescent women.

Foreword

Personal fitness training has become a popular profession, providing a host of services to consumers of all ages and levels of physical ability. The delivery of such services may well be the most profitable activity offered in health/fitness facilities. According to some accounts, over 4 million consumers in the United States may seek the services of personal fitness trainers each year.

Specific industry statistics are not available as to the actual number of personal trainers in the profession. However, according to the U.S. Department of Labor, over 200,000 professionals are believed to be employed in the fitness industry. Many of these individuals are personal fitness trainers.

Associated with the rise in personal fitness trainer service comes a concern regarding the level of skills and competencies mastered by those who profess to be "certified." To address consumer safety and raise the qualification bar for such professionals, AFAA and other industry education providers have joined with the National Board of Fitness Examiners (NBFE) to develop the industry's first formalized standards of practice. These standards will be used to test trainer competencies and qualifications through a national examination. According to AFAA's President, Linda Pfeffer, "The development of a uniform job task analysis for personal trainers bestows an important benefit on fitness trainers, health clubs, universities, certification organizations, and accrediting agencies. By using the same job task analysis in education, certification, accreditation, and for testing by the NBFE, there will be a consistency and continuity in the fitness industry that has not existed before."

As the nation's leader in education for fitness professionals, AFAA brings to the industry a beautifully written and comprehensive manual for personal fitness trainers around the world: *Personal Fitness Training: Theory & Practice*. This book provides the most up-to-date research and practical knowledge that have emerged for personal trainers over the past decade. Addressing wellness strategies, business and legal ethics and issues, exercise programming, fitness assessments, special populations, multitraining techniques, and more, AFAA provides the personal fitness trainer with an all-inclusive textbook detailing a professional role for success in the highly competitive and ever-changing world of fitness. AFAA's *Personal Fitness Training: Theory & Practice* should be the source for personal fitness trainers from this point forward.

Laura A. Gladwin, MS, MAFP
Director, You're in Charge!SM
Preferred Care/MVP Health Plan, Rochester, NY
AFAA Board of Certification and Training

Preface

This text, *Personal Fitness Training: Theory & Practice*, is primarily designed to accompany AFAA's Personal Fitness Trainer workshop and help prepare candidates for AFAA's Personal Fitness Trainer Certification as well as the National Board of Fitness Examiners' Exam. The information in this text is based on the most current and relevant research applicable to personal training. Numerous citations are provided to support the recommendations and guidelines outlined for fitness professionals. In areas where controversy exists, every attempt has been made to inform readers about the lack of consensus within the fitness industry.

Personal Fitness Training: Theory & Practice covers the major topic areas essential for effective and appropriate personal fitness training. As always, AFAA takes pride in a practical, hands-on approach as presented in this text. This is especially evident in the meticulously detailed "Applied Resistance Training Skills" chapter.

What do personal fitness trainers do? Practically speaking, they teach effective, individualized exercises to clients one-on-one, assisting them in achieving their personal fitness and wellness goals.

Personal trainers are responsible for screening clients and evaluating their ability to take part in fitness programs. Trainers have a duty to put safety first, to "do no harm." In order to follow this axiom, knowledge of industry guidelines for health screening, risk appraisal, and an understanding of injury prevention techniques are critical. To ensure the clients' welfare, personal fitness trainers need to recognize their own limitations and understand their scope of practice. Unless a trainer has specific training and/or licensing in subjects or domains, such as clinical exercise testing and programming, massage therapy, physical therapy, chiropractic, and nutrition, he/she should be cautious of appearing to provide service, practice, or give advice in these areas.

Personal fitness trainers individualize exercise programs to fit client goals. In order to understand the client's goals and provide appropriate motivation and education over time, personal fitness trainers need to have strong communication skills and understand principles of long-term lifestyle change. In addition, a broad knowledge base is necessary to adequately answer (or provide referrals to other professionals who can answer) the many questions clients have about exercise, calorie expenditure, healthy eating, weight loss, injuries, and the like.

Personal fitness trainers recognize that one of their duties is to enhance clients' feelings of self-efficacy, the feeling of "I can do it; I am capable!" Teaching clients that they are responsible for their own health, and that they can practice enhanced well-being and be independent are skills of quality trainers.

Personal fitness trainers must take seriously their responsibility to stay up to date on new research and medical findings. As the fitness field grows closer to medicine and science, trainers must continue to upgrade their education if they are to remain competent, and perhaps to obtain required licensure, state mandated certification, or registration when necessary. AFAA strongly advises trainers to seek higher education; a college degree may soon be necessary for entry into the fitness industry. A great deal of misinformation and folklore is still promoted by some media and individuals as fact. A qualified personal fitness trainer has the knowledge and the ability to think objectively and separate fact from fiction. At the same time, personal fitness trainers need to avoid providing any service that is reserved for provision by those who are licensed by state law in a variety of practice areas, including medicine, nursing, physical therapy, and dietetics/nutrition.

In summary, a personal fitness trainer is a skilled teacher, motivator, communicator, and continual student of fitness and positive lifestyle change. Trainers serve a valuable purpose in helping people become healthier and happier, and in improving the quality of many lives. It is our hope that this text will both inform and inspire you on your path toward enriching your own life and the lives of others!

Understanding Wellness

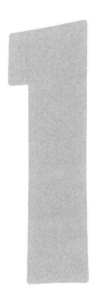

Outline

- Definition of Wellness

- Prevention of Coronary Heart Disease

- Prevention of Cancer

- Prevention of Diabetes

- Prevention of COPD

- Prevention of Cirrhosis

- Prevention of Osteoporosis and Osteoarthritis

- Prevention of Back Problems

- Prevention of Accidents

- Practical Strategies for Optimal Well-Being

To become a competent personal fitness trainer you must have a strong knowledge base as well as specific skills and abilities. The study of wellness, or optimal well-being, is a good starting point in the development of such a knowledge base. Personal fitness trainers are in an ideal position to help clients live their lives in a healthy manner, guiding them toward the ultimate goal of wellness. How can you help your clients understand the process of wellness and make behavior choices that will improve the quality of their lives? In this chapter, wellness will be defined and the major preventable diseases and disabilities will be discussed. Then practical strategies for helping your clients work toward optimal well-being will be outlined, with the ultimate goal of improving quality of life for as many individuals as possible. While unlicensed professionals can never permissibly provide health care services, fitness professionals can provide general health-related educational information, set standards for optimal living by example, and recommend client interaction with their physician.

Definition of Wellness

What is wellness and how can it be approached? Wellness, according to John Travis, MD, MPH (2004), was envisioned by the term's originators as a multidimensional concept incorporating the physical, mental, emotional, and spiritual aspects of a human being. Wellness can be approached from at least two related perspectives.

1. Prevention—the practice of behaviors that minimize the risk of lifestyle-related diseases and disabilities. One of the roles of a personal fitness trainer is to help clients identify risk factors and unhealthy behaviors, and in doing so to help enhance wellness and health.

2. Holism—the integration of the mind, body, and spirit for optimal functioning. Halbert Dunn, MD, identified **five dimensions** of the total person: emotional, social, intellectual, spiritual, and physical. When these aspects are fully developed and integrated, optimal well-being results, which he called a "zest for living" (Dunn, 1961). Bill Hettler, MD (2005) (cofounder of the National Wellness Institute, Inc.), incorporated a **sixth dimension**, occupational, recognizing the importance of work and career to personal satisfaction and enrichment.

Many people associate wellness with fitness, nutrition, or stress reduction; but it is much more. It is the self-empowered practice of prevention and full development of all the dimensions of life. But remember, wellness is a process, a way of life; it is not a state that can be achieved once and for all.

Good health depends to a great extent on the lifestyle choices you make, including what you eat, whether or not you are active, whether or not you smoke, and how you manage stress. Below is The Wellness Continuum adapted from the work of John Travis, MD, MPH (2004).

The Wellness Continuum

| Disability & Disease | Symptoms | Awareness | Education | Growth |

| Premature Death | Neutral Point (No discernible illness or wellness) | High Level Wellness (zest for life) |

A related approach to understanding the concept of wellness is shown below. This model helps identify major lifestyle diseases and disorders, which are often preceded by high-risk behaviors. Conversely, the practice of healthy behaviors can lead to high-level wellness and optimal well-being.

CONCEPT OF WELLNESS

DEATH ↔ DISEASE/ INJURY ↔ HIGH-RISK BEHAVIORS ↔		HEALTHY BEHAVIORS ↔	WELLNESS
Coronary Heart Disease	High-fat diet	Healthy diet	Physical
Osteoporosis	Smoking	Not smoking	Intellectual
Stroke	High stress	Meditation/Stress Management	Emotional
Cancer	Sedentary lifestyle	Regular exercise	Social
Obesity	Alcohol and drug abuse	Moderate or no alcohol	Spiritual
AIDS	Unsafe sex	Safe sex	
Hypertension	Drinking and driving	Not driving while impaired	
Diabetes	Excessive sun exposure	Moderate, protected sun exposure	
Cirrhosis	Poor body mechanics	Proper posture and body mechanics	
Low-back pain	Not wearing seatbelt	Always wears seatbelt	
Accidents			
Emphysema			

Many diseases and disabilities have been identified as preventable, or at least modifiable. One important role of the personal fitness trainer within permissible legal boundaries is to assist clients in identifying risk factors and practicing prevention, helping them to minimize illness and guiding them toward wellness. While such trainers cannot "treat" clients or engage in the unauthorized practice of those professions engaged in licensed health care activities, it is also important to emphasize to your clients that the same few risk factors can influence several diseases and conditions, as shown in the following table.

PLAN FOR PREVENTION

Condition/Injury	Preventive Behavior						
	Diet	Exercise	Avoid Smoking	Avoid Alcohol	Control Obesity	Control Stress	Use Seatbelt
Heart Disease	✔	✔	✔		✔	✔	
Cancer	✔	✔	✔	✔	✔	✔	
Diabetes	✔	✔			✔		
Emphysema			✔				
Cirrhosis				✔			
Osteoporosis	✔	✔	✔	✔	✔		
Back Problems		✔	✔		✔		
Accidents/Injuries		✔		✔			✔

Prevention of Coronary Heart Disease

Coronary heart disease (CHD, also referred to as coronary artery disease [CAD], and under the umbrella of cardiovascular disease [CVD]) is the leading cause of death in the United States and in most of the developed world. Since 1900, CVD (a general term for more than 20 different diseases of the heart and cardiovascular system) has been the No. 1 killer every year but 1918. Nearly 2,600 Americans die of CVD each day, an average of one death every 34 seconds. CVD claims about as many lives each year as the next five leading causes of death combined, which are cancer, chronic lower respiratory diseases, accidents, diabetes mellitus, influenza/pneumonia (American Heart Association, 2005). The three major cardiovascular disorders are heart attack, stroke, and hypertension. CHD is almost always the result of **atherosclerosis**, or narrowing (hardening) of the coronary arteries.

Atherosclerosis is a slow and progressive disease that gradually develops over decades. The rate of development depends on cholesterol and blood pressure levels, cigarette smoking, and other risk factors. Atherosclerosis of the coronary arteries can lead to myocardial **ischemia**, or lack of adequate blood flow to the heart muscle, which may lead to a **myocardial infarction** (MI), or a heart attack, which is the complete blockage of blood to the heart muscle. Also, stable **angina pectoris** is transient and predictable. Unstable angina (chest pain at rest) has graver consequences and can lead to sudden MI or cardiac arrest.

A **stroke** is often caused by atherosclerosis of the cerebral blood vessels, leading to ischemia in the brain, which then results in brain tissue death. Stroke can also result from a cerebral embolism, in which a blood clot (embolus) lodges in a cerebral artery. Stroke is a leading cause of serious, long-term disability in the United States. A "mini stroke," which produces stroke-like symptoms but no lasting damage, is termed a **transient ischemic attack** (TIA). The risk of stroke is greatly increased in persons with hypertension. Hemorrhagic stroke is due to severe hypertension in which blood leaks out of the weakened cerebral arteries (aneurysm), and thrombotic or embolic stroke is due to obstruction of the blood supply to the brain with clots. The treatment for these types of strokes is quite different. Fibrinolytic therapy (clot-dissolving drugs such as tPA) may be used in thrombotic stroke to reverse injury and prevent permanent damage, while careful blood pressure control is the treatment of choice for hemorrhagic strokes.

The tendency for **hypertension** (high blood pressure) may be inherited, but several lifestyle factors (e.g., excessive salt, fat, and alcohol in the diet, cigarette smoking, obesity, physical inactivity, and stress) strongly affect its development. Currently, nearly one in three adults has hypertension, with an even greater prevalence among African Americans (National High Blood Pressure Education Program, 2003). Hypertension is defined as systolic pressure of 140 mmHg or higher, or diastolic pressure of 90 mmHg or higher, or being on antihypertensive medication.

Risk factors that predispose individuals to CHD have been identified and may vary slightly according to the source. According to the American College of Sports Medicine (2006), positive risk factors for CHD are family history, cigarette smoking, hypertension, dyslipidemia (high cholesterol), impaired fasting glucose, obesity, and sedentary lifestyle. These will be further defined in Chapter 4 ("Health Screening and Risk Appraisal").

Prevention of Cancer

Cancer is a group of diseases characterized by uncontrolled growth and spread of abnormal cells. It can be caused by both external factors (smoking, chemicals, radiation, infectious organisms) and internal factors (inherited mutations, hormones, and immune conditions). Scientific evidence suggests that about one third of the 570,280 cancer deaths expected to occur in 2005 will be related to nutrition, physical inactivity, and overweight or obesity, and thus could also have been prevented (American Cancer Society, 2005a). Other cancers caused by infectious exposures (such as HIV and HPV) could be prevented by behavior changes, vaccines, or antibiotics, while skin cancer can be prevented by minimizing sun exposure. In short, approximately two thirds of all cancers are preventable. Cancer is the second leading cause of death, succeeded only by heart disease.

Cancers that are, or may be, preventable include the following.

- Cancer of the lung—the leading cause of cancer death in both men and women; more than 175,000 lung cancer deaths per year are caused by tobacco use and therefore could be prevented completely (National Cancer Institute, 2003).
- Cancer of the breast—the most common non-skin cancer and the second leading cause of cancer-related death in U.S. women (National Cancer Institute, 2005b); risk factors include age, family history, obesity, consumption of one or more alcoholic beverages per day, and a long menstrual history (periods that started early and/or ended late in life). Breastfeeding, moderate or vigorous physical activity, and maintaining a healthy body weight are all associated with a lower risk of breast cancer. Secondary prevention includes monthly breast self-exams and an annual medical examination.
- Cancer of the colon and rectum—colorectal cancer is the second leading cause of death from cancer in both sexes in the U.S. The risk of developing colorectal cancer rises after age 50. Dietary factors, especially a high consumption of red meat and/or saturated fat, account for about half of all colon cancers. Another important strategy for prevention is to eat enough dietary fiber (about 25–35 grams/day), as well as plenty of fruits and vegetables. An inverse relationship has also been found between colon cancer and physical activity (National Institutes of Health, 2005).
- Cancer of the pancreas—incidence of pancreatic cancer is more than twice as high for smokers as for non-smokers. Obesity, physical inactivity, and a diet high in fat have also been identified as risk factors (National Cancer Institute, 2002b).
- Leukemia—the risk of certain leukemias is increased by cigarette smoking, by exposure to chemicals such as benzene, and by exposure to radiation (American Cancer Society, 2005).
- Cancer of the skin—more than one million cases of basal cell or squamous cell skin cancers are diagnosed annually. Excessive sun exposure, particularly for fair skinned individuals, is the major risk factor. Malignant melanoma has been related to episodes of severe sunburn during the childhood years. Secondary prevention includes watching for changes in warts or moles and for small sores that don't heal ((National Cancer Institute, 2005b).
- Cancer of the bladder—much more common in men than in women. A primary risk factor is cigarette smoking, while drinking more fluids and eating more vegetables may lower the risk of bladder cancer (National Cancer Institute, 2002a).
- Cancer of the esophagus, pharynx, mouth, and tongue—cigarette, cigar, and pipe smoking, and chewing tobacco account for at least 90% of

these cancers. Heavy alcohol intake has also been implicated in cancers of the esophagus (American Academy Otolaryngology-Head and Neck Surgery [n.d.]).

- Cancer of the cervix—it is extremely important to follow physician recommendations for regular Pap smear exams and testing for human papillomavirus (HPV) (especially when there is evidence of cervical dysplasia) for secondary prevention (National Cancer Institute, 2005c).
- Cancer of the liver—more common in men than in women, the incidence of liver cancer is increasing in the U.S. Heavy alcohol intake greatly increases the risk of liver cancer (National Cancer Institute, 2002c).

No definite preventable risk factors have been identified for other types of cancer, such as bone, stomach, prostate, or brain cancer.

Prevention of Diabetes

Over 18.2 million Americans have diabetes (6.3%), of which 90–95% cases are type 2 (National Center for Chronic Disease Prevention and Health Promotion, 2003). Diabetes is the sixth leading cause of death in the United States, greatly increasing a person's risk of heart disease, stroke, blindness, kidney disease, nervous system disorders, and amputations (National Center for Chronic Disease Prevention and Health Promotion, 2004). Diabetes is a disease in which the body is unable to use **glucose** (blood sugar that comes from carbohydrates) for fuel, resulting in hyperglycemia. Insulin is necessary as the "gatekeeper," making the cell walls more permeable for glucose. People with diabetes either do not produce enough insulin (type 1) or their cells are not sensitive to the insulin that is produced (type 2). Type 2 diabetes (NIDDM, non-insulin dependent diabetes mellitus, also known as adult-onset diabetes) can often be managed or even avoided completely by implementing lifestyle modifications such as appropriate diet and exercise. A longitudinal epidemiologic study of adult men found that physical activity reduced the risk for developing diabetes, even when adjusted for obesity, hypertension, and family history (Helmrich, Ragland, Leung, and Paffenbarger, 1991). Physical activity and exercise help to improve a person's insulin sensitivity, thus making it easier for the body to utilize glucose; in other words, exercise has a beneficial insulin-like effect.

It should be noted that eating too much sugar is not the cause of diabetes. This misconception arises because diabetes is characterized by high levels of blood sugar. Excessive sugar consumption is indeed very dangerous for diabetics, who must curtail their sugar intake. However, sugar doesn't actually cause this disorder. Some studies have shown that the risk of developing diabetes is 2.5 times greater in individuals consuming refined and processed grain products that are low in fiber, as compared to those who eat a high-fiber diet that is also high in complex carbohydrates (Salmeron et al., 1997). Obesity, especially abdominal obesity, overwhelmingly appears to be the major risk factor in the development of adult onset diabetes (the causes of obesity are multifaceted, with physical inactivity and excessive caloric intake often playing a large part). While certain healthy lifestyle habits can help to prevent type 2 diabetes, family history of the disease and age are uncontrollable risk factors.

Finally, a condition called **Metabolic Syndrome** is linked to diabetes. Metabolic Syndrome (also referred to as Insulin Resistance Syndrome, and previously known as Syndrome X) is a cluster of disorders of the body's metabolism (including high blood pressure, high insulin levels, excess body weight, and abnormal cholesterol levels) that increase the chance of developing diabetes, heart disease, and/or stroke. Metabolic Syndrome is highly likely in individuals who have at least four of the following six conditions: high blood pressure, low HDL (good) cholesterol, high triglyceride levels, a medical diagnosis of insulin resistance, excessive abdominal obesity, and high fasting blood glucose. If a client has two or three of these conditions, then he/she has a high risk for developing the syndrome if he/she does not adopt a healthy lifestyle (National Institute of Diabetes, Digestive & Kidney Diseases, 2004). The best prevention against Metabolic Syndrome is to maintain a healthy weight, eat a proper diet, and exercise regularly.

Prevention of Chronic Obstructive Pulmonary Disease

Chronic obstructive pulmonary disease (COPD) is the fourth leading cause of death in the U.S. (behind heart disease, cancer, and stroke) (National Center for Health Statistics, 2004). Individuals suffering from this disease experience difficulty breathing due to the destruction of alveolar and parenchymal tissue with "air trapping." The main forms of the disease are chronic bronchitis and emphysema, with over 80–90% of cases caused by cigarette smoking (Petty, 1990). There is an ongoing debate about whether COPD includes asthma; those with asthma are much more likely to develop COPD in the long run. Other risk factors include age and excessive exposure to various pollutants (e.g., air pollution, dusts, and fumes).

Unfortunately, once the disease process is in place, lung damage does not reverse, although smoking cessation at any point is beneficial, and physical activity can make everyday activities easier. Smoking destroys the cilia (small hairs that move mucous toward the mouth), distends and destroys the alveoli (air cells of the lungs), decreases lung elasticity, and leads to airway collapse and increased airway resistance. This process results in slow oxygen starvation with a great limitation in daily functional activities. Smoking may also increase the thickness of blood, which is not necessarily a good thing. It also leads to higher risk of atherosclerosis. Smoking is unanimously identified as a major risk factor for heart disease, with smokers being more than twice as likely as non-smokers to die of a heart attack (National Cancer Institute, 2003). Additionally, passive or second-hand smoking carries a serious risk for children and others chronically exposed to cigarette smoke.

The U.S. Surgeon General lists several benefits for individuals who quit smoking, including lowered overall death rate, reduced heart disease risk, reduced lung cancer risk, and increased quality of life (fewer sick days, increased self-esteem, increased ability to exercise and play sports) (U.S. Department of Health and Human Services, 1990). If you have clients who continue to smoke, you can support them in quitting by providing them with educational materials and resources.

Prevention of Cirrhosis

Cirrhosis of the liver results from three factors: repeated injury to liver cells, fatty change and death of liver cells, and the accumulation of fibrous scar tissue. These factors prevent adequate blood flow through the liver and block the liver's ability to filter blood. Excessive alcohol intake is directly responsible for about 75% of cirrhosis cases. Alcoholic liver disease (cirrhosis) usually develops after more than a decade of heavy drinking; for women, two to three drinks per day appears to be linked with cirrhosis, and for men it may be as few as three to four drinks per day. After heavy scarring of the liver has occurred, cirrhosis is not reversible. Other kinds of liver injury, such as that caused by hepatitis C or hepatitis B, can also cause cirrhosis.

Prevention of Osteoporosis and Osteoarthritis

Osteoporosis (a condition of abnormally reduced bone density) compromises bone strength and can lead to easily fractured bones. One out of two women and one out of eight men over age 50 will have an osteoporosis-related fracture (primarily of the hip, spine, or wrist) in their lifetime. Physical inactivity has repeatedly been shown to reduce skeletal bone mass and increase the likelihood of the development of osteoporosis (American College of Sports Medicine, 1995). Other modifiable risk factors are inadequate calcium intake, vitamin D deficiency, cigarette smoking, and consumption of more than two alcoholic drinks daily. Unmodifiable risk factors include being a female Caucasian or Asian, having a family history of this condition, having a small, delicate frame size, and experiencing early menopause or amenorrhea. While there is no cure for osteoporosis, it can be reversed or slowed down with adequate weight-bearing exercise, proper diet with adequate calcium and vitamin D intake, and drug intervention (e.g., bisphosphonate medications such as risedronate [Actonel] and alendronate [Fosamax]).

According to the Centers for Disease Control and Prevention (2005a), **osteoarthritis** is the leading cause of disability in the U.S.; approximately 21 million Americans have osteoarthritis (Lawrence, Helmick, & Arnett, 1998). Osteoarthritis, or degenerative joint disease, is the erosion of articular cartilage, usually resulting from mechanical joint stress or trauma. This can eventually lead to bone-on-bone within the joint, and eventually result in the development of painful bone spurs or growths. Osteoarthritis is characterized by pain and stiffness within the joints, most commonly affecting the knees, hips, feet, and fingers. Osteoarthritis is much more common among individuals who are overweight or obese. It can be minimized to some extent by maintaining an active lifestyle, avoiding obesity, and by protecting the joints from injury.

Other rheumatic conditions include rheumatoid arthritis, gout, and fibromyalgia; these potentially serious disorders are, fortunately, much less common.

Prevention of Back Problems

Low-back pain is a common problem, often estimated to afflict 80% of adults at some point in their lives (Frymoyer & Cats-Baril, 1991). Back problems are the second leading cause of all office visits to primary care physicians (after colds) (Cohen, Chopra, & Upshur, 2001).

A majority of back problems are caused by weak or tight postural muscles and chronic poor body mechanics, such as slouching when sitting, driving in a hunched position, poor posture when standing, lifting or exerting incorrectly, sleeping on a sagging mattress, or being unfit and carrying excess weight. It is difficult to have proper body mechanics if the primary muscles affecting the spine are too tight or too weak. To prevent back pain and disability, strengthening the abdominals, spinal extensors, and scapular adductors, and stretching the spinal extensors, hip flexors, hamstrings and anterior chest muscles are helpful. Weight-bearing exercise is necessary to keep the bone mineral content high and maintain bone density. Body awareness and proper lifting techniques need to be practiced; most people need movement retraining since back pain can be the result of years of bad habits. Since back problems frequently occur in overweight individuals, maintaining an appropriate weight is important.

Prevention of Accidents

Most serious traumatic injuries are the result of automobile accidents. Seat belt use reduces the risk of sustaining a serious injury by about one half and represents a choice to stay safe and healthy. Failure to wear a seat belt contributes to more fatalities than any other single traffic safety-related behavior. Alcohol and/or drug intoxication is responsible for nearly one half of all accidents. Always wear a seat belt, and do not drive when under the influence of drugs or alcohol or ride with anyone who is so impaired (National Center for Injury Prevention and Control, 2005a; National Center for Injury Prevention and Control, 2005b).

Practical Strategies for Optimal Well-Being

As a personal fitness trainer, after you have screened clients in accordance with the prevailing standard of care and, if indicated, obtained physician clearance of them, consider educating clients (those for whom one or more of the strategies are indicated) through the following seven strategies for wellness maintenance and promotion. While you should never engage in practices that are reserved for provision by those who are licensed health care providers, you should encourage clients to be proactive in caring for themselves; the end result is an improved quality of life.

1. **Become Active**

    More and more Americans have become highly sedentary; studies show that almost 40% of adults have sedentary jobs and do not engage in any leisure-time physical activity (Schoenborn & Barnes, 2002). In fact, in 1996 the U.S. Surgeon General declared that there was "an epidemic of inactivity," with a resulting increase in disability and disease (U.S. Department of Health and Human Services, 1996).

    The American College of Sports Medicine (ACSM) differentiates physical activity from exercise and defines physical activity as "bodily movement that is produced by the contraction of skeletal muscle and that substantially increases energy expenditure" (American College of Sports Medicine, 2006). There are at least 50 well-documented benefits of physical activity as well as aerobic exercise, resistance training, and flexibility work. Clients typically can list many negatives involved with exercising (sweat, need to shower, no time, etc.), but they can rarely list more than one or two benefits. Adherence will be better and motivation will be higher if clients understand how much there is to gain from an active lifestyle.

    According to the 1996 report from the U.S. Surgeon General on physical activity and health, "regular physical activity that is performed on most days of the week reduces the risk of developing or dying from some of the leading causes of illness and death in the United States"

(U.S. Department of Health and Human Services, 1996). Regular physical activity improves health in the following ways.

- Reduces the risk of dying prematurely
- Reduces the risk of dying from heart disease
- Reduces the risk of developing diabetes
- Reduces the risk of developing high blood pressure
- Helps reduce blood pressure in people who already have high blood pressure
- Reduces the risk of developing colon cancer
- Reduces feelings of depression and anxiety
- Helps control weight
- Helps maintain healthy bones, muscles, and joints
- Helps older adults become stronger and better able to move about without falling
- Promotes psychological well-being

In addition, the Surgeon General's report (U.S. Department of Health and Human Services, 1996) makes three key points.

1. People who are usually inactive can improve their health and well-being by becoming even moderately active on a regular basis.
2. Physical activity need not be strenuous to achieve health benefits.
3. Greater health benefits can be achieved by increasing the amount (duration, frequency, or intensity) of physical activity.

A moderate amount of physical activity can be achieved in a variety of ways, and doesn't necessarily have to be in the form of a formalized, structured exercise session in order to help reduce the risk of disease or premature death. Following are some examples of moderate amounts of activity.

- Washing and waxing a car for 45–60 minutes
- Washing windows or floors for 45–60 minutes
- Gardening for 30–45 minutes
- Wheeling self in wheelchair for 30–40 minutes
- Walking 1 3/4 miles in 35 minutes (20 minute/mile)
- Dancing fast (social) for 30 minutes
- Pushing a stroller 1 1/2 miles in 30 minutes
- Raking leaves for 30 minutes
- Shoveling snow for 15 minutes

The Centers for Disease Control and Prevention (CDC) (2005b) and ACSM (American College of Sports Medicine, 1998) have issued recommendations for physical activity that include the following.

- Every U.S. adult should accumulate 30 minutes or more of moderate-intensity physical activity on most, and preferably all, days of the week.
- Physical activity can be accumulated in relatively short bouts.
- Adults who expend approximately 200 calories per day in moderate-intensity physical activity can expect many health benefits.
- Moderate physical activity is activity performed at an intensity equivalent to brisk walking at 3-4 mph for most healthy adults.
- Physical activity is closely related to, but distinct from, exercise and physical fitness.

- Physical activity and exercise are central ingredients of good health. Fitness professionals should realize that some activity is better than none, and that initial low-to-moderate levels of "activity" may enhance adherence with sedentary individuals, whereas higher levels of strenuous "exercise" may lead to injury and drop-out with previously inactive people.

2. **Become Physically Fit**

Although physical activity yields many health benefits, physical fitness carries additional benefits, such as higher levels of cardiovascular fitness and prevention of unhealthy weight gain. If an individual is already physically active, then personal fitness trainers can guide him/her towards physical fitness. **Physical fitness** is said to have skill-related, health-related, and physiologic components (President's Council on Physical Fitness, 2000). Skill-related components include agility, balance, coordination, speed, and power; these skills are primarily used in sports-specific activities and competition, and may not have a profound effect on health. **Health-related components of physical fitness** are cardiorespiratory endurance, muscular fitness (strength and endurance), flexibility, and body composition. Physiologic components include metabolic fitness (blood pressure measurements, cholesterol levels, blood glucose levels, etc.), morphologic fitness (body fat distribution, circumferences, etc.), and bone integrity.

To become physically fit, it is necessary to increase the intensity, duration, and frequency of physical activity; and therefore, true exercise becomes important. Exercise is defined as "planned, structured, and repetitive bodily movement done to improve or maintain one or more components of physical fitness" (American College of Sports Medicine, 2006). Exercise and physical fitness will be discussed in much greater detail in later portions of this book.

3. **Eat a Proper Diet**

While the development of individualized nutritional or diet programs may come within the provision of licensed nutritionists/dietitians and should not, therefore, be provided by unlicensed professionals, the American Heart Association, the American Cancer Society, the National Cancer Institute, and the American Dietetic Association all basically agree on the dietary changes that individuals must make to reduce their risk of disease. The dietary guidelines for Americans, published every five years since 1980, reflect a consensus of the above organizations along with the most current research available. Following are the current major guidelines (U.S. Departments of Agriculture and Health and Human Services, 2005).

- Consume a variety of nutrient-dense foods and beverages within and among the basic food groups while choosing foods that limit the intake of saturated and **trans fats,** cholesterol, added sugars, salt, and alcohol.
- Keep total fat intake between 20–35% of calories, with most fats coming from sources of polyunsaturated and monounsaturated fatty acids.
- Consume less than 10% of calories from saturated fatty acids and less than 300 mg/day of cholesterol, and keep trans fatty acid consumption as low as possible.

- Consume less than 2,300 mg of sodium (approximately 1 teaspoon of salt) per day. At the same time, consume potassium-rich foods, such as fruits and vegetables. Sodium consumption should be further limited in individuals with hypertension and congestive heart failure. However, iodized salt is important for prevention of thyroid disease.
- Those who choose to drink alcoholic beverages should do so sensibly and in moderation—defined as the consumption of up to one drink per day for women and up to two drinks per day for men.
- Choose a variety of fruits and vegetables each day. Be sure to include vegetables from all five subgroups (dark green, orange, legumes, starchy vegetables, and other vegetables) throughout each week.
- Consume 3 or more ounce-equivalents of whole-grain products per day, with the rest of the recommended grains coming from enriched or whole-grain products. In general, at least half the grains you consume should come from whole grains.
- Consume 3 cups per day of fat-free or low-fat milk or equivalent milk products.

4. **Prevent Obesity**

   Obesity is a rapidly increasing problem in the United States and in other industrialized countries, with approximately 65% of Americans over-weight and 31% obese (Flegel, Carroll, Ogden, & Johnson, 2002). Obesity is a condition characterized by excess body fat and is associated with an increased incidence of hypertension, hyperlipidemia (excess fat or cholesterol in the blood), diabetes, degenerative arthritis, certain cancers, reduced life expectancy, and early death (Pi-Sunyer, 2002). It increases the likelihood of hernias, hemorrhoids, gallbladder disease, varicose veins, and makes breathing more difficult. Excess weight can make everyday activities problematic. Obese people are hospitalized more frequently than are people of average weight, and they have more surgical complications. **Obesity** is defined as a level of excess body fat that increases the risk of disease. Other characteristics of obesity include: having a body mass index (BMI) of > 30 kg/m², or a waist girth > 102 cm for men and > 88 cm for women, or a waist/hip ratio of ≥ 0.95 for men and ≥ 0.86 for women. Weight control is a two-fold process: weight reduction and weight maintenance, with weight maintenance being the most difficult aspect. Many researchers believe that overeating and an environment that encourages sedentary living are the primary causes of the increasing incidence of obesity (Hill, Wyatt, Reed, & Peters, 2003).

5. **Do Not Smoke**

   In the United States, an estimated 26.3 million men (25.2%) and 21.2 million women (20.7%) are smokers (National Center for Health Statistics, 2004). Cigarette smoking is the leading cause of preventable death and disease according to the U.S. Surgeon General. Lung cancer and emphysema are perhaps the best-known outcomes associated with smoking. However, heart disease is statistically the most serious problem resulting from smoking. The risk and frequency of heart attacks are greater in individuals who smoke, and increase according to the number of cigarettes smoked. In addition, the rate of heart attacks is lower among those who have given up smoking as compared with current smokers. Smoking accelerates atherosclerosis, damages the lining of the arteries, increases total cholesterol, decreases HDL, and increases the stickiness of platelets, thereby increasing the risk of clotting. Smoking increases heart rate and blood pressure, causing the heart to require more oxygen. However, oxygen availability is compromised as carbon monoxide decreases the ability of the blood to carry oxygen. Smoking harms not only the smoker, but also family members, co-workers, and others who breathe the secondhand smoke.

The benefits of smoking cessation start almost immediately. Within 2 years, much of the risk of heart disease disappears, and within 5–10 years, the risk is about the same as a non-smoker. Bronchitis and emphysema sufferers can expect an improvement in breathing almost at once. Nothing an individual can do, including diet and exercise, is as important as giving up smoking.

6. **Practice Stress Management**

A high-stress lifestyle has been implicated in a number of diseases and disorders, including CHD, hypertension, stroke, heart arrhythmias, headaches, backaches, rheumatoid arthritis, asthma, ulcers, irritable bowel syndrome, eczema, acne, impaired immune system, overeating, and insomnia. In addition, symptoms of stress may overlap more serious psychological problems such as depression and anxiety disorders, which can also be linked to increased disease (Barefoot & Schroll, 1996).

Recent evidence suggests that acute negative emotional states, such as anger, anxiety, and frustration, are associated with heart attack (Gullette et al., 1997), and the chronically angry, suspicious, and mistrustful individual (as measured by objective tests) appears to be twice as likely to have coronary artery blockages. This type of behavior pattern, often seen in type A personalities, is characterized by hostility, depression, chronic stress, and social isolation (Almeda et al., 1991).

Anxiety disorders (e.g., panic disorder, phobias, obsessive-compulsive disorder, and posttraumatic stress disorder) are the most common adult mental disorders (Regier et al., 1990). Severe anxiety and hostility are significant predictors of CVD and risk of future overall illness (Russek, King, Russek, & Russek, 1990).

There are two major ways to break the stress/tension cycle: physical and intellectual/cognitive. Physical methods include, but are not limited to: regular aerobic exercise, deep breathing techniques, stretching exercises, progressive muscle relaxation, biofeedback (a device is used that gives feedback about physiological processes such as heart rate or blood pressure with the goal of gaining conscious control of them), imagery and visualization, autogenic training (use of visual imagery and body awareness to promote a state of deep relaxation), and meditation. These techniques all help to produce measurable physiological effects such as the relaxation response, which is characterized by decreased oxygen consumption, slowed metabolism, decreased resting heart rate and blood pressure, and increased alpha brain waves.

Intellectual or cognitive methods reducing stress and tension include: improving communication skills, consciously choosing to change negative internal voices, and developing adaptive techniques for dealing with stressors (taking action against the stressors within your control, and changing thoughts about the stressors beyond your control).

Other strategies for managing stress include seeking support from friends, family, or qualified health professionals, becoming active in charitable work, and adopting healthier behaviors such as increased sleep, physical activity, and a better diet.

7. **Practice Self-Care**

It is important to advocate self-responsibility to our clients. Individuals should appreciate and understand that they are in charge of their own health care management, working for prevention of diseases before they appear and for early detection and treatment of already existing illnesses. In general, healthy adults should have an annual physical and blood pressure check (blood pressure should be checked more often if there is a family history of CHD); glaucoma tests should be implemented every few years after age 40 (especially if there is a family history); dental checkups should be carried out annually; and women over age 25 should have a Pap smear annually and should practice breast self-examination monthly.

The following are government guidelines for prevention. Such guidelines should be used for educational purposes with clients—never to diagnose.

What is Preventive Care for Women Age 19+?

Checklist

What can you do for clients? You can set the stage by example. You can practice healthy behaviors, take medicines as prescribed, and get certain screening tests. When you go for your next checkup, talk to your primary care physician about how you can stay healthy no matter what your age.

Screening Tests: What You Need and When

Screening tests, such as mammograms and Pap smears, can find diseases early when they are easier to treat. Some women need certain screening tests earlier, or more often, than others. Talk to your doctor about which of the tests listed below are right for you, when you should have them, and how often.

- Mammograms: Begin with a baseline mammogram at age 35, followed by mammograms every 1–2 years starting at age 40.
- Pap Smears: Have a Pap smear every 1–3 years if you have been sexually active or are older than age 21.
- Cholesterol Checks: Have your cholesterol checked every 5 years starting at age 20.
- Blood Pressure: Have your blood pressure checked at least every 2 years.
- Colorectal Cancer Tests: Have a test for colorectal cancer starting at age 50. Your doctor can help you decide which test is right for you.
- Diabetes Tests: Have a test to screen for diabetes if you have high blood pressure or high cholesterol.
- Depression: If you've felt "down," sad, or hopeless, and have felt little interest or pleasure in doing things for 2 weeks straight, talk to your doctor about whether he or she can evaluate you for depression.

- Osteoporosis Tests: Have a bone density test at age 65 to screen for osteoporosis (thinning of the bones). If you are between the ages of 60–64 and weigh 154 lb. or less, talk to your doctor about whether you should be tested.
- Chlamydia Tests and Tests for Other Sexually Transmitted Diseases: Have a test for chlamydia if you are age 25 or younger and sexually active. If you are older, talk to your doctor to see whether you should be tested. Also, talk to your doctor to see whether you should be tested for other sexually transmitted diseases.
- Eye Exam: An eye (vision) examination should be performed once every 2 years.
- Dental Care: Dental examination and routine cleaning should be a part of your overall preventive care plan.

Should You Take Medicines To Prevent Disease?

- Hormones: According to recent studies, the risks of taking the combined hormones estrogen and progestin after menopause to prevent long-term illnesses outweigh the benefits. Talk to your doctor about whether starting or continuing to take hormones is right for you.
- Breast Cancer Drugs: If your mother, sister, or daughter has had breast cancer, talk to your doctor about the risks and benefits of taking medicines to prevent breast cancer.
- Aspirin: Talk to your doctor about taking aspirin to prevent heart disease if you are older than age 45 and have high blood pressure, high cholesterol, diabetes, or if you smoke.
- Immunizations: Stay up to date with your immunizations. Ask your health care provider about having the following.
  - A flu shot every year starting at age 50
  - A tetanus-diphtheria shot every 10 years (or a single booster at age 50)
  - A pneumonia shot once at age 65 (or earlier if you have certain health problems such as lung disease)
  - Hepatitis B shots

  (For immunization information, contact the National Immunization Information Hotline supported by CDC's National Immunization Program. It provides vaccination information for health care providers and the public. Available 8:00 am-11:00 pm, Monday-Friday. For English: [800] 232-2522; for Spanish [800] 232-0233; for the deaf [800] 243-7889.)

(Agency for Healthcare Research and Quality, 2004b; National Heart Lung and Blood Institute, National Institutes of Health, 2002)

What is Preventive Care for Men Age 19+?

Checklist

As with female clients, personal fitness trainers can set the example for their male clients. You can practice healthy behaviors, take medicines as prescribed, and get certain screening tests. When you go for your next checkup, talk to your primary care physician about how you can stay healthy no matter what your age.

Screening Tests: What You Need and When

Screening tests, such as colorectal cancer tests, can find diseases early when they are easier to treat. Some men need certain screening tests earlier, or more often, than others. Talk to your doctor about which of the tests listed below are right for you, when you should have them, and how often.

- Cholesterol Checks: Have your cholesterol checked every 5 years, starting at age 20.
- Blood Pressure: Have your blood pressure checked at least every 2 years.
- Colorectal Cancer Tests: Begin regular screening for colorectal cancer starting at age 50. Your doctor can help you decide which test is right for you. How often you need to be tested will depend on which test you have.
- Diabetes Tests: Have a test to screen for diabetes if you have high blood pressure or high cholesterol.
- Depression: If you've felt "down," sad, or hopeless, and have felt little interest or pleasure in doing things for 2 weeks straight, talk to your doctor about whether he or she can evaluate you for depression.
- Sexually Transmitted Diseases: Talk to your doctor to see whether you should be screened for sexually transmitted diseases, such as HIV.
- Prostate Cancer Screening: Talk with your doctor about the need for prostate gland screening for prostate cancer and benign prostatic hyperplasia (BPH) using PSA (prostate specific antigen blood testing) and the digital rectal examination (DRE) starting at the age of 40.
- Abdominal Aortic Aneurysm Screening: If you have ever smoked, an ultrasound is recommended between ages 65–75 to check for aneurysms. (An aneurysm is a bulge in an artery wall.)
- Eye Exam: An eye (vision) examination should be performed once every 2 years.
- Dental Care: Dental examination and routine cleaning should be a part of your overall preventive care plan.

Should You Take Medicines To Prevent Disease?
- Aspirin: Talk to your doctor about taking aspirin to prevent heart disease if you are older than age 40, or if you are younger than age 40 and have high blood pressure, high cholesterol, diabetes, or if you smoke.
- Immunizations: Stay up to date with your immunizations. Ask your health care provider about having the following.
  - A flu shot every year starting at age 50
  - A tetanus-diphtheria shot every 10 years (or a single booster at age 50)
  - A pneumonia shot once at age 65 (or earlier if you have certain health problems such as lung disease)
  - Hepatitis B shots
  (For immunization information, contact the National Immunization Information Hotline supported by CDC's National Immunization Program. It provides vaccination information for health care

providers and the public. Available 8:00 am–11:00 pm, Monday-Friday. For English: [800] 232-2522; for Spanish [800] 232-0233; for the deaf [800] 243-7889.)
(Agency for Healthcare Research and Quality, 2004a; National Heart Lung and Blood Institute, National Institutes of Health, 2002)

What Else Can Men and Women Do To Stay Healthy?

- Don't Smoke: But if you do smoke, talk to your doctor about quitting. You can take medicine and get counseling to help you quit. Make a plan and set a quit date. Tell your family, friends, and co-workers you are quitting. Ask for their support.
- Eat a Healthy Diet: Eat a variety of foods, including fruit, vegetables, animal or vegetable protein (such as meat, fish, chicken, eggs, beans, lentils, tofu, or tempeh) and grains (such as rice). Limit the amount of saturated fat you eat.
- Be Physically Active: Walk, dance, ride a bike, rake leaves, or do any other physical activity you enjoy. Start small and work up to a total of 20–30 minutes most days of the week.
- Stay at a Healthy Weight: Balance the number of calories you eat with the number you burn off by your activities. Remember to watch portion sizes. Talk to your doctor if you have questions about what or how much to eat.
- Drink Alcohol Only in Moderation: If you drink alcohol, one drink a day is safe for women, unless you are pregnant. If you are pregnant, you should avoid alcohol. Since researchers don't know how much alcohol will harm a fetus, it's best not to drink any alcohol while you are pregnant. Men should have no more than two drinks a day. A standard drink is one 12-ounce bottle of beer or wine cooler, one 5-ounce glass of wine, or 1.5 ounces of 80-proof distilled spirits.

(Agency for Healthcare Research and Quality, 2004a, 2004b; National Heart Lung and Blood Institute, National Institutes of Health, 2002)
Note: For regular updates addressing immunization and preventive care, visit The American Academy of Family Physicians http://www.aafp.org/online/en/home.html

---

Additionally, the American Diabetes Association (2004) and the National Institute of Diabetes, Digestive & Kidney Diseases (NIDDK) (2004) recommend the following.

1. Testing for diabetes should be considered for all individuals at age 45 years and above, particularly for those with a BMI 25 kg/m² and, if normal, should be repeated at 3-year intervals.
2. Testing should be considered at a younger age or be carried out more frequently for individuals who are overweight (BMI 25 kg/m² though this may not be correct for all ethnic groups) and have additional risk factors as follows. Ask your health care provider about testing and the frequency of testing if you have the following risk factors.
   - Habitual physically inactivity
   - Family history of diabetes (i.e., parents or siblings with diabetes)

- Member of a high-risk ethnic population (e.g., African American, Hispanic American/Latino, Native American, Asian American, Pacific Islander)
- History of gestational diabetes mellitus or delivery of a baby weighing > 9 lb.
- Hypertension (140/90 mmHg)
- HDL cholesterol level 35 mg/dl (0.90 mmol/L) and/or a triglyceride level ≥ 250 mg/dl (2.82 mmol/L)
- Polycystic ovary syndrome
- Previously identified impaired fasting glucose or impaired glucose tolerance
- Other clinical conditions associated with insulin resistance (e.g., acanthosis nigricans)
- History of vascular disease

Please check with your health care provider regarding insurance coverage of these tests.

Summary

In this chapter, wellness was defined and steps for good health were outlined. Measures were considered for the prevention of CHD, cancer, diabetes, COPD, cirrhosis, osteoporosis and osteoarthritis, back problems, and accidents. Seven strategies were offered for helping clients practice prevention. Client educational materials should be provided but without individualized advice to treat, cure, or alleviate specific medical conditions.

References

Agency for Healthcare Research and Quality. (2004a). *Men: Stay healthy at any age.* Retrieved December 2, 2005, from http://www.ahrq.gov/ppip/healthymen.htm.

Agency for Healthcare Research and Quality. (2004b). *Women: Stay healthy at any age.* Retrieved December 2, 2005, from http://www.ahrq.gov/ppip/healthywom.htm.

Almeda, S.L., Zonderman, A.B., Shekelle, R.B., Dyer, A.R., Daviglus, M.L., Costa Jr., P.T., et al. (1991). Neuroticism and cynicism and risk of death in middle-aged men: The Western Electric study. *Psychosomatic Medicine, 53*(2), 165-175.

American Academy of Otolaryngology–Head and Neck Surgery. (n.d.). *Head and neck cancer.* Retrieved November 20, 2005, from http://www.entnet.org/healthinfo/tobacco/cancer.cfm.

American Cancer Society. (2005a). *Cancer facts and figures.* Atlanta, GA: American Cancer Society.

American Cancer Society. (2005b). *What are the risk factors for leukemia?* Retrieved November 20, 2005, from http://www.cancer.org/docroot/CRI/content/CRI_2_4_2X_What_are_the_risk_factors_for_leukemia_24.asp.

American College of Sports Medicine. (1995). ACSM position stand on osteoporosis and exercise. *Medicine & Science in Sports & Exercise, 21*, i-vii.

American College of Sports Medicine. (2006). *ACSM's guidelines for exercise testing and prescription* (7th ed.). Baltimore: Lippincott Williams & Wilkins.

American College of Sports Medicine and Centers for Disease Control and Prevention. (1998). Joint position stand: The recommended quantity and quality of exercise for developing and maintaining cardiorespiratory and muscular fitness, and flexibility in healthy adults. *Medicine & Science in Sports & Exercise, 6*(30), 975-991.

American Diabetes Association. (2004). Screening for type 2 diabetes: Clinical practice recommendations. *Diabetes Care, 24*(Suppl.1), S5-S19.

American Heart Association. (2005). *Heart disease and stroke: 2005 update.* Retrieved July 6, 2005, from http://www.americanheart.org/downloadable/heart/110539091811 9HDSStats2005Update.pdf

Barefoot, J.C., & Schroll, M. (1996). Symptoms of depression, acute myocardial infarction, and total mortality in a community sample. *Circulation, 93,* 1976-1980.

Centers for Disease Control and Prevention. (2005a). *Bone health: Home.* Retrieved November 20, 2005, from http://www.cdc.gov/nccdphp/dnpa/bonehealth/.

Centers for Disease Control and Prevention (2005b). *Physical activity for everyone: Recommendations.* Retrieved November 20, 2005, from http://www.cdc.gov/nccdphp/dnpa/physical/recommendations/index. htm.

Cohen, R.I., Chopra, P., & Upshur, C. (2001). Primary care work-up of acute and chronic symptoms. *Geriatrics, 56*(11), 26-38.

Dunn, H. (1961). *High level wellness.* Washington, DC: Mt. Vernon.

Flegel, K.M., Carroll, M. D., Ogden, C. L., & Johnson, C. L. (2002). Prevalence and trends in obesity among U.S. adults, 1999-2000. *Journal of the American Medical Association, 288*(14), 1723-1727.

Frymoyer, J.W., & Cats-Baril, W.L. (1991). An overview of the incidence and costs of low back pain. *Orthopedic Clinics of North America, 22,* 263.

Gullette, E.C., Blumenthal, J.A., Babyak, M., Jiang, W., Waugh, R.A., Frid, D.J., et al. (1997). Effects of mental stress on myocardial ischemia during daily life. *Journal of the American Medical Association, 277*(19),1521-1526.

Helmrich, S.P., Ragland, D.R., Leung, R.W., & Paffenbarger, R.S. (1991). Physical activity and reduced occurrence of non-insulin-dependent diabetes mellitus. *New England Journal of Medicine, 325,* 147-152.

Hettler, B. (2005). National Wellness Institute, Inc.: 6 dimensional wellness model. Retrieved July 14, 2005, from http://www.nationalwellness.org/aboutus/index.php?id=167&id_tier=1.

Hill, J.O., Wyatt, H.R., Reed, G.W., & Peters, J.C. (2003). Obesity and the environment: Where do we go from here? *Science, 299*(5608), 853-855.

Joint National Committee on Prevention, Detection, Evaluation, and Treatment of High Blood Pressure. (2003). *The Seventh Report of the Joint National Committee on Prevention, Detection, Evaluation, and Treatment of High Blood Pressure (JNC 7).* [Electronic Version]. Washington, DC: National Heart Lung and Blood Institute. Retrieved July 6, 2005, from http://www.nhlbi.nih.gov/guidelines/hypertension/jnc7full.pdf.

Lawrence, R.C., Helmick, C.G., & Arnett, F.C. (1998). Estimates of the prevalence of arthritis and selected musculoskeletal disorders in the United States. *Arthritis and Rheumatism, 41*(5), 778-799.

National Cancer Institute. (2002a). *Bladder cancer: Who is at risk?* Retrieved November 20, 2005, from http://www.cancer.gov/cancertopics/wyntk/bladder/page4.

National Cancer Institute. (2002b). *Pancreatic cancer: Who is at risk?* Retrieved November 20, 2005, from http://www.cancer.gov/cancertopics/wyntk/pancreas/page4.

National Cancer Institute. (2002c). *Liver cancer: Who is at risk?* Retrieved November 20, 2005, from http://www.cancer.gov/cancertopics/wyntk/liver/page4.

National Cancer Institute. (2003). *Tobacco statistics snapshop.* Retrieved November 20, 2005, from http://www.cancer.gov/cancertopics/tobacco/statisticssnapshot.

National Cancer Institute. (2005a). *What you need to know about breast cancer.* Retrieved November 20, 2005, from http://www.cancer.gov/ cancertopics/wyntk/breast/.

National Cancer Institute. (2005b). *What you need to know about skin cancer.* Retrieved November 20, 2005, from http://www.cancer.gov/cancertopics/wyntk/skin/page1.

National Cancer Institute. (2005c). *Cervical cancer: Prevention.* Retrieved November 20, 2005, from http://www.cancer.gov/cancertopics/wyntk/cervix/page6.

National Center for Chronic Disease Prevention and Health Promotion. (2003). *National diabetes fact sheet.* Atlanta, GA: Centers for Disease Control and Prevention. Retrieved July 6, 2005, from http://www.cdc.gov/diabetes/pubs/pdf/ndfs_2003.pdf.

National Center for Chronic Disease Prevention and Health Promotion. (2004). *Chronic disease overview.* Retrieved November 20, 2005, from http://www.cdc.gov/nccdphp/overview.htm.

National Center for Health Statistics. (2004). Summary health statistics for U.S. adults: National health interview survey, 2002. [Electronic version]. *Vital and Health Statistics, 10*(222). Atlanta, GA: Centers for Disease Control and Prevention. Retrieved July 6, 2005 from http://www.cdc.gov/nchs/data/series/sr_10/sr10_222.pdf.

National Center for Injury Prevention and Control. (2005a). *Community-based interventions to reduce motor vehicle-related injuries: Evidence of effectiveness from systematic reviews.* Retrieved November 20, 2005, from http://www.cdc.gov/ncipc/duip/mvsafety.htm.

National Center for Injury Prevention and Control. (2005b). *Impaired driving fact sheet.* Retrieved November 20, 2005, from http://www.cdc.gov/ncipc/factsheets/drving.htm.

National Heart Lung and Blood Institute, National Institutes of Health (2002). *Third report of the National Cholesterol Education Program Expert Panel on detection, evaluation, and treatment of high blood cholesterol in adults (adult treatment panel III) final report.* Retrieved December 2, 2005, from http://www.nhlbi.nih.gov/guidelines/cholesterol/atp3full.pdf.

National Institute of Diabetes, Digestive & Kidney Diseases. (2004). *Am I at risk for type 2 diabetes? Taking steps to lower the risk of getting diabetes.* Retrieved July 14, 2005, from http://www.diabetes.niddk.nih.gov/dm/pubs/riskfortype2/index.htm.

National Institutes of Health. (2005). *NIH senior health: Colorectal cancer.* Retrieved November 20, 2005, from http://nihseniorhealth.gov/colorectalcancer/faq/faq3a.html.

Petty, T.L. (1990). Definitions in chronic obstructive pulmonary disease. *Clinics in Chest Medicine, 11,* 363-373.

Pi-Sunyer, F.X. (2002). The obesity epidemic: Pathophysiology and consequences of obesity. *Obesity Research; 10*(Suppl. 2), 97S-104S.

President's Council on Physical Fitness. (2000, March). Definitions: Health, fitness, and physical activity. PCPFS Research Digests. Retrieved July 6, 2005, from http://www.fitness.gov/digest_mar2000.htm.

Regier, D.A., Farmer, M.E., Rae, D.S., Locke, B.Z., Keith, S.J., Judd. L.L., et al. (1990). Comorbidity of mental disorders with alcohol and other drug abuse. Results from the epidemiologic catchment area study. *Journal of the American Medical Association. 264*(19), 2511-2518.

Russek, L.G., King, S.H., Russek, S.J., & Russek, H.I. (1990). The Harvard mastery of stress study—35-year follow-up: Prognostic significance of patterns of psychophysiological arousal and adaptation. *Psychiatric Medicine, 52,* 271-285.

Salmeron, J., Manson, J.E., Stampfer, M.J., Colditz, G.A., Wing, A.L., & Willett, W.C. (1997). Dietary fiber, glycemic load, and risk of non-insulin-dependent diabetes mellitus in women. *Journal of the American Medical Association, 277,* 472-477.

Schoenborn, C.A., & Barnes, P.M. (2002). Leisure-time physical activity among adults: United States, 1997-98. [Electronic version]. *Advanced Data from Vital and Health Statistics, 7*(325), 1-24. Retrieved July 6, 2005 from http://www.cdc.gov/nchs/data/ad/ad330.pdf.

Travis, J.W., & Ryan, R.S. (2004). *Wellness Workbook* (3rd ed.). Berkeley, CA: Celestial Arts.

U.S. Departments of Agriculture and Health and Human Services. (2005). *Nutrition and your health: Dietary guidelines for Americans* (6th ed.). Washington, DC: Government Printing Office.

U.S. Department of Health and Human Services. (1990). *The health benefits of smoking cessation* (DHHS, PHS, Office on Smoking and Health, DHHS Publication No. [CDC] 90-8416). Washington, DC: Superintendent of Documents.

U.S. Department of Health and Human Services. (1996). *Physical activity and health: A report of the Surgeon General.* Atlanta, GA: U.S. Department of Health and Human Services, Centers for Disease Control and Prevention, National Center for Chronic Disease Prevention and Health Promotion.

Suggested Reading

American College of Sports Medicine. (2006). *ACSM's resource manual for guidelines for exercise testing and prescription* (5th ed.). Baltimore: Lippincott Williams & Wilkins.

Blair, S.N., Kohl, H.W., Barlow, C.E., Paffenbarger, R.S., Gibbons, L.W., & Macera, C.A. (1995). Changes in physical fitness and all-cause mortality: A prospective study of healthy and unhealthy men. *Journal of the American Medical Association, 273*, 1093-1098.

Dickman, S.R. (1988). *Pathways to wellness.* Champaign, IL: Human Kinetics.

Expert Committee on the Diagnosis and Classification of Diabetes Mellitus. (2003). Follow-up report on the diagnosis of diabetes mellitus. *Diabetes Care, 26*, 3160-3167.

Lee, I.M. (1995). Exercise and physical health: Cancer and immune function. *Research Quarterly for Exercise and Sport, 66*, 286-291.

Nieman, D.C. (1998). *The exercise health connection.* Champaign, IL: Human Kinetics.

NIH Consensus Development Panel on Physical Activity and Cardiovascular Health. (1996). *Physical activity and cardiovascular health. Journal of the American Medical Association, 276*, 241-246.

Travis, J.W., & Ryan, R.S. (1991). *Wellness: Small changes you can use to make a big difference.* Berkeley, CA: Ten Speed Press.

Resources

- Action on Smoking and Health—(202) 659-4310
- American Association of Diabetes Educators—www.aadenet.org
- American Cancer Society—www.cancer.org
- American College of Sports Medicine—www.acsm.org
- American Diabetes Association—www.diabetes.org
- American Heart Association—www.americanheart.org
- American Liver Foundation—www.liverfoundation.org
- American Lung Association—www.lungusa.org
- Arthritis Foundation—www.arthritis.org
- Centers for Disease Control and Prevention—www.cdc.gov
- Dietary Guidelines—www.healthierus.gov/dietary guidelines
- National Coalition for Promoting Physical Activity—www.ncppa.org
- National Institute of Arthritis and Musculoskeletal and Skin Diseases—www.niams.nih.gov
- National Osteoporosis Foundation—www.nof.org
- NIH Osteoporosis and Related Bone Disease—www.osteo.org
- Smoking cessation Web sites:
  — www.smokefree.gov
  — www.quitTobacco.org
  — www.quitnet
  — www.endsmoking.org
- World Health Organization—www.who.int/hpr/physactiv/index.shtml

Exercise Physiology

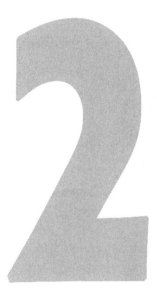

Outline

- Cardiorespiratory System
- Basic Principles of Energetics
- Anaerobic Energy Systems
- Aerobic (Oxidative) Energy System
- Comparison of the Energy Systems
- Fat versus Carbohydrate Utilization
- Cardiorespiratory Responses to Exercise
- Basic Neuromuscular Physiology

Exercise physiology is the science of how the body operates during exercise and at rest. In this chapter, you will first learn about the anatomy and function of two of the body's major systems: the circulatory system and the respiratory system. Next, there will be a discussion of the basic principles of energy metabolism; exactly how does the body make, store, and utilize energy for work and exercise? Finally, the anatomy and function of the body's neuromuscular system will be addressed, exploring how messages are conveyed and how muscle contractions are produced at the cellular level. Understanding the fundamentals of exercise physiology is essential for proper exercise programming. Clients frequently ask questions about topics such as heart rate, lactic acid and lactate, and fat burning, and a qualified trainer should be able to give accurate answers.

Cardiorespiratory System

Structure and Function of the Heart

The heart is a muscular organ located in the chest diagonally behind the breastbone, or sternum. About the size of a fist, this relatively small organ performs a tremendous amount of work to maintain life processes. Even at rest, the amount of blood pumped by the heart per minute (cardiac output) averages 5 liters. During vigorous exercise this level can increase to as much as 20–30 liters per minute (Wilmore & Costill, 2004).

The heart is divided into right and left sides by a wall, or septum. The right side of the heart receives deoxygenated blood as it is returned from the body by the venous system. It then pumps blood to the lungs where gas exchange occurs and oxygen is taken up by the hemoglobin molecules in the red blood cells. The left side of the heart receives the oxygenated blood from the lungs and pumps it, via the arterial system, throughout the body. Because the heart performs two distinct functions, it is often referred to as a double-pump.

The heart is further broken down into upper and lower chambers, respectively called the **atria** (atrium, singular) and the **ventricles**. The superior atria (left and right) are the blood-receiving units of the heart. After entering the atria, blood is forced through a one-way system of valves, known as AV (atrioventricular) valves, into the inferior ventricles. The contraction of the ventricles then forces blood through the semilunar valves and into the great arteries, delivering blood to the lungs (from the right ventricle) or to the rest of the body (from the left ventricle). The familiar "lub-dub" sounds of the heart are produced by the closing of the atrioventricular and semilunar valves. (The left AV valve is also known as the mitral valve).

The heart is entirely contained within a loose yet protective sac, called the pericardium, which prevents the beating heart from brushing against the chest wall. The heart itself is composed of three specialized layers of tissue: the epicardium, the myocardium, and the endocardium. The epicardium is a thin membrane located on the outermost layer of the heart. The primary work of the heart is performed by the next layer of muscular tissue, the **myocardium**. The myocardium is thickest and strongest in the walls of the left ventricle, the chamber responsible for pumping blood throughout the body. The endocardium is the smooth membrane that lines the chambers of the heart.

Both the epicardium and the myocardium of the heart are nourished primarily by the coronary arteries; therefore, it is essential that these important vessels be as healthy as possible. A **myocardial infarction** (MI), or heart attack, occurs due to a lack of blood flow (**ischemia**) through the coronary arteries to the heart muscle. This causes permanent damage to cardiac muscle fibers referred to as an infarction (blockage of blood flow). When infarction occurs, those portions of the myocardium that are affected die.

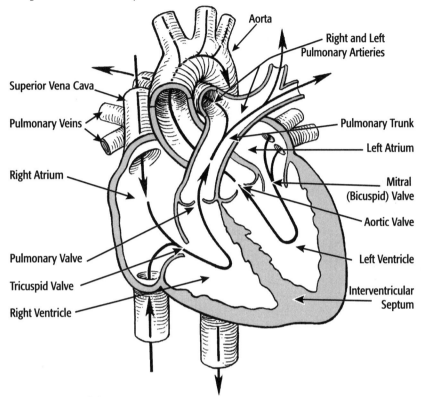

Fig. 2-1. Structure of the Heart
NOTE: The pulmonary and tricuspid valves are collectively known as the semilunar valves; the aortic and mitral valves are collectively known as the atrioventricular valves.

Cardiac Cycle

The contraction/relaxation pattern produced by the heart is known as the cardiac cycle. The ventricular contraction phase is called the systole and the relaxation phase is called the diastole. A rhythmic squeezing action of the heart pumps blood continuously through the arteries to all the tissues of the body, and the amount of blood pumped with each beat, or systole, is called the **stroke volume**. The number of times the heart beats each minute is known as the heart rate. Heart rate multiplied by stroke volume equals the amount of blood pumped per minute, or the cardiac output (heart rate x stroke volume = cardiac output). **Cardiac output** is usually measured in liters (or milliliters) of blood pumped per minute.

Conduction System

The conduction system of the heart is autorhythmic in nature and is controlled by a specialized nerve center in the brain called the medulla. Conduction in the heart begins with an electrical impulse of the sinoatrial (SA) node within the right atrium. The SA node dictates regulation of the contractions of the heart and is therefore referred to as the pacemaker. On average, an adult's resting heart rate beats approximately 60–80 times per minute (McArdle, Katch, & Katch, 2003). The electrical impulse of the SA node causes both atria to contract synchronously and, as a result, blood is forced into the ventricles. Almost immediately after the SA node fires, the electrical charge travels through specialized conduction tissue to reach the atrioventricular (AV) node. The AV node consists of slow-conducting muscle cells, which delay the impulse slightly before it excites the ventricular conductors, the bundle of His, the right and left bundle branches, and, finally, the Purkinje fibers. This chain of electrical events results in a simultaneous and powerful contraction of the ventricles, which forces blood out into the major arteries. Note that the electrical activity of the heart described above can be recorded on an ECG (EKG), or electrocardiogram, a device used to diagnose potential cardiac problems.

Circulatory System

The circulatory system consists of the blood-carrying vessels: the arteries, capillaries, and veins that produce a circuit of blood flow throughout the body. This circuit is shown in Figure 2-2 and can basically be explained as follows. Deoxygenated blood enters the right atrium from the vena cava and then flows into the right ventricle. The right ventricle pumps the blood through the pulmonary artery into the lungs, where carbon dioxide is exchanged for oxygen. The newly oxygenated blood leaves the lungs and returns to the heart via the pulmonary veins, entering the left atrium. From the left atrium the blood flows into the left ventricle, and with a powerful contraction it is forced into the aorta, the largest artery in the body. From the aorta the blood enters a network of arteries; the primary arteries include the carotid arteries in the neck and head, the abdominal arteries of the trunk, and the axillary and iliac arteries of the arms and legs, respectively. A great number of smaller arteries branch off the large arteries, yielding smaller and smaller units until the blood passes into the smallest arteries, called arterioles. Arteries are capable of expansion and contraction, helping to maintain a smooth and continuous blood flow, due to their elastic, muscular walls. After leaving the arterioles, blood passes into the capillaries, microscopic vessels where the exchange of oxygen and nutrients with tissue waste products takes place.

It is notable that the single-celled structure of the capillary walls allows for an easy transfer of materials to and from the tissue cells. Here, the blood gives up its oxygen, nutrients, and fluids to the tissues, and in return the tissues give up carbon dioxide and other wastes to the blood.

As the blood leaves the capillaries, it enters the venous system, which returns blood back to the heart (**venous return**). Here, the veins complement the arteries in function. Structurally, veins resemble arteries; however, they have thinner walls and are less muscular. Venous blood is returned to the heart under low pressure and is often forced to move against gravity. To keep a steady blood flow to the heart, veins contain a one-way system of valves that prevent the backflow of blood. Additionally, the massaging action of contracting muscles in the legs and arms helps move blood back to the heart; this is called the muscle pump. Blood return actually begins in the smallest units of the venous system, the venules, and then gradually branches into larger and larger vessels, eventually entering the largest veins, the superior and inferior vena cava, and from there back into the right atrium of the heart.

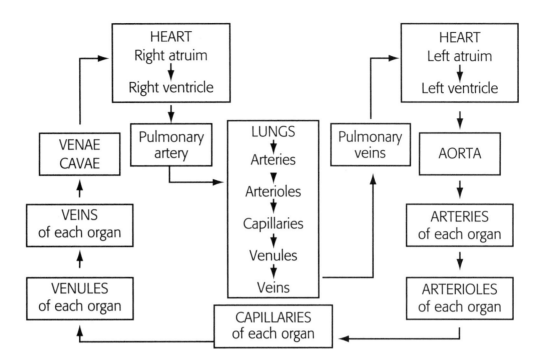

Fig. 2-2. Blood Flow Patterns of the Circulatory Vessels

Respiratory System

The respiratory, or pulmonary, system is responsible for providing two major functions: air distribution and gas exchange. Additionally, the respiratory system filters, warms, and moisturizes the air being breathed. Organs associated with the respiratory system also produce sound and speech, and provide a sense of smell.

Air enters the body through the mouth or nostrils and passes into the nasal cavity where it is warmed and humidified. The oral and nasal passages lead to the throat, or pharynx. After passing through the pharynx, the inspired air enters the larynx. The larynx is composed of pieces of cartilage, the largest of which is known as the Adam's apple. The larynx, or voice box, produces sound as air passes the vocal cords, located inside the larynx itself. Another cartilaginous structure found in the larynx is the epiglottis, which partially covers the opening in the larynx and closes during swallowing to prevent food from passing into the trachea. The epiglottis, or glottis, is the structure involved in the potentially dangerous Valsalva maneuver.

The **Valsalva maneuver** occurs when a person holds his or her breath during strenuous activity, such as lifting weights or shoveling snow. The glottis is closed against pressure, which causes an increased thoracic pressure leading to an interruption of the venous return to the heart, reducing blood flow to the coronary arteries, and decreasing oxygen supply to the brain. In healthy individuals, this may result in dizziness, slowing of the heart rate, or possibly even fainting. For the person predisposed to heart disease, the Valsalva maneuver could trigger arrhythmias and potentially serious complications. Proper breathing techniques are, therefore, essential during heavy exercise. Personal fitness trainers must consistently remind their clients to breathe!

Air flows from the larynx into the trachea, or windpipe, which connects the larynx to the lungs. The trachea is structurally protected by cartilaginous rings. Sometimes, however, a blockage of the trachea occurs, as in choking. The life-saving Heimlich maneuver can be used to free the trachea of obstructions caused by food or other foreign bodies. The Heimlich maneuver is an easily acquired skill and, like CPR, should be learned by all health/fitness professionals. (See Appendix A, "Emergency Protocol: Standard First Aid, CPR, and AED").

In the chest cavity, the trachea branches into two main bronchi, the right and left bronchus, which travel into the respective lung. In the lungs, each bronchus branches into smaller passageways called bronchioles. The walls of the bronchioles are formed with smooth, elastic muscle tissue. (Excessive spasm in the smooth muscles of the bronchioles creates breathing difficulties and associated diseases, such as asthma). The bronchioles lead to tiny tubes, or alveolar ducts, which attach to a cluster of grape-like structures called alveolar sacs. These alveolar sacs are composed of millions of alveoli, which have extremely thin walls. The thin walls of the alveoli permit an exchange of gases, into and out of the capillaries, through a process known as pulmonary diffusion. It is here that inhaled oxygen passes through the walls of the alveoli and into the blood in the nearby capillaries. Some of the oxygen is absorbed into the blood, but most of it combines with hemoglobin in the red blood cells; red blood cells then carry oxygen to the tissues of the body. In the tissues, oxygen is exchanged for carbon dioxide, which is then transported back to the alveoli for removal during exhalation.

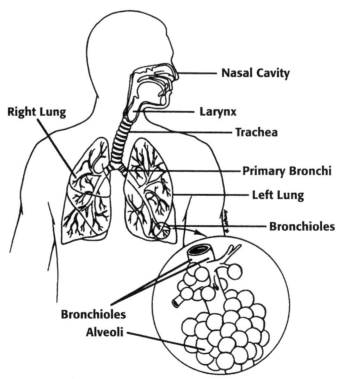

Fig. 2-3. Structures of the Pulmonary Systems

The entire breathing process is controlled in the respiratory center of the brain where nerve impulses signal the primary muscles of respiration, the diaphragm and the intercostal muscles, to contract. (Other muscles involved in respiration include the sternocleidomastoid, scalenes, and transverse abdominis). The diaphragm is a dome-shaped muscle that separates the chest cavity from the abdominal cavity, rising and falling with each breath. The total amount of air breathed per minute is called the **minute ventilation**; at rest, approximately 6 liters of air are exchanged per minute. Other useful pulmonary physiology terms include the residual lung volume, forced vital capacity, and total lung capacity. **Residual lung volume** refers to the amount of air remaining in the lungs after a complete and total forced exhale. This residual volume is necessary to prevent the lungs from collapsing in upon themselves. **Forced vital capacity** is a value measured during some fitness assessments (a spirometer is required); it is the amount of air that can be forcefully exhaled after a maximal inhale. Finally, **total lung capacity** is the sum of the residual volume and the forced vital capacity.

Basic Principles of Energetics

The source of all biological energy is the sun. In order to sustain human life, the sun's energy needs to be transformed from light into a form of chemical energy that can be used by the body. How does this happen? The transformation of light energy begins with its absorption by green plants through the process of photosynthesis. Plants produce complex food molecules that contain large supplies of stored chemical energy. Plants can form and store various types of carbohydrates, fats, and proteins. Animals and humans can derive energy by ingesting plants and using them as sources of fuel. Vegetarians obtain all their energy from plant sources alone, while those who eat meat derive a portion of their energy from the protein, carbohydrate, and fat stored in the meat of other animals.

Once eaten, **macronutrients** (protein, carbohydrate, and fat) are either stored or used for the energy necessary to live and perform biological work. Exactly how are macronutrients used for energy? Food energy is transformed in the body by entering one of three metabolic pathways, or energy systems, which will be described below. The primary purpose of these **metabolic pathways** is to transform food energy into adenosine triphosphate (ATP), a form of stored energy that can be directly utilized by the cells of the body. This energy flow is illustrated in Figure 2-4.

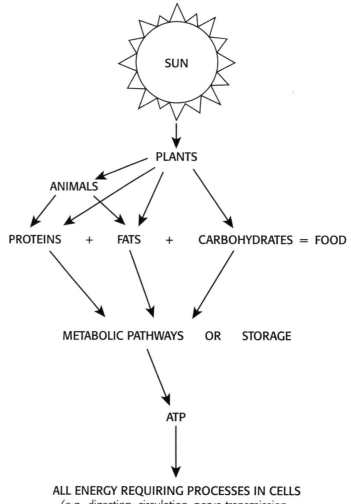

Fig. 2-4. Energy Flow Chart

Adenosine Triphosphate

Before discussing the metabolic pathways and energy storage, it is important to understand **ATP**, or **adenosine triphosphate**. ATP is a molecule, found in every cell in the body, that is composed of adenosine (a nitrogen-containing base), ribose (a five-carbon sugar), and three phosphate groups. This important chemical compound is the form in which food energy is stored in your cells. Any energy stored in the body in the form of carbohydrate or fat must first be converted into ATP before it can be used. ATP is necessary for cellular work and is needed in especially large quantities during exercise.

Adenosine – P ~ P ~ P = ATP   (~ = high-energy bond)

When ATP is broken down, a high-energy bond is broken and a phosphate group is released. This yields a significant amount of energy that can be used for cellular work.

ADP (Adenosine   ~   P   ~   P) + P are the end result.

Fig. 2-5. Breakdown of ATP

Note that the three phosphate groups in the ATP molecule are connected by high-energy bonds. Energy is released, allowing the cell to perform work, when the last phosphate group breaks off. The remaining compound is now called adenosine diphosphate (ADP) since only two phosphate groups are left. New ATP can be resynthesized from the ADP, the remaining phosphate, and the addition of more energy. This process of ATP breakdown and ATP resynthesis occurs nearly simultaneously in a coupled reaction. But where does the additional energy necessary to resynthesize ATP come from? Muscle cells have three methods of resynthesizing ATP, utilizing the three metabolic pathways or energy systems:

1. The phosphagen (ATP-PC) system
2. The anaerobic glycolytic (lactic acid) system
3. The aerobic (oxidative) system

These energy pathways will be discussed beginning with the simplest and moving toward the most complex. The phosphagen system is a simple system of coupled reactions; the anaerobic glycolytic system is more complex involving a sequence of reactions; and finally, the aerobic system is a complex and intricate combination of several pathways. In terms of their significance in everyday life, however, the order of discussion would be reversed. Most energetic needs throughout the day (and night) are met by the aerobic system alone. In fact, most cells primarily function aerobically, in particular the cells of the heart and brain. Anaerobic pathways are used primarily by muscle cells, as in activities that require a significant amount of muscular effort, such as moderate to intense exercise, heavy manual labor, climbing several flights of stairs, carrying a baby, or changing a tire. These types of activities require the recruitment of the anaerobic pathways: the anaerobic glycolytic and phosphagen systems.

Anaerobic Energy Systems

There are two energy systems in the body that can operate without oxygen—the phosphagen system and the anaerobic glycolytic system. Because of this, they are referred to as anaerobic energy systems. It is probably more important, however, to identify them as systems that can resynthesize ATP at a high rate. As you will see, the aerobic energy system is simply too slow to produce ATP at the speed required for short, intense activities. For these activities, the anaerobic energy systems are necessary.

Phosphagen (ATP-PC) System

The phosphagen system supplies energy very quickly and is the primary source of energy for very high-intensity exercise. Biochemically, the phosphagen system is by far the simplest of the three systems. Energy for the resynthesis of

ATP comes by way of a coupled reaction involving the breakdown of creatine phosphate (CP). The compound CP, also known as phosphocreatine (PC), is similar to ATP. Because of this similarity, CP and ATP are referred to collectively as phosphagens. CP consists of a creatine molecule connected to a phosphate group by a high-energy bond. When CP is split into creatine (C) and phosphate (P), enough energy is released to resynthesize ATP.

Creatine ~ P = CP   (~ = high-energy bond)

When CP is broken down, a high-energy bond is broken and enough energy is released to resynthesize ATP.

Adenosine ~ P ~ P + energy from the breakdown of CP + P = ATP

Fig. 2-6. Phosphagen System

The enzyme most responsible for helping to speed up the chemical reaction in the phosphagen system is called creatine kinase (CK). An enzyme is a protein molecule that speeds up a chemical reaction in the body; each energy system has its own specific regulatory enzymes. Any condition that stimulates or speeds CK will increase the rate at which the phosphagen system produces energy. Conversely, any condition that inhibits or slows CK will reduce the rate of energy production. The most significant stimulatory factor is the rapid accumulation of ADP within the muscle cell. This is a signal to the muscle that ATP is being consumed rapidly. In an attempt to maintain the concentration of ATP, creatine kinase is activated, and CP is rapidly broken down. The energy released from CP is used to replace the ATP being consumed.

The ATP-PC, or phosphagen, system is extremely important in activities that require energy very quickly for a very short period of time. Such activities include sprinting, jumping, throwing, kicking, and lifting heavy weights. Sports that include these activities rely at least in part on the phosphagen system. If the activity can be sustained for no more than 15–20 seconds, the phosphagen system is the primary source of energy. Good examples of specific events that primarily rely on the ATP-PC system include 100- and 200-meter running sprints, 50-meter swimming sprints, high jump and long jump, shot put and discus, and power lifting. With the limited supply of CP (remember, PC is the same thing) in muscle cells, the capacity of the phosphagen system is limited to approximately 1 mole or less of ATP (a **mole** is a unit of measurement used for counting extremely large numbers of atoms—1 mole of a substance is 6.022×10^{23} units of that substance). This is equivalent to about 10 kcal or less of energy, which is a very small amount; barely enough to sprint 200 meters (20–30 sec.) before it is exhausted. To summarize the phosphagen system: it can produce very small amounts of ATP extremely quickly, it is the primary energy source for very short, highly intense activities, and it is limited by the small supplies of CP stored within the cells.

Anaerobic Glycolytic (Lactic Acid) System

The body's other anaerobic pathway, the glycolytic system, also provides a rapid source of energy. Instead of CP, however, the fuel source for this system is

glucose, the body's usable form of carbohydrate. Carbohydrates are the only form of food that can be used as fuel in the anaerobic glycolytic system. The glucose used for fuel can come either from blood glucose or from stored glycogen (the storage form of carbohydrate) within the muscle. Inside the sarcoplasm of the cell, the glucose is broken down in a series of nine or more reactions called glycolysis, leading to the formation of pyruvic acid. If the intensity level is high, and the body is unable to provide enough oxygen, the pyruvic acid (pyruvate) is transformed into lactic acid (lactate). Under these circumstances, the process is called anaerobic glycolysis.

NOTE: "Lactic acid and lactate are not the same compound. Lactic acid is an acid…[and] lactate is any salt of lactic acid. When lactic acid releases H+, the remaining compound joins with Na+ or K+ to form a salt. Anaerobic glycolysis produces lactic acid but it quickly dissociates and the salt, lactate, is formed. For this reason, the terms are often used interchangeably" (Wilmore & Costill, 2004).

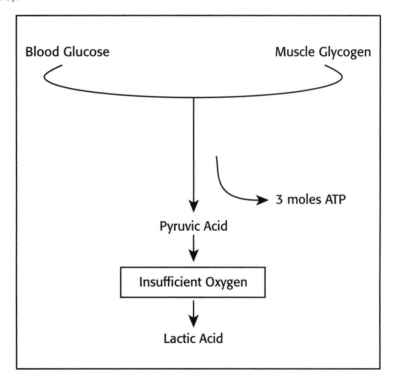

Fig. 2-7. Anaerobic Glycolytic (Lactic Acid) System

The most important enzyme that helps regulate the anaerobic glycolytic system is PFK, or phosphofructokinase. PFK, and hence the anaerobic glycolytic system, is stimulated by the rapid accumulation of ADP and the depletion of CP in the phosphagen system during high-intensity exercise. In the average person, 1 mole of glucose yields 2 ATP, while 1 mole of glycogen results in 3 ATP. Although the capacity of the anaerobic glycolytic system is greater than that of the phosphagen system, 2–3 moles of ATP are sufficient to provide only enough energy for short-duration exercise.

The primary limiting factor in the anaerobic glycolytic system is the build-up of lactic acid, causing fatigue, breathlessness, and a burning sensation in the muscles, which literally become too acidic to operate. The capacity of a person's glycolytic system is also determined by his or her ability to neutralize and tolerate lactic acid. Research suggests that the level of lactic acid that can be tolerated by the untrained person would allow for only about 1 minute of high-intensity exercise (Spencer & Gasti, 2001). In competitive athletes who have developed a tolerance for lactic acid, ATP may be produced during anaerobic glycolysis for as much as 2–3 minutes of high-intensity exercise.

The anaerobic glycolytic system is very important in prolonged sprints (400–800 meters running, 100–200 meters swimming, or 1,000–2,000 meters cycling). It also provides much of the energy for sustained, high-intensity rallies in soccer, field hockey, ice hockey, lacrosse, basketball, volleyball, tennis, badminton, and other sports. The floor routine in gymnastics relies in part on this system, with intermittent bursts of higher energy production from the phosphagen system. The common denominator in all of these activities is a sustained, high-intensity effort lasting from 1–2 minutes. To summarize the anaerobic glycolytic system: energy is produced rapidly via the breakdown of glucose into lactic acid. Lactic acid production results in fatigue, which explains why this pathway is typically the primary source of energy for only 45–90 seconds or so. It is utilized during high-intensity, short-duration activities.

Aerobic (Oxidative) Energy System

Unlike the anaerobic systems, the aerobic system has a virtually unlimited capacity for making ATP, primarily because it can use carbohydrates, fats, and proteins for fuel, and because it produces only carbon dioxide and water as its end products. The major limitations of the aerobic system are its many complex steps and its reliance on a constant supply of oxygen. It's important to understand that the aerobic system supplies all of the energy for most activities of daily living (including sleeping), and for low- to moderate-intensity exercise. As the activity or exercise becomes more intense, to the point that it can only be sustained for a matter of a few minutes, the aerobic system can no longer provide energy at a sufficient rate. At this stage, ATP production is supplemented by the anaerobic glycolytic and phosphagen systems.

The aerobic, or oxidative, system refers to a complex series of reactions that can be divided into three components. The first component can actually be one of three pathways depending upon whether the source of fuel is carbohydrate, fat, or protein. When carbohydrate is used, the first component is aerobic glycolysis; when fat is used, the first component is fat (beta) oxidation; and, if the source of fuel is protein, the first component pathway is protein metabolism. The second component is a cyclical process called the Krebs cycle, which leads to the third component, the electron transport system.

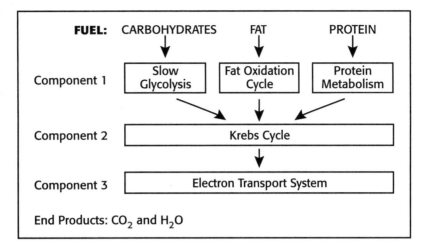

Fig. 2-8. Components of the Aerobic Energy System

Aerobic System: First Component

In order to describe the first component of the aerobic system, it is important to first consider the different ways that carbohydrates, fats, and proteins are metabolized aerobically. The aerobic production of ATP from carbohydrates starts with **aerobic glycolysis** in the sarcoplasm of the cell. The major difference between aerobic glycolysis and the anaerobic glycolysis described previously is the presence of sufficient oxygen. If the intensity is low enough that sufficient oxygen is available, lactic acid is no longer the end product. The process of glycolysis is exactly the same, beginning with a molecule of glucose, which is broken down through a series of nine or more reactions, resulting in pyruvic acid. In the presence of sufficient oxygen, the pyruvic acid does not degrade into lactic acid, but instead enters the **mitochondria**, a subcellular structure where oxidation takes place. Here, acetyl groups (acetyl CoA) are formed from the pyruvic acid, ready to enter the second component, the Krebs cycle.

Fats, on the other hand, are stored in the body in adipose tissue and within skeletal muscle in the form of triglycerides. Fat is a highly efficient fuel for storing energy; whereas, muscle and liver glycogen may only supply about 1,200–2,000 kcal of energy, fat can supply as much as 70,000–75,000 kcal of energy (Wilmore & Costill, 2004). For fat stored in adipose tissue to be used for exercise, it must first be converted into a usable form of fat called a free fatty acid (FFA). Within the mitochondria, free fatty acids are activated and made ready for the second component in a process called **beta oxidation**, which results in the conversion into acetyl CoA.

Finally, a brief word is in order about the use of protein as a fuel and **protein metabolism**. Protein usually provides no more than 5–15% of the total energy requirement of an activity (even this amount is only under extreme conditions, such as a prolonged endurance event). Therefore, protein is not as important a fuel as carbohydrate or fat during exercise. The main source of stored protein in the body is muscle. It is obviously not advantageous to use this source for fuel during exercise. Under special circumstances (e.g., severe glycogen depletion) protein can actually be converted into glucose by a process called gluconeogenesis. When protein is used directly, it is broken down into amino acids, a simpler, more usable form of protein, eventually producing small amounts of acetyl CoA.

Aerobic System: Second Component

The acetyl CoA formed in the first component of aerobic metabolism enters into the citric acid cycle, better know as the **Krebs cycle**. The Krebs cycle was named after the Nobel Prize winning biochemist Sir Hans A. Krebs who discovered the process in the 1930's. The combination of the acetyl with other compounds results in the production of citric acid; once citric acid is formed it goes through a series of reactions, including several oxidations in which hydrogen ions and electrons are removed. These electrons are important because they are the driving force for the electron transport system, the next step. Carbon molecules remain at the end of the Krebs cycle, but these readily combine with oxygen to form carbon dioxide, which is eventually exhaled through the lungs.

Aerobic System: Third Component

The final sequence of reactions in the aerobic production of ATP is the **electron transport system**. An electrical gradient (difference) exists between the beginning and the end of the electron transport system. The gradient created by this arrangement allows the electrons to "flow" through the system. This flow supplies the energy necessary to make a tremendous amount of ATP. The remaining hydrogen ions combine with oxygen to form water.

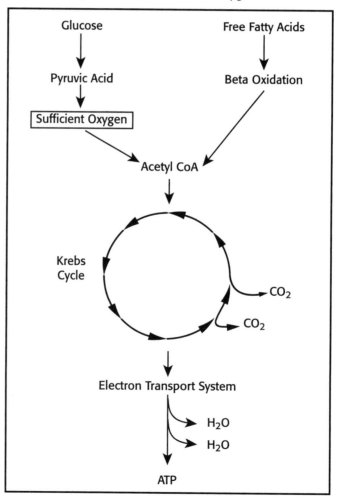

Fig. 2-9. Aerobic System Flow Chart

In terms of the amount of energy produced, the aerobic energy system is far more efficient than either the phosphagen system or the anaerobic glycolytic system. For example, 1 mole of carbohydrate produces 38 ATP; 1 mole of fat produces 147 ATP; and 1 mole of protein produces 15 ATP when combusted by the aerobic system. The major limiting factors of the aerobic system are its complexity and need for oxygen. Due to the many complex steps involved in aerobic metabolism, any rapid increase in intensity will necessitate supplementation from the anaerobic pathways, at least temporarily. If the increase in intensity is sustained at a high level (above 80–85% of maximum heart rate), then the limit of the aerobic system will eventually be reached and the anaerobic glycolytic system will provide ATP until exhaustion. The best examples of exercises relying primarily on the aerobic system for energy include distance running (> 5,000 meters), distance swimming (> 1,500 meters), distance cycling (> 10 kilometers), cross-country skiing (> 5,000 meters), and 40–60 minutes of cardiorespiratory group exercise. Any activity using large, major muscle groups repetitively for a minimum of 5 minutes at a low to moderate intensity, relies primarily on the aerobic system.

Comparison of the Energy Systems

COMPARISON OF THE ENERGY SYSTEMS					
System	**Fuel**	**ATP Production**	**ATP Capacity**	**Limiting Factor(s)**	**Intensity**
Phosphagen System	CP	very fast	< 1 mole	small supply of CP	very high
Anaerobic Glycolytic (Lactic Acid) System	glucose	fast	2–3 moles	anaerobic glycolytic causes fatigue	high
Aerobic System	glucose, fat, protein	slow	~ 147 moles	complexity, slow	low to moderate

Fat versus Carbohydrate Utilization

At rest, since oxygen is easily supplied to the cells, ATP is produced by the breakdown of both carbohydrate and fat in approximately equal measure. The average person burns about 1 calorie per minute at rest, and about 50% of this calorie is supplied from carbohydrate; the other 50% of the calorie comes from fat. During low- to moderate-intensity exercise, this 50:50 ratio persists, as both fat and carbohydrate are burned fairly evenly for fuel. As the level of intensity increases, however, changes occur that begin to inhibit the use of fats and increase the use of carbohydrates. A significant inhibitor is the lactic acid produced. Also, a person's aerobic fitness level determines the point at which the cardiorespiratory system can no longer supply sufficient oxygen. At higher intensities, less and less fat is used as fuel, and more and more carbohydrate is therefore used for energy production. It should be noted that for clients with weight management issues, it is most important to burn large numbers of calories, creating a negative energy balance. It is not correct to suggest that a client train at a lower intensity in order to burn more fat. This suggestion will result in the client simply burning fewer total calories, even though a greater percentage of fat is expended at lower intensities.

Cardiorespiratory Responses to Exercise

Anaerobic Threshold

The anaerobic or lactate threshold, also known as the onset of blood lactate accumulation (OBLA), is the point during exercise at which the work becomes so intense that muscle cells cannot produce the additional energy aerobically, and so begin to rely more and more on the anaerobic glycolytic system to produce ATP. At this level, lactic acid begins to accumulate and the so-called lactate or anaerobic threshold is reached. With cardiorespiratory training, the regular exerciser can work at high levels of activity without reaching the anaerobic threshold. For example, an untrained client may reach his/her anaerobic threshold at 50–60% of his/her VO_2 max, but a high-ranking competitive athlete may not reach his/her threshold until 70–80% of VO_2 max.

Maximal Oxygen Uptake

Maximal oxygen uptake, also known as maximal oxygen consumption or **VO_2 max**, is another important indicator of aerobic fitness. It refers to the maximum amount of oxygen consumed and utilized by the body during an all-out effort to exhaustion. It is assumed that this measurement represents the maximal capacity to resynthesize ATP aerobically. The more aerobically fit an individual is, the greater his/her ability to resynthesize ATP, and the higher his/her VO_2 max or ability to consume and process oxygen. VO_2 max is measured in either liters of O_2 consumed per minute (an absolute value), or in milliliters of O_2 consumed per kilogram of body weight per minute (a relative value).

EPOC

EPOC, or excess post-exercise oxygen consumption, refers to the additional oxygen consumed immediately after an exercise bout when the body is no longer exercising. Imagine sprinting up a couple of flights of stairs, only to stand still and breathe heavily for a few moments. The extra oxygen consumed is now termed EPOC, and was formerly known as oxygen debt.

Basic Neuromuscular Physiology

Nervous System Overview

The nervous system consists of the brain, spinal cord, and a complex network of nerves, all responsible for controlling and communicating with the rest of the body. The brain and spinal cord make up the **central nervous system** (CNS), while the cranial and spinal nerves comprise the peripheral nervous system (PNS). The **peripheral nervous system** is further divided into the two major types of nerves: (1) **sensory**, or afferent, neurons that bring messages back to the brain and spinal cord from the muscles, skin, and other areas of the body; and (2) **motor**, or efferent, neurons that send messages from the brain and spinal cord to the muscles, causing a neuromuscular response.

Motor neurons themselves are divided into two types: voluntary and involuntary. The voluntary nerves make up the somatic nervous system, the system that causes muscular action. Involuntary nerves, on the other hand, comprise the autonomic nervous system, which has two more divisions of its own: the sympathetic and the parasympathetic nerves. Sympathetic nerves provide physiologic (flight or fight) responses, such as increased heart rate, blood pressure, and metabolic rate, as well as vasodilated blood vessels, which allow more blood to be delivered to the working muscles. Parasympathetic nerves, however, are more active when the body is resting, providing effects such as decreased heart rate and vasoconstricted blood vessels.

Muscle Structure

There are three types of muscle found in the human body: skeletal, smooth, and cardiac muscle. **Skeletal muscle** is attached to bone via tendons and allows voluntary movement of the body. Because of its striped or band-like appearance under the microscope, skeletal muscle is also known as striated muscle tissue. **Smooth muscle** is not striated and is found in the walls of organs, such as the stomach and intestines. Because it does not require conscious control for a contraction, smooth muscle is also called involuntary muscle. **Cardiac muscle** forms the walls of the heart. While cardiac muscle is striated in appearance, it does not require our conscious thought to contract and pump blood through the body. The cardiac muscle consists of an entire structure of interconnected cardiac fibers that contract involuntarily as a unit.

Skeletal muscle, composed of contractile tissue including muscle fibers, is surrounded by fascial sheaths and connected to bone via tendons. The muscle fibers shorten or contract during muscular contractions, while tendons are noncontractile and connect the muscle to the bony attachment. **Fascia** is the thin, translucent connective-tissue covering that forms a sheath for an individual muscle or muscle group.

Sliding Filament Theory

Skeletal muscles contain bundles of muscle fibers. Each muscle fiber is a muscle cell. Muscle fibers contain myofibrils that have a basic functional unit known as a **sarcomere**. Within each sarcomere are thin myofilaments that cause muscle action. These are the proteins **actin** and **myosin**. The Huxley sliding filament theory is the most widely accepted theory explaining muscle shortening. Cross-bridges, or myosin heads, are thought to attach to specialized sites along the actin filaments, causing the myosin and actin to slide past each other in opposite directions. ATP provides the energy needed for the cross-bridges to attach. As multiple myosin cross-bridges simultaneously pull the actin inward, the entire sarcomere shortens. The shortening of the sarcomeres causes the muscle fibers to shorten and a muscle contraction occurs.

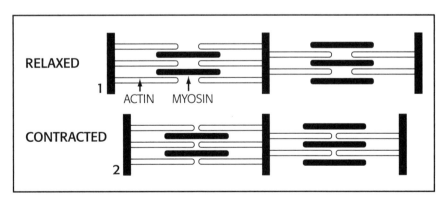

Fig. 2-10. Sliding Filament Theory

Muscle Fiber Types

There are two major muscle fiber types: **slow twitch** (ST) fibers and **fast twitch** (FT) fibers. Most skeletal muscles have both types of fibers. However, the percentages of ST and FT fibers are not the same in all muscles of the body, or from person to person. ST (also known as Type I or slow oxidative, SO) fibers are slow to fatigue and have a high level of aerobic endurance. These ST fibers are characterized by a high number of mitochondria and are perfused with blood; thus the fibers have a reddish color. The ST fibers are used for long-term, low-to-moderate intensity activities ranging from maintaining proper posture to long-distance running. FT fibers, on the other hand, have poor aerobic endurance. FT fibers have two broad subdivisions: fast twitch a (also known as Type IIa or fast oxidative glycolytic, FOG), and fast twitch b (also known as Type IIb or fast glycolytic, FG). Both types of fast twitch fibers tend to produce ATP anaerobically, have fewer mitochondria, and are pale in color. Fast twitch IIa fibers are used in short-duration, high-intensity activities and fatigue quickly. Unlike Type IIb, Type IIa fibers have the capacity to use both aerobic and anaerobic energy systems. Fast twitch IIb fibers are not used often and are stimulated by extremely high-intensity, maximum-strength, explosive-type events, using the anaerobic energy systems almost exclusively.

Different clients will have differing percentages of these fiber types in their various muscles. Some clients will have higher percentages of fast twitch fibers (and may therefore excel in activities that rely heavily on the anaerobic energy systems), while other clients will have a higher percentage of slow twitch fibers (enabling them to excel in long-duration, aerobic-type events). In general, an individual's fiber type distribution is genetically predetermined.

Muscle Innervation

Muscles contract when stimulated by a **motor neuron**, or specialized nerve cell. A typical neuron has a cell body, dendrites (information receivers), and an axon (the structure that sends messages). The axon is surrounded by a covering known as a myelin sheath, which helps speed messages along the axon's length. A motor neuron can transmit signals to a number of muscle fibers; one motor neuron and all the muscle fibers it stimulates are called a **motor unit**. In areas needing fine muscle control, such as the eye, a motor neuron may only connect with 5–10 muscle fibers. In larger muscles that require greater contractions, a single motor unit may be connected to as many as 500 muscle fibers. Each motor unit follows the all-or-none principle. When the motor neuron is stimulated, all the muscle fibers in the unit will fire simultaneously. A contraction of only a portion of the fibers in an individual motor unit is not possible. However, to allow for uniform muscle contractions and to avoid fatigue, all the motor units in a muscle will not contract at the same time.

Fibers are always recruited for exercise according to the size of the motor unit, with the smaller motor units being utilized first (the size principal). FT fibers have very large motor units when compared to ST fibers. Therefore, FT fibers are the last to be recruited since they are more difficult to stimulate. Recruitment order begins with the ST fibers, then the FT fibers (fast twitch IIa and then fast twitch IIb). FT fibers are stimulated whenever a large amount of total force is needed, as in lifting very heavy weights or in high-speed movements.

Proprioceptors

Proprioceptors in the muscle and tendon sense the degree of tension and the length of the muscle. **The muscle spindle**, the proprioceptive receptor that attaches to the sheaths of the surrounding muscle fibers, is parallel to the muscle. It sends afferent (sensory) information to the brain about changes in muscle length and the speed at which the changes are occurring. When stimulated, the muscle spindles relay a message to the spinal cord to cause a contraction in the same muscle. The afferent, or sensory, neurons in the muscle spindle communicate with the motor neurons of the target muscle through interneurons in the spinal cord without requiring any conscious thought. This spinal reflex is known as the **stretch reflex**. When ballistic (bouncing) movements are used, the muscle spindles will sense the quick changes in muscle length and cause a protective muscular contraction. A physician checks the spinal reflex of the quadriceps by tapping on the patellar tendon, causing a sudden lengthening of the muscle, which causes the knee to extend.

The **Golgi tendon organ**, located in the tendon, is the proprioceptor that protects the muscle from excessive shortening or lengthening. It senses tension caused by muscular contraction or extreme stretching. When stimulated by excessive tension or stretching, the Golgi tendon organ inhibits contraction of the muscle from which it originates. This reflex inhibition is used in the proprioceptive neuromuscular facilitation (PNF) stretching technique known as hold-relax.

Summary

In this chapter, the cardiorespiratory system was described, and fundamental principles of bioenergetics were introduced, including mechanisms of energy production in the body. Basic exercise physiology terms were covered. Finally, the nervous system was outlined, followed by basic muscle structure and the physiology of neuromuscular contraction.

References

McArdle, W., Katch, F., & Katch, V. (2003). *Exercise physiology: Energy, nutrition and human performance* (5th ed.). Baltimore: Lippincott Williams & Wilkins.

Spencer, M.R., & Gasti, P.B. (2001). Energy system contribution during 200 to 1,500 meter running in highly trained athletes. *Medicine & Science in Sports & Exercise, 33*(1), 157-162.

Wilmore, J.H., & Costill, D.L. (2004). *Physiology of sport and exercise* (3rd ed.). Champaign, IL: Human Kinetics.

Suggested Reading

American College of Sports Medicine. (2005). *ACSM's resource manual for guidelines for exercise testing and prescription* (4th ed). Baltimore: Lippincott Williams & Wilkins.

Fox, S.I. (1996). *Human physiology* (5th ed.). Dubuque, IA: Wm. C. Brown Pub.

Gardiner, P.F. (2001). *Neuromuscular aspects of physical activity.* Champaign, IL: Human Kinetics.

McArdle, W., Katch, F., & Katch, V. (2003). *Exercise physiology: Energy, nutrition and human performance* (5th ed.). Baltimore: Lippincott Williams & Wilkins.

Sharkey, B.J. (1990). *Physiology of fitness* (3rd ed). Champaign, IL: Human Kinetics.

Wilmore, J.H., & Costill, D.L. (2004). *Physiology of sport and exercise* (3rd ed.). Champaign, IL: Human Kinetics.

Anatomy and Kinesiology

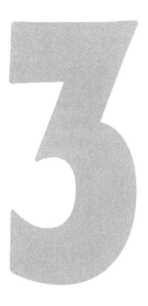

Outline

- Anatomical Position
- Cardinal Planes of Movement
- General Joint Action Terms
- Positions and Directional Terms
- Musculoskeletal Structures
- Major Joints and Muscles of the Body
- Roles Muscles Play
- Muscle Actions
- Types of Muscle
- Levers
- Opposing Muscle Groups
- Kinesiology Charts

Kinesiology is the study of human movement, a discipline with a language all its own. Knowing kinesiological and anatomical terms makes it much easier to talk about the body, discuss positions and movements for exercise, and communicate with other health and fitness professionals. In this chapter, you will learn the basic terminology used in kinesiology and functional anatomy. You will also be studying major joint actions and joint function; this will help you to plan safe exercise and minimize client injuries. Additionally, you will be learning which muscles perform which joint actions, and this will help you to provide clients with effective exercises that work.

Anatomical Position

The definitions of joint actions that follow assume that the actions are taking place from the anatomical position, an arbitrary starting position for the body. Notice in Figure 3-1 that the anatomical position is a standing position with the hands down and palms facing forward.

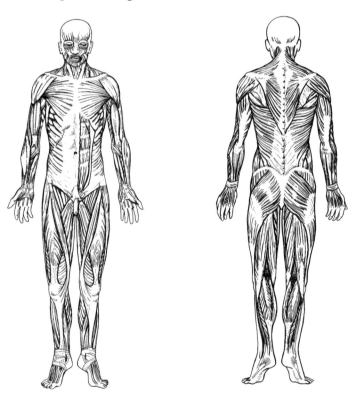

Fig. 3-1. Anatomical Position

Cardinal Planes of Movement

Planes geometrically bisect the body and help describe bodily movements. (Movements take place alongside or next to the planes). There are an infinite number of parallel planes to the cardinal, or primary, planes shown below (Figure 3-2a). These three cardinal planes are as follows.

1. **Horizontal plane**—(sometimes called transverse) divides the body into upper and lower portions. Rotation occurs within the horizontal plane.
2. **Frontal plane**—(sometimes called coronal) divides the body into front and back. Abduction and adduction occur within the frontal plane.
3. **Sagittal plane**—(sometimes called medial) divides the body into right and left portions. Flexion and extension occur within the sagittal plane.

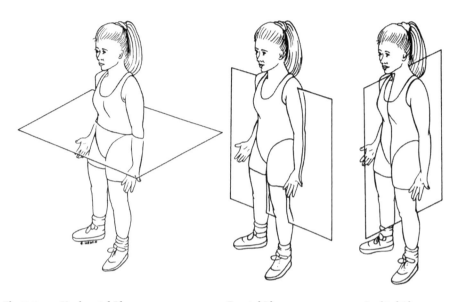

Fig. 3-2a.   Horizontal Plane   **Frontal Plane**   **Sagittal Plane**

General Joint Action Terms

Take a look at the following common joint action terminology before you begin to study the body joint by joint.

- **Flexion**—the most common definitions include: characterized by the joint angle diminishing, and/or movement that shortens the angle between two bones. Another easy way to remember flexion is to note that most flexion movements are forward movements, with the major exception of the knee joint (knee flexion is a backward movement from anatomical position).
- **Extension**—common definitions include: the return from flexion, and/or movement that increases the angle between two bones. Most extension movements are backward movements, although, once again, knee extension is the exception (knee extension is the return from flexion).
- **Abduction**—movement away from the midline of the body
- **Adduction**—movement toward the midline of the body
- **Rotation**—movement around an axis or pivot point
- **Circumduction**—movement in which an extremity describes a circle (360°)

Positions and Directional Terms

In the next section, you'll learn kinesiology terms that are helpful in describing body positions, body part locations, and direction of movements. Standard terms include the following.

- **Anterior**—to the front
- **Posterior**—to the back
- **Lateral**—away from the midline
- **Medial**—toward the midline
- **Superior**—above
- **Inferior**—below
- **Superficial**—on or near the surface of the body
- **Deep**—further from the surface of the body
- **Proximal**—closer to the trunk
- **Distal**—further from the trunk
- **Supine**—lying on the spine (on the back)
- **Prone**—lying face down

Musculoskeletal Structures

Bones

The basic functions of bones are to: (1) provide a supportive framework for the body; (2) protect the body's vital organs; (3) act as levers in conjunction with the muscles to cause movement; (4) produce red blood cells; and (5) store minerals such as calcium and phosphorus.

While bones are often thought of as lifeless, dry objects, they are actually living organs in the body that change as people age. They have an outer shell of compact bone encasing spongy bone that surrounds a medullary cavity. The spaces in the spongy bone and the medullary cavity are filled with bone marrow. Red bone marrow is where blood cells are made in a process known as hematopoiesis. As people mature, much of the red marrow is replaced with fatty yellow marrow except in parts of the ribs, skull, sternum, and vertebrae. The red marrow in these areas will continue to produce red blood cells throughout a person's lifetime. Like other organs of the body, bones also contain blood vessels, lymph vessels, and nerves.

The basic structure of bone can be studied by looking at the anatomy of a long bone, such as the femur (thigh bone), shown in Figure 3-2b.

The main parts of the femur are the diaphysis (shaft or long portion), the epiphyses (ends of the bone), the metaphysis (area between the diaphysis and epiphysis), and the articular cartilage and the periosteum. The articular cartilage covers the epiphyses and reduces the friction at the joint. The periosteum is a thin tissue-like covering around the surface of the bone that serves several purposes, including serving as the point of attachment for ligaments and tendons. Blood vessels and nerves supplying the bone are in the periosteum.

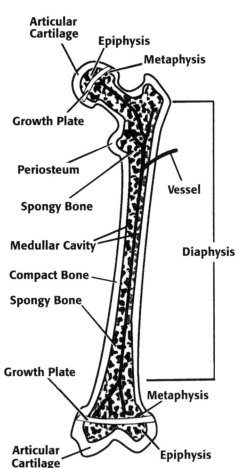

Articular Cartilage
Epiphysis
Metaphysis
Growth Plate
Periosteum
Vessel
Spongy Bone
Medullar Cavity
Diaphysis
Compact Bone
Spongy Bone
Growth Plate
Metaphysis
Articular Cartilage
Epiphysis

Fig. 3-2b. Anatomy of Femur

The metaphysis is one of the areas that changes with age. In a child, the metaphysis is cartilaginous, like columns of spongy tissue, joining the growth plate to the diaphysis. This is the area where the bone lengthens as the child increases in height. Once the bone reaches its adult length, the metaphysis ossifies and connects the diaphysis and epiphysis. If an injury to the growth plate causes premature fusion of the diaphysis and epiphysis, the bone will not grow to its normal length. This is one of the reasons why lifting heavy weights is controversial for children whose growth plates have not yet closed. While the diaphysis and epiphysis fuse at varying rates in different parts of the body, most of the bones are fused by about the age of 20 years. X-rays, however, provide the most accurate method of determining whether or not the growth plates have closed.

The 206 bones in the human body are often grouped into two broad categories: the **axial skeleton** (the skull, vertebral column, ribs, and sternum), and the **appendicular skeleton** (the upper extremities, including the scapulae and clavicles, and the lower extremities, including the pelvic girdle). The axial skeleton provides the framework for the trunk and head while the appendicular skeleton consists of both arms and legs, including the bones that connect these extremities to the axial skeleton. The appendicular skeleton contains trabecular bone, which has a faster turnover rate than the cortical bone found in the axial skeleton and ends of the long bones of the appendicular skeleton.

Fig. 3-2c. Skeleton Anterior View

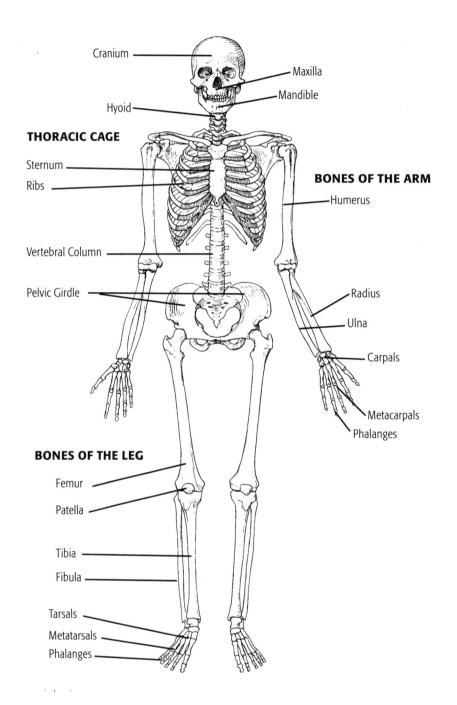

Cranium

Maxilla

Mandible

Hyoid

THORACIC CAGE

Sternum

Ribs

BONES OF THE ARM

Humerus

Vertebral Column

Pelvic Girdle

Radius

Ulna

Carpals

Metacarpals

Phalanges

BONES OF THE LEG

Femur

Patella

Tibia

Fibula

Tarsals

Metatarsals

Phalanges

Fig. 3-2d. Skeleton Posterior View

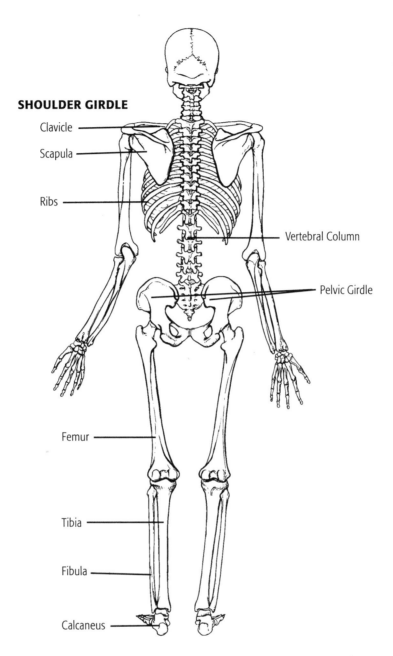

SHOULDER GIRDLE
Clavicle
Scapula
Ribs
Vertebral Column
Pelvic Girdle
Femur
Tibia
Fibula
Calcaneus

Joints

A joint is the point at which two or more bones meet, or articulate, and where movement occurs. There are several different methods of classifying joints, but here, two general categories will be considered: nonsynovial and synovial. **Nonsynovial joints** experience limited movement, while synovial joints move freely. The joints between the bones of the skull are examples of nonsynovial joints. **Synovial joints** (also known as **diarthrodial joints**) are the most common type of joint. They have a small space between the articulating bones that allows for a greater range of motion. Cartilage covers the weight-bearing surface of the bones, and the entire joint is typically enclosed by a joint capsule. **Cartilage** is a white, semi-opaque, fibrous connective tissue that cushions the joints and prevents wear on the joint surfaces. The **joint capsule** has two layers—the outer fibrous layer and the inner synovial membrane. The **synovial membrane** secretes synovial fluid, which provides nourishment, lubrication, and hydrostatic cushioning for the joint. **Bursae** are also liquid-filled membranes that protect soft tissues as they pass by bony projections.

Connective Tissues

- **Ligament**—band of fibrous tissue that connects bone to bone and provides joint stability. Ligaments are nonelastic; once stretched, they remain stretched, thereby compromising joint integrity. Personal fitness trainers must be aware of positions and exercises that can overstretch ligaments and avoid them whenever possible.
- **Tendon**—dense, fibrous connective tissue that forms the end of a muscle and attaches muscle to bone
- **Aponeurosis**—a wide, flat type of tendon or fibrous membrane that connects some muscles (e.g., the rectus abdominis) to bone
- **Fascia**—fibrous connective tissue that forms sheaths for individual muscles

Major Joints and Muscles of the Body

Shoulder (Glenohumeral) Joint

The shoulder joint is the junction of the head of the humerus (arm bone) with the glenoid fossa (cup-like projection) of the scapula, or shoulder blade. The shoulder joint is a ball-and-socket joint with a larger range of motion than any other part of the body. The shoulder girdle, discussed below, must provide a stable base for the mobile shoulder joint and the rest of the upper extremity.

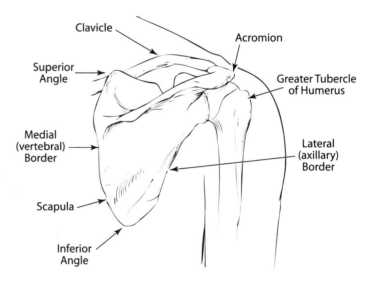

Fig. 3-3. Shoulder (Glenohumeral) Joint: Posterior View

There are nine primary **joint actions** of the shoulder joint.

1. Shoulder flexion
2. Shoulder extension
3. Shoulder abduction
4. Shoulder adduction
5. Shoulder horizontal adduction/shoulder horizontal flexion (these terms are synonymous)—movement toward the midline of the body when the arms are in the horizontal plane
6. Shoulder horizontal abduction/shoulder horizontal extension (these terms are synonymous)—movement away from the midline of the body when the arms are in the horizontal plane
7. Shoulder internal (medial or inward) rotation—inward rotation of the humerus
8. Shoulder external (lateral or outward) rotation—outward rotation of the humerus
9. Shoulder circumduction

NOTE: In order to be an effective personal fitness trainer, it is important to understand exactly what all the major muscles do; only then will you be able to design intelligent exercises that produce results for your clients. In this chapter, major muscles and their joint actions are listed under each joint. For further study purposes, there are also kinesiological joint action charts placed at the end of the chapter. In Chapter 8 ("Applied Resistance Training Skills"), you will find additional individual muscle illustrations followed by yet another list of applicable major muscles and their joint actions. Finally, in Chapter 10 ("Injury Prevention"), the major joints will be covered in greater depth so that you can better understand common mechanisms of injury. By utilizing these various learning formats and by studying the different kinesiology sections in the text, you will hopefully find it easier to learn and integrate this valuable information.

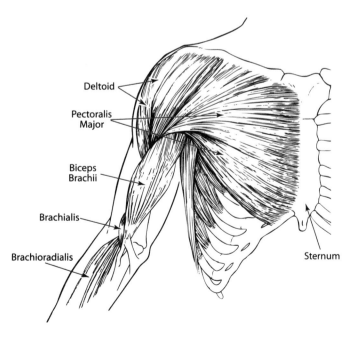

Fig. 3-4. Anterior Muscles of the Shoulder Joint

Deltoid

Pectoralis Major

Biceps Brachii

Brachialis

Brachioradialis

Sternum

Major Muscles of the Shoulder Joint

There are nine major muscles that cross the shoulder joint and, therefore, cause shoulder joint movement.

1. **Pectoralis major.** This large, anterior muscle performs several actions, most notably **shoulder horizontal flexion**, a movement that utilizes both the clavicular and sternal portions of the muscle. (The clavicular and sternal portions both cross the shoulder joint and insert onto the greater tubercle of the humerus). Additionally, the clavicular portion performs shoulder flexion, while the sternal portion performs shoulder extension and shoulder adduction. The pectoralis major is opposed by the posterior deltoids, and functionally, by the middle trapezius and rhomboids as well. Note that these sets of muscles are directly opposite each other on the upper body.

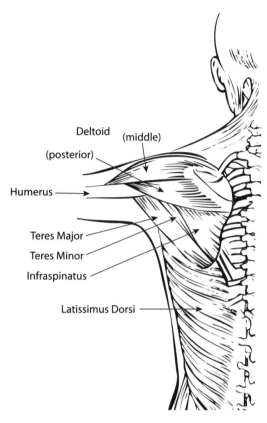

Deltoid   (middle)

(posterior)

Humerus

Teres Major

Teres Minor

Infraspinatus

Latissimus Dorsi

Fig. 3-5. Posterior Muscles of the Shoulder Joint

2. **Deltoids.** This muscle, which is directly on top of the shoulder, has three portions: anterior, medial, and posterior. All three portions insert onto the deltoid tubercle of the humerus. The anterior deltoid is a prime mover for shoulder flexion; the medial deltoid is a prime mover for shoulder abduction and shoulder horizontal abduction; and the posterior deltoid is responsible for shoulder horizontal abduction. The anterior and medial portions are opposed by the latissimus dorsi.

3. **Latissimus dorsi.** Although the latissimus dorsi muscle (lats) appears to be a large, superficial back muscle, the joint that is moved when the lats contract is actually the shoulder. The large mass of latissimus dorsi fibers twist and wrap under the arm, attaching to the anterior medial side of the intertubercular groove of the humerus. The lats are responsible for shoulder adduction and shoulder extension. Due to the anterior medial insertion point, the lats also act as an internal rotator of the shoulder joint.

4–7. **Rotator cuff muscles.** There are four rotator cuff muscles: supraspinatus, infraspinatus, teres minor, and subscapularis (sometimes remembered as the SITS muscles). These relatively small muscles form a cuff-type arrangement around the shoulder joint: supraspinatus above, subscapularis in front, and the infraspinatus and teres minor in back. All four muscles are important in providing stability to the shoulder joint; the infraspinatus and teres minor are especially important in holding the head of the humerus down and maintaining proper shoulder biomechanics. The supraspinatus is a prime mover in shoulder abduction; the subscapularis performs shoulder internal rotation, and the teres minor and infraspinatus are prime movers for shoulder external rotation. Note that there is a fundamental imbalance between the internal and external rotators: there are many more internal rotators of the shoulder (subscapularis, latissimus dorsi, pectoralis major, anterior deltoid, and biceps), but only a few, relatively small and weak external rotators (teres minor, infraspinatus, and posterior deltoid). As a result, most clients are encouraged to focus more on strengthening the external rotators of the shoulder for optimal joint conditioning.

8. **Biceps brachii.** The biceps, a muscle with two heads (points of origin), also crosses the shoulder joint. Both the long head and the short head of the biceps only assist with shoulder joint actions.

9. **Triceps brachii.** Only the long head of the triceps crosses the shoulder joint; the triceps, like the biceps, is an assistor at the shoulder.

NOTE: A tenth shoulder joint muscle, the **coracobrachialis**, is generally not considered a major muscle, although most kinesiology texts list it as a prime mover for shoulder horizontal adduction. Likewise, the **teres major**, also known as the "lats little helper," is a lesser muscle that always acts with the latissimus dorsi, performing the actions of shoulder adduction, shoulder extension, and shoulder internal rotation.

Shoulder Girdle

The clavicles and the scapulae (shoulder blades) form the shoulder girdle. The movements of the scapulae along the back of the rib cage are considered to be motions of the scapulothoracic joint, whereas anteriorly, the clavicles attach to the sternum and form the sternoclavicular joint.

There are eight primary **joint actions** of the shoulder girdle/scapulothoracic joint (NOTE: these are often called scapular joint actions).

1. Scapular elevation—upward movement of the shoulder girdle
2. Scapular depression—downward movement of the shoulder girdle
3. Scapular retraction/scapular adduction (these terms are synonymous)—backward movement of the shoulder girdle with scapulae pulled toward the midline
4. Scapular protraction/scapular abduction (these terms are synonymous)—forward movement of the shoulder girdle with scapulae pulled away from the midline
5. Scapular upward rotation—rotation (or upward turning) of the scapulae in the frontal plane with the glenoid fossa facing upward
6. Scapular downward rotation—return from upward rotation
7. Scapular upward tilt—a turning of the scapula on its frontal-horizontal axis so that the superior border turns slightly forward-downward and the inferior border moves slightly backward-upward (and away from the rib cage)
8. Scapular reduction of upward tilt—return movement from upward tilt

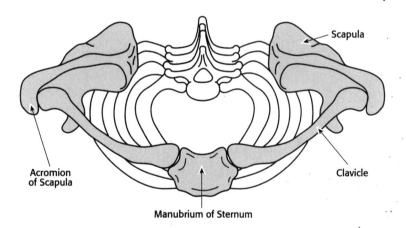

Fig. 3-6. Shoulder Girdle: Superior View

Major Muscles of the Shoulder Girdle

Movements of the arm on the trunk generally involve the cooperative actions of the shoulder joint and shoulder girdle, as well as the attached muscles. Additional movement of the scapula can further increase the available range of motion of the humerus. Pure isolation of the shoulder complex muscles is often not possible. Joint actions in this area are frequently caused by muscles acting as a force couple (equal parallel forces pulling in opposite directions), e.g., the trapezius II and serratus anterior act together to cause upward rotation.

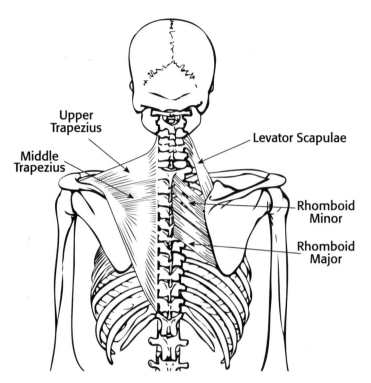

Fig. 3-7. Posterior Muscles of the Shoulder Girdle

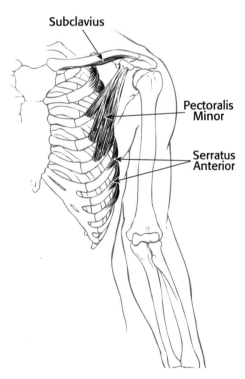

Fig. 3-8. Anterior Muscles of the Shoulder Girdle

- **Trapezius.** This unique, trapezoidal-shaped muscle is responsible for several different scapular joint actions. Depending on which text you read, the trapezius may be divided into three (upper, middle, and lower) or four (I, II, III, IV) parts. In this text, the actions of the four parts are listed in the chart at the end of this chapter ("Shoulder Girdle Muscles and Their Actions"), but the upper, middle, and lower portions will be referred to in Chapter 8 ("Applied Resistance Training Skills"). The upper trapezius (parts I and II) is responsible for scapular elevation; the middle trapezius (part III) is a prime mover for scapular retraction; and the lower trapezius (part IV) is a prime mover for both scapular depression and upward rotation. In many clients, the upper trapezius may be shortened and tight, while the middle and lower trapezius are weak and/or over-stretched. In this case, you would recommend stretching and relaxing the upper trapezius and strengthening and shortening the middle and lower trapezius.
- **Rhomboids.** The rhomboids lie underneath the trapezius and are prime movers for scapular retraction, downward rotation, and elevation. For good posture, it is critical for the rhomboid and middle trapezius muscles to have adequate muscle endurance.
- **Serratus anterior.** This muscle, with its sawtooth-shaped origin on the ribs, is a prime mover for scapular protraction and upward rotation.
- **Pectoralis minor.** A relatively small muscle lying underneath the pectoralis major and inserting onto the coracoid process of the scapula, the pectoralis minor performs scapular depression, protraction, and downward rotation. The serratus anterior and pectoralis minor, as protractors, oppose the middle trapezius and rhomboids, as retractors.
- **Levator scapulae.** As its name implies, the levator scapulae is responsible for scapular elevation.
- **Subclavius.** This small muscle helps to stabilize the clavicle and assists with scapular depression.

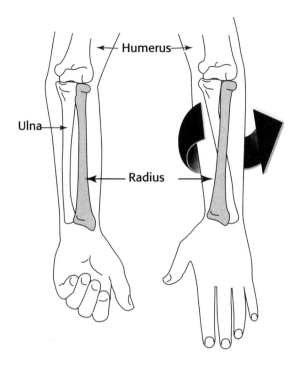

Fig. 3-9. Radioulnar Joint

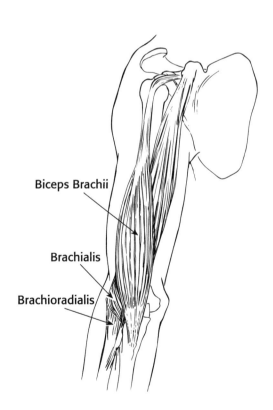

Fig. 3-10. Anterior Muscles of the Elbow

Elbow and Radioulnar Joints

The elbow (humeroulnar) joint is a hinge joint in which the ulna bone of the forearm forms an articulation with the humerus bone of the upper arm. There are two **joint actions** of the true elbow joint.

1. Elbow flexion
2. Elbow extension

The proximal radioulnar joint, the humeroulnar joint, and the humeroradial joint all share the same joint capsule at the elbow; the joint mechanics are somewhat complex. The radioulnar joints comprise both the proximal and distal articulations of the radius and ulna bones of the forearm. These bones rotate and cross each other in two **joint actions**.

1. Radioulnar supination—a lateral rotation of the forearm that brings the palm of the hand upward. In this position, the radius and ulna are parallel.
2. Radioulnar pronation—a medial rotation of the forearm, with the palm in a downward position so the radius lies diagonally across the ulna.

Major Muscles of the Elbow Joint

There are three flexors and two extensors of the elbow joint.

1. **Biceps brachii.** This is the largest and most familiar anterior elbow joint muscle. It is a two-joint muscle and is a prime mover for elbow flexion (the biceps also assists with shoulder flexion). The biceps and triceps oppose each other.
2. **Brachialis.** The brachialis lies under the biceps and is a prime mover in elbow flexion.
3. **Brachioradialis.** This narrow forearm muscle is a prime mover in elbow flexion.
4. **Triceps brachii.** The triceps is the major muscle of the posterior upper arm; it has three heads (long, short, and lateral), or origins, with a common insertion on the olecranon process of the ulna. All three heads of the triceps strongly perform elbow extension. The long head of the triceps is a two-joint muscle that assists with shoulder extension and adduction. See Fig. 3-11.
5. **Anconeus.** This muscle is a small posterior muscle behind the elbow and is responsible for elbow extension.

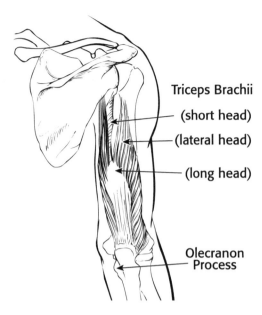

Fig. 3-11. Posterior Muscles of the Elbow

Triceps Brachii

(short head)

(lateral head)

(long head)

Olecranon
Process

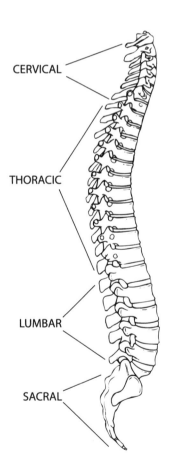

Fig. 3-12. The Spine

CERVICAL

THORACIC

LUMBAR

SACRAL

There is one primary muscle of the forearm for radioulnar supination, and two primary muscles for radioulnar pronation.

1. **Supinator.** A small lateral muscle of the forearm responsible for supination
2. **Pronator quadratus.** A deep muscle of the lower forearm responsible for pronation
3. **Pronator teres.** A small muscle of the forearm responsible for pronation

Spine

The spine, or vertebral column, is typically composed of 33 vertebrae: 7 cervical (neck), 12 thoracic (where the ribs attach), 5 lumbar (lower back), 5 sacral (fused to form the sacrum), and approximately 4 coccygeal (fused to form the coccyx, or tailbone). The ideal vertebral column, when viewed from the side, forms four natural curves. When these curves are in their proper relationship to each other, the spine is said to be in neutral. Located between the vertebral bodies (flat bony plates) of the vertebrae are the intervertebral discs, spongy disc-shaped tissues that permit spinal movement. There are four primary **joint actions** of the spine.

1. Spinal flexion
2. Spinal extension
3. Spinal rotation
4. Spinal lateral flexion—bending of the spine to the side

NOTE: Spinal joint actions can refer to movement of the entire spine or to specific areas of the spine, such as cervical spinal extension or lumbar flexion.

Major Muscles of the Spine/Torso

- **Rectus abdominis.** A long, flat, superficial muscle that originates on the pubic bone and inserts on the fifth, sixth, and seventh ribs, the rectus abdominis is a prime mover for spinal flexion. It is opposed by the erector spinae.
- **External and internal obliques**. These anterior muscles consist primarily of oblique, or diagonal, fibers. Therefore, the best exercises to effectively challenge the obliques are those that involve a diagonal action. The obliques are prime movers for spinal flexion with rotation. Most kinesiology textbooks state that the obliques only assist with spinal lateral flexion; they are not prime movers. The external obliques are superficial, whereas the internal obliques lie underneath and are deep. The fibers of the internal obliques run in the opposite diagonal direction to the external obliques.

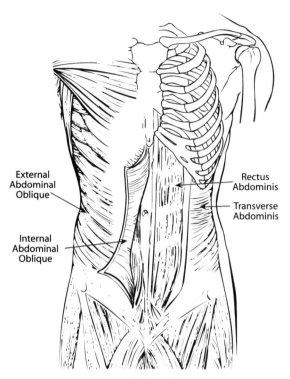

Fig. 3-13. Anterior Muscles of the Torso

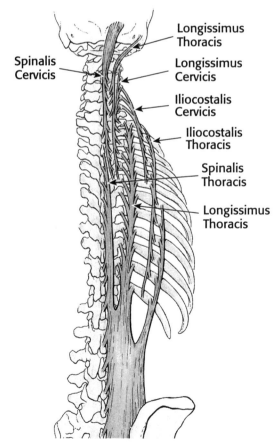

**Fig. 3-14. Erector Spinae
Posterior Muscles of the Torso**

- **Transverse abdominis.** The deepest abdominal muscle, the transverse abdominis is responsible for abdominal compression, as well as vigorous exhalation and expulsion. Many professionals describe the compressive action of the transverse abdominis as the "drawing in" or "hollowing" maneuver, imagining that the navel is drawn in towards the spine. The transverse abdominis is unique in that it causes no actual joint action.

- **Erector spinae.** The erector spinae is a large, superficial muscle that consists of three pairs of muscles: the iliocostalis, longissimus, and spinalis (each muscle has fibers on both the right and left sides of the vertebral column). The erector spinae is the prime mover for spinal extension.

- **Multifidus.** The multifidus (multifidi—plural) is one of several deep spinal muscles, located under the erector spinae. It has been identified as an important posterior stabilizer of the spine (Norris, 2000), connecting adjacent vertebrae or spanning two to three segments at a time on each side. When the multifidi contract bilaterally (on both sides), they help extend the spine, and when they contract unilaterally (on one side only), they rotate the spine to the opposite side.

- **Quadratus Lumborum.** This is a deep, vertical muscle that essentially connects the lowest ribs to the pelvis on each side. It is a prime mover for spinal lateral flexion.

Pelvic Girdle and Hip Joint

The pelvic girdle is the connecting link between the spine and the lower extremities. Unlike the shoulder girdle, in which the scapulae can move independently, the pelvic girdle moves as a unit. Pelvic movements cause movements in both the vertebral column and the hip joint, and vice versa. Note that the pelvic girdle is attached to the sacrum at the sacroiliac joint, a joint with little to no movement. The pelvic girdle has three **joint actions.**

1. Anterior pelvic tilt
2. Posterior pelvic tilt
3. Lateral pelvic tilt

Major Muscles of the Pelvic Girdle

The muscles of the pelvic girdle are also muscles that cause spinal and hip joint actions. As such, they are only listed here, but individually described under the spinal and hip joints, respectively.

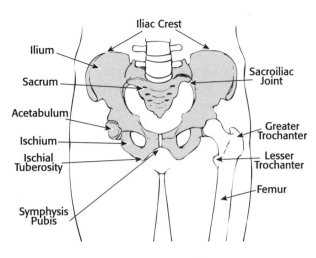

Iliac Crest
Ilium
Sacrum
Acetabulum
Ischium
Ischial Tuberosity
Symphysis Pubis
Sacroiliac Joint
Greater Trochanter
Lesser Trochanter
Femur

Fig. 3-15. Pelvic Girdle and Hip Joint

- **Hip flexors and erector spinae.** Together, these muscles cause an anterior pelvic tilt.
- **Gluteus maximus, hamstrings, and rectus abdominis.** These muscles are responsible for a posterior pelvic tilt.
- **Quadratus lumborum, gluteus medius, hip adductors.** Working together, these muscles cause a lateral pelvic tilt.

The hip joint is a large ball-and-socket joint, formed by the articulation of the acetabulum (cup-shaped indentation) of the pelvis and the head of the femur. Similar to the shoulder joint, the hip joint is capable of nine primary **joint actions**.

1. Hip flexion
2. Hip extension
3. Hip abduction
4. Hip adduction
5. Hip horizontal adduction/hip horizontal flexion (these terms are synonymous)
6. Hip horizontal abduction/hip horizontal extension (these terms are synonymous)
7. Hip internal (medial or inward) rotation
8. Hip external (lateral or outward) rotation
9. Hip circumduction

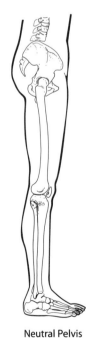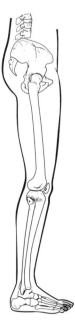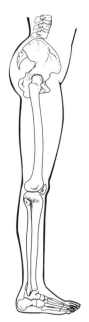

Neutral Pelvis   Posterior Pelvic Tilt   Anterior Pelvic Tilt

Fig. 3-16. Pelvic Alignment

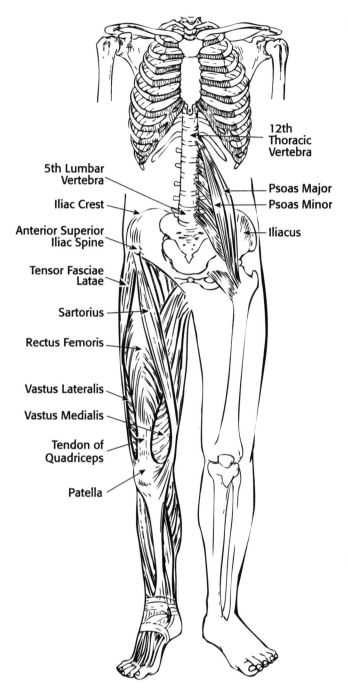

5th Lumbar
Vertebra

Iliac Crest

Anterior Superior
Iliac Spine

Tensor Fasciae
Latae

Sartorius

Rectus Femoris

Vastus Lateralis

Vastus Medialis

Tendon of
Quadriceps

Patella

12th
Thoracic
Vertebra

Psoas Major
Psoas Minor

Iliacus

Fig. 3-17. Major Muscles of the Anterior Leg and Hip

Major Muscles of the Hip Joint

- **Iliopsoas.** The iliacus and psoas major act as one muscle and are commonly grouped together, performing the action of hip flexion. Along with the rectus femoris (one of the four quadriceps), they are also known simply as the **hip flexors**. The iliopsoas is especially notable due to the origin of the psoas muscles on the lumbar vertebrae; when these muscles are very strong and/or tight, they can cause the lumbar spine to be misaligned and potentially lead to back problems. For injury prevention, care must be taken with excessive hip flexor strengthening. The hip flexors are opposed by the gluteus maximus and the hamstrings.

- **Gluteus maximus.** This muscle is the largest and most superficial of the buttock muscles; it is a prime mover for hip extension and hip external rotation.

- **Hamstrings.** The hamstrings are actually three muscles: biceps femoris, semitendinosus, and semimembranosus. All three muscles are two-joint muscles, crossing both the hip and the knee. At the hip, the hamstrings are prime movers, with the gluteus maximus, for hip extension. The hamstrings originate on the ischial tuberosities (sitting bones), a site where hamstring pulls or tears are often felt.

- **Gluteus medius.** This muscle, according to most texts, is the primary abductor of the hip (a few sources include the gluteus minimus and/or the tensor fasciae latae as prime movers as well). It is an important muscle for hip stabilization when standing or walking. The gluteus medius is opposed by the hip adductors.

- **Hip adductors.** There are five hip adductors: adductor longus, adductor brevis, adductor magnus, gracilis, and pectineus. All five adductors lie on the inside of the thigh and are prime movers for hip adduction; the pectineus is also a prime mover for hip flexion.

- **Gluteus minimus.** Situated beneath the gluteus medius, this muscle is a prime mover for hip internal rotation and a strong assistor for hip abduction. Note that there are a large number of assistors for hip internal rotation (all five adductors, two of the hamstrings, and the tensor

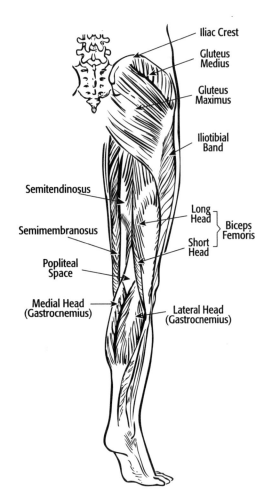

Fig. 3-18. Major Muscles of the Posterior Leg and Hip

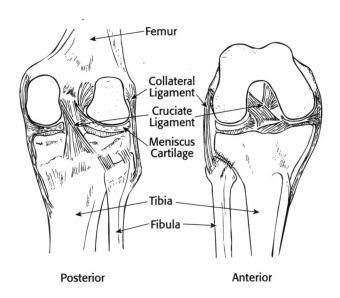

Fig. 3-19. Knee Joint

fasciae latae); these muscles may together contribute to hip tightness, e.g., when sitting on the floor cross-legged in external rotation.

- **Hip outward rotators.** There are six small muscles known as the outward rotators: piriformis, obturator internus, obturator externus, quadratus femoris, gemellus superior, and gemellus inferior. All six of these muscles lie deep to the gluteus maximus and are prime movers for hip external rotation. The piriformis is notable due to the proximity of the sciatic nerve, which may pass very near or even through the piriformis. An excessively tight piriformis muscle may cause sciatica-like symptoms.

Knee Joint

The knee joint is the articulation between the femur (thigh bone) and the tibia bone of the lower leg. The unique design of the knee allows for high levels of stability, mobility, and compression. The patella, or kneecap, lies in front of the knee joint and moves up and down along a groove between the condyles (large bony protrusions) of the femur during knee movements. Within the knee joint, and between the femur and the tibia bones, are the menisci, or semilunar cartilages, which act to minimize shock and compressive forces. The knee is classed as a hinge joint, although it is capable of a slight amount of rotation in certain circumstances. There are two primary **joint actions** of the knee joint.

1. Knee extension
2. Knee flexion

Major Muscles of the Knee Joint

- **Quadriceps.** The quadriceps muscle group actually consists of four muscles: the vastus lateralis, vastus medialis, vastus intermedius, and the rectus femoris. All four of these muscles cross the knee joint via the patella; they unite into a broad tendon just above the patella, and then insert onto the tibial tuberosity just below the patella via the patellar "ligament." All four muscles are prime movers for knee extension. One of the quadriceps, the rectus femoris, crosses the hip joint as well, performing the action of hip flexion along with the iliopsoas. The quadriceps is opposed by the hamstrings.
- **Hamstrings.** The hamstrings, described above under "Major Muscles of the Hip Joint," also cross the knee, inserting onto the tibia and fibula just below the knee joint. They are prime movers for knee flexion.

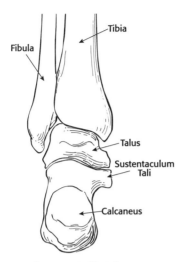

Fig. 3-20. Ankle Joint

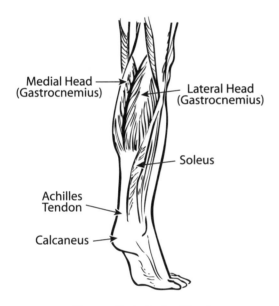

Fig. 3-21. Posterior Leg Muscles

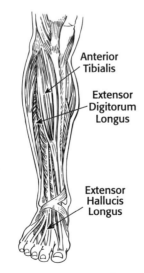

Fig. 3-22. Anterior Leg Muscles

- **Popliteus.** This small muscle, located just behind the knee, is also a prime mover for knee flexion. It is said to be an important stabilizer for the back and lateral side of the knee.

Ankle Joint

The ankle joint actually refers to two different sets of articulations, the talocrural and subtalar joints. The **talocrural joint** is a hinge joint and is the junction of the distal ends of the tibia and fibula with the talus. It is worth noting that the medial side of this joint is buttressed by an extremely strong ligament, making ankle sprains in which the ankle rolls toward the midline (eversion sprains) fairly uncommon. The lateral side of the ankle, however, has three rather small ligaments that provide less structural support for the ankle joint. As a result, ankle sprains in which the ankle rolls away from the midline (inversion sprains) are much more common. There are two **joint actions** of the talocrural joint.

1. Ankle dorsiflexion—movement that brings the top of the foot toward the shin
2. Ankle plantar flexion—movement that brings the sole of the foot downward (pointing the toes)

The subtalar joint is the articulation of the talus with the heel bone, or calcaneus. There are also two **joint actions** of the subtalar joint.

1. Ankle eversion (pronation)—movement of the ankle in which the sole turns or lifts outward and the medial border of the foot (the arch) tends to flatten
2. Ankle inversion (supination)—movement of the ankle in which the sole turns or lifts inward and the medial border of the foot (the arch) tends to lift

Major Muscles of the Ankle Joint

- **Anterior tibialis.** Just as its name implies, this long shin muscle lies in front of the tibia bone, inserting onto the medial side of the foot. It is a prime mover in ankle dorsiflexion and inversion. The anterior tibialis is opposed by the gastrocnemius and soleus.
- **Gastrocnemius.** This is the largest and most obvious calf muscle; it is a two-joint muscle, crossing both the knee joint (where it is an assistor for knee flexion) and the ankle joint. The gastrocnemius has two heads that fuse distally to form the Achilles tendon, which attaches to the calcaneus or heel bone. It is a prime mover for ankle plantar flexion.
- **Soleus.** The soleus lies under the gastrocnemius, however, unlike the gastrocnemius, it does not cross the knee joint. The soleus connects to the calcaneus via the Achilles tendon. It is a prime mover for ankle plantar flexion.

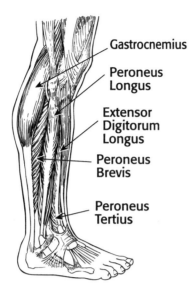

Gastrocnemius

Peroneus
Longus

Extensor
Digitorum
Longus

Peroneus
Brevis

Peroneus
Tertius

Fig. 3-22. Lateral Leg Muscles

- **Posterior tibialis.** This muscle is the deepest posterior muscle and is responsible for ankle inversion when the ankle is plantar flexed. It inserts onto the medial underside of the foot, helping to maintain the longitudinal arch.
- **Extensor digitorum longus.** Responsible for ankle dorsiflexion and ankle eversion, the extensor digitorum longus also lifts the four smaller toes.
- **Peroneus tertius, peroneus longus, and peroneus brevis.** The three peroneal muscles are all prime movers for ankle eversion; the peroneus tertius is also responsible for ankle dorsiflexion.

Roles Muscles Play

Depending on the work being performed, muscles can assume different roles or functions. For example, when performing a biceps curl, the biceps muscle performs the role of the agonist, or prime mover. Yet during a triceps kickback exercise, the biceps assumes the role of the antagonist, or opposing muscle (the triceps is now the agonist). The biceps can act as an assistor during shoulder front raises (the anterior deltoids are the agonist muscles) and as a stabilizer when holding the elbow at 90° of flexion while performing wrist exercises. Most muscles have the potential to perform these various roles, depending on the exercise and the position of the body. Note the following definitions.

- **Agonist**—prime mover, or the contracting muscle that is responsible for the movement that you see
- **Antagonist**—the muscle that works in opposition to the prime mover and reflexively elongates to allow the agonist to contract and move the joint
- **Assistor**—the muscle that assists in performing a movement, but is not a prime mover; sometimes called a secondary mover
- **Stabilizer**—the muscle that maintains a static or isometric contraction to anchor or support the movement of other primary movers. Torso muscles, for example, are important stabilizers of the spine during daily activities; ideally, they help maintain proper posture and aid in the prevention of back problems.
- **Synergist**—textbooks disagree on the definition of a synergist. Some describe it as a stabilizer; some describe it as an assistor. The muscle is contracting synergistically along with the prime mover in some way.

Muscle Actions

When muscles work, or develop force or tension, they are said to contract. However, this implies that the muscles shorten. Muscles sometimes shorten when they work, but they can also lengthen or even stay the same length and still produce tension. There are three main types of muscle actions.

1. **Isometric**—a held, static muscle action in which there is no change in the joint angle or muscle length. Strength gains that result from isometric contractions are joint-angle specific. A disadvantage of an isometric contraction is the tendency for breath holding (Valsalva maneuver), leading to a rise in blood pressure, which may be dangerous for some clients.

2. **Isotonic or Dynamic**—muscle actions that are not held, but that have movement. In most exercise settings this is the most common type of action. Muscle tension varies throughout the range of motion depending on mechanical factors. There are two types of isotonic muscle actions.
   - **Concentric**—shortening contraction of a muscle as it develops tension against a resistance (often called a positive contraction)
   - **Eccentric**—lengthening action of a muscle as it develops tension against a resistance (often called a negative contraction)

3. **Isokinetic**—muscle actions performed on special equipment in which speed is controlled, and any force applied against the machine results in an equal reaction force. This type of contraction is considered by many practitioners to be very safe; consequently, this equipment is most often found in the clinical rehabilitation setting.

Types of Muscle

- **Smooth muscle**—a type of muscle tissue that is present in many organs (e.g., intestines) and is generally not under voluntary control
- **Cardiac muscle**—an entire structure of interconnected cardiac fibers that contracts involuntarily as a unit
- **Skeletal muscle** (striated muscle)—muscle tissue that is composed of contractile tissue, causes joint movement, and is under voluntary control. Skeletal muscles have several types of fiber arrangements, including the following.
  - **Fusiform muscle**—fibers are arranged parallel to the line of pull, usually in a spindle shape, tapering at each end (e.g., biceps brachialis)
  - **Longitudinal muscle**—a long, strap-like muscle with parallel fibers (e.g., rectus abdominis)
  - **Fan-shaped or triangular muscle**—a flat muscle whose fibers radiate from a narrow end to a broad end (e.g., pectoralis major)
  - **Pennate muscle**—densely packed muscle fibers are arranged oblique to the line of pull in a feather-like arrangement. May be unipennate (e.g., tibialis posterior), bipennate (e.g., rectus femoris), or multipennate (e.g., deltoid).

Levers

When looking at the forces required to perform a joint action, it is necessary to understand the three basic types of levers. Levers are rigid rods that move about a fulcrum or pivot point. Acting on the lever are two different types of forces—resistance and effort. In the human body, the levers are the bones, the fulcrum is the joint, the effort force comes from the muscle, and the resistance force comes from gravity. The resistance force may also be increased with the use of training aids, such as weights or elastic bands or tubes.

The three types of levers are first-class, second-class, and third-class (see Figure 3-23). They are classified according to the placement of the fulcrum, the effort or applied force, and the resistance force on the lever. A first-class lever exists when the fulcrum is in between the applied force (AF) and the resistance (R). The classic example of a first-class lever is the see-saw. A second-class lever describes when the fulcrum or axis is at one end of the lever, resistance is in the middle, and the applied force is at the opposite end. The wheelbarrow is an example of a second-class lever. A third-class lever also has the axis at one end, but now the applied force is in the middle and the resistance is at the end. Using a hammer to drive a nail into a piece of wood is an example of a third-class lever.

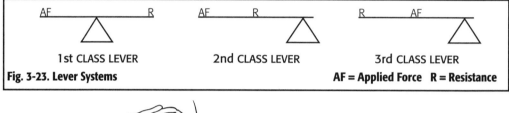

Fig. 3-23. Lever Systems   **AF = Applied Force   R = Resistance**

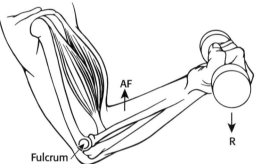

Fig. 3-24. Typical Third-Class Lever System

Opposing Muscle Groups

Knowing your opposing muscle groups is an important first step in proper exercise programming and in the correction of common muscle imbalances.

Opposing Muscle Groups		
Joint	**Muscle**	**Muscle**
Elbow	Biceps	Triceps
Shoulder	Pectoralis Major	Posterior Deltoid
Shoulder	Deltoids	Latissimus Dorsi
Shoulder	Subscapularis, Teres Major	Infraspinatus, Teres Minor
Scapulae	Upper Trapezius, Levatator Scapulae	Lower Trapezius, Pectoralis Minor
Scapulae	Serratus Anterior, Pectoralis Minor	Middle Trapezius, Rhomboids
Hip	Iliopsoas, Rectus Femoris	Gluteus Maximus, Hamstrings
Hip	Gluteus Medius	Hip Adductors
Knee	Quadriceps	Hamstrings
Ankle	Anterior Tibialis, Extensor Digitorum Longus	Gastrocnemius, Soleus
Ankle	Tibialis Anterior, Tibialis Posterior	Extensor Digitorum Longus, Peroneals

(Rasch & Burk., 1989)

Kinesiology Charts

Shoulder Joint Muscles and Their Actions								
	Flexion	**Extension**	**Abduction**	**Adduction**	**Internal Rotation**	**External Rotation**	**Horizontal Adduction**	**Horizontal Abduction**
Anterior deltoid	P.M.		Asst.		Asst.		P.M.	
Medial deltoid			P.M.					P.M.
Posterior deltoid		Asst.				Asst.		P.M.
Supraspinatus			P.M.					
Pectoralis major, clavicular	P.M.		Asst.*		Asst.		P.M.	
Pectoralis major, sternal		P.M		P.M	Asst.		P.M	
Coracobrachialis	Asst.			Asst.*	Asst.*	Asst.+	P.M.	
Subscapularis	Asst. ^		Asst. ^	Asst.*	P.M.		Asst.	
Latissimus dorsi		P.M.		P.M.	Asst.			Asst.
Teres major		P.M.		P.M.	P.M.			Asst.
Infraspinatus						P.M.		P.M.
Teres minor						P.M.		P.M.
Biceps, long head			Asst.					
Biceps, short head	Asst.			Asst.	Asst.		Asst.	
Triceps, long head		Asst.		Asst.				
* Indicated action takes place only when arm is above the horizontal.								
+ Indicated action takes place only from a position of rotation to the neutral point.								
^ Assistant actions vary with joint position and activity of synergistic muscles.								
P.M. = Prime Mover; Asst. = Assistant Mover								

(Rasch & Burk., 1989)

Shoulder Girdle Muscles and Their Actions						
	Elevation	**Depression**	**Protraction**	**Retraction**	**Upward Rotation**	**Downward Rotation**
Subclavius		Asst.				
Pectoralis minor		P.M.	P.M.			P.M.
Serratus anterior			P.M.		P.M.	
Trapezius I	P.M.					
Trapezius II	P.M.			Asst.	P.M.	
Trapezius III				P.M.		
Trapezius IV		P.M.		Asst.	P.M.	
Levator scapulae	P.M.					
Rhomboids	P.M.			P.M.		P.M.

NOTE: Movements of the arm on the trunk involve the cooperative actions of the shoulder joint and the shoulder girdle, as well as the attached muscles. Pure isolation of these muscles is often not possible. For instance, joint actions in this area are frequently caused by muscles acting as a force couple (equal parallel forces pulling in opposite directions), e.g., trapezius II and serratus anterior act together to cause upward rotation.

Elbow and Radioulnar Joint Muscles and Their Actions				
	Flexion	**Extension**	**Pronation**	**Supination**
Biceps brachii	P.M.			Asst.
Brachialis	P.M.			
Brachioradialis	P.M.		Asst.*	Asst.*
Pronator teres	Asst.		Asst.	
Pronator quadratus			P.M.	
Triceps brachii		P.M.		
Anconeus		Asst.		
Supinator				P.M.
Flexor carpi radialis	Asst.		Asst.	
Flexor carpi ulnaris	Asst.			
Palmaris longus	Asst.			
Extensor carpi radialis longus		Asst.		Asst.
Extensor carpi radialis brevis		Asst.		
Extensor carpi ulnaris		Asst.		
Flexor digitorum superficialis	Asst.			
Extensor digitorum		Asst.		
Extensor digiti minimi		Asst.		
Extensor pollicis longus				Asst.
Abductor pollicis longus				Asst.

*To the mid position

(Rasch & Burk., 1989)

Spinal Muscles and Their Actions				
Spinal Muscles	**Flexion**	**Extension**	**Rotation**	**Lateral Flexion**
Rectus Abdominis	P.M.			Asst.
External Oblique	P.M.		P.M.	Asst.
Internal Oblique	P.M.		P.M.	Asst.
Quadratus Lumborum				P.M.
Erector Spinae Group		P.M.	P.M.	P.M.
Multifidus		P.M.	P.M.	P.M.

Hip Joint Muscles and Their Actions						
	Flexion	**Extension**	**Abduction**	**Adduction**	**Inward Rotation**	**Outward Rotation**
Psoas	P.M.		Asst.			Asst.
Iliacus	P.M.		Asst.			Asst.
Sartorius	Asst.		Asst.			Asst.
Rectus femoris	P.M.		Asst.			
Pectineus	P.M.			P.M.	Asst.	
Gluteus maximus		P.M.	Asst.*	Asst.+		P.M.
Gluteus minimus	Asst.~	Asst.*	Asst.		P.M.	Asst.*
Gluteus medius	Asst.~	Asst.*	P.M.		Asst.~	Asst.*
Tensor fasciae latae	Asst.		Asst.		Asst.	
Biceps femoris		P.M.				Asst.
Semitendinosus		P.M.			Asst.	
Semimembranosus		P.M.			Asst.	
Gracilis	Asst.			P.M.	Asst.	
Adductor longus	Asst.			P.M.	Asst.	
Adductor brevis	Asst.			P.M.	Asst.	
Adductor magnus	Asst.*	Asst.+		P.M.	Asst.	
The six outward rotators #						P.M.
# Piriformis, Obturator internus, Obturator externus, Quadratus femoris, Gemellus superior, Gemellus inferior * Upper fibers + Lower fibers ~ Anterior fibers • Posterior fibers						
NOTE: Three less common hip joint actions include: horizontal adduction, horizontal abduction, and circumduction.						

(Rasch & Burk., 1989)

Knee Joint Muscles and Their Actions				
	Flexion	**Extension**	**Inward Rotation**	**Outward Rotation**
Biceps femoris	P.M.		P.M.	
Semitendinosus	P.M.		P.M.	
Semimembranosus	P.M.			P.M.
Rectus femoris		P.M.		
Vastus lateralis		P.M.		
Vastus intermedius		P.M.		
Vastus medialis		P.M.		
Sartorius	Asst.		Asst.	
Gracilis	Asst.		Asst.	
Popliteus*	Asst.		P.M.	
Gastrocnemius	Asst.			
Plantaris	Asst.			
* "Unlocks" the knee at the start of knee flexion				

Ankle Joint Muscles and Their Actions				
Extrinsic Muscles	**Dorsiflexion**	**Plantar Flexion**	**Inversion**	**Eversion**
Tibialis anterior	P.M.		P.M.	
Extensor digitorum longus	P.M.			P.M.
Peroneus tertius	P.M.			P.M.
Extensor hallucis longus	Asst.		Asst.	
Gastrocnemius		P.M.		
Plantaris		Asst.		
Soleus		P.M.		
Peroneus longus		Asst.		P.M.
Peroneus brevis		Asst.		P.M.
Flexor digitorum longus		Asst.	Asst.	
Flexor hallucis longus		Asst.	Asst.	
Tibialis posterior		Asst.	P.M.	

(Rasch & Burk., 1989)

Summary

In this chapter, kinesiological terms were introduced, major joint structures and joint actions were covered, and major muscles were described. Muscle roles, actions, and types were listed; opposing muscles were organized according to joint and opposing actions.

References

Norris, C.M. (2000). *Back stability.* Champaign, IL: Human Kinetics.

Rasch, P.J., & Burke, R.K. (1989). *Kinesiology and Applied Anatomy* (7th ed.). Philadelphia: Leah & Febiger.

Suggested Reading

Aaberg, E. (1993). *Muscle mechanics.* Champaign, IL: Human Kinetics.

Behnke, R.S. (2001). *Kinetic anatomy.* Champaign, IL: Human Kinetics.

Calais-Germain, B. (2003). *Anatomy of movement.* Seattle, WA: Eastland Press.

Clemente, C. (1997). *A regional atlas of the human body* (4th ed.). Philadelphia: Lippincott Williams & Wilkins.

Delavier, F. (2001). *Strength training anatomy.* Champaign, IL: Human Kinetics.

Enoka, R.M. (2001). *Neuromechanics of human movement.* Champaign, IL: Human Kinetics.

Floyd, R.T., & Thompson, C.W. (2003). *Manual of structural kinesiology* (15th ed.). New York: McGraw-Hill Co.

Golding, L.A., & Golding, S.M. (2003). *Musculoskeletal anatomy and human movement.* Monterey, CA: Healthy Learning.

Guyton, A.C., & Hall, J.E. (2005). *Textbook of medical physiology* (11th ed.). Philadelphia: W.B. Saunders Co.

Luttgens, K. (1996). *Kinesiology: Scientific basis of human motion.* New York: McGraw-Hill Co.

Norkin, C.C., & Levangie, P.K. (2005). *Joint structure and function: A comprehensive analysis* (4th ed.). Philadelphia: F. A. Davis Co.

Rasch, P.J., & Burke, R.K. (1989). *Kinesiology and Applied Anatomy* (7th ed.). Philadelphia: Leah & Febiger.

Tortora, G. (1999). *Principles of human anatomy* (8th ed.). New York: John Wiley & Sons.

Smith, L.K., Weiss, E.L., & Lehmkuhl, L.D. (1996). *Brunnstrom's clinical kinesiology* (5th ed.). Philadelphia: F.A. Davis Co.

Health Screening and Risk Appraisal

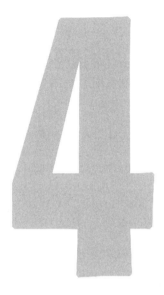

Outline

- Medical History Form
- Steps for Evaluating the Medical History Form
- Physician's Clearance Form
- Physical Activity Readiness Questionnaire
- Informed Consent
- Agreement and Release of Liability
- Other Health/Fitness Screening Tools
- Case Study Evaluation

When you first meet with a new client for an initial interview or consultation, you'll want to accomplish several things.

- Get acquainted.
- See if you are compatible.
- Acquire important health screening information and utilize various procedures and forms to meet the required standard of care you owe the client, while also laying the foundation for your delivery of service, and at the same time providing protection for you and your program.

Health screening information includes the client's medical history form and any other health/fitness screening devices or questionnaires. Such information is acquired and used, not for medical diagnosis or treatment, but to assist you in meeting your duties and responsibilities to the client regarding his/her participation in exercise activities. Based on your client's responses to such inquiries, and according to certain criteria established by the American College of Sports Medicine (ACSM), you may: (1) begin providing service, (2) need to require a physician's clearance, or (3) decide that your potential client belongs in a medically supervised and/or professionally guided program. In some circumstances you may even decide to deny service for a client who will not obtain medical clearance when deemed necessary. If considering such a course, you should obtain individualized legal advice. If your new client is cleared to exercise under your service, then certain legal forms must be completed and executed, such as an informed consent if testing is to be performed for exercise recommendation purposes, and a release or waiver absolving you and your organization of liability if permissible in your state. If such documents are not permissible in your state, express assumption of risk documents might be considered (see Chapter 14 and Appendix C). This must be done prior to fitness testing of the client or exercise programming. This chapter describes the forms and techniques used during the initial interview and consultation, and Appendix C has sample forms for reference. Finally, a method for evaluating the health screening process through a case study is offered at the end of this chapter.

Medical History Form

The medical history form is an essential part of any client's entry procedure for screening purposes into an activity program because it helps identify individuals at risk for cardiovascular, pulmonary, metabolic, musculoskeletal, or other potential problems. This health-screening process helps protect the client from unnecessary harm and is important for the personal fitness trainer (or club) from a legal and insurance perspective. Applicable forms and procedures should be carefully reviewed with your client by obtaining and analyzing information about age, risk factors, possible symptoms of heart disease, pregnancy, orthopedic problems, medications, as well as other health issues. If your client has risk factors requiring medical clearance, you will need to postpone fitness assessment activities and exercise programming with the client until a personal physician has cleared him/her and provided authorization for the client to participate (in writing) and returned the client's clearance form to you. In some cases, it may be necessary to refer the client to a facility where both the fitness assessment and the exercise sessions can be performed under medical supervision. It is important to take appropriate action (e.g., refer for further evaluation or recommend an appropriate exercise program as deemed necessary) on any medical history information you obtain. A sample medical history form can be found in Appendix C.

Steps for Evaluating the Medical History Form

Step 1: Determine the Client's Age.

It is recommended that men age 45 years or over and women age 55 years or over be cleared by their personal physicians. According to the American Heart Association (AHA), the risk of cardiovascular disease increases progressively with age (American Heart Association, 2005a). (Note, however, that age is not listed as an ACSM risk factor in Table 4-1.)

Step 2: Analyze Coronary Heart Disease (CHD) Risk Factors.

By definition, a health risk factor is any factor that increases the chance that an individual will develop a disease or condition. The more risk factors a person has, the greater the likelihood that he/she will have or develop a particular disease (on the other hand, a "negative" risk factor, such as the one identified below for HDL cholesterol > 60 mg/dl, helps to reduce the risk of disease). Risk factors for CHD identified by the ACSM (2006) are found in Table 4-1.

Table 4-1.	ACSM Coronary Heart Disease Risk Factors
Positive* Risk Factors	**Defining Criteria**
1. Family history	Myocardial infarction, coronary revascularization, or sudden death before 55 years of age in father or other male first-degree relative, or before 65 years of age in mother or other female first-degree relative
2. Cigarette smoking	Current cigarette smoker or those who quit within the previous 6 months
3. Hypertension	Systolic blood pressure ≥ 140 mmHg or diastolic ≥ 90 mmHg, confirmed by measurements on at least two separate occasions, or on antihypertensive medication
4. Dyslipidemia	Low-density lipoprotein (LDL) cholesterol > 130 mg/dl (3.4 mmol/L) or high-density lipoprotein (HDL) cholesterol < 40 mg/dl (1.03 mmol/L), or on lipid-lowering medication. If total serum cholesterol is all that is available, use > 200 mg/dl (5.2 mmol/L) rather than low-density lipoprotein (LDL) > 130 mg/dl.
5. Impaired fasting glucose	Fasting blood glucose ≥ 100 mg/dl (5.6 mmol/L) confirmed by measurements on at least two separate occasions
6. Obesity	Body mass index > 30 kg/m^2 or waist girth > 102 cm for men and > 88 cm for women or waist/hip ratio ≥ 0.95 for men and ≥ 0.86 for women
7. Sedentary lifestyle	Persons not participating in a regular exercise program or not meeting the minimal physical activity recommendations from the U.S. Surgeon General's Report
Negative* Risk Factor	**Criteria**
1. High-serum HDL cholesterol	> 60 mg/dl (1.6 mmol/L)
* In this case, positive risk factors can lead or contribute to CHD, while negative risk factors help to protect against CHD.	

(American College of Sports Medicine. [2006]. *ACSM's guidelines for exercise testing and prescription* [7th ed.]. Baltimore: Lippincott Williams & Wilkins. Reprinted with permission.)

AHA Coronary Heart Disease Risk Factors

1. Age (Risk for cardiovascular disease increases progressively with age. About four out of five people who die of CHD are age 65 or older.)
2. Male gender
3. Heredity (Parents or siblings with a heart or circulatory problem prior to age 55; African Americans have a higher percentage of hypertension than whites and their risk of heart disease is greater.)
4. Tobacco smoking
5. High blood cholesterol
6. High blood pressure
7. Physical inactivity
8. Obesity and overweight
9. Diabetes mellitus

(© 2005, American Heart Association. www.americanheart.org. Reproduced with permission.)

Step 3: Ask if the Client Has Any Signs or Symptoms Suggestive of Cardiovascular, Pulmonary, or Metabolic Disease.

If the client says yes, require medical clearance as ACSM recommends.

Major Signs or Symptoms Suggestive of Cardiovascular, Pulmonary, or Metabolic Disease

- Chest pain (or neck, jaw, or arm pain that may suggest ischemia)
- Shortness of breath at rest or with mild exertion (dyspnea)
- Dizziness or fainting (syncope)
- Dyspnea when lying down or sleeping (also orthopnea—a form of dyspnea in which the person can breathe comfortably only when standing or sitting erect; associated with asthma, emphysema, and angina pectoris)
- Ankle swelling (edema)
- Palpitations or irregular heartbeat
- Cramping pains in legs or feet when exercising
- Known heart murmur
- Unusual fatigue or shortness of breath with usual activities

(American College of Sports Medicine. [2006]. *ACSM's guidelines for exercise testing and prescription* [7th ed.]. Baltimore: Lippincott Williams & Wilkins. Reprinted with permission.)

NOTE: Women have been shown to exhibit very subtle or atypical signs and symptoms (when compared to men) while experiencing cardiac ischemia.

Step 4: Decide if the Client is Low, Moderate, or High Risk.

ACSM Risk Stratification Categories	
1. Low risk	Men < 45 years old and women < 55 years old who have no symptoms and zero or one risk factor
2. Moderate risk	Men ≥ 45 years old and women ≥ 55 years old, or those who have two or more risk factors
3. High risk	Individuals with one or more signs and symptoms of cardiovascular, pulmonary, or metabolic disease, or with known cardiovascular, pulmonary, or metabolic disease
NOTE: Cardiovascular disease includes cardiac, peripheral vascular, or cerebrovascular disease; pulmonary disease includes chronic obstructive pulmonary disease (COPD), asthma, or cystic fibrosis; metabolic disease includes insulin dependent diabetes mellitus (IDDM), non-insulin dependent diabetes mellitus (NIDDM), thyroid disorders, or renal or liver disease.	

(American College of Sports Medicine. [2006]. *ACSM's guidelines for exercise testing and prescription* [7th ed.]. Baltimore: Lippincott Williams & Wilkins. Reprinted with permission.)

Step 5: Determine Whether You Need to Recommend a Medical/Physician's Clearance and/or Refer the Client to a Medically Supervised Program According to the ACSM.

A physician's clearance is recommended if the client is moderate or high risk, according to the ACSM risk stratification categories. In other words, a physician's clearance is recommended if:

1. there are two or more risk factors for CHD present.
2. there are symptoms of cardiovascular, pulmonary, or metabolic disease.
3. there is known cardiac, pulmonary, or metabolic (including diabetes) disease.
4. your client is male and age 45 years or over.
5. your client is female and age 55 years or over.

Please be aware that the ACSM makes more detailed recommendations than those outlined above, including the following (American College of Sports Medicine, 2006).

- A distinction is made between clients exercising at low-to-moderate intensities and those exercising at vigorous intensities. The ACSM recommends that clients in the high-risk category have medical supervision if they wish to exercise vigorously. (Vigorous exercise is defined as ≥ 60% of heart rate reserve or ≥ 77% of maximal heart rate.)
- The higher risk the client, the more important it is that the client's personal fitness trainer be highly qualified, with advanced certifications and, preferably, a degree in the health/fitness field. Do not exceed the limits of your knowledge, skills, and abilities. When in doubt, refer a higher risk client to a more highly credentialed or degreed fitness professional.

Step 6: Ascertain if Your Client is Pregnant.

The American College of Obstetricians and Gynecologists (ACOG) (2002) recommends that all pregnant clients be cleared for exercise by their physicians prior to starting an exercise program. Such recommendations should be followed by fitness professionals.

Step 7: Decide if there are Any Other Reasons to Recommend a Medical Clearance.

Although there may be no unanimously accepted guidelines from professional organizations to be used in clearing clients for participation, it is advisable to request a physician's clearance for clients who have been recently hospitalized for any reason, who have chronic or acute muscle or joint injury, or who are on prescription medications. Additionally, such a clearance may be prudent for clients with asthma, epilepsy, multiple sclerosis, or other diseases and disorders.

If a client does not fall into any of the above categories, the client is then classified as low risk and does not generally need medical clearance prior to fitness testing or exercise. In the event that a client has several risk factors, known disease, or medical complications or injuries, you may decide that your level of knowledge is insufficient to provide the safest monitoring and exercise programming for his/her condition. Know your limitations. It may be more prudent to recommend that client activity be carried out in a cardiac rehabilitation facility or under the supervision of a physical therapist, depending on the nature of the client's problem.

Medications

Since many of your clients (especially those who are moderate or high risk) will be on medications, it is important that you understand the effects of various medications on exercise. For example, several drugs can increase or decrease the heart rate and make a client's target heart rate inaccurate. A brief list of common medications and their exercise effects can be found in Appendix B. When in doubt about a client's medication, always consult with his or her physician. Do not attempt to administer or advise your client about any drug. If you do so, you run the risk of being charged with the unauthorized practice of medicine or some other health care domain reserved for practice by licensed health care providers. In addition, such acts may well increase the level of care you are expected to provide, thereby increasing your risk of potential legal liability if a problem occurs.

Physician's Clearance Form

The physician's clearance process is important for several reasons. First, compliance with the process, where indicated, protects the client from harm. Second, it assists you in complying with the required standard of care. Third, it helps reduce your liability and your client's risk of an untoward event. Lastly, it opens up communication between you and the physician. Always adhere to physician specified limitations.

Your client may need a diagnostic graded exercise stress test (GXT) prior to beginning an exercise program. This decision should be made by the physician. A sample physician's clearance form can be found in Appendix C.

Physical Activity Readiness Questionnaire

The Physical Activity Readiness Questionnaire, also known as the PAR-Q, is a basic and well-known health history screening tool, a sample of which can be found in Appendix C. Even though the PAR-Q is widely used, it does not, for example, identify CHD risk factors. AFAA recommends that you use a more thorough medical history form (see Appendix C) and obtain more detailed screening information from your client. In this way you'll be able to provide safer and more appropriate fitness testing and exercise programming while helping to protect both your client from harm and yourself from potential legal pitfalls.

Informed Consent

Informed consent should be obtained from every client prior to exercise testing or programming. Failure to inform and warn clients about potential risks involved in testing and/or exercise may be judged as legally inadequate and below the required standard of care. If harm to the client should proximately result, claim or suit arising from such negligence may be instituted. The informed consent process and form should explain in reasonable detail the exercise test and/or program, outline potential risks, dangers, and discomforts, and describe the expected benefits. The form should let the client know that he or she is free to stop the exercise test or program at any time. Clients should be advised of their responsibility to disclose all relevant information and ask any questions necessary to ensure a safe exercise experience. Check with an attorney for further information on this process and to develop, or at least review, any form you utilize for this purpose.

Agreement and Release of Liability

The exercise waiver may be used for clients who refuse to obtain medical clearance or if you wish to secure an added potential measure of legal protection for yourself from lawsuit. It may be appropriate to obtain an exercise waiver/release of liability from all participants, even those who are apparently healthy and low risk, and for whom an exercise program may provide substantial benefits (American College of Sports Medicine, 1997). Using such signed in advance waivers is an attempt to limit your liability for injuries sustained by your client as a result of personal training and, in some circumstances, even in cases in which the personal fitness trainer may have caused harm through his/her own negligent act or omission. (It should be noted, however, that such fitness waivers are not valid in all states, that the law changes over time, and that no form should be developed or used without the assistance of, or at least review by, your individual legal counsel.)

Other Health/Fitness Screening Tools

A variety of questionnaires and lifestyle evaluation tools have been developed in order to help you further understand your clients' needs and goals. Following are a few information-gathering devices (see sample forms in Appendix C).

The Exercise and Activity Quiz

The exercise and activity quiz gives you specific information about your client's activity level, exercise goals, past exercise history, and beliefs about exercise. It helps open the lines of communication between you and your client.

The Nutrition and Weight Profile

The nutrition and weight profile develops your client's awareness of his/her eating habits and helps educate him/her regarding healthy food choices. Relevant weight-loss issues are raised, helping you better understand your client.

The Self-Assessment Quiz

The self-assessment quiz helps your client begin to understand wellness and the key benefits of wellness promotion. This quiz may be completed privately by the client and does not necessarily have to be returned to you. Its purpose is to educate and inform.

Case Study Evaluation

A case study is a practical exercise based upon hypothetical facts and circumstances that helps personal fitness trainers apply various concepts discussed in this text. The one presented here will be based upon your evaluation of an individual from an examination and evaluation of his/her responses to the questions in the forms discussed in this chapter, as well as the results of his/her fitness assessment. You will need to determine risk factors and health status, decide whether or not to perform exercise testing, obtain information from the fitness assessment and counseling sessions, and then formulate a plan for exercise programming.

When evaluating this case study, you will want to proceed according to the following steps.

1. How many CHD risk factors does your client have according to the ACSM?
2. Has your client communicated to you any symptoms of CHD or does he/she readily show any such symptoms or signs potentially suggestive of CHD that need to be evaluated by a health care provider?
3. Is your client low, moderate, or high risk according to the ACSM?
4. Do you need to recommend a medical clearance according to the ACSM?
5. Are there any other reasons to recommend a medical clearance (e.g., back pain, asthma, or pregnancy)?
6. Should you perform a fitness assessment on this client or not? If so, what type of tests will you choose? (Decide for each test whether the benefit outweighs the risk and complete the informed consent process and forms for all such tests.) Consider cardiorespiratory, muscle strength and/or endurance, flexibility, postural, and body composition assessments. Be familiar with test endpoints and think about signs of fatigue that your client might exhibit.
7. Evaluate and interpret the results of the fitness assessment. Was everything normal?
8. Consider the client's interests, needs, goals, and level of motivation.
9. Have you formulated an exercise program based on all of the data collected? Be sure to incorporate the components of fitness: cardiorespiratory conditioning, muscular fitness, flexibility, and body composition. Have you considered mode, frequency, intensity (including target heart rate range [THRR] and rate of perceived exertion [RPE] range), duration, and the rate of exercise progression over time?
10. When will you retest your client?
11. What suggestions do you have for the client in terms of lifestyle modifications? What kind of counseling approach might work best with this client?

Sample Case Study

Ralph M., age 57. Ralph has not exercised since college and works as a financial analyst. He weighs 197 pounds and is 6'0". He was an all-American football player in college and is interested in getting back in shape. However, he has arthritis pain in both knees that he feels is associated with his football days. He has smoked on and off for 40 years and currently smokes 5–10 cigarettes per day. About one year ago, he was diagnosed with mild hypertension. He scored in the average category on the push-up test, the fair category on the crunch test, and the poor category on the Sit and Reach Test.

Evaluation

1. Ralph has three risk factors according to the ACSM (smoker, hypertension, sedentary lifestyle).
2. He has no known symptoms of CHD.
3. He is moderate risk according to the ACSM.
4. Yes, a medical clearance is recommended on the basis of his CHD risk factors and age.
5. Ralph's knee pain indicates that it would also be prudent to recommend a medical clearance for musculoskeletal reasons as well.
6. Ralph may need improvement in his abdominal endurance as well as his hamstring and low-back flexibility, according to his history. Physician input into these matters should be solicited during the physician clearance process.
7. He wants to "get back in shape"—a nonspecific goal. Further discussion with Ralph is needed to understand what exactly this means to him.
8. After clearance, potential exercise programming recommendations might include:
   - beginning a cardiorespiratory program to help reduce his risk of CHD based upon recommendations from his physician, and possibly lower his blood pressure—3x per week, 15–20 minutes duration, 40–50% heart rate reserve, walking (initial level of progression).
   - beginning a resistance training program with emphasis on increasing abdominal endurance—2x per week, 15–20 minutes duration, all major muscle groups, 1 set, 8–12 repetitions.
   - beginning a flexibility program, with emphasis on hamstring and low-back flexibility—5x per week, all major muscle groups, static stretching to the point of tightness, hold 15–30 seconds each.
9. Reassess in 3–4 months.
10. Lifestyle modifications could include increasing daily physical activity (e.g., parking farther from work, taking stairs instead of elevators) and exploring options for smoking cessation (e.g., online or health insurance company programs, physician suggestions).

Summary

In this chapter, initial steps for client health screening and risk appraisal were outlined. This important process must take place prior to fitness assessment and/or exercise programming. The medical history form, physician's clearance, PAR-Q, informed consent form, exercise waiver, and other health/fitness screening tools were presented, as well as the ACSM and AHA CHD risk factors, and ACSM risk stratification categories. Methods for evaluating a case study were also described.

References

American College of Obstetricians and Gynecologists. (2002). Exercise during pregnancy and the postpartum period, ACOG Committee Opinion No. 267. *Obstetrics and Gynecology, 99,* 171-173.

American College of Sports Medicine. (1997). *ACSM's health fitness facility standards & guidelines* (2nd ed.). Champaign, IL: Human Kinetics.

American College of Sports Medicine. (2006). *ACSM's guidelines for exercise testing and prescription* (7th ed.). Baltimore: Lippincott Williams & Wilkins.

American Heart Association. (2005a). *Risk factors I can't change.* Retrieved August 29, 2005, from http://www.americanheart.org/presenter.jhtml?identifier=2646.

American Heart Association. (2005b). *Primary prevention in the adult.* Retrieved August 29, 2005, from http://www.americanheart.org/presenter.jhtml?identifier=4726.

Suggested Reading

American College of Sports Medicine. (2003). *ACSM fitness book* (3rd ed.). Champaign, IL: Human Kinetics.

Balady, G. J., Chaitman, B., Driscoll, D., Foster, C., Froelicher, E., Gordon, N., et al. (1998). Joint position statement: AHA/ACSM joint statement: Recommendations for cardiovascular screening, staffing, and emergency policies at health/fitness facilities. *Medicine & Science in Sports & Exercise, 30*(6), 1009-1018.

Canadian Society for Exercise Physiology. (1994). *PAR-Q and you.* Gloucester, Ontario: Canadian Society for Exercise Physiology.

Resources

- American College of Sports Medicine—www.acsm.org
- American Heart Association—www.americanheart.org
- International Health, Racquet and Sportsclub Association—www.ihrsa.org

Fitness Assessment

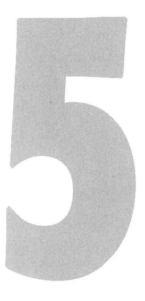

Outline

- Benefits of a Fitness Assessment
- Preliminary Testing Information
- Components of a Fitness Assessment
    - Step 1: Assess resting heart rate and blood pressure
    - Step 2: Assess body composition
    - Step 3: Assess cardiorespiratory fitness
    - Step 4: Assess muscular fitness
    - Step 5: Assess flexibility and posture
    - Step 6: Optional fitness assessment components

This chapter will cover basic fitness assessment information, including the most commonly performed fitness assessment tests and protocols. You will learn how to administer a complete fitness assessment, addressing all the components of health-related fitness. Since no one test is perfect for all clients, you are encouraged to learn more about other assessments than those covered in this text. In this way you will eventually be able to adapt your fitness assessment sessions to the needs of each client. Remember that for some clients a particular fitness test may pose an unnecessary risk; the risk may in fact be greater than the benefit. In such a case it is important to avoid a test that is problematic, substitute an assessment that is more appropriate, or refer for health care provider assessment.

After your client has filled out the appropriate forms, including informed consent documents, and returned a signed physician's clearance form to you (if necessary), you are ready to begin.

Benefits of a Fitness Assessment

Benefits of a fitness assessment include the following.
- Establishing the client's current fitness status and providing you with baseline information. This information is valuable when developing your client's individualized exercise recommendations.
- Utilizing this information for comparison later as the client progresses and improves.
- Serving as a powerful educational and motivational tool, and increasing the likelihood of adherence.
- When performed along with the prerequisite health screening, demonstrates your professional prudence and knowledge, which can be important if potential legal issues arise.

Limitations regarding a fitness assessment include the fact that you are only predicting, or estimating, your client's fitness level. Avoid focusing on the absolute numerical values. What's important is to evaluate your client's progress; look at change over time or **percent improvement**.

Below are the necessary steps to calculate percent improvement and quantify change over time.
1. After reassessing your client (3–4 months after the initial assessment) with the exact same test and protocol, find the difference between the two test results.
2. Divide this difference by the previous, or initial, test result.
3. Multiply by 100.

Example: A client performed 20 push-ups on the push-up test in January. In April, this same client was able to perform 32 push-ups on the test. 32 - 20 = 12. 12 ÷ 20 = 0.60. 0.60 x 100 = 60% improvement!

Some clients will be much more motivated by seeing tangible proof of change over time than by having themselves compared to norms, which can be discouraging for clients with poor initial fitness levels. On the other hand, some clients will enjoy seeing the normative data. You will need to use your professional judgment when deciding which approach works best with which clients. The bottom line, however, is to use the fitness assessment process to help your client focus on continued improvement in his or her well-being and fitness. A "Fitness Assessment Data Sheet" is provided in Appendix C.

Preliminary Testing Information

Remember that prior to the actual exercise tests, your client needs to be informed about appropriate footwear and clothing, and instructed to avoid drinking caffeinated or alcoholic beverages, smoking, or consuming a heavy meal for at least 3 hours before the fitness assessment. Nicotine, alcohol, a large meal and/or caffeine can all alter resting and exercising heart rate and blood pressure responses. Conversely, not eating anything for several hours prior to testing may cause a drop in blood sugar levels after the tests, leaving the client feeling dizzy, lightheaded, or nauseous. In addition, have your client avoid exercising prior to the fitness assessment. Finally, if your client is ill or has recently had a viral infection, it is probably best to postpone the assessment. Following is a summary of the pre-test information according to the American College of Sports Medicine (ACSM) (2006).

General Pre-Test Instructions
- Wear comfortable clothing.
- Avoid a heavy meal, alcohol, and caffeine for at least 3 hours before the test.
- Drink plenty of fluids during the 24 hours preceding the test.
- Avoid strenuous exercise on the day of the test.
- Get plenty of sleep (6–8 hours) on the night before the test.

General Test Environment
- The room temperature should be 68–72°F (20–22°C) and humidity should be less than 60%.
- The room should be quiet and private.
- The room should be well ventilated.

NOTE: Remember that the informed consent process must be completed prior to all testing activities.

Components of a Fitness Assessment

The components of a standard fitness assessment reflect the major components of health-related fitness: body composition, cardiorespiratory endurance, muscular strength and endurance (muscular fitness), and flexibility. The recommended test order places resting measurements (e.g., heart rate, blood pressure, weight, body composition) first, followed by cardiorespiratory assessment. Cardiorespiratory tests should come before muscular fitness testing because assessments of muscle strength and endurance can affect heart rate. The recommended fitness assessment components are as follows.

1. Assess resting heart rate and blood pressure (if possible).
2. Assess body composition (e.g., skinfolds, waist-to-hip ratio and girths).
3. Assess cardiorespiratory fitness (3-Minute Step Test or Rockport Walking Test).
4. Assess muscular strength and/or endurance (e.g., push-up test and partial curl-up test).
5. Assess flexibility (e.g., Sit and Reach Test) and posture.
6. Optional fitness assessment components

Step 1: Assess resting heart rate and blood pressure

Resting heart rate—A true resting heart rate is obtained first thing in the morning when you are completely relaxed but conscious, before getting out of bed. Since even a true resting heart rate fluctuates, it's best to perform measurements on three consecutive days and take the average. In the fitness assessment setting, try to obtain as accurate a resting heart rate as possible by having the client sit quietly for 5–10 minutes prior to palpation. Heart rates fluctuate depending on the time of day, anxiety, stress, temperature, medication, smoking, eating, and drinking (especially caffeine).

Resting heart rate may be palpated at the **radial artery** at the wrist for 1 full minute or for 30 seconds (multiply by 2 for the minute value). It is normal for some individuals (especially athletes) to have respiratory sinus arrhythmia at rest, meaning that the pulse speeds up during inhalation and slows during exhalation. For this reason, counting for 30 or 60 seconds at rest is more accurate than counting for 6, 10, or 15 seconds. It is also acceptable to palpate the pulse at the **carotid artery** at the side of the larynx on the neck, although it may not be as accurate if too much pressure is applied. Baroreceptors in the carotid artery detect pressure and may reflexively cause the heart rate to decrease. As a result, many professionals prefer that heart rate measurement be taken at the radial pulse.

An accurate resting heart rate is important for three reasons.

1. It is often used in the calculation of exercise target heart rate (Karvonen formula) for graded exercise tests and exercise prescription.

2. It can provide a baseline value for comparison as cardiovascular fitness improves. (With training, an individual's resting heart rate usually decreases as his/her stroke volume increases.)

3. Normal resting heart rates are usually regular (no palpitations), and are between 60–100 beats/minute. If your client's resting heart rate is over 100 bpm, under 60 bpm, or is irregular, a physician should be consulted. An exception is the aerobically trained athlete; it is not unusual for athletes to have resting heart rates as low as 40 bpm.

Resting blood pressure—Since high blood pressure, or hypertension, is one of the alterable risk factors for heart disease, and since an estimated one in three Americans has borderline or high blood pressure, routine measurement of resting blood pressure is very important (National High Blood Pressure Education Program, 2003). However, check your state's laws and regulations as some states may require that blood pressure only be taken by licensed health care providers. It is recommended that all fitness professionals, particularly personal trainers, learn to monitor blood pressure. This becomes increasingly important should you decide to work with higher risk clients. During the fitness assessment, if your client has high resting blood pressure readings after three measurements, and has another risk factor (e.g., family history), then the client should be regarded as moderate risk and further testing or exercise should be postponed until he/she is cleared by a physician.

Resting blood pressure can be affected by the same factors as resting heart rate (e.g., caffeine, stress, time of day). In addition, since many clients become anxious about having their blood pressure measured, relaxing quietly for 5–10 minutes prior to measurement may help.

Normal, or average, blood pressure is usually thought to be around 120/80 mmHg. See Table 5-1 for classification of blood pressure measurements.

Table 5-1. Classification and Management of Blood Pressure for Adults

BP Classification	Systolic	Diastolic	Lifestyle Modification
Normal	< 120 mmHg	And < 80 mmHg	Encourage
Prehypertension	120–139 mmHg	Or 80–89 mmHg	Yes
Stage 1 Hypertension	140–159 mmHg	Or 90–99 mmHg	Yes
Stage 2 Hypertension	≥ 160 mmHg	Or ≥ 100 mmHg	Yes

(National High Blood Pressure Education Program, 2003. Reprinted with permission.)

ACSM defines the risk factor for hypertension as systolic blood pressure ≥ 140 mmHg, and/or diastolic blood pressure ≥ 90 mmHg, on at least two separate occasions, or if the individual is on high blood pressure medication (American College of Sports Medicine, 2006). The top number, or higher value, is referred to as the **systolic pressure**, or the amount of pressure or force exerted against the arterial walls immediately after the heart has contracted. The bottom number or **diastolic pressure**, may be thought of as the "run off" force, or the amount of pressure still remaining against the arterial walls as the heart relaxes before the next contraction.

Measuring Blood Pressure—(NOTE: In some states, blood pressure may only be taken by a licensed health care provider. Always check with the given state's laws and regulations before taking such measurements. If you may permissibly take a blood pressure reading, always remember that you are not doing so for diagnostic or other medical purposes but rather for an assessment of fitness levels only!)

Blood pressure is measured with a stethoscope and a blood pressure cuff connected to a manometer (column or dial) from which the numerical values are read. (This device is called a sphygmomanometer.) Cuffs are available in child, adult, and large-adult sizes. Size is important because too small a cuff on a large arm can result in a falsely elevated reading. Although the following is not a substitute for professional training in blood pressure measurement, it is the generally used procedure for taking blood pressure. (NOTE: No such procedure should be performed by any trainer except with adequate professional training and only where permissible under state law.) Normally, blood pressure measurement is completed by:

1. placing the cuff firmly around the upper arm (under clothing) with the lower edge approximately 1 inch above the bend in the elbow, or antecubital fossa. The middle of the cuff bladder should be over the brachial artery on the inner part of the arm and the cuff bladder should surround at least 80% of the upper arm.
2. placing the bell of the stethoscope 1 inch below the cuff, directly over the brachial artery. (Sometimes it is necessary to first palpate the brachial pulse at this site to be sure of placement.)
3. inflating the cuff pressure to 200 mmHg while listening through the stethoscope.
4. slowly releasing the pressure at approximately 2–3 mmHg per second. The point at which the first rhythmic sound (called the first Korotkoff sound) is heard is the top number, or systolic pressure.

5. continuing to steadily release the pressure and note the point at which the sound or pitch changes (fourth Korotkoff sound) and/or the point at which the sound completely disappears (fifth Korotkoff sound). Usually the point at which the sound disappears is considered to be the diastolic reading, although in some individuals the sound is occasionally heard all the way down to zero during exercise. In that case, the change in pitch signifies the diastolic pressure.

6. waiting approximately 60 seconds or more, if a measurement needs repeating, with the cuff completely deflated to allow circulation to return to normal.

At rest, the client should have both feet flat on the floor and be in a relaxed sitting position with the arm supported. During aerobic exercise, it is normal for the systolic blood pressure (along with the heart rate) to increase with increasing work. The normal response of the diastolic blood pressure during exercise is to lower slightly (no more than 10 mmHg), or to stay the same. However, if systolic blood pressure fails to increase, or if the diastolic blood pressure increases rapidly with increased work, then the exercise should be stopped and a physician should be consulted. Exercising blood pressure should be measured with the client's arm relaxed and not grasping a treadmill bar or cycle handlebar.

NOTE: These blood pressure measurement steps are illustrative only and should not be performed unless you have been trained in such measurement by a health care provider or qualified professional previously trained in such procedures. Performance of such measurement may be limited by law to licensed health care providers. The process described above is illustrative only.

Step 2: Assess body composition

Although many clients may be interested in learning about their estimated percent body fat for cosmetic reasons, a primary reason for assessing body composition is to educate your client about the risks involved with excessive body fat. It is well established that too much body fat is a hazard and increases the risk of heart disease, diabetes, high blood pressure, some forms of cancer, low-back pain, and other musculoskeletal problems (Flegal, Carroll, Ogden, & Johnson, 2002).

Body composition refers to the percentage of body weight that is fat and is based on the assumption that body weight can be divided into various components. Most equations use the two-compartment model: fat mass and lean body mass (lean body mass is assumed to include, but is not limited to, muscles, bones, organs, and internal fluids). The norms for body composition are based on equations that assume the densities for fat and lean body mass are the same for everyone. Therefore, the norms that you use to estimate your client's percent (%) body fat should ideally have been developed on a population with your client's same age, gender, race, and physical activity level; specific protocols and norms are available (see Heyward & Wagner, 2004). The Aerobics and Fitness Association of America's (AFAA's) (2002) current recommendation for acceptable % body fat for men is 15%, and for women is 25%. These "standards" essentially represent the average percent fat for young adults. See Tables 5-2 and 5-3 for population-specific percentile values on men and women.

Table 5-2.	Body Composition (% body fat) for Men*				
	Age				
Percentile	**20–29**	**30–39**	**40–49**	**50–59**	**60+**
90	7.1	11.3	13.6	15.3	15.3
80	9.4	13.9	16.3	17.9	18.4
70	11.8	15.9	18.1	19.8	20.3
60	14.1	17.5	19.6	21.3	22.0
50	15.9	19.0	21.1	22.7	23.5
40	17.4	20.5	22.5	24.1	25.0
30	19.5	22.3	24.1	25.7	26.7
20	22.4	24.2	26.1	27.5	28.5
10	25.9	27.3	28.9	30.3	31.2

*Data provided by the Institute for Aerobics Research, Dallas, TX (1994). Study population for the data set was predominantly White and college educated. The following may be used as descriptors for the percentile rankings: well above average (90), above average (70), average (50), below average (30), and well below average (10).

Table 5-3.	Body Composition (% body fat) for Women*				
	Age				
Percentile	**20–29**	**30–39**	**40–49**	**50–59**	**60+**
90	14.5	15.5	18.5	21.6	21.1
80	17.1	18.0	21.3	25.0	25.1
70	19.0	20.0	23.5	26.6	27.5
60	20.6	21.6	24.9	28.5	29.3
50	22.1	23.1	26.4	30.1	30.9
40	23.7	24.9	28.1	31.6	32.5
30	25.4	27.0	30.1	33.5	34.3
20	27.7	29.3	32.1	35.6	36.6
10	32.1	32.8	35.0	37.9	39.3

*Data provided by the Institute for Aerobics Research, Dallas, TX (1994). Study population for the data set was predominantly White and college educated. The following may be used as descriptors for the percentile rankings: well above average (90), above average (70), average (50), below average (30), and well below average (10).

(Fitness norms used with permission of the Cooper Institute, Dallas, TX)

Methods of Body Composition Assessment

Several methods of estimating % body fat have been developed and are included below.

- **Hydrostatic (underwater) weighing**—This method, traditionally known as the gold standard of body composition assessment, is based on the Archimedes' principle. Since muscle mass is more dense than water, and fat mass is less dense than water (fat floats), a highly muscular person will weigh more in the water than a person with a high percentage of body fat. Although this method is said to be the most accurate, it still has a standard error of estimate of ± 2.7% (Lohman, 1992).

- **Dual-energy X-ray absorptiometry (DEXA)**—Available primarily in clinical settings, the DEXA machine uses low-level radiation and is also used for measurements of bone density. Although more research is needed, the standard error of estimate is ± 1.8% (Lohman, 1992).

- **Plethysmography**—This technique requires the client to enter a dual-chamber device that measures the air displaced inside the chamber. Expensive, and not yet thoroughly researched, this body composition assessment method has a standard error of estimate of approximately ± 2.2–3.7% (Fields, Goran, & McCory, 2002).

- **Near-infrared interactance**—This method uses a portable, easy-to-use device (e.g., the Futrex 5000) that attempts to assess the absorption of an infrared beam placed on the biceps. The standard error of estimate is high (≥ +5.0%) and only limited research has been carried out on this device (Eckerson, Stout, Evetovich, Housh, Johnson, & Worrell, 1998).

- **Bioelectrical impedance analysis**—Many clubs have invested in bioelectrical impedance equipment, which attempts to estimate % lean body mass based on its ability to conduct a mild electrical current (lean tissue contains mostly water and electrolytes, and is, thus, a good conductor of electricity). The greatest disadvantage of this method is that it is not very accurate unless you adhere to numerous conditions. These include controlling the client's hydration status (fluid intake, alcohol intake, meal timing, time of last urination, diuretic or caffeine use, recent exercise, date of last menstrual period), as well as the room temperature, humidity, and use of the appropriate population-specific equation (Hendel, Gotfredsen, Højgaard, Andersen, & Hilsted, 1996). Remember that the result that comes out of the computer is only as accurate as the information that went into the computer, and this includes using the right equation for the right client. Standard error of estimate is approximately ± 3.5–5%.

- **Skinfold caliper analysis**—The skinfold method of body composition assessment has been widely used and validated; when properly performed by experienced examiners it is relatively accurate, with a standard error of estimate of approximately ± 3.5% (differs with each equation) (Heyward & Wagner, 2004). Calipers are used to measure the skin and subcutaneous fat thicknesses at selected sites (sites vary depending on the equations used). Calipers range in price from $25–350 with the more expensive models being more accurate and long lasting. The major disadvantage and source of error in the skinfold method is incorrect technique and/or lack of experience on the part of the examiner. It takes a great deal of time and practice as well as proper training to develop accurate technique. Always adhere conscientiously to the standardized procedures found in Table 5-4.

Table 5-4.	Standardized Procedures for Skinfold Analysis

- All measurements should be made on the right side of the body with the subject standing upright.
- Caliper should be placed directly on the skin surface, 1 cm away from the thumb and finger, perpendicular to the skinfold, and halfway between the crest and the base of the fold.
- Pinch should be maintained while reading the caliper.
- Wait 1–2 seconds (not longer) before reading caliper.
- Take duplicate measurements at each site and retest if duplicate measurements are not within 1–2 mm.
- Rotate through measurement sites or allow time for skin to regain normal texture and thickness.
- Meticulously identify the site using anatomical landmarks.

(American College of Sports Medicine, 2006)

Other tips for skinfold accuracy include the following.

- Try grasping the skinfold at the site to be measured with the thumb and forefinger of the left hand (the more subcutaneous fat a client has, the further apart the tester's thumb and forefinger will need to be to grasp an adequate skinfold). The tester's left elbow should be angled up.
- The grasp should be 1 centimeter (1/2 inch) above the site where the calipers will be placed to ensure that pressure from the fingers does not affect the measurement.
- To be certain that only skin and fat have been grasped, the tester may, at some sites, have to ask the client to contract the underlying muscle while the tester continues holding the skinfold with his/her left hand. If the tester has inadvertently pinched muscle as well as fat, the muscle tissue will separate from the rest of the skinfold as the client contracts.
- While holding the calipers in his/her right hand, the tester should take the measurement 1 centimeter (1/2 inch) below his/her left thumb and forefinger. The calipers should be held level and perpendicular to the direction of the skinfold. The jaws of the calipers should be released completely (with the tester still holding the skinfold with his/her left hand) for no more than 2 seconds while a reading is obtained. (If the calipers remain pinching the skinfold for longer than 2 seconds, intracellular fluids will be forced out of the tissues and result in an inaccurate, lower value.)

Many population-specific equations have been developed to predict body fat from skinfold measurements. Two of the most widely used equations appropriate for the general adult population (approximate ages 17–65) are those by Durnin and Womersley (1974) and those by Jackson and Pollock (1978). In this text the commonly used Jackson and Pollock (1978) protocol is presented below; norms for this equation can be found in Appendix C. See Photographs 5-1a–e.

Skinfold Measuring

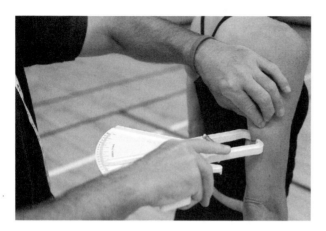

Photo 5-1a. Triceps Skinfold

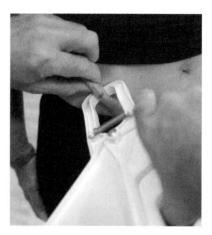

Photo 5-1b. Suprailiac Skinfold

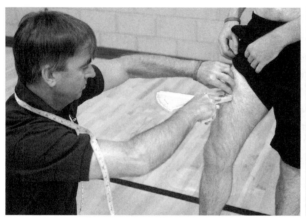

Photo 5-1c. Thigh Skinfold

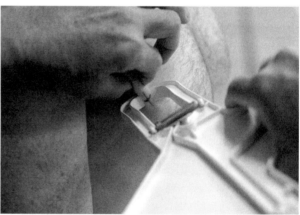

Photo 5-1d. Pectoral Skinfold

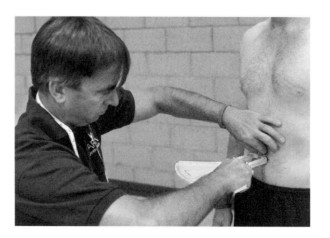

Photo 5-1e. Abdominal Skinfold

- Standardized sites for women
  1. **Triceps**—a vertical fold measured in the midline of the posterior arm over the triceps muscle. Anatomical landmarks are the lateral projection of the acromial process and the inferior border of the olecranon process with the elbow flexed at a 90° angle. A tape measure should be stretched between these two landmarks and the midpoint located on the lateral aspect of the arm. The actual site is at this level, only on the posterior aspect. During measurement, the right elbow should be extended and relaxed.
  2. **Suprailiac**—a 45°-angle diagonal fold immediately above the iliac crest along the anterior axillary line (This is different from the site used in the Durnin and Womersley [1974] protocol.)
  3. **Thigh**—a vertical fold in the midline of the anterior aspect of the thigh, midway between the inguinal crease (fold in the hip during hip flexion) and the proximal border of the patella. Body weight should be placed on the left leg, allowing the right thigh to relax.

- Standardized sites for men
  1. **Chest** (pectoral)—a diagonal fold taken one half the distance between the anterior axillary line (underarm crease) and the nipple
  2. **Abdomen**—a vertical fold taken at a distance of 2 centimeters (1 inch) to the right of the umbilicus (This fold is horizontal in some other protocols.)
  3. **Thigh**—same as for females (see above)

- Calculating estimated % body fat
  1. Carefully measure the appropriate sites two to three times each, following the directions outlined above.
  2. Find the average value for each site and then add all the sites together.
  3. Using the norm tables titled "Percent Fat Estimations" in Appendix C, note where the sum of the skinfolds and your client's age intersect. This is the estimated % of body fat.
  4. When counseling a client, a personal fitness trainer should emphasize improvement and progressive change of body fat levels over time. Personal fitness trainers should avoid allowing clients to become fixated on a specific estimated number. In many cases, and especially with clients who already know they are obese, it may be more appropriate to simply look at change over time for each skinfold site, and avoid giving the client an overall body fat % number. Pronouncing a client to be "obese" or "well below average" may cause the client to become less motivated and more discouraged. On the other hand, lean, competitive individuals may be motivated by knowing their % body fat number.

- **The body mass index (BMI)**—BMI was developed as a simple ratio of height to weight to use as an easy way to estimate body composition (and to classify degrees of obesity) for large groups. Note that it does not take into account % body fat or lean body mass and so it is a less accurate way of estimating body composition. BMI is calculated by dividing body weight (in kilograms) by body height (in meters) squared (weight/height^2). You can also use the nomogram and the table for classification of obesity in Appendix C. Studies have shown the higher the BMI, the greater the risk of negative health outcomes. The Expert Panel on the Identification, Evaluation, and Treatment of Overweight and Obesity in Adults (1998) lists a BMI of 25.0–29.9 kg/m^2 for overweight and a BMI of $\geq$ 30.0 kg/m^2 for obesity.

- **Waist-to-hip ratio**—Where body fat is distributed is important. Studies have shown that when a greater amount of fat is stored in the abdominal area relative to the extremities, a person is at a higher risk for heart disease, diabetes, and metabolic disorders. An easy method for assessing this risk is the waist-to-hip ratio—simply divide the waist circumference by the hip circumference (Bray & Gray, 1988). If the ratio is $\geq$ 0.95 for younger men (< 60 years old) or $\geq$ 0.86 for younger women (< 60 years old), the client is considered to be obese and should be counseled about fat-loss methods. Additionally, older clients (60–69 years old) with waist-to-hip ratios $\geq$ 1.03 for men and $\geq$ 0.90 for women are considered obese (American College of Sports Medicine, 2006).

- **Girth (circumference) measurements**—Clients are often interested in changes in their measurements as a result of an exercise program. Placement of a tape measure on the right side of the body can be used for limb measurements; while doing so, a client should stand erect but relaxed; two measurements should be taken at each site (measurements should be within 1/4 inch of each other); pulling the tape too tight or not tight enough should be avoided. Consistency is key. (Special cloth tapes, known as Gulick tapes, are available to help standardize the tension.)

  - **Abdominal**—horizontal measure at level of umbilicus
  - **Waist**—horizontal measure taken at the level of the narrowest part of torso (above the umbilicus and below the xiphoid process)
  - **Hips**—maximum posterior protrusion of the buttocks
  - **Thigh** (proximal)—just below the fold of the buttocks
  - **Upper arm**—midway between the acromion and olecranon processes
  - **Forearm**—maximum circumference with elbow extended and palm supinated
  - **Calf**—maximum circumference between knee and ankle

  Of particular interest is the waist circumference; because of the higher risk associated with abdominal obesity, a large waist circumference may be used alone as an indicator of unhealthy body composition. According to the ACSM, a waist girth > 102 cm for men and > 88 cm for women is a risk factor for coronary heart disease (CHD) (American College of Sports Medicine, 2006). See Table 5-5 for waist circumference criteria.

Table 5-5.	Criteria for Waist Circumference in Adults		
Waist Circumference cm (in)			
Risk category	**Females**	**Males**	
Very low	< 70 cm (< 28.5 in.)	< 80 cm (31.5 in.)	
Low	70–89 (28.5-35.0)	80-99 (31.5-39.0)	
High	90-109 (35.5-43.0)	100-120 (39.5-47.0)	
Very High	> 110 (> 43.5)	> 120 (47.0)	

(Bray, 2004. Reproduced with permission by the *American Journal of Clinical Nutrition.* © Am J Clin Nutr. American Society for Clinical Nutrition.)

Step 3: Assess cardiorespiratory fitness

Cardiorespiratory endurance, or aerobic capacity, is one of the most important components of fitness. Low levels of cardiorespiratory endurance have been associated with increased risk of premature death from all causes, most specifically from cardiovascular disease. In addition, greater aerobic fitness usually means that an individual is regularly active, and this has been linked with many health benefits (Blair, Kohl, Barlow, Paffenberger, Gibbons, & Macera, 1995); Sesso, Paffenberger, & Lee, 2000). You will find a list of these benefits in Chapter 6 ("Cardiorespiratory Programming").

Aerobic or **cardiorespiratory fitness** is defined as the ability to perform repetitive, moderate- to high-intensity, large-muscle movement for a prolonged period of time. (See Chapter 2, "Exercise Physiology," for more information). Cardiorespiratory fitness can be evaluated with either maximal or submaximal exercise tests, and can be assessed either directly (with oxygen consumption equipment) or estimated (no oxygen consumption equipment is used).

- **Maximal exercise tests**—These fall generally into two categories: diagnostic and functional. The purpose of a **diagnostic exercise test** (sometimes called a "stress" test or GXT) is to diagnose the presence and/or the extent of CHD in addition to evaluating ability to perform work (this is the type of test that a physician may recommend be performed on higher risk clients). The subject will be continuously monitored during exercise via a multi-lead ECG (electrocardiogram), and may or may not be using oxygen consumption equipment. This test usually takes place on a treadmill or cycle ergometer, and the patient is pushed to achieve maximum work effort. By evaluating the ECG (especially at higher intensities), the physician or technologist can discern heart function abnormalities as well as cardiorespiratory endurance. Obviously, this kind of test should only be administered by a licensed health care provider, authorized to perform such tests, in a clinical setting and only for medical or diagnostic purposes.

  The purpose of a **functional maximal exercise test** is simply to assess cardiorespiratory fitness. It is often used to evaluate athletes and is important in research. VO$_2$ max is usually directly measured with oxygen consumption equipment as the subject exercises to exhaustion, most commonly on a treadmill or cycle.

The **advantages** of max tests include the following.

- The large amount of information gathered, including the actual measurement of a person's ability at high levels (however, there is still about a 2% range of error due to equipment and other factors) versus the estimated level obtained in submaximal testing.
- Specific cardiorespiratory responses to stress and high intensity enable the diagnosis of heart disease.

The **disadvantages** of max tests include the following.

- The need for special, expensive equipment and highly trained test administrators. It is recommended that a physician be present.
- Maximal testing is riskier than submaximal testing due to the potential for heart wave abnormalities at higher workloads.
- A high level of motivation on the part of the subject is necessary for exercise to exhaustion.

All forms of testing are affected by the principle of **specificity**. Your clients will usually achieve higher test results when they are assessed performing an exercise with which they are familiar. For example, a cyclist will perform better on a cycle ergometer test than a client who never cycles, even though they may both be aerobically fit. However, on any piece of equipment it is still possible to assess a person's progress over time.

Another type of test requiring a maximal effort is the **field test**. The 1.5-mile run and the 12-minute run tests are widely used in college-type settings where it is necessary to test large groups of young athletes all at once. Although inexpensive and easy to administer, these tests are higher risk due to their less supervised nature, and are not recommended for general population assessment. Norms are available (see Pollock & Wilmore, 1990).

- **Submaximal exercise tests**—There are many types of submaximal tests. Here the purpose is not to diagnose heart disease (ECGs are rarely used), but to assess the client's functional aerobic fitness, show improvement of that fitness level over time, and to help you develop an appropriate level of exercise intensity. Submaximal tests may be used to predict or estimate VO_2 max, but the tests are concluded when a predetermined submaximal level has been reached (usually 85% of the estimated maximum heart rate), or when the subject has exercised for a specified time period (e.g., 3-Minute Step Test). The premise underlying submaximal testing is that the more fit an individual is, the lower his/her heart rate will be at any given level of intensity or workload.

The **advantages** of submaximal testing (as compared with maximal testing) include the following.

- Submaximal testing is less expensive.
- Submaximal testing is less risky since the test ends at or before 85% of maximum heart rate or 70% of heart rate reserve.
- Less specialized equipment is required.
- Testing personnel does not have to be as highly trained or qualified.

The major **disadvantages** of submaximal testing include the following.

 - Less information is obtained.
 - Since maximum is only estimated and not actually achieved, submaximal testing is less accurate if the purpose is to measure VO_2 max.

There are two basic types of submaximal tests: **multi-stage** (graded) and **single stage** (fixed load). A multi-stage, or graded, submaximal exercise test is based on three assumptions: (1) there is a linear relationship between VO_2, heart rate, and workload; (2) that mechanical efficiency (the amount of oxygen utilized at a given workload) is the same for everyone; and (3) that max heart rate can be predicted from the formula 220 - age = max heart rate. (In fact, this commonly used formula is accurate for only about 75% of the population. In the remaining 25%, max heart rate can vary from the formula by as much as 10–15 bpm, resulting in either an under or over prediction of max heart rate (McArdle, Katch, & Katch, 1990). Even with these limitations, a multi-stage submaximal test will provide you with valuable information about the client's cardiorespiratory responses and ability to perform work at various intensities, and therefore enable you to recommend appropriate and accurate workloads during exercise sessions. Also, during follow-up re-tests, heart rate, rate of perceived exertion (RPE), and blood pressure responses to various workloads can be compared, allowing clients to see measured change in their cardiorespiratory fitness from the recommended program.

Multi-stage tests can be performed on treadmills, cycle ergometers, or steps, and there are a variety of different protocols (testing formats) available. At many commercial and corporate fitness facilities, the submaximal cycle ergometer test is the preferred form of aerobic fitness assessment. Advantages of the test are that the ergometer is easy to calibrate, relatively inexpensive and portable (as compared to a treadmill), non-intimidating to clients, and that heart rate and blood pressure are easier to assess during cycling exercise than during walking or running exercise. Also, in a multi-stage test, more information can be obtained than during a single-stage test. Disadvantages are that it may be difficult to maintain a constant speed or workload, and localized muscle fatigue may limit performance.

Advantages of treadmill testing include the fact that more muscle mass is involved, resulting in potentially higher estimated VO_2 max values; additionally, walking is an activity that is familiar to almost everyone.

A multi-stage submaximal test typically involves the following scenario.
 • Warm-up
 • Stage 1: 3 minutes at a workload eliciting ~65% HRR
 • Stage 2: 3 minutes at a workload eliciting ~75% HRR
 • Stage 3: 3 minutes at a workload eliciting ~85% HRR
 • Cool-down

Heart rates are taken at the end of each minute; blood pressure and RPE are taken at the end of each 3-minute stage. As you can see, considerably more data is collected, allowing for a more accurate estimation of VO$_2$ max as well as more points for comparison in future reassessments. Note that special training is required to administer multi-stage tests. This can be obtained through university courses or through certification programs such as those offered by the ACSM (Health Fitness Instructor Certification) or the YMCA.

An alternative to the multi-stage test is the **single-stage** (fixed load) test. This test usually takes even less training to administer and requires less equipment. However, since there is only one stage, or workload, less information is obtained about your client. Heart rate, blood pressure, and RPE are usually not monitored during the actual exercise, which makes the test less useful for exercise prescription. Two popular types of submaximal fixed-load tests are the 3-Minute Step Test and the Rockport 1-Mile Walking Test.

• **The 3-Minute YMCA Step Test**—The premise underlying the step test is that if a client has a low-recovery heart rate 1 minute after stepping, he/she is in better physical condition and therefore has a higher VO$_2$ max and a higher level of aerobic fitness. Advantages of the step test are that it requires inexpensive pieces of equipment (step, metronome, and watch), the client does not have to be skilled, the test is short, and large numbers of people can be tested at once. Major disadvantages of the step test are that it can be relatively strenuous for deconditioned clients, and may be harmful or dangerous for those with bad knees or balance problems. The protocol for administering the 3-Minute Step Test, after the informed consent process has been completed, is as follows.

1. Explain the purpose of the test to your client and describe the procedure. It is a good idea to suggest that clients refrain from conversation since talking, laughing, etc. may elevate their heart rate (although they must be encouraged to report any pain or discomfort). Static stretching of the gastrocnemius, hamstring, and iliopsoas muscles may be advised; and a short practice session is allowed (two- or three-step cycles). Make certain to tell your client that he/she may stop the test at any time if he/she feels pain or discomfort. There is no active warm-up.

2. Set the metronome at 96 bpm (24-step cycles per minute), and when the client begins stepping, start your timer or stopwatch. For this test, stepping must be performed on a 12-inch (30.5 cm) bench with a basic step pattern of up, up, down, down. The lead foot may change if necessary during the test (no continuous alternating lead). Have your client step for 3 full minutes, and let him/her know when 1 minute has passed, 2 minutes have passed, and when 10 seconds are remaining.

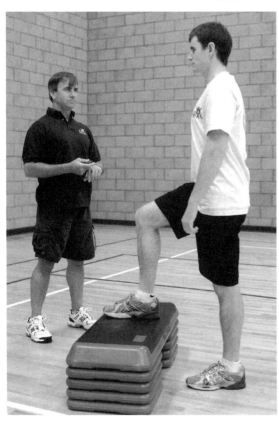

Photo 5-2. 3-Minute Step Test

3. When the 3 minutes are up, remind the client to sit down immediately; within 5 seconds palpate the recovery heart rate (preferably on the radial artery at the wrist). Count the recovery heart rate for 1 full minute.

4. Use the minute value for the recovery heart rate and consult the norms appropriate for the client's age and sex in Appendix C. (Norms are also available that estimate VO_2 max based on recovery heart rate [Golding, 1989]). Note that the ACSM currently recommends that an ECG, heart rate monitor, or stethoscope be used to assure the most accurate heart rate measurement (American College of Sports Medicine, 2006).

- **The Rockport Walking Test**—In 1986, the Rockport Walking Institute developed a test appropriate for the general population, including older and/or sedentary clients. The protocol for the test, after the informed consent process has been completed, is as follows.

1. Precede the test with a light warm-up consisting of rhythmic limbering and static stretching. Advise your client to stop at any time if he/she feels pain or discomfort, but that this test requires the most vigorous walk he/she can maintain for 1 mile.

2. The walking course needs to be smooth and flat, ideally a 1/4-mile track. As your client walks, announce the distance remaining with each lap.

3. After a mile has been completed, immediately palpate the pulse for 10 seconds (preferably on the radial artery). Allow your client to cool down.

4. Multiply the 10-second count by 6 and consult the norms for the client's age and sex in Appendix C (use both heart rate and completion time). Note that these norms are for men weighing 170 pounds and for women weighing 125 pounds. If your client weighs significantly more, then his/her aerobic fitness will be over-predicted; if he/she weighs significantly less, aerobic fitness will be under-predicted. Other factors that can influence the results are the client's level of motivation, ability to set a consistent pace, and level of body fat. VO_2 max may be estimated using a generalized equation (Kline et al., 1987).

When consulting clients about the results of cardiorespiratory testing, remember that, for them, VO_2 max numbers may have little meaning. They may be more interested in their increased stamina and enhanced ability to perform daily activities. Help them to see tangible proof of their improvement over time.

- **The Rockport Walking Treadmill Test**—This test is very similar to the one outlined above. The testing protocol is as follows.

1. Precede the test with a warm-up consisting of static stretching and walking on the treadmill. Find the exact pace at which the client can walk vigorously for 1 mile.

2. Have the client walk at the established pace for 1 mile. Record the time.

3. Immediately palpate the pulse for 10 seconds and then allow the client to cool down.

4. Multiply the 10-second count by 6 and consult the norms for age and sex in Appendix C.

NOTE: All of the foregoing testing procedures must be preceded by the informed consent process, documented in writing, signed by the client, and disclosing risks/benefits associated with such procedures. These testing procedures should never be performed by personal fitness trainers for diagnostic-type purposes, but rather, only for fitness assessment.

Step 4: Assess muscular fitness

Muscle strength (the ability of a muscle or muscle group to exert maximal force for one repetition) and **muscle endurance** (the ability of a muscle or muscle group to exert submaximal force for several repetitions, or to hold a contraction for a sustained length of time) are both important components of fitness for your client's physical well-being. Without adequate muscle strength and endurance, clients are more likely to suffer from low-back pain and/or poor posture, as well as other musculoskeletal problems. Performing weight-bearing exercises that promote muscular fitness is a primary way to enhance or maintain bone mass, helping to prevent osteoporosis. The development of muscle strength and endurance leads to an increase in lean body mass and an improvement in body composition, which in turn causes an elevation in resting metabolic rate. In addition, maintaining muscle strength and endurance is an important factor (especially for elderly clients) in performing everyday essential tasks adequately and without undue risk of injury.

- **Assessing muscular strength**—Muscle strength can be assessed either statically (isometrically) or dynamically (isotonically). Note that no one test can assess total body muscle strength or muscle endurance; all muscle fitness tests are specific to the muscle group being tested. For example, a bench press test is specific to the upper body, in particular the pectoralis major, anterior deltoids, and triceps.

  Static strength tests are most often performed on dynamometers. Dynamometers are available to assess hand grip strength and back and leg extensor strength, with the hand grip dynamometer being most widely used (keep in mind, this test does not measure a major muscle group and is therefore of limited predictive value). The procedure is simple—after adjusting the handgrip size for your client, have the client stand, holding the dynamometer in one hand with the elbow flexed. Instruct him/her to exhale while squeezing as hard as possible (maximal voluntary contraction) for 2–3 seconds. Allow three trials for each hand and compare to the published norms (Canadian Society for Exercise Physiology, 2003). Keep in mind that static strength tests are specific to the muscle group being tested and measure strength only at the particular angle at which the test is performed. Also, since clients tend to hold their breath and "bear down" (Valsalva maneuver) during isometric contractions, they must be instructed to exhale during exertion in order to prevent possible cardiovascular problems.

  Muscular strength can also be assessed **dynamically** by the **one-repetition maximum (1 RM) test**. Frequently performed 1 RM tests are the bench press, which assesses the strength of the pectoralis major, anterior deltoid, and triceps muscle groups, and the leg press, which tests the strength of the upper leg muscles. The client's maximum amount of strength for one repetition is found through trial and error. Following are the steps for basic 1 RM testing for the bench press (Australian Sports Commission, 2000).

1. Have your client warm up by statically stretching and limbering up the muscle groups to be tested.

2. Familiarize the client with the equipment and have him/her start with a weight that can be comfortably lifted (about 50–70% of his or her perceived capacity). Then progressively add weights (by about 2.5–20 kg at a time) until the weight can be lifted with proper form just one time (try to find the maximum amount within four attempts to avoid excessive fatigue). Allow the client to rest 3-5 minutes between trials. Perform all repetitions at the same speed and through the same range of motion for consistency.

3. After finding the 1 RM for the bench press, divide the 1 RM weight (in pounds) by the client's body weight (in pounds) in order to find the client's percentile ranking (upper body strength norms can be found in Appendix C).

Disadvantages of 1 RM testing include the potential for injury that exists with any maximal effort, the fact that clients may perform the Valsalva maneuver, the lack of portability of the equipment, and the "intimidation factor" for clients unfamiliar with weights. In addition, some research indicates that the 1 RM test is not appropriate for beginners and is best used for strength athletes. To minimize a few of these disadvantages, some coaches recommend measuring a percentage of the client's 1 RM. For example, if your client can perform six but not seven repetitions of a bench press at 80 pounds, then he/she has a 6 RM of 80 pounds. Tables exist that allow you to then estimate the 1 RM value (Hoeger, Hopkins, & Bareete, 1990).

- **Assessing muscular endurance**—The most commonly performed tests for muscle endurance include the push-up test, the YMCA Dynamic Bench Press Test, the sit-up test, and the partial curl-up test.

The **push-up test** measures upper body (pectoralis, anterior deltoid, and triceps) endurance, is easy to administer, and needs no special equipment. A disadvantage of the test is that performing even one push-up for deconditioned clients may require a maximal effort, and then the test no longer measures the ability to perform repeated contractions over time. Additionally, the standard protocol and associated norms imply that all men can perform a sufficient number of full push-ups and that all women cannot. A solution to these problems is to simply measure change over time, and calculate percent change if desired; you can then disregard the norms. The standard protocol is as follows.

1. After explaining the purpose of the test to your client, have your client assume the appropriate position: men on hands and toes (regular push-up), women on hands and knees (modified push-up). Instruct your client to breathe with each repetition and to repeat as many as possible with proper form. Assure your client that he/she may stop if he/she feels any pain or discomfort.

2. Count the number of push-ups performed correctly without rest. The spine should remain in proper alignment supported by the abdominals, with the neck continuing as a natural extension of the spine. The chest should come within 3 inches of the floor (you may use your fist as a guide or use a 3-inch Nerf®-type or foam soft ball or half-foam roller for clients to touch with each repetition).

3. The test is over when correct form can no longer be maintained or when your client is unable to complete another repetition. Push-up endurance norms are available in Appendix C. See Photographs 5-3a-b.

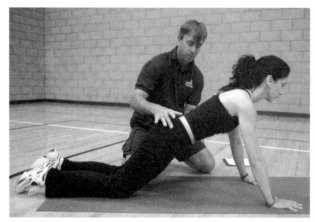

Photo 5-3a. Push-Up Test on Knees

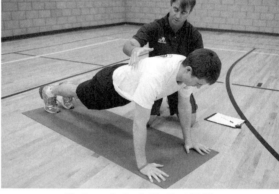

Photo 5-3b. Push-Up Test (Full)

The **Dynamic Bench Press Test**, developed by the YMCA, uses an external, standardized weight (barbell) of 35 pounds for women and 80 pounds for men. The barbell is lifted to a metronome count of 60 bpm (30 repetitions per minute). The test is concluded when your client can no longer keep pace, begins to break form, or cannot complete another repetition. Published norms are available for ranking your client's upper body muscle endurance on the bench press (Golding, 1989).

The **sit-up test** is also frequently used to assess the endurance of the trunk muscles. This test has been criticized because it involves not only the rectus abdominis but the iliopsoas muscle group. The client is asked to perform as many full sit-ups (elbows touching the knees) as possible in 1 minute while the feet are held in place by the personal fitness trainer. This test may aggravate existing low-back pain and relies on an exercise (the full sit-up) that is not recommended for training.

The **partial curl-up test** has been recently developed as a safer modification of the sit-up test (Canadian Society for Exercise Physiology, 2003; American College of Sports Medicine, 2006). It is important to include some assessment of abdominal endurance when evaluating clients, since weak abdominal muscles with poor endurance have been linked with the development of low-back pain (Diener, Golding, & Diener, 1995). The protocol is as follows.

1. After explaining the purpose of the test to your client, have the client lie supine with knees comfortably bent at 90°, arms at sides, palms down, with fingers pointing toward feet and finger-

tips touching a piece of masking tape. A second piece of masking tape is placed 10 cm away. The low back should remain on the floor at all times, including during the actual curl-ups.

2. Set a metronome for 50 bpm and start the timer; the test is performed for one full minute. Have your client perform slow, controlled curl-ups in time with the metronome, at a rate of 25 per minute. The goal is for the trunk to flex to a 30° angle with each repetition. Remind the client to exhale with each repetition.

3. After your client has performed as many repetitions as possible without pausing, to a maximum of 25 or until the end of 1 minute, you may compare the score with the percentile norms for partial curl-up test, listed by age and sex, in Appendix C. See Photographs 5-4a-b.

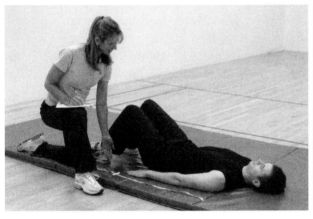 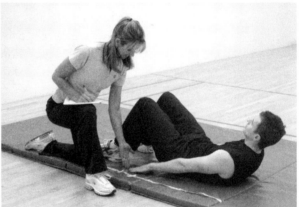

Photo 5-4a. Partial Curl-Up Test   **Photo 5-4b. Partial Curl-Up Test**

NOTE: Alternative positions and protocols have been identified, including: (1) having the hands held across the chest, with the head activating a counter when the trunk reaches a 30° position (Diener et al., 1995), and (2) placing the hands on the thighs and curling up until the hands reach the knee caps (Faulkner, Sprigings, McQuarrie, & Bell, 1989). Elevation of the trunk to 30° is the most important criteria for the test. You may also evaluate change over time or percent improvement instead of using the norms.

Other muscular fitness tests

Isokinetic testing—This form of assessment is used primarily in rehabilitation centers, and measures a muscle's tension throughout the full range of motion at a constant speed. It involves specialized, expensive equipment and is not widely available in commercial facilities.

Anaerobic power tests—These tests measure a person's short-term, power-generating capabilities and are primarily used for performance athletes and for research purposes. Examples include the Sargent jump and reach test (measuring vertical jump), the standing broad jump test, running sprint tests, and cycling "sprint" or power tests (e.g., the Wingate power test). These tests are very intense and typically last only 1 minute or less; they are usually not appropriate for the general mixed population interested in health-related fitness.

NOTE: As with other testing procedures, all strength-related testing procedures should be preceded by a documented informed consent process.

Step 5: Assess flexibility and posture

Flexibility is defined as the range of motion possible around a joint. Like muscle strength and endurance, flexibility level is specific to each joint and its surrounding muscles. There is no single test that assesses total body flexibility. Flexibility assessment is important for clients; when range of motion is limited around a joint due to muscular tightness, that joint is more susceptible to injury. This is especially evident for proper functioning of the spine; tight erector spinae, hamstring, and iliopsoas muscles have all been implicated as possible causes of low-back pain. Also, ability to comfortably perform activities of daily living (such as bending over and picking up a piece of paper) is limited if the body is inflexible.

Flexibility is assessed directly by goniometers and flexometers. These tools actually measure the individual joint angle in degrees as the body part is moved through its range of motion, and texts are available that describe specific protocols (Clarkson, 2000). Remember that flexibility is joint and joint-angle specific; no one test can measure total body flexibility.

In most commercial and corporate fitness settings, it is more common to assess flexibility indirectly, and perhaps the most widely performed assessment is the **Sit and Reach Test** used by the YMCA (Golding, 1989). This trunk-flexion test primarily measures the flexibility of the hamstring and erector spinae muscles, as well as the calf and upper back muscles (the flexibility of all of these groups is important for healthy low-back functioning). Advantages of this test include: (1) it is easy to administer; (2) it requires a minimum of equipment; and (3) it has widely validated norms. Disadvantages include: (1) the slight risk of injury due to the position required (seated unsupported forward flexion); and (2) the fact that a person's score may be influenced by the length of his/her body segments (e.g., a long trunk and short legs). The procedure is as follows.

1. After explaining the purpose of the test to your client, have him/her actively warm up (if he/she is not already warm from the cardiorespiratory assessment) and perform some static stretching, particularly of the hamstrings, low back, and calf muscles.

2. Instruct your client to remove his/her shoes and sit on the floor with knees straight (pressed to the floor), feet approximately 12 inches apart, and ankles dorsiflexed. The heels should be aligned at the 15-inch mark on a yardstick or tape, with the zero end toward the body (the yardstick or tape can be secured to the floor with masking tape placed at a right angle to the 15-inch mark).

3. Have your client place his/her hands on top of each other with fingers aligned, and slowly exhale, stretch out, and touch the tape or yardstick without bouncing. Make sure your client's knees do not flex during the trials. Allow your client to relax and then perform two more trials (total of three).

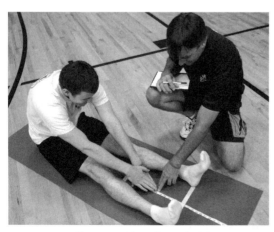

Photo 5-5. Sit and Reach Test

4. Your client's score is the best of the three trials and may be compared to the norms for his/her age and sex in Appendix C, listed under "Standard Values for Trunk Flexion in Inches." See Photograph 5-5.

Other Flexibility Tests

There are several other tests for specific joint range of motion and muscle flexibility, including the following.

Trunk extension ability—Have your client lie prone with hands on the floor beneath shoulders. Attempt to push upper body up while maintaining hip contact with floor (good flexibility of lumbar spine is evident when elbows fully extend and hips remain on the floor; fair flexibility of lumbar spine is evident when hips rise from ground up to 2 inches; poor flexibility is evident when hips rise from ground 2 inches or more). Use caution when performing this stretch; move slowly and stop immediately if there is any pain.

Hamstring flexibility—Have your client lie supine and lift one leg straight up while keeping the other pressed flat to the floor. Passing, or adequate, hamstring flexibility is the ability to lift the leg to a 90° angle, or to a vertical position, without straining. Assess both legs.

Hip flexor (iliopsoas) flexibility—Have your client lie supine. Clasp hands behind right knee and pull it in to the chest as far as possible. Keeping low back pressed to floor, extend the left leg and attempt to press back of left knee to floor. Adequate flexibility exists if the back of the knee and the low back can both be pressed to the floor simultaneously. Check both sides.

Quadriceps flexibility—Have your client lie prone with knees together. With right hand, gently pull right heel directly to middle of right buttock. Heel should comfortably touch buttock for passing flexibility. Repeat on left side.

Calf (gastrocnemius and soleus) flexibility—Have your client stand with his/her back, hips, and heels against a wall. Attempt to raise (dorsiflex) the right forefoot while keeping both knees straight. Passing, or adequate, flexibility is attained if the forefoot is able to elevate by at least 1 inch. Repeat with the left forefoot.

Shoulder (deltoid, latissimus dorsi, triceps, rotator cuff muscles) flexibility—Have your client stand and raise left arm overhead and bend left elbow so that left hand points down the upper spine between the shoulder blades (hand should also be able to touch the opposite shoulder blade). Have your client bring his/her right arm behind the back, and bend the right elbow so the fingers point up the spine between the scapulae. Good flexibility of the right shoulder exists if fingertips of both hands can touch. Change sides.

Shoulder (latissimus dorsi, teres major, and pectoralis major) flexibility—Have your client lie supine, knees comfortably bent, feet flat on floor, and maintain a neutral spine. Flex both shoulders as far overhead as possible. Passing, or adequate, flexibility exists if both arms lie flat overhead on or near the floor.

See Photographs 5-6a-g. In addition to assessing muscle-specific flexibility, these tests are valuable as a teaching tool, and they may all be used as stretches to enhance flexibility.

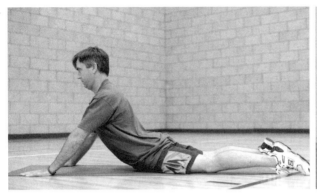

Photo 5-6a. Trunk Extension Assessment

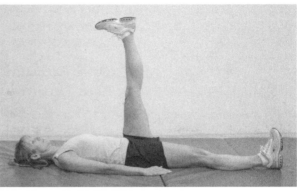

Photo 5-6b. Hamstring Flexibility Assessment

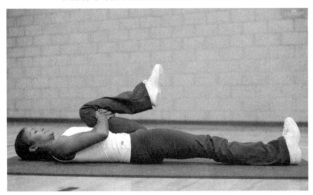

Photo 5-6c. Hip Flexor Flexibility Assessment

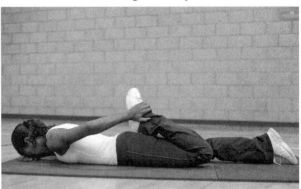

Photo 5-6d. Quadriceps Flexibility Assessment

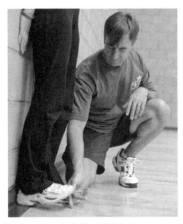

Photo 5-6e. Calf Flexibility Assessment

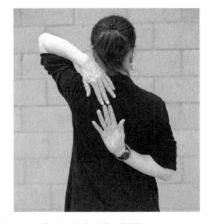

Photo 5-6f. Shoulder Flexibility Assessment

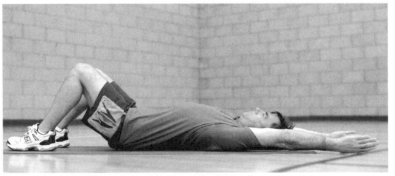

Photo 5-6g. Shoulder Flexibility Assessment

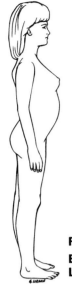

**Fig. 5-1.
Excessive
Lordosis**

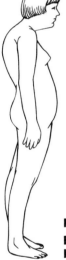

**Fig. 5-2.
Excessive
Kyphosis**

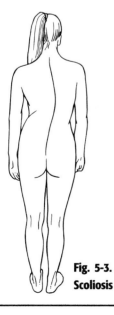

**Fig. 5-3.
Scoliosis**

Postural Screening

Many individuals have postural deviations that can predispose them to low-back pain and/or other musculoskeletal problems. It's important to understand that a postural deviation in one part of the body's kinetic chain can predispose your client to pain or dysfunction in another part of the kinetic chain. (The kinetic chain refers to the interrelationship between the body's skeletal, muscular, and neurological systems that produces movement.) The following postural assessments are simple, easy to administer, and help to develop client awareness.

Excessive lordosis (swayback) assessment—Have your client stand in normal alignment with shoulders and hips against a wall, feet hip-width apart, and heels 1 inch from wall. Have client relax, breathe normally, and avoid consciously pressing low back to wall. Normal lumbar curvature exists if you can slide your palm between client's lower back and the wall without forcing. If a large gap (greater than one palm depth) is found, your client may have a tendency towards lordosis and an anterior pelvic tilt, and should strengthen the abdominals and stretch the iliopsoas and erector spinae muscles. (Also observe client's bony anatomy: the anterior superior iliac spine of the ilium should not be in front of [anterior to] the pubic bone.) See Figure 5-1.

Excessive kyphosis and forward head assessment—Have your client march in place for a few seconds and then ask him/her to stand normally (without altering his/her natural posture) and observe him/her from the side. There is a tendency toward kyphosis if the upper back appears hunched or slouched forward. Note if the shoulders appear protracted or rounded. "Forward head" may or may not accompany this position. Forward head stance is indicated if the ears are not in line with the shoulders and/or the chin juts forward. If these tendencies exist, clients will need to strengthen scapular adductors (mid-trapezius and rhomboids) and stretch shoulder horizontal adductors (pectoralis major and anterior deltoids). See Figure 5-2.

Hip and shoulder height discrepancies—If a significant hip and/or shoulder height discrepancy exists, your client may have scoliosis, or lateral curvature of the spine. If this condition is accompanied by back pain or discomfort, further evaluation by a physician is needed. Also, it may be inappropriate for clients with scoliosis to participate in high-impact activities, such as running or high-impact aerobics, due to increased risk of injury. (NOTE: Such clients must be referred to a health care professional for clearance for a particular activity before that activity is recommended to them.)

To measure hip height/leg length discrepancy, have your client remove his/her shoes and stand normally with feet a comfortable hip-width apart. Place one end of tape measure on iliac crest (top of hip bone), and bring other end down outside of leg to the floor, past the lateral malleolus (outside ankle bone). Measure both sides, making sure to be consistent from right to left sides in terms of tape placement.

To measure shoulder height discrepancy, tape a large piece of paper at shoulder height on wall. Have your client stand normally against wall with shoulders pressed against paper, hips back, and heels 1 inch from wall. Place a level clipboard or notebook on right shoulder and draw a horizontal line on the paper. Repeat with left shoulder, making sure to be consistent in terms of clipboard placement. Measure distance from each horizontal line to floor with tape measure.

For both hip and shoulder height assessments, a discrepancy of 1⁄4 inch or greater between right and left sides may suggest a misalignment, or possibly scoliosis. (Misalignments may be due to many causes, including improper footwear, muscle imbalances, or habitually carrying a handbag, baby, or small child on one side.)

Finally, you will find a "Postural Analysis Guide" in Appendix C, which may be used along with the above specific postural screening techniques or alone. Many such guides exist, and all are designed to help you become familiar with your client's musculoskeletal imbalances so that you can design an appropriate exercise program. If your client experiences pain around these imbalances, do not hesitate to refer him or her to a physician.

Step 6: Optional fitness assessment components

Optional assessment components, depending on your client, skill, equipment, and knowledge base, might include a stress management/coping strategy questionnaire, three-day dietary recall, lung function tests, and cholesterol testing. Additionally, power and agility assessments for athletes are available, as well as specific protocols for seniors.

Lung function can be assessed with a portable spirometer. Two values are usually obtained: forced vital capacity (FVC), the total volume of air that can be moved through the lungs in one breath from full inhalation to a maximum exhalation, and forced expiratory volume (FEV1), the percentage of the vital capacity that can be expired in 1 second (indicating the speed that the air can be moved through the lungs). In average healthy people, approximately 85% of the vital capacity can be expired in 1 second. Less than 70% FEV1 would indicate some type of airway obstruction difficulty (such as with emphysema or bronchial asthma).

Several types of cholesterol tests are available. Some facilities offer their clients relatively inexpensive, fasting blood lipid profiles performed by an outside laboratory. This is the most accurate test, as it requires the client to fast for 12 hours, and the blood is returned to the lab for LDL, HDL, triglyceride, and total cholesterol analysis. Some facilities have on-site equipment for cholesterol testing, such as Reflotron, Vision, or Kodak DT-60™. Although the initial purchase of these machines is costly and the person operating the machine needs some training, this type of basic cholesterol screening can be a valuable adjunct to other forms of fitness and wellness assessment. The test is quick, no fasting is required, immediate results are available, and the results are relatively accurate. Disadvantages include the fact that only total cholesterol is assessed, lengthy calibration and quality control procedures are essential to ensure accuracy, and some states require that only phlebotomists or other medical personnel may use finger sticks to draw blood due to the possibility of contamination from blood borne pathogens if correct procedures are not followed.

A large battery of assessments for seniors has been developed (Rikli & Jones, 2001). These fitness tests address the major components of fitness, with specific adaptations for the typical functional impairments found in older adults. Some of the suggested assessments include: the 30-second chair stand test, the 8-foot up-and-go test, the 6-minute walk test, and the chair sit-and-reach test. If you intend to work with seniors, you would be well advised to become familiar with these educational, motivational, and appropriate assessments specific to that group.

Finally, consider developing "functional" fitness tests that are specific to your individual client's goals. Assessing physiological parameters, such as heart rate and RPE, after climbing a flight of stairs or taking a routine walk with the dog, can be a very practical way to measure change over time. When you choose activities that the client performs regularly and in which the client wants improvement, functional fitness tests can provide yet another way to validate the client's exercise program and enhance adherence.

PUTTING IT ALL TOGETHER	
Procedure	**Materials needed**
I. The Initial Interview	
Tell the client about yourself, and ask what she/he is looking for. Perform a screening procedure:	
a. Have client fill out the medical history form.	Medical history form
b. Review form and determine need for a signed physician's clearance form prior to testing and/or exercise.	
c. Give client the physician's clearance form if necessary.	Physician's clearance form
d. Have client read (and/or read it to him/her) and sign informed consent form (including delineated risks/benefits), and answer questions.	Informed consent form
e. Give client other forms to fill out (depending on client).	E.g., self-assessment quiz, exercise and activity quiz
f. Discuss payment and business arrangements.	
g. Give information about clothing, footwear, abstaining from caffeine, smoking, etc. prior to fitness test.	
II. Fitness Assessment (If a signed physician's clearance is necessary, postpone fitness assessment until form is returned.)	
a. Assess resting values.	
- Take a 30- or 60-second resting HR.	Stopwatch
- Take a resting blood pressure.	BP cuff and stethoscope
b. Assess body composition.	
- Estimate % body fat with skinfold calipers, and/or calculate body mass index, and/or take tape measurements for comparison at re-tests.	Calipers, calculator, tape measure, norms, nomogram for BMI
- Assess waist-to-hip ratio.	
c. Assess cardiorespiratory fitness.	Stopwatch, 12-in. bench, metronome, OR smooth, flat 1/4-mile track
- Perform either the 3-Minute Step Test or the Rockport 1-Mile Walking Test.	
d. Assess muscle strength and/or endurance.	
- Options include: 1 RM tests, push-up test, and partial curl-up test	Machines, mat, tape, norms, metronome, watch
e. Assess flexibility and posture.	
- Options include: Sit and Reach Test, muscle- specific tests, posture tests	Tape measure or yardstick, masking tape, mat, paper taped to wall
f. Perform other optional assessments.	
III. Interpretation and Goal-Setting Session	
Depending on time factors, you may or may not decide to present the results of the fitness assessment at the same session as the actual testing. Results should always be presented in a positive manner. No matter how your client scored on a particular test, encourage him/her not to focus on a specific numerical score, but instead to focus on the fact that if he/she adheres to an exercise program, there will be change and improvement over time (see the information on percent improvement presented earlier in this chapter under "Benefits of a Fitness Assessment"). Review the five components of fitness and the importance of reducing risk factors, and encourage a larger view of health and wellness. Educate and motivate!	
Help your client to have a reasonable expectation about his/her exercise program and its expected results. Both preparing for a realistic experience and establishing achievable goals have been proven to help with exercise adherence and long-lasting behavior change (see "Secrets of Goal Setting" in Chapter 13, "Behavior Modification and Communication Skills"). Help the client define specific, focused goals that are measurable and attainable. Short-term goals of 4 weeks or so are more effective than long-term goals (e.g., lose 50 pounds). At the end of each goal period, reevaluate client progress and give appropriate feedback. During the goal-setting session, create a game plan for exactly how your client will reach his/her goal and be specific with exercise dates, times, places, attire, and dietary modifications (a goal-setting form is provided in Appendix C). Specify the date for fitness test reassessment. Allow approximately 3–4 months for measurable benefits, such as decreased resting heart rate, increased aerobic capacity, and decreased % body fat. Be sure to encourage the less quantifiable internal reinforcements of progress, such as enhanced self-esteem, decreased stress, and increased energy. Consider using a behavior contract to enhance compliance (see Appendix C).	
Based on client feedback during this session, the next task is to develop an appropriate exercise program for your client. See "Exercise Session Recording Form" in Appendix C.	

Summary

In this chapter, benefits and limitations of fitness assessment were discussed. The following components of the fitness assessment were covered: (1) assess resting values; (2) assess body composition; (3) assess cardiorespiratory fitness; (4) assess muscular fitness; (5) assess flexibility and posture; and (6) optional fitness assessment components. The use of an interpretation and goal-setting session was briefly discussed and recommended for increased client education, motivation, and adherence to exercise. Adherence to informed consent procedures and documentation were also stressed.

References

Aerobics and Fitness Association of America. (2002). *Fitness: Theory and practice* (4th ed., L.A. Gladwin, Ed.). Sherman Oaks, CA: Aerobics and Fitness Association of America.

American College of Sports Medicine. (2006). *ACSM's guidelines for exercise testing and prescription* (7th ed.). Baltimore: Lippincott Williams & Wilkins.

Australian Sports Commission. (2000). Protocols for the assessment of isoinertial strength. In C.J. Gore (Ed.), *Physiological tests for elite athletes*. Champaign, IL: Human Kinetics.

Blair, S.N., Kohl, H.W., Barlow, C.E., Paffenberger, R.S., Gibbons, L.W., & Macera, C.A. (1995). Changes in physical fitness and all-cause mortality: A prospective study of healthy and unhealthy men. *Journal of the American Medical Association, 273*, 1093-1098.

Bray, G.A. (2004). Don't throw the baby out with the bath water. *American Journal of Clinical Nutrition, 70*(3), 347-349.

Bray, G.A., & Gray, D. S. (1988). Obesity. Part I. Pathogenesis. *Western Journal of Medicine, 149*, 429-441.

Canadian Society for Exercise Physiology. (2003). *The Canadian physical activity, fitness & lifestyle approach: CSEP-health & fitness program's health-related appraisal & counseling strategy* (3rd ed.). Ottawa, Ontario, Canada: Canadian Society for Exercise Physiology.

Clarkson, H.M. (2000). *Musculoskeletal assessment: Joint range of motion and manual muscle strength*. Champaign, IL: Human Kinetics.

Diener, M.H., Golding, L.A., & Diener, D. (1995). Validity and reliability of a one-minute half sit-up test of abdominal muscle strength and endurance. *Sports Medicine Training and Rehabilitation, 6*, 5-119.

Durnin, J.V.G.A., & Womersley, J. (1974). Body fat assessed from total body density and its estimation from skinfold thicknesses: Measurements on 481 men and women aged 16-72 years. *British Journal of Nutrition, 32*, 77-97.

Eckerson, J.M., Stout, J.R., Evetovich, T.K., Housh, T.J., Johnson, T.O., & Worrell, N. (1998). Validity of self-assessment techniques for estimating percent body fat in men and women. *Journal of Strength and Conditioning Research, 12*(4), 243-247.

Expert Panel. (1998). Executive summary of the clinical guidelines on the identification, evaluation, and treatment of overweight and obesity in adults. *Archives of Internal Medicine, 158*, 1855-1867.

Faulkner, R.A., Sprigings, E.J., McQuarrie, A., & Bell, R.D. (1989). A partial curl-up protocol for adults based on an analysis of two procedures. *Canadian Journal of Sport Sciences, 14*(3), 135-14.

Fields, D.A., Goran, M.I., & McCory, M.A. (2002). Body composition assessments via air displacement plethysmography in adults and children: A review. *American Journal of Clinical Nutrition, 75*, 453-467.

Flegal, K.M., Carroll, M.D., Ogden, C.L., & Johnson, C.L. (2002). Prevalence and trends in obesity among U.S. adults, 1999-2000. *Journal of the American Medical Association, 288*, 1728-1732.

Golding, L.A. (1989). *YMCA fitness testing and assessment manual.* Champaign, IL: Human Kinetics.

Hendel, H.W., Gotfredsen, A., Højgaard, L., Andersen, T., & Hilsted, J. (1996). Change in fat-free mass assessed by bioelectrical impedance, total body potassium and dual energy X-ray absorptiometry during prolonged weight loss. *Scandinavian Journal of Clinical and Laboratory Investigation, 56*(8), 671-679.

Heyward, V.H., & Wagner, D.R. (2004). *Applied body composition assessment.* Champaign, IL: Human Kinetics.

Hoeger, W.W., Hopkins, D.R., & Bareete, S.L. (1990). Relationship between repetitions and selected percentages of one repetition maximum: A comparison between untrained and trained males and females. *Journal of Applied Sport Science Research, 4*(2), 47-54.

Institute for Aerobics Research. (1994). Body composition percentile values in men and women. (Available from the Institute for Aerobics Research, Dallas, Texas)

Jackson, A.S., & Pollock, M.L. (1978). Generalized equations for predicting body density of men and women. *British Journal Nutrition, 40*, 407-504.

Kline, G.M., Porcari, J.P., Hintermeister, R., Freedson, P.S., Ward, A., McCarron, R.F., et al. (1987). Estimation of VO₂ max from a one-mile track walk, gender, age, and body weight. *Medicine & Science in Sports & Exercise, 19*(3), 253-259.

Lohman, T.G. (1992). *Advances in body composition assessment.* Champaign, IL: Human Kinetics.

McArdle, W.D., Katch, F.I., & Katch, V.L. (1990). *Exercise physiology, energy, nutrition and performance* (3rd ed.). Philadelphia: Lea & Febiger.

National High Blood Pressure Education Program. (2003). *The seventh report of the joint national committee on prevention, detection, evaluation, and treatment of high blood pressure* (JNC7). 03-5233.

Pollock, M.L., & Wilmore, J.H. (1990). *Exercise in health and disease: Evaluation and prescription for prevention and rehabilitation* (2nd ed.). Philadelphia: W.B. Saunders, Co.

Rikli, R.E., & Jones, C.J. (2001). *Senior fitness test manual.* Champaign, IL: Human Kinetics.

Sesso, H.D., Paffenbarger, R.S., & Lee, I.M. (2000). Physical activity and coronary heart disease in men: The Harvard alumni health study. *Circulation, 102*, 975-980.

**Suggested
Reading**

American College of Sports Medicine. (1998). Position stand: The recommended quantity and quality of exercise for developing and maintaining cardiorespiratory and muscular fitness, and flexibility in healthy adults. *Medicine & Science in Sports & Exercise, 30,* 975-991.

American College of Sports Medicine. (2006). *ACSM's resource manual for guidelines for exercise testing and prescription* (5th ed.). Baltimore: Lippincott Williams & Wilkins.

Bryant, C.X., Franklin, B.A., & Conviser, J.M. (2002). *Exercise testing and program design.* Monterey, CA: Healthy Learning.

Griffin, J.C. (1998). *Client-centered exercise prescription.* Champaign, IL: Human Kinetics.

Heyward, V. (2002). *Advanced fitness assessment and exercise prescription* (4th ed.). Champaign, IL: Human Kinetics.

Howley, E., & Franks, B. (1997). *Health fitness instructor's handbook* (3rd ed.). Champaign, IL: Human Kinetics.

Kendall, F.P., McCreary, E.K., & Provance, P.G. (1993). *Muscles: Testing and function* (4th ed.). Baltimore: Lippincott Williams & Wilkins.

Cardiorespiratory Programming

Outline

- Benefits of Cardiorespiratory Fitness

- Guidelines for Cardiorespiratory Programming

- Warming Up and Cooling Down

- Cardiorespiratory Training Systems

- Cardiorespiratory Modalities and Equipment

Cardiorespiratory fitness is defined as the ability to perform repetitive, moderate- to high-intensity, large-muscle movement for a prolonged period of time. In this chapter the benefits of cardiorespiratory fitness will be presented, and principles of cardiorespiratory training will be introduced. You will learn how to select an appropriate intensity, duration, frequency, and type of exercise for your clients. Finally, various aerobic training systems and cardio equipment usages will be discussed, so that you'll be familiar with the best ways to help your clients attain fitness in this important area.

Benefits of Cardiorespiratory Fitness

Many benefits and training adaptations have been associated with cardiorespiratory or aerobic fitness (see Table 6-1) (American College of Sports Medicine, 2006a). Personal fitness trainers should be familiar with these benefits; and letting clients know about the positive changes they can expect with training is educational and motivational.

Table 6-1. Benefits of Cardiorespiratory Fitness

Reduction in coronary heart disease (CHD) risk factors
- Reduced resting blood pressure
- Increased HDL cholesterol
- Decreased triglycerides
- Reduced body fat and intra-abdominal fat
- Reduced insulin needs, and improved glucose tolerance
- Reduced blood platelet adhesiveness and aggregation

Improvement in cardiovascular and respiratory function
- Increased VO_2 max (maximal oxygen uptake)
- Increased stroke volume
- Stronger heart
- Decreased heart rate (HR) and blood pressure at submaximal workloads
- Increased capillary density in skeletal muscle
- Increased anaerobic threshold
- Increased stamina, endurance, energy

Other benefits
- Decreased anxiety and depression
- Enhanced feelings of well-being
- Enhanced performance of work and sport activities
- Enhanced function and independent living in older persons
- Improved sleep
- Improved immune function
- Increased quality of life
- Decreased morbidity and mortality

(American College of Sports Medicine. [2006]. *ACSM's guidelines for exercise testing and prescription* [7th ed.]. Baltimore: Lippincott Williams & Wilkins. Reprinted with permission.)

In Chapter One ("Understanding Wellness"), a distinction was made between becoming more physically active and becoming physically fit. Because so many Americans are sedentary, everyone should assume responsibility to adopt a physically active lifestyle in order to begin experiencing some of the benefits listed in Table 6-1, as per *The U.S. Surgeon General's Report on Physical*

Activity and Health (United States Department of Health and Human Services, 1996). However, increased benefits are linked with higher levels of activity, or exercise, in a phenomenon known as a dose-response relationship (Bouchard, 2001), and these higher levels of exercise may be recommended for more active clients. Yet another way to place various types and levels of activity into a visual context is the Activity Pyramid (Figure 6-1).

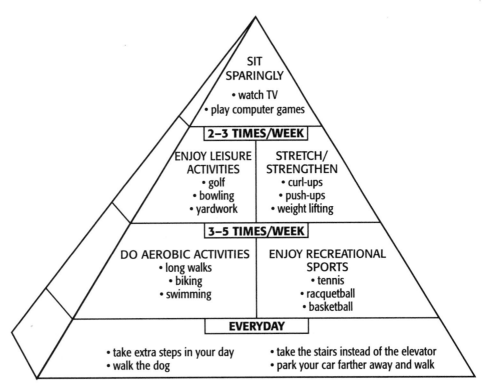

Start your weekly activity plan with the daily activities at the base of the pyramid.
Enhance your fitness by choosing other activities on the pyramid. Move more, sit less.

Fig. 6-1. The Activity Pyramid
(*The Activity Pyramid* © 2003 Park Nicollet Health*Source*, Minneapolis, U.S.A. 1-888-637-2675. Reprinted with permission.)

The American College of Sports Medicine (ACSM) (1998, 2006a) has published guidelines and position statements about health maintenance and for the development of cardiorespiratory fitness. In general, ACSM notes that the guidelines for health improvement are at a slightly lower threshold than those for cardiorespiratory fitness. In other words, individuals may exercise at lower levels (40–50% of heart rate reserve [HRR]) and still see reductions in various risk factors. This is especially important for very deconditioned or inactive clients for whom any activity is better than no activity. For these clients, adopting a moderately active lifestyle may significantly improve their well-being and may be a more attainable goal than achieving a very high level of fitness. As clients become more fit, ACSM's 1998 position stand recommendations should be followed in order to see significant changes in VO$_2$ max and body composition. The ACSM guidelines are summarized below.

ACSM 2006 Guidelines for Cardiovascular Stimulus

- **Mode/Type** Any activity that uses large muscle groups, can be maintained continuously, and is rhythmical and aerobic in nature
- **Frequency** 3–5 days/week
- **Intensity** 40–85% (40–50% for the deconditioned) of HRR OR 64–94% (64–70% for the deconditioned) of maximum heart rate (max HR)
- **Duration/Time** 20–60 minutes of continuous or intermittent (10-minute bouts accumulated throughout the day) aerobic activity
- **Progression (rate)** Depends on functional capacity, health status, age, and client preferences and goals; three stages: initial, improvement, and maintenance

NOTE: ACSM also recommends 150–400 kcal of physical activity and/or exercise energy expenditure per day, or a minimum of approximately 1,000 kcal per week from physical activity (which would mean averaging 150 calories per day or 200 x 5 days per week). Clients should be encouraged to work towards a caloric expenditure of 300–400 kcal per day. And, to achieve optimal weight control, the goal is to bring the weekly expenditure closer to 2,000 kcal as health and fitness progresses. (American College of Sports Medicine. [2006]. *ACSM's guidelines for exercise testing and prescription* [7th ed.]. Baltimore: Lippincott Williams & Wilkins. Reprinted with permission.)

To improve the cardiorespiratory system, **overload** must occur, which means that the body must be given an appropriate challenge greater than it has been used to. Manipulating frequency, intensity, duration, and mode are all ways to overload and cause improvement to the cardiorespiratory system. It should be noted that too much of a challenge can cause injury, drop-out, and decreased fitness; trainers must strike the right balance between too much and too little overload in order to keep clients safe and satisfied.

Another important principle in training is **specificity**. The body's systems adapt quite specifically to what is practiced, or, in other words, you get good at what you do, and not at what you don't do. So, if your client wants to run fast, he or she will need to follow a training program that involves running at faster and faster speeds. Running speed will not be improved, for example, by swimming, weight training, or even by running slowly.

Guidelines for Cardiorespiratory Programming

Mode

Mode refers to the type of activity that is used for cardiorespiratory improvement. The greatest improvement in VO_2 max results from repetitive and rhythmical use of the large muscle groups for a prolonged period of time (>20 minutes). Activities that are considered to be aerobic include, but are not limited to: walking, running, cycling, swimming, stepping, aerobic dancing, rowing, and cross-country skiing. Some activities are useful for developing aerobic endurance if the individual has the skill to perform them continuously. These include such activities as: skating, jumping rope, tennis, racquetball, and basketball. However, keep in mind that since high-impact activities (e.g., running, jumping rope, and high-impact aerobic dance) have been linked with high risk of injuries, low-impact activities are recommended for beginners and those vulnerable to orthopedic problems.

Recently, a greater emphasis has been made on walking as a preferred mode of activity. This is because walking is a functional activity, necessary for many activities of daily living (ADLs); walking is also relatively inexpensive, accessible, and easy to do for most clients. A number of studies have shown that regular walking programs have resulted in benefits, and, at higher speeds, improved fitness (e.g., Franklin et al., 1983; Spelman, Pate, Macera, & Ward, 1993).

Beyond choosing safe, appropriate activities for your client, it is important to find a type of activity (or several activities) that your client enjoys and will actually participate in. This is essential for long-term adherence and behavior change.

Intensity

Intensity is the most complex of the training variables. It is interrelated with duration; together, intensity and duration determine the total calorie cost of an exercise session. Intensity and duration are also said to be inversely related. If intensity is very high, then duration is shortened; whereas if intensity is low, then duration can be long.

The total amount of work performed is one of the most significant factors in improving cardiorespiratory fitness. Improvement is similar for low-intensity, long-duration activities versus high-intensity, short-duration activities if the total energy costs of the activities are equal. However, high-intensity exercise carries a higher risk of cardiovascular complications, orthopedic injuries, and decreased adherence. Low- to moderate-intensity training programs with longer durations are recommended for most adults (American College of Sports Medicine, 1998).

As noted in ACSM's position stand (1998), the American Heart Association (AHA), the National Institutes of Health (NIH), and the Office of the Surgeon General have issued statements on the health benefits of activity and exercise. These statements have noted that even lower levels of exercise intensity than those recommended in ACSM's position stand may be sufficient to reduce CHD risk factors and enhance health. In 2006 ACSM recommended an intensity of 40–85% (40–50% for the deconditioned) of HRR.

Programming Exercise Intensity

Methods for figuring how hard your client should exercise are nearly the same as those used to assess intensity (discussed later in this chapter) while exercising. Methods of programming intensity include the following.

- **HR methods:** percentage of maximum HR and the **Karvonen** or HRR method
- **Rate of perceived exertion** (RPE scale/Borg scale)
- Using **METS** to establish the proper workload

Heart Rate Methods

Programming and measuring intensity by taking a pulse is very common and convenient. However, this method has some limitations, including the following.

- All maximum HR prediction formulas contain large standard errors of estimate (Robergs & Landwehr, 2002; Whaley, Kaminsky, Dwyer, Getchall, & Norton, 1992); the formula,

220 – age = maximum HR, is accurate for only about 75% of the population (McArdle, Katch, & Katch, 1990). This limitation can be overcome, to some extent, by combining the HRR method with the RPE method.

• The effect of medications (may decrease or increase the HR)

• The effect of the **pressor response** (a phenomenon in which the HR is elevated due to upper body exercise, but oxygen consumption and calorie expenditure are not elevated along with HR, thus giving a false impression of the actual exercise intensity)

• The initial difficulty teaching clients to take an accurate pulse

NOTE: Many commercial HR monitors make it easier to take a client's pulse, but their programmed target HR zones may be inaccurate for your client.

Heart Rate Method Formulas

• Percentage of maximal HR

  This method is simple and is used in the ubiquitous target HR charts found in most fitness clubs. It will yield a more conservative target HR than the Karvonen formula. There are two steps:
  1. 220 - age = estimated max HR
  2. Estimated max HR x percentage (e.g., 70%) = target HR

• Karvonen Formula (HRR method)

  This method, which factors in resting HR, yields training ranges that correspond more closely to percentage of VO_2 max, and is therefore considered more accurate throughout all intensity levels. (If a client performs a graded maximal exercise test, VO_2 max can be measured and a training range can be determined as a percentage of VO_2 max. This is not practical for most clients, and the Karvonen formula is recommended instead.) The Karvonen, or HRR, formula has four steps:
  1. 220 - age = estimated max HR
  2. Estimated max HR - resting HR = HRR
  3. HRR x percentage (e.g., 60%) = percent of HRR
  4. Percent of HRR + resting HR = target HR

In both of the above methods only one target HR is obtained. Since clients need a target HR range (e.g., 60–70%), the calculation should be repeated for the second percentage as well (e.g., 70%).

Finally, since both HR methods yield a target HR in beats per minute (e.g., 160 bpm), a final step should be added to make it easier for clients to count their pulse: divide the target HR by 6 to get a 10-second value (AFAA recommends taking the pulse for 10 seconds at the radial artery). Generally, the 10-second values are what you'll give your client. For example, you might tell Ms. Novice Exerciser that her target HR is 21–23 beats per 10 second count, or 126–138 for a full minute.

RPE (Borg) Scale	
6	
7	Very, very light
8	
9	Very light
10	
11	Fairly light
12	
13	Somewhat hard
14	
15	Hard
16	
17	Very hard
18	
19	Very, very hard
20	

Revised RPE (Borg) Scale	
0	Nothing at all
0.3	
0.5	Extremely weak
0.7	
1	Very weak
1.5	
2	Weak
2.5	
3	Moderate
4	
5	Strong
6	
7	Very strong
8	
9	
10	Extremely strong
*	Absolute maximum

(© Gunnar Borg, 1985, 1994.
For correct usage of the Borg scales see
*Borg's Perceived Exertion and Pain
Scales*, Champaign, IL. Human Kinetics,
1998. Reprinted with permission.)

Selecting Appropriate Intensity or Target Heart Rate Percentages
How do you select the appropriate HR range percentages? This is an arbitrary decision based on at least four factors.

1. **Client's risk factors and/or any orthopedic limitations**—if your client is moderate to high risk, then training, especially in the early stages, should be low intensity.
2. **Client's level of fitness** (estimated during the fitness assessment)—clients with low fitness levels can improve their fitness with lower intensity programs. Clients with high-fitness levels will need to work at higher intensities for improvement.
3. **Client's goals**—weight loss, decreased CHD risk factors, and achieving a better time in a 10K run are different goals that demand different training intensities.
4. **Client's level of motivation**—a highly motivated client may be more likely to adhere to a high-intensity program, whereas a client with a low level of motivation may drop out of a high-intensity program, but adhere to one that is low intensity. Some experts have stated that when inactive people are arbitrarily given an intensity that they perceive to be very stressful, they may be less likely to continue exercising (Dishman, 1994).

Rate of Perceived Exertion (RPE) Method
This method is valuable for assessing and recommending intensity for several reasons, including the following.

- RPE may be used even if clients are taking HR-altering medications.
- RPE helps clients to "listen to their bodies."
- RPE can provide an accurate gauge of approaching fatigue.
- RPE is useful for clients who have trouble taking their HR.

When teaching a client about RPE, you should take care to match his or her perceived level or exertion to each specific mode of training; studies have shown that the HR/RPE relationship varies from mode to mode (Whaley, Brubaker, Kaminsky, & Miller, 1997). RPE can be used in conjunction with the HR methods.

Using the original Borg scale, a rate of 12–13 approximates 40–59% of HRR and a rate of 16 approximates 84% of HRR. Therefore, the ACSM recommends that clients exercise within an RPE range of 12–16 (meaning, to the clients, that the intensity subjectively feels somewhat hard to hard). On the revised scale (sometimes referred to as the 10-point scale), this would be between 2.5 and 5. Clients can be given a RPE range (e.g., 12–14) as part of their recommended program. Most people will need instruction to help them understand how to use the RPE scale; extremely unfit or inactive clients may need two to three sessions before they use the scale properly. The following table shows the correlation between RPE and the two HR methods discussed above.

Table 6-2. Classification of Exercise Intensity for Cardiorespiratory Endurance			
Intensity	**% of HRR or VO$_2$R**	**% of HR$_{max}$ %**	**RPE**
Very light	< 20	< 35	< 10
Light	20–39	35–54	10–11
Moderate	40–59	55–69	12–13
Hard	60–84	70–89	14–16
Very hard	> 85	> 90	17–19
Maximal	100	100	20
HRR = heart rate reserve; VO$_2$R = oxygen uptake reserve; HR$_{max}$ = maximum heart rate; RPE = rating of perceived exertion			

(American College of Sports Medicine. [2006]. *ACSM's guidelines for exercise testing and prescription* [7th ed.]. Baltimore: Lippincott Williams & Wilkins. Reprinted with permission.)

Using METS to Establish the Proper Workload

A MET (metabolic equivalent) is a unit of energy expenditure often used by physiologists and cardiologists. Most people, on a pound per pound basis, consume approximately the same amount of oxygen at rest (VO$_2$ ~ 3.5 ml of O$_2$/kg of BW/min.$^{-1}$, with BW = body weight). This resting oxygen uptake value is equivalent to 1 MET. In other words, having an energy expenditure of 1 MET means that an individual is expending only a resting level of energy (calories). If a person exercises at a 5-MET level of energy expenditure, that means he/she is consuming 5 times more oxygen and calories than at rest. (5 x 3.5 ml/kg/minute would equal 17.5 ml of O$_2$ consumed per kg of body weight per minute.) Therefore, 10 METS equals 10 times resting, and so on.

If your client performed a graded exercise stress test, MET values, which are useful when deciding what intensity is appropriate, can be obtained. For example, if your client reached maximum, a percentage (e.g., 50–85%) of the maximal MET level can be used. If your client had symptoms of heart disease at a certain MET level, then exercise programming would obviously take place below that MET level. Also, many cardiologists specify the MET levels at which they want their patients to exercise. The energy cost (MET level) of most daily activities and exercises is known (see Table 6-3). Equations exist that allow you to calculate the MET levels for various running, walking, cycling, and stepping workloads (American College of Sports Medicine, 2006a).

HR and RPE recommendations stay relatively constant as your client's fitness level improves; with training adaptation, a given workload feels easier (and HR decreases) and, therefore, your client has to work harder to stay in his/her target HR range. MET levels (workloads) need to be increased as aerobic endurance progresses. Following are the MET levels of selected activities.

Table 6-3. Estimated MET levels for Selected Activities

METS	Activity
4.0	Bicycling, < 10 mph, leisure, to work or for pleasure
8.0	Bicycling, 12–13.9 mph, leisure, moderate effort
10.0	Bicycling, 14–15.9 mph, racing or leisure, fast, vigorous effort
16.0	Bicycling, > 20 mph, racing, not drafting
7.0	Bicycling, stationary, 150 watts, moderate effort
10.5	Bicycling, stationary, 200 watts, vigorous effort
3.0	Weight lifting, light or moderate effort
6.0	Weight lifting, power lifting, body-building, vigorous effort
7.0	Rowing, stationary, 100 watts, moderate effort
7.0	Ski machine, general
6.5	Aerobic dance, general
8.5	Step aerobics, 6–8 inch step
3.0	Fishing, general
3.3	Carpet sweeping, sweeping floors
2.0	Making bed
5.0	Spreading dirt with a shovel
1.0	Watching TV
2.5	Mowing lawn with a riding mower
4.3	Raking lawn
6.0	Shoveling snow by hand
4.0	Playing drums
2.5	Playing piano
8.0	Running, 5 mph (12 min./mile)
10.0	Running, 6 mph (10 min./mile)
12.5	Running, 8 mph (7.5 min./mile
15.0	Running, 9 mph (6.5 min./mile)
3.0	Walking, 2.5 mph
3.8	Walking, 3.5 mph, level, brisk, walking for exercise
6.3	Walking, 4.5 mph, level, very brisk pace
7.0	Swimming laps, freestyle, slow, moderate or light effort
10.0	Swimming laps, freestyle, fast, vigorous effort
3.0	Bowling
10.0	Racquetball, competitive
6.0	Tennis, doubles
9.0	Tennis, singles
8.0	Skiing, cross-country, 4.0–4.9 mph, moderate effort
6.0	Skiing, downhill, moderate effort

(Adapted from Ainsworth, B.E., et al. [2006]. *ACSM's resource manual for guidelines for exercise testing and prescription* [5th ed.]. Baltimore: Lippincott Williams & Wilkins. Reprinted with permission.)

Methods of programming intensity have just been presented. Methods of assessing intensity (finding out if your client is working at an appropriate level) include the following.

1. Measuring HR to determine if your client is in his/her target HR range.
2. Asking your client to rate his/her perceived exertion.
3. Using the talk test (or breathlessness test). Your client should be able to talk and breathe comfortably during aerobic exercise. A possible exception might be the highly fit and motivated client who is performing sprint-type work above the anaerobic threshold.

Duration

The ACSM recommends 20–60 minutes of continuous or intermittent aerobic activity (10 minute bouts accumulated throughout the day). Studies have shown that VO2 max can be improved when the multiple short bouts are equivalent to a single 30-minute bout of exercise (Murphy & Hardman, 1998). This does not include warm-up and cooldown. Duration is inversely related to intensity—the lower the intensity, the longer the duration may be. For very deconditioned clients, several low-intensity, short-duration (< 10 minutes) sessions may be preferable. Duration can then be gradually increased as your client adapts to training.

Frequency

The ACSM recommends a frequency of 3–5 days per week. For weight-reduction purposes, 4–5 days per week are better than 3 due to increased caloric expenditure. Extremely deconditioned clients may benefit from several short, low-intensity daily exercise sessions, and/or may also need rest days interspersed between exercise days. At the other end of the continuum, research shows that exercising more than 5 days per week has little effect on VO2 max, and increases the risk of injury and burnout. High-impact activities are associated with higher risk of injury and probably should be avoided on a daily basis by non-conditioned individuals. Remember, according to *The U.S. Surgeon General's Report on Physical Activity and Health* (United States Dept. of Health and Human Services, 1996), an accumulation of 30 minutes per day of moderate physical activity is recommended, but moderate to vigorous exercise has a recommended frequency of 3–5 days per week.

Progression

There are three stages of progression depending on your client's functional capacity, health status, age, needs, and goals. These are the initial, improvement, and maintenance stages.

1. **Initial conditioning stage**—This stage is especially critical for the less fit and/or inactive client. The foundation is laid for long-term, increased physical activity and healthy lifestyle changes, with the main purpose of establishing an exercise habit. For these clients in particular, it is important not to be too aggressive in programming, to find activities they enjoy, minimize injury and soreness, and encourage a sense of inner satisfaction with the exercise process. Set them up for success with realistic goals and an appropriate initial exercise program. This stage should include a thorough warm-up, light muscular endurance exercises, low-level aerobic activities (40–60% of HRR), and an extended cool-down. Duration may begin with 12–15 minutes or less and gradually progress. Three non-consecutive days per week are desirable (American College of Sports Medicine, 2006a). This stage typically lasts 4–6 weeks for the less fit client.

2. **Improvement stage**—In this stage, progression is more rapid, and intensity is gradually progressed into a range of 50–85% of HRR. Frequency, intensity, duration and mode may be manipulated to cause progressive, yet gradual, **overload** to the cardiorespiratory system. Many trainers systematically increase one or more of these factors every 2–3 weeks depending on the client's ability to adapt. Note that adaptation may take longer in older adults (American College of Sports Medicine, 1998).

3. **Maintenance stage**—When a client reaches his/her fitness goals, maintenance and adherence can become goals in themselves. Cross-training and variety in programming are two important strategies to help your client with compliance. Use your creativity to help make exercise fun and keep your client motivated.

Warming Up and Cooling Down

All exercise sessions should be preceded by a **warm-up**. A proper warm-up increases blood flow, oxygen, and energy substrates to the working muscles, increases core temperature, gradually increases HR, and helps increase the metabolic rate from resting to exercising levels (Gutin, Stewart, Lewis, & Kruper, 1976). Additionally, some studies have shown that a thorough warm-up may help prevent heart problems (Foster, Dymond, Carpenter, & Schmidt, 1982). According to AFAA guidelines, a general 8-12-minute warm-up should consist of a balanced combination of limbering (i.e., large, full-body movements that increase body temperature and increase blood flow to the heart and muscles) and static stretching (held, sustained preparatory stretches lasting 8–10 seconds for major muscle groups) (Aerobics and Fitness Association of America, 2002).

For personal fitness trainers, this can mean asking your client to walk or cycle at an easy to moderate pace (10–30% HRR) for 5–10 minutes, followed by light, short-duration preparatory static stretches of muscles that will be targeted during the exercise session and/or that are commonly tight (10 seconds each). See Chapter 9 ("Flexibility Programming") for a thorough review of stretching exercises.

Cardiorespiratory activity should be followed by a post-cardio **cool-down** phase, a 3–5-minute period (or longer if needed) of gradually decreasing intensity (e.g., slower walking) that helps prevent blood pooling in the extremities, reduces feelings of dizziness, lowers HR and BP to near-resting levels, helps dissipate lactic acid, and helps minimize potentially threatening cardiac arrythmias. Stretches may be repeated and held for longer periods of 10–20 seconds or more each, for an additional total of 5 or more minutes of stretching.

Cardiorespiratory Training Systems

There are several options in training methods, or systems, for cardiorespiratory fitness, including the following.

- Continuous training
- Interval training
- Fartlek training
- Super circuit training
- Cross-training

Continuous Training

Often called long, slow, distance training (LSD), this type of program involves exercising at the same workload for a prolonged period of time (20–60 minutes) without a rest interval. For example, Mr. C. walks on the treadmill at 4 mph, 3% grade continuously for 25 minutes. This protocol is safe and easy to teach to clients, and beginners may prefer this type of training. The major disadvantage is that it is highly repetitive and may become boring.

Interval Training

Interval training may be used for all levels of participants. It involves repeated bouts of harder work interspersed with periods of easier work (or, occasionally, rest periods). For less fit clients on the treadmill, this may mean three minutes of "easy" work at 3 mph and 0% grade, then 1 minute of "hard" work at 3.5 mph and 0% grade. This might be repeated five times for a total of 20 minutes. The client could be encouraged to work at 12 on the RPE scale during the easy bout, and at 14 on the RPE scale during the hard bout.

Interval training can be utilized all the way up the fitness ladder. For extremely fit clients, the program may consist of 4 minutes of running at 9 mph, alternated with 1 minute of relief at 8 mph, and so on. Ratios of 2 minutes hard: 2 minutes easy (2:2), or 3 minutes hard: 2 minutes easy (3:2), for example, can be established depending on your client's goals. Advantages of this type of training include: (1) the total amount of work performed may be greater than continuous training; (2) clients may find it less boring and thus be more likely to adhere; and (3) it is easy to systematically cause progressive overload.

Fartlek Training

Similar to interval training (but less structured), Fartlek, or speed play training, is very demanding and is therefore more appropriate for fit, low-risk, motivated clients. It involves free form, non-systematic alternations between high-speed, high-intensity, anaerobic work and low-intensity, relief-type periods.

Super Circuit Training

Super circuit, or aerobic circuit, training alternates aerobic exercise stations with resistance exercise stations. For example, 3 minutes on the treadmill, then 1 minute of leg presses, 3 minutes on the stairclimber, 1 minute of lunges, 3 minutes on the cycle, 1 minute of lat pull-downs, 3 minutes on rower, 1 minute of bench presses, etc. Advantages of this type of format include: (1) it is fun; (2) it helps eliminate boredom; (3) it can work equally well for class-type settings as well as one-on-one; and (4) it allows a large amount of total work in a short period of time. Clients need to be familiar with the exercises and equipment that will be used, as they will need to move quickly from one station to the next.

Cross-Training

Aerobic cross-training can be applied in several different ways.

- Using a variety of cardiorespiratory equipment within one workout, e.g., 10 minutes on the cycle, 10 minutes on the treadmill, 10 minutes on the stairclimber
- Using a variety of equipment (or modalities) throughout the week, e.g., Monday: run 30 minutes; Wednesday: cycle 40 minutes; Friday: cross-country ski 25 minutes; Saturday: play singles tennis for 1 hour
- Periodizing cross-training involves the use of different modalities across large blocks of time or seasons, e.g., summer: emphasize swimming and training for windsurfing; fall: versa-climber, outdoor rock-climbing, and tennis; winter: cross-country and downhill skiing; spring: running and canoeing.

Advantages of cross-training include decreased risk of injury and reduced risk of burnout due to boredom.

Cardiorespiratory Modalities and Equipment

Cardiorespiratory modalities include, but are certainly not limited to, walking, running, cycling, swimming, water aerobics, rowing, cross-country skiing, stair-climbing, elliptical machines, and cardio group activities, such as step, kickboxing, and high-low impact. In this section basic skills and techniques for utilizing selected modalities will be briefly covered.

Walking is one of the safest, and most accessible and functional of the cardiorespiratory modes. It can be done outdoors or indoors on a track, at the mall, or on a treadmill. It is an excellent activity for most deconditioned clients; initial walking programs can be very low intensity and short duration, allowing for a safe and gradual progression. Recently, a goal of 10,000 steps per day has been promoted in an effort to stimulate the population to be moderately active for at least 30 minutes daily. Wearing a pedometer can be a helpful motivator for your clients, who may find that they fall considerably short of 10,000 steps on an average day. The average person takes approximately 2,000 steps per mile of walking. Personal fitness trainers may need to exercise some care when recommending walking in areas that may be inaccessible to emergency response or are located in certain areas, such as "high-crime" locales.

Proper footwear is essential for both walking and running; shoes should be supportive and have adequate traction. Proper posture is key for a comfortable walking experience; clients should stand tall and take special care to maintain a neutral pelvis throughout all phases of the walking gait. A common mistake is to let the pelvis anteriorly tilt, which may eventually lead to backache. Chest should be lifted with shoulder blades depressed. Make certain clients "roll through" the feet from heel, to ball, to toe with each footstrike. Teach your clients basic stretches for walking that can be performed right on the (stopped) treadmill: calves, hip flexors, hamstrings, quadriceps, and low back can all be stretched while standing.

When using a **treadmill**, make certain clients straddle the belt prior to starting the machine. Instruct them to hold the handrails initially, but with the eventual goal of hands off and allowing arms to swing naturally at the sides. Leaning or hanging on the handrails causes a reduction in caloric expenditure. Of course, if a client is extremely deconditioned, frail, and/or has balance problems, then holding the handrail is advised. Have your client experiment with a 1% incline instead of zero; a 1% grade often feels more comfortable. On a treadmill, intensity can be progressed either by increasing the speed or by increasing the elevation. Clients who want to avoid the impact of running can still increase the intensity significantly by changing the elevation. Treadmills, as with other forms of exercise equipment, can sometimes present certain dangers and may be subject to some unintended events when used. Always instruct clients in the proper use of such devices. Placement of such devices away from other pieces of equipment or walls, furniture, etc. is prudent should falls occur.

Cycling is an excellent modality, especially for clients with lower body issues, such as foot or ankle pain. Overweight clients may also welcome the fact that cycling is weight-supported. Stationary indoor cycling can be performed in a group setting with music, or individually. You will need to help your client find the proper settings on his or her bike. Generally, there are up to three adjustments: seat height, saddle position, and handlebar height. The seat height should be high enough to allow only a slight bend in the client's knee when the pedal is in its lowest position (ball of the foot is on the pedal). Positioning the seat too low can cause anterior knee pain. Conversely, positioning the seat too high may cause the knee to hyperextend and result in posterior knee pain. Some seats (saddles) can slide forward or backward; in this case, the seat should be aligned so that the front kneecap is directly over the ball of the foot when the pedal shaft is horizontal; the shin should be vertical. Handlebar placement is largely a matter of personal preference; a low handlebar more closely simulates a racing posture, but is usually more stressful for the back and neck. Clients with back problems will do better with higher handlebars and maintenance of a neutral spine. Semi-recumbent cycles are also popular, especially with deconditioned clients. However, exercising on a semi-recumbent cycle results in a lower energy expenditure than the same level of exercise on a traditional upright bike (Bonzheim, Franklin, Dewitt, Marks, Goslin, Jarski, et al., 1992).

Stair climbing machines are also popular in many clubs. Make certain your client stands upright and avoids leaning or hanging on the machine, which can reduce the number of calories burned and lower the exercise intensity. Rounding over or leaning forward on the machine may also create problems for the lower back, as can taking excessively deep steps, which causes the hips to rock side to side; this has the potential to aggravate the sacroiliac joint as well as the lower back. Similar to stair climbers, **elliptical machines** combine an up and down movement with the forward motion of walking or running. Feet move in an elliptical, or oval-like, pattern on the machine, without actually leaving the pedals; thus, impact is minimized. As with stair climbers, your client should stand with upright posture and avoid leaning on the machine. Most ellipticals also allow a backward motion, which can provide variety and a slightly different muscle stimulus for clients. In addition, some machines incorporate an arm-pumping action as well, providing a total body workout.

Cross-country ski machines are somewhat less common, even though the cardiorespiratory stimulus can be excellent due to the large amount of muscle mass involved (upper and lower body). Unfortunately, cross-country ski machines require some skill and practice in order for most clients to feel comfortable. Feet slide back and forth (as in skiing), while the hands and arms pull ropes, simulating poling. The hips are braced against an adjustable, supportive pad, but the exerciser must maintain balance and not allow the feet to slide too far forward or backward, risking a fall.

Rowing machines provide a nice contrast to most other cardiorespiratory equipment, as the upper body musculature is much more heavily recruited. It should be noted though, that much or most of the pulling action is powered by the lower body muscles. Since clients are seated, the workout is non-impact and non-weight bearing—a plus for many clients with orthopedic problems. Care should be taken not to flex or round the back; the spine should stay in neutral throughout the entire rowing action while the hips perform flexion and extension.

Upper body ergometers (arm bikes) are found in some clubs, and are particularly useful for clients with lower body injuries. Be aware that HRs will be higher for upper body ergometry than for lower body exercise at the same workload. Clients are usually seated with the pivot point of the handle adjusted to shoulder height.

The ultimate goal in providing your clients with cardiorespiratory programming is to help them adhere to and maintain a lifelong habit of exercise and physical activity. To that end, variety and fun are key aspects of training. Help your clients to find modalities or activities that they enjoy and want to participate in on a long-term basis. So what's the best exercise? The activities your clients will actually do!

Summary

In this section, the benefits of cardiorespiratory fitness are listed and the ACSM guidelines and position stand for enhancement of well-being and cardiorespiratory fitness were discussed. Specifics of intensity programming were covered, including HR methods, RPE, and METS. Frequency, duration, mode, and progression were discussed, as well as several cardiorespiratory training systems and equipment activities.

References

Aerobics and Fitness Association of America. (2002). *Fitness: Theory and practice* (4th ed., L.A. Gladwin, Ed.). Sherman Oaks, CA: Aerobics and Fitness Association of America.

Ainsworth, B.E., Haskell, W.L., Whitt, M.C., Irwin, M.L., Swartz, A.M., Strath, S.J., et al. (2006). Compendium of physical activities: An update of activity codes and MET intensities (Appendix A). In American College of Sports Medicine, *ACSM's resource manual for guidelines for exercise testing and prescription* (5th ed.) (pp. 667-698). Baltimore: Lippincott Williams & Wilkins.

American College of Sports Medicine. (1998). Position stand: The recommended quantity and quality of exercise for developing and maintaining cardiorespiratory and muscular fitness, and flexibility in healthy adults. *Medicine & Science in Sports & Exercise, 30,* 975-991.

American College of Sports Medicine (2006a). *ACSM's guidelines for exercise testing and prescription* (7th ed.). Baltimore: Lippincott Williams & Wilkins.

American College of Sports Medicine. (2006b). *ACSM's resource manual for guidelines for exercise testing and prescription* (5th ed.). Baltimore: Lippincott Williams & Wilkins.

Bonzheim, S.C., Franklin, B.A., Dewitt, C., Marks, C., Goslin, B., Jarski, R., et al. (1992). Physiologic responses to recumbent versus upright cycle ergometry and implications for exercise prescription in patients with coronary artery disease. *American Journal of Cardiology, 69*(1), 40-44.

Borg, G. (1998). *Borg's perceived exertion and pain scales.* Champaign, IL: Human Kinetics.

Bouchard, C. (2001). Physical activity and health: Introduction to the dose-response symposium. *Medicine & Science in Sports & Exercise, 33,* S347-350.

Dishman, R.K. (1994). Prescribing exercise intensity for healthy adults using perceived exertion. *Medicine & Science in Sports & Exercise, 26*(9), 1087-1094.

Foster, C., Dymond, D.S., Carpenter, J., & Schmidt, D.H. (1982). Effect of warm-up on left ventricular response to sudden strenuous exercise. *Journal of Applied Physiology, 53*(2), 380-383.

Franklin, B.A., Pamatmat, A., Johnson, S., Scherf, J., Mitchell, M., & Rubenfire, M. (1983). Metabolic cost of extremely slow walking in cardiac patients: Implication for exercise testing and training. *Archives of Physical Medicine and Rehabilitation, 64*(11), 564-565.

Gutin, B., Stewart, K., Lewis, S., & Kruper, J. (1976). Oxygen consumption in the first stages of strenuous work as a function of prior exercise. *Journal of Sports Medicine and Physical Fitness, 16*(1), 60-65.

McArdle, W.D., Katch, F.I., & Katch, V.L. (1990). *Exercise physiology, energy, nutrition, and performance* (3rd ed.). Philadelphia: Lea & Febiger.

Murphy, M.H., & Hardman, A.E. (1998). Training effect of short and long bouts of brisk walking in sedentary women. *Medicine & Science in Sports & Exercise, 30,* 152-157.

Robergs, R.A., & Landwehr, R. (2002). The surprising history of the "Hrmax = 220 – age" equation. *Journal of Exercise Physiology Online, 5*(2), 1-10.

Spelman, C.C., Pate, R.R., Macera, C.A., & Ward, D.S. (1993). Self-selected exercise intensity of habitual walkers. *Medicine & Science in Sports & Exercise, 25,* 1174-1179.

U.S. Department of Health and Human Services. (1996). *Physical activity and health: A report of the Surgeon General.* Atlanta, GA: U.S. Department of Health and Human Services, Centers for Disease Control and Prevention, National Center for Chronic Disease Prevention and Health Promotion.

Whaley, M.H., Brubaker, P.H., Kaminsky, L.A., & Miller, C.R. (1997). Validity of rating of perceived exertion during graded exercise testing in apparently healthy adults and cardiac patients. *Journal of Cardiopulmonary Rehabilitation, 17*(4), 261-267.

Whaley, M.H., Kaminsky, L.A., Dwyer, G.B., Getchell, L.H., & Norton, J.A. (1992). Predictors of over and underachievement of age-predicted maximal heart rate. *Medicine & Science in Sports & Exercise, 24,* 1173-1179.

Suggested Reading

American College of Sports Medicine. (2000). *ACSM's metabolic calculations tutorial* CD-ROM. Philadelphia: Lippincott Williams & Wilkins.

Fletcher, G.F., Balady, G., Amsterdam, E.A., Chaitman, B., Eckel, R., Fleg, J., et al. (2001). Exercise standards for testing and training by the American Heart Association Science Advisory and Coordinating Committee. *Circulation, 104,* 1694-1790.

Karvonen, M., Kentala, K., & Mustala, O. (1957). The effects of training on heart rate: A longitudinal study. *Annales Medicinae Experimentalis et Biologiae Fenniae, 35,* 307-315.

Sleamaker, R., & Browning, R. (1996). *Serious training for endurance athletes* (2nd ed.). Champaign, IL: Human Kinetics.

Muscular Strength and Endurance Programming

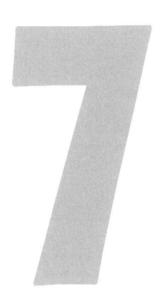

Outline

- Benefits and Definitions of Muscular Fitness
- Guidelines for Muscular Strength and Endurance Programming
- Strength Training Specifics
- Designing a Resistance Training Program
- Resistance Training Systems
- Resistance Training Equipment and Methods
- Other Resistance Training Methods
- Common Training Errors and Safety Considerations
- Muscle Soreness
- Resistance Training Sports
- Ergogenic Aids
- Important Factors in the Development of Strength
- Overtraining, Detraining, and Retraining Issues
- Women and Resistance Training
- Children and Resistance Training
- Common Weight-room Exercises Grid
- Sample Programs for Resistance Training

Muscular strength and endurance, also known as muscular fitness, are components of fitness (along with cardiorespiratory fitness, flexibility, and appropriate body composition) that are important for overall health and well-being. In this chapter, issues related to muscular fitness, such as benefits of resistance training, programming guidelines, resistance training equipment, factors in the development of strength, and gender and age concerns, will be discussed. Personal fitness trainers need to be familiar with this information in order to choose appropriate resistance training exercises and to provide accurate and motivating information to clients.

Benefits and Definitions of Muscular Fitness

There are a number of documented benefits that can result from resistance training (Winnett & Carpinelli, 2001; Pollock, Franklin, & Balady, 2000; American College of Sports Medicine, 1998). See Table 7-1 for a list of these potential benefits. Resistance training should not be offered by non-health-care licensed personnel in efforts to treat, cure, alleviate, etc. any applicable conditions in clients. However, educational activities and the provision of information, in an effort to increase clients' knowledge of resistance training and its benefits, are generally permissible.

Table. 7-1. Benefits of Muscular Fitness
- Increased physical work capacity (increased functional ability) resulting in improved ability to perform activities of daily living
- Increased bone density
- Increased fat-free mass resulting in decreased sarcopenia (age-related muscle mass loss) and potentially resulting in increased metabolism
- Increased strength of connective tissue
- Decreased risk of injury
- Increased motor performance
- Enhanced feelings of well-being and self-confidence
- Improved quality of life

In addition, **circuit weight training** (resistance exercises performed one after the other without rest for approximately 20 minutes or more) may result in the following benefits.
- Modest improvements in cardiorespiratory fitness (about 6%)
- Improved glucose tolerance
- Modest reductions in resting blood pressure
- Improved blood lipid profiles

It should be noted that the idea of a significant increase in metabolism due to resistance training is controversial, with a few recent studies showing little, if any, increase (Lemmer et al., 2001; Van Etten, Westerterp, & Verstappen, 1995). It appears that it may be difficult for the general population, and especially women, to acquire enough new muscle mass to have much of an effect on metabolism and weight loss. Even so, the benefits of resistance training (as listed above) on the overall improvement of a client's quality of life are significant.
- **Muscular strength** is defined as the maximum force a muscle or muscle group can generate at one time.

- **Muscular endurance** is the capacity to sustain repeated muscle actions, as in push-ups or sit-ups, or to sustain fixed, static muscle actions for an extended period of time.
- **Muscle power** is the explosive aspect of strength, and is the product of strength and speed of movement. Power = (force x distance)/time. Power is especially important for improved athletic performance.
- **Muscle stability** refers to the ability of a muscle or muscle group to stabilize a joint and maintain its position without movement; in other words, to be able to perform a sustained **isometric**, or held, contraction. Stability training is especially important for postural muscles, such as the erector spinae, middle trapezius and rhomboids, and the abdominals, since these muscle groups stabilize the spine. Many resistance exercises require movements of the extremities while the core, or torso, stays completely still. Furthermore, in most activities of daily living, such as sitting, standing, and bending over, it is important to be able to maintain a torso that is in proper alignment in order to prevent injury and back pain.
- **Muscle hypertrophy** refers to an increase in the muscle fiber size, specifically in an increased cross-sectional area resulting from increased myofibrils (American College of Sports Medicine, 2002).
- **Muscular fitness** is developed by using the **overload principle**: increasing the intensity (resistance), frequency, or duration of the training above the levels normally experienced.
- **Specificity** is an important concept in fitness training. It refers to the specific adaptations in the metabolic and neuromuscular systems depending on the type of program or exercises that are performed. The principle of specificity is also known as the SAID (specific adaptations to imposed demands) principle. In strength training, for example, research shows that results are specific to the range of motion trained (Graves, Pollock, Jones, Colvin, & Leggett, 1989). It is recommended that exercises be performed through the full range of motion for maximum benefit. Also, the effect of exercise training is specific to the area of the body being trained; training the upper body has very little effect on the lower body, and vice versa. In athletic performance, the muscles must be trained with movements as close as possible to the desired movement or skill for optimal results.
- **Volume** is a weight-training concept defined as the total number of repetitions performed multiplied by the total amount of weight, or resistance, used during a single training session (American College of Sports Medicine, 2006). In other words: reps x weight = volume. Volume can be varied by changing the number of repetitions, the number of sets, the number of exercises performed, or the amount of weight used.

Guidelines for Muscular Strength and Endurance Programming

The American College of Sports Medicine (ACSM) (2006a) recommends the following guidelines for resistance training for the average healthy adult.
- Perform one set of each exercise to the point of volitional fatigue, while maintaining proper form.

Major muscle groups listed in opposing pairs
Quadriceps/Hamstrings
Hip abductors/Hip adductors
Pectoralis major/Posterior deltoid, Mid-trapezius, and Rhomboids
Anterior and Medial deltoids/ Latissimus dorsi
Biceps/Triceps
Abdominals/Erector spinae

- Most people should complete 8–12 repetitions for each exercise, although a range of repetitions within 3–20 (e.g., 3–5, 8–10, 12–15) may also be appropriate.
- Perform both the concentric and eccentric phases of the exercises in a controlled manner (~ 3 sec. concentric, ~ 3 sec. eccentric).
- Exercise each muscle group 2–3 non-consecutive days per week, and, if possible, perform a different exercise for the muscle group every two to three sessions.
- Perform a minimum of 8–10 exercises that condition the major muscle groups, with a primary goal of developing total body strength and endurance in a relatively time-efficient manner. Muscle imbalance occurs and risk of injury increases if only a few muscle groups are trained.

Strength Training Specifics

- **Sets**—A large majority of studies show that performing a single-set program to fatigue results in improvements in strength, endurance, and muscle hypertrophy (increased size) similar to a multiple-set program (American College of Sports Medicine, 1998; Hass, Garzarella, de Hoyos, & Pollock, 2000; Stone & Coulter, 1994). Single sets may help with exercise adherence since several exercises can be performed in a short amount of time. Programs lasting more than 60 minutes per session are associated with higher drop-out rates. However, there are a few studies that show better results with a multi-set program (Rhea, Alvar, & Burkett, 2002), and clients who enjoy weight training and/or need additional calorie expenditure may prefer a multi-set routine (although aerobic conditioning activities are more efficient at calorie expenditure than weight training, per unit of time). One way to address the set controversy is to recommend a single-set program for novice exercisers and for more experienced exercisers with time restraints. For intermediate and advanced exercisers with sufficient time, multiple-set programs may be necessary for optimal gains in muscular fitness.
- **Repetitions and intensity**—ACSM makes a distinction between high-intensity and submaximal-intensity resistance training (American College of Sports Medicine, 2006a). High-intensity or maximal training occurs whenever momentary muscle failure occurs; this can happen at 3 RM, 10 RM, 15 RM, etc. Submaximal training occurs by ending the set when the client fatigues and noticeably slows down the speed of the movement, or when one to three more repetitions could still potentially be performed. Clients with high blood pressure, diabetes, or at risk of stroke should not perform high-intensity resistance training exercises. Another way to gauge resistance training intensity is by using the rate of perceived exertion (RPE) scale. On the 20-point RPE scale (see Chapter 6, "Cardiorespiratory Programming," for more information on the Borg RPE scale), a suggested range is 12–13 initially, and then 15–16 near the end of the set for submaximal training, and up to 19–20 for high-intensity training (Faigenbaum, Pollock, & Ishida, 1999).

  The traditional strength-endurance continuum model has become controversial, as few scientific studies support its validity (Campos, Luecke, & Wendeln, 2002). Apparently both muscle strength and muscle endurance can be developed to a high degree within common repetition ranges, such as 3–6, 6–10, or 10–12 (Stone & Coulter, 1994; Weiss, Coney, & Clark, 1999). However, for optimal strength development, high-intensity training at or near maximal effort (RPE of 19–20 on the 20-point scale) should occur.

- **Frequency**—Although somewhat greater strength gains can be made by training 3 days per week, studies show that 2 days per week also elicits a significant improvement in strength and may be more practical for the general population. Since resistance training can produce cellular microtrauma that can lead to muscle soreness and temporary reductions in strength, adequate rest and recovery time is necessary. Waiting 48 hours between resistance training sessions is a good guideline (longer recovery time may be necessary after very intense workouts). For those who prefer to train every day (as in a split routine system), avoid working the same muscle groups on consecutive days.

- **Variety**—Providing clients with a large variety of exercises for individual muscle groups helps maintain interest and may promote better adherence. Additionally, different exercises stimulate the muscle fibers in different ways and help to create more adaptive responses (Kramer et al., 1997). Challenge your client's muscles by providing exercises in not only the sagittal plane (this is the most common), but also the frontal and horizontal planes. As your client becomes more skilled, consider varying the speed of movement as well, always keeping safety in mind. You can provide variety by changing your client's routine from session to session, or by alternating exercise choices from week to week. Use a variety of large equipment, including machines and free weights, as well as small equipment such as stability balls, wobble boards, foam rollers, medicine balls, elastic resistance, and the BOSU. As your client becomes more advanced, change his or her program by varying the resistance training system (see "Resistance Training Systems" later in this chapter). While full-range-of-motion training is recommended, some muscle groups (notably muscles of the core or torso) may benefit from static/isometric or stability training.

- **Order of exercises**—Training the larger muscle groups first is recommended when working with the general public. For example, if the biceps (smaller muscles) were fatigued first, the ability to fatigue the latissimus dorsi (larger muscles) would be limited since the biceps are needed in most latissimus dorsi exercises. Many advocate performing structural exercises (e.g., squats) before isolated body part exercises (e.g., knee extensions) to enhance safety and effectiveness. Abdominal and erector spinae muscles are needed as stabilizers in many exercises, so it makes sense not to exercise them to the point of fatigue until the end of a workout.

- **Progression**—Progressive resistance exercise (PRE) means that resistance must be gradually, progressively increased (overloaded) as the muscles adapt to a given exercise. The double-progressive approach works well with most clients: for example, begin with a resistance the client can lift 8 times to fatigue, and as he/she improves, gradually increase the number of repetitions up to 12. When the client can easily perform 12 repetitions, increase the weight (usually about 5%), and that will reduce the number of repetitions back to about eight. Progression can also refer to overloading the body's systems by providing harder and less stable exercises over time (Yoke & Kennedy, 2004). For example, beginner exercises place the body in a stable, supported position (such as a supine triceps extension) in which the focus is on muscle isolation and stability. As the client's skill and muscular fitness improve, exercises can be chosen that focus more on strength and require an increased ability to stabilize the body (e.g., a bent-over triceps kickback). At advanced or performance levels, clients are challenged with unstable surfaces (e.g., BOSU or core board) and exercises that focus more on power, speed, or rotation (e.g. an overhead ball toss with triceps extension on one leg).

- **Speed**—Although fast lifting may be appropriate for some competitive athletes, risk of injury is increased and it is more difficult to monitor form. For most clients, slow, controlled movement is recommended, especially in the initial stages of training. High-intensity work and rapid movement during the eccentric phase have been linked to muscle soreness. ACSM recommends approximately 3 seconds for the concentric phase, and approximately 3 seconds for the eccentric phase for general training (American College of Sports Medicine, 2006a). For variety, another technique is to pause for 1–3 seconds (adding an isometric component) between the concentric and eccentric contractions.

- **Breathing**—To avoid the Valsalva maneuver and the accompanying rise in blood pressure, regular, continuous breathing is important. "Exhaling on the exertion" (or concentric phase) is a good recommendation for most exercises. Studies have shown that high-intensity weight-training exercise combined with the Valsalva maneuver can raise blood pressure to dangerously high levels ((MacDougall, McKelvie, & Moroz, 1992) and should be avoided, especially for high-risk clients.

- **Functional exercise**—The concept of functional exercise simply refers to the idea that muscles should be trained and developed in such a way as to make the performance of everyday activities easier, smoother, safer, and more efficient. In other words, attention should be given to exercises that enhance everyday movements, and thereby improve a client's ability to "function independently" in the real world. Functional training tends to be associated with **closed kinetic chain** (CKC) exercise; in CKC exercises, feet are generally on the floor or are connected to a resistance (as on a leg-press machine). CKC exercises often resemble activities of daily living. For example, a squat is a closed chain (foot is on the floor and weight-bearing), multi-muscle, and multi-joint exercise that closely resembles the lower body movement patterns in everyday, real-life activities (e.g., getting up and down out of a chair, into and out of a car, and lifting objects off the floor). Many experts advocate moving from **open kinetic chain** (OKC) isolation-type exercises (e.g., knee extensions) to functional exercises (e.g., squats) as fitness and body awareness improves. A related concept in functional exercise is training the core for stability, since stability of the core or torso is necessary for proper posture and alignment in everyday life.

Designing a Resistance Training Program

When formulating an individualized resistance training exercise program, the following steps are helpful.

1. **Determine your client's short- and long-term goals for muscular fitness.** Does your client have a specific area of the body on which he or she wants to focus? Are there chronic injury issues, such as a history of low-back pain or ankle sprains, or previous shoulder problems that should be avoided while completing fitness-related goals? Is your client preparing for a bodybuilding competition or is this his/her first experience in the weight room? Does he/she desire muscle strength (e.g., power lifter), muscle endurance (e.g., long-distance runner), muscle hypertrophy (bodybuilder), or general training?

2. **Identify which muscle groups will be trained.** Consider the following two steps.
   - Create a balanced program that addresses all major muscle groups. Keep in mind that opposing muscle groups and/or muscles on both sides of a joint need to be challenged for muscle symmetry and injury prevention. See the box, "Major muscle groups listed in opposing pairs," earlier in this chapter for a list of the major and opposing muscle groups.
   - Add exercises that specifically work the client's target areas. For example, if your client wants to focus on abdominals, add exercises that will challenge the abdominals in a variety of ways. For athletes, utilizing the principle of specificity is important: select exercises that train the muscle(s) with the same joint action, range of motion, speed, intensity, and type of contraction that will be needed during the athlete's sport.

3. **Identify areas of injury, or potential injury, that need special attention.** For instance, has your client suffered from back pain in the past? Does he or she feel a "clicking" and mild pain in the knees when going down stairs? Does he or she play vigorous singles tennis several times a week? Is there a muscle imbalance? Are the muscles evenly strengthened and stretched on all sides of the joint? In all these examples, there are resistance exercises that may be helpful and/or should be avoided. Remember, if your client has persistent pain or disability in any area, you must recommend that he/she seeks medical advice before proceeding.

4. **Identify the type of muscle training to be used.** Isometric (good for injured areas and for stabilization training), isotonic (free weights or machines), eccentric (negative training), plyometric, power, or speed training (appropriate for some athletes and for sports-specific goals) are some of your options.

5. **Select the specific exercises**. Keep in mind muscle balance, symmetry, the client's goals and fitness level, and specificity if appropriate. Also, you'll need to consider the type of equipment available, whether or not the client will need to take the exercises "on the road" or perform them at home, and whether or not a spotter will be needed. Initially, the exercises you select may be traditional machine-type exercises, so your client becomes familiar with a basic routine. However, over time, you'll want to provide variety, incorporating exercises that use free weights, stability balls, elastic resistance, and other pieces of small equipment.

6. **Select the exercise order.** In general, large muscle groups are worked first. Other options include: core exercises before non-core exercises, alternating push with pull exercises, alternating upper with lower body exercises, and so on.

7. **Determine the frequency of training.** Is your client available to weight train two to three times a week? Does he/she want daily (split routine) training and is he/she committed enough to maintain such a schedule?

8. **Determine the number of sets and repetitions.** This depends on your client's fitness level, goals, and time available for weight training.

9. **Determine the intensity (load or amount of resistance).** There are two major methods for determining the weight load.
   - Trial and error (probably the most common method used for the general public)—for example, after establishing the desired number of repetitions, say 8–12, find the resistance that your client can lift 8 times, but no more than 12. This method can also be used to determine a client's number of repetition maximum for a particular load, i.e., if muscle failure occurs on the sixth repetition, that is the 6 RM load. It's a good idea to err on the side of caution, however, especially with novice exercisers; start with a relatively low weight, see that he or she can perform the exercise with proper form, and gradually increase the weight load.
   - Percent of 1 RM—this method requires 1 RM (maximal lift) testing in order to figure the desired percentage. For example, if your client can press 100 pounds, then 75% or 75 pounds would be a good load for the development of both strength and endurance (~ 10 repetitions). Following are the percentages of 1 RM and the range of repetitions that are typically used in training.

% 1 RM	Repetition Range
100	1
95	2–4
90	4–6
85	6–8
80	8–10
75	10–12
70	12–14
65	14–16
60	16–18

   NOTE: 1RM testing is not recommended for the average client due to the intimidation factor and the risks inherent in any type of maximal test (see Chapter 5, "Fitness Assessment").

10. **Determine the length of the rest period between sets and/or between exercises.** With high-intensity or maximal training (to momentary muscle failure), a longer rest period is generally needed (2–3 minutes). Some studies indicate that a longer rest/recovery time enables greater phosphagen repletion within the muscle, potentially enabling it to generate greater force (Kraemer & Ratamess, 2004). With low-intensity or submaximal training (to the point of fatigue), no rest (or a very short rest) may be needed. Yet another viewpoint is to provide a rest period of

2–3 minutes for multi-joint exercises, while only 1–2 minutes may be necessary for single joint exercises that do not produce as much fatigue (Sorace & Lafontaine, 2005). For sports-specific needs, the rest period may be manipulated to encourage better lactic acid tolerance.

11. **Plan ahead for progressive overload.** For general strength and endurance goals, review the double-progressive approach discussed earlier in this chapter. When deciding how much to increase the weight, the following recommendations may be useful: for beginners, increase the weight by 2.5–5%; for intermediate to advanced clients, increase the weight by 5–10%. In both cases, lower body weights can be increased to a greater degree than upper body weights.

12. **Determine how the training program will be varied over time.** This may be either a within-the-week-type variation (e.g., Monday—heavy weights, Wednesday—light weights, Friday—medium to heavy weights), or a longer term-type cycling called periodization.

    Periodization refers to variations in the training program over the course of several months or a year that help to improve performance and prevent injury, staleness, and burnout. (Rhea, Alvar, & Burkett, 2002). The concept of periodization is supported by Hans Selye's General Adaptation Syndrome (GAS) theory, which suggests that the body goes through three phases of adaptation: (1) alarm or shock—muscle soreness develops and performance may decrease as a result of a bout of resistance training; (2) adaptation—the body adapts to resistance training and strength increases; (3) exhaustion or staleness—the body has adapted, reached a plateau, and no new changes take place, or the body is not given a chance to adapt, and injury and burnout result (Selye, 1976). With training variations over time (periodization), staleness, burnout, and injury are less likely; the body's potential for increased strength (adaptation to training) is enhanced.

    There are a number of ways in which authorities have qualified periodization. Some periodization literature divides the time frames into cycles: (1) a microcycle—the shortest time frame (1–4 weeks) in which short-term goals are set, such as training in the gym three times per week; (2) a mesocycle—(3–4 months), which entails achieving a longer-term goal such as measurably increased muscle power; and (3) a macrocycle—(6–12 months), which includes a long-term goal such as competing in a sports event. According to Fleck and Kraemer (1997), periodization consists of four phases: (1) training for hypertrophy, (2) training for strength, (3) training for power, and (4) training at peak intensity. The whole cycle is followed by a period of active rest (a fifth phase). In addition, ACSM (2006b) presents the following model of periodization: (1) general preparation phase (6–8 weeks) wherein basic fitness levels are acquired; (2) preparation phase (2–4 weeks) with high-volume and low-intensity training; (3) strength phase (2–4 weeks) incorporating lower volumes, higher intensities, and longer rest durations; (4) power phase (2–4 weeks) consisting of speed training and low volumes and very high intensities; and (5) transition phase (several days to 2 weeks), also called active recovery.

    You can create your own periodization cycle, arranging phases and/or methods of resistance training to suit client needs. Although the concept may sound complex, it's really just about changing your client's program over time in order to stimulate the greatest positive changes, and minimize any negative changes such as injury and drop-out. Below is a sample program appropriate for a strength athlete.

Phase	Level	Sets	Repetitions	Weight	Training Methods
1	Hypertrophy	4–6	8–20	Low weight	High-volume training, such as super-sets, giant sets, light to heavy pyramids
2	Strength	3–5	3–8	Heavy weight	More intense training methods, such as heavy to light pyramids, priority muscle training, full (double) pyramids
3	Power	3–5	2–3	Heavier weight	More intense training methods utilizing speed
4	Peak	1–3	1–3	Very heavy weight	Blitz training, forced reps, power drills
5	Active rest	1–2	8–12	Low to moderate weight	Circuit weight training, single sets

Resistance Training Systems

Many clients reach a point where further increases in strength become difficult and progress seems to stop. This is called a **plateau**. There are several strategies for overcoming strength plateaus, including: choosing different exercises, increasing rest and recovery time, varying the number of sets or repetitions, varying the intensity or speed, and/or choosing a different training system.

A knowledge of various systems of resistance training is useful in helping clients to overcome plateaus and optimize results. Although no multiple-set system has been conclusively shown in research studies to be better than any other system, varying the method of training can help prevent injuries, overtraining, and boredom. Resistance training systems can be part of every personal fitness trainer's "toolbox," and include the following.

- **Single-set system**—This is the basic system (one set of 8–12 repetitions for each muscle group) that is widely recommended and used for beginners and those interested in an effective, time-efficient workout (most of the general public).
- **Multiple-set system**—This system is also widely used. It consists of three to six sets of an exercise (usually with the same weight load throughout).
- **Super-set system**—A super-set is any combination of two different exercises immediately following one another without a rest (this may be repeated for several sets). This system is popular with bodybuilders and is said anecdotally to produce hypertrophy. There are several different types of super-sets.
  - Two exercises for the same muscle group: e.g., military press, lateral raises, military press, lateral raises
  - Two exercises for opposing muscle groups, e.g., military press, lat pull-down, military press, lat pull-down
  - Two exercises alternating upper body with lower body, e.g., military press, barbell squat, military press, barbell squat

- **Tri-set system**—Tri-sets are similar to super-sets except that three different exercises immediately follow one another (usually for the same muscle group). There is no rest between exercises or between sets. An example might be: barbell incline bench press, flat bench dumbbell fly, standing cable crossovers.
- **Giant set** (also known as a compound set)—These are similar to super-sets and tri-sets except that four to six different exercises may follow one another without a rest. These are often used for muscle groups (such as abdominals) where many different variations of an exercise are possible.
- **Pyramids**—There are three major types of pyramid training.
  - Light to heavy or ascending pyramid (modified DeLorme method)—here the weight is increased and the repetitions are decreased with each set.
  - Heavy to light or descending pyramid (two types): (1) the Oxford technique, which is simply the reverse of the ascending pyramid above (adjusting for the 1 RM start)—the weight decreases while the repetitions increase; or (2) decreasing weights and decreasing repetitions. This second type is also known as breakdown training.
  - Complete pyramid or triangle program—an exhaustive, intense training method combining light-to-heavy with heavy-to-light, first increasing the resistance and then decreasing it.

Pyramids

For ex., start with 1 RM	For ex., start with 12 RM	
25 lb / 1 rep	40 lb / 1 rep	25 lb / 12 rep	25 lb / 1 rep
20 lb / 5 reps	35 lb / 2 reps	20 lb / 8 reps	20 lb / 5 reps
15 lb / 10 reps	30 lb / 4 reps	15 lb / 5 reps	15 lb / 10 reps
10 lb / 15 reps	25 lb / 6 reps	12 lb / 1 rep	10 lb / 15 reps

For ex., start with 15 RM   Oxford Technique   Decreasing Weights/Reps   For ex., start with 15 RM

Ascending Pyramid   Descending Pyramid   Complete Pyramid
(Light to Heavy)   (Heavy to Light)   (Triangle Program)

- **Pre-exhaustion system**—This widely used technique simply means performing exercises that isolate large muscles first, prior to exercises that work both large and small muscles simultaneously. For example, if your client is super-setting bench presses with dumbbell flys, perform the flys first for pre-exhaustion of the large pectoralis major and anterior deltoid group. This helps ensure that the smaller triceps group (needed for elbow extension during the bench press) won't fatigue before the larger chest muscles and, thereby, limit the potential for overload.
- **Priority training**—This simple concept entails training weaker, less developed muscles first during workouts while the client is most energetic. Strong, developed muscles are not emphasized, but are put on maintenance during this kind of training.
- **Split routine system**—This is a common method of organizing exercises so that clients can train more frequently during a week. Exercises are arranged so that no body part is worked 2 days in a row; each muscle group is allowed sufficient recovery time. Because the client weight

trains four to six times per week, this system allows for greater volume and higher intensity workouts than would be possible if all exercises were performed together on alternate days.

- 4-day split example: Monday/Thursday—train legs, gluteals, lower back, and abdominals; Tuesday/Friday—train chest, upper back, shoulders, and arms
- 6-day split example: Monday/Thursday—train lower body (thighs, gluteals, and calves); Tuesday/Friday—train chest, shoulders, and triceps; Wednesday/Saturday—train latissimus dorsi, trapezius muscles, and biceps

- **Blitz system**—This intense system is a variation of the split routine. In this case, a single body part is isolated each day, keeping the duration and volume of the workout the same. Blitz training is often used by bodybuilders and athletes before a competition. For example: Monday—chest, Tuesday—back, Wednesday—shoulders, Thursday—arms, Friday—legs, Saturday—trunk.

- **Circuit training**—With this program, your client moves quickly from one resistance training exercise to another with very little rest between exercises. Only one set is performed with 8–20 repetitions at 40–60% of 1 RM. The circuit can be repeated several times. Advantages of this system are its time efficiency and the fact that it has also been shown to cause modest aerobic conditioning (Gettman & Pollock, 1981). Note that improvements in cardiovascular fitness are substantially less (4–12% increase in VO_2 max) than those derived from running-type programs (15–20% increase).

- **Super-circuit training**—This system is popular in group exercise classes. It alternates approximately 1–3 minutes of aerobic-type training (e.g., step, cycling, treadmill running) with approximately 1 minute of resistance training for a particular body part. Several different stations or exercises may be used for the resistance training segments.

- **Partial repetitions** (or burn system)—After a set of full-range-of-motion exercises are completed to exhaustion, partial-range-of-motion exercises are performed, also to the point of exhaustion. Strict form must be maintained.

- **Forced repetitions**—Similar to the burn system, forced repetitions are those that are performed after a full set of range-of-motion exercises are completed to exhaustion. Forced repetitions, however, are assisted. The trainer assists the client to force out additional repetitions with proper form and spotting technique.

- **Eccentric (negative) training**—Similar to forced repetitions, this type of training emphasizes the "negative" or eccentric phase of the contraction. This can be done with special types of equipment (such as Keiser) in which the resistance can be increased with the push of a button during the eccentric phase, and decreased during the concentric phase; or with the trainer assisting during the concentric phase and allowing the client to lower the weight unassisted. Muscles are approximately 30–40% stronger during the eccentric phase, and some studies have shown that eccentric training helps maximize strength and hypertrophy gains (Dudley, Tesch, Miller, & Buchanan, 1991). However, it should be noted that eccentric training has also been shown to be a primary instigator of delayed onset muscle soreness and is somewhat controversial.

- **Super-slow training**—In this type of training, repetitions are performed very slowly: concentric contractions may take as long as 10 seconds to move through full range of motion. Once in the fully contracted position, there is a pause (isometric contraction), and then a slow return (about 4–6 seconds) to the starting position.

- **Cheat system**—Although this system is popular with bodybuilders, it is not recommended because of the high risk of injury. It involves performing a set of exercises to exhaustion, then performing a few more repetitions by breaking proper form and allowing momentum and other muscle groups to assist.

Resistance Training Equipment and Methods

Resistance training equipment falls into three main categories:
- dynamic constant resistance
- dynamic variable resistance
- isokinetic

With **dynamic constant resistance** equipment the external resistance or weight does not vary through the range of motion. Barbells and dumbbells are examples of constant resistance; if you lift a 20-pound dumbbell, it remains 20 pounds throughout the exercise.

Dynamic variable resistance equipment attempts to match the external resistance to the exerciser's strength curve. Strength varies throughout the range of motion for each muscle. For example, the biceps brachii can exert maximal strength at approximately 100° of elbow flexion, but is much weaker at 60° and at 180° (the end ranges) (Wilmore & Costill, 2004). This is due both to the angle of pull of the muscle and to the muscle's length-tension relationship. (Maximal tension can be produced when the sarcomeres are at an optimal length and all myosin cross-bridges connect with actin filaments.) Because of the differences in strength throughout the range of motion, the heaviest constant weight that can be lifted can be no heavier than the weight that can be lifted at the weakest point of the muscle. Variable resistance equipment is designed to compensate for this problem. Such equipment as cams, moving levers, pulleys, and air resistance are used to alter the resistance through the range of motion, ideally providing maximal tension at all joint angles. Nautilus®, Bodymaster®, Icarion®, Camstar®, Cybex®, and Keiser® are a few examples of manufacturers who make variable resistance equipment.

It should be noted that traditional weight-room equipment is often designed to isolate a specific muscle or muscle group, and is usually manufactured to move the body in a single plane or single path. Some newer equipment designs (e.g., Freemotion™), however, promote a more functional, multi-joint, multi-planar exercise program. This type of equipment attempts to duplicate real-world movements, incorporating "free" paths of motion and core stabilization principles.

Isokinetic resistance equipment maintains constant muscle tension at a steady speed or velocity. This preset speed cannot be suddenly increased; any force applied against the equipment results in an equal reaction force. Theoretically, muscles could contract maximally through the full range of motion. This premise, as well as the fact that the controlled speed enhances safety, makes isokinetic equipment popular with both elite athletes and physical therapists (it is usually found in rehabilitation centers).

Advantages and disadvantages of the three major types of resistance training equipment are shown in Table 7-2.

Table 7-2.	Types of Resistance Training Equipment		
Equipment Examples	**Constant Resistance**	**Variable Resistance**	**Isokinetic Resistance**
Advantages	• simple; easy to use • relatively inexpensive • requires balance resulting in better coordination and greater muscle utilization • provides for greater variability • easy to maintain • takes up very little space • exercises resemble real-life movements • both multi-and single-joint exercises	• safe; easy to use • good for beginners because less balance is required • productivity in a short amount of time • requires less supervision • ideal for circuit training-isolates muscle groups	• safe; easy to use • excellent for rehabilitation • intense workout in a short amount of time • detailed performance feedback
Disadvantages	• requires strength to maintain balance and coordination • accidents are more likely to happen • spotters are required • complete workouts may take up more time • inability to train through full range of motion in many exercises • poor matching of resistance to strength curve	• lack of development of balance and coordination • constrained movement patterns • machines are expensive • machines take up a lot of space • machines do not adjust for all sizes	• lack of development of balance and joint strength • lack of variety • muscles are worked in isolation • machines are very expensive • machines take up a lot of space • lack of accessibility • some lack ability to perform eccentric contractions

Equipment Inventory

In order to familiarize yourself with weight-room equipment, review the equipment in as many facilities as possible. Identify whether the machines provide constant or variable resistance, what exercises can be performed on which machines, types of free weights, etc. Typical weight-room equipment might include the following.

Constant Resistance	
• Bench press bench (wide uprights for Olympic bar)	• Flat benches
• Incline bench (adjustable)	• Slant board
• Decline bench	• Roman chair
• Preacher curl	• Set-up for pull-ups and dips
• Olympic bar with plates	• Smith machine
• Standard bar with plates	• Squat rack
• Collars for bars	• Lunge box
• EZ curl bar	• Leg press
• Dumbbells	• Calf machines (standing, seated, donkey)
• Cable set-ups with high and/or low pulleys	• Gravitron

Variable Resistance	
• Chest press machine	• Abdominal curl machine (note whether machine targets abdominals or hip flexors)
• Pec dec machine	
• Scapular adduction machine	
• Lateral raise machine	• Seated rotary torso machine
• Military press machine	• Back extension machine
• Lat pull-down machine	• Leg press machine
• Lat pull-over machine	• Knee extension machine
• Biceps curl machine	• Knee curl machine
• Triceps extension machine	• Standing multi-hip machine
	• Seated abduction/adduction machine

In addition to the major types of resistance equipment listed in the equipment inventory boxes above, many other options are available to personal fitness trainers, including the following.

- Elastic resistance—tubes and bands are portable, inexpensive, available in several thicknesses, and can provide a wide variety of exercise options. A number of studies show that resistance training with elastic can be a valuable supplement or alternative to traditional weight training (Page & Ellenbecker, 2003).
- Manual resistance—applying skillful, careful, and appropriate hands-on resistance to your client
- Small equipment, such as stability balls, medicine balls, foam rollers, BOSU, slides, ankle weights, wobble boards, and core boards.

Other Resistance Training Methods

Isometric (static) resistance training involves contracting a muscle in a held position (no change in the joint angle), usually against a wall, weight machine, or against another part of the body. Increases in strength and endurance have been shown from isometric training, especially when the contractions are held for at least 6 seconds with a maximal effort, and several contractions per day are performed (American College of Sports Medicine, 2006b). Isometric training is a common modality in rehabilitation, as it helps maintain strength without excessive joint movement. However, there are several training factors to be considered when utilizing isometric exercises: strength gains will be greatest closest to the joint angle at which the exercise is performed; isometric exercise may not increase specific motor performance skills; and if performed without proper breathing technique, may cause blood pressure elevation. The rise in blood pressure occurs when the held contraction is accompanied by the Valsalva maneuver (breath holding while bearing down on the glottis). This may create a potentially dangerous situation for cardiac patients, hypertensives, and pregnant women. All clients must be consistently reminded to breathe if isometric exercises are performed.

The word "core" has different meanings, according to the context in which it is applied. The National Strength and Conditioning Association (2004) states that a **core exercise** is any exercise that is multi-joint and recruits one or more large muscle groups or areas with the synergistic help of one or more smaller muscle groups. Examples of core exercises include the bench press, shoulder press, and back squat. It is suggested that personal fitness trainers move their clients toward skilled and regular performance of core exercises.

Alternatively, the word "core" is often applied to **core training**, or core stabilization exercises; in this case, core refers to the center of the body, or torso. Specifically, core training most often incorporates stabilization exercises for the muscles of the spine, neck, pelvis, and scapulae. In addition to training more familiar muscles, such as the rectus abdominis, obliques, and erector spinae, personal fitness trainers are encouraged to include exercises that train the transverse abdominis, multifidus, diaphragm, pelvic floor muscles, scapular retractors, and scapular depressors. Several studies show that training these muscles may help to reduce the incidence of low-back pain and back dysfunction (Hodges & Richardson, 1996; O'Sullivan et al., 1997). See Chapter 8, "Applied Resistance Training Skills," for some examples of exercises in which the core is specifically challenged to remain in neutral alignment.

Balance is the ability to maintain a position without moving for a certain period of time, and can also be defined as a state of bodily equilibrium, or the ability to maintain the center of body mass over the base of support without falling (Irrgang, Whitney, & Cox, 1994). In sports and activities of daily living, muscles and neurological pathways need to work together to create dynamic, or functional, balance; for example, when going down or up stairs, balance is required for short periods of time on each step. Balance is also required with each step during walking or running. In older adults, as balance abilities decline, functional independence also declines. In order to improve balance, proprioceptors (organelles that send messages to the brain regarding movement and spatial positioning) must be trained. You can help clients become better at balance by training them on less stable surfaces. For example, you could move from standing on two feet to standing on one foot, then progress to standing on a balance board, half foam roller, core board, BOSU, Dyna Disc, or wobble board. Stability balls are excellent for training balance in a variety of positions, such as prone, supine, seated, or side-lying. Dynamic balance can be trained by stepping or hopping up to a one-leg balance (on a step bench) and other sports-type drills, such as zig-zags with a balance on one leg at the end of each change of direction. Additional balance exercises are suggested in Chapter 8, "Applied Resistance Training Skills."

Plyometric training involves using the stretch reflex to increase muscle fiber recruitment (Wilk et al., 1993). Known also as jump, rebound, reactive, or power training, plyometric exercises eccentrically load the muscle, and require muscles to explosively contract on the rebound. This type of training is more appropriate for athletes as it helps develop speed and power. However, it should be avoided for deconditioned clients due to the need for increased levels of coordination and the high potential for injury. Examples of plyometric-type exercises include: squat jumps, horizontal jumps, tuck jumps, medicine ball passes, depth/plyo push-ups, and abdominal curl-ups with a medicine ball pass.

Common Training Errors and Safety Considerations

It is helpful to be aware of the most common errors that clients, especially new clients, make when performing exercises. You will find common errors listed for each exercise in Chapter 8, "Applied Resistance Training Skills." However, the most general **common training errors** include the following.

- The client uses too much weight, resulting in poor alignment and technique and an increased risk of injury.
- The client performs an improper warm-up, or none at all, leading to injury.
- The client is unable to keep his/her core stabilized, leading to injury (most commonly of the back).
- Safety devices (clips, collars) are not used.
- The client holds his or her breath (Valsalva maneuver).
- The client has range-of-motion problems (e.g., excessive range of motion may cause joints to hyperextend, resulting in poor alignment, whereas inadequate range of motion may not cause an appropriate training stimulus).
- The client performs the exercise too quickly, leading to an increased risk of injury.

Additionally, clients often have predictable problems depending on their skill and fitness levels.

Beginners often:

- have trouble with core and scapular stabilization. Therefore, in the initial stages of training, you'll want to focus on basic stabilization exercises (such as those suggested in the "Torso Stability Exercises" section of Chapter 8, "Applied Resistance Training Skills") and on basic scapular retraction and depression exercises (also in Chapter 8) for scapular stability. Usually, it is best to provide beginner clients with basic machine exercises because most machines place the exerciser in a stable and supported position.
- need to move slowly to develop body, or kinesthetic, awareness. For this reason, single joint, isolation-type exercises are recommended in

order to help novice exercisers understand how to consciously contract specific muscles.

- do not know their limits, and often push beyond appropriate levels in the belief that "more is better," or "no pain, no gain." This kind of thinking can lead to injury and drop-out. The paradigm "no pain, no gain," if appropriate at all, belongs in the military or for highly skilled and competitive athletes—it is never appropriate for novice exercisers!

- have difficulty telling the difference between muscle soreness and inappropriate joint pain. Here again, if the operating motto is "no pain, no gain," a client may think that knee pain, back pain, foot pain, etc. are a necessary part of becoming fit. Your job, in this case, is to provide education to your client without diminishing his or her motivation or crossing the line in providing advice reserved for provision by licensed health care providers.

- need simple, direct, and short cues. A novice exerciser is often distracted by the sights and sounds of the gym and the novelty of the situation.

Intermediates often:

- are better at maintaining core and scapular stability all the way through a set.

- can perform more complex exercises. During this stage you'll start moving your client towards free-weight exercises and less stable surfaces; you'll also incorporate more multi-joint, multi-muscle exercises.

- have better kinesthetic awareness; they are in better control of their bodies.

- can begin to utilize more advanced training systems, such as super-sets or super-slow techniques.

- need more detailed cues. More skilled exercisers may enjoy understanding the "why" and the "how" of various exercises. For example, when giving the cue to keep the scapulae depressed during a lat pull-down, you may find yourself stopping and explaining how an unstable shoulder girdle can contribute to shoulder injuries.

- may plateau (see "Resistance Training Systems" earlier in this chapter).

Advanced exercisers often:

- can maintain stability throughout the entire workout.

- can perform sports-specific exercises. Advanced exercises are often performed on an unstable surface (such as a half-foam roller, BOSU, or wobble board), involve speed or plyometric movements, require balance (may be performed on one leg), or add rotational movements (such as the reverse wood-chopper exercise, where a medicine ball may be lifted from ground on the left side of the body and rotated up to the ceiling on the right side of the body). Such movements increase the risk of injury, and should therefore be carefully applied only to highly skilled and fit exercisers. Additionally, if the exercise is truly high risk, consider whether its benefit outweighs the risk for your client. A client may need to perform a high-risk exercise (such as a dead lift) if he or she is competing in an upcoming event that requires that exercise (such as a power-lifting competition).

- know their bodies well enough to know when to stop before injury occurs.
- tend to approach all aspects of their workout with patience and thoroughness.

Using the AFAA Five Questions

The AFAA Five Questions were developed to help you decide whether an exercise is appropriate for your client, taking into consideration an exercise's purpose, effectiveness, and level of safety (Aerobics and Fitness Association of America, 2002). This system of questioning an exercise is an excellent method for you to analyze, on a case-by-case basis, the exercises you choose at any given time. The AFAA Five Questions are as follows.

1. What is the purpose of this exercise?
   Consider: muscular strength or endurance, cardiorespiratory conditioning, flexibility, warm-up or activity preparation, skill development, and stress reduction
2. Are you doing that effectively?
   Consider: proper range, speed, or body position against gravity
3. Does the exercise create any safety concerns?
   Consider: potential stress areas, environmental concerns, or movement control
4. Can you maintain proper alignment and form for the duration of the exercise?
   Consider: form, alignment, or stabilization
5. For whom is the exercise appropriate or inappropriate?
   Consider: risk-to-benefit ratio, whether the exerciser is at a beginner, intermediate, or advanced level

Safety Factors

Safety factors are specifically covered for each exercise given in Chapter 8 ("Applied Resistance Training Skills"), and are also addressed joint by joint in Chapter 10 ("Injury Prevention"). Because it is so important for personal fitness trainers to understand safety and mechanism of injury, another list of common injuries and injury mechanisms with exercise examples is provided below.

Body Part	Common Injuries/ Mechanisms of Injuries	Exercise Example
Cervical spine	ballistic hyperextension	fast, full head circles
	ballistic or loaded hyperflexion	yoga plow
Lumbar spine	ballistic hyperextension	Roman chair extensions, uncontrolled cable hip extensions
	ballistic or loaded extreme flexion	stiff-legged dead lifts, good mornings
	rotation combined with the above	windmills, bar twists
	hip flexor traction on lumbar spine	bilateral supine leg lifts, full sit-ups
Shoulder	impingement	upright rows, lateral raises with > 90° abduction
	rotator cuff problems	behind-the-neck lat pull down, military press, snatch and power clean
	dislocation	supine DB flys with excessive ROM
Knee	hyperflexion	deep squats, deep lunges

Muscle Soreness

There are two main types of muscle discomfort and soreness: acute and delayed-onset. **Acute muscle soreness** occurs during and immediately after exercise and is due to the accumulation of lactate, decreased oxygen, and tissue swelling within the muscle. This type of discomfort or soreness is usually short-lasting and disappears immediately after the exercise is over. **Delayed onset muscle soreness** (DOMS) occurs 24–48 hours post-exercise. Theories that explain DOMS include: damage (ruptures and structural changes) to the muscle fibers themselves; inflammation with accompanying increased white blood cell count; and the stimulation of nerve endings as a result of tissue repair activity. DOMS appears to be even more likely after eccentric exercise, during which large forces are distributed over relatively small cross-sectional areas of muscle (Clarkson & Sayers, 1999). Training methods that focus on eccentric (negative) muscle actions should be avoided in the initial stages of training, especially with inactive populations. DOMS may be perceived as unpleasant and contribute to noncompliance. Strategies for managing DOMS may include stretching, ice, rest, and nutritional supplementation, although none of these methods have been shown conclusively to help. There are definite legal risks associated with the recommendation of any form of nutritional supplements. AFAA's Nutritional Supplement Policy should be consulted in this regard; see Appendix D. Such supplements should **never** be used to treat or cure any medical condition.

From a behavioral standpoint, many trainers have observed that some clients want to feel sore after a workout; these clients may believe that they haven't had a good workout unless they're sore afterwards. Still other clients, however, do not want to be sore from their personal training sessions; this type of client may include seniors, beginners, those with some type of injury, or deconditioned persons wary of exercise. As a personal fitness trainer, you need to be sensitive to the outcomes expected by your various clients and adjust their programs accordingly. Often the simplest thing to do is ask your client directly if he/she wants to feel muscle soreness after a workout or not. If a client is quite deconditioned, explaining to him/her that a little muscle soreness is normal can be helpful. However, as the trainer, you should attempt to minimize exercises and routines that typically cause soreness in order to avoid discouraging your client from continuing.

Resistance Training Sports

There are three main resistance training sports; some personal fitness trainers specialize in training clients for these events.

- **Bodybuilding**—Competitive bodybuilders are judged according to muscle hypertrophy, definition, and symmetry. Posing ability is also important. A typical bodybuilding routine involves performing several exercises per muscle group to maximize fiber recruitment and stress the muscle from a number of angles. Many sets (four to six) of several repetitions are performed with very brief rests (~ 15–45 seconds) between sets. The brief rest periods are said to produce a "muscle pump." Split routines and super setting are popular training systems. Prior to competition, dietary manipulations are sometimes used by some competitors in attempts to reduce body fat and allow the developed musculature to be visible.
- **Power lifting**—Power lifters compete in three lifts: the bench press, squat, and the dead lift. The winner must lift the most weight in all three lifts for their weight class. Since the goal is to lift the most weight possible, competitors train for strength with heavy loads (1–6 RM), several sets, and long rest periods (2–5 minutes, depending on the resistance). Training revolves around the competition exercises with assistor and stabilizer muscle groups worked last.
- **Olympic lifting**—This Olympic sport involves two events: the snatch and the clean and jerk. The winner totals the most weight between the two lifts for his/her weight class. Skill and technique are very important in the execution of the lifts. Competitors train for strength and power with heavy loads (1–6 RM), many sets, and lengthy rest periods, with a special emphasis on pulling-type movements.

Ergogenic Aids

An **ergogenic aid** is a substance or device that improves, or is thought to improve, an athlete's performance (some so-called ergogenic aids actually detract from performance). There is a long list of possible ergogenic aids, including: alcohol, drugs, hormones, blood doping, oxygen, vitamins and minerals, creatine, protein supplements, carbo-loading, and certain kinds of equipment or clothing. Following is a brief discussion of several common ergogenic aids.

- **Anabolic steroids**—synthetic derivatives of the male sex hormone testosterone, taken to increase muscle mass and strength. Studies have shown that steroids are effective for this purpose at high dosages, but that the risks of taking steroids are very serious. In addition to being illegal and unethical, the risks include: testicular atrophy, reduced sperm count, breast enlargement in men and breast regression in women, prostate gland enlargement in men, masculinization in women, liver damage, cardiovascular disease, and personality changes (Clark & Henderson, 2003). Anabolic steroids can also increase the growth of cancer cells.

- **Human Growth Hormone (hGH)**—a hormone secreted by the anterior pituitary gland that has been shown to increase lean body mass and decrease fat mass (Nindl, Kraemer, Marx, Tuckow, & Hymer, 2003). However, as with other steroids, there are several potential risks. These include: acromegaly (enlargement of the hands, feet, and face, and skin thickening), edema (fluid retention that may result in carpal tunnel syndrone), glucose intolerance, hypertension, muscle and joint pain, cardiomyopathy, and benign intracranial pressure resulting in headaches.

- **Blood doping**—an artificial increase in a person's total volume of red blood cells (via transfusion), enhancing endurance performance. Risks include: blood clotting, heart failure, and the potential for injections of improperly labeled blood, leading to the transmission of hepatitis and human immunodeficiency virus (HIV, the virus that causes AIDS).

- **Creatine**—an extremely popular supplement, creatine has been shown to enhance high-intensity, short-duration exercise (Becque, Lochmann, & Melrose, 2000). However, no effect has been shown on long duration, endurance-type exercise such as distance running and cycling. Scientists are concerned about the long-term effects of creatine supplementation; some studies have shown kidney function deterioration. Note that without simultaneous exercise training, creatine taken alone has no measurable benefit.

- **Caffeine**—a central nervous system stimulant that is sometimes used to enhance energy levels, endurance, and reaction time. Although not all studies agree, most recent studies show that caffeine does improve endurance performance (Bell & McLellan, 2002). Risks include: nervousness, restlessness, insomnia, and tremors in those consuming high doses and/or who are sensitive to caffeine. It also acts as a diuretic, increasing the risk of dehydration and heat stress.

Important Factors in the Development of Strength

The influence of genetics on training can scarcely be overemphasized. The goal of proper training is to optimize results within the limits set by each client's genetic potential. In order to avoid unnecessary frustration and discouragement, it is important to help clients understand the following strength factors over which they have no control.

Biomechanical Factors

- **Limb length**—Shorter limbs mean shorter levers, and a shorter lever has a biomechanical advantage (the resistance, or weight, is closer to the fulcrum, or joint, and is easier to lift than a weight that is farther away). In general, clients with shorter limbs will be able to lift more weight than clients with longer limbs, all other factors being equal.

- **Tendon insertion**—The further the muscle tendon attaches from the joint, or axis, the greater the mechanical advantage affecting muscle strength.

Muscular Factors
- **Muscle belly length**—This is the length of the muscle fibers, not including the attached tendons. Clients with greater muscle tissue (as opposed to tendon, or connective tissue) apparently have a greater ability to develop muscle size and strength.
- **Muscle fiber composition**—Fast twitch (FT) fibers tend to hypertrophy more readily than slow twitch (ST) fibers. (A muscle that hypertrophies increases in fiber size, and strength production is directly related to a muscle's size or cross-sectional area.) Clients who inherited a high percentage of FT fibers will be more successful at strength and power activities, all other factors being equal.

Hormonal Factors
- **Testosterone**—This male sex hormone has a positive influence on the ability of a muscle to hypertrophy; the higher levels of testosterone in men lead to greater muscle size (and greater strength production) and account for the major difference between men and women in strength training. Women typically experience much less muscle growth than men; the average woman has about one tenth the testosterone of the average man. (Testosterone levels are on a continuum with both men and women; a few women do normally possess higher levels.)

Neurological Factors
The most rapid gains in a strength training program are usually at the beginning (1–2 months) as the following neurological adaptations take place.
- Recruitment of additional motor units (thus increasing the muscle's ability to produce force)
- Increased synchronization of the motor units (more motor units fire at one time)
- More efficient recruitment order
- Decreased activity from inhibitory Golgi tendon organs

(Note that the factors listed above are not completely under voluntary control.)

Resistance Training Strength Gains
Early gains in strength appear to be more influenced by neural factors, but later long-term gains are almost solely the result of hypertrophy (Wilmore & Costill, 2004). Neural factors may include the following.
- Recruitment of additional motor units (increasing a muscle's ability to generate force)
- Decreased activity from inhibitory Golgi tendon organs
- Improved coordination
- Improved motor learning

Chronic muscle hypertrophy (increase in fiber size) appears to be related to the following.
- Increased myofibrils
- Increased actin and myosin filaments
- Increased connective tissue
- Increased capillary density
- Increased muscle protein synthesis
- High levels of testosterone
- Intense resistance training

Whether or not strength gains result from muscle hyperplasia (increase in the number of muscle fibers) remains controversial. Hyperplasia has been shown in animal studies, but human studies have been inconclusive (Antonio & Gonyea, 1993). There seems to be a definite need for further research addressing hyperplasia in humans.

In the early stages of resistance training, strength gains are usually more dramatic because of the large genetic potential to be realized. After this period of rapid initial strength gain, improvement continues, but at an increasingly slower rate as an individual gets closer to realizing his/her genetic potential.

Overtraining, Detraining, and Retraining Issues

Overtraining occurs when physical performance decreases, even with continued training (Fry & Kraemer, 1997), and is a mixture of emotional, behavioral, and physical symptoms caused by excessive training and not enough rest. Symptoms of overtraining syndrome include the following.

- Decline in physical performance
- Loss of muscle strength, coordination, and maximal working capacity
- Decreased appetite and body weight loss
- Muscle tenderness and joint soreness
- Increased number of minor injuries, muscle strains, etc.
- Occasional nausea
- Sleep disturbances
- Elevated resting heart rate
- Elevated blood pressure
- Emotional instability (apathy, depression, irritability)
- Loss of motivation to exercise

Overtraining also suppresses normal immune function and causes increased susceptibility to infections. Counseling and complete rest may be necessary to help athletes obsessed with training overcome symptoms. Overtraining syndrome may be avoided by following periodization or cyclical training-type programs, alternating hard, easy, and moderate periods of training. In addition, allowing adequate time for recovery between bouts of intense exercise is critical. Be cautious if your client is highly motivated and engages in high levels of exercise intensity, duration, and frequency. This type of client combined with an overly aggressive trainer can easily result in overtraining. Help your client to respect his or her body and know when to reduce the level of training.

Detraining is a deconditioning process that occurs as a result of inactivity and/or the cessation of regular physical training. It is the opposite of what a client experiences during the training program. Complete inactivity, or immobilization, causes the most severe responses to detraining. Skeletal muscle atrophy results from inactivity, with a resulting decline in muscle strength and power. However, this decline is relatively small during the first few months, especially if there is no complete immobilization. Several studies have shown that strength can be maintained with only minimal stimulation (exercise once every 10–14 days). In contrast, muscle and cardiorespiratory endurance decrease much more rapidly. This is thought to be due to: decreased oxidative enzyme activities, decreased muscle glycogen storage, disturbance of the acid-base balance, and decreased blood supply to the muscles. Training at least three times per week at 70% of regular training intensity is necessary to maintain cardiorespiratory endurance (Wilmore & Costill, 2004).

Retraining refers to the concept that the more fit clients are, the more they have to lose during periods of detraining. As a result, they also have more to recover during periods of retraining, and the process of regaining peak fitness will take longer. Retraining, therefore, is influenced by the client's fitness level and the duration of the inactivity. Note, however, that the neurological pathways of an individual who was once fit are already "primed" for retraining.

Women and Resistance Training

Women tend to be weaker than men primarily because of their lower quantity of muscle. However, given the same amount of muscle, there are no differences in strength between the sexes (Wilmore & Costill, 2004). Some studies show that when strength is expressed relative to lean body mass, men are 45% stronger than women in the bench press, but that women are 6% stronger than men in the leg press (Wilmore, 1974). The large discrepancy between upper and lower body strength may be due to the fact that both men and women walk, run, and climb stairs, but that men usually lift heavy objects with their arms more frequently as compared to women.

Since female muscle tissue has the same physiological characteristics as male muscle tissue, it responds to training in the same manner. Many women are afraid that they will develop large bulky muscles from weight training, but research shows that this is unlikely for the average female. Athletic women who are able to develop significant muscle hypertrophy typically have: (1) higher than normal testosterone levels; (2) a lower than normal estrogen-to-testosterone ratio; (3) a genetic disposition to develop a greater muscle mass; and (4) a very intense resistance training program (Fleck & Kraemer, 1997). In any event, the principle of reversibility states that all exercise adaptations are transient (temporary) and reversible.

Children and Resistance Training

Resistance training for children has been the subject of controversy in the past due to concerns regarding injury to the epiphyseal growth plates of the long bones. However, medical and fitness organizations now agree that preadolescent strength training following recommended guidelines may be appropriate and beneficial; these organizations include the American College of Sports Medicine, the American Academy of Pediatrics, the American Orthopaedic Society for Sports Medicine, and the National Strength and Conditioning Association.

Preadolescence usually describes girls, age 11 or younger, and boys, age 13 or younger. Resistance training may provide many potential benefits for children, including: increased strength of muscles, tendons, and ligaments, increased bone density, improved body composition, reduced risk of injuries, improved motor coordination and performance, and increased likelihood the child will participate in other physical activities. Although concerns exist regarding potential injury to the epiphyseal growth plates, the risk of undue stress can be minimized by avoiding prolonged periods of repetitive impact, and by providing an appropriate frequency, duration, and intensity of exercise (Faigenbaum et al., 1996). A synopsis of the major resistance training guidelines for children follow.
  • All participants should be able to accept and follow directions.
  • The program should be fun, educational, challenging, and safe.

- For apparently healthy children a pre-participation medical exam is desirable, but not necessary.
- Avoid competition in the weight room.
- Strength training should complement and not neglect other components of physical fitness.
- Young or small children should not use weight machines designed for adults.
- Exercises for all major muscle groups should be incorporated.
- Five to 10 minutes of warm-up should precede the resistance training session.
- Exercises should be performed through a full range of motion.
- Use no-load repetitions during the initial learning phase.
- One to three sets of 6–15 repetitions may be used.
- Two to 3 days per week is recommended.
- Qualified adults should provide supervision.
- Participants who continually want to lift maximal weights should be redirected towards developing proper form and technique using submaximal loads on a variety of exercises.
  (Vehrs, 2005)

Common Weight-Room Exercises Grid

Muscles Worked	Exercise	Muscles Worked	Exercise
Chest	Bench press	Mid-trapezius, rhomboids, posterior deltoids	Reverse fly
	Incline/decline press		Horizontal (high) row
	Dumbbell fly		Reverse fly machine
	Bilateral cable cross-over		Prone reverse pec dec
	Push-up		
	Pec dec		
Trapezius (upper)	Shrugs	Trapezius (lower)	Depression dips
			High pulley depression
Deltoids (anterior and medial)	Front raises	Latissimus dorsi	Lat pull-down
	Lateral raises		Bent-over row
	Overhead press		Seated low row
	Upright row		Lat pull-over
	Shoulder press machine		Prone shoulder ext.
Rotator cuff (external)	External rotation with tube		
	Side-lying external rotation		
Biceps	Alt. biceps curls	Triceps	Triceps kickback
	Concentration curl		Standing press-down
	Preacher curl		Overhead/French press
	Standing barbell curl		Supine elbow ext.
	Reverse curl		Triceps dips
	Hammer curl		
Abdominals	Curl-up/crunch	Erector spinae	Back ext. machine
	Hip lift		Prone back ext.
	Supine crunch twist		Roman chair back ext.
	Abdominal machine		
Quadriceps	Knee extension machine	Hamstrings	Knee curl machine
	Supine knee extension		All-fours hip/knee lift
	Leg press machine		Leg press machine
	Squats		Squats
	Lunges		Lunges
Abductors	Abductor machine	Adductors	Adductor machine
	Side-lying abduction		Side-lying adduction
Anterior tibialis	Dorsiflexion with band	Calves	Heel raises

Sample Programs for Resistance Training

Novice

A basic resistance training session for a novice exerciser (weeks 1–4) might include the following.

> - 5-minute warm-up
> - 40–45 minutes of resistance training, 1 set each, 8-12 repetitions to fatigue
>   - Wall squat with stability ball
>   - Smith press squat with no added weight
>   - Leg press machine
>   - Knee extension machine
>   - Knee curl machine
>   - Chest press machine
>   - Reverse fly machine
>   - Shoulder press machine
>   - Seated low row
>   - Triceps machine
>   - Biceps machine
>   - Abdominal machine
>   - Erector spinae machine
> - 5–10 minutes of flexibility training

Intermediate/Advanced

A more complex resistance training session for an intermediate/advanced exerciser (8–12 months into the program) might include the following.

> - 5-minute warm-up
> - 40–45 minutes of upper body super-set resistance training (lower body on another day), 3 sets total per muscle group, 8–12 repetitions to fatigue
>
> | | |
> |---|---|
> | - Latissimus dorsi: | prone shoulder extensions on stability ball
seated low row
lat pull-down |
> | - Deltoids: | lateral raises
front raises
overhead press seated on stability ball |
> | - Chest: | dumbbell flys
bilateral cable cross-over
bench press |
> | - Mid-trapezius, Rhomboids: | reverse flys
reverse cable cross-over
seated high row |
> | - Triceps: | dips
overhead triceps extension
press-down |
> | - Biceps: | alternating dumbbell curls
low-pulley curl with EZ curl bar
concentration curl |
> | - Abdominals: | decline crunch (head lower than hips)
incline hip lift (hips lower than head)
crunch twists on stability ball |
>
> - 5–10 minutes of flexibility training

Summary

This chapter covered benefits of strength and endurance training, strength training guidelines, advantages and disadvantages of different types of resistance training equipment, steps for creating an individualized strength training exercise program, periodization, plateaus, systems of resistance training, and common training errors. Additionally, popular ergogenic aids were briefly discussed. Factors influencing strength were listed, and principles of overtraining, detraining, and retraining were described. Strength training, as it relates to women and children, was also discussed.

References

Aerobics and Fitness Association of America. (2002). *Fitness: Theory and practice* (4th ed., L.A. Gladwin, Ed.). Sherman Oaks, CA: Aerobics and Fitness Association of America.

American College of Sports Medicine. (1998). American College of Sports Medicine position stand: The recommended quantity and quality of exercise for developing and maintaining cardiorespiratory and muscular fitness, and flexibility in healthy adults. *Medicine & Science in Sports & Exercise, 30,* 975-991.

American College of Sports Medicine. (2002). Position stand: Progression models in resistance training for healthy adults. *Medicine & Science in Sports & Exercise, 34*(2), 364-380.

American College of Sports Medicine. (2006a). *ACSM's guidelines for exercise testing and prescription* (7th ed.) Baltimore: Lippincott Williams & Wilkins.

American College of Sports Medicine. (2006b). *ACSM's resource manual for guidelines for exercise testing and prescription* (5th ed.). Baltimore: Lippincott Williams & Wilkins.

Antonio, J., & Gonyea, W.J. (1993). Skeletal muscle hyperplasia. *Medicine & Science in Sports & Exercise, 25*(12), 1333-1345.

Becque, M.D., Lochmann, J.D., & Melrose, D.R. (2000). Effects of oral creatine supplementation on muscular strength and body composition. *Medicine & Science in Sports & Exercise, 32*(3), 654-658.

Bell, D.G., & McLellan, T.M. (2002). Exercise endurance 1, 3, and 6 h. after caffeine ingestion in caffeine users and nonusers. *Journal of Applied Physiology, 93*(4), 1227-1234.

Campos, G.E., Luecke, T.J., & Wendeln, H.K. (2002). Muscular adaptations in response to three different resistance-training regimens: Specificity of repetition maximum training zones. *European Journal of Applied Physiology, 88,* 50-60.

Clark, A.S., & Henderson, L.P. (2003). Behavioral and physiological responses to anabolic-androgenic steroids. *Neuroscience and Biobehavioral Reviews, 27,* 413-436.

Clarkson, P.M., & Sayers, S.P. (1999). Etiology of exercise induced muscle damage. *Canadian Journal of Applied Physiology, 24,* 234-248.

Dudley, G.A., Tesch, P.A., Miller, B.J., & Buchanan, P. (1991). Importance of eccentric actions in performance adaptations to resistance training. *Aviation, Space, and Environmental Medicine, 62,* 543-550.

Faigenbaum, A.D., Kraemer, W.J., Cahill, B., Chandler, J., Dziados, J., Elfrink, L., et al. (1996). Youth resistance training: Position statement paper and literature review. *Strength and Conditioning, 18*(6), 62-75.

Faigenbaum, A., Pollock, M.L., & Ishida, Y. (1999). Prescription of resistance training for health and disease. *Medicine & Science in Sports & Exercise, 31*, 38-45.

Fleck, S.J., & Kraemer, W.J. (1997). *Designing resistance training programs* (2nd ed.). Champaign, IL: Human Kinetics.

Fry, A.C., & Kraemer, W.J. (1997). Resistance exercise overtraining and over-reaching. *Sports Medicine, 23*,106-129.

Gettman, L.R., & Pollock, M.L. (1981). Circuit weight training: A critical review of its physiological benefits. *Physician and Sports Medicine, 9*, 44-60.

Graves, J.E., Pollock, M.L., Jones, A.E., Colvin, A.B., & Leggett, S.H. (1989). Specificity of limited range of motion variable resistance training. *Medicine & Science in Sports & Exercise, 21*, 84-89.

Hass, C.J., Garzarella, L., de Hoyos, D., & Pollock, M.L. (2000). Single versus multiple sets in long-term recreational weightlifters. *Medicine & Science in Sports & Exercise, 32*, 235-242.

Hodges, P.W., & Richardson, C.A. (1996). Inefficient muscular stabilization of the lumbar spine associated with low back pain. *Spine, 21*(22), 2640-2650.

Irrgang, J.J, Whitney, S.L., & Cox, E.D. (1994). Balance and proprioceptive training for rehabilitation of the lower extremity. *Journal of Sport Rehabilitation, 3*, 68-83.

Kraemer, W.J., & Ratamess, N.A. (2004). Fundamentals of resistance training: Progression and exercise prescription. *Medicine & Science in Sports & Exercise, 36*(4), 674-688.

Kramer, J.B., Stone, M.H., O'Bryant, H.S., Conley, M.S., Johnson, R.L., Nieman, D.C., et al. (1997). Effects of single vs. multiple sets of weight training: Impact of volume, intensity, and variation. *Journal of Strength and Conditioning Research, 11*(3), 143-147.

Lemmer, J.T., Ivey, F.M., Ryan, A.S., Martel, G.F., Hurlbut, D.E., Metter, J.E., et al. (2001). Effect of strength training on resting metabolic rate and physical activity: Age and gender comparisons. *Medicine & Science in Sports & Exercise, 33*, 532-541.

MacDougall, J.D., McKelvie, R.S., & Moroz, D.E. (1992). Factors affecting blood pressure during heavy weight lifting and static contractions. *Journal of Applied Physiology, 73*,1590-1597.

National Strength and Conditioning Association. (2004). *National Strength and Conditioning Association's essentials of personal training* (R.W. Earle & T.R. Baechle, Eds.). Champaign, IL: Human Kinetics.

Nindl, B.C., Kraemer, W.J., Marx, J.O., Tuckow, A.P., & Hymer, W.C. (2003). Growth hormone molecular heterogeneity and exercise. *Exercise & Sport Sciences Reviews, 31*(4), 161-166.

O'Sullivan, P.E., Twomey, L., Allison, G., Sinclair, J., Miller, K., & Knox, J. (1997). Altered patterns of abdominal muscle activation in patients with chronic low back pain. *Australian Journal of Physiotherapy, 43*(2), 91-98.

Page, P., & Ellenbecker, T.S. (2003). *The scientific and clinical application of elastic resistance.* Champaign, IL: Human Kinetics.

Pollock, M.L., Franklin, B.A., & Balady, G.J. (2000). AHA Science Advisory. Resistance exercise in individuals with and without cardiovascular disease: Benefits, rationale, safety, and prescription: An advisory from the Committee on Exercise, Rehabilitation, and Prevention, Council on Clinical Cardiology, American Heart Association; Position paper endorsed by the American College of Sports Medicine. *Circulation, 101*, 828-833.

Rhea, M.F., Alvar, B.A., & Burkett, L.N. (2002). Single versus multiple sets for strength: A meta-analysis to address the controversy. *Research Quarterly for Exercise and Sport, 73*, 485-488.

Selye, H. (1976). *The stress of life.* New York: McGraw Hill.

Sorace, P., & LaFontaine, T. (2005). Resistance training muscle power: Design programs that work! *ACSM's Health & Fitness Journal, 9*(2), 6-12.

Stone, W.J., & Coulter, S.P. (1994). Strength/endurance effects from three resistance training protocols with women. *Journal of Strength and Conditioning Research, 8*(4), 231-234.

Van Etten, L.M., Westerterp, K.R., & Verstappen, F.T. (1995). Effect of weight-training on energy expenditure and substrate utilization during sleep. *Medicine & Science in Sports & Exercise, 27*, 188-193.

Vehrs, P.R. (2005). Strength training in children and teens: Implementing safe, effective, and fun programs—part two. *ACSM's Health & Fitness Journal, 9*(4), 13-18.

Weiss, L.W., Coney, H.D., & Clark, F.C. (1999). Differential functional adaptations to short-term low, moderate, high-repetition weight training. *Journal of Strength and Conditioning Research, 13*(3), 236-241.

Wilk, K.E., Voight, M.L., Keirns, M.A., Gambetta, V., Andrews, J.R., & Dillman, C.J. (1993). Stretch-shortening drills for the upper extremities: Theory and clinical application. *Journal of Orthopaedic and Sports Physical Therapy, 17*, 225-239.

Wilmore, J.H. (1974). Alterations in strength, body composition, and anthropometric measurements consequent to a 10-week weight training program. *Medicine & Science in Sports & Exercise, 6*, 133-138.

Wilmore, J.H., & Costill, D.L. (2004). *Physiology of sport and exercise* (3rd ed.). Champaign, IL: Human Kinetics.

Winnett, R.A., & Carpinelli, R.N. (2001). Potential health-related benefits of resistance training. *Preventive Medicine, 33*, 503-513.

Yoke, M.M., & Kennedy, C.A. (2004). *Functional exercise progressions.* Monterey, CA: Healthy Learning.

Suggested Reading

Alway, S.E., Grumbt, W.H., Gonyea, W.J., & Stray-Gundersen, J. (1989). Contrasts in muscle and myofibers of elite male and female bodybuilders. *Journal of Applied Physiology, 67*(1), 24-31.

Baechle, T.R., & Earle, R.W. (2000). *Essentials of strength training and conditioning* (2nd ed.). Champaign, IL: Human Kinetics.

Baechle, T., & Groves, B. (1998). *Weight training—Steps to success.* Champaign, IL: Human Kinetics.

Bompa, T.O. (1999). *Periodization training for sports.* Champaign, IL: Human Kinetics.

Bompa, T.O., & Cornacchia, L.J. (1998). *Serious strength training; Periodization for building muscle power and mass.* Champaign, IL: Human Kinetics.

Brooks, D.S. (2004). *The complete book of personal training.* Champaign, IL: Human Kinetics.

Brooks, D.S., & Brooks, C.C. (1995). *Resist-a-ball: Programming guide for fitness professionals.* Indianapolis, IN: Ground Control, Inc.

Brzycki, M. (1995). *A practical approach to strength training* (3rd ed.). New York: McGraw-Hill.

Chu, D.A. (1992). *Jumping into plyometrics* (2nd ed.). Champaign, IL: Human Kinetics.

Ellenbecker, T.S., & Davies, G.J. (2001). *Closed kinetic chain exercise: A comprehensive guide to multiple-joint exercise.* Champaign, IL: Human Kinetics.

Faigenbaum, A., & Westcott, W. (2000). *Strength and power for young athletes.* Champaign, IL: Human Kinetics.

Graves, J.E., & Franklin, B.A. (Eds.). (2001). *Resistance training for health and rehabilitation.* Champaign, IL: Human Kinetics.

Kraemer, W., & Fleck, S. (1993). *Strength training for young athletes.* Champaign, IL: Human Kinetics.

Kreider, R.B., Fry, A.C., & O'Toole, M.L. (Eds.). (1998). *Overtraining in sport.* Champaign, IL: Human Kinetics.

McArdle, W.D., Katch, F.I, & Katch, V.L. (2001). *Exercise physiology: Energy, nutrition, and human performance* (5th ed.). Philadelphia: Lippincott Williams & Wilkins.

Sjöström, M., Lexell, J., Eriksson, A., & Taylor, C.C. (1992). Evidence of fiber hyperplasia in human skeletal muscles from healthy young men? *European Journal of Applied Physiology, 62,* 301-304.

Tippet, S., & Voight, M. (1995). *Functional progressions for sports rehabilitation.* Champaign, IL: Human Kinetics.

Westcott, W.S. (1995). *Strength fitness: Physiological principles and training techniques* (4th ed.). Dubuque, IA: Brown.

Yesalis, C.E., & Cowart, V.A. (2001). *The steroids game: An expert's inside look at anabolic steroid use in sports.* Champaign, IL: Human Kinetics.

Zatsiorsky, V.M. (1995). *Science and practice of strength training.* Champaign, IL: Human Kinetics.

Applied Resistance Training Skills

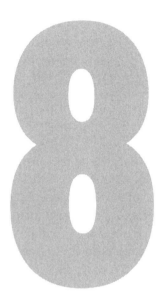

Outline

- General Spotting Guidelines
- Hands-On Techniques
- Effective Cueing
- Proper Lifting
- Exercise Teaching Method
- Teaching Specific Weight-Room Exercises
- Stability Ball Exercises
- Balance Exercises
- Pilates

A primary responsibility of personal fitness trainers on a day-to-day basis is to teach, supervise, spot, and cue appropriate resistance-training exercises. To better understand how to best provide resistance exercises for clients, it's helpful to consider the client's perspective. Below are some of the common reasons why a client might hire a trainer.

- The client wants to be motivated to exercise.
- The client isn't sure what to do in the "weight room."
- The client wants to be sure he/she is exercising correctly.
- The client wants the trainer's help to avoid getting hurt.
- The client already knows the basics, and now wants to learn different and/or harder exercises.

This chapter is designed to help you become more knowledgeable and skilled as a personal fitness trainer in the weight room, or wherever you might teach and supervise resistance-training exercises.

General Spotting Guidelines

As a client's personal fitness trainer, one of your professional/legal responsibilities is to provide proper spotting to the client. Spotting is important in enhancing client safety, as well as in guiding proper alignment and exercise technique. High-risk exercises, such as barbell squats, and bench and incline presses, demand particular awareness. Under some circumstances, failure to spot has been judged "tantamount to willful and wanton conduct." Therefore, it is very important for you to adhere to safe-spotting guidelines for your clients. Follow these general spotting guidelines whenever you work with clients on resistance training.

- It is your responsibility to keep loose plates, barbells, dumbbells, and other equipment in their place and out of your client's way.
- Be sure that you are strong enough to assist your client if needed. Some exercises, such as a back squat, may need more than one spotter.
- Practice injury prevention. When spotting, keep your knees flexed, back in neutral alignment, and abdominals tight in case you have to suddenly assist.
- Keep hands as close to the weights as possible without obstructing the movement. When assisting with a bar, use the appropriate closed grip for the lift.
- Make sure the bar is evenly loaded, and always use collars or clips.
- Communicate with your client about how many more repetitions will be performed and whether or not you are going to assist.
- Assist any time the predetermined movement speed decreases.

You will find spotting guidelines for specific exercises outlined later in this chapter.

Hands-On Techniques and Trainer Body Position

Another less defined type of spotting is the use of hands-on techniques when training your clients. Most, but not all, clients will benefit from skilled hands-on spotting and cueing. Since some clients may be uncomfortable being touched, always ask permission first and explain why such touching is necessary or desirable. If necessary and the client refuses, move on to another exercise. If desirable but not necessary, explain to the client the shortcomings of doing the activity without touching. Document your records accordingly. A simple, "Do you mind if I put my hands here, so I can help you get better results with this exercise?" is appropriate. When working with a client for the first time, it may be helpful to make a general statement about touch, such as, "I want to help my clients achieve better results from their exercise session, and so I often use hands-on palpation techniques to help them feel proper alignment and muscle contractions more effectively. Will this be OK with you? If not, please let me know." Be aware that a few clients may find touch distracting, intrusive, or simply uncomfortable. Be sensitive not only to their words, but also to their body signals. If a client pulls away or flinches as your hands approach him/her, you'll know that your client is uncomfortable with physical cues. Be respectful and provide a variety of verbal and visual cues instead.

Hands-on techniques can be of great value for most clients. Various types of palpation can increase clients' body awareness and help them perform exercises more safely and effectively. However, because of cultural, religious, gender-based differences and individual hypersensitivities, touch can be easily misunderstood. Therefore, it is important to observe the following guidelines when using hands-on techniques with clients (Rothenberg, 1995).

- Explain to your client the benefits of hands-on techniques and what they are designed to accomplish.
- Always ask the client's permission before using hands-on techniques.
- Advise your client of his/her right to decline the use of hands-on techniques or to withdraw permission at any time.
- Discuss with your client his/her touch boundaries, hypersensitivities, and touch comfort level.
- If working with minors (under age 18), require parents/guardians to sign a consent form and consider having parents/guardians physically present for training sessions.
- Be extremely sensitive to gender-related issues. A male trainer touching a female client, especially, may be subject to sexual harassment charges unless the touch is always construed as purely professional. Consistently conduct yourself in a respectful, considerate, and professional manner. Stay away from gender-specific areas of the body, and avoid groping types of touch.

Due to a lack of disciplinary boards or regulation for personal fitness trainers, it may be prudent to work with a lawyer to develop a consent form for use of hands-on technique training. For an example of such a consent form, see Appendix C.

Consider using your hands in various appropriate ways depending on the exercise or goal. Below are several specific types of touch to use when training clients (Rothenberg & Rothenberg, 1995).

- **Maintained touch**—This technique can be used to help your clients identify the working muscle, or to remind them of proper alignment. For example, while your client is performing lateral raises, you could stand behind him/her and maintain a gentle downward pressure on the shoulder blades, providing a physical reminder to keep shoulder blades depressed.
- **Palpation**—Palpating the working muscle with one to three fingers can help your client locate the focus area. This technique is particularly good with new clients, many of whom have low body awareness and can't

seem to feel which muscle is supposed to be working. You could say, for example, "I'd like you to feel this here," as you palpate the triceps with two fingers during a triceps kickback exercise.

- **Knife-edge**—Again, with the goal of heightening your client's body awareness, the knife-edge technique involves simply using the outer edge of your hand to stroke along the line of pull, or border, of a particular muscle. Running the outer edges of both your hands, for instance, along the line of pull of your client's latissimus dorsi muscles helps the client to feel the direction of the contraction during a lat pull-down.

Additionally, other ways to use your hands include the following.

- **Move-away**—With this method, you place your hand on or near a particular body part, then ask your client to move that body part away from your hand. For example, when training clients on hands and knees in the quadruped position, many clients will allow their abdominals to sag. In order to help them to hollow, or lift, their abdominals, you might place your open hand or fist under their abdominals and ask them to move their abdominal wall away from your hand without changing the neutral position of the spine.

- **Move-towards**—In this technique, you direct your client to move toward your hand; this works especially well when you are trying to help the client lengthen a body segment. A good example is to position your hand just slightly above the crown of your client's head and ask him/her to lengthen and stretch the spine upward until he/she touches your hand.

When training clients, be sensitive to body position differences. A client lying supine on the floor performing abdominal curls, for example, may be intimidated by a trainer standing over him or her barking directions. A better choice for the trainer would be to kneel or sit next to the client. In this position, hands-on techniques may be used if necessary, communication is easier, and the client feels more comfortable. Ask yourself the following questions with regard to positioning your body and hands.

- How can I best ensure my client's safety in this exercise?
- How can I help my client stay in the best alignment?
- How can I help my client to feel the proper muscles working?
- How can I position my body so my client feels the most comfortable and successful?

Consider also that your spotting techniques will vary depending on the skill level of your client and on the amount of weight being lifted. If the weight is light and the chance of injury occurring from a dropped weight is minimal, the more appropriate it is to use the hands-on techniques described above and to view your client's alignment from different angles. On the other hand, if your client already has proper technique and alignment and is lifting heavy weights, then you will need to provide appropriate spotting of the weights themselves in order to protect your client from injury.

Effective Cueing: Motivating Your Clients With Appropriate Verbal Cues

What you say while your clients are performing their sets and repetitions can make all the difference. The best cueing is specific (what exactly is correct and what needs improvement), provides the information necessary for correction, and is worded positively. Negative cueing includes words such as "don't," "can't," "difficult," "doubt," and "ought to." These words have been shown to decrease motivation and positive feelings (Jampolsky, 1979). A positive cue helps the client by suggesting what to do instead of what not to do. For example, "Keep your abdominals tight throughout the lift" is more effective than "Don't let your belly hang out, or your back arch." When you cue in a positive manner, you use the client's name frequently and recognize his/her effort. Your body language and verbal cues should be congruent for maximum effectiveness, which means that what you say matches your body signals. (You send a mixed message if you look distractedly around the room while praising your client.)

Inspire and help your clients to believe in themselves by using affirmations and promoting a positive attitude and self-acceptance. You may affirm a positive quality in someone by stating a quality that he/she currently possesses or is capable of attaining in the near future. Always word the affirmation as if it were a fact now, in the present. For example, "Susan, you are really powerful when you do those push-ups." "Paul, you are certainly full of energy!" "Liz, you are consistent and dedicated." Comments such as these help clients to realize the best in themselves.

Learning Styles

A number of texts have described three main types of learning styles: visual, auditory, and kinesthetic (Knowles, Holton, and Swanson, 1998). As a personal fitness trainer, you will be a more effective communicator if you can connect with your clients in these three ways. Some clients will be primarily visual learners (around 65% of the population), others will be auditory learners (about 30%), and still others will be more kinesthetic in their learning style. Visual learners generally learn best by seeing; they will benefit from watching you demonstrate proper alignment and technique when cueing. Auditory learners learn through listening; they enjoy verbal lectures and discussions and will listen carefully to all your verbal cues and voice inflections. Kinesthetic or tactile learners learn best with a hands-on approach; they need to do the movement themselves to fully understand it.

Types of Cues

Many trainers seem to struggle for words when training clients. Novice trainers, especially, tend to count repetitions and say little else. Remember, your clients already know how to count; continuous counting is unlikely to help them perform their exercises as safely and effectively as possible. While some clients dislike nonstop talking and continuous cueing, others will not appreciate long silent gaps in a training session. You will need to find the balance that works best with each client. Increase your effectiveness as a trainer by becoming adept at giving several types of cues for each exercise. This is particularly important when working with a client for a prolonged period of time; you will lose effectiveness if you keep saying the same thing over and over in the same way. In fact, a skilled trainer works at saying the same thing in a number of different ways. For example, how many different cues can you give to help a client find ideal posture? Remember to cue visually, verbally, and kinesthetically (including the use of touch). Try experimenting with the following different types of cues.

- **Alignment cue**—Detail the proper alignment of each joint: knees, hips, pelvis, spine, shoulders, scapulae, neck, elbows, wrists, etc. An alignment cue might also clearly state which joints are moving and which joints are still. Example: "Be sure to keep your wrists still and in a straight, neutral line during the biceps curl."

- **Educational/informational cue**—This type of cue educates your client about the working muscle, the purpose of the exercise, how it relates to activities of daily living, etc. Example: "This exercise is for your triceps, the muscle on the back of your arms. You use this muscle every time you push up and out of a chair."

- **Safety cue**—Similar to an educational cue, this type of cue lets your client know about a potential injury risk and how it can be minimized. Example: "In the down phase of a squat, you will want to avoid over-shooting your toes with your knees. Allowing this to happen frequently can cause stress to your patellar tendon and lead to knee problems."

- **Breathing cue**—This cue is simple: remind your clients to breathe! In most weight-room exercises the general rule is to exhale on the exertion phase of the movement. Example: "Be sure to exhale each time you're pushing up."

- **Motivational/affirmational cue**—Affirmational cues were described above, early on in "Effective Cueing." Motivational cues can be fun, silly, upbeat, energizing, commanding, and encouraging. Examples: "Go!" "You can do it!" "Alright!" "Fantastic job!" "Super!" "This rep is perfect; let's see four more just like it!"

- **Imagery cue**—Popular in Pilates and yoga teaching, an imagery cue can help the client to think about or feel the move in a new way; many clients will appreciate a creative and pithy imagery cue. Example: "Pretend you're trying to zip yourself into a pair of jeans that are one size too small." (This cue can help your clients learn to hollow, or draw in, their abdominal wall.)

- **Visual cue**—This may mean actually demonstrating a move, pointing to a part of your own body, or focusing on a demonstration of a specific body part. Example: "Do you see how I'm keeping my knees behind my toes?" (While demonstrating a squat movement, stop and point to your knees, drawing an imaginary plumb line down to your foot with your hand).

- **Wrong/right cue**—In this cueing technique, you may move your own body into and out of correct alignment, or you may ask your clients to do the same. The objective is to help them kinesthetically feel when they are in alignment and using proper form. Example: In order to help your clients find and feel the neutral wrist position, have them move their wrist into and out of neutral, reinforcing the correct position.

- **Tactile cue**—When you use one of the hands-on techniques described at the start of this chapter under "Hands-on Techniques and Trainer Body Position," you are using a tactile cue. Alternatively, have clients place their hands on their body or on your body to feel a specific movement pattern. Example: Have your clients place their hands on your retracting scapulae in order to aid in their understanding of the scapular retraction movement during a reverse fly.

Proper Lifting

Proper lifting technique is one of the most important skills you can teach your client. Lifting is a functional activity of daily living, and when performed improperly, can lead to back pain or other serious injury. See Figure 10-9b-c in Chapter 10 ("Injury Prevention") for illustrations of proper lifting techniques. Clients who make a habit of lifting with these practical techniques during daily activities can minimize their risk of low-back pain. Lifting a bar off of the floor properly demands even greater skill.

- **Use the correct grip.** Always use a closed (thumbs wrapped around the bar) grip. Grips may be underhand (supinated), overhand (pronated), or alternate (mixed). Be sure to place hands on the bar in such a way that it is balanced. Grip width on the bar may be shoulder-width apart (common), narrow, or wide.
- **Position the body correctly.** Feet should be far enough apart that the body has an adequate base of support and is balanced (usually shoulder-width apart). Knees and feet should be aligned in the same direction. When lowering the body to grasp the bar, heels need to stay in contact with the floor, and hips need to press backwards and stay low. Practice hip flexion, not spinal flexion, on the descent. The pelvis should be in neutral, with the tailbone pointing backwards, and the natural curvature of the spine should be maintained. Do not drop hips below knee level as this stresses knee ligaments and tendons. Scapulae are adducted, head is up, and eyes look straight ahead.
- **Tighten the abdominals and keep the bar close when lifting.** Use the leg muscles, not the back, and straighten to full extension of the hips and knees (avoid hyperextension). Exhale as the knees extend.
- **When lifting bar up to shoulders, keep the upward movement of the bar smooth and continuous.** Do not let the bar rest on the thighs. As the knees and hips extend, flex the elbows, abduct the shoulders, keep wrists as neutral as possible, and "rack" the bar in front of the shoulders. If the bar is heavy, it may be necessary to rise up on the balls of the feet as legs straighten, elevate the scapulae when abducting the shoulders, and flex the knees slightly when the bar makes contact with the collarbone.

Exercise Teaching Method

How do you teach clients new exercises and/or refine their performance on exercises they already know? The whole-part-whole and the demo-detail-demo methods of teaching are modified below. This method will help you give clear, specific instructions and will help sharpen your awareness of proper technique.

Step 1: Identify:
- name of exercise.
- equipment used.
- major muscles worked.
- purpose of the exercise.

Step 2: Demonstrate the exercise yourself (show the "whole" movement).

Step 3: Detail the exercise (break down the "parts").
- Describe the **starting** or **set-up** position, including the proper grip.
- Detail the proper **alignment** of each major joint; include which joints are stabilized and which joints should move.
- Describe the **movement** or the specific technique involved in the performance of the exercise.

- Go over **safety** and injury factors; discuss common errors.
- Consciously "**engage**" or contract the working muscle(s).

Step 4: Demonstrate the exercise again ("whole").

Step 5: Have your client perform the exercise. A good strategy during the set-up phase is to walk around your client, viewing his or her alignment from all sides, correcting any errors you observe. If you detail the exercise (Step 3) while you demonstrate, you'll probably need to detail it again as your client experiences the movement. Use some of the additional spotting and cueing techniques discussed above, including various hands-on techniques, proper positioning of your body for client comfort and safety, using your client's name, addressing the three learning styles (as appropriate), as well as alignment, educational, safety, breathing, motivational, imagery, visual, wrong/right, and tactile types of cueing.

Step 6: As your client performs the exercise, be alert for common errors and provide appropriate corrections in a polite, unthreatening manner. Remember to word the corrective comment positively. When your client successfully makes the correction, give genuine praise.

Step 7: Be prepared to modify, or progress, the exercise if necessary. If your client is unable to perform the exercise correctly or safely, or has any pain or disability that affects his or her performance, then you'll need to show an easier modification or perhaps even a completely different exercise that is more appropriate. On the other hand, a skilled and experienced client may need to be progressed, either by increasing the sets, reps, or weight, or by giving a harder and more challenging variation or exercise. A method of categorizing exercises according to level of difficulty has been developed using an **exercise continuum** (Yoke and Kennedy, 2004), shown below.

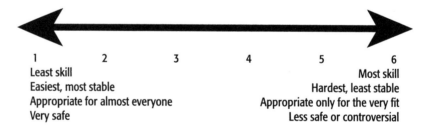

1	2	3	4	5	6
Least skill					Most skill
Easiest, most stable					Hardest, least stable
Appropriate for almost everyone					Appropriate only for the very fit
Very safe					Less safe or controversial

Obviously, a beginner exerciser or less conditioned client needs to perform exercises from the left side of the continuum, while a highly skilled and fit exerciser may be able to safely and appropriately perform exercises from the right side. A great number of exercises fall somewhere in the middle, and you will need to decide which exercises are suitable for each client.

Teaching Specific Weight-Room Exercises

The remainder of this chapter will cover a number of resistance-training exercises using most of the steps outlined above for each exercise. For further clarification of joint actions and terminology, see Chapter 3 ("Anatomy and Kinesiology"). For strength training principles and recommendations, see Chapter 7 ("Muscular Strength and Endurance Programming"). Keep in mind that joint actions always describe the concentric phase. **Modification** = easier; **progression** = harder.

Chest Exercises

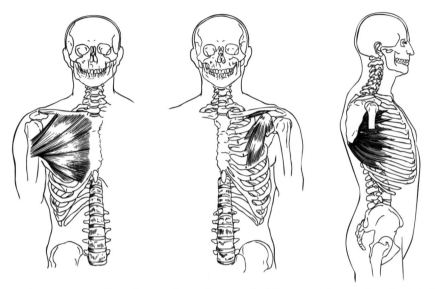

Fig. 8-1a. Pectoralis Major   **Fig. 8-1b. Pectoralis Minor**   **Fig. 8-1c. Serratus Anterior**

Muscle	Prime Mover for:	Assists with:
Pectoralis Major	shoulder flexion (clavicular portion) shoulder horizontal adduction (both parts) shoulder adduction (sternal portion) shoulder extension (sternal portion)	shoulder internal rotation
Pectoralis Minor	scapular depression scapular abduction scapular downward rotation	
Serratus Anterior	scapular abduction scapular upward rotation	

1 - Bench Press

Equipment used: barbell or dumbbells, flat bench

Moving joints	Joint action	Muscles worked
shoulders	horizontal adduction	pectoralis major, anterior deltoid, coracobrachialis
elbows	extension	triceps
Optional: shoulder girdle	protraction	pectoralis minor, serratus anterior

Exercise purpose: to develop muscle strength and endurance of the chest, fronts of shoulders, and backs of the arms.

1. Starting/set-up position: Lie supine, feet flat on floor or on bench, spine and pelvis in neutral, OR lumbar spine pressed flat with pelvis posteriorly tilted (may be better for beginners or those with back pain). Use wide, closed, pronated grip (narrow grip = greater triceps involvement) with evenly spaced hands. Elevate the feet onto low boxes or the bench itself if client is unable to maintain proper spinal alignment. Starting position is up.

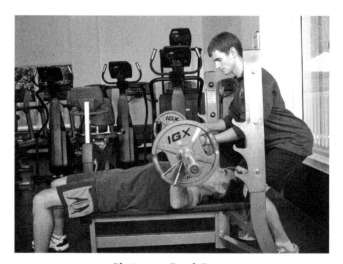

Photo 8-1a. Bench Press

2. Alignment: Upper arm is angled 80–90° out from torso; forearms are perpendicular to floor, wrists as neutral as possible. Shoulders and elbows move, but other joints should be stabilized, including the scapulae, which should remain pressed to the bench. Keep spine and wrists stabilized.

3. Movement: Contracting the abdominals, lower the weight with control; do not allow the shoulder joints to roll forward as the elbow lowers. Press up, fully extending, but not hyperextending, the elbows. Exhale on the upward phase; inhale on the downward phase.

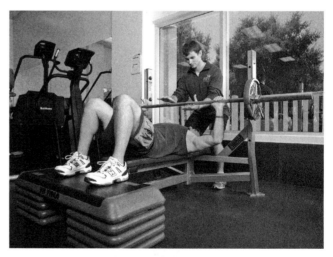

Photo 8-1b. Bench Press

4. Safety factors: Watch for uncontrolled descent; avoid extreme end range of motion (red/danger zone) in order to decrease shoulder joint stress. Avoid wrists rolling, back arching, hips pressing up, and bouncing the bar off the sternum. Many exercisers attempt to lift too much weight to maintain proper form.

5. Engage and contract the pecs, anterior deltoids, and triceps.

Spotting guidelines for trainers: Assist with unracking and racking the bar. Stand behind bench with flexed knees and neutral spine (abdominals in). Use alternate grip inside the client's hands and spot the bar on both descent and ascent. Have client let you know when he/she's performing the final repetition. Use three spotters for heavy loads.

Common Errors

- Uncontrolled descent of bar or dumbbells
- Bouncing bar off chest
- Arching the spine off the bench
- Hyperextending the elbows
- Breath holding on the up phase

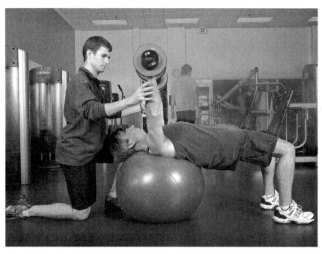

Photo 8-1c. Bench Press on Stability Ball

Modifications	Progressions
• For clients who express a **history** of low-back pain* and are **cleared by physician**: elevate feet onto boxes or up onto bench, press lower back flat, and perform posterior pelvic tilt. • For clients who express a **history** of shoulder pain* and are **cleared by physician**: shorten range of motion, especially on the down phase, and bring elbows in towards ribs (more into the sagittal plane)	• Perform an optional scapular movement at the end of the up phase: a "plus" may be performed by protracting, then retracting, the scapulae back to neutral, then performing the down phase of the bench press. This optional four-count movement requires greater coordination and is therefore appropriate for more advanced exercisers; however, this move is not appropriate if client has round shoulders or excessive kyphosis. • Unilateral dumbbell press • Bench press on a stability ball

*NOTE: Any client who expresses or demonstrates pain during any activity, including those for which modifications are suggested in this text, may need to be referred to a health care provider.

2–3 - Incline Press, Decline Press

Equipment used: barbell or dumbbells, incline bench or decline bench

The moving joints, working muscles, and joint actions are akin to those used in the standard flat bench press (see exercise #1, "Bench Press," above). However, keep in mind the following information.

For the incline press:
- Due to the increasingly vertical line of pull (depending on the incline), the clavicular fibers of the pectoralis major are targeted.
- The greater the incline, the greater the anterior and medial deltoid involvement (the shoulder joint action becomes more like abduction).
- The greater the incline, the greater the tendency to elevate the shoulder girdle and involve the upper trapezius fibers, as well as the levator scapulae and rhomboids (responsible for elevation). See training tips below under exercise #17, "Overhead Press."

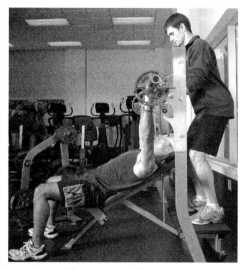

Photo 8-2a. Incline Press

For the decline press:
- With the head lower than the chest, the sternal fibers of the pectoralis major are emphasized.
- The greater the decline, the more the shoulder joint movement becomes like adduction. Prime movers for adduction are the latissimus dorsi, teres major, and sternal portion of the pecs.
- Depending on client goals, there is an opportunity for resisted shoulder girdle depression at the end of the range of motion. This would utilize the pectoralis minor and the lower trapezius fibers.

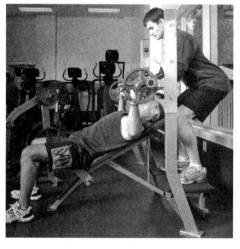

Starting position, alignment, movement, safety factors, spotting guidelines, and common errors are all similar to those for the bench press (see exercise #1 above).

Photo 8-2b. Incline Press

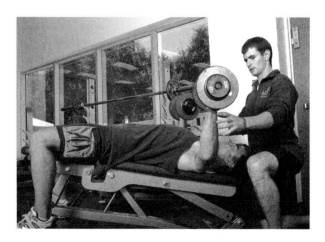

Photo 8-3a. Decline Press

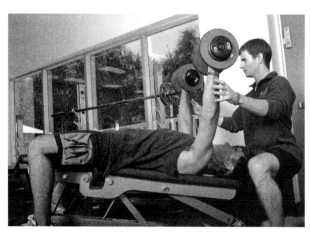

Photo 8-3b. Decline Press

4 - Dumbbell Fly (Flat, Incline, or Decline)

This exercise provides more isolation for the pectorals than the bench press since the elbows are held stable and the triceps are not involved (except as stabilizers).

Equipment used: dumbbells and flat, incline, or decline bench

Moving joints	Joint action	Muscles worked
shoulders	horizontal adduction	pectoralis major, anterior deltoid, coracobrachialis
Optional: shoulder girdle shoulders	protraction internal rotation	pectoralis minor, serratus anterior subscapularis, teres major

Exercise purpose: to develop strength and endurance of the chest and fronts of shoulders

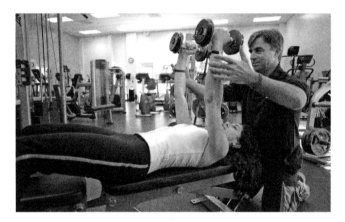

Photo 8-4a. Dumbbell Fly

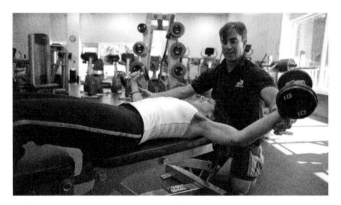

Photo 8-4b. Dumbbell Fly

1. Starting/set-up position: Lie supine, feet flat on floor or on bench, spine and pelvis in neutral, OR lumbar spine pressed flat with pelvis posteriorly tilted (may be better for beginners or those with back pain). Start in up position, elbows slightly flexed, palms facing each other (mid pronated).

2. Alignment: Elbows maintain slightly flexed position throughout exercise. Wrists are in neutral; spine, neck, and pelvis are stabilized. Shoulders are the only moving joints; maintain scapular stabilization.

3. Movement: Contracting the abdominals, lower the weights until upper arms are parallel with chest, keeping elbows in a slightly flexed, stable position. Palms face up, although some trainers prefer to horizontally abduct the shoulders and move into external rotation, and then finish the movement with shoulders internally rotated (minimizing radioulnar joint movement). Exhale on upward phase; inhale on the downward phase.

4. Safety factors: Some professionals place this exercise on their "high-risk" list because of the potential for an out-of-control descent and excessive range of motion, leading to shoulder injuries. Dumbbells should go no lower than chest level. Watch for problems with wrist breaking and elevated shoulders as well.

5. Engage and contract the pecs and anterior deltoids. Keep the contraction throughout both the concentric and the eccentric phases.

Spotting guidelines for trainers: Kneel or stand behind client's head and spot the forearms, wrists, or dumbbells.

Common Errors
- Uncontrolled descent (eccentric phase)
- Unstable wrist leading to potential for dropped dumbbell
- Arching the spine off the bench

Modifications	Progressions
• For clients who express a **history** of low-back pain and are **cleared by physician**: elevate feet onto boxes or up onto bench, press lower back flat, and perform posterior pelvic tilt. • For clients who express a **history** of shoulder pain and are **cleared by physician**: it would be prudent to avoid this exercise.	• Perform an optional scapular movement at the end of the up phase: a "plus" may be performed by protracting, then retracting the scapulae back to neutral, then performing the down phase of the fly. This optional four-count movement requires greater coordination and is therefore appropriate for more advanced exercisers; however, this move is not appropriate if client has round shoulders or excessive kyphosis. • Unilateral dumbbell fly • Dumbbell fly on a stability ball

5 - Bilateral Cable Cross-Over

Equipment used: high pulleys, cable cross-over set-up

Moving joints	Joint action	Muscles worked
shoulders	horizontal adduction	pectoralis major, anterior deltoid, coracobrachialis
Optional: shoulder girdle shoulders	protraction internal rotation	pectoralis minor, serratus anterior subscapularis, teres major

Exercise purpose: to develop strength and endurance of the chest and fronts of shoulders

1. Starting/set-up position: Stand with feet slightly wider than hip-width apart, OR feet can be staggered. Knees are flexed, abdominals contracted, scapulae depressed and adducted, elbows slightly flexed. Start with arms in open position.

2. Alignment: Shoulders are the only moving joint. Stabilize elbows and wrists, with elbows slightly flexed and wrists in neutral. Pay particular attention to maintaining a neutral, stable position with the torso. Depress and stabilize scapulae unless pec minor and serratus anterior strengthening is a goal.

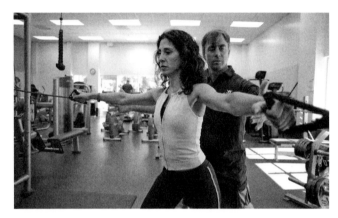

Photo 8-5a. Cable Cross-Over

3. Movement: Contracting the abdominals, exhale as arms are brought forward in horizontal plane. Palms may stay in mid-pronated position, or shoulders can internally rotate so that at full concentric contraction the thumbs are touching and palms are pronated (hands may also cross). Inhale as arms return (eccentric phase), controlling the movement. Variations include bringing the arms below the horizontal plane (from a high pulley), or bringing the arms above the horizontal plane (from a low pulley). Another variation is to perform a multi-joint press movement to the front (elbows extend and flex) instead of the single-joint cross-over movement.

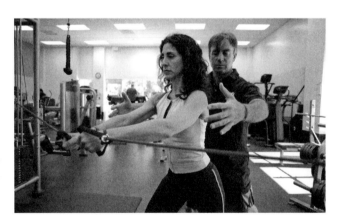

Photo 8-5b. Cable Cross-Over

4. Safety factors: Too much weight can make this exercise very difficult to control. The potential for excessive range of motion and too much speed on the eccentric phase increases shoulder joint risk. Perform the eccentric phase slowly and keep shoulders and scapulae down.

5. Engage and contract the pectoralis major and the anterior deltoids.

Spotting guidelines for trainers: Stand in back of client and spot wrists/forearms.

Common Errors
- Rocking or pushing with the torso
- Uncontrolled eccentric phase
- Unstable wrists
- Arching the spine and/or hyperextending the knees, especially if feet are parallel

Modifications	Progressions
• Staggered foot stance is slightly easier.	• Unilateral arm movement
• Seated position is easier to stabilize.	• Stand on single leg.

6 - Push-Up

Equipment used: mat, aerobic (low) step, bench, wall

Moving joints	Joint action	Muscles worked
shoulders	horizontal adduction	pectoralis major, anterior deltoid, coracobrachialis
elbows	extension	triceps

NOTE: Muscles that work strongly as stabilizers (due to antigravity position) are the abdominals, erector spinae, gluteus maximus, trapezius, rhomboids, serratus anterior, and pectoralis minor.

Exercise purpose: to develop strength and endurance of the chest, front of shoulders, and triceps muscles, and to promote core stability

1. Starting/set-up position for flat (hands-on-floor) push-up: Distribute body weight on hands and knees or hands and toes. Start in up position. Neck, spine, and pelvis stabilized in neutral position. For standard push-up, hands are slightly wider than shoulder-width apart with fingers facing straight ahead.

2. Alignment: Shoulders and elbows are the only moving joints. Stabilization of all other joints is very important for injury prevention. There should be no movement of the spine, neck, scapulae, or pelvis.

3. Movement: Perform the exercise smoothly, contract the abdominals, and avoid sagging through the back. Avoid hyperextending the elbows on the way up; lower until the chest is approximately a fist's width from the floor. Exhale on the way up, inhale down. Avoid looking up as this stresses the cervical vertebrae.

4. Safety factors: Turning the hands inward or outward increases stress to the wrists and elbows. If neutral spinal alignment is difficult to maintain, modify the exercise. The most common error is the loss of core stabilization, which may lead to back injury. Control the descent and avoid bringing the chest to the floor as this may cause stress to the shoulder joint.

5. Engage and contract the pecs, anterior deltoids, and the triceps. Maintain a constant awareness of abdominals contracting.

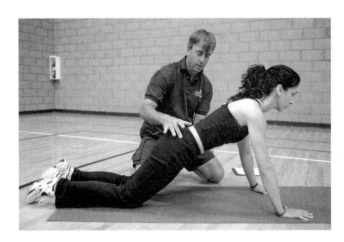

Photo 8-6a. Knee Push-Up

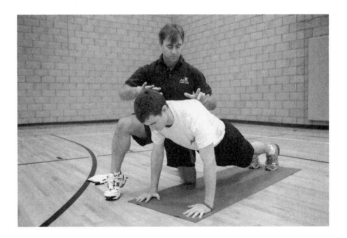

Photo 8-6b. Full Push-Up

Spotting guidelines for trainers: Kneel or sit next to client where you can observe spinal alignment from the side.

Common Errors
- Letting the back arch (hyperextend) and abdominals sag
- Flexing at the hips so the hips are "piked" up
- Hyperextending the elbows on the up phase
- Hyperextending, or flexing, the neck (cervical spine)
- Inability to keep the scapulae stable

Modifications	Progressions
• For clients who express a **history** of back pain and are **cleared by physician**: if moving to an easier variation (see below) doesn't help, avoid this exercise and train the chest muscles on a seated chest-press machine. • For clients who express a **history** of shoulder pain and are **cleared by physician**: bring elbows in closer to ribs, or avoid this exercise.	• From easiest to hardest: wall push-up, hands and knees (table-top) push-up, knee push-up with hands on weight-room bench, knee push-up with hands on aerobic step, knee push-up with hands on floor, knee push-up with knees elevated (decline), full-body push-up with hands on bench, full-body push-up with hands on floor, full-body push-up with feet elevated (decline), full-body decline push-up with weights on back • Use of unstable equipment in any of the above positions will make that position more difficult. For more skilled clients, consider: hands on wobble board, core board, flat side of BOSU, foam roller, medicine balls; feet on stability ball or foam roller • Plyometric push-up • Intersperse each push-up with another move, such as a side plank NOTE: In any position, the closer the hands are together, the greater the triceps involvement.

7–8 - Chest Exercise Machines

Chest press: flat, incline, or seated

- Muscles worked, joint actions, etc. are the same as those for exercise #1, "Bench Press."

- When adjusting machine, be sure the bar handles are aligned with or slightly above nipples.

- Alignment, joints stabilized, movement, etc. are the same as those for exercise #1, "Bench Press." Exhale on the way up (or out).

Pec dec: flat, incline, or seated

- Muscles worked, joint actions, etc. are the same as those for exercise #4, "Dumbbell Fly."

- Adjust machine so that the upper arms are perpendicular to the torso. Keep wrists, forearms, and elbows in contact with the pads; use forearms when pushing.

- Keep in mind that this exercise is high risk for clients with shoulder problems since most machines take the shoulder joint to an extreme range of external rotation and horizontal extension (red zone). This places the shoulder in a vulnerable position. Have clients move slowly through the eccentric phase and assist them when entering and leaving the machine if necessary. Avoid spinal or hip flexion; keep head, shoulders, and buttocks pressed against the pad.

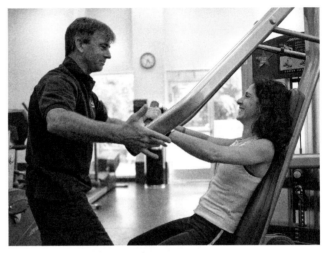

Photo 8-7. Chest Press Machine

Upper Back Exercises

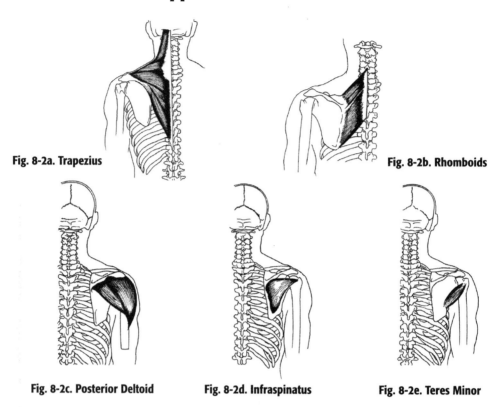

Fig. 8-2a. Trapezius **Fig. 8-2b. Rhomboids**

Fig. 8-2c. Posterior Deltoid **Fig. 8-2d. Infraspinatus** **Fig. 8-2e. Teres Minor**

Muscle	Prime Mover for:	Assists with:
Trapezius I	scapular elevation	
Trapezius II	scapular elevation scapular upward rotation	scapular adduction
Trapezius III	scapular retraction	
Trapezius IV	scapular depression scapular upward rotation	scapular adduction
Rhomboids	scapular retraction scapular elevation scapular downward rotation	
Posterior Deltoid	shoulder horizontal extension	shoulder extension shoulder external rotation
Teres Minor and Infraspinatus	shoulder horizontal extension shoulder external rotation	

From a functional perspective, it is very important to train the upper back using the following upper back exercises (#9–14). Common weight-room exercises for the pectoralis major (e.g., bench press, flys, push-ups) may result in postural misalignment if performed excessively without working the opposing muscle groups. Specifically, tight anterior muscles may cause excessive scapular abduction (protraction) and shoulder internal rotation (the powerful latissimus dorsi is also an internal rotator of the shoulder joint). In addition, kyphosis (rounded, hunched back) is a common postural misalignment among non-exercisers, and the following exercises are useful as a corrective measure.

9 - Reverse Fly

Equipment used: dumbbells, and flat or incline bench

Moving joints	Joint action	Muscles worked
shoulders	horizontal abduction	posterior deltoid, infraspinatus, teres minor
scapulae	retraction	trapezius III, rhomboids

Exercise purpose: to develop the muscle strength and endurance of the upper back and the back of the shoulders, as well as to promote better posture

1. Starting/set-up position: Lie prone on flat or incline bench, or seated on bench (bend over, flexing at hips). Support back either on bench (prone), or on thighs (seated). Start with arms down, palms facing each other.

2. Alignment: Spine and neck are in neutral. Elbows are stabilized in a slightly flexed position; wrists in neutral. Stabilize spine (no spinal rotation with extension) and neck. Shoulders and scapulae are the only moving joints. Avoid looking up and hyperextending neck.

3. Movement: Keep upper arm perpendicular to torso, lead with elbows and move up slightly beyond the shoulder joint range of motion and into conscious scapular retraction. Another variation is to start with scapular retraction, and then perform the shoulder joint movement (horizontal abduction). Stay in the horizontal plane. Exhale on the upward movement and control the descent.

4. Safety factors: Keep movement slow and controlled to avoid shoulder injury. Watch for tendency to extend the shoulder joint in the sagittal plane, especially if weights are too heavy (this allows the latissimus dorsi to help out). Most clients will need to start this exercise with little or no weight. Avoid the seated, hip-flexed position if clients are unable to adequately support the torso either with the abdominals and erector spinae, or on thighs.

5. Engage and contract the posterior deltoid, and especially the mid-trapezius and rhomboids.

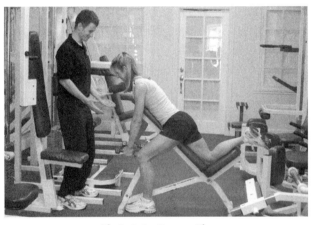

Photo 8-9a. Reverse Fly

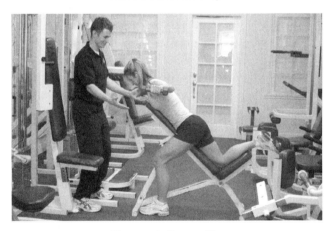

Photo 8-9b. Reverse Fly

Spotting guidelines for trainers: If client is seated, spot from behind. If client is prone, trainer may kneel in front of bench and spot forearms or wrists. Alternatively, spotting from behind and palpating the scapular retractors and posterior deltoids may help clients stay focused and promote awareness.

Common Errors

- Hunched shoulders (elevated scapulae)
- Failure to keep neck in neutral
- Tendency to perform shoulder extension instead of shoulder horizontal abduction
- Failure to finish the up phase with scapular retraction
- Using weight that is too heavy to finish with scapular retraction

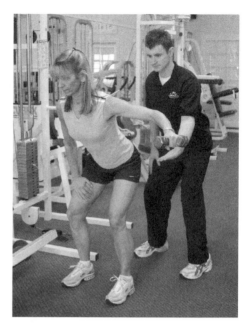

Photo 8-9c. Standing Unilateral Reverse Fly

Modification
- For clients who express a **history** of shoulder pain and are **cleared by physician**: avoid the movement of shoulder horizontal abduction. Instead, allow the arms to hang down towards the floor, elbows straight, and ask client to perform scapular retraction only.

Progressions
- Standing reverse fly with unilateral arms
- Reverse fly with a "plus" (four-count move): (1) reverse fly—up phase, (2) scapular retraction, (3) scapulae return to neutral, (4) reverse fly—down phase
- Reverse fly on stability ball
- Reverse fly on stability ball with unilateral arms
- Reverse fly on stability ball, one leg up

10 - Horizontal Seated (High) Row

Equipment used: low pulley machine, horizontal seated row machine, or tubing

Moving joints	Joint action	Muscles worked
shoulders	horizontal abduction	posterior deltoid, infraspinatus, teres minor
scapulae	retraction	trapezius III, rhomboids
elbows	flexion	biceps, brachialis, brachioradialis

Exercise purpose: to develop muscle strength and endurance of the upper back and the back of the shoulders, as well as to promote better posture

1. Starting/set-up position: Sit with hips flexed at 90°, spine in neutral alignment. If seated on floor, flex knees slightly to assist with proper seated posture. Use grips or a bar that allows palms to pronate and face down. Start with elbows extended and arms in horizontal plane (out phase).

2. Alignment: Contracting the abdominals, keep entire spine in neutral, including neck. Maintain scapular depression, elbows slightly lower than shoulders, wrists slightly lower than elbows. Keep wrists neutral. The only moving joints are the shoulders, scapulae, and elbows.

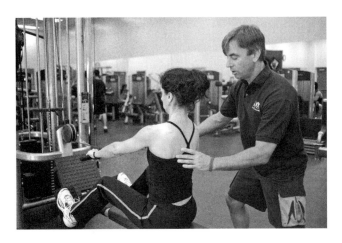

Photo 8-10a. Horizontal Seated (High) Row

3. Movement: When rowing, lead backwards with elbows. Keep upper arm in horizontal plane and consciously go back into scapular movement (or scapular movement can precede the arm/shoulder movement). Pull the bar directly into the chest. Exhale when pulling (in phase), and control the eccentric (out) phase.

4. Safety factors: Watch for wrist breaking (pulling with the wrists) and rocking with the lower spine. Avoid elevating the shoulder girdle.

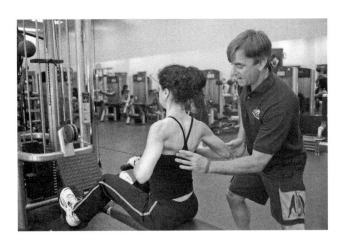

Photo 8-10b. Horizontal Seated (High) Row

5. Engage and contract the posterior deltoids and consciously contract the mid-trapezius muscles and the rhomboids.

Spotting guidelines for trainers: Spot from behind, holding forearms if necessary. As the client brings his/her elbows back, guide elbows into horizontal plane. Palpating the scapular retractors is helpful to focus client awareness.

Common Errors
- Extending hips or spine instead of maintaining stability
- Confusing the high-row movement with the low-row movement
- Elevating the shoulder girdle
- Not controlling the return

Modification	Progressions
• For clients who express a **history** of shoulder pain and are **cleared by physician**: avoid the action of shoulder horizontal abduction and have client perform scapular retraction only.	• High row on stability ball • High row on stability ball on one leg • Standing high row at mid-pulley • Standing high row on one leg

11 - Bent-Elbow Reverse Fly Machine

Equipment used: reverse fly/row machine

Moving joints	Joint action	Muscles worked
shoulders	horizontal abduction	posterior deltoid, infraspinatus, teres minor
scapulae	retraction	trapezius III, rhomboids

Exercise purpose: to develop muscle strength and endurance of the upper back and the back of the shoulders, as well as to promote better posture

1. Starting/set-up position: Sit with hips flexed at 90°, feet on floor, spine in neutral, and abdominals contracted. Adjust seat so that upper arms are perpendicular to torso and movement occurs in the horizontal plane. Forearms are crossed; palms face floor.

2. Alignment: Keep spine and neck in neutral; maintain scapular depression throughout. Shoulders and scapulae move. Neck, spine, and elbows are stabilized.

3. Movement: Exhale on backward movement, taking scapulae through full range of retraction. Inhale and control the forward movement (eccentric phase).

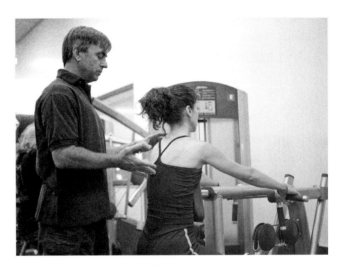

Photo 8-11. Bent Elbow Reverse Fly Machine

4. Safety factors: Make certain torso is in contact with pad, and the neck and upper trapezius muscles are relaxed.

5. Engage and contract the middle trapezius and rhomboids, as well as the posterior deltoids, through both concentric and eccentric phases.

Spotting guidelines for trainers: Depending on the configuration of the machine, it is often helpful to stand behind your client and maintain contact with his or her shoulders, encouraging scapular depression throughout the move.

Common Errors
- Arching the back
- Elevating the shoulder girdle

12 - Shoulder Shrugs

Equipment used:

Moving joints	Joint action	Muscles worked
scapulae (shoulder girdle)	elevation	trapezius I and II, rhomboids, and levator scapulae

Exercise purpose: to develop muscle strength and endurance of the upper trapezius/scapular elevators

1. Starting/set-up position: Sit or stand with feet shoulder-width apart for stability. If using a barbell, place hands directly in line with shoulders (some trainers recommend holding the barbell behind the body for the optimal line of pull). If standing, maintain proper alignment; start with shoulder girdle depressed.

2. Alignment: Sit or stand with pelvis, spine, and neck in neutral alignment, abdominals contracted, scapulae down. If standing, have knees slightly flexed; if sitting, flex hips at 90°. The only moving joint is the shoulder girdle; all other joints are stabilized. Elbows and wrists have no independent movement.

3. Movement: Elevate the shoulder girdle in a straight line up towards ears; feel the scapulae sliding up and down the ribcage in the back. Many strength training experts recommend inhaling when elevating shoulders and exhaling on the descent.

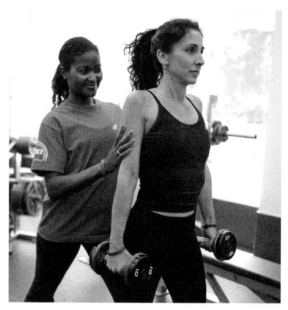

Photo 8-12. Shoulder Shrug

4. Safety factors: With the exception of body builders, football players, and wrestlers, this may not be an important exercise for most clients. From a functional perspective, many clients need to stretch the scapular elevators and relax tight neck muscles, and they need to strengthen the scapular depressors. Many clients are unable to maintain sufficient scapular depression throughout the day and/or during standard exercises. It is suggested that trainers focus more on scapular depression than scapular elevation for most clients.

5. Engage and contract the upper trapezius muscles, levator scapulae, and rhomboids.

Common Errors
-   Swinging the weights back and forth
-   Ducking the head forward
-   Jerking the head backward
-   Using momentum of the torso or legs to assist the lift

Scapular Depressor Exercises

13 - Depression Dip

Equipment used: bench or dip stand

Moving joints	Joint action	Muscles worked
scapulae	depression	trapezius IV, pectoralis minor

Exercise purpose: to develop muscle strength and endurance of the scapular depressors; to promote scapular stability and better shoulder joint mechanics and posture; and to help reduce the incidence of neck fatigue and muscle spasm

1. Starting/set-up position: If using a bench, support torso with heels of hands on bench, fingers pointing forward. Allow spine and pelvis to hang in a neutral line, hips and knees flexed, feet flat on floor. Start with scapulae elevated up towards ears.

2. Alignment: Elbows slightly flexed (not hyperextended), with neck, spine, and pelvis in neutral. The only moving joints are the scapulae; keep elbows, spine, pelvis, and neck still.

3. Movement: Feel the shoulder blades sliding down the back of the ribcage as the scapulae are "shrugged down" (depressed) on an exhale. Inhaling, allow gravity to pull them back up to the ears (scapular elevation).

4. Safety factors: In order to avoid wrist stress, experiment with placing the heels of the hands close to the edge of the bench, maintaining as neutral a wrist as possible. Keep elbows slightly flexed in order to avoid elbow stress.

5. Engage and contract the scapular depressors. Triceps act only as elbow stabilizers.

Spotting guidelines for trainers: At first this may be a difficult exercise to cue—clients not familiar with the exercise typically want to perform standard triceps dips. You may need to help stabilize their elbows to prevent elbow movement. Many clients benefit from palpation of the lower traps; this is a good time to use the knife-edge technique to create increased awareness.

Common Errors

- Mistaking this exercise for a standard triceps dip and using the elbows
- Thrusting the spine or pelvis away from the bench
- Using leg muscles to lift and lower the body

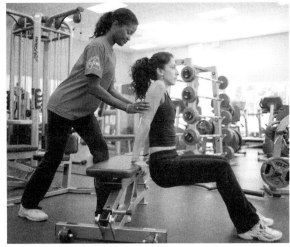

Photo 8-13a. Depression Dip

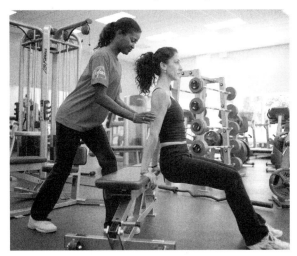

Photo 8-13b. Depression Dip

Modification
- For less fit or less skilled clients: have them simply stand and elevate and depress the shoulder girdle until they become familiar with the movement.

Progression
- Depression dips on a dip stand utilizing the entire body weight as resistance

14 - High-Pulley Scapular Depression

Equipment used: high-pulley cable column

Moving joints	Joint action	Muscles worked
scapulae	depression	trapezius IV, pectoralis minor

Exercise purpose: to develop muscle strength and endurance of the scapular depressors; to promote scapular stability and better shoulder joint mechanics and posture; and to help reduce the incidence of neck fatigue and muscle spasm

1. Starting/set-up position: Sit at high pulley (lat pull-down machine) using a bar with a wide grip. With feet on floor, secure the legs under the stabilizing pad. Allow the bar attached to the high pulley to pull the scapulae up into elevation; starting position is up.

2. Alignment: Hips flexed at 90°, with pelvis, spine, and neck in neutral, and abdominals contracted. Elbows are straight without being hyperextended; wrists are in neutral, palms pronated, wide grip. The scapulae are the only moving joints; shoulders and elbows do not move (unlike a lat pull-down).

3. Movement: Starting with the scapulae elevated, slide and depress the scapulae down the ribcage, exhaling. Smoothly return to scapular elevation.

4. Safety factors: Avoid elbow hyperextension.

5. Engage and contract the scapular depressors.

Spotting guidelines for trainers: This may be a difficult exercise to cue, as clients may confuse the movement with the standard and familiar lat pull-down. You may need to stabilize the elbows in order to prevent elbow flexion. The knife-edge hands-on technique is helpful in directing client awareness to the lower traps.

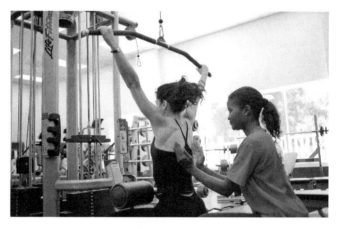

Photo 8-14a. High-Pulley Scapular Depression

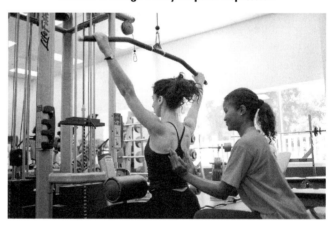

Photo 8-14b. High-Pulley Scapular Depression

Common Errors
*   Attempting to perform a lat-pull down instead of pure scapular depression
*   Leaning away from the cable column in order to gain assistance from the spinal or hip extensors

Modification
*   For clients who express a **history** of shoulder pain and are **cleared by physician**: avoid this exercise. Instead, try depression dips, prone propping, or standing, unresisted scapular elevation and depression to increase body awareness.

Shoulder Exercises

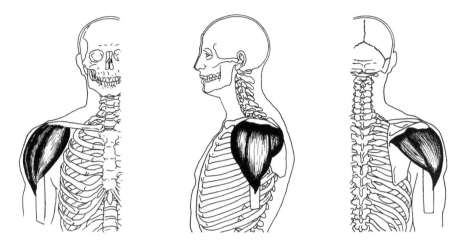

Fig. 8-3. Deltoids: Anterior, Medial, and Posterior Views

Muscle	Prime Mover for:	Assists with:
Anterior Deltoid	shoulder flexion shoulder horizontal adduction	shoulder internal rotation
Medial Deltoid	shoulder abduction shoulder horizontal abduction	
Posterior Deltoid	shoulder horizontal abduction	shoulder extension shoulder external rotation

15 - Front Raises

Equipment used: dumbbells, barbell, low pulley, or tubing, bench

Moving joints	Joint action	Muscles worked
shoulders	flexion	anterior deltoid, pectoralis major (clavicular portion)

Exercise purpose: to develop muscle strength and endurance of the front of the shoulders and the upper chest

1. Starting/set-up position: Stand or sit in proper alignment, feet shoulder-width apart. Starting position is down.

2. Alignment: In standing position, feet are shoulder-width apart, knees slightly flexed, with neck, spine, and pelvis in neutral alignment, abdominals contracted. Elbows are fully extended but not hyperextended; palms are pronated with dumbbells or barbell against thighs. In seated position, feet are flat on floor, hips are flexed at 90°, and spine and neck are in neutral. Scapulae are depressed and in neutral in both positions, wrists and elbows are stabilized; abdominals are contracted to stabilize spine. The only moving joints are the shoulders.

3. Movement: May be performed bilaterally or unilaterally. Palms remain pronated throughout movement. Flex shoulders until arms are above shoulder height (some experts recommend flexing until arms are overhead). Exhale during the upward movement.

4. Safety factors: Seated, unilateral front raises are safer for the back than standing, bilateral raises. If client is standing, take care to ensure that the torso is stable and that there is no momentum. Watch that the neck maintains a neutral position. Avoid wrist breaking. Be aware that the anterior deltoids tend to be overworked in activities of everyday living and are generally much stronger than the posterior deltoids; be cautious with too much emphasis on the anterior deltoids.

5. Engage and contract the anterior deltoids and the upper pectorals throughout both the concentric and eccentric phases.

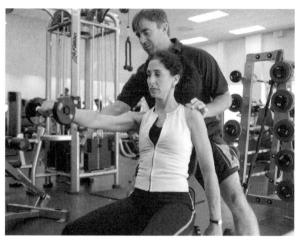

Photo 8-15a. Seated Front Raise

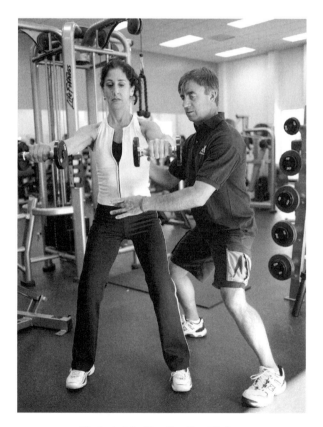

Photo 8-15b. Standing Front Raise

Spotting guidelines for trainers: Stand in front of client, spotting the weights if heavy. Alternatively, stand behind client, with maintained touch on tops of shoulders; remind client to depress and maintain neutral scapulae throughout movement.

Common Errors
- Hyperextended knees
- Hyperextended spine
- Inability to maintain core stability
- Elevated scapulae

Modifications	Progressions
• For clients who express a **history** of shoulder pain and are **cleared by physician**: shorten range of motion, perform exercise with thumbs up • For clients who express a **history** of back pain and are **cleared by physician**: perform exercise seated in weight-room chair or standing, knees flexed, with back stabilized against a wall	• Front raise facing away from low pulley • Front raise seated on stability ball • Front raise seated on stability ball, one foot up • Front raise standing on one leg • Front raise while performing a front or back lunge

16 - Lateral Raises

Equipment used: dumbbells or tubing, bench

Moving joints	Joint action	Muscles worked
shoulders	abduction	medial deltoid, supraspinatus
scapulae	upward rotation	trapezius II and IV, serratus anterior

Exercise purpose: to develop muscle strength and endurance of the shoulder muscles

1. Starting/set-up position: Stand or sit, holding dumbbells or tubing down at sides.

2. Alignment: In standing position, feet are shoulder-width apart, knees slightly flexed, with neck, spine, and pelvis in neutral alignment. In seated position, feet are flat on floor, hips are flexed at 90°, and neck and spine are in neutral. In both positions, abdominals are contracted; scapulae are depressed and in neutral; elbows are slightly flexed, and wrists are neutral (arms hang down at sides, palms facing thighs). The only moving joints are the shoulders. Wrists and elbows are stabilized. Scapulae remain depressed and in neutral, neck stays in neutral. There should be no movement of the spine or legs. Note that some experts recommend a slight flexion at the hips (spine in neutral) in order for the medial deltoid to receive optimal resistance against gravity.

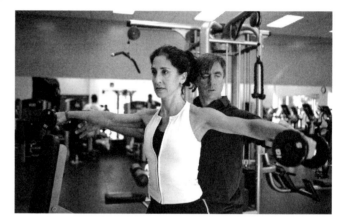

Photo 8-16. Lateral Raise

3. Movement: As the shoulders are abducted, maintain partial shoulder external rotation (palms should face the floor), and abduct shoulders only to 90° (the greater the abduction, the more important the external rotation). Lead with the elbows, not the wrists. Exhale on the way up (concentric phase).

4. Safety factors: Abducting the shoulders beyond 90° while maintaining internal rotation may lead to impingement syndrome (the greater tubercle of the humerus abuts the acromion process and irritates soft tissue structures, especially the supraspinatus tendon). Some experts recommend performing the entire exercise in external rotation (thumbs point up); others recommend starting as described above, then moving into full external rotation as the shoulders abduct to 90°. Also, if standing in slight hip flexion as mentioned above, there is increased risk to the spine unless abdominals are sufficiently strong to maintain core stability throughout the set.

5. Engage and contract the deltoids throughout both the concentric and the eccentric phases.

Spotting guidelines for trainers: Stand behind client and spot the forearms, wrists, or weights. Remind client to lead with the elbows, not the wrists. If weights are relatively light, maintain touch on tops of shoulders, reminding client to keep scapulae depressed.

Common Errors
- Initiating movement with legs or torso
- Hyperextending knees in standing
- Inability to maintain core stability
- Ducking the head forward during shoulder abduction
- Elevating the scapulae
- Wrist breaking

Modifications	Progressions
• For clients who express a **history** of shoulder pain and are **cleared by physician**: decrease weights and range of motion to < 30°, if pain persists, discontinue exercise and perform front raises instead. Try bringing lateral raise in front of the frontal plane (yellow zone). • For clients who express a **history** of back pain and are **cleared by physician**: perform exercise seated on weight-room chair.	• Perform lateral raises unilaterally. • Unilateral raise at low pulley • Lateral raise on stability ball, one foot up • Lateral raise standing on one leg • Lateral raise while performing standing, one-leg hip abduction

17 - Overhead Press (Military or Standing Press)

Equipment used: dumbbells or barbell, bench

Moving joints	Joint action	Muscles worked
shoulders	abduction	deltoids, supraspinatus
scapulae	upward rotation	trapezius II and IV, serratus anterior
elbows	extension	triceps

Exercise purpose: to develop muscle strength and endurance of the shoulder muscles and the backs of the arms

1. Starting/set-up position: Sit or stand in proper alignment. Starting position is down, with shoulders externally rotated and palms pronated (if using dumbbells, palms may be also be mid-pronated, facing ears).

2. Alignment: In the seated position, feet must be flat on floor, hips flexed at 90°, spine neutral, scapulae depressed and adducted. In the standing position, knees are slightly flexed with pelvis, spine, and neck in neutral, and scapulae depressed and adducted. In both positions, abdominals are contracted; hands are slightly wider than shoulder-width apart. The moving joints are the shoulders, scapulae (in upward rotation only), and elbows. Spine and neck should be stabilized. Wrists stay in neutral, and shoulder elevation is minimized.

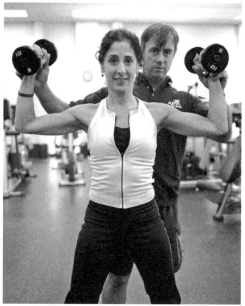

Photo 8-17a. Overhead Press

3. Movement: Exhale when pressing up. Fully extend elbows without hyperextending; may be performed bilaterally or unilaterally. Try to lift weights up over the top of the head while maintaining scapular adduction and depression. With a barbell, lightly touch the clavicle and press up in front of the face. Lower with control, inhaling on the way down.

4. Safety factors: The behind-the-neck military press has become controversial due to the vulnerable position of the shoulder joint (horizontally abducted and externally rotated behind the frontal plane) and is not recommended. To reduce the risk of injury, perform the exercise in front of the head. Encourage your client to utilize proper shoulder joint mechanics with humeral head depression (see Chapter 10, "Injury Prevention").

5. Engage and contract the deltoids and triceps. Isometrically contract the scapular retractors, as well as the pectoralis minor and lower trapezius to maintain depression.

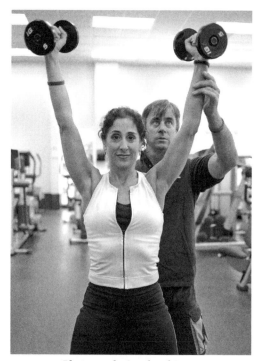

Photo 8-17b. Overhead Press

Spotting guidelines for trainers: With dumbbells, stand or sit behind client and cup the elbows or spot the forearms. With barbell, stand behind and track the barbell with hands. Encourage client to maintain shoulder girdle depression.

Common Errors
- Leaning backward, especially with heavy weights
- Excessive shoulder girdle elevation
- Ducking the head and neck forward
- Lack of core stability
- Wrist breaking

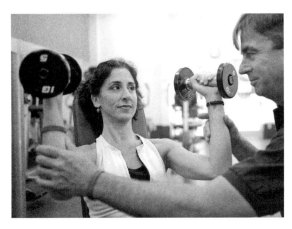

Photo 8-17c. Overhead Press Modification

Modifications	Progressions
• For clients who express a **history** of shoulder pain and are **cleared by physician**: move arms in front of the frontal plane and more into the sagittal plane (the joint action becomes less shoulder abduction and more shoulder flexion); continue to press weights straight up, although for some clients range of motion will need to be decreased. Reduce the weight. Another strategy is to perform the overhead press slightly inclined (about 20°) on an inclined chair, which helps take the shoulder away from the riskier position of shoulder abduction and external rotation. • For clients who express a **history** of back pain and are **cleared by physician**: perform exercise seated on weight-room chair.	• Sit on stability ball with one foot up. • Perform overhead press standing on one leg. • Combine overhead press with squat. • Combine overhead press with Russian lunge.

18 - Upright Row

Equipment used: dumbbells or barbell

Moving joints	Joint action	Muscles worked
shoulders	abduction	deltoids, supraspinatus
scapulae	upward rotation	trapezius II and IV, serratus anterior
elbows	flexion	biceps
Optional: scapulae	elevation	trapezius I and II, rhomboids, and levator scapulae

Exercise purpose: to develop muscle strength and endurance of the shoulder muscles and the biceps

1. Starting/set-up position: Stand with feet shoulder-width apart in proper alignment. Hands are in a pronated, narrow grip in front of thighs. Starting position is down.

2. Alignment: Stand with knees slightly flexed, and pelvis, spine, and neck in neutral position; abdominals contracted. Moving joints: Shoulders, scapulae and elbows move. Elevation of the scapulae at the beginning or at the end of the range of motion is an option if upper trapezius strengthening is a goal (otherwise, keep scapulae depressed). Wrists stay as neutral as possible. Stabilize lower body, keeping abdominals contracted.

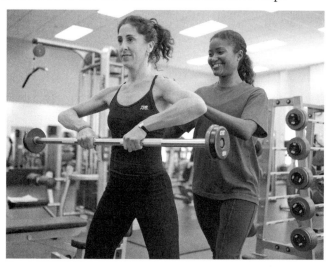

Photo 8-18. Upright Row

3. Movement: Lead with elbows, not wrists. Keep barbell or dumbbells close to the body. If upper trapezius work is a goal, lift elbows above shoulder level and elevate scapulae; otherwise, shoulder abduction occurs only to 90° or less. Exhale when lifting up.

4. Safety factors: A typical problem with this exercise is the tendency to lead with the wrists and keep elbows down, placing great stress on the wrists. This exercise has become controversial because shoulder abduction above 90° coupled with internal shoulder rotation may lead to shoulder impingement or rotator cuff problems (see Chapter 10, "Injury Prevention"). For optimal shoulder safety, keep abduction less than 90° and minimize shoulder girdle elevation.

5. Engage and contract the deltoids, biceps, and, optionally, the upper trapezius muscles.

Spotting guidelines for trainers: Stand behind client, hands tracking close to bar in a wide grip. Remind client to lead with elbows. Alternatively, maintain palpation on the shoulder girdle as a reminder to maintain scapular depression.

Common Errors
- Leaning backwards on the up phase
- Bringing wrists higher than elbows
- Abducting arms higher than 90°, placing stress on the shoulder joint
- Inability to stabilize the torso

Modifications
- For clients who express a **history** of shoulder pain and are **cleared by physician**: avoid this exercise.
- For clients who express a **history** of back pain and are **cleared by physician**: avoid this exercise.

Progression
- Perform upright row from low pulley.

19–20 - Shoulder Exercise Machines

Overhead Press

- The exerciser is usually in seated position. Machine may be part of a multi-unit setup, or may be a variable resistance single station-type machine.

- Muscles worked, joints stabilized, alignment, safety factors, etc. are the same as those for the free-weight "Overhead Press" (exercise #17).

- Adjust seat height so that handles are level with shoulder joint.

- If machine has a back pad, press hips, shoulders, and head against the pad and maintain contracted abdominals. If there is no back pad, take care to keep the torso and neck in neutral alignment, and avoid leaning backwards.

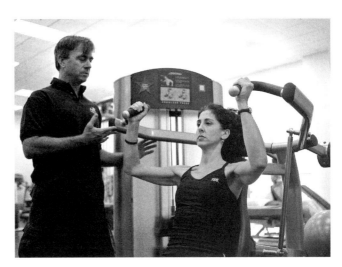

Photo 8-19. Overhead (Shoulder) Press Machine

- Multi-unit shoulder presses may be used facing either toward or away from the weight stack. Depending on where the stool is placed, facing away may be riskier for the shoulder joint (if shoulders are horizontally extended and externally rotated behind the frontal plane).

- Avoid hyperextending or snapping the elbows during extension.

Lateral Raise

- The exerciser is in a seated position.

- Muscles worked, joints stabilized, alignment, safety factors, etc. are the same as those for free-weight "Lateral Raises" (exercise #16).

- Adjust seat height so that the cam or pivot point is aligned with the shoulder joint.

- Press hips, shoulders, and head back against pad.

- Maintain pressure against arm pads with the lateral aspect of the arms and lead with the elbows. Avoid lifting with the wrists.

Rotator Cuff Exercises

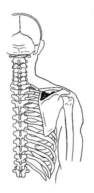

Fig. 8-4a. Supraspinatus

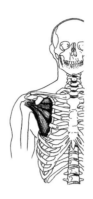

Fig. 8-4b. Subscapularis

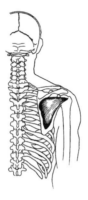

Fig. 8-4c. Infraspinatus

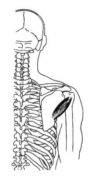

Fig. 8-4d. Teres Minor

Muscle	Prime Mover for:	Assists with:
Supraspinatus	shoulder abduction	
Subscapularis	shoulder internal rotation	
Infraspinatus	shoulder external rotation shoulder horizontal abduction	
Teres Minor	shoulder external rotation shoulder horizontal abduction	

21 - External Rotation with Tube

Equipment used: rubber tube or band

Moving joints	Joint action	Muscles worked
shoulders	external rotation	infraspinatus, teres minor (posterior deltoid assists)

Exercise purpose: to develop strength and endurance of the external rotator cuff muscles, to provide muscle balance against the powerful internal rotators of the shoulder, and to promote healthy shoulder joint functioning

1. Starting/set-up position: Sit or stand. Elbow on working side is pressed against ribs and is flexed at 90° (a towel may be placed under the arm for more comfortable alignment). Palm may be either supinated or mid-pronated. Start with palm in front of body and forearm perpendicular to torso.

2. Alignment: Keep pelvis, spine, and neck in neutral, and abdominals contracted. Shoulders are the only joint moving. Elbow is stabilized against ribs and fixed at 90°, wrist is locked in neutral, and scapulae are depressed.

3. Movement: With elbow anchored against side, externally rotate shoulder (forearm will visibly move through horizontal plane at hip height). Movement should be slow and controlled during both concentric and eccentric phases. Keep humerus depressed throughout range of motion. Make band tighter or looser as necessary to fatigue the muscles and maintain proper form. Exhale on backward movement. May be performed unilaterally or bilaterally.

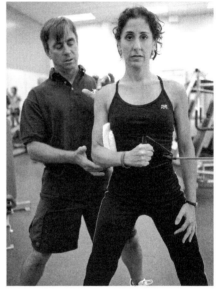

Photo 8-21a. Shoulder External Rotation

4. Safety factors: Shoulder external rotation should be performed frequently in order to help maintain healthy shoulders and prevent injury. Avoid forcing a large range of motion; it is not necessary for the forearm to move completely into (or behind) the frontal plane.

5. Engage and contract the external rotators.

Spotting guidelines for trainers: Stand behind your client where you may maintain palpation on the tops of the shoulders, guide the forearm, and/or help create an awareness of wrist stabilization.

Common Errors
- Shoulder hiking
- Moving the wrist instead of performing external rotation

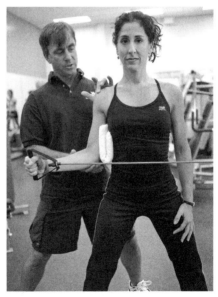

Photo 8-21b. Shoulder External Rotation

NOTE: It is probably not as important to perform isolation-type exercises for the internal rotator cuff muscles. These muscles (subscapularis and teres major) are assisted by many other powerful muscles, including: anterior deltoid, pectoralis major, biceps, and the latissimus dorsi.

Middle Back Exercises

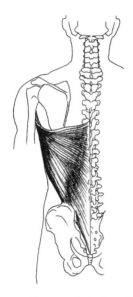

Fig. 8-5a. Latissimus Dorsi

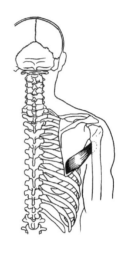

Fig. 8-5b. Teres Major

Muscle	Prime Mover for:	Assists with:
Latissimus Dorsi	shoulder extension shoulder adduction	shoulder internal rotation shoulder horizontal abduction
Teres Major	shoulder extension shoulder adduction shoulder internal rotation	shoulder horizontal abduction

22 - Lat Pull-Down (Wide Grip)

Equipment used: high pulley or lat pull-down machine

Moving joints	Joint action	Muscles worked
shoulders	adduction	latissimus dorsi, teres major, sternal portion of pectoralis major
scapulae	downward rotation	pectoralis minor, rhomboids
elbows	flexion	biceps, brachialis, brachioradialis

Exercise purpose: to develop strength and endurance of the middle back and biceps muscles

1. Starting/set-up position: Sit or kneel. If seated, knees are placed under knee pad with hips flexed at 90°. If kneeling, pelvis should be held in neutral position (avoid hip or spinal flexion). Start in up position, hands in wide, pronated grip.

2. Alignment: Stabilize scapulae to avoid elevation and protraction. Keep head and neck in a natural extension of the spine, with spine stabilized, abdominals contracted, elbows straight but not hyperextended, and wrists in neutral. The only moving joints are the shoulders, scapulae, and elbows.

3. Movement: Pull bar in front of the head, towards the sternum, exhaling. Elbows should stay away from the body during pull-down. Release bar upwards slowly, with control, keeping the scapulae depressed.

4. Safety factors: The behind-the-neck lat pull-down is no longer recommended; this exercise places the shoulder joint in the vulnerable position of horizontal extension and external rotation behind the frontal plane and is therefore on the "high risk" list for many sports medicine practitioners. In addition, many clients don't have adequate shoulder flexibility to stay in proper alignment; they hunch over and duck their neck during back lat pull-downs. Using the pull-down in front is safer for your clients.

5. Engage and contract the latissimus dorsi prior to the pull-down, maintaining a conscious contraction on the way down and on the way up.

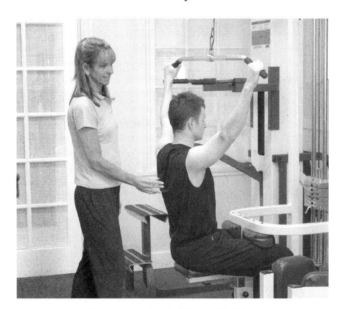

Photo 8-22a. Lat Pull-Down Machine

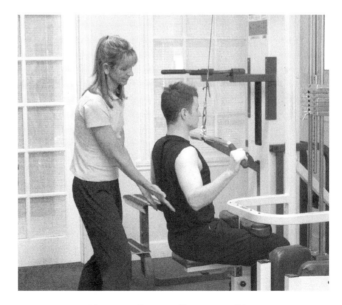

Photo 8-22b. Lat Pull-Down Machine

Spotting guidelines for trainers: Stand behind client with hands pronated above the bar. Encourage client to depress scapulae throughout. Using the knife-edge hands-on technique helps focus client awareness.

Common Errors

- Leaning backwards and rocking the pelvis
- Leaning forwards and flexing the spine
- Wrist breaking
- Uncontrolled eccentric phase with scapulae elevating
- Hyperextended elbows

Modification	Progressions
• For clients who express a **history** of shoulder pain and are **cleared by physician**: avoid this exercise and substitute a low row instead.	• A kneeling lat pull-down is harder to stabilize than a seated lat pull-down. • Standing lat pulls from high pulleys in a two-cable column set-up; progress to unilateral lat pulls.

23 - Bent-Over Row (Unilateral)

Equipment used: dumbbell, bench

Moving joints	Joint action	Muscles worked
shoulder	extension	latissimus dorsi, teres major, sternal portion of pectoralis major (posterior deltoid and long head of triceps assist)
elbow	flexion	biceps, brachialis, brachioradialis

NOTE: Trapezius III and rhomboids contract strongly isometrically as stabilizers due to antigravity position.

Exercise purpose: to develop strength and endurance of the mid-back muscles and the biceps

1. Starting/set-up position: Half-kneel on bench. Same side hand and knee are on bench; working side has extended leg with foot on floor. Dumbbell is held with mid-pronated palm (facing bench). Starting position is straight down.

2. Alignment: Spine should be in neutral and parallel to floor, with head and neck in a natural extension of the spine (neither looking up nor down). Scapulae are depressed and retracted. The only moving joints are the shoulder and elbow. Unless the goal is to work the mid-trapezius muscles and rhomboids, the scapulae should remain stabilized. Spine and neck are stabilized, abdominals are contracted.

3. Movement: Exhale as the weight is lifted; keep the working arm close to the body. Lower the weight slowly, with control, maintaining scapular retraction.

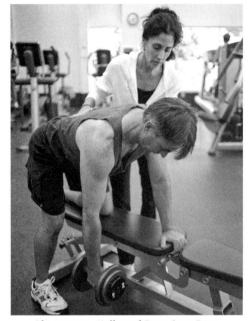

Photo 8-23a. Unilateral Bent-Over Row

4. Safety factors: Avoid dropping the weight too quickly, causing a dislocation force at the shoulder and hyperextending the elbow.

5. Engage and contract the latissimus dorsi and the biceps. Consciously contract the mid-trapezius and rhomboids isometrically throughout the exercise.

Spotting guidelines for trainers: Stand or kneel at client's side, spotting forearm or weight. Remind client to keep scapulae retracted and spine in neutral.

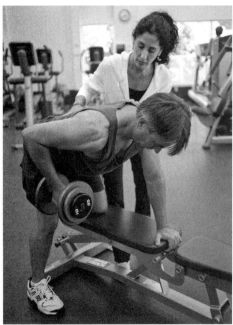

Photo 8-23b. Unilateral Bent-Over Row

Common Errors

- Uncontrolled eccentric phase
- Loss of scapular stabilization; hunched shoulders
- Ducking head towards the weight as it is lifted
- Hyperextended elbow
- Rotation of the spine on the way up
- Loss of spinal stabilization

Modification	Progressions
• For clients who express a **history** of back pain and are **cleared by physician**: a seated low row is a more conservative version of a bent-over low row; it is easier to stabilize the spine in this position.	• Unilateral bent-over row from a low pulley • Unilateral bent-over row from a low pulley on one leg • Standing bilateral bent-over row (advanced clients only)

24 - Seated Lat Row (Low Row)

Equipment used: low pulley or seated row machine, tubing

Moving joints	Joint action	Muscles worked
shoulders	extension	latissimus dorsi, teres major (posterior deltoid and long head of triceps assist)
elbows	flexion	biceps, brachialis, brachioradialis
Optional: scapulae	retraction	trapezius III, rhomboids

Exercise purpose: to develop strength and endurance of the mid-back and biceps muscles

1. Starting/set-up position: Sit in proper alignment with hips flexed at 90°. If seated on floor or low pad, knees should be flexed. Start with arms out in shoulder flexion, elbows soft, and palms in mid-pronation (facing each other, thumbs up). If using a bar, take a narrow, pronated grip.

2. Alignment: Depress and retract scapulae. Hold the lower back still, lift the chest, and stabilize the torso and neck in neutral for optimal latissimus dorsi isolation. Moving joints: Shoulders and elbows. Scapulae can either be stabilized (mid-trapezius muscles and rhomboids contract isometrically), or can actively abduct and adduct, depending on goals.

3. Movement: Exhale when pulling back; pull handles to lower chest, leading with elbows. Make sure torso remains upright through both concentric and eccentric phases.

4. Safety factors: Many clients tend to perform "low-back" rows. This is not appropriate if the goal is to work the latissimus dorsi and/or trapezius muscles. Locked knees in the low-sit position increases stress to the low back. Avoid fly-away weights, especially on the return.

5. Engage and contract the latissimus dorsi and biceps. Focus on either contracting the scapular retractors isometrically (to help isolate the latissimus dorsi), or isotonically through full range (if goal is to work the middle trapezius and rhomboid muscles).

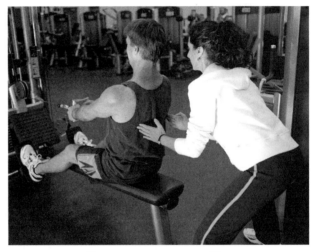

Photo 8-24a. Low Row Machine

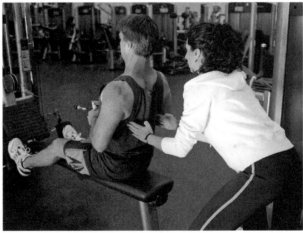

Photo 8-24b. Low Row Machine

Spotting guidelines for trainers: Kneel behind client and spot forearms. Make certain client maintains erect, stable torso throughout.

Common Errors
- Rounding the back on the return phase
- Hyperextending the spine on the concentric phase
- Hyperextending the elbows
- Elevating the scapulae

Progressions
- Seated low row on stability ball
- Standing low row
- Standing low row on one leg
- Low row with anchored tubing while performing a back lunge

---

25 - Lat Pull-Over

Equipment used:

Moving joints	Joint action	Muscles worked
shoulders	extension	latissimus dorsi, teres major, sternal portion of pectoralis major (posterior deltoid and long head of triceps assist)
scapulae	depression	pectoralis minor, trapezius IV
	downward rotation	pectoralis minor, rhomboids
	upward tilt	pectoralis minor

Exercise purpose: to develop strength and endurance of the mid-back muscles

1. Starting/set-up position: Lie supine on bench, feet flat on floor or on bench (depending on leg length and on ability to keep spine in neutral). The end of the bench should support the head; neck should maintain natural alignment. Hold barbell with narrow, pronated grip over the lower chest; elbows are flexed at sides with wrists locked. If holding dumbbell, cup end of dumbbell with both hands, positioning it over lower chest.

2. Alignment: Pelvis, spine, and neck are in neutral with option to press lumbar spine down and perform posterior pelvic tilt. Abdominals are contracted to maintain spinal stability throughout exercise. Moving joints: Shoulders and scapulae. Stabilize spine, neck and pelvis. Stabilize elbows in flexed position.

3. Movement: Stay in sagittal plane and move weight over face, behind head, and toward the floor. Exhale as elbows are pulled back toward sides of chest. Keep movement slow and controlled.

4. Safety factors: Be very cautious with heavy weights; proper spotting is essential to prevent shoulder injury. Perform the exercise slowly and use great control during the eccentric phase. Also, since the weight passes over the client's face, care is required. Avoid arching the lower back; contract abdominals. Keep arms in sagittal plane; avoid flaring the elbows out.

5. Engage and contract the latissimus dorsi and lower pectorals. Keep abdominals isometrically contracted throughout the exercise.

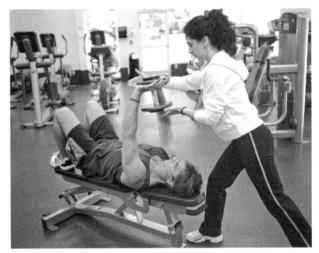

Photo 8-25a. Lat Pull-Over

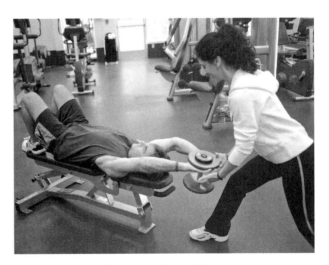

Photo 8-25b. Lat Pull-Over

Spotting guidelines for trainers: Kneel or stand behind client's head, tracking barbell or dumbbell with hands. Encourage client to maintain abdominal tightness.

Common Errors

- Inability to maintain spinal stability; back hyperextends
- Uncontrolled eccentric phase; too much range of motion
- Elbows flare out

Modifications	Progressions
• For clients who express a **history** of shoulder pain and are **cleared by physician**: avoid this exercise. • For clients who express a **history** of back pain and are **cleared by physician**: avoid this exercise.	• Lat pull-over on stability ball • Plyometric lat pull-over with medicine ball on stability ball; during concentric phase, dynamically return to sitting and toss ball to partner; then catch ball and return back to lat pull-over position

Arm (Triceps and Biceps) Exercises

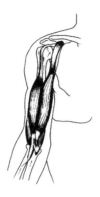

Fig. 8-6a. Biceps

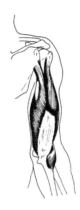

Fig. 8-6b. Triceps

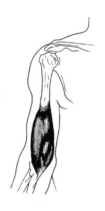

Fig. 8-6c. Brachialis

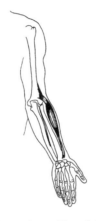

Fig. 8-6d. Brachioradialis

Muscle	Prime Mover for:	Assists with:
Biceps Brachii	elbow flexion	radioulnar supination shoulder flexion shoulder internal rotation shoulder horizontal adduction shoulder abduction (long head) shoulder adduction (short head)
Brachialis	elbow flexion	
Brachioradialis	elbow flexion	
Triceps Brachii	elbow extension	shoulder extension shoulder adduction

26 - Triceps Kickback/Extension (Unilateral)

Equipment used: dumbbell, bench, tubing

Moving joints	Joint action	Muscles worked
elbow	extension	triceps

NOTE: Latissimus dorsi, teres major, mid-trapezius muscles, and rhomboids all contract strongly isometrically due to antigravity position.

Exercise purpose: to develop strength and endurance of the backs of the arms

1. Starting/set-up position: Half kneel on bench. Same-side hand and knee are on bench; working side has extended leg with foot flat on floor. Dumbbell is held at side with elbow flexed at 90°.

2. Alignment: Abdominals are contracted so that the spine maintains neutral alignment and the head and neck maintain a natural extension of the spine (neck neither flexes down nor extends up). Maintain "rectangle" of torso parallel to floor. Keep scapulae depressed and retracted; shoulder joint is extended so that upper arm is parallel to floor. Elbow is flexed at 90° with wrist straight, mid-pronated palm facing bench. Moving joints: Elbow moves while shoulder joint and shoulder girdle are stabilized. Wrist is stabilized in neutral (straight) position.

3. Movement: Exhale as the elbow extends. Elbow should extend fully without hyperextension. Movement should be slow and controlled. Optional radioulnar joint movement to full pronation may provide more gravitational resistance for long head of the triceps. Return elbow to 90° flexed position.

4. Safety factors: Watch for "slamming" elbow joint into full extension; movement should always be smooth and controlled.

5. Engage and contract the triceps. Isometrically contract the latissimus dorsi, teres major, posterior deltoid, mid-trapezius, and rhomboids.

Spotting guidelines for trainers: Spot client from side; assist forearm or weight if necessary. Alternatively, palpate working upper arm, shoulders, and/or scapulae to assist client in maintaining stability.

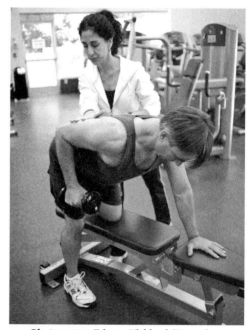

Photo 8-26a. Triceps Kickback/Extension

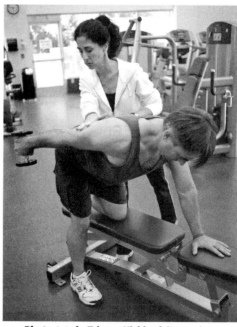

Photo 8-26b. Triceps Kickback/Extension

Common Errors
- Unnecessary wrist movement
- Hunching shoulders
- Neck hyperextension
- Unstable torso; spine rotating with extension
- Hyperextending elbow
- Inability to maintain upper arm parallel to floor

Modification	Progressions
• If client is unable to maintain proper alignment, try standing triceps press-down or supine unilateral triceps extension instead.	• Standing bilateral bent-over triceps kickbacks • Standing triceps kickback on one leg • Prone triceps extensions on stability ball

27 - Standing Triceps Press-Down

Equipment used: high pulley cable column

Moving joints	Joint action	Muscles worked
elbows	extension	triceps

Exercise purpose: to develop strength and endurance of the triceps (back of arms)

1. Starting/set-up position: Stand in proper alignment. Bring lat bar or ropes down to shoulder level; elbows are flexed approximately 90° and touch sides of ribs. Hands are approximately 6 inches apart and pronated if using bar, or mid-pronated if using ropes. Starting position is up.

2. Alignment: Torso is stabilized with abdominals contracted; pelvis, spine, and neck are in neutral. Elbows remain pressed into sides of body. Shoulders are stabilized so that neither flexion nor abduction is possible. Scapulae are depressed throughout exercise. Wrists are neutral. The only moving joints are the elbows.

3. Movement: Exhale as elbows extend and bar is pressed down. Elbows should fully extend without hyperextending. Slowly return to start, flexing elbows to about 90° and maintaining contact with sides of body.

4. Safety factors: Using momentum on the concentric phase and hyperextending the elbows may cause elbow problems.

5. Engage and contract the triceps. Isometrically contract the lower trapezius muscles and the pectoralis minor to maintain scapular depression; keep the latissimus dorsi contracted to maintain a neutral shoulder position.

Spotting guidelines for trainers: Stand behind client, ready to assist with pronated, wide grip. Remind client to depress scapulae, stabilize upper arms, and to use only triceps.

Common Errors
- Inability to stabilize torso; torso rocks back and forth
- Inability to stabilize shoulder joints
- Scapular elevation
- Wrist breaking

Progressions
- Press-down on one leg
- Press-down on one leg balanced on half-foam roller

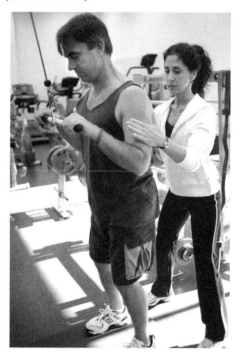

Photo 8-27a. Triceps Press-Down

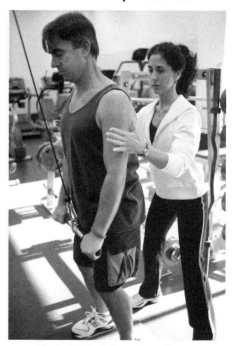

Photo 8-27b. Triceps Press-Down

28 - Seated Triceps Extension (French/Overhead Press)

Equipment used: barbell or dumbbell

Moving joints	Joint action	Muscles worked
elbows	extension	triceps

Exercise purpose: to develop strength and endurance of the triceps (back of arms)

1. Starting/set-up position: Sit or stand in proper alignment. Hold barbell with pronated, close grip (hands no more than 6 inches apart). If using dumbbell, cup one end of the dumbbell with both hands. Alternatively, this exercise may be performed unilaterally: hold dumbbell with one hand and use other hand to support working arm. Start with weight overhead and elbows extended; elbows are held close to ears.

2. Alignment: If standing, knees must be flexed and abdominals contracted, with pelvis, spine, and neck in neutral. If sitting, keep hips flexed at 90° with feet on floor. Scapulae should be depressed throughout exercise; wrists are neutral. Moving joints: Elbows. All other joints are stabilized, including shoulders, wrists, neck, spine, and pelvis.

3. Movement: Flexing the elbows, slowly lower the barbell behind the head to the tops of shoulders. Maintain the upper arm position: elbows point straight to ceiling and are pressed in (towards sides of head). Exhale as elbows extend. May be performed bilaterally or unilaterally.

4. Safety factors: Shoulder flexibility is required to place the upper arm in the proper position. Clients who are unable to stay in correct alignment should be given another exercise. Due to lack of flexibility, scapulae may elevate, shoulders may not fully flex, and it may be difficult to keep elbows close to head.

5. Engage and contract the triceps throughout both concentric and eccentric phases. Maintain lower trapezius and pectoralis minor isometric tension, as well as tight abdominals.

Spotting guidelines for trainers: Stand behind client, tracking bar with alternate grip. If client is performing the exercise unilaterally, maintain hand support on upper working arm (if necessary), while tracking dumbbell with other hand.

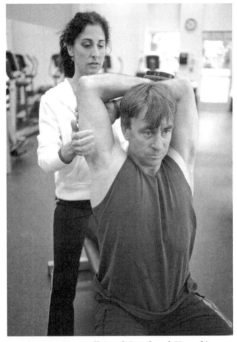

Photo 8-28a. Unilateral Overhead (French) Triceps Press

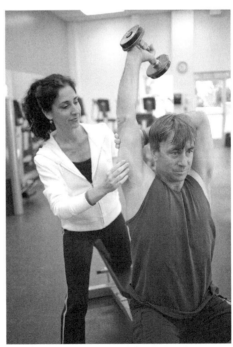

Photo 8-28b. Unilateral Overhead (French) Triceps Press

Common Errors

- Flexing and/or extending the spine
- Inability to maintain stable torso
- Hunching over, failing to maintain vertical upper arms
- Hyperextending elbows

Modifications	Progressions
• For clients who express a **history** of shoulder pain and are **cleared by physician**: avoid this exercise.	• Sit on stability ball.
• For clients with insufficient shoulder flexibility: provide shoulder stretches to increase flexibility; until shoulder flexibility is acquired, provide more appropriate triceps exercises (such as the standing press-down).	• Sit on stability ball with one leg up.

29 - Supine Elbow Extension

Equipment used: barbell or dumbbells, bench

Moving joints	Joint action	Muscles worked
elbows	extension	triceps

Exercise purpose: to develop strength and endurance of the triceps (back of arms)

1. Starting/set-up position: Lie supine on bench with feet flat on floor or up on bench, depending on client leg length and/or ability to maintain a neutral spine. Barbell is held with pronated, close grip (hands no more than 6 inches apart), and shoulders are flexed at 90° with forearms, wrists, and hands in straight line. Single dumbbell is cupped on one end with both hands. If using two dumbbells, start in pronation. If exercise is performed unilaterally, non-working hand provides support to working upper arm. Starting position is up.

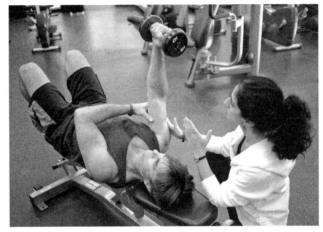

Photo 8-29a. Unilateral Supine Elbow Extension

2. Alignment: Pelvis, spine, and neck are in neutral. Press scapulae down into bench. Elbow(s) are the only moving joints. Shoulders and upper arms are held stable, wrists are neutral, and spine is stabilized on bench.

3. Movement: Slowly lower the weight to forehead or top of head (dumbbell is lowered just behind head) with elbow(s) pointed toward ceiling. Exhale as elbow(s) extend. If using two dumbbells, lower weights into mid-pronated grip so that palms face ears. Extend and return to full pronation.

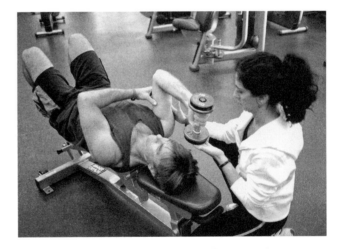

Photo 8-29b. Unilateral Supine Elbow Extension

4. Safety factors: Emphasize control during the eccentric phase to prevent potential head injuries. Do not let the elbow(s) hyperextend.

5. Engage and contract the triceps. Maintain a secure abdominal contraction (isometric) throughout the exercise.

Spotting guidelines for trainers: Stand behind client's head, with knees flexed. Be prepared to kneel during client's eccentric phase as you spot the weight in order to prevent head injuries. Use an alternate grip on the barbell.

Common Errors

- Extending the shoulders and using the latissimus dorsi (confusing this exercise with a lat pull-over)
- Flaring the elbows
- Moving the upper arm
- Wrist breaking
- Unstable torso

Modification	Progressions
• For clients who express a **history** of back pain and are **cleared by physician**: elevate feet onto bench or other low boxes; lie supine on floor.	• Perform supine extension on stability ball. • Perform supine extension on foam roller. • Perform supine extension on foam roller with one leg up.

30 - Triceps Dip

Equipment used: dip bars, bench or triceps dip machine

Moving joints	Joint action	Muscles worked
elbows	extension	triceps
shoulders	flexion	anterior deltoid, pectoralis major

NOTE: Trapezius IV and pectoralis minor contract isometrically quite strongly to keep shoulder girdle from elevating.

Exercise purpose: to develop strength and endurance of the triceps (back of arms)

1. Starting/set-up position: Hands are placed on bars (or bench) with elbows straight but not hyperextended. If using bench, hands should be on edge of bench with hips close in front. Knees may be bent or straight. Starting position is up.

2. Alignment: Abdominals are contracted and body hangs from shoulders in neutral with knees bent. Scapulae are depressed and adducted. Moving joints: Elbows and shoulders. All other joints should be stabilized, with special focus on scapular stabilization. If using bench, stabilize lower body so that the work is performed by the triceps and shoulder flexors. Let lower body hang so that all the weight is lifted by the appropriate muscles.

3. Movement: Lower the body until the elbows are flexed at 90° and the upper arms are parallel to the floor. Exhale as elbows extend and lift body. Keep the elbow and shoulder movement in the sagittal plane; do not let the elbows flare out.

4. Safety factors: Avoid over-bending (hyperflexing) or hyperextending the elbow joint in a weight-bearing position as this causes joint stress. Be cautious with extreme range of motion at the shoulder joint as well; very deep dips may lead to anterior shoulder joint instability. Weight-bearing wrist extension may lead to wrist stress; keep wrists in as neutral a position as possible.

5. Engage and contract the triceps, anterior deltoids, and pectorals. Engage the lower trapezius muscles and the pectoralis minor to keep scapulae depressed.

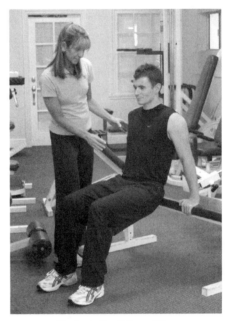

Photo 8-30a. Triceps Dip

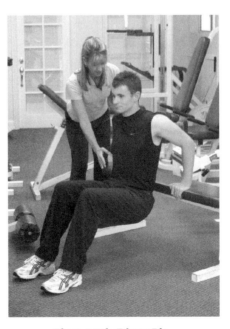

Photo 8-30b. Triceps Dip

Common Errors

- Scapular elevation/shoulder hunching
- Letting elbows flare out
- If using bench: "cheating" by lifting and lowering with legs instead of triceps

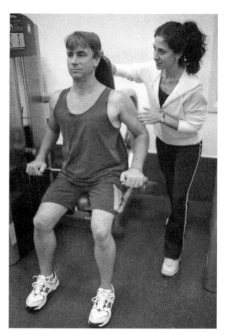

Photo 8-30c. Triceps Dip Machine

Modifications

- For clients who express a **history** of shoulder pain and are **cleared by physician**: avoid this exercise.

Progressions

- Dips off a foam roller
- Dips off a stability ball
- Dips off a stability ball with one leg up

31 - Alternate Dumbbell Biceps Curl

Equipment used: dumbbells

Moving joints	Joint action	Muscles worked
elbows	flexion	biceps, brachialis, brachioradialis
radioulnar	supination	supinator

Exercise purpose: to develop strength and endurance of the biceps (front of arms)

1. Starting/set-up position: Stand or sit in proper alignment. Palms face sides of body (mid-pronation). Starting position is down.

2. Alignment: In standing position, the knees are slightly flexed, with pelvis, spine, and neck in neutral. If seated, hips are flexed 90°, with spine and neck in neutral. Abdominals are contracted and shoulder girdle is depressed and retracted. The elbow and radioulnar joints move. Shoulders do not move; scapulae, neck, spine, etc. are stabilized. Wrists stay neutral.

3. Movement: Exhale as one elbow slowly flexes. Palm supinates gradually as weight is lifted. Inhale and gradually return back to mid-pronation as weight is lowered. Repeat with other side.

4. Safety factors: Avoid wrist breaking (no flexing or extending); this may lead to tennis elbow and/or carpal tunnel syndrome. Be aware that slowly alternating heavy weights in this exercise creates increasing tension in forearm muscles, which isometrically contract to maintain grip on dumbbells.

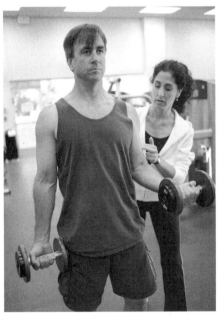

Photo 8-31. Alternate Dumbbell Curl

5. Engage and contract the biceps. Maintain the contraction throughout both concentric and eccentric phases.

Spotting guidelines for trainers: Stand behind client, spotting forearms if necessary. Touch backs of elbows as a reminder to stabilize.

Common Errors
- Wrist breaking
- Swinging upper arm/using momentum
- Pulling arms backward (shoulder extension) while lifting
- Inability to keep torso stable
- Hyperextended knees
- Hunching or lifting shoulders with movement

Modification
- For clients who express a **history** of back pain and **are cleared by physician:** sit instead of stand, or, position spine against a wall with knees bent.

Progressions
- Perform curls on incline bench; start with arms hanging straight down.
- Perform curls on stability ball.
- Perform curls on stability ball with one leg up.
- Perform curls standing on one leg.

32 - Concentration Curl

Equipment used: dumbbells, bench

Moving joints	Joint action	Muscles worked
elbows	flexion	biceps, brachialis, brachioradialis

Exercise purpose: to develop strength and endurance of the biceps (front of arms)

1. Starting/set-up position: Sit, placing elbow of working arm on inside of thigh. Opposite hand is placed either on opposite thigh or behind working arm for support. Feet are flat on floor and hips are flexed. Dumbbell is held with a supinated grip and neutral wrist. Start with elbow extended.

2. Alignment: Flexion should occur at hips only (perform a hip hinge); spine and neck are in neutral with scapulae depressed. Moving joints: Elbows. Wrist is kept straight; shoulder is stabilized. Spine and neck are stabilized.

3. Movement: Exhale as elbow flexes; bring weight up towards shoulder. Slowly lower, inhaling. This exercise may place slightly more emphasis on the short head of the biceps due to the internally rotated position of the shoulder (the short head assists with internal shoulder rotation).

4. Safety factors: As with all biceps exercises, wrist breaking is a concern (flexing and or extending). Maintain neutral wrist.

5. Engage and contract the biceps, brachialis, and the brachioradialis throughout the entire exercise.

Spotting guidelines for trainers: Kneel and guide weight if necessary. Palpate shoulder and lower back to create awareness of neutral spine.

Common Errors
- Rounded shoulders; hunching over
- Spinal flexion instead of hip flexion
- Protracted scapulae
- Wrist breaking
- Hyperextending elbow

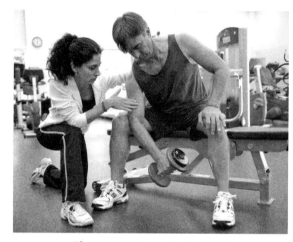
Photo 8-32a. Concentration Curl

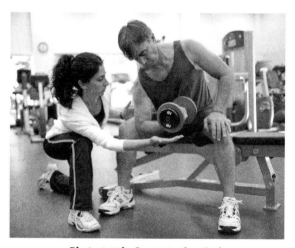
Photo 8-32b. Concentration Curl

Modification
- For clients who express a **history** of back pain and are **cleared by physician**: avoid this exercise. Instead provide biceps exercises on a weight-room chair to help stabilize the spine

33 - Preacher Bench Curls

Equipment used: preacher curl bench with barbell (may use EZ curl bar) or dumbbells, machine

Moving joints	Joint action	Muscles worked
elbows	flexion	biceps, brachialis, brachioradialis

Exercise purpose: to develop strength and endurance of the biceps (front of arms)

1. Starting/set-up position: Sit facing preacher bench. Bench should be adjusted so that shoulders are flexed about 45°. Upper arms rest on pad. Sit so that rib cage rests against pad. Grip barbell or dumbbells with supinated palms and start with elbows extended.

2. Alignment: Sit in a hip hinge without flexing or rounding the spine. Spine and neck are in neutral, scapulae depressed and retracted. Moving joints: Elbows. Stabilize shoulder girdle, neck, and spine. Keep wrists in neutral.

3. Movement: Exhale as elbows flex through as full a range of motion as possible. Slowly lower, inhaling.

4. Safety factors: In order to avoid elbow hyperextension and undue stress on elbows and wrists, it's probably a good safety precaution to stop short of full elbow extension when performing this exercise.

5. Engage and contract the biceps, brachialis, and brachioradialis. Isometrically contract the lower trapezius muscles and pectoralis minor to prevent scapular elevation.

Spotting guidelines for trainers: Kneel in front of client, tracking weights with hands.

Common Errors
- Hunching the shoulders/protracted scapulae
- Collapsing forward into spinal flexion
- Hyperextending the elbows on the eccentric phase
- Wrist breaking

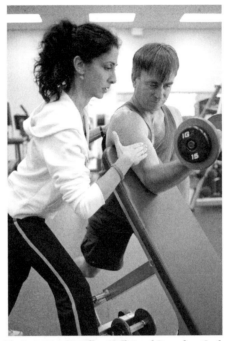

Photo 8-33a. Standing Unilateral Preacher Curl Using Incline Bench

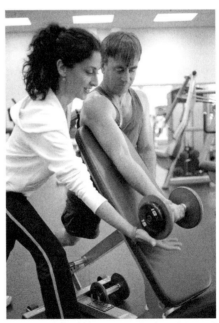

Photo 8-33b. Standing Unilateral Preacher Curl Using Incline Bench

34 - Standing Barbell Curl

Equipment used: barbell or EZ curl bar, may use low pulley

Moving joints	Joint action	Muscles worked
elbows	flexion	biceps, brachialis, brachioradialis

Exercise purpose: to develop strength and endurance of the biceps (front of arms)

1.   Starting/set-up position: Standing in proper alignment (may be performed with back against a wall), hold bar with supinated, shoulder-width grip. Starting position is down.

2.   Alignment: Knees are slightly flexed; pelvis, spine, and neck are in neutral; scapulae are depressed and retracted. Elbows are extended with upper arms tight against body. Moving joints: Elbows. All other joints are stabilized, including the knees, pelvis, spine, shoulders, scapulae, and wrists.

3.   Movement: Exhale as elbows flex. Keep upper arms pressed against ribs at all times. Inhale and lower slowly with control.

4.   Safety factors: When weight is too heavy, many clients will rock torso back and forth, swinging the weights up (increasing risk of injury to the low back). Keep torso absolutely still and anchor the upper arms against the sides of the rib cage. Be sure client goes through full range of motion.

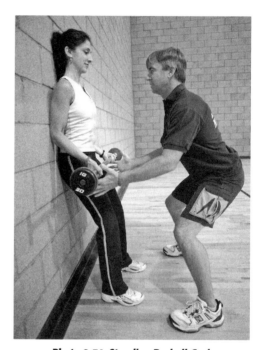

Photo 8-34. Standing Barbell Curl

5.   Engage and contract the biceps, brachialis, and brachioradialis through both concentric and eccentric phases. Many strength experts recommend a slight pause (isometric contraction) at the top.

Spotting guidelines for trainers: Stand in front of client, tracking bar with hands. Alternatively, may stand behind and maintain palpation on tops of shoulders or upper arms.

Common Errors
   •   Wrist breaking
   •   Inability to stabilize torso
   •   Hyperextended elbows
   •   Hyperextended knees
   •   Elevation of scapulae as weight is being lifted

Modification	Progressions
• For clients who express a **history** of back pain and **are cleared by physician**: stand against wall.	• Stand on one leg. • At low pulley stand on one leg on half-foam roller.

35 - Reverse Curl

Equipment used: dumbbells or barbell (EZ curl may be used), bench

Moving joints	Joint action	Muscles worked
elbows	flexion	biceps, brachialis, brachioradialis

Exercise purpose: to develop strength and endurance of the front of the arms, with a greater emphasis on the brachialis

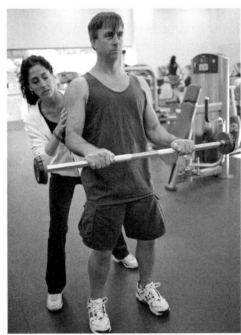

Photo 8-35. Reverse Curl

1. Starting/set-up position: Assume the same as for barbell curl except that palms are pronated on barbell or dumbbells. This places much more stress on the brachialis. If using dumbbells, exercise may be performed seated.

2. Alignment: Knees are slightly flexed; pelvis, spine, and neck are in neutral; scapulae are depressed and retracted. Elbows are extended with upper arms tight against body. Moving joints: Elbows. All other joints are stabilized, including the knees, pelvis, spine, shoulders, scapulae, and wrists.

3. Movement: Exhale as elbows flex. Keep upper arms pressed against ribs at all times. Inhale and lower slowly with control.

4. Safety factors: When weight is too heavy, many clients will rock torso back and forth, swinging the weights up (increasing risk of injury to the low back). Keep torso absolutely still and anchor the upper arms against the sides of the rib cage. Be sure client goes through full range of motion.

5. Engage and contract the biceps, brachialis, and brachioradialis through both concentric and eccentric phases. Many strength experts recommend a slight pause (isometric contraction) at the top.

Spotting guidelines for trainers: Stand in front of client, tracking bar with hands. Alternatively, may stand behind and maintain palpation on tops of shoulders or upper arms.

Common Errors
*   Wrist breaking
*   Inability to stabilize torso
*   Hyperextended elbows
*   Hyperextended knees
*   Elevation of scapulae as weight is being lifted

Modification	Progressions
• For clients who express a **history** of back pain and **are cleared by physician**: stand against wall.	• Stand on one leg. • At low pulley stand on one leg on half-foam roller.

36 - Hammer Curl

Equipment used: dumbbells, bench

Moving joints	Joint action	Muscles worked
elbows	flexion	biceps, brachialis, brachioradialis

Exercise purpose: to develop strength and endurance of the front of the arms, with a greater emphasis on the brachialis

1. Starting position: Assume the same position as that for "Standing Barbell Curl" (exercise #34), except that dumbbells are held at sides in mid-pronated position—this places slightly more stress on the brachioradialis. Weights may be lifted simultaneously or alternating. Exercise may be performed seated.

2. Alignment: Knees are slightly flexed; pelvis, spine, and neck are in neutral; scapulae are depressed and retracted. Elbows are extended with upper arms tight against body. Moving joints: Elbows. All other joints are stabilized, including the knees, pelvis, spine, shoulders, scapulae, and wrists.

3. Movement: Exhale as elbows flex. Keep upper arms pressed against ribs at all times. Inhale and lower slowly with control.

4. Safety factors: When weight is too heavy, many clients will rock torso back and forth, swinging the weights up (increasing risk of injury to the low back). Keep torso absolutely still and anchor the upper arms against the sides of the rib cage. Be sure client goes through full range of motion.

5. Engage and contract the biceps, brachialis, and brachioradialis through both concentric and eccentric phases. Many strength experts recommend a slight pause (isometric contraction) at the top.

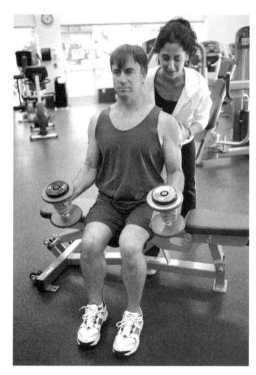

Photo 8-36. Hammer Curl

37 - Palms-Up (Supinated) Wrist Curl

Equipment used: dumbbells or barbell, bench

Moving joints	Joint action	Muscles worked
wrist	flexion	flexor carpi radialis, flexor carpi ulnaris

Exercise purpose: : to develop strength and endurance of the forearm (wrist flexor) muscles

1. Starting/set-up position: Sit on bench with forearms on thighs, holding dumbbells with palms up (supinated). Wrist starts in extension (down position). Alternatively, client may kneel and place forearms on a bench for support.

2. Alignment: Sit in a hip hinge with spine and neck in neutral (no rounding), feet flat on floor. Contract abdominals and keep chest lifted as much as possible, scapulae depressed. Elbows and forearms rest on thighs.

3. Movement: Perform the actions of wrist flexion and extension, exhaling on the way up. Keep movement slow and controlled.

4. Safety factors: Avoid gripping the weights too tightly as this may exacerbate carpal tunnel syndrome and/or tennis elbow.

5. Engage and contract the wrist flexors on both the concentric and eccentric phases.

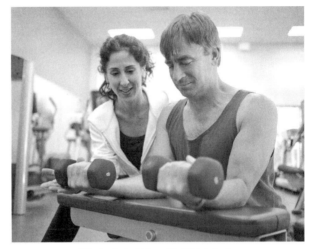
Photo 8-37. Palms-Up Wrist Curl

Common Errors
- Clenching the weights too tightly
- Rounding the spine
- Hunching the shoulders/scapular elevation

38 - Palms-Down (Pronated) Wrist Curl

Equipment used: dumbbells or barbell, bench

Moving joints	Joint action	Muscles worked
wrist	extension	extensor carpi radialis longus, extensor carpi radialis brevis, extensor carpi ulnaris

Exercise purpose: : to develop strength and endurance of the forearm (wrist flexor) muscles

1. Starting/set-up position: Sit on bench with forearms on thighs, holding dumbbells with palms down (pronated). Wrist starts in flexion (down position). Alternatively, client may kneel and place forearms on a bench for support.

2. Alignment: Sit in a hip hinge with spine and neck in neutral (no rounding), feet flat on floor. Contract abdominals and keep chest lifted as much as possible, scapulae depressed. Elbows and forearms rest on thighs.

3. Movement: Perform the actions of wrist extension and flexion, exhaling on the way up. Keep movement slow and controlled.

4. Safety factors: Avoid gripping the weights too tightly, as this may exacerbate carpal tunnel syndrome and/or tennis elbow.

5. Engage and contract the wrist extensors on both the concentric and eccentric phases.

Common Errors
- Clenching the weights too tightly
- Rounding the spine
- Hunching the shoulders/scapular elevation

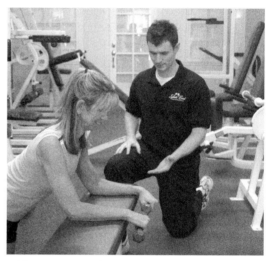

Photo 8-38a. - Palms-Down (Pronated) Wrist Curl

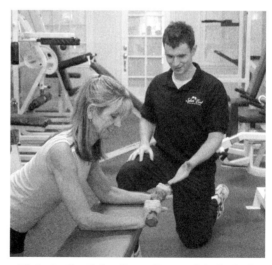

Photo 8-38b. - Palms-Down (Pronated) Wrist Curl

Abdominal Exercises

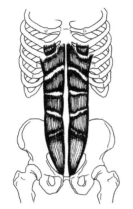

Fig. 8-7a. Rectus Abdominus

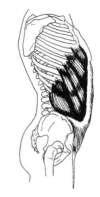

Fig. 8-7b. Internal Obliques

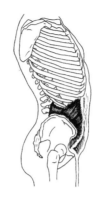

Fig. 8-7c. External Obliques

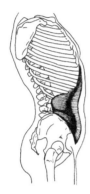

Fig. 8-7d. Transverse Abdominus

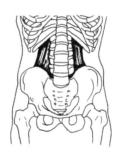

Fig. 8-7e. Quadratus Lumborum

Muscle	Prime Mover for:	Assists with:
Rectus Abdominus	spinal flexion	spinal lateral flexion
Internal and External Obliques	spinal flexion spinal rotation	spinal lateral flexion
Transverse Abdominis	exhalation, expulsion, compression	
Quadratus Lumborum	spinal lateral flexion	

39 - Pelvic Tilt and Hollowing/Drawing-In for Abdominals

Equipment used: mat

Moving joints	Joint action	Muscles worked
lower spine	lumbar flexion	rectus abdominis
pelvis	posterior pelvic tilt	rectus abdominis
Recommended: Muscle action	exhalation, compression	transverse abdominis

Exercise purpose: The pelvic tilt exercise may be used as a beginner exercise to train two muscle groups: the hip extensors (gluteus maximus and hamstrings), and/or the abdominals. In Pilates, posteriorly tilting the pelvis and pressing the lumbar spine into the mat while "hollowing" or "drawing in" the transverse abdominis is called imprinting the spine. An imprinted spine has been shown to provide greater spinal stability for beginners and those with back issues (Richardson et al., 2002). The purpose of the following exercise is to develop body awareness, teach neutral spine and abdominal hollowing, and provide a mild stimulus for the abdominal muscles.

1. Starting/set-up position: Lie supine on mat with knees flexed, feet flat on floor, and arms at sides.

2. Alignment: Pelvis, spine, neck, and scapulae are all in neutral. There should be a very slight lift under the lower back—a natural lordotic curve. Allow the upper body to relax. Moving joints: Lower spine and pelvis.

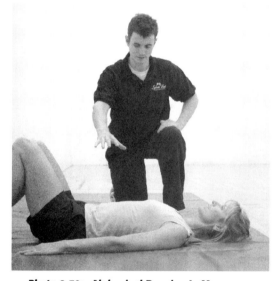

Photo 8-39a. Abdominal Drawing-In Maneuver

3. Movement: Posteriorly tilt the pelvis through its full range, about 10°, using only the abdominals (this is a small movement); press low back and sacrum to floor. Touch gluteals to see if they are relaxed. Try to avoid hip extension and/or pressing into the floor with the feet if the purpose is to work the abdominals. Exhale as the pelvis tilts posteriorly and perform a diaphragmatic (abdominal) breath; the abdominal wall should pull in towards the spine on the exhale. Navel should appear to drop in toward floor and should attempt to be lower than the pubic bone. This is the drawing-in maneuver, also called abdominal hollowing. An isometric contraction may be performed at the end of the range of motion. Inhaling, return the spine to neutral (a small movement).

4. Safety factors: Avoid anteriorly tilting the pelvis and arching the low back on the return. The spine should return only to neutral after the posterior pelvic tilt. Note that many clients will breathe "backwards," and push the abdominal wall out on the exhale. This is an ideal exercise to develop awareness of proper breathing (the abdomen should pull in on the exhale).

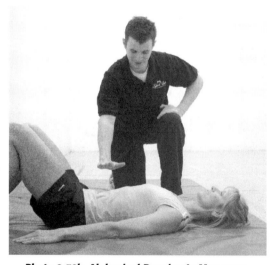

Photo 8-39b. Abdominal Drawing-In Maneuver

5. Engage and contract the transverse and the rectus abdominis. Encourage your client to focus on the area between the navel and pubic bone, to feel a tug on the pubic bone from the rectus abdominis.

Spotting guidelines for trainers: Kneel or sit next to your client. If your client is comfortable with palpation, it is often helpful to gently press down on the abdominal area during the exhale/drawing-in portion of the exercise, releasing your hand on the client's inhale.

Common Errors

- Performing hip extension with the buttocks instead of using the abdominals
- Incorrect breathing: abdominals push out on the exhale
- Allowing the spine to arch (hyperextend) on the return

Progressions
- Perform pelvic tilt/abdominal hollowing on an incline board.
- Perform pelvic tilt/abdominal hollowing inclined on stability ball.

---

40 - Hip Lift

The hip lift (also known as the reverse curl) is simply a more difficult version of the pelvic tilt.

Equipment used: mat, slant board

Moving joints	Joint action	Muscles worked
lower spine	lumbar flexion	rectus abdominis, internal and external obliques
pelvis	posterior pelvic tilt	rectus abdominis
Recommended: Muscle action	exhalation, compression	transverse abdominis

Exercise purpose: to develop strength and endurance of the abdominal muscles

1. Starting/set-up position: Lie supine with legs elevated. Hips are flexed at 90° or greater. Knees may be flexed or straight. Hands may be at sides, crossed on chest, behind head, etc.

2. Alignment: Hips are stabilized and kept in one position throughout exercise (no hip flexion or extension). Knees are stabilized. Moving joints: lower spine and pelvis. Upper spine movement (spinal flexion) increases the difficulty and is optional. Neck stays in line with the spine.

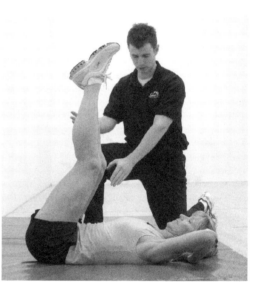

Photo 8-40. Hip Lift

3. Movement: Posteriorly tilt the pelvis using only the abdominal muscles and curl the lower torso up. Exhale when tilting up and pull the abdominals in (diaphragmatic breath) so that the pubic bone rises higher than the navel; tip the tailbone upwards. Keep legs and hips locked into a stable position (hip flexors are isometrically contracted). Most clients will only be able to curl the lower torso up about 10° unless they are very strong and/or have favorable biomechanics (a long torso and flat gluteals help make flexion more visible).

4. Safety factors: Controlled spinal flexion must be performed in order to work the abdominals through full range of motion. Dropping the legs away from the torso (toward the floor) greatly increases the shearing stress on the lumbar spine as the hip flexors exert a pull on the lumbar vertebrae.

5. Engage and contract the abdominals. Concentrate on pulling the lower area in (hollowing) and feeling a pull on the pubic bone.

Spotting guidelines for trainers: Kneel or sit next to your client. If your client is comfortable with palpation, gently press the abdominals down on the lift phase. Another good cue is to draw the hip bones closer to the ribs.

Common Errors
- Use of momentum/swinging legs back and forth to mimic the appearance of a lift (this allows the hip flexors to become the prime movers instead of the abdominals)
- Pressing down on the floor with the arms
- Breath holding

Modification
- For clients who express a **history** of back pain and are **cleared by physician**: avoid this exercise. Perform abdominal curls with the feet on the floor or elevated on a bench instead.

Progression
- Incline the body on a slant board, hands holding on above head

41 - Abdominal Curl (Torso Curl or Crunch)

Equipment used: mat, slant board

Moving joints	Joint action	Muscles worked
spine	flexion	rectus abdominis, internal and external obliques
Recommended: Muscle action	exhalation, compression	transverse abdominis

Exercise purpose: to develop strength and endurance of the abdominal muscles

1. Starting/set-up position: Lie supine (can be inclined on slant board for an easier variation, or declined with head lower than spine for a harder variation). Knees are flexed with feet flat on the floor at a comfortable distance from hips (feet may be supported up on a wall or on a bench). Starting position is down.

2. Alignment: Spine and neck are in neutral alignment, although some beginners and those with back pain may feel better in the imprint position (see "Pelvic Tilt," exercise #39). Hands and arms may be in a variety of positions (e.g., at the sides, on the chest, fingers behind ears, etc. The closer the hands and arms are to the trunk, the easier the lift is biomechanically; the longer the lever, the more difficult). The moving joint: entire spinal column, which curves into flexion.

3. Movement: Exhale as spinal flexion is performed; use a correct diaphragmatic breath (abdomen pulls in and hollows on the exhale). Pull ribs toward pubic bone and pull pubic bone toward ribs (posterior pelvic tilt). Full range of spinal flexion is about 40° (30° with upper torso, 10° with pelvis). Shoulder blades should lift off floor. Neck is stabilized and continues the line of the spine (since the spine is flexed, also flex the neck slightly), but should have no independent movement of its own. To optimally isolate the abdominals, hips should be stabilized.

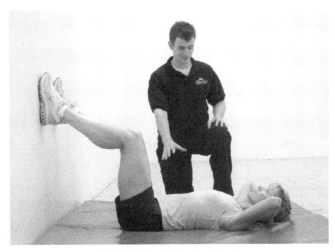

Photo 8-41a. Abdominal Curl

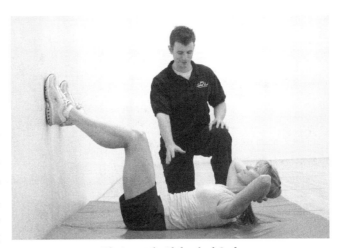

Photo 8-41b. Abdominal Curl

4. Safety factors: Avoid jerking or yanking on head or neck; this decreases the exercise's effectiveness and increases the risk of injury. Hyperextending the cervical spine (looking at the ceiling while crunching) also places stress on the neck. Many clients do their curl-ups too quickly, using momentum. Keep movements slow and controlled with focused awareness. Avoid arching the low back as the upper torso is lowered.

5. Engage and contract the abdominals, pulling them in hard on the exhale/lift. Adding an isometric contraction at the top (keep exhaling) increases the difficulty.

Spotting guidelines for trainers: Kneel or sit next to your client. If your client is comfortable with palpation, gently press the abdominals down during spinal flexion. Another good cue is to draw the ribs and hip bones closer together.

Common Errors

- Performing "neck-ups" (excessive neck flexion) instead of lower spinal flexion
- Breath holding
- Using momentum
- Allowing the abdominal wall to bulge outwards during spinal flexion

Modifications	Progressions
• For clients who express a **history** of back pain and are **cleared by physician**: supporting feet up on bench or wall (knees flexed at 90°) may be the safest and most comfortable position for clients with a history of back pain. Most clients with back pain feel best working from the imprint position (see "Pelvic Tilt," exercise #39) with the lumbar spine pressed down and the pelvis posteriorly tilted. • For clients who express a **history** of neck pain and are **cleared by physician**: gently support the head with one or both hands behind ears. Remind client to relax the neck muscles and put his/her focus on contracting the abdominals. Encourage client to stop and rest the head on the floor, turning the neck from side to side, whenever necessary.	• Perform curls on a declined slant bench (head lower than hips). • Perform curls on a stability ball, either flat or declined. • Perform curls on a stability ball, one leg up. • Perform curls on stability ball, holding tubing anchored on wall behind head. • Perform curls, adding lower body movement.

42 - Supine Crunch Twist (Rotational Curl-Up)

Equipment used: mat, slant board

Moving joints	Joint action	Muscles worked
spine	flexion with rotation	internal and external obliques
Recommended: Muscle action	exhalation, compression	transverse abdominis

Exercise purpose: to develop strength and endurance of the abdominal muscles

1. Starting/set-up position: Lie supine. There are many variations for both lower and upper body: legs may be elevated, ankles crossed, feet flat on floor, hands behind head, reaching toward legs, etc. Spine and neck start in neutral alignment.

2. Alignment: Neck is stabilized and has no independent movement. If one or both hands are behind head, shoulder and elbow joints are stabilized (elbow remains in peripheral vision). Lower body is stabilized in order to isolate the obliques. The moving joint is the entire spinal column, which curves into flexion and rotation.

3. Movement: Exhale when lifting. Cross one side of upper torso diagonally across toward opposite hip. Shoulder blade lifts up off floor. Movement is slow and controlled. Inhale on the return.

4. Safety factors: As in the basic crunch, avoid yanking on neck, which may cause neck problems. Some clients will perform shoulder horizontal flexion (moving the elbow forward) to mimic the correct action. Avoid momentum.

5. Engage and contract the obliques. Add an isometric contraction at the top to increase the difficulty.

Spotting guidelines for trainers: Kneel or sit next to your client, directing him/her to pull the ribs across toward the opposite hip.

Common Errors
- Rocking side to side without stabilizing the hips
- Pulling on the neck/loss of neck stability
- Excessive shoulder or arm movement
- Too much momentum
- Breath holding

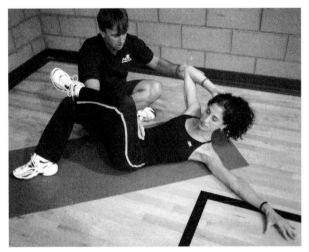

Photo 8-42. Abdominal Cruch Twist

Modifications
- For clients who express a **history** of back pain and are **cleared by physician**: support feet up on bench to facilitate lumbar flexion and to help prevent spinal extension on the down phase.
- For clients who express a **history** of neck pain and are **cleared by physician**: gently support head with one or both hands behind ears. Rest head and neck frequently.

Progressions
- Perform crunch twist on a decline slant board.
- Perform crunch twist on stability ball.
- Perform crunch twist on stability ball, one leg up.
- Perform crunch twist adding lower body movement.

43 - Abdominal Exercise Machines

Many seated abdominal exercise machines are designed in such a way that it is much more likely that the exerciser will perform hip flexion instead of spinal flexion. In order to work the abdominals effectively, spinal flexion must be performed through the full range of motion, and the hips must be stabilized.

- Sit so that the axis of rotation, or cam, is aligned with the lower part of the sternum.

- Flex the spine so that the rib cage and pubic bone tilt towards each other. Exhale during flexion, pulling the abdominals in.

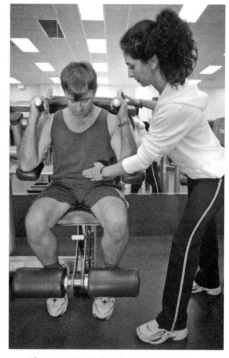

Photo 8-43. Abdominal Curl Machine

Standing Roman Chair

In order to effectively train the abdominals on this apparatus, the exerciser needs to already have very strong abdominals as well as good body awareness. A very common mistake that many exercisers make is to perform rapid hip flexion (with either straight or bent knees) with a great deal of momentum. The correct method is as follows.

- Bring hips in to about 90° of flexion (knees bent) and stabilize them at that degree. This takes a great deal of isometric hip flexor strength.

- Maintaining the isometric contraction of the hip flexors, slowly curl the pubic bone up toward the ribs, exhaling. For most clients, the movement will be small. The moving joint actions are posterior pelvic tilt and lower spinal flexion.

Lower Back Exercises

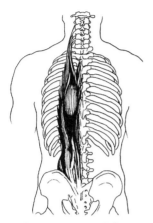

Fig. 8-8a. Erector Spinae

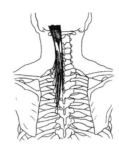

Fig. 8-8b. Semispinalis and Multifidus

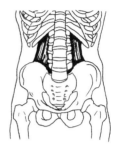

Fig. 8-8c. Quadratus Lumborum

Muscle	Prime Mover for:	Assists with:
Longissimus	cervical and thoracic spinal extension, lateral flexion and rotation	
Spinalis	cervical and thoracic spinal extension, lateral flexion and rotation	
Iliocostalis	cervical, thoracic, and lumbar spinal extension, lateral flexion and rotation	
Semispinalis	cervical and thoracic spinal extension, lateral flexion and rotation	
Multifidus	cervical, thoracic, and lumbar spinal extension, lateral flexion and rotation	
Quadratus Lumborum	spinal lateral flexion	

44 - Seated Back Extension Machine

Equipment used: seated back extension machine

Moving joints	Joint action	Muscles worked
lower spine	extension	erector spinae
hips	extension	gluteus maximus and hamstrings

Exercise purpose: to develop strength and endurance of the lower back muscles. This may be done by isotonically challenging the erector spinae through its full range of motion or by isometrically challenging the erector spinae when the spine is maintained in neutral.

1. Starting position: Sit with belt across hips, hands on thighs or handles for support. To challenge the spinal extensors isotonically, adjust the machine so that the axis of rotation is near the lower thoracic spine. Most back extension machines also allow for hip extensor focus, depending on where the axis of rotation is set; if the goal is to work the hip extensors and train the erector spinae muscle as a stabilizer, align the axis of rotation near the hips.

2. Alignment: If spinal movement and an isotonic challenge is the goal, stabilize the hips, start in spinal flexion (hands on thighs), and move into spinal extension. Moving joints: spine. If only hip joint movement is used, spine should be stabilized in neutral, contracting the abdominals. Neck should be stabilized in both cases.

3. Movement: Exhale as spine and/or hips extend. Movement should be slow and controlled at all times. Return slowly to start while inhaling.

4. Safety factors: This exercise may be risky for clients with back problems. In this case, discuss appropriate exercises with their physician. Be conservative, use lighter weight with more repetitions, and avoid exercising the low-back muscles to failure. Hands should be on thighs when the spine is flexed and weight bearing.

5. Engage and contract the targeted muscle group (erector spinae or gluteus maximus and hamstrings). Isometrically contract abdominals and erector spinae if hip extensor work is desired. Isometrically contract hip extensors if erector spinae work is the goal.

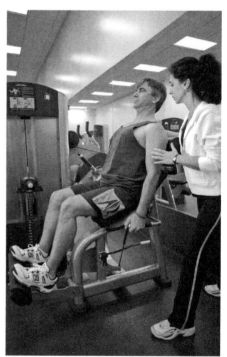

Photo 8-44. Back Extension Machine

Common Errors
-   Use of momentum
-   Incorrect setting of machine axis
-   Using too much weight
-   Breath holding

45 - Prone Back Extension

Equipment used: mat

Moving joints	Joint action	Muscles worked
lumbar and thoracic spine	extension	erector spinae

Exercise purpose: to develop strength and endurance of the lower back muscles

1. Starting/set-up position: Lie prone with forehead on mat, and neck in neutral alignment. Hips are pressed into floor with gluteals contracted. For modified cobra, elbows are flexed and pressed into sides with palms on floor. For other variations, arms may be in neutral at sides, or flexed overhead and resting on mat.

2. Alignment: spine and neck are in neutral position; scapulae are depressed and retracted. Moving joints: lumbar and thoracic spine. Cervical spinal extensors contract isometrically, maintaining neutral alignment. Hips are stabilized.

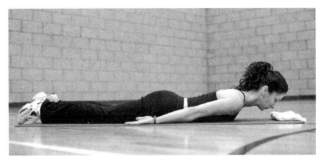

Photo 8-45. Prone Back Extension

3 Movement: This exercise has several variations. Perhaps the safest and most conservative is the supported, modified cobra position: move smoothly and slowly up onto elbows, hold for a few seconds, and slowly return; perform 8–12 repetitions. Other variations include extending spine with both arms at sides, one arm at side and one arm overhead, both arms overhead, etc. In all cases the extension is smooth and controlled, with pelvis and neck in neutral. For many clients, breathing feels most natural when inhaling on the way up, and exhaling on the return.

4. Safety factors: This exercise may not be appropriate for all clients. If it seems to trigger pain, don't do it (discuss back exercises with the client's physician). Avoid hyperextending the neck; it should have no independent movement.

5. Engage and contract the erector spinae muscles. Isometrically contract the cervical spinal extensors, the scapular retractors, and the buttocks.

Spotting guidelines for trainers: Kneel or sit next to your client, using palpation to help him/her feel the contraction of the erector spinae.

Common Errors
- Hyperextending the neck/thrusting the chin forward
- Using momentum
- Forcefully hyperextending the lower back

Modification
- For clients who express a **history** of low-back pain and are **cleared by physician**: try significantly reducing the range of motion; have your client lie prone and lift the head, neck, and chest only an inch or two off the floor; hold and breathe. If this still triggers pain, avoid the exercise.

Progressions
- Perform spinal extension on a stability ball.
- Perform spinal extension on a stability ball with one leg up.
- Perform spinal extension, adding rotation.

46 - Back Extension on Roman Chair

Equipment used: Roman chair (back-extension bench)

Moving joints	Joint action	Muscles worked
lower spine	extension	erector spinae
hips	extension	gluteus maximus, hamstrings

Exercise purpose: to develop strength and endurance of the lower back muscles. However, this exercise device may be used to work either the hip extensors or the spinal extensors or both, depending on the placement of the hips on the pad.

1. Starting/set-up position: To isolate the erector spinae, lay over the front pad so that the edge of the pad is slightly above the iliac crest. Flex the spine with head down. As with abdominal crunches, hand position can vary, depending on client goals and muscular strength. Biomechanically, keeping arms at sides is the easiest variation, while arms overhead is the hardest. (For increased hip-extensor work, slide hips forward on the front pad so that the edge of the pad is below the iliac crest or even under the upper thighs.)

2. Alignment: Cervical spine stays in line with the rest of the spine: if the spine is flexed, the cervical spine is slightly flexed as well; if the spine is extended, the cervical spine also has very slight extension. Moving joints: Lower spine. Stabilize hips if the goal is erector spinae strengthening.

3. Movement: Inhale as spine extends upward. Experts are divided on whether or not the spine should extend just to neutral (parallel to floor), or move beyond neutral into increased extension. All movements, concentric and eccentric, should be very smooth and controlled. Exhale as the spine slowly flexes.

4. Safety factors: This exercise has been considered controversial in the past according to several major fitness organizations. It is still advisable to use caution, since extending the spine up above parallel is especially risky for some clients. Carefully consider the client's goals and past history of back problems. Never continue back-extension work if it causes pain; and avoid exercising these muscles to failure.

5. Engage and contract the erector spinae muscles. Isometrically contract the cervical spinal extensors, the scapular retractors, and the gluteals and hamstrings.

Common Errors
*   Excessive range of motion
*   Jerky movement/momentum
*   Hyperextending the neck

> **Modification**
> *   For clients who express a **history** of back or neck pain and are **cleared by physician**: avoid this exercise.

Torso Stability Exercises

In this section, exercises will be shown in which the core muscles are challenged isometrically as stabilizers; in all cases, the goal is to maintain the spine and the scapulae in neutral. A neutral spine maintains the four curves of the spine in their ideal alignment; neutral scapulae are fully depressed and mid-way between retraction and protraction. The torso muscles challenged have already been presented in this text.

- rectus abdominis
- external and internal obliques
- transverse abdominis
- quadratus lumborum
- erector spinae
- multifidus

Scapular muscles challenged have been previously discussed as well:

- trapezius
- rhomboids
- pectoralis minor
- serratus anterior
- levator scapulae

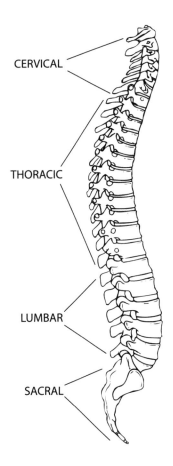

CERVICAL

THORACIC

LUMBAR

SACRAL

47 - Supine Heel Slides and Dead Bug

Equipment used: mat

Muscles used: see torso and scapular muscles listed above under "Torso Stability Exercises"

Exercise purpose: to learn to maintain neutral alignment in the supine position while the extremities are moving

1. Starting/set-up position: Lie supine on mat in ideal alignment, both knees bent, feet flat on floor, arms at sides, palms down.

2. Alignment: Carefully position spine (including neck) in neutral, maintaining the four curves in their proper relationship to each other. Hips are level, and scapulae are depressed and completely in contact with the mat. Hollow (draw in) the abdominals.

3. Movement: While stabilizing core, slowly slide one heel out along the floor, exhaling, pause and inhale, then slide it back in, exhaling. Repeat with other heel. Abdominals remain hollowed throughout. If client successfully maintains ideal alignment, more difficult variations may be shown; see "Progressions" below.

4. Safety factors: This exercise is conservative and safe; however, loss of spinal stability may be problematic for clients with back pain.

5. Engage and contract all spinal and scapular stabilizing muscles simultaneously and isometrically.

Spotting guidelines for trainers: Sit or kneel next to client. If client is comfortable, palpation techniques are important for enhanced body awareness; your hands may be placed on client's abdomen, under the lumbar spine, on both hips, on both shoulders, etc. Help client become aware of the slightest inappropriate core movement.

Common Errors

- Back arches off floor during heel slide
- Neck does not stay in neutral
- Scapulae protract off floor
- Abdominals bulge out during heel slide
- One hip presses up higher than the other

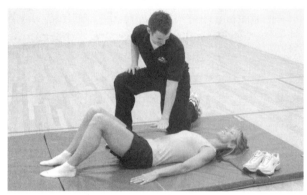

Photo 8-47a. Supine Heel Slide Stability Exercise

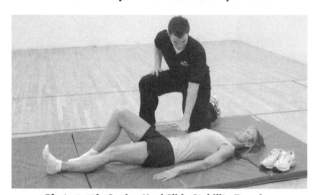

Photo 8-47b. Supine Heel Slide Stability Exercise

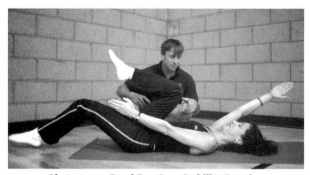

Photo 8-47c. Dead Bug Core Stability Exercise

Progressions

- Perform knee lifts instead of heel slides: slowly alternate knees, lifting first one up, then the other. Tips of toes just touch the floor on the way down. Goal is to keep torso perfectly still.
- Perform knee lifts and add straight-arm movements (this is the dead bug), with same-side arm and leg moving together. Goal is to keep torso perfectly still.

48 - Quadruped

Equipment used: mat

Muscles used: see torso and scapular muscles listed above under "Torso Stability Exercises"

Exercise purpose: to learn to maintain neutral alignment in the all-fours position; to promote balance

1. Starting/set-up position: On hands and knees in ideal alignment on a mat

2. Alignment: Pelvis, spine, neck, and scapulae are all in neutral. Hips and shoulders are level, forming an even rectangle when viewed from above. Abdominals are lifted and contracted without causing spinal flexion. Hands are directly under shoulders; knees are directly under hips; elbows are slightly flexed with fingers pointed straight ahead.

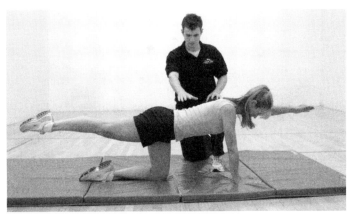

Photo 8-48. Quadruped

3. Movement: This exercise is typically performed completely statically: one leg lifts so that the leg is in line with the spine; the opposite arm is lifted also in line with the spine, parallel to the floor. This position is then held for several seconds. Maintain even, regular breathing. Switch sides. Alternatively, the static quadruped can progress to very slow and mindful movement: opposite arm and leg can lift and lower 5–10 times, maintaining torso absolutely still.

4. Safety factors: Abdominals must remain lifted and contracted to protect the spine. Avoid neck hyperextension.

5. Engage and contract all spinal and scapular stabilizing muscles simultaneously and isometrically.

Spotting guidelines for trainers: Kneel next to client and use your hands to create enhanced body awareness if necessary, e.g., place your hand under the abdominal wall and ask him or her to lift the navel away from your hand.

Common Errors
- Abdominals aren't contracted, leading to spinal misalignment.
- Scapulae are either excessively retracted or protracted.
- Hyperextended elbows
- Knees aren't in line with hips.
- Neck hyperextension

Modification
- For clients with poor core stability and/or balance problems: place an appropriately sized stability ball under the torso (it should be small enough that torso is still parallel to floor); allow the core to "rest" on the ball while performing the quadruped.

Progression
- Perform quadruped with one knee balancing on a BOSU while the opposite hand balances on a medicine ball.

49 - Planks

Equipment used: mat

Muscles used: see torso and scapular muscles listed above under "Torso Stability Exercises"

Exercise purpose: to learn to maintain neutral alignment in the plank position and provide a significant challenge to the core stabilizer muscles

1. Starting/set-up position: There are several options, depending on your client's fitness level and on the variation desired. The starting position for the basic plank is on hands and toes with the torso in neutral alignment. Alternatively, a side plank may be performed.

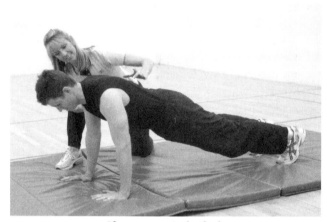

Photo 8-49a. Basic Plank

2. Alignment for basic plank: Hands under shoulders, fingers spread wide, elbows just slightly flexed (not hyperextended). Pelvis, spine, and neck are all in neutral alignment with abdominals contracted. Hips and shoulders are level. Scapulae are depressed and in neutral (neither protracted nor retracted). A straight line is maintained from the heels to the head. For a modified side plank, support body on the side, up on one elbow, hip on floor, knees bent. Form a straight line from the hips through the head. When viewed from the side, pelvis, spine, and neck are in neutral. Scapulae are depressed, with especial attention to the weight-bearing scapula.

3. Movement: If a plank is performed for stability-training purposes, it is usually held without movement for several seconds (e.g., 10-60). There are no moving joints; everything is stabilized and perfectly immobile.

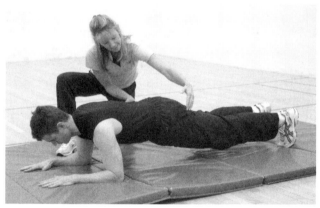

Photo 8-49b. Modified Plank

4. Safety factors: Care must be taken not to hyperextend the spine. Prolonged holding in this pose without sufficient abdominal support may compromise the back. For less skilled exercisers, it is much safer to perform the plank on the knees, maintaining a straight line from the knees to the head. Make certain your client continues to breathe while holding in the abdominals.

5. Engage and contract all spinal and scapular stabilizing muscles simultaneously and isometrically.

Spotting guidelines for trainers: Kneel next to client and use your hands to create enhanced body awareness if necessary, e.g., place your hand under the abdominal wall and ask him/her to lift the navel away from your hand.

Common Errors

- Abdominals aren't contracted, leading to spinal misalignment.
- Scapulae are either excessively retracted or protracted.
- Hyperextended elbows
- Neck hyperextension or flexion
- Weight-bearing scapula is elevated in side plank.

Modifications	Progressions
• For clients who express a **history** of back pain and are **cleared by physician**, or beginners: perform basic plank on knees. • For clients who express a **history** of wrist pain and are **cleared by physician**: perform planks on elbows and forearms.	• Perform basic plank, one leg up. • Perform basic plank, lower into "hover" position (elbows flexed) and hold. • Perform side plank on one hand with legs straight, feet stacked up top of each other. • Perform side plank on one hand with one leg straight, other leg held in abduction. • Perform basic plank, move to side plank on one side; repeat other side.

Lower Body Exercises
(Quadriceps, Hamstrings, Gluteals, Abductors, Adductors)

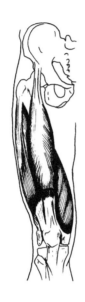
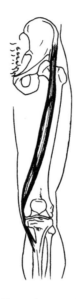
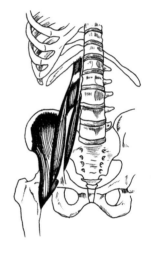

Fig. 8-9a. Quadriceps   **Fig. 8-9b. Sartorius**   **Fig. 8-9c. Psoas and Iliacus**

Muscle	Prime Mover for:	Assists with:

Quadriceps:
    Rectus Femoris
    Vastus Lateralis
    Vastus Intermedius
    Vastus Medialis
	hip flexion and knee extension
	knee extension
	knee extension
	knee extension	

Psoas	hip flexion	
Iliacus	hip flexion	
Sartorius		hip flexion hip abduction hip outward rotation knee flexion

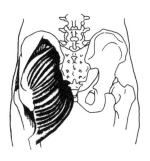

Fig. 8-10a. Gluteus Maximus

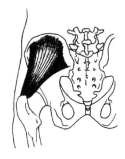

Fig. 8-10b. Gluteus Medius

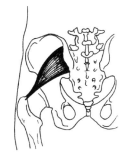

Fig. 8-10c. Gluteus Minimus

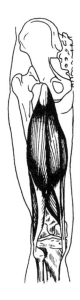

Fig. 8-10d. Hamstrings

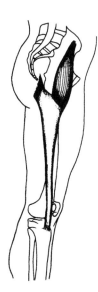

Fig. 8-10e. Tensor Fasciae Latae

Muscle	Prime Mover for:	Assists with:
Gluteus Maximus	hip extension hip outward rotation	
Gluteus Medius	hip abduction	
Gluteus Minimus	hip inward rotation	

Hamstrings
  Biceps Femoris
 	
  Semitendinosus
 	
  Semimembranosus
	hip extension
	knee flexion
	hip extension
	knee flexion
	hip extension
	knee flexion	

Tensor Fasciae Latae		hip abduction, flexion, and inward rotation

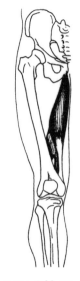

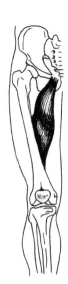

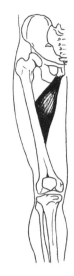

Fig. 8-11a. Adductor Magnus   **Fig. 8-11b. Adductor Longus**   **Fig. 8-11c. Adductor Brevis**

Fig. 8-11d. Pectineus   **Fig. 8-11e. Gracilis**

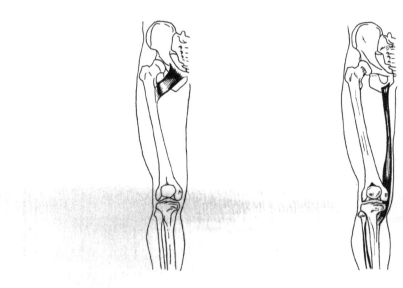

Muscle	Prime Mover for:	Assists with:
Adductor Magnus	hip adduction	hip flexion and inward rotation
Adductor Longus	hip adduction	hip flexion and inward rotation
Adductor Brevis	hip adduction	hip flexion and inward rotation
Pectineus	hip adduction hip flexion	inward rotation
Gracilis	hip adduction	hip flexion and inward rotation

50 - Knee Extensions

Equipment used: knee extension machine or bench with ankle weights

Moving joints	Joint action	Muscles worked
knees	extension	quadriceps: rectus femoris, vastus lateralis, vastus intermedius, vastus medialis

Exercise purpose: to develop strength and endurance of the quadriceps muscles

1. Starting/set-up position: Adjust machine so that axis of rotation lines up with knee joint. Knees should be flexed at slightly more than 90°. If using bench with ankle weights, place hands at sides for support, keeping spine in neutral alignment.

2. Alignment: Press back into pad, contract abdominals, and maintain spine, neck, and scapulae in neutral alignment. Moving joints: Knees. Keep hips, spine, and neck stabilized.

3. Movement: Exhale as knees extend. Movement should be smooth and slow. A one- to two-second isometric contraction may be added at the top. Many experts recommend full extension of the knee (including pulling the patella proximally), although there is some controversy. Physical therapists often use terminal knee extension exercises (flexing the knee only about 10–20° and moving to full extension) to target the vastus medialis. Inhaling, lower the weight slowly.

4. Safety factors: Use caution with heavy knee extension loads; some experts fear that using heavy weight, especially when the knee is flexed greater than 90° (as in the starting position), is harmful to the knee joint.

5. Engage and contract the quadriceps. Isometrically contract the abdominals to help press the back towards the pad.

Spotting guidelines for trainers: Make certain your client's back is pressed to the back of the seat; direct client's attention to the quadriceps action.

Common Errors
- Using rapid, jerky, sudden movements that rely on momentum to accomplish the exercise
- Allowing hips to move
- Arching low back away from the seat

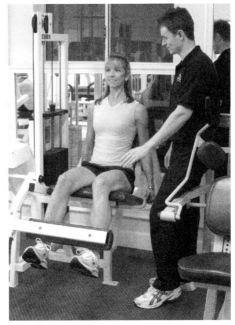

Photo 8-50. Knee Extension Machine

Modification
- For clients who express a **history** of knee pain and are **cleared by physician:** reduce the weight. Some knee extension machines have range-of-motion limiters; use these to keep knees from moving into painful or deeply flexed ranges. If clients still experience pain, avoid this exercise and try short-arc quad exercises (shown in Chapter 10, "Injury Prevention," Figure 10-12).

Progressions
- Seated unilateral knee extension on stability ball with elastic band around ankle
- Standing unilateral knee extension with elastic band around ankle

51 - Knee Flexion Machine

Equipment used: knee-flexion (knee-curl) machine

Moving joints	Joint action	Muscles worked
knees	flexion	hamstrings: biceps femoris, semitendinosus, semimembranosus

Exercise purpose: to develop strength and endurance of the hamstrings muscles

1. Starting/set-up position: May sit, stand, or lie prone, depending on machine. In all cases, hip action should be neutralized. If lying prone on a flat bench, gluteals should be contracted to press hips down and kneecaps should be just off the bench; if standing, neutral pelvis and spine should be maintained. In sitting position, press back, neck, and head against pad.

2. Alignment: Regardless of the position required by the machine, care should be taken to keep the pelvis, spine, neck, and scapulae in neutral with abdominals contracted. The only moving joints are the knees.

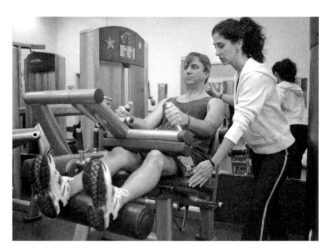

Photo 8-51. Knee Flexion Machine

3. Movement: Exhale as knees flex. Bring heels as close as possible to the buttocks. Inhaling, slowly lower.

4. Safety factors: Keep knees from hyperextending; some machines have a pad that stabilizes the thighs but may press the knees into an uncomfortable, hyperextended range. In this case, use range-of-motion limiters if available.

5. Engage and contract the hamstrings, maintaining contraction through both concentric and eccentric phases.

Spotting guidelines for trainers: Use your hands, if necessary, to stabilize client's spine and create increased awareness of stable core.

Common Errors
- Allowing the hips to move
- Core instability
- Back hyperextension
- Knee hyperextension
- Excessive momentum

Modification
- For clients who express a **history** of back pain and are **cleared by physician**: prone and standing hamstring machines pose a higher risk to the spine than does a seated machine. If only prone and/or standing hamstring machines are available, substitute a more conservative exercise on the floor, such as supine buttock squeezes or supine knee flexion with feet on a stability ball, knees flexing and extending.

Progression
- Standing unilateral knee flexion with elastic band around ankles

52 - Leg Press or Leg Sled Machine

The leg-press movement is similar to a squat; however, because the body is much more supported, it is safer and easier for beginners to learn.

Equipment used: leg press machine

Moving joints	Joint action	Muscles worked
hips	extension	gluteus maximus, hamstrings
knees	extension	quadriceps
ankles	plantar flexion	gastrocnemius, soleus

Exercise purpose: to develop strength and endurance of the lower body muscles

1. Starting/set-up position: Sit, or lie supine (most "supine" machines are actually inclined). Adjust the seat or the footpad so that the knees are flexed at 90°. Feet should be flat on the footpad.

2. Alignment: Pelvis, spine, neck, and scapulae are in neutral with abdominals contracted. Moving joints: Hips, knees, and ankles. Pelvis is stabilized in neutral; spine and neck do not move.

3. Movement: Exhale as the hips and knees extend. Knees may come to full extension in a controlled manner without hyperextending. Inhale and slowly return to flexion.

4. Safety factors: Rapid, uncontrolled movement with knee snapping and jerking increases risk of knee injury. Help clients to feel the difference between full extension of the knee and a forceful "locking" or hyperextending of the knee. Avoid hyperflexion of the knee in a weight-bearing position; do not allow the knees to go much beyond 90° of flexion. Avoid arching or flexing the back or anteriorly or posteriorly tilting the pelvis. Take care to maintain a proper foot position so that slipping off the footpad is not a problem.

5. Engage and contract the gluteus maximus, hamstrings, and quadriceps. Isometrically contract the abdominals to maintain the back against the seat.

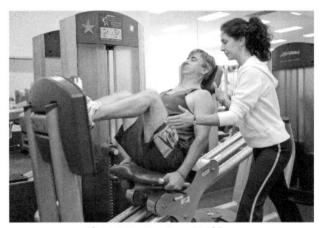

Photo 8-52a. Leg Press Machine

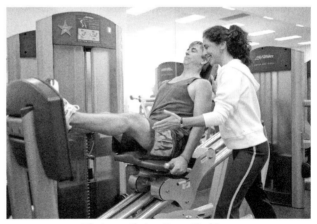

Photo 8-52b. Leg Press Machine

Spotting guidelines for trainers: Sit or kneel by your client's side in order to check alignment and knee hyperextension tendencies. Alternatively, for heavy loads, two spotters may be required to assist with the weights if necessary.

Common Errors

- Hyperextending the knees
- Excessive momentum
- Back hyperextension
- Lumbar flexion when the hips and knees are flexing; spine should not flex or extend

Modification	Progressions
• For clients who express a **history** of knee and/or back pain and are **cleared by physician**: decrease range of motion and reduce the weight.	• Perform leg press unilaterally. • When knees and hips extend, perform the additional movement of ankle plantar flexion and dorsiflexion; flex knees and hips back to starting position.

53 - Squats

The weight-room style squat is an excellent functional exercise; it is needed in activities of daily living, such as lifting heavy objects and getting in and out of chairs. In addition to the ballet-style squat, or plié (modified squat), there are many variations of the weight-room squat, including (from easiest to hardest) the following.

- Sit-back squat supported by a barre, railing, or other fixed object; sit to chair (may raise seat with a cushion so clients with knee pain can perform a partial squat)
- Sit-back squat to chair without sitting down
- Wall squat using stability ball
- Squat with hands on thighs to chair or bench without sitting down
- Squat with light dumbbells resting on thighs
- Squat with dumbbells held at sides
- Back squat using Smith press
- One-leg back squat using Smith press
- Back squat using barbell
- Front squat using Smith press
- Front squat using barbell
- Squat to overhead press (using dumbbells or barbell)

Equipment used: may need a barre, bench, stability ball, dumbbells, barbell, Smith press machine, power rack, etc.

Moving joints	Joint action	Muscles worked
hips	extension	gluteus maximus, hamstrings
knees	extension	quadriceps
ankles	plantar flexion	gastrocnemius, soleus

Exercise purpose: to develop strength and endurance of the lower body muscles

1. Starting/set-up position for back squat: Stand with feet shoulder-width apart, toes straight ahead. Hands have a slightly wider-than-shoulder-width grip (pronated) on the barbell; barbell rests on posterior deltoids (not on base of cervical spine). Starting position is up.

2. Alignment: Pelvis, spine, neck, and scapulae are stabilized in neutral; abdominals are contracted and knees are soft. Moving joints: Hips, knees, and ankles. Spine, neck, and shoulders must be stabilized in a fixed position without any independent movement during both concentric and eccentric phases.

3. Movement: Inhale as weight is lowered and hips and knees flex. Shift middle third of body (hips and pelvis) back so that knees don't overbend and overshoot the toes. Lower until thighs are almost parallel to floor, keeping torso erect, chest lifted, and head in line with spine. Exhale and extend knees and hips, bringing pelvis fully back into neutral alignment. Lift with legs and buttocks, not back. Keep heels down.

4. Safety factors: Always use collars and evenly load the bar. Avoid dropping the hips below the knees as this places tremendous stress on the knee joint. Overshooting the toes with the knee also stresses knee ligaments. Pushing or jerking with the low back should be avoided. Watch for proper breathing.

5. Engage and contract the gluteus maximus, hamstrings, and quadriceps. Remind your client to be especially conscious on the way up, so as not to lift with the back. Erector spinae and abdominals remain strongly isometrically contracted throughout movement.

Spotting guidelines for trainers: For back squats, stand close behind client in order to reinforce proper spinal alignment and/or help support the barbell if necessary. For heavy loads, squat with client and track bar with hands (two spotters, one on each end, are often necessary). For front squats, stand in front of client and track bar with hands.

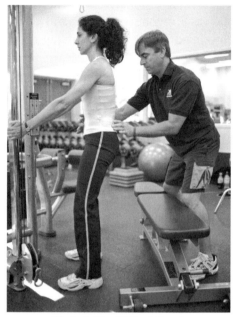

Photo 8-53a. Sit-Back Squat

Common Errors
- Hyperextended neck
- Knees overshooting toes
- Knees failing to stay in line with toes (torque)
- Inability to stabilize core/spine flexing forward
- Inability to perform proper hip hinge with tailbone pointing back
- Failure to bring pelvis back into neutral at end of lift
- Heels lift off floor

Modifications
- For frail or deconditioned clients: sit-back squat
- For clients who express a **history** of knee pain and are **cleared by physician**: sit-back squat with partial range; wall squat with stability ball
- For clients who express a **history** of back pain and are **cleared by physician**: wall squat with stability ball

Progressions
- Squat followed by heel raise
- Squat followed by hip abduction on one side, alternate
- Single-leg squat
- Plyometric squat

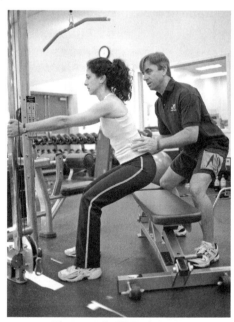

Photo 8-53b. Sit-Back Squat

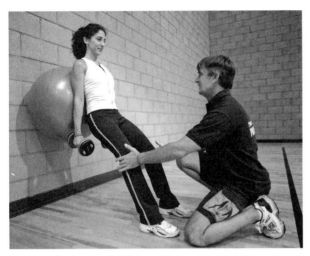

Photo 8-53c. Wall Squat Using Stability Ball

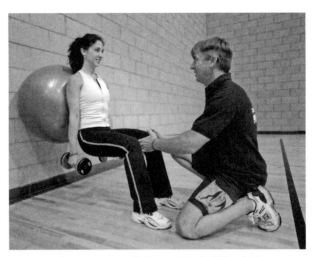

Photo 8-53d. Wall Squat Using Stability Ball

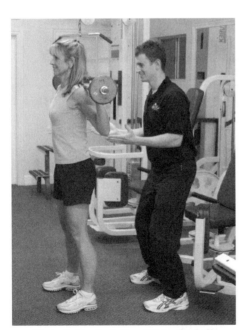

Photo 8-53e. Back Squat Using Barbell

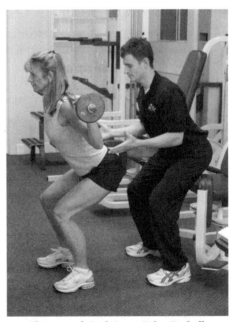

Photo 8-53f. Back Squat Using Barbell

54 - Lunges

The many variations of a lunge include the following (from easiest to hardest).
- Stationary (squat) lunge with wall support
- Stationary lunge at Smith press
- Step-back lunge with wall support
- Step-back lunge with dumbbells
- Forward lunge (back knee bent or back knee straight) onto box or slant board
- Forward lunge flat (back knee bent or back knee straight)
- Forward lunge with dumbbells, then barbell
- Side lunge onto box
- Side lunge flat
- Side lunge with dumbbells
- Split lunge with back shin on stability ball
- Crane lunge (back lunge up to knee-lift balance)
- Russian lunge (traveling front lunge with knee-lift balance; when down in lunge arms perform weighted overhead press)

NOTE: Even the easiest lunge is still difficult for most novice exercisers due to the balance, flexibility, strength, and coordination required. It may be wise to postpone lunges until your client has progressed to a more intermediate skill level.

Equipment used: Smith press, dumbbells, barbell, slant board, stability ball, etc., depending on the lunge variation

Moving joints	Joint action	Muscles worked
hips	extension	gluteus maximus, hamstrings
knees	extension	quadriceps
ankles	plantar flexion	gastrocnemius, soleus

NOTE: Side lunges require more hip abduction and adduction.

Exercise purpose: to develop strength and endurance of the lower body muscles.

1. Starting/set-up position for forward lunge: Stand in proper alignment. Dumbbells may be held at sides with palms facing body. Barbell is held in same place as for squats (on posterior deltoids, slightly wider than shoulder width, pronated grip). Feet are shoulder-width apart with toes pointing straight ahead.

2. Alignment: Pelvis, spine, neck, and scapulae are in neutral with abdominals contracted and knees slightly flexed. Moving joints: Hips, knees, and ankles. Torso goes along for the ride, but has no independent movement of its own. Pelvis stays in neutral, as do the spine and neck. Shoulders remain level with head up.

3. Movement: Lead leg takes big step forward, landing heel first, and flexes knee until the front thigh is parallel to the floor. Front knee should flex no more than 90°; knee should never extend beyond toes. Back knee may be bent at 90° with thigh perpendicular to floor (this is easier), or may be nearly straight with hip fully extended (this takes more balance, coordination, and iliopsoas flexibility). Stay on the ball of the back foot with heel up. Torso stays completely upright and stabilized throughout both concentric and eccentric phases. Exhale on the return; push off with front foot, balancing, and return feet to neutral. If balance is difficult, one or two small "stutter" steps are acceptable on the return.

4. Safety factors: The lunge is a difficult exercise for many clients (using a slant board or bench is helpful for beginners). Because of the difficulty with balance, coordination, and poor flexibility, a common error is understriding (taking too small a step). This results in the front knee overshooting the toes and creating increased knee stress. Avoid using torso momentum to initiate the backward movement; this places stress on the spine (use the front foot and leg instead). Back knee should not touch the floor. Watch for hips, knees, and ankles all pointing the same direction; torquing is a common problem.

5. Engage and contract the quadriceps, gluteus maximus, and hamstrings. Isometrically contract the abdominals, scapular adductors, and erector spinae.

Spotting guidelines for trainers: This is a difficult exercise to spot. For heavy loads, two spotters are recommended, one at each end of barbell.

Common Errors
- Front knee overshoots toes
- Leaning forward with spine flexed
- Back hip not fully extended (this takes iliopsoas flexibility)
- Placing feet in a single straight line (tightrope), making it difficult to balance (think of feet being on parallel tracks instead)
- Trying to keep the back heel down instead of up

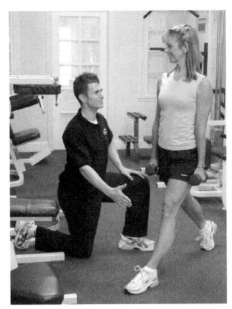
Photo 8-54a. Stationary Lunge with Dumbbells

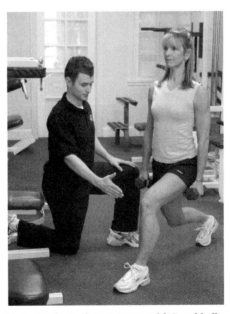
Photo 8-54b. Stationary Lunge with Dumbbells

Modifications	Progressions
• For clients who express a **history** of knee pain and are **cleared by physician**: avoid this exercise. • For clients who express a **history** of back pain and are **cleared by physician**: try a stationary lunge at the Smith press with no additional weight. If back pain persists avoid this exercise.	• Traveling front, back, side, or Russian lunges • Lunge with back foot on slideboard. • Lunge with front foot on slideboard. • Plyometric lunge

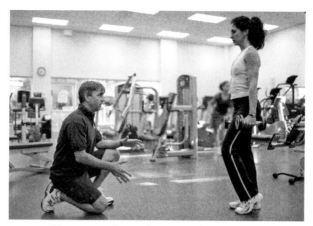
Photo 8-54c. Forward Lunge with Dumbbells

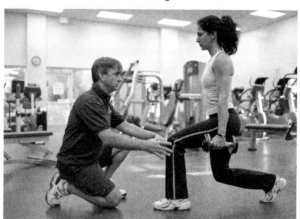
Photo 8-54d. Forward Lunge with Dumbbells

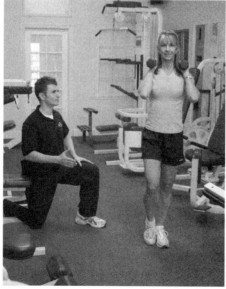
Photo 8-54e. Side Lunge with Dumbbells

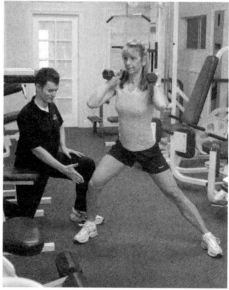
Photo 8-54f. Side Lunge with Dumbbells

55 - Multi-Hip Machine

Many gyms have multi-hip machines that may be used for hip flexor, abductor, adductor, or hip extensor strengthening.

Equipment used: multi-hip machine

Moving joints	Joint action	Muscles worked
hips	flexion abduction adduction extension	iliopsoas and quadriceps gluteus medius adductors, gracilis, pectineus gluteus maximus, hamstrings

Exercise purpose: to develop strength and endurance of the lower body muscles

1. Starting/set-up position: Adjust floor pad so that when a client stands on it, one hip lines up with the machine's pivot point or axis of rotation. Adjust machine for desired exercise (e.g., hip abduction). Thigh pad should rest against middle part of thigh, and body should be positioned so that the appropriate joint action can be performed through full range of motion.

2. Alignment: Supporting knee is slightly flexed, while pelvis, spine, neck, and scapulae are in neutral with abdominals contracted. Moving joints: Hips. All other joints are stabilized, including the knees, spine, shoulders, and neck. Pelvis maintains neutral pelvic alignment throughout the exercise; hips and shoulders are level.

3. Movement: Exhale as the hip abducts (or flexes, adducts, or extends). Move the leg through its full range of motion, lifting it as high as possible within the context of a stable pelvis. There should be no pelvic movement.

4. Safety factors: Lack of core (pelvic) stabilization can lead to back or hip injury. If clients are unable to maintain a neutral stable torso and/or knee, choose an alternative exercise (such as side-lying hip abduction and adduction) where core stabilization is easier. Avoid momentum and initiating the movement with the torso. Keep movements slow and controlled.

5. Engage and contract the prime movers. Isometrically contract the abdominals and the hip and thigh muscles of the support leg (pelvic stabilizers).

Spotting guidelines for trainers: Move around and view your client's alignment from different angles. It may be necessary to provide hip and/or spinal stabilization cues with your hands (e.g., holding the hips level).

Common Errors
- Inability to stabilize the spine; back hyperextends or laterally flexes
- Inability to stabilize the pelvis
- Hyperextended support knee and/or knee torque
- Excessive momentum

Modification
- For clients who express a **history** of back pain and are **cleared by physician**: avoid this exercise. Instead, perform hip abduction and hip adduction in a stable side-lying position, and perform hip extension in the prone position. Avoid weight-bearing hip flexion.

Progressions
- Standing hip abduction, adduction, extension, or flexion at a low pulley; step away from the cable unit so that hands cannot be used on the machine for balance.
- Same as above, add a greater balance component by standing on a half-foam roller.

56 - Hip Abduction and Adduction Machine

Equipment used: seated abductor/adductor machine(s)

Moving joints	Joint action	Muscles worked
hip	horizontal abduction/ horizontal extension	gluteus medius (assisted by the tensor fasciae latae, hip flexors, sartorius, and gluteus minimus)
hip	horizontal adduction/ horizontal flexion	adductors longus, magnus and brevis, gracilis, and pectineus

Exercise purpose: to develop strength and endurance of the outer and inner thigh muscles

Horizontal Abduction: Lateral movement away from the midline of the body in a horizontal plane; moving the thighs outward with hips bent.

1. Starting/set-up position: Sit on the machine and place the outside (lateral) side of knees against the pads.
2. Alignment: Maintain neutral spine. Head and neck should continue the line of the spine with shoulders relaxed down away from the ears; contract the abdominals.
3. Movement: Contract and resist against the knee pads while moving the knees away from each other to shoulder-width apart, exhaling on effort. Maintain resistance against knee pads while moving back, inhaling. Do not let the weight set all the way back to the start position.
4. Safety: Exhale as legs move apart; inhale as legs move toward the midline.
5. Engage the hip abductors through both concentric and eccentric phases.

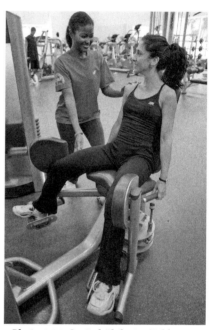

Photo 8-56. Seated Abductor/Adductor Machine

Horizontal Adduction: Medial movement toward the midline of the body in a horizontal plane; moving the thighs inward with hips bent.
1. Starting/set-up position: Sit on the machine and move the lever to increase the range of motion, bringing the knees shoulder-width apart.
2. Alignment: Maintain neutral spine. Head and neck should continue the line of the spine with shoulders relaxed down away from the ears; contract the abdominals.
3. Movement: Contract and resist against the knee pads while moving the knees together, exhaling on the effort. Maintain resistance against the pads while moving knees back to shoulder-width apart, inhaling. Do not let the weight set all the way back to the start position.
4. Safety: Exhale as legs come together; inhale as legs move apart.
5. Engage the hip adductors through both concentric and eccentric phases.

Common Errors
- Collapsing in the core
- Not taking movement through a full range of motion
- Tensing in the shoulders; jutting the head and neck forward

57 - Side-Lying Hip Abduction and Adduction

Equipment used: mat, ankle weights

Moving joints	Joint action	Muscles worked
hip	abduction	gluteus medius (assisted by the tensor fasciae latae, hip flexors, sartorius, and gluteus minimus)
hip	adduction	adductors longus, magnus and brevis, gracilis, and pectineus

Exercise purpose: to develop strength and endurance of the outer and inner thigh muscles

1. Starting/set-up position: Lie on one side. For abduction: rest head on arm and stack hips. Legs may be extended in a straight line or flexed at the hip about 45°; knees may be extended or flexed depending on the variation. Top arm may be used to stabilize torso. For adduction: rest head on arm and stack hips. Move top leg out of the way of the working bottom leg by flexing the top hip and positioning the top leg so that the hips remain stacked (top leg can rest on a low bench, or knee can be slightly elevated or on the floor, depending on client's hip width and femur length). Bottom (working) leg may have either a flexed or extended knee.

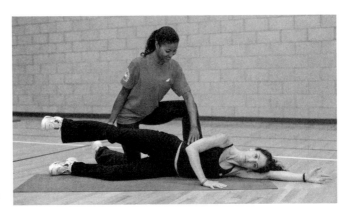

Photo 8-57a. Side-Lying Hip Abduction

2. Alignment: For both hip abduction and hip adduction, maintain stacked hips, with neutral pelvis, spine, neck, and scapulae. Head and neck should continue the line of the spine. Contract abdominals. Moving joints: Hips. Stabilize pelvis, knees, and ankles. To best isolate the hip abductors and adductors, stabilize the hips so that no active hip flexion or extension takes place. (Hips may be stabilized in a flexed position depending on the variation.)

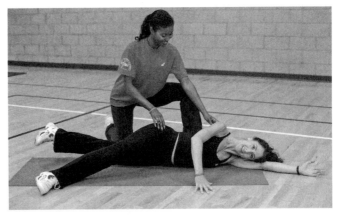

Photo 8-57b. Side-Lying Hip Adduction

3. Movement: Move the working leg through its full range of motion, as high as possible without distorting or changing the hips. Keep the knee of the working leg facing forward for both abduction and adduction. Exhale as leg lifts; inhale as leg lowers.

4. Safety factors: Avoid flexing the hips 90° for abduction; this places stress on the gluteus medius tendon. Avoid the couch-potato neck position (head resting in hand while the neck is severely laterally flexed) as this places stress on the neck.

5. Engage and contract the hip abductors or the hip adductors, depending on the exercise. Maintain a conscious contraction through both concentric and eccentric phases.

Spotting guidelines for trainers: Sit or kneel next to your client, making certain that hips are stacked and the torso is in neutral. If ankle weights are not used, you may provide manual resistance if appropriate.

Common Errors

- Allowing the hips to roll backward or forward
- Lifting the leg so high that core stability cannot be maintained
- Assuming a position (such as rolling the hips backward) that allows the hip flexors to become the prime movers instead of the hip adductors or abductors
- Resting the head on the hand (couch-potato position)

Modification	Progressions
• For clients who express a **history** of back pain and are **cleared by physician**: make certain head is down on arm and knees are bent. Avoid rolling hips back and using hip flexors; this may place stress on the back.	• Use ankle weights. • Use elastic band around thighs for hip abduction. • Use bodybar against lower leg for hip adduction. • Perform hip abduction planked on stability ball. • Perform side-lying hip adduction with stability ball held between lower legs; lift both legs laterally simultaneously.

Lower Leg/Ankle Exercises

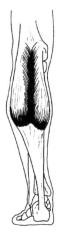

Fig. 8-12a. Gastrocnemius

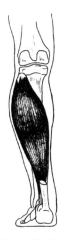

Fig. 8-12b. Soleus

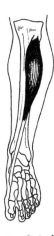

Fig. 8-12c. Anterior Tibialis

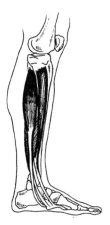

**Fig. 8-12d. Peroneals
(Peroneus Longus, Brevis, and Tertius)**

Muscle	Prime Mover for:	Assists with:
Gastrocnemius	ankle plantar flexion	
Soleus	ankle plantar flexion	
Anterior Tibialis	ankle dorsiflexion ankle inversion	
Extensor Digitorum Longus	ankle dorsiflexion ankle eversion	
Tibialis Posterior	ankle inversion	
Peroneus Tertius	ankle dorsiflexion ankle eversion	
Peroneus Longus	ankle eversion	
Peroneus Brevis	ankle eversion	

58 - Heel Raises

Equipment used: step or board, dumbbells or barbell

Moving joints	Joint action	Muscles worked
ankles	plantar flexion	gastrocnemius and soleus

Exercise purpose: to develop strength and endurance of the calf muscles

1. Starting/set-up position: Stand with feet hip-width distance apart and toes pointing straight ahead. Balls of feet are on the edge of the step or board with heels hanging down. If using dumbbells, hold with mid-pronated grip (palms face sides). If using barbell, rest it across shoulders on the posterior deltoid, hands in pronated, wide grip.

2. Alignment: Stand with knees slightly flexed, pelvis, spine, neck, and scapulae in neutral, and shoulders level. Contract abdominals. Moving joints: Ankles. Entire rest of body should be stabilized with no other joints moving. Although knees are soft, they have no independent movement of their own.

3. Movement: Exhale and raise up on balls of feet as high as possible. Inhale and slowly lower as far as possible.

4. Safety factors: Avoid rapid lifting and sudden lowering, which may strain the Achilles tendon. Avoid lowering so far that pain is felt. Watch that the hips and knees remain stable throughout the movement. Balance may be an issue. The exercise may be performed holding onto a rail or wall with no weight or with a weighted belt.

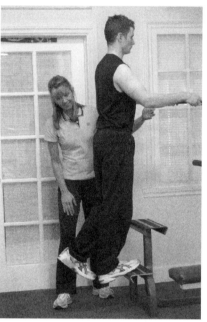

Photo 8-58a. Unilateral Heel Raise

5. Engage and contract the gastrocnemius and soleus. Maintain an isometric contraction of the abdominals, quadriceps, etc.

Spotting guidelines for trainers: Observe client from all sides to see that proper alignment is maintained. If client is holding a barbell, stand behind and spot the barbell, tracking with both hands.

Common Errors
- Lowering the heels rapidly and straining the Achilles tendon
- Not lowering the heels far enough
- Flexing and extending the knees instead of moving the ankles
- Swaying the torso back and forth

Modification	Progressions
• For novice clients: hold onto barre or other sturdy equipment for balance and support.	• Perform heel raise unilaterally. • Perform heel raise on half-foam roller or BOSU.

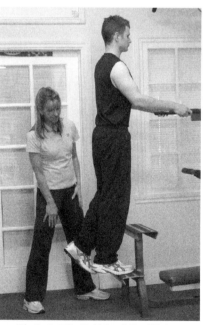

Photo 8-58b. Unilateral Heel Raise

59 - Dorsiflexion and Eversion

Equipment used: elastic resistance band, weighted boot, or T-bar device, bench

Moving joints	Joint action	Muscles worked
ankle	dorsiflexion	anterior tibialis, extensor digitorum longus, peroneus tertius
tarsal	eversion	peroneus tertius, peroneus longus, peroneus brevis, extensor digitorum longus

Exercise purpose: to develop strength and endurance of the lower leg muscles. Training the everters is especially important to minimize the risk of ankle sprain.

1. Starting/set-up position: Sit on bench or floor in proper sitting alignment. Hands may be at sides or slightly behind for support; alternatively, client may sit with back against wall. If seated on bench, rest working leg lengthwise on bench, foot off the end. For both dorsiflexion and eversion, rubber band is placed over top of foot, trainer holds other end.

2. Alignment: Sit in hip hinge, weight on sitting bones. Pelvis, spine, neck, and scapulae are in neutral; knees are extended without hyperextension. Moving joints: Ankles and/or tarsal joints. Knees, hips, spine, neck, etc. must be kept stable.

3. Movement: For dorsiflexion, exhale and pull forefoot toward body as far as possible and slowly return to starting position. For eversion, exhale and evert the foot against the resistance of the band (lift up the outside edge of the foot). An isometric contraction may be added.

4. Safety factors: Keep movement smooth and controlled. Avoid locking (hyperextending) the knees.

5. Engage and contract the dorsiflexors and the everters, respectively.

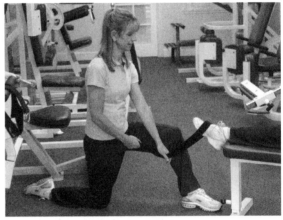
Photo 8-59a. Ankle Dorsiflexion (Shin)

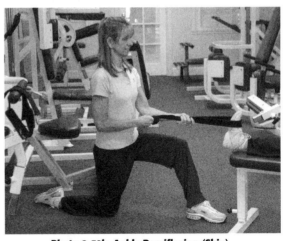
Photo 8-59b. Ankle Dorsiflexion (Shin)

Spotting guidelines for trainers: Hold the anchor end of the band. For some clients, you may need to palpate the working muscles and/or assist the foot into the appropriate concentric contraction. (Weaker clients or those with low levels of body awareness will have a difficult time understanding the required movement and may need assistance).

Common Errors
- Minimizing the range of motion
- Failure to maintain proper seated posture

Stability Ball Exercises

In many weight rooms, stability balls (also known as Swiss balls or physioballs) are now standard equipment, along with other small training devices, such as foam rollers, weighted medicine balls, wobble boards, core boards, slideboards, elastic bands and tubing, air discs, and the BOSU. These and other pieces of small equipment can greatly expand your repertoire of exercises and increase the variety of your programming, and they are especially useful for in-home personal training.

Choose the right size stability ball for your client's height. When sitting on the ball, your client's knees should form a 90° angle with the hips just slightly higher than the knees. A person 4'6" – 5'0" tall should use a 45 cm ball; a person 5'1" – 5'7" needs a 55 cm ball; 5'8" – 6'2" in height takes a 65 cm ball; and someone over 6'2" should use a 75 cm ball.

Virtually every major muscle group can be trained using a stability ball; many of these exercises were mentioned in the preceding pages under the "Progressions" subheading. Generally, performing an exercise utilizing a stability ball is harder than carrying out the same exercise without the ball, as more muscles are required to stabilize the body. Using a ball is an excellent strategy for skilled clients who need to develop greater core stability, coordination, and balance.

Listed below are examples of stability ball exercises for the major muscle groups.

- **Pectoralis major, anterior deltoids**
  Supine dumbbell flys, supine bench press (stability ball supports upper back, neck, and head), decline push-ups with feet on ball

- **Posterior deltoids, middle trapezius, rhomboids**
  Prone reverse flys (stability ball supports abdomen and chest), seated high row (sit on ball facing mid-pulley)

- **Deltoids**
  Seated lateral raises, seated overhead press (sit on ball with only one foot on floor to increase difficulty)

- **Latissimus dorsi**
  Prone shoulder extension, seated lat row using mid-pulley, seated unilateral lat pull-down using tubing

- **Triceps**
  Prone bilateral kick-backs, supine unilateral elbow extension, dips with hands on ball

- **Biceps**
  Seated biceps curls (one foot on floor to increase difficulty)

- **Rectus abdominis**
  Supine curls (may be performed inclined, parallel to floor, or declined), supine curls holding tubing anchored behind head

- **Obliques**
  Supine crunch twists (may be performed inclined, parallel to floor, or declined)

- **Erector spinae**
  Prone spinal extension (may lift one leg for increased difficulty)

- **Quadriceps**
  Seated knee extension, wall squat with ball behind back

- **Hamstrings**
  Supine hip extension and knee flexion (feet on ball), prone hip extension with partner resistance (ball supports abdominals and chest, hands must be anchored)

- **Hip abductors**
  Side-plank position (ball supports middle torso) with top leg abducting

- **Hip adductors**
  Side-lying position with ball between lower legs—lift both legs, supine position squeezing ball between thighs

- **Gastrocnemius, soleus**
  Seated heel raises

Balance Exercises

Balance is defined as a state of bodily equilibrium, or the ability to maintain the center of body mass over the base of support without falling (Irrgang, Whitney, and Cox, 1994). As a personal fitness trainer, you will want to provide your clients with balance-training exercise as part of a complete program. Balance exercise is especially important for seniors and those with neuromuscular disorders such as Parkinson's disease or multiple sclerosis. One way to progress your clients is by lessening the degree of hand support during balance exercise. For example, a progression from easiest to hardest may go as follows: hold with both hands, hold with one hand, touch tips of fingers to support, drum fingers on support while balancing, hands off but just above support, hands at sides, etc. Below are several ideas for standing-balance exercises.

- Balance on one leg.
- Balance on one leg while swinging the free leg back and forth.
- Balance on one leg while pedaling the free leg.
- Balance on one leg while catching and throwing a ball.
- Balance one leg on a half-foam roller, BOSU, or wobble board (progression to an unstable surface).
- Hop and balance on one leg.
- Walk a "tightrope" (this can be a simple line of masking tape on the floor, progressing to a 2-inch-high balance beam). Walk forward, backward, and sideways.
- Perform standard weight-room exercises with the feet staggered on a "tightrope."

Pilates

Pilates exercise, named after Joseph Pilates, is a growing trend in most fitness centers. This method of exercise is briefly included in this chapter because it has been shown to be a valid method of resistance training (Otto et al., 2004). In addition, Pilates promotes flexibility, core stability, balance, and coordination. Pilates exercise may be performed using only a mat, or on special equipment, called Pilates apparatus. The various primary pieces of equipment are known as the Reformer, Cadillac, Chair, and Barrel; hundreds of different exercises can be performed on this specialized equipment. Resistance is provided mostly with spring-loaded tension and/or the exerciser's own body weight. A hallmark of most Pilates exercise is that the entire body is worked as a unit, and muscle groups are rarely worked in isolation. Breathing, control, mental focus, abdominal hollowing, and impeccable alignment are some of the other key concepts of Pilates movement. Being able to train clients in both the traditional weight room and on Pilates apparatus can greatly add to your knowledge, skills, marketability, and the programming options you offer your clients.

Summary

In this chapter, critical information for more than 59 major weight-room exercises was outlined, including the equipment used, exercise purpose, what muscles were worked, what joint actions took place, starting position, alignment and technique, safety factors, spotting tips, common errors, modifications, and progressions for each particular exercise. Spotting guidelines, hands-on techniques, personal training cues, and proper lifting techniques were discussed. Additionally, brief segments on stability ball training, balance exercise, and Pilates exercise were included.

References

Irrgang, J.J., Whitney, S.L., & Cox, E.D. (1994). Balance and proprioception training for rehabilitation of the lower extremity. *Journal of Sport Rehabilitation, 3*, 68-83.

Jampolsky, G.G. (1979). *Love is letting go of fear.* Berkeley, CA: Celestial Arts.

Knowles, M.S., Holton, E.F., & Swanson, R.A. (1998). The adult learner (5th ed.). Houston, TX: Gulf Publishing Co.

Otto, R.M., Yoke, M.M., Morrill, J., Lail, A., McLaughlin, K., Viola, A., et al. (2004). The effect of twelve weeks of Pilates vs. resistance training on trained females. *Medicine & Science in Sports & Exercise, 36*(Suppl.), 5.

Richardson, C.A., Snijders, C.J., Hides, J.A., Damen, L., Pas, M.S., Storm, J., et al. (2002). The relation between the transverse abdominis muscles, sacroiliac joint mechanics, and low back pain. *Spine, 27*(4), 399-405.

Rothenberg, O. (1995). Professional and legal concerns related to the use of Systematic T.O.U.C.H. Training[sm]. *The Exercise Standards and Malpractice Reporter, 9*(1), 8-11.

Rothenberg, B., & Rothenberg, O. (1995). *Touch training for strength.* Champaign, IL: Human Kinetics.

Yoke, M., & Kennedy, C. (2004). *Functional exercise progressions.* Monterey, CA: Healthy Learning.

Suggested Reading

Aaberg, E. (1998). *Muscle mechanics.* Champaign, IL: Human Kinetics.

Aaberg, E. (1999). *Resistance training instruction.* Champaign, IL: Human Kinetics.

American Council on Exercise. (2002). *Stability ball training.* Monterey, CA: Healthy Learning.

Earle, R.W., & Baechle, T.R. (Eds.). (2004). *NSCA's essentials of personal training.* Champaign, IL: Human Kinetics.

Goldenberg, L., & Twist, P. (2002). *Strength ball training.* Champaign, IL: Human Kinetics.

Chaitow, L. (2004). M*aintaining body balance, flexibility, and stability.* Philadelphia: Elsevier Limited.

Page, P., & Ellenbecker, T.S. (2003). *The scientific and clinical application of elastic resistance.* Champaign, IL: Human Kinetics.

Perkins-Carpenter, B. (1999). *How to prevent falls: A comprehensive guide to better balance.* Penfield, NY: Senior Fitness Productions.

Pilates, J. (2003). *Return to life through contrology.* Miami, FL: Pilates Method Alliance.

Rothenberg, B., & Rothenberg, O. (1995). *Touch training for strength.* Champaign, IL: Human Kinetics.

Yoke, M., & Kennedy, C. (2004). *Functional exercise progressions.* Monterey, CA: Healthy Learning.

Flexibility Programming

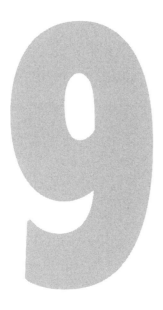

Outline

- Benefits of Flexibility Training

- Guidelines for Flexibility Programming

- Physiology of Stretching

- Types of Stretching

- Factors Influencing Flexibility

- Props and Equipment for Stretching

- Common Flexibility Exercises

Flexibility is a key component of physical fitness. It is defined as the range of motion possible around a joint (such as the shoulder), or around a series of joints (such as the spine). This range of motion is dependent on the extensibility of the soft tissues (e.g., muscles, tendons) around the joint itself (Alter, 1996). Flexibility is joint and joint-action specific, which means that you may be flexible in one joint but not in another. It is also possible to flexible in, for example, hip external rotation but not in hip extension. In this chapter the important concepts and principles involved in flexibility programming will be discussed, and common stretches for all major muscle groups will be detailed.

Benefits of Flexibility Training

A number of benefits have been identified for flexibility training; these benefits are presented in Table 9-1.

Table 9-1. Benefits of Flexibility Training

- Decreased risk of injury
- Decreased chronic muscle tension
- Decreased low-back pain
- Improved posture
- Increased motor performance
- Decreased stress
- Relief of muscle soreness
- Increased mind/body connection
- Improved ability to perform activities of daily living (increased functional ability)

Maintenance of and improvement in flexibility is especially important for older adults; declining flexibility coupled with reduced muscle mass and decreased muscle strength and endurance can result in less independence and loss of function. Stretching exercises have been shown to increase flexibility even as age increases (Feland, Myrer, Schulthies, Fellingham, & Measom, 2001).

Guidelines for Flexibility Programming

A major goal of stretching is to change the resting length of the muscles around a joint; in order to accomplish this, excessive muscle tension must be reduced. Many experts believe that changes such as a longer resting length and reduced tension in a muscle are temporary. There is little research to support a long-lasting effect from stretching. Consequently, daily stretching may be best, especially if the goal is to improve flexibility. The American College of Sports Medicine (ACSM) (2006a) recommends the following guidelines for flexibility training for the average healthy adult.

- Precede stretching with a warm-up to elevate muscle temperature.
- Perform a static stretching routine that exercises the major muscle-tendon units.
- Focus on muscle groups (joints) that have a reduced range of motion.
- Perform stretching a minimum of 2–3 days per week, and ideally 5–7 days per week.
- Stretch to the end of the range of motion, to the point of tightness, without inducing discomfort.

- Hold each stretch for 15–30 seconds.
- Perform 2–4 repetitions for each stretch.
- Perform stretches in a slow, controlled manner with a gradual progression to greater ranges of motion.

A practical tip for helping your clients know how long to hold a stretch is to have them count their breaths. Slow, deep diaphragmatic breathing with the emphasis on the exhale is very relaxing and helps facilitate the mind/body connection. Try having your clients count three to five deep, slow breaths as they hold each stretch, visualizing the muscles letting go on each exhale, and allowing the range of motion to gently increase with each breath.

Chapter 5 ("Fitness Assessment") includes assessment procedures for flexibility. It is recommended that you assess your clients for specific muscle tightness and provide appropriate stretches. Additionally, you should be familiar with stretches for the muscles that are commonly tight; including these stretches in your client's programming can help prevent muscle imbalances that can lead to postural dysfunction and joint injury. See Table 9-2 for a list of muscles that are commonly tight.

Table 9-2.	Commonly Tight Muscles
Upper trapezius	Pectoralis major, anterior deltoid
Erector spinae (lumbar portion)	Iliopsoas (hip flexors)
Hamstrings	Gastrocnemius and soleus

Physiology of Stretching

Muscle structure was described in Chapter 2 ("Exercise Physiology"). When stretching, the basic contractile unit (the sarcomere) relaxes and elongates, and the myofilaments (actin and myosin) pull away from each other.

Muscles are protected by neurological commands carried out by reflexes. A reflex is a response that bypasses the brain and is transmitted directly from muscles to the spinal cord and back to the muscles. Embedded in the musculotendinous unit are two intrinsic receptors, the proprioceptors known as the **muscle spindles** and the **Golgi tendon organs** (GTO). The function of these receptors is to detect when a muscle has been extended or stretched and to respond by cueing the muscle to contract or release. Anytime a muscle is stretched, a signal is sent to contract that same muscle. This reaction is called the myotatic or **stretch reflex**.

The muscle spindle lies parallel and between the contractile fibers in muscles. It is a very small receptor responsible for activating the stretch reflex. The spindle is sensitive to length changes in a muscle and responds to the speed at which the length change occurs. The faster you stretch, the greater the response. Stretching with fast, bouncy movements will cause the stretch reflex to fire and will immediately send a signal to the muscle being stretched to contract. However, stretching slowly and holding the stretch allows the muscle spindles to reset (to become sensitive at a longer length) and shuts off the stretch reflex signal that causes a reflexive muscle contraction. Resetting a spindle allows a muscle to be stretched further before it fires.

The GTO is located at the musculotendinous junction. This receptor is a protective device that detects changes in muscle tension. When the muscle tension is great enough, the GTO is activated, overriding the stretch reflex and causing a relaxation of the stretched muscle. This is called the inverse myotatic reflex.

Types of Stretching

Ballistic Stretching

Ballistic stretching is characterized by bouncing-, pulsing-, rapid-, or uncontrolled-type movements. Although ballistic stretching may be appropriate for certain athletic warm-ups as preparation for specific performance movements, the risk of injury outweighs the benefit for most exercisers. Ballistic stretching has the potential of invoking the stretch (myotatic) reflex. Muscle spindles (sensitive to sudden changes in muscle length) can trigger a reflex contraction after being rapidly, suddenly stretched. This creates more tension in the muscle and may lead to injuries such as muscle tears.

Static Stretching

Static stretching is characterized by low-intensity, long-duration muscle elongation, ideally in a supported position that allows the muscle fibers to relax. Static stretching has been shown to help provide relief from delayed onset muscle soreness and to have a much lower risk of injury. Static stretching is the most commonly recommended method of stretching, and is safe, effective, and appropriate for almost all clients. Studies disagree on the exact length of time a static stretch should be held, but the general recommendation is to hold a stretch at least 15 seconds and progress toward a duration of 30 seconds or more (American College of Sports Medicine, 2006b).

Active and Passive Stretching

Some professionals categorize stretching according to what muscles are contracting and whether or not another person is assisting the stretch. **Active or unassisted stretching** can be either static or ballistic, and is a type of stretching you perform alone, using the concentric contraction of the opposing muscles. For example, one way to stretch the pectoral muscles is to actively contract the scapular adductors (mid-trapezius and rhomboids) and the posterior deltoids. In **passive or assisted stretching**, the stretch is initiated by another person or outside force (i.e., traction), and the person being stretched is passive. This type of stretching carries a greater risk of injury because the person applying the force cannot feel the sensations of the person being stretched, and therefore, is generally not recommended for personal fitness trainers to perform. (If you have special training in physical therapy, massage therapy, or chiropractic, passively stretching your clients may be more appropriate.)

Proprioceptive Neuromuscular Facilitation (PNF)

PNF is defined as a flexibility technique that promotes or hastens the neuromuscular response through stimulation of the proprioceptors. PNF utilizes several complex principles, including reciprocal inhibition (when the agonist contracts, the antagonist relaxes), as well as the reflex responses of the proprioceptors, especially the GTOs. By isometrically contracting the muscle that is to be stretched, the GTOs (which are sensitive to changes in tension) allow the muscle to relax and move through an increased range of motion. Proponents of PNF cite research showing that PNF is more effective than other types of stretching, may help "reset" the stretch reflex level, and creates more strength, balance, and stability around a joint (Funk, Swank, Mikla, Fagan, & Farr, 2003). Disadvantages of PNF include the possibility of the Valsalva maneuver (during the isometric contraction), the increased risk of injury when a partner (or trainer) is used, and the increased risk of injury even when performed individually due to the increased tension occurring in the muscles.

PNF was originally used to describe a method of therapy using spiral-diagonal patterns of movement. PNF stretching involves a variety of techniques. Some of the most common methods include the following.

- **Hold-relax (HR)**—The muscle to be stretched is placed in its lengthened position and is isometrically contracted against a partner's immovable resistance. The stretcher then relaxes, and the limb is moved passively into the new range by the partner or by the stretcher.
- **Contract-relax (CR)**—This stretching technique is similar to hold-relax. The difference is that instead of an isometric contraction, there is a concentric action through a full range of motion before the relaxation phase.
- **Contract-relax, antagonist-contract (CRAC)**—Begin with the contract-relax method described above, and then, the stretcher, following the isometric contraction of the muscle being stretched, actively contracts the opposing muscle, moving the limb into the new range of motion.

Myofascial Release

Clients can perform myofascial release on themselves with a foam roller. The fascia (connective tissue within and around the muscles) can be a limiting factor in flexibility; after injury, in particular, the fascia can become distorted and tight (Alter, 1996). This technique involves applying pressure (with a foam roller) perpendicular to the muscle fibers in order to release connective tissue tightness. Generally, the client positions him or herself on top of the roller and rolls up and down across the muscle(s). Upon finding a tight or tender area, the position is held for 20 seconds or so, allowing the musculature and connective tissues to relax. For example, to perform myofascial release unilaterally on the hamstrings, have your client sit on the roller with the roller under and perpendicular to the upper thigh. Gently and slowly roll back and forth across the roller, causing a "stretch" to the hamstrings and the corresponding fascia. Several books and articles have been written on myofascial release (e.g., Cantu & Grodin, 1992), however, few studies have documented its effectiveness. Nevertheless, the popularity of foam roller self-myofascial release is growing.

Factors Influencing Flexibility

Many factors determine and influence our flexibility including the following.
- Genetic bony and connective tissue structure
- Tight or loose ligaments
- Muscular fascial sheaths and joint capsules
- Connective tissue structures
- Stress and muscular tension
- Injury, pregnancy, and age
- Core temperature

The first factor, genetic bony structure, is something you cannot alter. The shape and size of bones and the type of connective tissue in a given body is mainly determined by genetics, or the structure with which each person is born.

Knowing the natural limitations of individual anatomical structure allows a person to stretch safely. Every joint in the body has a different range of motion dictated by shape, size, and how the bones fit together. Different body types are built with varying degrees of joint range. For example, the pelvis and hip joints are often shaped differently in men and women. A wider pelvis allows for greater turn-out in the hip. Consequently, the range of motion at the joint is greater. If an individual is born with the anatomical disposition for greater external hip rotation, he/she will be able to develop a larger "stretch" at that joint. Each joint can have variations in structure that enhance or limit flexibility.

The second influence on flexibility is the quality of the connective tissues: ligaments, fascial sheaths, joint capsules, and the musculotendinous units. Connective tissue, such as fascia, can make up to 30% of a muscle's mass. Although muscles have great elastic properties, the fascial sheath covering muscle is composed of connective tissue that is rather non-elastic; in fact, fascia can be a major factor limiting a person's range of motion (Alter, 1996; Hedrick, 1993). Muscle tissue can stretch and return to its original shape and size, whereas connective tissue remains extended once it is stretched. The role of connective tissue, such as ligaments, is to bind bone to bone and provide stability to the joints. Some individuals have ligaments with a higher proportion of elastic fibers, making them seem "naturally flexible."

The condition of **ligament laxity** results from being born with ligaments that have a higher degree of elastic properties. A joint with ligament laxity is more mobile and can extend further. The term "double jointed" is sometimes used to describe ligament laxity because of the extreme positions that can be manipulated and held, forcing joints beyond their normal range. People with ligament laxity can be more prone to injury if they do not have adequate strength to support their joints. Stretching with this condition may be considered safe if the body is well-positioned in each stretch, and there is a balance of strength to flexibility. Moving a joint beyond the limit to which it can be actively controlled is a set-up for injury.

Stress and muscular tension keep muscles in a shortened, contracted state. When muscles relax, tension is released. High levels of muscular tension tend to decrease sensory awareness and can contribute to an elevation in blood pressure. Habitually tense muscles tend to cut off blood circulation. Reduced blood supply results in a lack of oxygen and essential nutrients, and causes toxic waste products to accumulate in the cells, leading to fatigue and pain.

Emotional tension and muscular tension are related; ailments from emotional tension can include headaches, joint and muscle pain, and even stomach ulcers. Chronic muscle tension (called contracture or hypertonicity) causes a muscle to be continually in a shortened state, resulting in tightness and reduced strength.

Pregnancy, injury, and age all influence the quality of our flexibility. During pregnancy, the hormone **relaxin** causes ligaments and connective structures to increase in their elastic properties. Although it can be helpful for some women to stretch, caution should be followed not to overstretch areas of the pelvis.

When performing a seated adductor stretch with the soles of the feet together, pregnant women should avoid pushing down and out on the inside of the knees, which may cause unintentional injury to the cartilage and supportive tissues of the symphysis pubis and the hip joints.

Musculoskeletal injury interferes with the functioning of the soft tissues. Often an injury, such as a sprained ankle, results in reduced range of motion. This is because there is a build-up of scar tissue resulting from the connective tissue repairing itself. Stretching can help or hinder the healing from an injury; therefore, it is always wise to consult with a client's medical caregiver.

With aging, connective tissue, which is made up primarily of collagen fibers, forms cross-links in areas that have restricted motion. Age is often associated with a sedentary lifestyle. The older and less active an individual is, the more rapidly muscles and joints tighten up. If the joints are not extended through various ranges, collagen cross-links are laid down in the tissues, restricting movement potential and making the body feel stiff and less flexible.

Range of motion is also affected by core temperature; when the body is warm it is easier and safer to stretch because the tissues are more extensible (Wirth, Van Luten, Mistry, Saliba, & McCue, 1998).

Props and Equipment for Stretching

Flexibility equipment and props are available that may increase your client's enjoyment of stretching, and include the following.

- **Stability balls**—stretches for virtually every major muscle can be performed on the standard stability (physio) ball.
- **Straps and bands**—these simple props are especially useful for less flexible clients. Placing a strap around the foot when performing the supine hamstring stretch, for example, helps individuals with tight hamstrings to maintain alignment and stretch in a pain-free zone.
- **Blocks**—used primarily in yoga and Pilates, a foam block can help less flexible clients avoid unsupported forward flexion; instead of bending over and dangling, hands can rest on a block. This protects the spine and helps the hamstring muscles to relax.
- **Foam rollers**—usually 6 inches in diameter, these hard-foam rollers are useful for myofascial release techniques.
- **Calf-stretch devices**—these pieces of small equipment place the ankle in dorsiflexion with the heel lower than the forefoot, thus increasing the stretch for the gastrocnemius and soleus muscles.
- **Hip adductor-stretch machines**—several manufacturers make seated adductor stretch devices that hold the legs apart and allow the exerciser to gradually increase the length of the adductors.
- **BackSystem 3 device, StretchMate Flexibility System, Precor Stretch Trainer**—these, and other pieces of large flexibility equipment, are found in some commercial fitness centers. All are designed to allow various stretches for several muscles and muscle groups.

Common Flexibility Exercises

Figuring out how to stretch your muscles is easy when you know basic kinesiology. If you know the concentric joint action for each major muscle or muscle group, then you simply perform the opposite joint action in order to stretch the muscle(s). For example, the concentric joint actions of the hamstrings are hip extension and knee flexion; this is when the contractile units are shortened and tightened—clearly not a position of stretch. Therefore, to stretch the hamstrings you must do the opposite of hip extension and knee flexion; in other words, you must flex the hip and extend the knee, and then ideally place the leg in a supported position for a static stretch.

In this section, you will find some of the most common stretches for the major muscles and muscle groups.

Chest (Pectoralis Major and Anterior Deltoid) Stretches

Joint actions: shoulder horizontal abduction/extension

1 - Butterfly Chest Stretch

1. Sit or stand in proper alignment.

2. Placing hands behind ears, gently draw the elbows backward.

3. Feel the stretch in the pectoralis major and anterior deltoid.

4. Hold 15–30 seconds or 3–5 slow breaths.

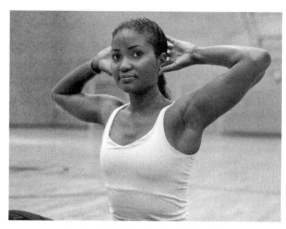

Photo 9-1. Butterfly Chest Stretch

2 - Standing Chest Stretch

1. Stand in proper alignment with arms reaching behind the body (this stretch can also be performed seated).

2. Hands may clasp together or remain unclasped, depending on flexibility.

3. Feel the stretch in the pectoralis major and anterior deltoid.

4. Hold for 15–30 seconds or 3–5 slow breaths.

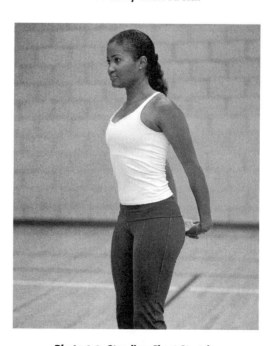

Photo 9-2. Standing Chest Stretch

3 - Standing Unilateral Wall/Door Stretch for the Chest

1. Stand in proper alignment with one hand holding onto a wall, doorway, or other piece of equipment.

2. Slowly turn the body away from the out-stretched arm.

3. Feel the stretch in the pectoralis major and anterior deltoid.

4. Hold for 15–30 seconds or 3–5 slow breaths.

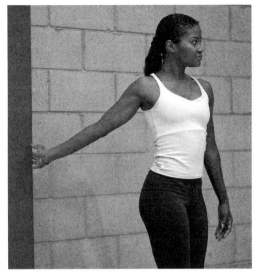

Photo 9-3. Standing Wall Chest Stretch

Safety precaution for all chest stretches: if shoulder pain exists, move the arm down and away from the horizontal plane.

Upper Back and Neck
(Trapezius, Rhomboid, and Posterior Deltoid) Stretches

Joint actions: scapular depression, cervical spinal lateral flexion, cervical spinal flexion, scapular protraction, and shoulder horizontal adduction

4 - Lateral Flexion (Neck) Stretch

1. Stand or sit in proper alignment.

2. Gently tilt head to side.

3. Feel the stretch on the side of the neck and in the upper trapezius.

4. Hold for 15–30 seconds or 3–5 slow breaths.

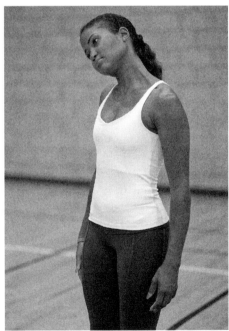

Photo 9-4. Lateral Flexion Neck Stretch

5 - Cervical Spinal Flexion (Neck) Stretch

1. Stand or sit in proper alignment.

2. Gently tilt head forward, looking down.

3. Feel the stretch in the back of the neck in the upper trapezius.

4. Hold for 15–30 seconds or 3–5 slow breaths.

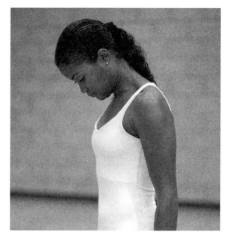

Photo 9-5. Cervical Flexion Neck Stretch

6 - Upper Back Stretch

1. Stand or sit in proper alignment.

2. Clasping hands together in front of the body, allow shoulders to round forward and feel the shoulder blades pulling apart in the back.

3. Feel the stretch in the muscles between the shoulder blades and in the back of the shoulders (mid-trapezius, rhomboids, and posterior deltoids).

4. Hold for 15–30 seconds or 3–5 slow breaths.

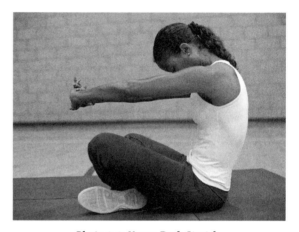

Photo 9-6. Upper Back Stretch

Deltoid (Anterior, Medial, and Posterior) Stretches

Joint actions: shoulder adduction

7 - Deltoid Stretch in Front

1. Stand or sit in proper alignment.

2. Gently pull arm in front of body; maintain shoulder girdle depression; lightly support arm with opposite hand.

3. Feel the stretch in the medial and posterior deltoids.

4. Hold for 15–30 seconds or 3–5 slow breaths.

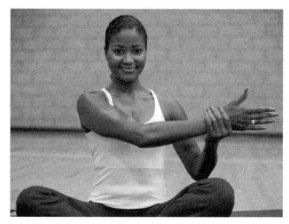

Photo 9-7. Deltoid Stretch In Front

8 - Deltoid Stretch in Back

1. Stand or sit in proper alignment.

2. Gently pull arm in back of body (elbow may be bent or straight), maintain shoulder girdle depression; lightly support arm with opposite hand.

3. Feel the stretch in the medial and anterior deltoids.

4. Hold for 15–30 seconds or 3–5 slow breaths.

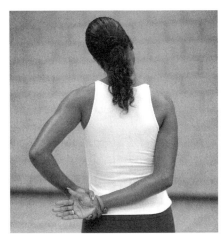

Photo 9-8. Deltoid Stretch in Back

Latissimus Dorsi Stretches

Joint actions: shoulder flexion and shoulder abduction

9 - Arms Reach Forward Lat Stretch

1. Bend over with one hand on thigh; contract abdominals for support.

2. Reach opposite arm forward and diagonally off to opposite side; keep spine flexed.

3. Feel the stretch in the latissimus dorsi on one side (erector spinae is unilaterally stretched also).

4. Hold for 15–30 seconds or 3–5 slow breaths.

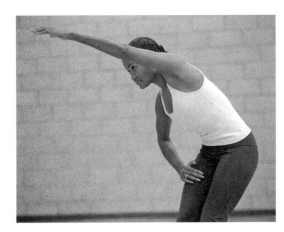

Photo 9-9. Arms Reach Forward Lat Stretch

10 - Unilateral Side Stretch for Lats

1. Sit or stand in proper alignment.

2. Reach one arm up and over; adding lumbar spinal lateral flexion is optional. Keep opposite hand on floor or on thigh for support.

3. Feel the stretch in the latissimus dorsi on one side (obliques, rectus abdominis, and erector spinae are unilaterally stretched as well).

4. Hold for 15–30 seconds or 3–5 slow breaths.

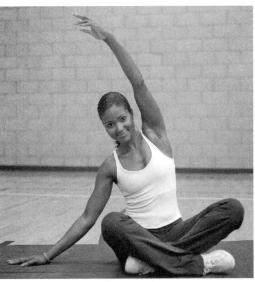

Photo 9-10. Unilateral Side Stretch for Lats

Triceps Stretches

Joint actions: elbow flexion (also shoulder flexion)

11 - Triceps Stretch with Arm Overhead

1. Sit or stand in proper alignment

2. Reach one arm overhead and bend (flex) the elbow with hand reaching down the spine. Ideally the elbow should point straight up. Support the upper arm with the opposite hand.

3. Feel the stretch in the triceps.

4. Hold for 15–30 seconds or 3–5 slow breaths.

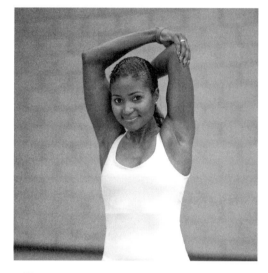

Photo 9-11. Triceps Stretch with Arm Overhead

12 - Triceps Stretch with Arm in Front

1. Sit or stand in proper alignment.

2. Cross one arm in front of the chest and bend (flex) the elbow with the hand reaching over the opposite shoulder. Support the upper arm with the opposite hand.

3. Feel the stretch in the triceps.

4. Hold for 15–30 seconds or 3–5 slow breaths.

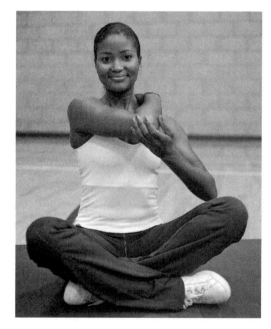

Photo 9-12. Triceps Stretch with Arm in Front

Biceps Stretches

Joint actions: elbow extension (also shoulder extension)

13 - Biceps Stretch with Arms Behind

1. Sit or stand in proper alignment.

2. Reach arms behind body with elbows straight (extended).

3. Feel the stretch in the biceps.

4. Hold for 15–30 seconds or 3–5 slow breaths.

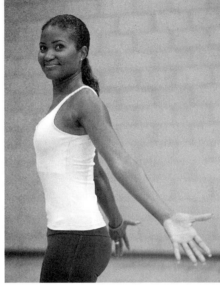

Photo 9-13. Biceps Stretch with Arms Behind

14 - Biceps Stretch with Arm in Front

1. Sit or stand in proper alignment.

2. Reach one arm forward with elbow straight (extended) and palm supinated; support arm with opposite hand.

3. Feel the stretch in the biceps.

4. Hold for 15–30 seconds or 3–5 slow breaths.

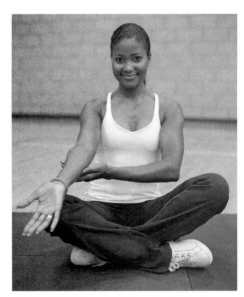

Photo 9-14. Biceps Stretch with Arm in Front

Wrist Stretches

Joint actions: wrist flexion and wrist extension

15 - Forearm "Tennis Elbow" Stretch

1. Sit or stand in proper alignment.

2. Reach one arm forward with palm pronated, gently maintaining wrist flexion with opposite hand.

3. Feel the stretch in the wrist extensor muscles.

4. Hold for 15–30 seconds or 3–5 slow breaths.

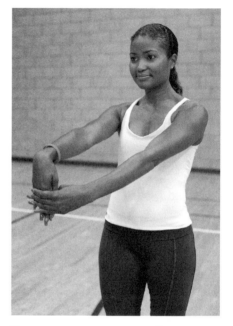

Photo 9-15. Forearm "Tennis Elbow" Stretch

16 - Forearm "Golfer's Elbow" Stretch

1. Sit or stand in proper alignment.

2. Reach one arm forward with palm supinated, gently maintaining wrist extension with opposite hand.

3. Feel the stretch in the wrist flexor muscles.

4. Hold for 15–30 seconds or 3–5 slow breaths.

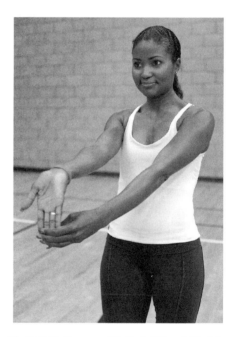

Photo 9-16. Forearm "Golfer's Elbow" Stretch

Rectus Abdominis Stretches

Joint actions: spinal extension

17 - Prone Modified Cobra Stretch

1. Lie prone, propped up on elbows.

2. Pressing pubic bone down, extend spine upward allowing neck to continue the line of the spine. Press shoulder blades down and away from ears.

3. Feel the stretch in the abdominal muscles.

4. Hold for 15–30 seconds or 3–5 slow breaths.

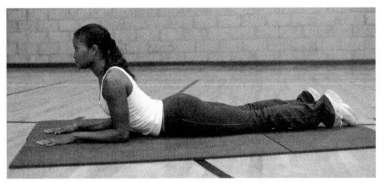

Photo 9-17. Prone Modified Cobra Stretch

18 - Supine Pencil Stretch for Abdominals

1. Lie supine.

2. Reach arms overhead and lengthen body, reaching toes and fingers as far as possible in opposite directions.

3. Feel the stretch in the abdominal muscles.

4. Hold for 15–30 seconds or 3–5 slow breaths.

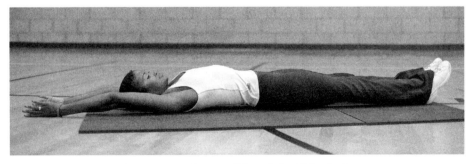

Photo 9-18. Supine Pencil Stretch for Abdominals

Oblique Stretches

Joint actions: spinal rotation and spinal extension

19 - Supine Knee Down Twist

1. Lie supine.

2. Pull knees toward torso and slowly rotate torso, lowering knees to the floor on one side. Reach opposite arm away and press opposite shoulder toward floor.

3. Feel the stretch in the obliques. (Several other muscles are being stretched as well, including the gluteus medius and the chest muscles on one side.)

4. Hold for 15–30 seconds or 3–5 slow breaths.

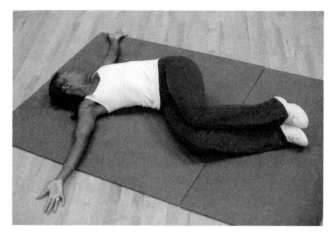

Photo 9-19. Supine Knee Down Twist

20 - Seated Knee to Chest Twist

1. Sit in proper alignment.

2. Cross one knee over the opposite leg and place the foot flat on the floor. Hug knee to chest with opposite arm. Lengthening the spine upwards, rotate the spine in the direction of the bent knee, looking over the back shoulder.

3. Feel the stretch in the obliques. (Several other muscles are being stretched as well, including the gluteus medius and gluteus maximus on one side.)

4. Hold for 15–30 seconds or 3–5 slow breaths.

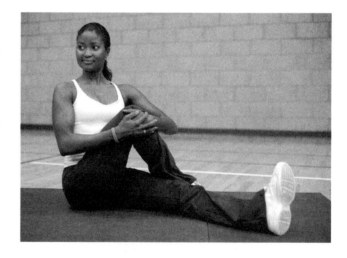

Photo 9-20. Seated Knee to Chest Twist

Lower Back (Erector Spinae) Stretches

Joint actions: spinal flexion

21 - Supine Double Knee to Chest Stretch

1. Lie supine.

2. Pull both knees toward chest, holding behind the knees. Allow the pelvis to posteriorly tilt and the lower spine to flex.

3. Feel the stretch in the erector spinae (gluteus maximus is also stretched).

4. Hold for 15–30 seconds or 3–5 slow breaths.

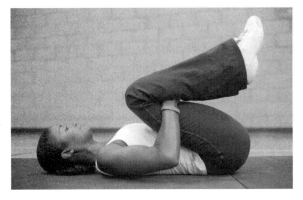

Photo 9-21. Supine Double Knee to Chest Stretch

22 - All-Fours Angry Cat Stretch

1. Kneel on hands and knees in tabletop position.

2. Flex spine (especially the lumbar spine), with head and tailbone down and abdominals lifted.

3. Feel the stretch in the erector spinae.

4. Hold for 15–30 seconds or 3–5 slow breaths.

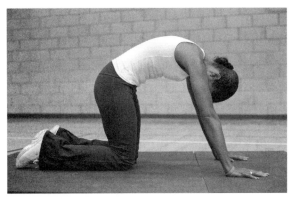

Photo 9-22. All-Fours Angry Cat Stretch

23 - Standing Angry Cat Stretch

1. Bend over with hands on thighs.

2. Flex spine (especially the lumbar spine), with head and neck continuing the line of the spine; contract abdominals.

3. Feel the stretch in the erector spinae.

4. Hold for 15–30 seconds or 3–5 slow breaths.

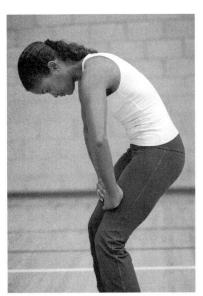

Photo 9-23. Standing Angry Cat Stretch

Hip Flexor (Iliopsoas and Rectus Femoris) Stretches

Joint actions: hip extension and posterior pelvic tilt

24 - Standing Hip Flexor Stretch

1. Stand in proper alignment with feet staggered.

2. Lift back heel up and bend both knees. Tilt pelvis posteriorly, maintaining a neutral spine, with abdominals contracted.

3. Feel the stretch in the hip flexor muscles on one side.

4. Hold for 15–30 seconds or 3–5 slow breaths.

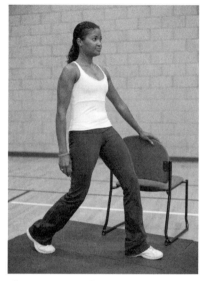

Photo 9-24. Standing Hip Flexor Stretch

25 - Runner's Lunge

1. Lunge with one foot forward, front knee bent at a 90° angle, and shin vertical.

2. Back leg may be either straight with knee off floor, or bent with the back knee on the floor. Hands are on either side of the front foot; hips are pressed evenly down, with spine in neutral and head in line with the spine.

3. Feel the stretch in the hip flexor muscles on the extended side.

4. Hold for 15–30 seconds or 3–5 slow breaths.

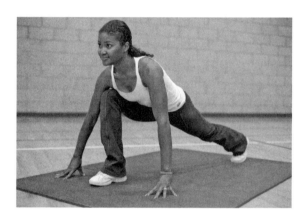

Photo 9-25. Runner's Lunge

26 - Supine Hip Flexor Stretch

1. Lie supine.

2. Hug one knee all the way into the chest; stretch the other leg out along the floor, pressing the straight knee gently down.

3. Feel the hip flexor muscles stretching on the extended side. Note that if reasonable hip flexor flexibility exists, your client may not feel this stretch. In that case, use one of the two stretches described above.

4. Hold for 15–30 seconds or 3–5 slow breaths.

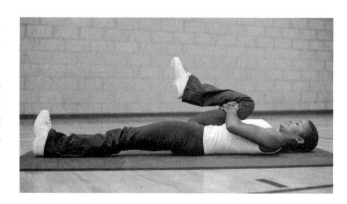

Photo 9-26. Supine Hip Flexor Stretch

Gluteus Maximus Stretches

Joint actions: hip extension and knee flexion

27 - Supine Double Knee To Chest Stretch

This stretch has already been shown and described in "Supine Double Knee to Chest Stretch" (stretch #21) under "Lower Back (Erector Spinae) Stretches."

28 - Seated Knee to Chest Twist

This stretch has already been shown and described in "Seated Knee to Chest Twist" (stretch #20) under "Oblique Stretches."

Quadriceps Stretches

Joint actions: hip extension and knee flexion

29 - Prone Quadriceps Stretch

1. Lie in the prone position with hand under forehead.

2. Grasp foot or ankle with same-side hand and gently pull foot towards the buttock in a straight line.

3. Feel the stretch in the quadriceps.

4. Hold for 15–30 seconds or 3–5 slow breaths.

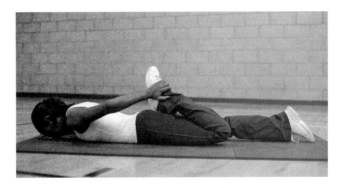

Photo 9-29. Prone Quadriceps Stretch

30 - Side-Lying Quadriceps Stretch

1. Lie on side with head supported on upper arm.

2. Grasp top ankle with top hand and gently pull foot towards the buttock in a straight line. Keep hips stacked and contract the abdominals.

3. Feel the stretch in the quadriceps.

4. Hold for 15–30 seconds or 3–5 slow breaths.

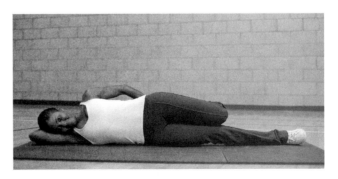

Photo 9-30. Side-Lying Quadriceps Stretch

31 - Standing Quadriceps Stretch

1. Stand in proper alignment, near a wall if balance is an issue.

2. Grasp one foot with same-side hand and gently pull foot towards the buttock in a straight line. Keep the support knee slightly flexed, and maintain the pelvis and spine in neutral with abdominals contracted.

3. Feel the stretch in the quadriceps.

4. Hold for 15–30 seconds or 3–5 slow breaths.

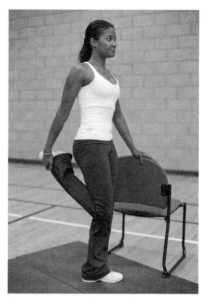

Photo 9-31. Standing Quadriceps Stretch

Hamstring Stretches

Joint actions: hip flexion and knee extension

32 - Standing Hamstring Stretch

1. Stand with one foot on a chair, bench, or bar. This stretch is safest if one hand can be placed on a nearby object or on the leg for support.

2. Square the hips and torso in the direction of the leg to be stretched, and slowly hinge the hips in the direction of the leg. Maintain a neutral spine and neck as long as possible, contracting the abdominals. Avoid flexing the spine if possible. Avoid hyperextending the knees.

3. Feel the stretch in the hamstrings.

4. Hold for 15–30 seconds or 3–5 slow breaths.

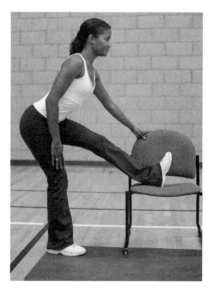

Photo 9-32. Standing Hamstring Stretch

33 - Supine Hamstring Stretch

1. Lie supine with spine and neck in neutral alignment.

2. Bend one knee and place foot flat on floor. Raise other leg up towards ceiling, keeping knee as straight as possible without hyperextension. Hold behind the thigh or calf; if hamstrings are tight, use a strap or band around the foot.

3. Feel the stretch in the hamstrings.

4. Hold for 15–30 seconds or 3–5 slow breaths.

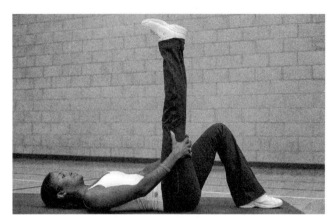

Photo 9-33. Supine Hamstring Stretch

34 - Seated Unilateral Hamstring Stretch

1. Sit in proper alignment with one leg straight in front, the other knee bent with foot against the opposite thigh.

2. Hinging at the hips, lengthen the spine and fold the torso towards the outstretched leg, maintaining a neutral spine. Hands may be placed on the floor at the sides for less flexible clients, holding toes or ankle for more flexible clients. Alternatively, a strap around the foot may be used.

3. Feel the stretch in the hamstrings.

4. Hold for 15–30 seconds or 3–5 slow breaths.

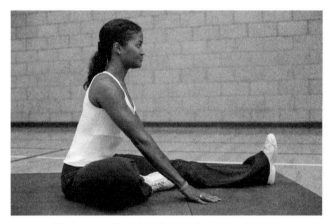

Photo 9-34. Seated Unilateral Hamstring Stretch

Gluteus Medius and Gluteus Minimus Stretches

Joint actions: hip adduction and hip external rotation

35 - Figure Four Stretch

1. Lie supine with one knee bent and foot in air.

2. Place opposite foot on thigh, allowing hip to turn out (externally rotate) and flex. Gently reach through space between thighs and pull the leg towards the torso.

3. Feel the stretch in the gluteus minimus (outside of hip).

4. Hold for 15–30 seconds or 3–5 slow breaths.

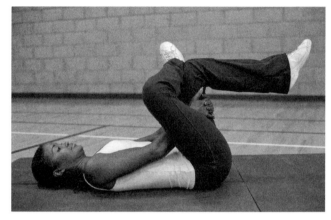

Photo 9-35. Figure Four Stretch

36 - Side-Lying Abductor Stretch

1. Lie on side with head resting on upper arm.

2. Bring bottom leg forward on floor with knee bent. Place top thigh directly in line with the torso (in the frontal plane) and bend top knee at a 90° angle. Gently lower top knee toward floor without flexing at the hip (keep thigh in line with the torso).

3. Feel the stretch in the gluteus medius (hip abductors).

4. Hold for 15–30 seconds or 3–5 slow breaths.

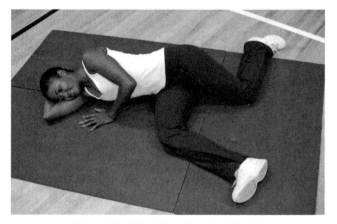

Photo 9-36. Side-Lying Abductor Stretch

Hip Adductor Stretches

Joint action: hip abduction

37 - Seated Straddle Stretch

1. Sit on floor in proper alignment with spine neutral.

2. With legs comfortably apart, hinge at hips. Avoid flexing the spine forward. For less flexible clients, hands may remain slightly behind the body, helping to maintain an erect and neutral spine. For more flexible clients, hands are in front, supporting the spine as the hips flex forward.

3. Feel the stretch in the inner thigh muscles (hip adductors).

4. Hold for 15–30 seconds or 3–5 slow breaths.

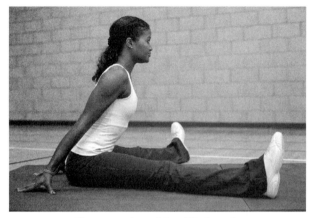

Photo 9-37. Seated Straddle Stretch

38 - Standing Side Lunge Stretch

1. Stand with feet wide apart.

2. Bend one knee, keeping knee in line with toes. Hinge at hips and press tailbone out and behind. Maintain spine in neutral with abdominals lifted. One hand (or elbow) may be on bent knee for support, or hands may be on floor if client is flexible.

3. Feel the stretch in the inner thigh muscles.

4. Hold for 15–30 seconds or 3–5 slow breaths.

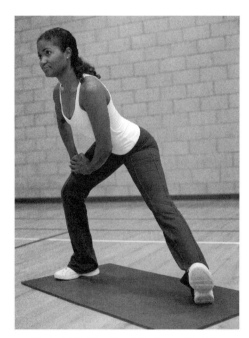

Photo 9-38. Standing Side Lunge Stretch

Calf (Gastrocnemius and Soleus) Stretches

Joint action: ankle dorsiflexion

39 - Standing Calf Stretch

1. Stand in proper alignment with feet staggered.

2. Bend front knee and make certain toes of both feet are pointing in the same direction; back knee is straight. Back heel should be down and the distance between the feet adjusted so that a comfortable stretch is felt. Hands can be on a wall, bar, or on the thigh for support. Abdominals are contracted and spine is in neutral alignment.

3. Feel the stretch in the calf muscles on one side.

4. Hold for 15–30 seconds or 3–5 slow breaths.

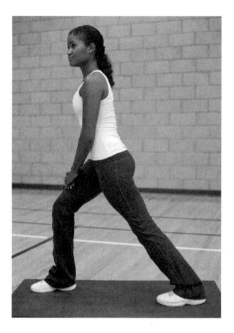

Photo 9-39. Standing Calf Stretch

40 - Seated Calf Stretch

1. Sit in proper alignment with one or both legs straight in front.

2. Maintain proper posture by keeping hands on floor at sides. Dorsiflex ankles, bringing toes towards knees and pushing heels away. Alternatively, a strap may be used to pull forefeet towards knees.

3 Feel the stretch in the calf muscles.

4. Hold for 15–30 seconds or 3–5 slow breaths.

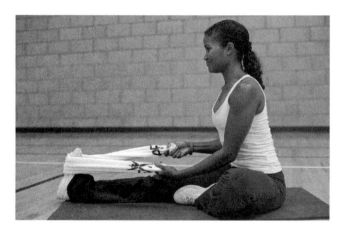

Photo 9-40. Seated Calf Stretch

41 - Standing Soleus (Achilles Tendon) Stretch

1. Stand in proper alignment with feet staggered.

2. Bend front knee and make certain toes of both feet are pointing in the same direction. Back heel should be down and the distance between the feet adjusted so that a comfortable stretch is felt. The difference between the soleus stretch and the standing calf stretch described above is that the back knee is bent (heel still stays down). Hands can be on a wall, bar, or on the thigh for support. Abdominals are contracted and spine is in neutral alignment.

3. Feel the stretch in the lower calf muscle (soleus) on one side.

4. Hold for 15–30 seconds or 3–5 slow breaths.

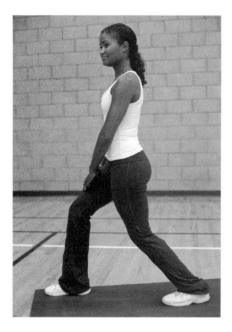

Photo 9-41. Standing Soleus (Achilles Tendon) Stretch

Shin (Anterior Tibialis) Stretches

Joint action: ankle plantar flexion

42 - Standing Shin Stretch

1. Stand in proper alignment with feet staggered.

2. Bend front knee slightly. Point the toes of the back foot, keeping toes, ankle, knee, and hip in a straight line. Hands can be on a wall or bar for support. Abdominals are contracted and the spine is in neutral alignment.

3. Feel the stretch in the shin (anterior tibialis) muscles.

4. Hold for 15–30 seconds or 3–5 slow breaths.

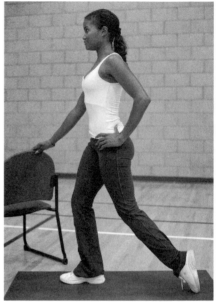

Photo 9-42. Standing Shin Stretch

43 - Seated Shin Stretch

1. Sit in proper alignment with legs straight in front.

2. Maintain proper posture by keeping hands on floor at sides. Point (plantar flex) toes, keeping ankles straight.

3. Feel the stretch in the shin (anterior tibialis) muscles.

4. Hold for 15–30 seconds or 3–5 slow breaths.

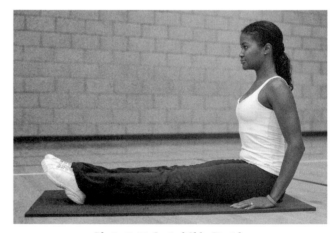

Photo 9-43. Seated Shin Stretch

Table 9-3.	Range of Motion of Select Single-Joint Movements (in degrees)		
Shoulder Joint			
Flexion	90–120	Extension	20–60
Abduction	80–100		
Horizontal Abduction	30–45	Horizontal Adduction	90–135
Internal Rotation	70–90	External Rotation	70–90
Elbow			
Flexion	135–160		
Supination	75–90	Pronation	75–90
Spine			
Flexion	30–45	Extension	20–45
Lateral Flexion	10–35	Rotation	20–40
Hip			
Flexion	90–135	Extension	10–30
Abduction	30–50	Adduction	10–30
Internal Rotation	30–45	External Rotation	45–60
Knee			
Flexion	130–140	Extension	5–10
Ankle			
Dorsiflexion	15–20	Plantar Flexion	30–50
Inversion	10–30	Eversion	10–20

(Norkin, C., & Levangie. P. [1992]. *Joint structure and function: A comprehensive approach* [2nd ed.]. Philadelphia: F.A. Davis. Reprinted with permission.)

NOTE: Range of motion of various joints can be measured with a goniometer.

References

Alter, M.J. (1996). *Science of flexibility* (2nd ed.). Champaign, IL: Human Kinetics.

American College of Sports Medicine. (2006a). ACSM's guidelines for exercise testing and prescription (7th ed.). Baltimore: Lippincott Williams & Wilkins.

American College of Sports Medicine. (2006b). ACSM's resource manual for guidelines for exercise testing and prescription (5th ed.). Baltimore: Lippincott Williams & Wilkins.

Cantu, R.I., & Grodin, A.J. (1992). Myofascial manipulation: Theory and clinical application. Gaithersburg, MD: Aspen.

Feland, J.B., Myrer, J.W., Schulthies, S.S., Fellingham, G.W., & Measom, G.W. (2001). The effect of duration of stretching of the hamstring muscle group for increasing range of motion in people aged 65 years or older. *Physical Therapy, 81,* 1110-1117.

Funk, D.C., Swank, A.M., Mikla, B.M., Fagan, T.A., & Farr, B.K. (2003). Impact of prior exercise on hamstring flexibility: A comparison of proprioceptive neuromuscular facilitation and static stretching. *Journal of Strength and Conditioning Research, 17,* 489-492.

Hedrick, A. (1993). Flexibility and the conditioning program. *National Strength and Conditioning Association Journal, 14*(5), 25-27.

Norkin, C., & Levangie. P. (1992). *Joint structure and function: A comprehensive approach* (2nd ed.). Philadelphia: F.A. Davis.

Wirth, V.J., Van Luten, B.L., Mistry, D., Saliba, E., & McCue, F.C. (1998). Temperature changes in deep muscles during upper and lower extremity exercise. *Journal of Athletic Training, 33*(3), 211-215.

Suggested Reading

Adler, S.S., Beckers, D., & Buck, M. (1993). *PNF in practice: An illustrated guide.* New York: Springer-Verlag.

Alter, J. (1983). *Surviving exercise.* Boston: Houghton Mifflin.

Alter, M.J. (1990). *Sport stretch.* Champaign, IL: Human Kinetics.

Anderson, B. (1980). *Stretching.* Bolinas, CA: Shelter.

Benson, H. (1980). *The relaxation response.* New York: Avon Books.

Blahnik, J. (2004). *Full-body flexibility.* Champaign, IL: Human Kinetics.

Chaitow, L. (2004). *Maintaining body balance, flexibility and stability.* Philadelphia: Elsevier Churchill Livingstone.

Couch, J. (1979). *Runner's world yoga book.* Mountain View, CA: World.

Enoka, R.M. (1988). *Neuromechanical basis of kinesiology.* Champaign, IL: Human Kinetics.

Iyengar, B.K.S. (1979). *Light on yoga.* New York: Schocken Books.

Kendall, H.O., Kendall, F.P., & Wadsworth, G.E. (1971). *Muscles testing and function.* Baltimore: Williams & Wilkins.

McAtee, R.E., & Charland, J. (1999). *Facilitated stretching.* Champaign, IL: Human Kinetics.

Injury Prevention

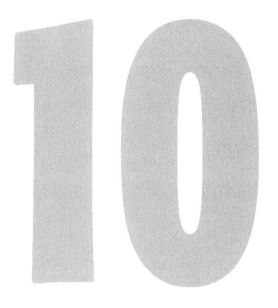

Outline

- Injury Risk Factors
- Types of Injuries
- Stages of Inflammation and Repair
- Basic Strategies for First Aid
- Common Muscle Imbalances
- Controversial High-Risk Moves
- Injury Prevention and Basic Rehabilitation Techniques

"First, do no harm" has long been one of the tenets of the medical profession; and it is an equally important principle for personal fitness trainers. All trainers should understand the most common mechanisms of injury for the major joints of the body; whenever possible, exercises that place the joints in a compromised position should be avoided. In this chapter, you will learn about risk factors, both intrinsic and extrinsic, that increase the risk of injury. Controversial movements and common training errors will be discussed. You will understand some of the basic types or classes of injuries, as well as the stages of injury and the phases of healing. Finally, we'll review, joint by joint, the most common musculoskeletal injuries and the safest strategies for their prevention and rehabilitation.

An important reminder: do not exceed your scope of practice! Although personal trainers are increasingly being asked to work with clients recently released from physical therapy and/or clinical rehabilitation, you must continue to work with your client's other health care providers. When in doubt about a client's injury or chronic pain, it is necessary to request a medical clearance and communicate with the appropriate physician or physical therapist for guidance. Exercise used to treat or rehabilitate is reserved for licensed health care providers.

Injury Risk Factors

Are there some general risk factors that increase a client's risk of injury? Studies have shown that some individuals are more likely to become injured due to the factors listed below (American College of Sports Medicine, 2005). However, doing "too much, too soon" (Pollock & Wilmore, 1990) has been suggested as the number-one cause of injury. Trainers would be wise to utilize the principle of shaping, or progression. This is the concept of slow, steady, gradual, one-step-at-a-time improvement. Apply overload conservatively, especially with beginners, and allow plenty of time for adaptation to occur. Typically, at least 2–3 weeks are necessary for the body to adapt and before continued overload should be applied. Also, be cautious when a client's exercise sessions exceed five sessions/week, exceed 60 minutes duration (45 minutes for beginners), exceed 85% of maximum heart rate, or are always high impact (as in running). Clients who train aggressively, with high frequencies, long durations, and at high intensities, are more likely to become injured.

Intrinsic Risk Factors for Injury	Extrinsic Risk Factors for Injury
Muscle imbalance	Improper or no warm-up
Bony alignment abnormalities	Excessive or uncontrolled speed
Previous injury	Fatigue
Obesity	High number of repetitions
Joint laxity	High intensity
Predisposing illness or disease	Poor alignment and/or technique
Leg-length discrepancy	Improper footwear
Restricted ROM/inflexibility	Inappropriate progression
Poor core stability	Environmental factors
	Confusion between muscle soreness and inappropriate joint pain

Types of Injuries

Musculoskeletal injuries fall into two basic categories: acute and overuse. An **acute injury** has a sudden onset due to a specific trauma, such as twisting the ankle. If the symptoms of an acute injury are ignored and the tissues continue to be stressed, the injury may become chronic. For example, without proper rehabilitation, a person with an ankle sprain is more likely to re-injure his or her ankle at another time. On the other hand, when excessive, repeated stress is placed on one area of the body over an extended period of time, the affected tissues may begin to fail. This failure results in a **chronic injury**, often called overuse syndrome. In this case, no single specific event causes the injury; it is, rather, the accumulation of repeated episodes of microtrauma that causes disease. Painful symptoms may persist for months with little change. Also, remember that repetitive overload stress can cause other problems besides injuries; and when this happens, overtraining syndrome can result. **Overtraining syndrome** symptoms include the following.

- Loss of muscle strength, coordination, and maximal working capacity
- Decreased appetite and body weight loss
- Muscle tenderness
- Increased number of minor injuries, muscle strains, etc.
- Occasional nausea
- Sleep disturbances
- Elevated resting heart rate
- Elevated blood pressure

Several studies have shown that overtraining suppresses normal immune system function and causes increased susceptibility to infections (Kuipers & Keizer, 1988). Counseling and complete rest may be necessary to help athletes obsessed with training overcome symptoms. Overtraining syndrome may be avoided by following periodization or cyclical training-type programs, and/or alternating hard, easy, and moderate periods of training. In addition, allowing adequate time for recovery between bouts of intense exercise is critical.

Other Basic Injury Terminology

- **Muscle strain**—an overstretching, overexertion, or overuse of soft tissue; less severe than a sprain. This may occur from a slight trauma or unaccustomed repeated trauma.
- **Sprain**—usually caused by a severe stress, stretch, or tear of soft tissues such as ligaments or joint capsules
- **Subluxation**—an incomplete or partial dislocation that often involves secondary trauma to the surrounding tissue
- **Dislocation**—the displacement of a bony part of a joint that leads to soft tissue damage, inflammation, pain, and muscle spasm
- **Muscle/tendon rupture or tear**—with a partial tear, pain is felt when the muscle is stretched or contracted against resistance. With a complete tear, the muscle is incapable of working.
- **Tendinitis** (technically known as tendinosis)—inflammation of a tendon leading to scarring or calcium deposits
- **Synovitis**—inflammation of a synovial membrane; an excessive amount of synovial fluid within a joint is usually caused by trauma
- **Bursitis**—inflammation of a bursa
- **Contusion**—bruising from a direct blow, resulting in capillary rupture, bleeding, edema, and inflammation

- **Adhesions**—abnormal adherence of collagen fibers to surrounding tissues during immobilization or after an injury, resulting in a loss of normal elasticity
- **Contractures**—a shortening or tightening of skin, fascia, muscle, or joint capsules that prevents normal mobility of that structure
- **Joint dysfunction**—mechanical loss of normal joint play in synovial joints, usually leading to pain and a loss of function; may be caused by trauma, immobilization, disuse, aging, etc.

Stages of Inflammation and Repair

- **Acute (inflammatory) stage**—usually lasts 4–6 days. Swelling (edema), redness, heat, pain, and loss of function are evident during the initial reaction to the injury.
- **Subacute (repair and healing) stage**—when repair of the injured site begins. Immature connective tissue is produced that is very fragile and easily injured. Most soft tissue cannot regenerate the exact, specific tissue that was damaged, so healing occurs with formation of scar tissue, in which the fibers are randomly formed. Signs of inflammation gradually decrease and eventually are absent. This stage may last 14–21 days after the injury.
- **Chronic (maturation and remodeling) stage**—a long-standing condition with recurring pain episodes often accompanied by dysfunctions resulting from the healing process. The connective tissue matures as collagen fibers and scar tissue continue to form and realign. These may limit normal range of motion or joint play. Often there is muscle weakness and decreased function of the injured part. Over time the scar tissue becomes stronger; strength of the connective tissues continues to increase for 3 months to 1 year post-injury; ligamental healing may take even longer. This stage begins between days 14–21 and lasts until there is pain-free functional use of the afflicted part.

Basic Strategies for First Aid

RICE

Response to an acute injury consists of RICE: Rest, Ice, Compression, and Elevation. As a personal fitness trainer, you should recommend RICE first to clients, both for acute and chronic injuries, except when referral to a health care practitioner is needed. While first aid may be provided, care beyond that is reserved for others.

Rest is necessary for proper healing to occur. Recommendations for rest depend upon the severity of the injury and vary from modifications of the exercise program to complete non-use.

Ice or other cold modalities are used to decrease swelling, lower tissue temperature, produce numbness and pain relief, decrease muscle spasm, and slow metabolic activity. Cold should not be applied to areas of reduced skin sensitivity, or to patients who have Raynaud's syndrome, sickle cell anemia, or peripheral vascular disease. Following are some of the ways to apply cold.

Durable, reusable, plastic cold packs contain silica gel. A wet towel should be applied between the pack and the skin to avoid nerve damage or frostbite. Endothermal cold packs are squeezed or crushed to activate; these are for single use only and are convenient for emergencies. Crushed ice bags are the most effective local application method as they mold easily to body parts; again, a wet towel should be used between the bag and the skin. Ice can be applied for 20 minutes approximately every 2 hours during the day, or according to a physician's recommendations.

Compression also helps to decrease swelling. Ace bandages and elastic wraps are examples of compression devices, and they may be used in conjunction with ice. The area above and below the injury should be included in the wrapping to ensure even compression.

Elevation of the injured area helps to decrease swelling; it is optimal if the afflicted area is raised above the level of the heart.

Other Strategies

Heat is often reserved for chronic injuries, as it helps relieve muscle spasm, and increase blood flow and flexibility. However, vigorous heating is contraindicated for acute inflammation! Various heat methods include heat packs, hot tubs, steam rooms, and saunas, in addition to various modalities used in physical therapy. If any of these modalities are recommended by clients' health care providers, personal fitness trainers should be aware of them.

Massage therapy can greatly assist in decreasing muscle spasm and stiffness and increasing local circulation.

Traction, both joint traction and spinal traction, are modalities that must be left to health care practitioners with specific training in these techniques. By providing a gentle and slight distraction of the joint surfaces, joint pain and muscle spasm can be reduced.

Finally, it can hardly be overstated that you must listen to your client in order to prevent injury or to minimize the recurrence of a pre-existing injury. As the trainer, you need to constantly ask your client for feedback with questions such as, "How does this feel?" "Are you feeling any pain throughout this move?" "Are you sure you're OK?" Many clients confuse normal muscle exertion and/or soreness with joint pain. While ordinary muscle soreness generally goes away within 24–48 hours and is therefore often manageable, joint pain is never acceptable. If a movement or exercise triggers "ouch" pain, then stop that move; clients should not push through this type of pain. The move or exercise should be modified and/or a completely different exercise should be given that doesn't trigger pain. This is especially important when recovering from an injury. A sharp, acute, "ouch" pain usually results in more inflammation and delayed healing and is a sign that something is wrong.

Common Muscle Imbalances

Our discussion of injury prevention would not be complete without mention of common muscle imbalances. Over time, these imbalances can lead to joint dysfunction, pain, and injury, so it is important for personal fitness trainers to address these imbalances as soon as possible within the exercise program, thus helping to prevent client injury. Many of these imbalances are due to a sedentary lifestyle, although some can result from an improper training program. See Chapter 5 ("Fitness Assessment") for helpful muscle screening techniques. Common muscle imbalances include the following.

- Tight pectoralis major and anterior deltoids
- Weak and overstretched middle trapezius and rhomboids
- Weak posterior deltoids
- Tight upper trapezius and levator scapulae
- Weak lower trapezius and pectoralis minor

- Tight internal rotators of the shoulder
- Weak external rotators of the shoulder
- Weak abdominals
- Tight and/or weak erector spinae
- Tight hip flexors
- Weak vastus medialis
- Tight hamstrings
- Tight calf muscles

To help correct these imbalances, the rule of thumb is to stretch the tight muscles and strengthen the weak or overstretched muscles. Now, consider the list of common imbalances in this way.

Muscles needing to be stretched	Muscles needing to be strengthened
Pectoralis major and anterior deltoids	Middle trapezius, rhomboids, and posterior deltoids
Upper trapezius and levator scapulae	Lower trapezius and pectoralis minor
Internal rotators of the shoulder	External rotator cuff muscles
Erector spinae	Abdominals
Hip flexors	Vastus medialis
Hamstrings	
Calves	

Controversial, High-Risk Moves

A number of exercises or moves listed below have been considered controversial or high risk for the general public by various organizations. Personal fitness trainers should be aware of these moves; having a client perform them without a valid rationale may increase your risk of legal liability. Note that many of these moves can be considered sport specific. Competitive athletes in various sports or activities may need to perform these moves because they constitute the "language" of that particular sport. For example, power lifters should practice dead lifts because they will perform this move during competition; hurdlers should practice the hurdler's stretch for the same reason. Ballet dancers practice deep-knee bends (grand pliés) as part of their daily practice regimen; a plié is an inherent part of the ballet "vocabulary." However, these and other competitive athletes assume physical risk as part of their sport, and most sports have some specific moves, when performed repetitively, that will eventually result in injury. As a trainer, you will need to evaluate whether your client needs to be exposed to these types of moves. If your client is not a competitive athlete and is interested in health-related fitness without injury, then you are encouraged to avoid and/or minimize the following high-risk moves.

- Ballistic stretching
- Hurdler's stretch
- Full straight-leg sit-ups
- Double straight-leg raises
- Forced high kicks
- Deep knee bends
- Plough (yoga)
- Full cobra (yoga)
- V sits
- Dead lifts
- Unsupported forward flexion of the lumbar spine
- Unsupported forward flexion with rotation (of the lumbar spine)
- Unsupported lateral flexion of the lumbar spine
- Hyperextension of the cervical spine
- Percussive (ballistic) lumbar hyperextension

Injury Prevention and Basic Rehabilitation Techniques

Shoulder

The shoulder, or glenohumeral, joint is a highly mobile joint and is subject to a number of injuries including the following.

- Rotator cuff tendinitis and/or tears
- Impingement syndrome
- Biceps tendinitis
- Shoulder dislocation/subluxation

It should be noted that in order for the shoulder joint to function optimally, the shoulder girdle must be capable of adequate stabilization. Therefore, trainers should train not only the muscles of the shoulder joint, but also the muscles of the shoulder girdle. Shoulder girdle muscles that are typically weak include the scapular retractors (middle trapezius and rhomboids) and the scapular depressors (lower trapezius and pectoralis minor). See Chapter 8 ("Applied Resistance Training Skills") for specific exercises for these muscle groups.

Rotator Cuff Tendinitis and/or Tears

Rotator cuff tendinitis and tears are common overuse injuries of the rotator cuff muscles and tendons (supraspinatus, subscapularis, infraspinatus, and teres minor). As the humerus abducts above the horizontal, it must externally rotate to clear the bony acromion. The infraspinatus and teres minor muscles are responsible for externally rotating and depressing the head of the humerus. If the greater tubercle of the humerus fails to properly clear the acromion, wear and tear of the supraspinatus tendon or the subacromial bursa can occur, leading to inflammation and possibly eventual tearing—the result is rotator cuff tendinitis. This, in turn, can result in restricted shoulder movement, especially abduction, and possible formation of bony spurs in people over age 40.

Keep in mind the following strategies for prevention of rotator cuff tendinitis.

- Keep the external rotator cuff muscles (infraspinatus and teres minor) strong. See Chapter 8 ("Applied Resistance Training Skills") for specific exercises.
- Teach humeral head depression; remind clients that "as the arm goes up (shoulder abduction or flexion), feel the top of the arm bone (humerus) going down in the socket."
- When abducting the humerus near or above 90°, make certain to perform shoulder external rotation (a good cue is to keep the thumbs up).
- Avoid exercises that place the shoulder joint in a vulnerable position in which the humerus may impinge the soft tissues under the acromial arch. Exercises that are problematic and/or high-risk include upright rows (especially with the elbows above 90°), behind-the-neck lat pull-downs, behind-the-neck overhead presses, full-range-of-motion pec decs, and deep bench presses in 90° shoulder abduction (Starkey & Ryan, 2001).

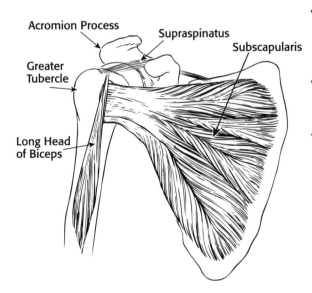

Fig. 10-1. Anterior View of the Shoulder Joint

Impingement Syndrome

Impingement is a pinching overuse injury of the shoulder tissues that leads to inflammation. The tendon of the long head of the biceps, the subdeltoid/subacromial bursa, and the tendons of the rotator cuff muscles (usually the supraspinatus and the infraspinatus) can all become impinged beneath the coracoacromial arch. This can cause rotator cuff tendinitis, biceps tendinitis, and subdeltoid bursitis. Repetitively lifting the arm with incorrect shoulder mechanics is a primary cause (often seen in swimmers). Prevention of impingement is similar to that for rotator cuff tendinitis.

Biceps Tendinitis

Biceps tendinitis is an inflammation of the long head of the biceps tendon as it passes through the shoulder joint bicipital groove. Pain is often felt along the tendon and biceps muscle and when flexing the elbow. Prevention is similar to that for rotator cuff problems. Heavy weight training or sudden, forceful contraction of the biceps muscle may precipitate a biceps tendon rupture, which causes immediate swelling and pain in the muscle.

Dislocation/Subluxation

The shoulder joint is capable of great mobility but is also rather unstable. Subluxation is a partial dislocation of the joint surfaces, whereas a dislocation implies complete separation of the glenohumeral joint. The cause is often trauma to the shoulder when there is excessive external rotation with horizontal abduction. Many individuals suffer recurring dislocations as the shoulder ligaments become more and more overstretched. Prevention means avoiding the vulnerable position of shoulder horizontal abduction and external rotation (including such exercises as behind-the-neck lat pull-downs and pull-overs and deep bench presses). Keeping the rotator cuff muscles strong is important, especially for those with congenitally hypermobile shoulders.

Major Mechanisms of Shoulder Injury

- **Extreme horizontal shoulder abduction while in external rotation** (the "red or danger zone"). Examples include behind-the-neck lat pull-downs, behind-the-neck overhead presses, excessive range of motion in pec decs, flys, or cable cross-overs. Even deep push-ups and bench presses can be troublesome, creating shearing forces on the joint structures. Avoid assisting clients with stretches in the red zone.
- **Internal rotation while abducting the shoulder joint.** Examples include traditional upright rows and lateral raises. Modify these moves as much as possible by abducting the shoulder no more than 90°. Ideally, the elbows should remain lower than the shoulders in both of these exercises.

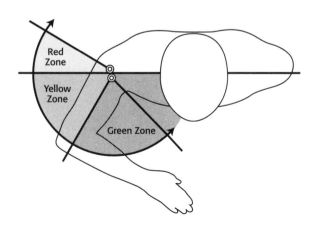

Fig. 10-2. Zones of Safe Shoulder Movement

- **Muscle imbalance between the powerful internal rotators and the weak external rotators.** The external rotators are responsible for holding the head of the humerus down in the shoulder socket; when they are weak the shoulder joint doesn't function properly.
- **Muscle imbalance between the scapular elevators and the scapular depressors** (the upper trapezius and levator scapulae versus the lower trapezius and pectoralis minor). Weak depressor muscles increase the risk of poor shoulder joint mechanics.

Activity Following Completion of Shoulder Treatment/Rehabilitation

If a client has been referred to a personal fitness trainer by a physical therapist after completion of shoulder treatment/rehabilitation, it is the responsibility of the personal fitness trainer to provide exercise programming that does not re-injure the shoulder. When working with a client with a previously injured shoulder:

- know what NOT to do. Avoid movements that require the shoulder to be flexed or abducted above 90°, that take the shoulder through a large range of motion or into the red zone, and/or that cause pain. Have the client keep his/her arms down in a neutral position initially. Help the client to avoid compensatory hunching or shoulder girdle elevation (this is not uncommon in an exercise such as biceps curls).
- never ask or allow your client to perform an exercise that causes pain. Stop any activity that causes twinges. Often, simply decreasing the resistance eliminates the pain. Always stay within a pain-free range of motion. Pain in the joint is never OK.
- gentle stretching is usually appropriate as long as it is pain free. Try "wall-walking" stretches in shoulder flexion against a wall. Avoid stretches in which the arm is in pure frontal plane abduction. Anterior deltoid and pectoralis major stretches with the arms kept low are generally acceptable.

Elbow

Tennis elbow (lateral epicondylitis) is a tendinitis of the wrist extensor muscles at their attachment to the lateral epicondyle of the humerus. Anyone who flexes, extends, or rotates their forearm excessively or improperly is at risk. Burning pain is usually felt on the lateral side (the thumb side) of the elbow, radiating to the wrist or shoulder. Gripping an object usually aggravates the pain. Strategies for prevention of tennis elbow include the following.

- Strengthen the forearm muscles: the wrist extensors, wrist flexors, pronators, and supinators.
- Stretch the wrist extensor and flexor muscle groups.
- Unless the forearm muscles are being specifically strengthened or stretched, keep the wrist in a neutral position whenever possible.
- Minimize repetitive and forceful wrist extension and flexion in activities of daily living.

Golfer's elbow (medial epicondylitis) results from overuse of the wrist and finger flexor muscles, causing tendinitis at the medial epicondyle of the humerus. Prevention is similar to that for lateral epicondylitis.

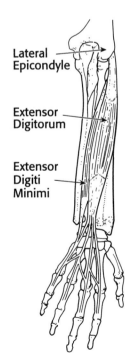

Lateral Epicondyle

Extensor Digitorum

Extensor Digiti Minimi

Fig. 10-3. Wrist Extensor Muscles

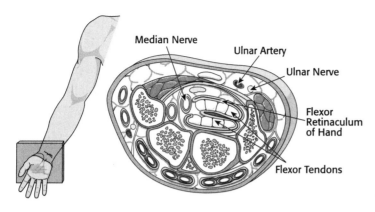

Fig. 10-4. Carpal Tunnel

Wrist

Carpal tunnel syndrome (CTS) may be caused by mechanical compression, which results in reduced blood flow to the median nerve (Crenshaw, 1992). Usually, flexor tenosynovitis, an inflammation and thickening of the wrist flexor tendons and their sheaths, causes the mechanical compression (or nerve entrapment) of the median nerve that leads to this overuse injury. Typists, hairdressers, carpenters, and others who perform repetitive motions involving wrist actions are particularly susceptible to carpal tunnel syndrome. Chronic carpal tunnel syndrome is also associated with pregnancy, diabetes, and thyroid disease. Symptoms include pain, numbness, or tingling in the fingers and thumb and, occasionally, an inability to flex and grasp with the fingers. Following are some preventive strategies.

- Keep wrists straight when working with the hands.
- Lift objects with the whole hand or with both hands in order to reduce wrist stress.
- Minimize working in cold temperatures, which can reduce blood flow to the wrists.
- When typing, use a soft touch.
- Take frequent breaks when working with the hands. Cut down on repetitive gestures as much as possible.
- Stretch the wrist flexors and extensors.

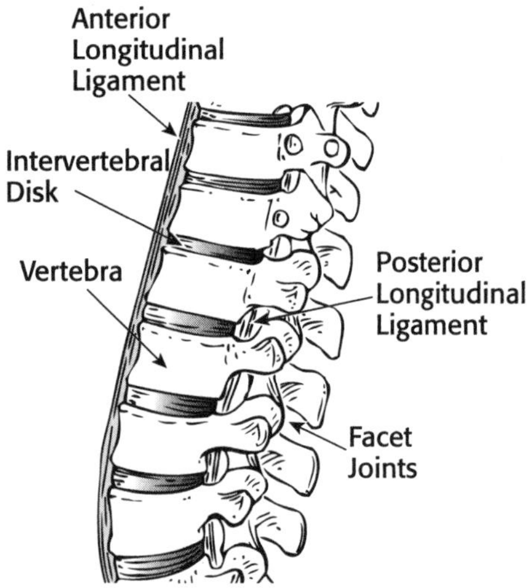

Fig. 10-5. Spinal Segment

Spine

Low-back pain (LBP) is a common problem, afflicting 80% of adults at some point in their lives (Frymoyer & Cats-Barile, 1991). A major factor in preventable back pain is poor body mechanics—how an individual sits, stands, walks, sleeps, lifts, and exercises, as well as performs all the other activities of daily living. It is difficult to have proper body mechanics if important major muscles are weak and/or tight. Common postural imbalances that contribute to back pain are excessive lordosis (swayback) and excessive kyphosis (hunchback); these imbalances often result from muscles that are too tight and/or too weak. Other risk factors for low-back pain are loss of flexibility, muscle endurance, and torso stabilization, poor posture and cardiovascular fitness, and excessive lifestyle forward flexion. Loosely linked to the development of low-back pain are: high mental stress or inadequate coping mechanisms, obesity, and smoking (Walsh & Fernyhough, 1995).

In order to provide effective, and appropriate exercises for your clients, it is important to first understand the basic anatomy of the spine. There are approximately 33 vertebrae in the spine, divided into cervical (7), thoracic (12), lumbar (5), sacral (5), and coccygeal (2–4) regions. When the spine is in **neutral** alignment it should have four curves: a lordotic curve in the cervical region, a kyphotic curve in the thoracic region, a lordotic curve in the lumbar spine, and a kyphotic curve in the sacral spine (see Figure 3-12 in Chapter 3,

"Anatomy and Kinesiology"). Each vertebra has an opening through which the spinal cord passes and several protrusions, or processes. There are two sets of articulations: between the vertebral bodies (and disks), and between the facet joints. Between each pair of vertebrae an opening, or foramen, is formed; nerves pass from the spinal cord through this opening. Disks have two parts: the outer fibers (annulus fibrosus) and the inner core (nucleus pulposus). Disks act as shock absorbers and permit compression and movement in several directions. Two long ligaments (anterior and posterior longitudinal ligaments) hold the vertebrae in place, top to bottom. The major muscles that support the spine are the rectus abdominis, obliques, transverse abdominis, multifidus, and erector spinae (including the longissimus, spinalis, and iliocostalis groups).

Neck and Cervical Spine

A very common postural misalignment of the cervical spine is known as **forward head** or chin jut (see Figure 10-6). This posture is characterized by increased flexion of the lower cervical and upper thoracic regions and by increased extension of the upper cervical vertebrae and of the occiput on the first cervical vertebra. Forward head is often accompanied by excessive kyphosis. Occupational or functional postures requiring leaning forward for extended periods, poor pelvic and lumbar spine posture, muscular imbalance, and poor body awareness may all be factors in forward head posture. Forward head may result in the following.

- Longitudinal ligament stress
- Excess tension of the supporting muscles leading to muscle fatigue
- Irritation of the facet joints
- Narrowing of the foramen in the upper cervical region, causing impingement of the blood vessels and nerves
- Impingement caused by a tight upper trapezius
- Temporomandibular joint (TMJ) pain, possibly leading to headaches
- Muscle imbalances, such as tight levator scapulae, scalenes, and sternocleidomastoids, and possibly tight upper trapezius, with stretched and weakened lower cervical and upper thoracic erector spinae muscles

In clients over age 50, neck pain may also be caused by degenerative changes in the cervical spine. When pain extends into the upper extremities it may indicate nerve root compression; refer clients with such symptoms to their primary care physician or a neurologist, orthopedist, or neurosurgeon. Strategies helpful in the avoidance of neck pain include the following.

- Stretch the upper trapezius, levator scapulae, and scalenes.
- Teach body awareness. Many clients don't realize they have a forward head posture.
- Help clients to feel a lengthening or traction-like effect of the upper spine. This may be done with the client lying supine or standing against a wall; give cues to gently tuck the chin in and lengthen the back of the neck towards the floor or wall.
- Avoid cervical hyperextension, which can exacerbate narrowing of the foramen and impingement of nerves.

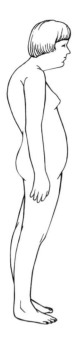

**Fig. 10-6. Forward Head Posture/
Excessive Kyphosis**

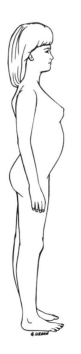

Fig. 10-7. Excessive Lordosis

Thoracic Spine

Round back or **excessive kyphosis** is the postural deviation most often seen in the thoracic area. It is characterized by an increased thoracic curve, protracted (abducted) scapulae, and often by an accompanying forward head. Internally rotated shoulders may also create the appearance of a rounded back. Excessive lifestyle flexion (especially continuous sitting and incorrect lifting) is a contributing factor in excessive kyphosis. In clients over age 50, degenerative changes in the spine resulting from **osteoporosis** may lead to increased thoracic flexion. The following strategies are helpful in the prevention and management of excessive kyphosis.

- Strengthen the middle trapezius and rhomboids.
- Strengthen the posterior deltoids.
- Strengthen the thoracic erector spinae.
- Strengthen the external rotator cuff muscles.
- Strengthen the scapular depressors.
- Stretch the pectoralis major and anterior deltoids.
- Stretch the latissimus dorsi.
- Stretch the internal rotators of the shoulder.
- Teach postural awareness.

Lumbosacral Spine and Low-Back Pain

One of the most common causes of lower back pain is the postural misalignment known as **excessive lordosis**. Excessive lordosis (swayback) is characterized by an increased lumbosacral angle, increased lumbar lordosis, increased anterior pelvic tilt, and hip flexion. It may be precipitated by obesity, pregnancy, weak abdominal muscles, and poor body awareness. Excessive lordosis typically causes pain by:

- stressing the anterior longitudinal ligament.
- narrowing the posterior disk space and the intervertebral foramen.
- compressing the related nerve root (e.g., sciatica).
- causing the facet joints to become weight bearing, with resultant synovial irritation and joint inflammation.
- producing muscle spasms and muscular fatigue, especially in the erector spinae and the deep posterior muscle groups.

Clients with excessive lordosis often have loose, weak abdominals, which contribute to poor posture and muscular imbalance. The back muscles, in contrast, tend to be short and tight, yet not necessarily strong. A good initial strategy with most clients is to strengthen and tighten the abdominals first, while providing stretches for the erector spinae. Then, after control of the abdominals has improved, begin to incorporate strength exercises for the spinal extensors. Additionally, due in part to sedentary lifestyles, hip flexors tend to be tight, causing the pelvis to be pulled into an anterior pelvic tilt and increasing the lumbar lordosis.

Tight hamstrings are very common in the general public and can be a contributor to low-back pain because they inhibit proper body mechanics. For example, it is more difficult to lift objects correctly and/or sit properly with shortened hamstring muscles. Hamstrings have their origin on the ischial tuberosities (sitting bones) of the pelvis; when tight, they exert a pull on the sitting bones, tugging the pelvis into a posterior pelvic tilt. This makes it difficult to sustain proper sitting posture for any length of time, and significantly lessens the likelihood of maintaining a neutral spine and pelvis while lifting.

Other causes of low-back pain include the following.

- A **herniated** or **ruptured disk** can cause considerable pain and disability. A herniated disk is usually the result of months or years of cumulative poor body mechanics. Excessive lumbar flexion, especially when accompanied by rotation, appears to be a factor in progressively tearing the rings of the annulus fibrosus. A herniated disk occurs when the innermost ring finally tears, or ruptures, and the nucleus pulposus presses out onto spinal nerves, potentially causing shooting, disabling pain in the back and legs.
- **Sacroiliac pain** is often seen in clients with significant leg-length discrepancy (more than a half inch). Overstretched ligaments of the SI joint (e.g., the iliolumbar ligaments) or weak musculature can lead to instability in the sacroiliac region, resulting in discomfort.
- **Spondylolysis** is a stress fracture of the pars interarticularis (vertebral neck), a site where the bone is not fully fused.
- **Spondylolisthesis** is a forward slipping of a lumbar vertebra on the vertebra immediately below it. This slipping occurs at the site of a lysis defect. It is classified into five types, with Type V being the most severe and pathologic (surgery may be necessary). Both spondylolysis and spondylolisthesis may be caused by moves involving prolonged or forceful spinal extension (e.g., a dismount in gymnastics).
- **Cancer** of the vertebral bones (with subsequent progression to the surrounding areas) is a less common cause of back pain.
- **Ankylosing spondylitis**, or rheumatoid arthritis of the spine, is a painful inflammatory disease in which the bones undergo decalcification and longitudinal ligaments of the spine become rigid, causing the patient to have a stooped, bent posture.
- **Osteoarthritis** (degenerative joint disease) in the spine affects two parts of the functional unit: the disk and the facet joints. Disks can be damaged and dehydrated, allowing the vertebral bodies to become closer together. The facet joints, which normally glide on each other without bearing weight, may begin to bear weight. Osteophytes (calcified bone spurs) may develop and encroach on the spinal canal.
- **Scoliosis** is a sideways or lateral curvature of the spine. Since this postural misalignment is often congenital and may have serious consequences (especially for developing children), a diagnosis should be made by a medical professional and corrective exercises should be prescribed by a physical therapist.

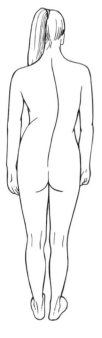

Fig. 10-8. Scoliosis

Activity Following Completion of Low-Back Pain Treatment/ Rehabilitation

If a client has been referred to a personal fitness trainer by a physical therapist after completion of low-back pain treatment/rehabilitation, it is the responsibility of the personal fitness trainer to provide exercise programming that does not lead to low-back pain and/or re-injury. Follow these strategies when working with a client with previous low-back pain.

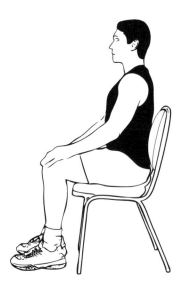

Fig. 10-9a. Proper Sitting

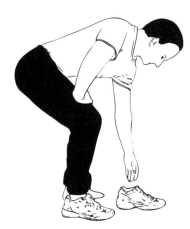

Fig. 10-9b. Proper One-Handed Lift

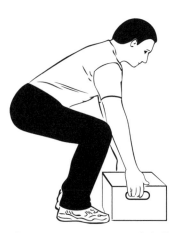

Fig. 10-9c. Proper Two-Handed Lift

- Avoid pain and muscle tension with muscle relaxation training and stretching.
- Maintain body awareness and continue to encourage proper neutral alignment. Emphasize abdominal hollowing (drawing in maneuver) and bracing (isometrically contracting abdominals while neither drawing in nor pushing out). Neutral alignment (core stability) exercises can be taught in the following positions.
  - Supine
  - All-fours
  - Prone
  - Side-lying
  - Seated
  - Standing
- Maintain range of motion with stretching and mobility exercises.
  - Erector spinae stretches
  - Quadratus lumborum stretches
  - Hip flexor (iliopsoas) stretches
  - Hamstring stretches
  - Mobility exercises for the spine (such as moving bridges)
- Strengthen weak or overstretched muscles.
  - Abdominals
  - Erector spinae
  - Quadratus lumborum
- Teach proper body mechanics in activities of daily living.
  - Sitting
  - Standing
  - Lifting:
    - one-handed lift
    - two-handed lift
  - Sleeping
  - Shoveling snow, raking leaves, vacuuming
- Encourage weight loss and smoking cessation if applicable.

Exercise Hazards for the Low Back

Personal fitness trainers should be aware of moves that pose a higher risk for the low back. Whenever possible these moves should be avoided or modified, especially for clients with pre-existing conditions.

- **Unsupported spinal flexion** overstretches the long ligaments of the spine, leading to loss of spinal stability.
  Examples: an incorrectly performed dead lift, good-morning exercise, bilateral bent-over rows, and/or bilateral bent-over reverse flys
  Solution: teach hip hinging, maintain spine in neutral, place one or both hands on thighs or shins for support, and/or avoid holding weights in this position
- **Unsupported spinal flexion with rotation** has the same problem described above, with the additional risk of potential disk herniation.
  Example: windmills
  Solution: place one hand on the thigh for support.

- **Unsupported lateral flexion** overstretches the long ligaments of the spine, leading to loss of spinal stability.
  Example: standing side stretch with both hands overhead
  Solution: place one hand on the thigh for support.
- **Extreme lumbar hyperextension** overstretches the long ligaments of the spine, leading to loss of spinal stability.
  Examples: cobra, upward-facing dog, donkey kicks on all fours
  Solution: modify cobras, perform donkey kicks on elbows and only to hip height
- **Long-lever traction** can produce shearing forces on the spine, leading to ligament overstretch and/or protruding (bulging) disks.
  Examples: double, straight leg-lifts; full sit-ups
  Solution: modify these exercises with bent knees, single-leg lifts, or perform crunches (partial sit-ups)

Exercise Protocols for the Low Back

Various exercise regimens are advocated for treatment of low-back pain. Some of the most widely recognized exercises come from Williams (1965) and McKenzie (Donelson, 1990).

Williams (1965) popularized **flexion** exercises with the rationale that back extensors need to be stretched, abdominals need to be strengthened, and the intervertebral foramen and facet joints need to be widened. This approach would allow the nucleus pulposus of the disks to shift **posteriorly** during flexion (assuming the nucleus pulposus position needs to be corrected).

In contrast, **extension** principles have been most widely advocated by McKenzie (Donelson, 1990). These exercises are intended to increase spinal mobility, restore a normal lumbar lordosis (in clients who spend much of their time in flexed positions), and shift the location of the nucleus pulposus **anteriorly** within the intervertebral disk. Extension exercises have been shown to cause a centralization of pain, reducing or eliminating leg or sciatica pain, and leaving only lumbar pain. Some specialists recommend finding the patient's directional preference, the direction that centralizes and minimizes pain. Flexion, rotation, and lateral gliding exercises may be used, as well as spinal extension-type movements.

More recently, progressive stabilization exercise protocols have been advocated for the prevention and rehabilitation of low-back pain (McGill, 2002, 2005; Norris, 2000). These protocols emphasize the maintenance of a neutral spine, preserving the normal low-back curve, especially when performing loading and lifting types of tasks. Some recent studies have called into question the safety of emphasizing large-range-of-motion spinal flexibility, made even more troublesome when the spine is loaded during mobility exercises. Remember—treatment and rehabilitation are limited for provision by those who are licensed, health care professionals.

Hip and Pelvis

The most common injuries to the hip and pelvis include the following.
- Iliotibial band tendinitis
- Piriformis syndrome
- Adductor and hamstring strains
- Osteoarthritis

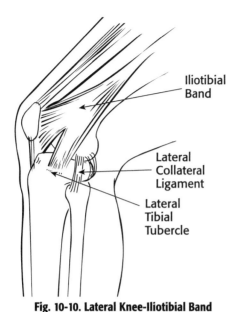

Iliotibial
Band

Lateral
Collateral
Ligament

Lateral
Tibial
Tubercle

Fig. 10-10. Lateral Knee-Iliotibial Band

Iliotibial band tendinitis, also known as ITB syndrome, is an overuse injury typically caused by a tight iliotibial band. The iliotibial band is aggravated by excessive or abnormal rotational movements of the femur and tibia while running or walking. Pain is usually felt laterally just above the knee joint and the lateral femoral epicondyle. Treatment provided by health care professionals may include rest, ice after exercise, stretching the iliotibial band, and strengthening the hip abductors. If the injury fails to respond, orthotics may be prescribed by such professionals. Preventive measures include avoiding running downhill or on banked surfaces, and performing regular iliotibial band stretching.

Piriformis syndrome is a tendinitis of the hip external rotators, which may cause sciatic-like pain. The sciatic nerve may also be squeezed by an excessively tight piriformis muscle, leading to pain in the hip and buttock. Massage and stretching of the hip external rotators usually relieves the buttock pain.

Adductor and **hamstring strains** are relatively common in weekend athletes. Immediately after the injury has occurred, it's important to rest and avoid stretching or strengthening the affected muscles in order to prevent further bleeding or muscle tearing. As the muscle heals, begin passive stretching and range-of-motion exercises, progressing to resistance exercise. These muscle strains are best prevented by performing a proper warm-up and by maintaining adequate flexibility of the adductors, hamstrings, and hip flexors.

Osteoarthritis (degenerative joint disease) commonly affects the hip as part of the aging process. Wearing away of cartilage, bone chipping and fragmentation, and bony spurs may develop in the hip. Pain is present when weight bearing, and eventually daily activities become difficult. Treatment includes range-of-motion exercises, joint-manipulation techniques (by a physical therapist), and strength and flexibility exercises. Once the client completes treatment/rehabilitation, strengthening of the hip muscles may be done using isometric contractions (making sure the client breathes), and progressing to dynamic training as the client tolerates movement. Muscles to be strengthened include the hip abductors, quadratus lumborum (hip hiker), hip extensors, and hip external rotators. Important muscles for stretching are the hip flexors, hip adductors, hip internal rotators, gluteus maximus, and hamstrings. If nonsurgical alternatives, such as those described above, fail to resolve a client's hip pain, his or her physician may recommend a total hip replacement. Personal fitness trainers need to follow physician guidelines for exercise after a hip replacement; patients are usually advised not to adduct the hip past neutral, and to avoid > 90° of hip flexion and/or hip internal rotation. For more information on osteoarthritis, see Chapter 11 ("Special Populations").

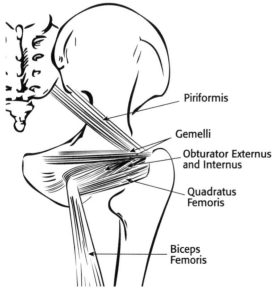

Piriformis

Gemelli

Obturator Externus
and Internus

Quadratus
Femoris

Biceps
Femoris

Fig. 10-11. Hip Outward Rotators

Knee

The major injuries and disorders of the knee include the following.

- Patellofemoral pain syndrome
- Patellar tendinitis
- Iliotibial band syndrome
- Ligament injuries
- Meniscus (cartilage) tears
- Knee osteoarthritis and bursitis

Patellofemoral Pain Syndrome

Patellofemoral pain syndrome is characterized by chronic anterior knee pain that may include chondromalacia patellae. Abnormal lateral tracking of the kneecap describes a lateral subluxation or malposition of the patella; this results in increased contact with the lateral femoral condyle, which can lead to articular cartilage softening, pain, and crepitation in the knee. Causes may include trauma, immobilization, excessive foot pronation, and muscle imbalances around the knee (and elsewhere), which can be especially problematic with impact activities. A typical muscle imbalance around the knee occurs when the vastus lateralis is larger and stronger than the vastus medialis obliquus (VMO, or more commonly known as vastus medialis), resulting in the kneecap being pulled laterally and therefore not tracking properly. Pain is often evident when descending stairs, and when sitting or squatting for prolonged periods, and may be accompanied by swelling or grinding. Treatment, as performed by licensed health care professionals, may include icing, bracing, and foot orthotics. Fitness professionals may assist clients after treatment/rehabilitation has been completed by following these useful strategies.

- Strengthening the vastus medialis with short-arc quadriceps exercises.
- Strengthening the muscles of the quadriceps isometrically with single straight-leg raises.
- Stretching the iliotibial band.
- Cross-training to minimize repetitive stress on the knee.
- Teaching clients proper knee mechanics.
- Avoiding positions and activities for clients that cause aching or pain.

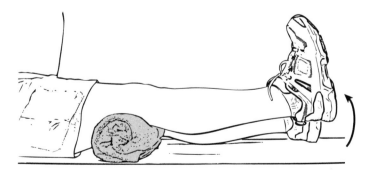

Fig. 10-12. Short-Arc Quadriceps Exercise

Patellar Tendinitis

Patellar tendinitis (jumper's knee) is an inflammation of the distal patellar tendon due to repetitive stress. Tenderness will be felt at the point where the patellar tendon attaches to the tibia, or at any point around the patella. It may be caused by improper shoe type, training surface, high-impact forces, weak quadriceps, and/or poor training strategies (e.g., too much, too soon). Treatment includes quadriceps strengthening, icing, and patellar tendon straps.

Iliotibial Band Syndrome

See above under "Hip and Pelvis."

Ligament Injuries

Ligament injuries, especially those involving the anterior cruciate ligament (ACL), are common. Approximately 70% of all traumatic knee injuries involve the anterior cruciate ligament. Athletes playing contact sports are at risk of sustaining blows to the knee, or of experiencing excessive torque when tripping or falling, both of which can cause a ligament sprain. Ligament injuries are graded according to severity, with a grade III sprain meaning the ligament is completely disrupted. The most common signal that a ligament injury has occurred is a loud pop that can be felt and heard, followed by the knee giving way. Tears, especially of the cruciate ligaments, warrant referral to an orthopedic surgeon, as surgery will probably be necessary. Depending on the severity of the injury, treatment by health care professionals may include immobilization, icing, cross-fiber massage, and range-of-motion and strengthening exercises for the knee flexors and extensors. A physician's clearance for exercise activity is prudent for any client who has had ligament reconstruction within the past year, as many doctors prefer the patient to wait at least a year for complete healing.

Meniscus Tears

Meniscus (cartilage) tears are caused by traumatic blows to the knee, rotary forces (torquing) within the joint, and by bending and straightening the knee too far. Menisci are highly vulnerable to injury from sudden rotations of the knee while it is weight bearing. Deep squatting also subjects the menisci to traumatic forces. A large meniscal tear can cause a piece of the meniscus to break loose and act as a foreign body within the joint, possibly causing the knee to catch and lock. If the meniscal piece catches between the femur and the tibia, severe pain results along with probable swelling and bleeding in the knee. Arthroscopic surgery is standard treatment for meniscal tears.

Knee Osteoarthritis and Bursitis

Osteoarthritis is a degenerative joint disorder caused by a gradual wearing away of the cartilage at the ends of the long bones. This leads to increased friction as bone rubs against bone, resulting in pain and disability. Obesity and abnormal joint stress (occurring, for example, in contact sports such as football) are contributing factors to an early onset of osteoarthritis. While treatment/rehabilitation may only be implemented by those who are appropriately licensed, experienced professionals may help clients to manage knee osteoarthritis by avoiding heavy impact activities such as running and racquetball, which shock the knee joints. Walking, cycling, and water aerobics, however, may be beneficial for reducing stiffness. Create better joint support by strengthening the muscles around the knee. Bursitis is a swelling of the bursae (small fluid-filled sacs) around the knee, causing pain and stiffness when kneeling or bending the knee. Health care treatment for bursitis is similar to that for arthritis.

Strategies to Avoid Knee Injuries
- Respect your client's pain and/or twinges. Do not perform any activity that causes pain and/or twinges!
- Stretch the hamstrings, calf muscles, and quadriceps.
- Strengthen the quadriceps and the hamstrings.
- Maintain muscle balance between the powerful vastus lateralis and the weaker vastus medialis. Quad sets and terminal knee extension exercises are good ways to target the vastus medialis.
- Perform both **open kinetic chain** exercises (OKC) and **closed kinetic chain** exercises (CKC). In an open kinetic chain exercise the terminal (end) joint is free; examples include quad sets and knee extension exercises. In a closed kinetic chain exercise the terminal joint is fixed; examples include leg presses, squats, and step-ups.
- For clients with a history of knee pain, modify the range of motion in traditional exercises; for example, perform partial or supported sit-back squats instead of full or regular squats.
- Teach your client proper knee mechanics. Help him/her to avoid: knee flexion > 90° (hyperflexion) in a weight-bearing position, knee torque (rotational force around the knee, especially when the foot is fixed to the ground), and knee hyperextension.
- When in doubt, always check with the client's medical caregiver prior to recommending activity!

Lower Leg
Shin splints and anterior compartment syndrome are relatively common injuries of the lower leg.

Shin splints is a catch-all term for pain in the shin due to repetitive impact-loading activities. This term may include tibial stress syndrome, tibial stress fractures, periostitis (inflammation of the covering of the bone), and anterior compartment syndrome. Pain is usually felt along the posteromedial border of the tibia, about two thirds of the way down the leg, when walking or running. Shin splints most often occur with changes in activity level or with a sudden change in running terrain. Clients who over-pronate are especially susceptible. Treatment by health care providers may include orthotics, icing, rest, calf stretches, and dorsiflexor strengthening. Following are some strategies for avoiding lower leg problems.
- Avoid or minimize running on hard surfaces.
- Wear shoes with a well-cushioned heel and forefoot.
- Perform thorough warm-ups and cool-downs.
- Stretch the plantar flexors (calf muscles).
- Strengthen the dorsiflexors (tibialis anterior).
- Avoid improper progression of training (too much, too soon).

Anterior compartment syndrome is usually characterized by pain on the lateral side of the tibia. This occurs when the leg muscles that perform dorsiflexion become so swollen that the fascia around the muscles restricts the blood supply, leading to pain, numbness, and paralysis. This condition can become a medical emergency. Surgical decompression (fasciotomy) of the anterior tibial compartment may be necessary.

Ankle and Foot

The most common ankle and foot injuries include the following.
- Achilles tendinitis
- Ankle sprains
- Plantar fasciitis
- Metatarsalgia

Achilles tendinitis is a term for a variety of injuries, including inflammation of the peritendinous sheath, of the tendon itself, or of the retrocalcaneal bursa. It is usually due to overuse and is found most often in runners, dancers, and participants in step classes. Achilles tendinitis can result from poor body mechanics, poorly cushioned shoes, excessive hill running, sudden stops and starts (as in basketball), and forceful eccentric loading (as in improperly performed lunges and repeaters on the step). Achilles tendinitis may be a precursor to Achilles tendon rupture. Medical treatment includes rest, ice, heel lifts, or orthotics, and slow, controlled stretching of the plantar flexors. Techniques to avoid such problems include the following.
- Stretch the calf muscles (gastrocnemius and soleus).
- Strengthen the calf muscles.
- Perform thorough warm-ups.
- Avoid excessive uphill running.
- Wear well-cushioned shoes.
- Use proper technique when stepping in group exercise (avoid pressing the back heel to the floor in lunges and repeaters, avoid stepping too far back, avoid bouncing on the "down" phase, etc.).

Ankle sprains are common in running, jumping, and sudden turning. Most sprains involve inversion and plantar flexion. Severe sprains often cause chronic instability with a high rate of recurrence due to the permanently overstretched ligaments of the lateral side of the ankle. Inversion sprains are graded according to the degree of injury, with a grade III sprain involving complete tearing of the anterior talofibular ligament. Immediate treatment consists of rest, ice, compression, and elevation. Depending on the degree of injury, the ankle may be immobilized in a cast, splint, or brace. Rehabilitation consists of cross-fiber massage, range-of-motion exercises, strengthening the peroneal muscles, and exercises to enhance ankle proprioception. You can help to avoid ankle sprains with the following strategies.
- Strengthen the ankle dorsiflexors (tibialis anterior, extensor digitorum longus, and peroneus tertius).
- Stretch the plantar flexors (gastrocnemius and soleus).
- Strengthen the ankle evertors (extensor digitorum longus, and the peroneus brevis, tertius, and longus).
- If there is a history of ankle sprain, consider wearing high-top shoes.
- Train the proprioceptors of the ankle. This may be done with balance exercises, agility drills, or rope skipping.

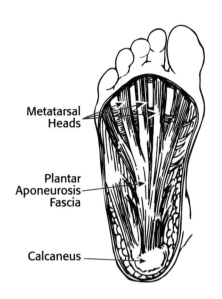

Metatarsal
Heads

Plantar
Aponeurosis
Fascia

Calcaneus

**Fig. 10-13. Anatomy of the Plantar Aspect
of the Foot**

Plantar fasciitis, or heel spur syndrome, is a chronic inflammation of the plantar fascia. Over time, a calcium build-up on the calcaneus (heel bone) may result in heel spurs secondary to the plantar fasciitis. Pain is usually felt in the medial arch near the heel, and is worse during a client's first steps in the morning. Walking on the toes or dorsiflexing the toes and forefoot increases the pain. Plantar fasciitis can occur in those with high arches and in those who overpronate. Flat, lightweight shoes with no arch support may also increase the risk in those with susceptible foot structure. Efforts to avoid such problems while clients are engaged in activity include the following.

- Wear shoes with adequate arch support, heel padding, and/or heel lifts. Orthotics may be needed.
- Ice the heel.
- Restrict weight-bearing activities.
- Stretch the calf muscles and Achilles tendon.
- Stretch the intrinsic muscles of the foot.
- Strengthen the intrinsic muscles of the foot.

Metatarsalgia is a term used for generalized pain and/or tenderness in the metatarsals, the heads of the long bones of the foot. Excessive or repeated forces on the ball of the foot (as in jumping) and/or degenerative changes in the arches of the feet are listed as possible causes. Wearing shoes with adequate forefoot cushioning and minimizing repetitive stress to the forefoot are the primary strategies for prevention.

Summary

This chapter provided a review of the most common musculoskeletal injuries, plus strategies for the avoidance of such problems. Injury risk factors and major types of injuries were presented. Stages of inflammation and repair were detailed, followed by strategies for management of clients after they have completed treatment/rehabilitation, as well as common muscle imbalances, and a list of high-risk moves. Avoidance of injuries is an area in which personal fitness trainers can be particularly instrumental; most clients seek fitness activities to improve their well-being, but need education and helpful strategies for minimizing the risk of injury while exercising.

References

American College of Sports Medicine. (2005). *ACSM's resource manual for guidelines for exercise testing and prescription* (4th ed.). Baltimore: Lippincott Williams & Wilkins.

Crenshaw, A. H. (Ed). (1992). *Campbell's operative orthopaedics* (8th ed.). St. Louis, MO: C.V.Mosby Co.

Donelson, R. (1990). The McKenzie approach to evaluating and treating low back pain. *Orthopedic Review, 19,* 681-686.

Frymoyer, J.W., & Cats-Baril, W.L. (1991). An overview of the incidences and costs of low back pain. *Orthopedic Clinics of North America, 22,* 263-271.

Kuipers, H., & Keizer, H.A. (1988). Overtraining in elite athletes: Review and directions for the future. *Sports Medicine, 6,* 79-92.

McGill, S. (2002). Low back disorders. Champaign, IL: Human Kinetics.

McGill, S. (2005). Low back exercises. In *ACSM's resource manual for guidelines for exercise testing and prescription* (4th ed.). Baltimore: Lippincott Williams & Wilkins.

Norris, C. (2000). *Back stability.* Champaign, IL: Human Kinetics.

Pollock, M.L., & Wilmore, J.H. (1990). *Exercise in health and disease: Evaluation and prescription for prevention and rehabilitation* (2nd ed.). Philadelphia: W.B. Saunders, Co.

Starkey, C., & Ryan, J. (2001). *Evaluation of orthopedic injury.* Philadelphia: F.A. Davis, Co.

Walsh, D.J., & Fernyhough, J.C. (1995). Back injury management. *Rehab Management, 8*(3): 30-34.

Williams, P.C. (1965). *The lumbosacral spine: Emphasizing conservative management.* NY: McGraw-Hill.

Suggested Reading

Arnhiem, D.D., & Prentice, W.E. (1997). *Principles of athletic athletic training* (9th ed.). Madison, WI: Brown and Benchmark.

Bloomfield, J., Ackland, T.R., & Elliott, B.C. (1994). Applied anatomy and biomechanics in sport. Champaign, IL: Human Kinetics.

Cailliet, R. (1981). *Low back pain syndrome* (3rd ed.). Philadelphia: F.A. Davis, Co.

Darrow, M. (2002). *The knee sourcebook.* New York: McGraw-Hill.

Ellenbecker, T.S., & Davies, G.J. (2001). *Closed kinetic chain rehabilitation.* Champaign, IL: Human Kinetics.

Galaspy, J., & May, J. (2001). *Signs and symptoms of athletic injuries.* New York: McGraw-Hill.

Goldberg, L., & Elliot, D.L. (1994). *Exercise for the prevention and treatment of illness.* Philadelphia: F.A. Davis, Co.

Hoppenfield, S. (1976). *Physical examination of the spine and extremities.* Norwalk, CT: Appleton-Century Crofts.

Kendall, F.P., & McCreary, E.K. (1993). *Muscles: Testing and function* (4th ed.). Baltimore: Lippincott Williams & Wilkins.

Norkin, C.C., & Levangie, P.K. (1992). *Joint structure and function: A comprehensive analysis* (2nd ed.). Philadelphia: F.A. Davis, Co.

Prentice, W.E. (1994). *Therapeutic modalities in sports medicine* (3rd ed.). St. Louis, MO: Mosby Year Book.

Smith, E.L., & Lehmkuhl, L.D. (1996). *Brunnstrom's clinical kinesiology* (5th ed.). Philadelphia: F.A. Davis, Co.

Whiting, W.C., & Zernicke, R.F. (1998). *Biomechanics of musculoskeletal injury.* Champaign, IL: Human Kinetics.

Special Populations

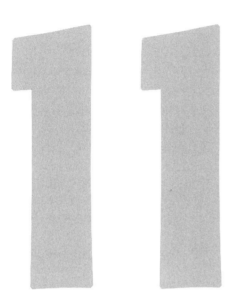

Outline

- Working with Pregnant Clients

- Training Older Adults

- Training Children and Youth

- Special Programming Recommendations

Much of the information in this text is directed toward helping you train lower risk, apparently healthy clients. However, eventually you will probably work with clients who have special needs and issues, and you will require additional knowledge and skills in order to train them safely and effectively. For most of the following special populations, it is recommended that you seek additional training and workshops, particularly if you plan to target a specific group (e.g., older adults). This chapter is intended to be only an introduction to some of the most relevant issues for each special population subgroup. Furthermore, be careful not to exceed your level of expertise; be aware that most of the following types of clients will require a physician's clearance prior to exercise testing or programming.

Working With Pregnant Clients

Most pregnant women can and should exercise. However, all pregnant clients should have clearance from their physicians prior to training, according to the American College of Obstetricians and Gynecologists (ACOG). Pregnancy causes profound changes in a woman's body, including the following.

- Increased lordosis and strain on the sacroiliac and hip joints resulting in increased potential for back pain and risk of falls
- Nerve compression syndromes, such as carpal tunnel syndrome due to increased fluid retention
- Total blood volume increase (30–50% increase over pre-pregnancy levels) with the major increase coming from plasma volume
- Increased heart rate, cardiac output, and blood pressure both at rest and during exercise
- Potential compression of the vena cava by the enlarging uterus (especially in the supine position)
- Displacement of the diaphragm upward, potentially causing discomfort and shortness of breath
- Lateral expansion of the rib cage
- Increased need for calories: ~ 300 additional calories per day (Artal Mittelmark, Wiswell, & Drinkwater [Eds.], 1991)
- Increased basal metabolic rate
- Increased heat production and decreased tolerance of heat
- Increased fatigue and nausea (especially in first trimester)
- Diastasis recti (split in the rectus abdominis)
- Tendency toward constipation and heartburn
- Tendency toward varicosities in legs and pelvic area
- Difficulty sleeping
- Fluctuating emotions
- Laxity of joints (Dumas & Reid, 1997)

Benefits of Exercise

There are several benefits of exercise during pregnancy including: improved circulation, sleep, digestion, elimination, as well as muscle tone to support joints; increased energy and endurance; better ability to regulate body temperature; improved posture, body image, and self-esteem; relief of discomforts, such as backaches, leg cramps, and fatigue; improved support of pelvic organs with pelvic floor strengthening; decreased stress; increased control of excessive weight gain (American College of Obstetricians and Gynecologists, 2002); and possible improved sense of control during labor. Recent studies indicate that pregnant women who are physically active have a significantly decreased incidence of gestational diabetes, while the risk of pregnancy-induced hypertension (PIH, also known as toxemia, a potentially life-threatening disorder of pregnancy) is also reduced (Dempsey, Butler, & Williams, 2005). Keep in mind, however, that there is little to no research supporting claims that exercise ensures a shorter, less painful labor, or that babies born to exercising mothers are healthier than those born to non-exercisers.

Risks and Concerns of Exercise During Pregnancy

Because it is extremely important not to compromise fetal or maternal well-being, there have been some special concerns regarding prenatal exercise. Personal fitness trainers should be aware of the following potential difficulties.

- Strenuous exercisers may gain less weight and deliver lighter babies than sedentary women. Under conditions of hard labor (work), nutritional stress, and prolonged standing, strenuous occupational exercise has been shown to adversely affect fetal growth (Clapp, 1996).
- There is concern that exercise may result in elevated body temperature to a degree that would cause negative effects on the fetus (especially to the sensitive neural cells). This has been shown in animal studies; and women exposed to heat in the first trimester (hot tubs, saunas, and fevers) have shown an increase in fetal neural tube defects (Milunsky, Ulcickas, Rothman, Willet, Jick, & Jick, 1992). However, there are no human studies showing that exercise can elevate core body temperature to the extent that the fetus would be affected. Most experts recommend that core temperature not exceed 38°C, or 101°F.
- Shunting of blood to the working muscles during exercise decreases utero-placental blood flow and may compromise fetal oxygen supply. In animal studies, this has resulted in altered fetal growth.
- There is a concern that exercising muscles will compete with the fetus for glucose. Throughout pregnancy, carbohydrates are utilized at a greater rate during exercise, and fluctuations in glucose levels are larger, both of which may put the mother and the fetus at greater risk of hypoglycemia (carbohydrate stores are the fetus's primary energy source for growth and development). Repeated hypoglycemic episodes may inhibit fetal growth (Wolf, Brenner, & Mottola, 1994).

Even though the above concerns persist, current studies show that healthy pregnant women without complications may perform appropriate exercise without fearing adverse effects (American College of Obstetricians and Gynecologists, 2002). To protect women at risk, be aware of the following contraindications for exercising during pregnancy, compiled by ACOG.

Relative Contraindications for Exercising During Pregnancy

- Severe anemia
- Unevaluated maternal cardiac dysrhythmia
- Chronic bronchitis
- Poorly controlled type 1 diabetes
- Extreme morbid obesity
- Extreme underweight (BMI < 12)
- History of extremely sedentary lifestyle
- Intrauterine growth restriction in current pregnancy

- Poorly controlled hypertension
- Orthopedic limitations
- Poorly controlled seizure disorder
- Poorly controlled hyperthyroidism
- Heavy smoker

Absolute Contraindications for Exercising during Pregnancy
- Hemodynamically significant heart disease
- Restrictive lung disease
- Incompetent cervix
- Multiple gestation at risk for premature labor
- Persistent second or third trimester bleeding
- Placenta previa after 26 weeks of gestation
- Premature labor during the current pregnancy
- Ruptured membranes
- Pregnancy-induced hypertension (PIH)

Conditions for Exercise Termination during Pregnancy
- Vaginal bleeding
- Dyspnea (shortness of breath) prior to exertion
- Dizziness
- Headache
- Chest pain
- Muscle weakness
- Calf pain or swelling (need to have health care provider rule out deep vein thrombosis [DVT])
- Preterm labor
- Decreased fetal movement
- Amniotic fluid leakage

(American College of Obstetricians and Gynecologists, 2002).

Guidelines and Recommendations

The 2002 ACOG Guidelines for Exercise during Pregnancy include the following.

- Pregnant women not only can, but should, exercise.
- When no medical or obstetric complications exist, pregnant women should aim for 30 minutes or more per day of moderate exercise.
- Moderate intensity is defined as 12-14 on the rate of perceived exertion (RPE) 6-20 scale (see "Intensity" in Chapter 6, "Cardiorespiratory Programming").
- Activities with a high risk of falling or abdominal trauma should be avoided (e.g., ice hockey, soccer, basketball, and downhill skiing).
- Scuba diving should be avoided, while care should be taken when exercising at altitudes > 6,000 feet (watch for signs of altitude sickness).
- Recreational and competitive athletes with uncomplicated pregnancies may stay active during pregnancy while modifying their usual exercise routines as medically indicated. Because information on strenuous exercise in pregnancy is scarce, women who participate in such activities should have close medical supervision.
- Exercise during pregnancy may provide additional benefits to women with gestational diabetes.

- Pregnancy is a unique time for behavior modification; healthy behaviors maintained or adopted during pregnancy may improve health for the rest of a woman's life. (American College of Obstetricians and Gynecologists, 2002)

Recommendations from the 1998 ACOG patient education pamphlet, "Exercise during Pregnancy," are included below for your interest.

- After 20 weeks of gestation, avoid doing any exercises on your back.
- Avoid brisk exercise in hot, humid weather or when you are sick with a fever.
- Wear comfortable clothing that will help you remain cool.
- Wear a bra that fits well and gives lots of support to help protect your breasts.
- Drink plenty of water to help keep you from overheating.
- Make sure you consume the extra 300 calories a day you need during pregnancy.
- While exercising pay attention to your body. Do not exercise to exhaustion.
- Be aware of warning signs that you may be exercising too strenuously (pain, vaginal bleeding, dizziness or feeling faint, increased shortness of breath, rapid heartbeat, difficulty walking, uterine contractions and chest pain, etc. (American College of Obstetricians and Gynecologists, 1998)

Other recommendations addressing exercise and pregnancy include the following.

- Sedentary pregnant women should not begin an exercise program in the first or third trimesters. When starting an exercise program, begin with light intensity (20–39% heart rate reserve [HRR]), and low- or non-impact activities, such as walking and swimming (American College of Sports Medicine, 2006a).
- Perform push-ups in a standing position against the wall after the first trimester.
- Weight training may be continued throughout pregnancy if the client has used weights regularly before, utilizes spotters when necessary, avoids maximal lifts, and has medical clearance to weight train.
- Pelvic floor exercises (Kegels) should be performed regularly; this may reduce the incidence of future urinary incontinence (Morkved, Bo, & Schei, 2003).
- Keep stretching exercises static.
- Moderate exercise during lactation does not affect the quantity or composition of breast milk or impact infant growth.
- Abdominal exercise is indicated for most pregnant clients as long as there is no Valsalva maneuver and as long as a position other than supine is used (side-lying, standing, or all-fours are acceptable). Check for diastasis (a split in the rectus abdominis) by having the client lie supine with knees bent (this only takes a few seconds), and curl up. If there is a diastasis, it will be near the navel, and will be vertically oriented. Assess the width of the split with fingertips (determine if it is one, two or three finger-widths wide). If the client has a separation, curl-ups should be performed while splinting the gap with the hands (this

applies primarily to women in the first trimester and/or who are post-partum). No oblique work should be performed with a diastasis, and regular curl-ups should be avoided if the separation is greater than three fingers in width (Aerobics and Fitness Association of America, 2004). Pregnancy is a time to maintain fitness, not strive for dramatic improvements.

- It is not recommended for pregnant women to undergo maximal exercise testing; submaximal testing can be performed with an endpoint of < 75% of HRR (American College of Sports Medicine, 2006a).

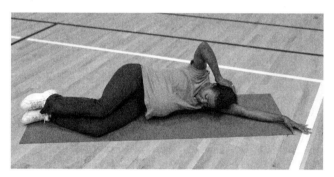

Photo 11b. Side-Lying Abdominal Exercise for Pregnancy

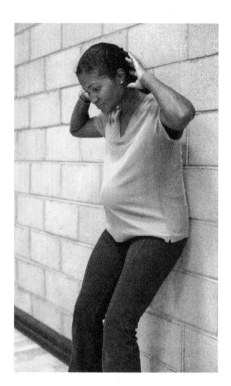

Photo 11a. Standing Abdominal Exercise for Pregnancy

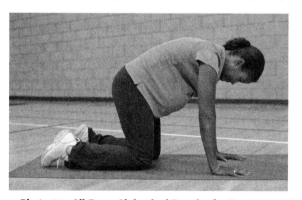

Photo 11c. All-Fours Abdominal Exercise for Pregnancy

Training Older Adults

The Administration on Aging (2003) released the following data. Older adults—persons 65 years or older—numbered 35.9 million in 2003 (the most recent year for which data are available), and represented 12.4% of the U.S. population, or about one in every eight Americans. The number of older Americans increased by 3.1 million or 9.5% since 1993, compared to an increase of 13.3% for the under-65 population. However, the number of Americans aged 45–64—who will reach age 65 over the next two decades–increased by 39% during this period. By 2030, there will be about 71.5 million older persons, more than twice their number in 2000. People over 65 represented 12.4% of the population in the year 2000 but are expected to grow to be 20% of the population by 2030. The age 85+ population is projected to increase from 4.6 million in 2002 to 9.6 million in 2030. This represents a significant marketing niche for personal fitness trainers.

Although there is a wide spectrum of ability and fitness levels among the elderly, there are a number of common characteristics of aging that affect exercise programming, including the following.

- Decreased maximal heart rate as a result of increased "stiffness" of the ventricular walls and slower ventricle filling (stroke volume also declines, leading to a reduced cardiac output)
- Decreased VO_2 max (about 1% per year between 25 and 75 years), largely due to the reduced cardiac output (American College of Sports Medicine, 2006a)
- Increasing blood pressure, primarily resulting from progressive arteriosclerosis
- Increased use of medications, especially those for hypertension and cardiac arrhythmias (there is an increased likelihood of underlying coronary heart disease [CHD] in older clients)
- Slower reaction time due to a slower velocity of nerve conduction (slows by about 10–15% by age 70)
- Progressive loss of bone mass (osteoporosis) and bone strength, especially in women, and the degeneration of joint cartilage causing an increase in osteoarthritis, which then increases the likelihood of back and knee problems
- Increasing percentage of body fat (creeping obesity), which is partly due to a slowing of the BMR (~ 2% per decade), as well as to increasing inactivity
- Loss of muscle strength due partly to declining muscle mass, which in turn is due to aging and inactivity (known as **sarcopenia**)
- Declining flexibility, particularly in the inactive, due to connective tissue changes in the muscles, ligaments, joint capsules, and tendons
- Increased tendency toward dehydration due to decline in kidney function
- Increased susceptibility to soreness and injury

It should be noted that several researchers are currently examining how much of the above factors are due to the natural aging process versus how much are contributed by inactivity.

There are many benefits of exercise for seniors, including: increased strength with mild to moderate muscle hypertrophy (this may occur even in persons as old as age 95 (Fiatarone et al., 1994)), increased bone density, improvements in joint range of motion, improved balance, increased VO_2 max, increased lean body mass, decreased percentage of body fat, improved glucose tolerance, improved cholesterol status, decreased stress, enhanced sense of well-being, and improved ability to carry out activities of daily living. New research continues to be published; for example, a recent study found that the risk of dementia (Alzheimer's disease) was significantly decreased in men who walked at least 2 miles per day (Abbott, White, Ross, Masaki, Curb, & Petrovich, 2004).

Basic recommendations for programming for older adults include the following.

- Obtain a medical history and a physician's clearance prior to fitness testing and/or exercise.
- Use fitness assessment protocols specific for older people. A number of resources exist (e.g., *Senior Fitness Test Manual* by Rikli & Jones, 2001, and *Position Stand: Exercise and Physical Activity for Older Adults* by American College of Sports Medicine, 1998).
- Recognize individual differences in senior fitness levels.

- Remember that too much, too soon is the major cause of injury and drop-out. Focus on safety with clients. Remember that many elderly are afraid they might overdo or become sore.
- Include a longer warm-up and cool-down.
- Consider minimal or non-weight bearing activities, such as cycling, swimming, and water, chair, and floor exercises for clients with significant musculoskeletal limitations.
- If arthritis flares up, reduce the intensity and duration of the workout. When arthritic joints are pain-free, concentrate on gentle range-of-motion-type movements.
- Emphasize functional exercises (those that relate to activities of daily living), such as walking, stair-climbing, and squats, whenever possible. Help clients maintain their ability to pick up grandchildren, garden, button clothing, open cans, and so on. Balance and coordination exercises are also beneficial for improved self-care.
- Moderate strength training is appropriate for clients without orthopedic problems. Keep repetitions slow and controlled.
- Emphasize flexibility work to help maintain joint range of motion. Mobility exercises for hands, wrists, and feet may be important.
- If the client has had a recent graded exercise stress test, consult with the physician and/or exercise test technologist to determine appropriate cardiovascular intensity (this is especially important for clients with CHD). Use the RPE method to assess intensity if the client is on blood pressure or cardiac medication.
- The longer a client has been sedentary and/or the more limitations he/she has, the lower the starting intensity.
- Older adults should be encouraged to be physically active for at least 30 minutes every day, as per the U.S. Surgeon General's recommendations (U.S. Department of Health and Human Services, 1996).
- Be alert for signs of joint pain, distress, or overtraining.
- Help build your client's confidence in his/her ability to exercise safely and enjoyably. Encourage long-term maintenance of an exercise habit.

American College of Sports Medicine (ACSM) Guidelines for Elderly People

Cardiorespiratory Fitness
- Walking is an excellent choice for many seniors; water exercise and stationary cycling are good for those who must limit weight-bearing exercise.
- Avoid excessive orthopedic stress.
- The activity should be accessible, convenient, and enjoyable.
- Intensity levels should start low (possibly as low as 40% of HRR).
- Avoid using age-predicted heart rates (220 - age) due to HR variability in older adults and increased risk of CHD. Instead, use rate of perceived exertion (RPE).
- Shorter bouts of exercise (e.g., 10 minutes) may be preferable.

Resistance Training
- Carefully supervise the first several sessions.
- Begin with minimal resistance.
- Perform one set of 8–10 exercises that involves all major muscle groups.

- Perform 10–15 repetitions at an RPE rating of 12-13 (somewhat hard).
- Perform all exercises within a pain-free range of motion.
- Machines are preferable to free weights for most older adults.

Flexibility Training

- Provide a well-rounded program of stretching and maintain range of motion of all joints.
- Consider devoting an entire session to flexibility for beginner older adult exercisers. (American College of Sports Medicine, 2006a)

Arthritis

Afflicting over one third of Americans, arthritis is the leading cause of disability in the United States (Clauw & Crofford, 2003). There are three main arthritic conditions: osteoarthritis, rheumatoid arthritis, and fibromyalgia.

Osteoarthritis, also known as degenerative joint disease, is quite common, affecting approximately 12% of adults, with the knee and the joints of the hand being the most common sites (Lawrence, et al., 1998). Osteoarthritis is caused by a wearing away of the articular cartilage, leading to bone-on-bone abrasion, possibly leading to bone chipping and/or bone spur development; this results in joint pain and stiffness. Mechanical stress, such as gravity or the repetitive impact or positioning found in certain activities (e.g., football, dance) is thought to be the cause of osteoarthritis; note that this condition is much more common in those who are overweight or obese. Typically, osteoarthritis has cycles of more and less pain. Your clients may have days when they are completely pain-free, and they may have days when everything seems to hurt and they are experiencing flare-ups. The best time to work with a client, obviously, is on a day when he or she is without pain.

Even though people with osteoarthritis seem to become less and less active, thinking that rest will relieve their symptoms, exercise and physical activity have, in fact, been found to be one of the best treatments. Walking, especially, has been shown to be beneficial (Kovar, Allegrante, Mackenzie, Peterson, Gutin, & Charlson, 1992); additionally, lower body resistance training appears to reduce pain and increase function, as does the loss of excess weight. Stronger muscles help support painful joints and prevent future disability.

Strategies for helping those with osteoarthritis to engage in exercise activities include the following.

- Start with short bouts of low-intensity, low- or non-impact exercise.
- Avoid higher levels of exercise on days when arthritis pain is severe.
- Stretch daily, if possible, always staying within a pain-free range of motion; if possible, gently move every joint every day, enhancing mobility of both muscles and joints.
- Perform strengthening exercises twice a week for unaffected joints.
- Strengthen affected joints on days when relatively pain-free.
- Isometric exercise may be preferable, especially for joints that are chronically painful.
- Be gentle with any joint that is hot or swollen.
- Stop any exercise that causes pain.

- If a client is sore 2 hours after an exercise session, reduce the intensity in the next few sessions.

Rheumatoid arthritis is, fortunately, less common. While exhibiting similar symptoms to osteoarthritis (such as joint pain and disability), rheumatoid arthritis is an inflammatory disease, not a degenerative joint disease. Classed as an autoimmune disorder (the person's own cells attack other healthy cells within the joint capsules), rheumatoid arthritis results in severe, often disabling pain, dysfunction, and potential joint deformity. It is characterized by swollen, inflamed, hot joints and decreased mobility; it is most common in the hands, wrists, and feet.

Exercise, particularly strength training, has been found to help manage pain symptoms, prevent muscle atrophy, and minimize disability. Since rheumatoid arthritis is such a painful and potentially disabling condition, it is recommended that personal fitness trainers refer clients to medically supervised programs.

Fibromyalgia is characterized by symptoms such as widespread pain in joints, muscles, and ligaments, heightened pain at "tender" points throughout the body, and possible insomnia, irritable bowel syndrome, fatigue, and psychological distress (Wolfe, Ross, Anderson, Russell, & Hebert, 1995). At present, the main medical treatment for fibromyalgia is to manage the pain, preferably, without medication; exercise therapy is a preferred form of treatment by some licensed health care providers. Cardiorespiratory exercise, especially, seems to result in decreased pain and improved mood and self-efficacy (Richards & Scott, 2002). It should be noted that most people with fibromyalgia are deconditioned, so a primary strategy is to address their muscle weakness and loss of stamina. Care should be taken to avoid making their pain worse, as overexertion can lead to decreased adherence.

Osteoporosis

Osteoporosis is a condition of abnormally reduced bone density, leading to fragile, porous bones and the increased risk of bone fractures. A precursor to osteoporosis, known as **osteopenia**, is defined as premature bone thinning, with a bone density 1-2.5 standard deviation units below average. Modifiable risk factors for osteoporosis include: physical inactivity, inadequate calcium intake, vitamin D deficiency, cigarette smoking, and consumption of more than two alcoholic drinks daily. Non-modifiable risk factors include being a female Caucasian or Asian, having a family history of this condition, having a small, delicate frame size, and experiencing early menopause or amenorrhea.

Exercise, particularly weight-bearing exercise, has been shown to be helpful in modifying some of the risk factors for osteoporosis (Liu-Ambrose, Khan, & McKay, 2001). Following are several exercise recommendations for clients with osteoporosis (American College of Sports Medicine, 2006a).

- Avoid all spinal flexion, especially cervical spinal flexion (this includes sit-ups and toe touches); perform as many exercises as possible in an upright position.

- Spinal extension (e.g., prone partial-range extension) may be beneficial in reducing the risk of vertebral fractures (Sinaki, Wollan, Scott, & Gelzer, 1996).
- If your client is pain-free, it is appropriate to recommend aerobic weight-bearing activity four times per week, resistance training two to three times per week, and flexibility training five to seven times per week.
- Perform resistance training with the load directed over the long axis of the bone or 8–10 repetitions at an RPE of 13–15 for one to two sets.
- Include balance training and functional exercises related to activities of daily living.
- Avoid high-impact activities and any activities with an increased risk of falling, such as crossover stepping, step aerobics, skating, and trampolines.

Training Children and Youth

Sadly, physical activity levels among most children and youth are significantly lower than in the past (U.S. Department of Health and Human Services, 1996), with physical education in schools on the decline; meanwhile, childhood obesity is on the rise, more than doubling in the past twenty years. Television viewing, combined with computer activity and video gaming, conspire to keep children and youth sedentary. Rarely has there been a more important time for personal fitness trainers to become involved in helping children and youth establish lifelong beneficial lifestyle habits. Helping children to exercise and eat healthfully now may prevent serious consequences later in life, such as adult obesity, adult onset diabetes, hypertension, osteoporosis, and CHD.

It is important to understand that children are not simply small adults. For example, their heart rates are higher and blood pressure is lower, both at rest and during exercise, and they are emotionally immature and may have difficulty staying focused or following directions. A number of fitness assessment protocols have been developed for children; these include the one-mile walk or run, curl-up test, pull-up or push-up test, and Sit and Reach Test (see Cooper Institute of Aerobic Research's FITNESSGRAM [1999] and President's Council on Physical Fitness and Sports' President's Challenge Test [1998] under "Suggested Reading" at the end of this chapter).

Several organizations and researchers have published statements and guidelines for exercising children and youth (Cavill, Biddle, & Sallis, 2001; Sallis & Patrick, 1994; Corbin, Pangrazi, & Welk, 1994). Following are some of the guidelines for children ages 5–12 from the National Association for Sport and Physical Education (2004).

- Discourage extended periods (> 2 hours) of inactivity, especially during the daytime.
- Provide a variety of age-appropriate physical activities.
- Children should accumulate at least 60 minutes (or up to several hours) of physical activity on all or most days of the week.
- Allow children to engage in intermittent activity; many children find this to be preferable to the continuous steady-state activity traditionally performed by adults. Several bouts of 15 minutes or so are ideal.

Recommendations from the American College of Sports Medicine (2006a) include the following.

- Emphasize active play and intermittent bouts of activity (rather than sustained exercise) for younger children.
- As children mature, 20–30 minutes of vigorous exercise at least 3 days per week is appropriate, with 30–60 minutes, 6–7 days per week recommended to reduce obesity.
- Heart rate monitoring is not necessary due to low cardiac risk; RPE is preferable and helps children to monitor themselves.
- Competition should be discouraged in the weight room.
- Avoid overly intense or 1 RM training.
- Focus on participation and proper technique rather than the amount of resistance.

(For additional information on children and resistance training, see Chapter 7, "Muscular Strength and Endurance Programming.")

Note that the thermoregulatory response of children is different from that of adults; in other words, their sweating rate is lower, meaning that it is easy for children to become overheated. You can prevent heat-related problems by keeping them hydrated and avoiding prolonged, strenuous exercise in hot and humid weather.

Always provide competent supervision and encourage children to talk about significant aches and pains; prevention of injuries is key for adherence to a healthy lifestyle. And remember, children will be more apt to exercise if adults, teachers, and other role models encourage them to participate in healthy and active lifestyles. Fitness should be a learning experience that encourages good habits, positive attitudes, and, most importantly for kids, fun!

Special Programming Recommendations

Hypertension and Stroke

Hypertension is a common health problem; currently, nearly one in three adults has hypertension, with an even greater prevalence among African Americans (National High Blood Pressure Education Program, 2003). It is a major risk factor for the development of heart disease, stroke, kidney failure, and congestive heart failure. Although the tendency for hypertension may be inherited, everyday health habits strongly affect the development of high blood pressure. Lifestyle factors influencing blood pressure include the following.

- High sodium intake (one third of all hypertensives are sodium sensitive)
- High dietary saturated fat intake
- Cigarette smoking
- Heavy alcohol consumption
- Obesity (The Framingham Heart Study indicates that nearly 75% and 65% of the cases of hypertension in men and women [respectively] are directly attributed to obesity [Garrison, Kannel, Stokes, & Castelli, 1987].)
- High-stress lifestyle
- Physical inactivity

Normal, or average, blood pressure is usually thought to be around 120/80 mmHg. Both the ACSM and the American Heart Association (AHA) define high blood pressure as starting at 140/90 mmHg (measured on at least two separate occasions), or on antihypertensive medication. See Table 5-1,

"Classification and Management of Blood Pressure for Adults," in Chapter 5, "Fitness Assessment," for the classification of blood pressure measurements. The top number is referred to as the systolic pressure, or the amount of pressure or force exerted against the arterial walls immediately after the heart has contracted. The bottom number, or diastolic pressure, may be thought of as the "run off" force, or the amount of pressure still remaining against the arterial walls as the heart relaxes before the next contraction.

Programming Recommendations for Hypertensives

- Personal fitness trainers working with hypertensive clients should learn to take blood pressure measurements where permitted. Hypertensives should have their blood pressure monitored frequently (ideally before, during, and after exercise). However, check your state's laws regarding determination of vital signs. In some states, blood pressure may only be taken by a licensed health care provider.
- Respect the limits of your expertise. There are some clients with hypertension and/or heart disease who need to be in a medically supervised program where emergency care may be more readily or completely available. These clients may include: those who have systolic BP decreases with exercise; those who frequently have resting systolic BP > 160 mmHg or resting diastolic BP > 90 mmHg; and those with an abnormal increase in BP > 200/100 mmHg.
- Be alert for symptoms of heart disease (see Chapter 4, "Health Screening and Risk Appraisal"), onset of angina (chest pain), or an inappropriate drop in heart rate. Notify a physician promptly.
- An intensity of 40–70% of HRR is recommended; studies have shown that mild- to moderate-intensity exercise may be better than high-intensity exercise at controlling hypertension (Fagard, 2001).
- Use the RPE method of assessing intensity if your client is on blood pressure medication.
- Be familiar with the exercise effects of blood pressure medications. Consult the client's physician or pharmacologist when in doubt.
- Use caution when recommending strength training to hypertensives. Avoid very heavy weights and clenched fists. Keep intensity low and increase the number of repetitions. Avoid resistance training to the point of failure, even if weights are light.
- Avoid isometric training due to the likelihood of straining with a closed throat (Valsalva maneuver), which may cause an elevation in blood pressure.
- Avoid positions in which the feet are higher than the head.
- Teach relaxation and stress management techniques.

A **stroke**, or **cerebrovascular accident** (CVA), is caused by a loss of blood flow to the brain, resulting in the death of affected brain tissue. Loss of blood flow is most often due to a thrombosis, or blood clot, which can form in arteries supplying the brain with blood. Individuals who have suffered a stroke may have a loss of muscle control, difficulty speaking, and an impaired ability to think; this can lead to profound disability. Of those who have suffered strokes, 15–30% are permanently disabled, with 20% requiring institutional care. Stroke is the third leading cause of death in the

United States (American Heart Association, 2005). Risk factors for stroke include hypertension, diabetes, carotid or other artery disease, heart disease, high cholesterol, smoking, obesity, excessive alcohol use, sickle cell disease, and physical inactivity. Recommendations for training people who have suffered strokes include the following.

- Be aware of the many issues that may affect exercise capabilities, such as impaired vision, spastic or flaccid muscles, loss of sensation, inability to follow or remember directions, etc.
- Seated cardiorespiratory exercise, such as stationary cycling, is preferable due to balance impairments.
- Weight machines are generally more appropriate than free weights.
- Include exercises for coordination and balance.
- Follow additional recommendations listed above at the start of this section, "Programming Recommendations for Hypertensives."

Clients who have had strokes will have varying degrees of disability, ranging from mild impairment to paralysis; it is extremely important not to exceed the limits of your expertise. If you decide to work with a client who has suffered a stroke, you must communicate closely with his or her physician and medical team.

Peripheral Vascular Disease

Peripheral vascular disease (PVD), also known as peripheral arterial disease (PAD), is a condition of atherosclerosis in the extremities, primarily affecting the calves. Because of the atherosclerotic lesions and reduced blood flow (ischemia) to the working muscles, a cramping, burning pain called **claudication** results in the legs. Claudication is most problematic during exercise or activities of daily living involving walking; it generally goes away as soon as the activity is stopped. Approximately 8–10 million Americans have PVD (Criqui, 2001). Many of these individuals manage their pain by walking more slowly, less often, and for shorter distances; such adjustments can affect quality of life and may eventually result in an increased sedentary lifestyle and a reluctance or inability to leave the home. Recommendations from the ACSM (2006b) for exercise and peripheral vascular disease include the following.

- Encourage risk factor modifications to reduce the risk of CHD.
- Clients with PVD may need to be in a medically supervised program; work closely with their physicians and medical team.
- Do not exceed the limits of your expertise.
- Provide warm-ups and cool-downs of at least 5–10 minutes each.
- Walking is the preferred form of exercise.
- Encourage walking in short bouts (3–5 minutes) or until moderate claudication symptoms occur; follow each bout with a period of rest to let the symptoms diminish. Repeat this pattern throughout the session.

Diabetes

Over 18.2 million Americans have diabetes (6.3%), of which 90–95% are diagnosed type 2 (National Center for Chronic Disease Prevention and Health Promotion, 2003). Diabetes mellitus is a metabolic disease caused by problems with blood sugar utilization. Blood sugar, or glucose, is necessary for both anaerobic and aerobic metabolic pathways. Insulin, a hormone released by the pancreas, helps make cell walls more permeable, and promotes the entry of the large glucose molecule into the cells, where it can be used for energy.

There are two types of diabetes: type 1 (juvenile onset), or IDDM (insulin dependent diabetes mellitus), and type 2 (adult onset), or NIDDM (non-insulin dependent diabetes mellitus). IDDM diabetics usually depend on daily injections of insulin, as their pancreas does not produce enough, if any, insulin. NIDDM diabetics do manufacture insulin, but their cells have decreased insulin sensitivity, and so do not accept glucose inside. In both cases, hyperglycemia (high blood sugar) results. The majority (about 90%) of diabetics are NIDDM (National Center for Chronic Disease Prevention and Health Promotion, 2003).

NIDDM diabetics may or may not need to take insulin, and may be able to manage their disease completely with diet and exercise. Exercise has an insulin-like effect, assisting the entry of glucose into the cells and enhancing insulin sensitivity. However, if exercise is excessive, or if the diet is inadequate, glucose levels may suddenly drop and the person with diabetes may become hypoglycemic. A hypoglycemic reaction (also known as insulin shock) is potentially life-threatening and you should help your client take steps for prevention, including the following.

- Work with your client's physician (a medical clearance is essential). Insulin dosage should be appropriate for an exercising person with diabetes.
- Keep the emergency medical number and your emergency response plan handy.
- For 1 hour after injection, avoid exercising muscles that have been injected.
- Do not have your client exercise at the time of peak insulin action.
- Have your client eat carbohydrate snacks before and during prolonged exercise, unless directed otherwise by his/her physician.
- Always have some form of sugar available for the prevention of a hypoglycemic reaction or when a client shows symptoms of low blood sugar, and help your client to stay hydrated.
- Monitor blood glucose frequently, especially when starting a program.
- Know the signs of hypoglycemia, including: excessive fatigue, nausea, lightheadedness, dizziness, profuse perspiration (diaphoresis), spots in front of eyes, confusion, shakiness, headaches, sudden rapid heart rate, and even seizures. Fainting, known as **syncope**, may occur, potentially progressing into a coma and life-threatening situation.

Other recommendations include the following.

- Promote aerobic exercise. Cardiovascular exercise is ideal for people with diabetes because it helps with weight control, increases insulin sensitivity, and increases glucose tolerance (American College of Sports Medicine, 2000). Regular, consistent, steady-state exercise as recommended by clients' health care providers, performed at the same time each day, may be best for helping to control clients' diabetes.
- Help clients to accumulate a minimum of 1,000 kcal/week of physical activity, progressing to 2,000 kcal/week if weight loss is a goal.
- Help clients practice proper foot hygiene. One outcome of diabetes is nerve damage (neuropathy) and accelerated atherosclerosis (resulting in poor circulation) in the extremities. Sores, blisters, and cuts may become

infected and gangrenous without the clients' knowledge, since they may have reduced sensation in their feet.
- Seek additional training if you plan to work with people with diabetes.

Chronic Obstructive Pulmonary Disease (COPD)

COPD is the fourth leading cause of death in the United States (behind heart disease, cancer, and stroke) (Centers for Disease Control and Prevention, 2003a). Traditionally, COPD has included any condition in which airway resistance is increased, making it difficult to breathe; the primary conditions have been identified as chronic bronchitis, emphysema, and asthma. More recently, the inclusion of asthma has been the subject of controversy, since asthma is usually completely reversible (Barnes, 2000). (NOTE: There is wide variability among individuals diagnosed with asthma, and their experience of the condition can range from very mild to severe. Reversibility is dependent on severity of the condition and the individual patient [Clark, 2003].)

With chronic bronchitis, the conducting airways are damaged and sputum is produced on a near daily basis for a prolonged period of time (> 2 years); emphysema, on the other hand, is characterized by destruction of the alveoli (air sacs) in the lungs and a narrowing of the airways. Both disorders are primarily caused by smoking and result in shortness of breath (dyspnea) with physical activity, limiting functional abilities. People with severe COPD need to be under a physician's care and should be referred to a pulmonary rehabilitation program; most likely they will be using supplemental oxygen. Basic exercise recommendations for COPD include the following.
- Walking is the preferred form of exercise since it is needed in activities of daily living.
- Avoid upper body ergometry as this tends to cause increased dyspnea (shortness of breath).
- Instead of assessing intensity with heart rate, use the scale for dyspnea; clients should keep intensity below 3.
  <u>Dyspnea Scale</u>
    1. Light, barely noticeable
    2. Moderate, bothersome
    3. Moderately severe, very uncomfortable
    4. Most severe or intense dyspnea ever experienced
- Duration, especially initially, may be very short; many COPD patients can only tolerate 2–3 minutes of exercise at first.
- Resistance training, especially of the upper body muscles, is important.
- Specific training of the muscles of respiration (especially the inspiratory muscles) is recommended.

Asthma

Asthma is a common disease, especially among children; it affects between 14-15 million Americans (National Heart, Lung, and Blood Institute, 1999) and can be caused by allergens, stress, cigarette smoke, air pollution, and exercise. It is characterized by hyperreactive airways with a tendency to develop bronchospasm or bronchoconstriction, or, sometimes both; it is usually completely reversible, especially in its early stages and depending on the severity of the condition. Personal fitness trainers should be aware of a somewhat separate type of asthma, called exercise-induced asthma (EIA). This type of asthma is triggered by exercising (usually early in the session) and leads to coughing and wheezing; fortunately, it is not life threatening. After the initial exercise-induced asthma attack, a refractory period occurs; this is the time when it is very unlikely that another asthma attack will happen. The refractory period can last anywhere from 1–4 hours. Many athletes with EIA take advantage of the refractory period by performing a longer warm-up prior to vigorous exertion; this can bring on the onset of mild asthma symptoms, followed by an extended symptom-free period. Note that intermittent exercise is much less likely to trigger an EIA attack. Following are some recommendations for exercising with asthma.

- Perform long warm-ups to take advantage of the refractory period.
- Exercise in warm, humid air.
- Avoid intense exercise that causes heavy breathing, or keep such workouts short.
- Try sports that involve short bursts of activity, such as tennis or football, rather than those with continuous activity.
- Breathe through the nose (rather than the mouth) as much as possible.
- Control breathing to prevent hyperventilation.
- Follow daily and pre-exercise medication schedules provided by the physician (an inhaler used before exercise may decrease the likelihood of an asthma attack).

Cancer

Regular physical activity appears to reduce the risk of developing certain cancers, especially those of the colon and breast (Fridenreich, 2001). When working with cancer patients, consider their current functional ability level, whether or not other diseases are present (e.g., CHD), status of the cancer (e.g., size of the tumor, extent of the spreading, lymph node involvement, and extent of metastasis), complications resulting from the tumor (such as spinal cord compression or increased intracranial pressure), type of therapy, and complications arising from the therapy.

Cancer chemotherapies may interfere with exercise due to the likelihood of fatigue, nausea, irregular heart rhythms and other side effects. Cancer medications may have potentially negative effects that must be taken into consideration, such as gastrointestinal bleeding, hearing loss, hypertension, heart arrythmias, and confusion. Radiation therapy may cause anorexia, nausea, diarrhea, and pneumonia, among other effects. The aftereffects of surgeries to eliminate cancer may also present unique limitations to certain forms of exercise.

Many cancer patients become weak and fatigued partially as a result of bed rest prescriptions. Moderate cardiorespiratory exercise may help maintain the ability to perform activities of daily living and improve quality of life, whereas low-intensity strength training may help cancer patients minimize the loss of lean body mass and maintain the strength needed for daily living.

Depending on the type of cancer, some precautions for exercise programming have been identified (Courneya, Mackey, & Jones, 2000), including the following.

- Avoid or minimize high-intensity cardiorespiratory exercise.
- Avoid or minimize activities that may increase the risk of bacterial infection, such as swimming.
- Avoid activities that increase the risk of bleeding, such as contact sports.

- If the patient has severe muscle mass loss (cachexia), only mild-intensity exercise should be performed.
- If the patient has bone metastases or pain, avoid activities that increase the risk of fracture at the site of bone pain or metastases.
- Use caution if the patient experiences dizziness, dyspnea, severe nausea, or extreme fatigue or muscle weakness; consult with his or her cancer-care providers.

General aerobic exercise recommendations for otherwise healthy cancer survivors have been identified (Courneya, Mackey, & Jones, 2000); these guidelines closely parallel the 2006 ACSM Guidelines discussed elsewhere in this text.

HIV/AIDS

The Centers for Disease Control and Prevention (CDC) (2003b) estimates that up to 900,000 people in the United States may be HIV (human immunodeficiency virus) infected. "HIV disease" and AIDS (acquired immune deficiency syndrome) are both caused by HIV, which damages macrophage cells (cells responsible for combating disease). The result is suppression of the immune system and a diminished ability to fight infection and disease. HIV infection causes many clinical symptoms including severe weight loss and wasting, chronic diarrhea, nonproductive cough with shortness of breath, dementia, fevers of unknown origin, chronic fatigue, and swollen lymph glands. The term "HIV disease" describes all the manifestations of infection prior to the development of AIDS, the final, fatal stage of HIV infection. The CDC estimates the average incubation period between HIV infection and full-blown AIDS to be 8–10 years.

Considerations when working with HIV/AIDS patients include: whether or not the patient needs direct medical supervision when exercising, confidentiality, medications used, weight loss and difficulty maintaining lean body mass (nutritional counseling is important), catheter use, and current functional level. Avoid having a client with HIV/AIDS exercise if he or she has nausea, uncontrolled diarrhea, dehydration, or a temperature greater than 100° (American College of Sports Medicine, 2002). Moderate cardiorespiratory exercise has been shown to increase the number of helper T cells and boost the immune system (Nixon, O'Brien, Glazier, & Tynan, 2001), but strenuous, exhaustive exercise suppresses the immune system and is not recommended. Benefits of exercise for HIV/AIDS patients include enhanced psychological coping skills, decreased fatigue, increased lean muscle mass, and increased cardiovascular fitness.

Neuromuscular Disorders

Multiple sclerosis (MS) is caused by gradual damage to the myelin sheath, or fatty coating, that surrounds motor neurons. The cause of MS is currently unknown, although scientists are exploring genetic, viral, and environmental factors. Symptoms of MS include numbness or tingling in one or more limbs, blurred vision, fatigue, muscle weakness, inability to tolerate heat, and muscle spasticity leading to loss of balance, coordination, and muscle function. There are four main types of MS, ranging from a benign form with little or no disability, to a progressive, disabling form characterized by acute attacks of dysfunction (Burks & Johnson, 2000).

Considerations when working with a person who has MS include the following.

- Chair aerobics, stationary cycling, or water exercise may be preferable to high-/low-impact or treadmill activity due to balance issues.
- "Foot drop," or weakness in the anterior tibialis, may increase the chance of stumbling or falling.
- Provide cool environments for exercise, as people with MS have a low tolerance for heat.
- Moderate strength training is appropriate; provide functional exercises such as squats whenever possible.
- Weight machines may be preferable due to the reduced need for balance.

Parkinson's disease (PD) is a disorder of the nervous system, specifically of the basal ganglia, a mass of nerve cells in the brain that is responsible for motor functions. With PD, the neurotransmitter dopamine is progressively lost, affecting the ability of the basal ganglia and its pathways to function effectively. Tremors, rigidity, slow and hesitant movements (known as bradykinesia), and postural instability are the four major signs of PD (Koller & Hubble, 1992). PD is most common in older adults, with about 1.5–2.5% of the population over 70 years of age affected (Tanner & Ben-Schlomo, 1999). Note the following considerations for exercise and Parkinson's.

- Provide cardiorespiratory activities that take balance issues into account. Swimming and stationary cycling are two good choices.
- Emphasize extensor muscles (e.g., erector spinae, middle trapezius and rhomboids, gluteus maximus, gastrocnemius) when strength training; promote postural awareness to combat the tendency to assume a stooped, bent-over posture.
- Simple plyometric or rebounding exercises may be appropriate in order to enhance neuromuscular functioning.
- Flexibility exercises are key as muscles are prone to contracture in PD.
- Provide functional exercises whenever possible.

Summary

In this chapter, physiological changes during pregnancy as well as exercise benefits, concerns, and guidelines for exercise during pregnancy were discussed. Characteristics of aging, exercise benefits, and guidelines for older adult programming were explored. This was followed by a discussion of common arthritic conditions and osteoporosis. Issues pertinent to exercise training of children and youth were covered. Finally, basic programming recommendations for hypertension, stroke, peripheral artery disease, diabetes, COPD, asthma, cancer, HIV/AIDS, multiple sclerosis, and Parkinson's disease were presented.

References

Abbott, R.D., White, L.R., Ross, G.W., Masaki, K.H., Curb, J.D., & Petrovich, H. (2004). Walking and dementia in physically capable elderly men. *Journal of the American Medical Association, 292,* 1447-1453.

Administration on Aging, U.S. Department of Health and Human Services. (2003). A statistical profile of older Americans aged 65+. *Snapshot.* Retrieved on November 16, 2005, from http://www.aoa.dhhs.gov/press/fact/pdf/ss_stat_profile.pdf.

Aerobics and Fitness Association of America. (2004). *Perinatal fitness workshop manual.* Sherman Oaks, CA: AFAA.

American College of Obstetricians and Gynecologists. (1998). *Exercise during pregnancy.* Patient Education Pamphlet. Washington, DC: American College of Obstetricians and Gynecologists.

American College of Obstetricians and Gynecologists. (2002). Exercise during pregnancy and the postpartum period. ACOG Committee Opinion No. 267. *Obstetrics and Gynecology, 99,* 171-173.

American College of Sports Medicine. (2000). Position stand: Exercise and type 2 diabetes. *Medicine & Science in Sports & Exercise, 32,* 1345-1360.

American College of Sports Medicine. (2002). *ACSM's resources for clinical exercise physiology: Musculoskeletal, neuromuscular, neoplastic, immunologic, and hematologic conditions.* Baltimore: Lippincott Williams & Wilkins.

American College of Sports Medicine (2006a). *ACSM's guidelines for exercise testing and prescription* (7th ed.). Baltimore: Lippincott Williams & Wilkins.

American College of Sports Medicine (2006b). *ACSM's resource manual for guidelines for exercise testing and prescription* (5th ed.). Baltimore, MD: Lippincott Williams & Wilkins.

American Heart Association. (2005). *Heart and stroke facts: 2005 statistical supplement.* Dallas, TX: American Heart Association.

Artal Mittelmark, R., Wiswell, R.A., & Drinkwater, B.L. (Eds.). (1991). *Exercise in pregnancy* (2nd ed.). Baltimore: Williams and Wilkins.

Barnes, P.J. (2000). Mechanisms in COPD: Differences from asthma. *Chest, 117*(Suppl.), 10S-4S.

Burks, J.S., & Johnson, K. P. (Eds.). (2000). *Multiple sclerosis: Diagnosis, medical management and rehabilitation.* New York: Demos Publications.

Cavill, N., Biddle, S., & Sallis, J.F. (2001). Health enhancing physical activity for young people. Statement of the United Kingdom Expert Consensus conference. *Pediatric Exercise Science, 13,* 12-25.

Centers for Disease Control and Prevention. (2003a). *National diabetes fact sheet: General information and national estimates on diabetes in the United States, 2002.* Atlanta, GA: U.S. Department of Health and Human Services, Centers for Disease Control and Prevention.

Centers for Disease Control and Prevention. (2003b). *HIV/AIDS; Surveillance report. Cases of HIV infection and AIDS in the United States, 15.* Retrieved October 20, 2005, from http://www.cdc.gov/hiv/stats/2003surveillancereport.pdf.

Clapp, J.F. (1996). Pregnancy outcome: Physical activities inside versus outside the workplace. *Seminars in Perinatology, 20,* 70-76.

Clark, C.J. (2003). Asthma. In J.L. Durstine & G.E. Moore (Eds.), *ACSM's exercise management for persons with chronic diseases and disabilities* (pp. 105-110). Champaign, IL: Human Kinetics Publishers.

Clauw, D.J., & Crofford, L.J. (2003). Chronic widespread pain and fibromyalgia: What we know, and what we need to know. *Best Practice and Research: Clinical Rheumatology, 17,* 685-701.

Corbin, C., Pangrazi, R., & Welk, G. (1994). Toward an understanding of appropriate physical activity levels of youth. *Physical Activity and Fitness Research Digest, 1*(8), 1-8.

Courneya, K.S., Mackey, J.R., & Jones, L.W. (2000). Coping with cancer: Can exercise help? *Physician and Sportsmedicine, 28,* 49-73.

Criqui, M.H. (2001). Peripheral arterial disease (epidemiological aspects). *Vascular Medicine, 6,* 3-7.

Dempsey, J.C., Butler, C.L., & Williams, M.A. (2005). No need for a pregnant pause: Physical activity may reduce the occurrence of gestational diabetes mellitus and preeclampsia. *Exercise and Sport Sciences Reviews, 33*(3), 141-149.

Dumas, G.A., & Reid, J.G. (1997). Laxity of knee cruciate ligaments during pregnancy. *Journal of Orthopeadic Sports Physical Therapy, 26*(1), 2-6.

Fagard, R. (2001). Exercise characteristics and the blood pressure response to dynamic physical training. *Medicine & Science in Sports & Exercise, 33,* S484-S492.

Fiatarone, M.A., O'Neill, E.F., Ryan, N.D., Clements, K.M., Solares, G.R., Nelson, M.E., et al. (1994). Exercise training and nutritional supplementation for physical frailty in very elderly people. *New England Journal of Medicine, 330,* 1769-1775.

Friedenreich, C.M. (2001). Physical activity and cancer prevention: From observational to intervention research. *Cancer Epidemiological Biomarkers Prevention, 10,* 287-301.

Garrison, R.J., Kannel, W.B., Stokes, J., & Castelli, W.P. (1987). Incidence and precursors of hypertension in young adults: The Framingham Offspring Study. *Preventive Medicine, 16,* 235-251.

Koller, W.C., & Hubble, J.P. (1992). Classification of Parkinsonism. In W.C. Koller (Ed.), *Handbook of Parkinson's Disease* (2nd ed.) (pp.59-103). New York: Marcel Dekker.

Kovar, P.A., Allegrante, J.P., MacKenzie, C.R., Peterson, M.G., Gutin, B., & Charlson, M.E. (1992). Supervised fitness walking in patients with osteoarthritis of the knee. A randomized, controlled trial. *Annals of Internal Medicine, 116,* 529-534.

Lawrence, R.C., Helmick, C.G., Arnett, F.C., Deyo, R.A., Felson, D.T., Giannini, E.H., et al. (1998). Estimates of the prevalence of arthritis and selected musculoskeletal disorders in the United States. *Arthritis and Rheumatology, 41,* 778-799.

Liu-Ambrose, T., Khan, K., & McKay, H. (2001). The role of exercise in preventing and treating osteoporosis. *International Sports Medicine Journal, 2*(4), 1-13.

Milunsky, A., Ulcickas, M., Rothman, K., Willet, W., Jick, S.S., & Jick, H. (1992). Maternal heat exposure and neural tube defects. *Journal of the American Medical Association, 268,* 882-885.

Morkved, S., Bo, K., Schei, B. (2003). Pelvic floor muscle training during pregnancy to prevent urinary incontinence: A single-blind, randomized, controlled trial. *Obstetrics and Gynecology, 101*(2): 313-319.

National Association for Sport and Physical Education. (2004). *Physical activity for children: A statement of guidelines* (2nd ed.). Reston, VA: National Association for Sport and Physical Education.

National Center for Chronic Disease Prevention and Health Promotion. (2003). *National diabetes fact sheet.* Atlanta, GA: Centers for Disease Control and Prevention. Retrieved July 6, 2005, from http://www.cdc.gov/diabetes/pubs/pdf/ndfs_2003.pdf.

National Heart, Lung, and Blood Institute. (1999). Asthma statistics: Data fact sheet. Bethesda, MD: U.S. Department of Health and Human Services, National Institutes of Health. Retrieved on November 7, 2005, from http://www.nhlbi.nih.gov/health/prof/lung/asthma/asthstat.pdf.

National High Blood Pressure Education Program. (2003). *The seventh report of the Joint National Committee on prevention, detection, evaluation, and treatment of high blood pressure* (JNC7). 03-5233.

Nixon, S., O'Brien, K., Glazier, R.H., & Tynan, A.M. (2001). Aerobic exercise interventions for adults living with HIV/AIDS. *Cochrane Database Systems Review, 2,* CD001796.

Richards, S.C., & Scott, D.L. (2002). Prescribed exercise in people with fibromyalgia: Parallel group randomized controlled trial. *British Medical Journal, 325,* 185.

Rikli, R.E., & Jones, C.J. (2001). *Senior fitness test manual.* Champaign, IL: Human Kinetics.

Sallis, J.F., & Patrick, K. (1994). Physical activity guidelines for adolescents: Consensus statement. *Pediatric Exercise Science, 6,* 302-314.

Sinaki, M., Wollan, P.C., Scott, R.W., & Gelczer, R.K. (1996). Can strong back extensors prevent vertebral fractures in women with osteoporosis? *Mayo Clinic Proceedings, 71,* 951-956.

Tanner, C.M., & Ben-Schlomo, Y. (1999). Epidemiology of Parkinson's disease. In G.M. Stern (Ed.), *Parkinson's disease: Advances in neurology,* vol. 80 (pp. 153-157). Philadelphia: Lippincott and Williams.

U.S. Department of Health and Human Services. (1996). *Physical activity and health: A report of the Surgeon General.* Atlanta, GA: U.S. Department of Health and Human Services, Centers for Disease Control and Prevention, National Center for Chronic Disease Prevention and Health Promotion.

Wolf, L.A., Brenner, I.K., & Mottola, M.F. (1994). Maternal exercise, fetal well-being and pregnancy outcome. In J.O. Hollowszy (Ed.), *Exercise and sports sciences reviews* (pp. 145-194). Baltimore: Williams & Wilkins.

Wolfe, F., Ross, K., Anderson, J., Russell, I.J., & Hebert, L. (1995). The prevalence and characteristics of fibromyalgia in the general population. *Arthritis and Rheumatology, 38,* 19-28.

Suggested Reading

Aerobics and Fitness Association of America. (2002). *Exercise standards & guidelines reference manual* (4th ed.). Sherman Oaks, CA: Aerobics and Fitness Association of America.

American College of Sports Medicine. (1998). Position stand: Exercise and physical activity for older adults. *Medicine & Science in Sports & Exercise, 30,* 992-1008.

American College of Sports Medicine. (2003). *ACSM's exercise management for persons with chronic diseases and disabilities* (2nd ed.) (J.L. Durstine & G.E. Moore, Eds.). Champaign, IL: Human Kinetics.

American Council on Exercise. (1998). *Exercise for older adults* (R.T. Cotton, Ed.). Champaign, IL: Human Kinetics.

American Council on Exercise. (1999). *ACE's clinical exercise specialist manual.* San Diego, CA: American Council on Exercise.

American Diabetes Association. (2003). Physical activity/exercise and diabetes mellitus: Position statement. *Diabetes Care, 26* (Suppl.), S73-S77.

American Senior Fitness Association. (1995). *Senior fitness instructor, personal trainer, and long-term care training manuals.* New Smyrna Beach, FL: American Senior Fitness Association.

Anthony, L. (2002). *Pre- and post-natal fitness.* San Diego, CA: American Council on Exercise.

Best-Martini, E., & Botenhagen-DiGenova, K.A. (2003). *Exercise for frail elders.* Champaign, IL: Human Kinetics.

Bonnick, S.L. (1997). *The osteoporosis handbook.* Dallas, TX: Taylor Publishing.

Brill, P.A. (2004). *Functional fitness for older adults.* Champaign, IL: Human Kinetics.

Cheung, W.Y., & Richmond, J.B. (Eds.). (1995). *Child health, nutrition, and physical activity.* Champaign, IL: Human Kinetics.

Clapp, J.F. (2002). *Exercising through your pregnancy.* Champaign, IL: Human Kinetics.

Clark, J. (1992). *Full life fitness: A complete exercise program for mature adults.* Champaign, IL: Human Kinetics.

Clark, J. (Ed.). (1996). *Exercise programming for older adults.* Binghamton, NY: Haworth Press, Inc.

Cooper Institute for Aerobics Research. (1999). *FITNESSGRAM.* Champaign, IL: Human Kinetics.

Evans, W., & Rosenberg, I.H. (1991). *Biomarkers: The 10 keys to prolonging vitality.* New York: Simon and Schuster.

Faigenbaum, A.D., & Westcott, W.L. (2001). *Youth fitness.* San Diego, CA: American Council on Exercise.

Goldberg, L., & Elliot, D.L. (1994). *Exercise for prevention and treatment of illness.* Philadelphia: Davis Co.

Gordon, N.F. (1992). *Arthritis: Your complete exercise guide.* Champaign, IL: Human Kinetics.

Gordon, N.F. (1992). *Diabetes: Your complete exercise guide.* Champaign, IL: Human Kinetics.

Gordon, N.F. (1992). *Stroke: Your Complete Exercise Guide.* Champaign, IL: Human Kinetics.

Hinson, C. (1995). *Fitness for children.* Champaign, IL: Human Kinetics.

Katz, J. (1995). *Water fitness during your pregnancy.* Champaign, IL: Human Kinetics.

Khan, K., McKay, H.A., Kannus, P., Bailey, D., Wark, J., & Bennell, K. (2001). *Physical activity and bone health.* Champaign, IL: Human Kinetics.

National Strength and Conditioning Association. (1996). Youth Resistance Training: Position Statement Paper and Literature Review: *Strength and Conditioning, 18* (6), 62–76.

Noble, E. (2003). *Essential exercises for the childbearing year* (4th ed.). Harwich, MA: New Life Images.

President's Council on Physical Fitness and Sports. (1998). *Get fit: A handbook for youth ages 6-17.* Washington, DC: President's Council on Physical Fitness and Sports.

Rikli, R.E., & Jones, C.J. (2001). *Senior fitness test manual.* Champaign, IL: Human Kinetics.

Roberts, S.O. (1996). *Strength and weight training for children.* Reston, VA: National Association for Sport and Physical Education.

Rowland, T. W. (1994). *Exercise and children's health.* Champaign, IL: Human Kinetics.

Ruderman, N.B., & Devlin, J.T. (Eds.) (1995). *The health professional's guide to diabetes and exercise.* Alexandria, VA: American Diabetes Association.

Shephard, R.J. (1990). *Fitness in special populations.* Champaign, IL: Human Kinetics.

Skinner, J.S. (1993). *Exercise testing and exercise prescription for special cases* (2nd ed.). Baltimore: Williams & Wilkins.

Sobel, D., & Klein, A.C. (1993). *Arthritis: What exercises work.* New York: St. Martin's Press.

Spirduso, W. (1995). *Physical dimensions of aging.* Champaign, IL: Human Kinetics.

Tupler, J., & Thompson, A. (1996). *Maternal fitness.* New York: Simon and Schuster.

Van Norman, K.A. (1995). *Exercise programming for older adults.* Champaign, IL: Human Kinetics.

Westcott, W.L., & Baechle, T.R. (1998). *Strength training past 50.* Champaign, IL: Human Kinetics.

YMCA (with Hanlon, T.W.). (1994). *Fit for two: The official YMCA prenatal exercise guide.* Champaign, IL: Human Kinetics.

Resources

- www.acog.org (American College of Obstetricians and Gynecologists)
- www.americanheart.org (American Heart Association)
- www.aoa.gov (Administration on Aging)
- www.arthritis.org (Arthritis Foundation)
- www.diabetes.org (American Diabetes Association)
- www.fitpregnancy.com
- www.lamaze.org
- www.nationalmssociety.org (National Multiple Sclerosis Society)
- www.nof.org (National Osteoporosis Foundation)
- www.parkinson.org (National Parkinson's Disease Foundation)

Nutrition and Weight Management

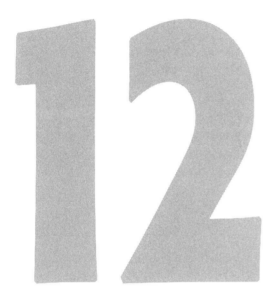

Outline

- Nutrition and Its Impact on Disease
- Nutrient Analysis
- Healthy Eating Guidelines
- Other Dietary Options
- Nutrition Concepts
- Pre- and Post-Exercise Eating
- Label Reading
- Eating Disorders
- Weight Management

Since poor nutrition and obesity are implicated in many chronic diseases, and since clients typically have many nutrition-related questions, personal fitness trainers have a responsibility to provide educational information about the fundamentals of appropriate diets. Clients with special dietary needs and problems, or those who need individualized advice to be provided by a licensed health care provider, nutritionist, or dietitian, must be referred to a registered dietitian or similar professional (trainers must not "prescribe a diet"). Otherwise, information that is educational in nature and in the public domain, such as that from the U.S. Department of Agriculture (USDA) Food Guide Pyramid, can and should be shared with clients. In this chapter, basic nutrition information is reviewed and strategies for weight management are discussed.

Nutrition and Its Impact On Disease

As mentioned in Chapter 1 ("Understanding Wellness"), eating a healthy diet and avoiding obesity are two important strategies in reducing your risk of developing several diseases, including coronary heart disease (CHD), some types of cancer, diabetes, and osteoporosis. Dietary factors that are critical in the management or prevention of these diseases follow.

Coronary Heart Disease

CHD risk factors related to nutrition include dyslipidemia (abnormal cholesterol profile), hypertension, impaired fasting glucose, and obesity. In order to manage these risk factors as effectively as possible from a nutritional standpoint, the following strategies are recommended (Kraus et al., 2000; American Heart Association, 2002).

- Eat a diet that is moderate or low in saturated fat (7–10% of daily calories) and cholesterol.
- Decrease trans fatty acid consumption.
- Increase omega-3 fatty acid consumption (e.g., at least two servings of fatty fish per week).
- Shift fat sources to include more monounsaturated fats (e.g., olive oil).
- Consume plenty of vitamins and antioxidants from food sources.
- Eat an appropriate amount of plant foods (e.g., fruits, vegetables, breads, cereals, nuts, and seeds) that provide fiber, plant sterols, and phytochemicals.
- Consider eating more protein from soy sources.
- For those who consume alcoholic beverages, lower consumption to moderate levels. Red wine, for example, has been shown to have cardiovascular protective effects.
- Limit daily sodium intake to less than 2,400 mg and even less for those with hypertension and congestive heart failure. When appropriate, increase sources of food with calcium, magnesium, and potassium.

Cancer

The most important dietary risk factor for cancer is obesity. Cancers associated with obesity include those of the breast, endometrium, kidney, colon, esophagus, gallbladder, and stomach (Calle, Rodriguez, Walker-Thurmond, & Thun, 2003). (Note that obesity will be discussed later in this chapter.) The American Institute of Cancer Research (1997) and the American Cancer Society (n.d.) basically agree on the following nutritional recommendations.

- Keep BMI between 18.5–25 (Centers for Disease Control and Prevention, n.d.).

- Consume a large variety of minimally processed plant foods, providing 45–60% of total calories. Limit refined sugars to less than 10% of total calories.
- Alcohol consumption is not recommended for the prevention of cancer.
- Limit red meat to less than 3 oz./day.
- Limit total fat intake to 15–30% of calories.
- Keep salt intake less than 6 g/day.
- Make certain that perishable foods are safely stored or refrigerated to minimize fungal contaminants and mycotoxins.
- Be cautious of foods with high levels of food additives, as well as contaminants and other residues, especially in developing countries where there may be insufficient regulation.
- Do not eat charred food or burned meat juices. Only occasionally consume meat or fish that has been grilled over direct flames.

Diabetes

Impaired fasting glucose ≥ 100 mg/dl (5.6 mmol/L) is an indicator of diabetes or prediabetes; additionally, obesity, especially abdominal obesity, may increase insulin resistance and predispose individuals to diabetes (Centers for Disease Control and Prevention Primary Prevention Working Group, 2004). Following are several nutritional recommendations from the American Diabetes Association (2004).

- Carbohydrates may be substituted with monounsaturated fats to reduce post-meal, high blood sugar and high triglycerides. However, care should be taken not to over-consume fats, since this may lead to weight gain.
- Limit saturated fat intake to 7–10% of total daily calories, and keep total fat intake to less than 30%.
- Keep cholesterol intake to less than 200 mg/day, especially if LDL level is > 100 mg/dl.
- High-protein diets are not recommended due to the increased stress on the kidneys (kidney disease is much more prevalent in people with diabetes). The recommended protein intake is 0.8 g/kg of body weight per day for prevention of kidney disease.

Metabolic Syndrome

This disorder, also known as Insulin Resistance Syndrome, is actually a group of disorders of the body's metabolism (including insulin resistance, high fasting blood glucose, abdominal obesity, abnormal cholesterol levels, and hypertension) that increases the chance of developing diabetes, heart disease, and/or stroke. The nutritional recommendations listed above for diabetes and CHD are important in the management of this syndrome. (Metabolic Syndrome is the new name for Syndrome X, which featured a broader category of ailments under its name.)

Osteoporosis

The National Institutes of Health (NIH) Consensus Development Panel on Osteoporosis Prevention, Diagnosis and Therapy (2001) states that risk of osteoporosis can be decreased by a prolonged high-calcium intake. Calcium supplementation studies have shown that additional calcium can cause an increase in bone density by about 2%, but increases above that level are not likely; also, bone density loss occurs when supplementation ends (Shea et al.,

2004). Following are some dietary recommendations with regard to osteo-porosis (Feskanich, Willett, & Colditz, 2003).

- The current Dietary Reference Intake (DRI) for calcium is 1,000 mg/day for adults under age 50, and 1,200 mg/day for adults age 50 and over. Sources include dairy products, kale, and broccoli.
- Vitamin D is important for calcium absorption; make certain to consume 5 μg/day for those under age 50, 10 μg/day for persons between ages 50–70, and 15 μg/day for those over age 70. Dietary sources include fortified milk and cereal products.
- High protein diets may increase calcium excretion through the kidneys; therefore, maintain a moderate protein intake.
- Consume alcohol moderately, if at all.
- Avoid excessive supplemental vitamin A (> 1.5 mg/day) since it has been linked to increased risk of hip fracture.

Nutrient Analysis

Before proceeding, a brief explanation is needed for the acronym DRI, Dietary Reference Intake, which was established for the Federal Government by the Institute of Medicine of the National Academies (2002). The DRI value provides an estimate of appropriate nutrient intakes for generally healthy people. The DRI value can stand alone or include the Recommended Dietary Allowance (RDA). In some cases, DRI may be used instead of RDA because there may not be enough research to establish RDA for that nutrient.

Carbohydrates

Carbohydrates are the body's main source of energy, providing fuel substrates for both anaerobic and aerobic metabolism. Glucose, the end result of carbohydrate digestion, is the sole source of energy for the brain under normal circumstances, and is essential in maintaining the functional integrity of nerve tissue. Carbohydrates are also necessary for the normal metabolism of fat (see Chapter 2, "Exercise Physiology"). A diet that is too low in carbohydrates may cause the body to utilize protein for fuel, seriously compromising protein's ability to build and maintain tissue. Also, a low-carbohydrate diet may cause ketones to form from an incomplete breakdown of fat; a buildup of ketones in the bloodstream can lead to a potentially fatal condition known as **ketosis**. For all these reasons, a proper balance of carbohydrates in the body is essential, and of course, many carbohydrates are loaded with vitamins, minerals, and fiber important for health and wellness.

There are two main types of carbohydrate: **simple carbohydrates** (sugars, including glucose and fructose from fruit and vegetables, lactose from milk, and sucrose from cane or beet sugar) and **complex carbohydrates** (e.g., carrots, broccoli, corn, potatoes, bread, cereal, pasta, rice and beans), which contain glucose, fiber, and many other nutrients. In recent years, low-carbohydrate diets have been widely advocated by best-selling authors. Unfortunately, studies show that in the average American diet, carbohydrates contribute about half of all calories, but most of these calories come from just eight sources (Block, 2004). (Note that the majority of these foods are made up of sugars and/or highly refined grains.)

- Soft drinks, sodas, and fruit-flavored drinks
- Cake, sweet rolls, doughnuts, and pastries
- Pizza

- Potato chips, corn chips, and popcorn
- White rice
- White bread, rolls, buns, English muffins, and bagels
- Beer
- French fries and frozen potatoes

This type of high-carbohydrate diet is obviously not recommended; it is low in vitamins, minerals, and fiber, and may lead to **insulin resistance** in some people (a condition in which the body is less able to use glucose for fuel, leading to eventual high blood sugar levels). Over time, this may lead to diabetes, especially in individuals who are obese and/or have a genetic predisposition. Even if the body doesn't develop insulin resistance, the repeated spiking and falling of insulin and blood sugar levels can set the stage for overeating as the brain sends out hunger signals in response to a sudden drop in blood sugar. A carbohydrate ranking, known as the **Glycemic Index**, has been developed to help define which carbohydrate foods may or may not contribute to the insulin surge and eventual resistance problem (this index will be discussed later in the chapter).

Personal fitness trainers should be aware of healthier sources of carbohydrate. Remember, fruits, vegetables, and whole grains are carbohydrates, and virtually all of the major health organizations recommend a diet high in a wide variety of these healthy and important foods. Some examples of naturally occurring carbohydrates loaded with nutrients include: blueberries, whole wheat bread, whole wheat spaghetti, broccoli, red peppers, spinach, oatmeal, and oranges.

The new USDA Food Guide Pyramid (U.S. Department of Agriculture and Health and Human Services, 2005) adjusts the number of carbohydrate servings needed per day to an individual's age, activity level, and total calories consumed per day. For example, if you consume 2,000 calories per day, then the Pyramid recommendations include six 1-ounce servings of grains (preferably whole), 2 1/2 cups of vegetables, and 2 cups of fruit per day. The USDA Food Guide Pyramid will be covered in more detail later in this chapter.

The National Academy of Sciences Food and Nutrition Board gives a recommended range of 45–65% of carbohydrates per day (Institute of Medicine of the National Academies, 2002), while the American Heart Association (AHA) (1996) recommends five servings of fruits and vegetables and six servings of grains (preferably whole) per day.

For lean and athletic exercisers, a high-carbohydrate diet is often recommended in order to ensure sufficient energy for training and competition. This is especially true for endurance athletes, those who exercise aerobically for more than 90 minutes per day. Some sources recommend up to 8–10 grams per kg of body weight (a substantial amount) for long-duration exercisers (Jacobs & Sherman, 1999). A high-carbohydrate diet is important for anyone who wants to have enough energy to train hard, day after day. Remember that 1 gram of carbohydrate is equal to 4 calories. You will find more about carbo-loading later in this chapter.

Fiber

Fiber is a primarily indigestible type of carbohydrate found in fresh fruits, vegetables, and grains. There are two types of fiber: soluble and insoluble. **Soluble fiber** is found in fruits, vegetables, seeds, brown rice, barley, and oats.

USDA (2005) Dietary Guidelines for Carbohydrates

- Choose a variety of fruits and vegetables each day. In particular, select from all five vegetable subgroups (dark green, orange, legumes, starchy vegetables, and other vegetables) several times a week.

- Consume three or more 1- ounce equivalents of whole grain products per day, with the rest of the recommended grains coming from enriched or whole grain products. In general, at least half the grains should come from whole grains.

It appears to lower blood cholesterol levels and retard the entry of glucose into the bloodstream. **Insoluble fiber** includes cellulose, and is found mainly in whole grains and on the outside of seeds, fruits, and legumes. Insoluble fiber is key in promoting more efficient elimination and may play a role in colon cancer prevention. Whole grains offer more fiber, vitamins, and minerals than their processed counterparts. Whole wheat bread, oatmeal, brown and wild rice, and barley are all examples of whole grains. The daily recommendation for fiber is 20–30 grams per day, or 14 grams per 1,000 calories (American Heart Association, 1996; U.S. Department of Agriculture, 2005a).

Protein

Protein is essential for building and repairing muscles, red blood cells, hair, and other tissues, and is necessary for synthesizing hormones. Next to water, proteins are the most abundant substances in most cells. Protein is digested into 22 amino acids, 13 of which the body manufactures. Since the human body cannot manufacture the other 9 amino acids, they are known as essential. A "complete" protein (such as animal- or fish-based foods) supplies these essential amino acids. An "incomplete" protein lacks one or more of the essential amino acids. These incomplete proteins are generally from plants (e.g., fruits, grains, and vegetables). By combining grains with legumes (e.g., dried beans with corn, tofu with brown rice, or peanut butter with bread), the nine essential amino acids can still be obtained without necessarily eating animal products. (Note that consumption of protein from meat products is much more stressful to the environment than consumption of protein from plant sources. As an example, it takes approximately 20 lb. of feed, most often corn, to make a pound of beef [Brower & Leon, 1999]).

The RDA for protein for adults is 0.8 grams of protein for each kg (2.2 lb.) of body weight; the RDA is set intentionally higher than necessary, in order to provide a wide safety margin for 97.5% of Americans. Further specifications state that an adult male, weighing about 79 kg (174 lb.), needs 63 grams of protein per day, while an adult female, weighing about 63 kg (139 lb.), needs about 50 grams of protein per day. The RDA for protein increases by 30 grams/day during pregnancy and by 20 grams/day during lactation (U.S. Department of Agriculture and Health and Human Services, 2005). Additionally, the AHA recommends consuming at least two servings of fatty fish (such as tuna or salmon) per week (American Heart Association, 1996). Note that there are 4 calories in 1 gram of protein.

To Calculate Protein Needs
1. Calculate your weight in kg: body weight in lb. x .45 = body weight in kg.
2. Multiply weight in kg by 0.8. The result is the grams of protein you should consume per day.
For example: client body weight is 160 lb. 1. 160 lb. x .45 = 72 kg body weight 2. 72 kg x 0.8 = 57.6 grams of protein per day

Government surveys show that Americans typically consume 3–5 times as much protein as they need, and that most of this protein comes from meat sources (American Heart Association, 1996). There are a number of problems associated with excessive meat and protein consumption. Meat is a primary source of saturated fat, which is the major culprit in elevated cholesterol levels, leading to an increased risk of CHD. The more protein you eat, the more calcium is excreted; this can compromise bone health. High-protein diets also stress the kidneys, and may cause diarrhea and worsen dehydration.

The RDA, as described above, is set to provide more than adequate protein for 97.5% of Americans. However, controversy remains regarding whether athletes have higher requirements for protein. Many authorities believe that an athlete's need for protein is greater due to the following reasons.

- A small percent (5–15%) of protein is used for fuel during exercise, with an increased percentage of protein utilized as carbohydrate stores become depleted. Carbohydrate (glycogen) depletion is most likely with prolonged endurance training.
- Microscopic muscle damage is likely during strenuous exercise, and protein is needed for tissue building and repair.
- Prolonged exercise has been shown to result in small amounts of protein being excreted in the urine.
- More protein may be necessary for maintenance of an athlete's greater lean body mass.

Even so, many athletes consume far more protein than necessary in hopes of better performance. Studies of athletes have not found that protein supplements improve strength, power, or endurance. There are no scientific studies showing that > 2.0 grams per kg of protein per day provide any additional advantage (Lemon, 1995). And remember, excess protein in the body is usually turned into fat, not muscle. However, there are some groups for whom protein consumption is a special concern, and these include the following.

- Young athletes who need extra protein for the reasons listed above as well as for age-related growth and maturation
- Athletes who are dieting in order to make a desired weight or body profile
- Vegetarian athletes

The American College of Sports Medicine (ACSM), American Dietetic Association (ADA), and the Dietitians of Canada, in a Joint Position Statement, agree that protein requirements for endurance athletes are 1.2–1.4 grams/kg of body weight per day, whereas requirements for strength-trained athletes may be as high as 1.6–1.7 grams/kg body weight per day. However, these organizations state that "these recommended protein intakes can generally be met through diet alone, without the use of protein or amino acid supplements, if energy intake is adequate to maintain body weight" (American College of Sports Medicine, 2000).

Fat

Fat adds flavor to food and is an important component of a healthy diet. Fat is necessary for producing energy, transporting fat-soluble vitamins, protecting internal organs, providing insulation, maintaining healthy skin and hair, and for supplying the "essential" fat, linoleic acid. However, a high-fat diet has been linked in numerous studies to increased risk of heart disease, cancer, diabetes, and other problems. It is also a major contributor to obesity and all its associated ills. Fat is more than twice as fattening as proteins or carbohydrates, with 9 calories in 1 gram of fat. The 2005 USDA Dietary Guidelines for Americans include the following statements regarding fat.

- Consume less than 10% of calories from saturated fatty acids and less than 300 mg/day of cholesterol, and keep **trans-fatty acid** consumption as low as possible.
- Keep total fat intake between 20–35% of calories, with most fats coming from sources of polyunsaturated and monounsaturated fatty acids, such as fish, nuts, and vegetable oils.
- When selecting and preparing meat, poultry, dry beans, and milk or milk products, make choices that are lean, low-fat, or fat-free.
- Limit intake of fats and oils high in saturated and/or trans-fatty acids, and choose products low in such fats and oils (U.S. Department of Agriculture and Health and Human Services, 2005).

Types of Fat

Triglycerides (fats and oils) are the main type of fat found in the diet and in adipose tissue. Desirable serum levels are under 150 mg/dl (National Cholesterol Education Program Expert Panel, 2001).

Saturated fats come primarily from animal sources and include: butter, whole milk dairy products, and meats. Hamburger is the largest contributor to saturated fat intake in the American diet, with cheese ranking second. Coconut and palm oils are also highly saturated. Vegetable oil margarines become partially saturated when they are hydrogenated, making them solid at room temperature (which is why liquid oils and soft tub margarines are preferable to stick margarines). Healthy adults should follow a diet with less than 10% of daily calories coming from saturated fat sources, while those with high LDL cholesterol levels are urged to cut saturated fats to less than 7% of daily calories.

Unsaturated fats include the following.

- **Monounsaturated fats** have been shown to reduce LDL cholesterol without affecting the beneficial HDL cholesterol, and are therefore the preferred form of fat in the diet. Good sources include olive oil, canola oil, peanut oil, and avocado oil. The 2005 USDA Dietary Guidelines for Americans suggest that a diet may include up to 35% fat if the majority of the fat is monounsaturated(U.S. Department of Agriculture and Health and Human Services, 2005) and if weight loss is not an issue.
- **Polyunsaturated fats** are divided into the omega-6 vegetable oils and the omega-3 fish oils. The vegetable oils include sunflower, corn, soybean, and sesame. Omega-3 fatty acids come primarily from fish, especially mackerel, halibut, salmon, albacore tuna, and whitefish. **Omega-3 fatty acids** have been shown to suppress atherosclerosis by decreasing the stickiness of platelets, and by reducing blood pressure, cholesterol, triglycerides and blood clotting (Harper & Jacobson, 2001). Studies have also shown a strong link between fish consumption and a significant reduction in CHD (Whelton, He, Whelton, & Muntner, 2004).

Trans-fatty acids have received much attention in recent years. They are formed during food processing when manufacturers change the chemical structure of unsaturated fats to make them semi-solid at room temperature. This process is called **hydrogenation** and it increases the stability of the product, which increases shelf life. Unfortunately, trans-fatty acids behave like saturated fats, increasing LDL cholesterol; even worse, they act to decrease the "good" HDL cholesterol level (Whelton, He, Whelton, & Muntner, 2004). The 2005 USDA Dietary Guidelines recommend that trans-fatty acid consumption be ≤ 1% of daily caloric intake (U.S. Department of Agriculture and Health and Human Services, 2005). Major sources of trans-fatty acids are stick margarine, shortening, commercial frying fats, high-fat baked goods, and salty snacks.

All fats and oils have 9 calories per gram of fat and contain about 14 grams of fat, which equals approximately 120 calories per tablespoon. "Healthful oils" have the highest proportions of unsaturated fat to saturated fat. While some athletes may have a fixation on an excessively low-fat diet, the majority of Americans still need to make a concerted effort to avoid fat over-consumption; diets high in fat are typically high in calories. Since the majority of Americans are overweight (65%) and/or obese (31%) (Flegel, Carroll, Ogden, & Johnson, 2002), decreasing fat consumption is an important issue.

To figure the maximum amount of fat your client should be eating, estimate how many calories he or she consumes each day and multiply by 30%. Divide that number by 9 to figure grams of fat per day.

Total Caloric Intake	Maxiumum Total Calories from Fat	Maxiumum Grams of Fat
1,200	360	40
1,500	450	50
1,800	540	60
2,000	600	66
2,500	750	83

Help clients to reduce fat in their diets. Teach them to:
- read labels. Determine both the amount and type of fats in foods. To determine the number of calories that come from fat, multiply the grams of fat in a serving by 9. Divide this number by the total calories in the serving to find the percentage of calories coming from fat.

  For example, a cup of 2% milk has 120 calories and 5 grams of fat. To find the percent fat, multiply 5 grams by 9, which equals 45 calories from fat. Divide 45 by 120 (the total number of calories in 1 cup of 2% milk) and you will find that 2% milk is actually 38% fat! The 2% label refers to the fact that fat accounts for 2% of the weight of the product, not 2% of the calories; this discrepancy in advertising is very misleading to consumers.
- substitute fish or chicken (skinless) for some red meat.
- eat more meatless meals. Use vegetables, grains, and legumes as the main dish.
- select lean meats and eat smaller portions (3–5 oz.) Trim off all visible fat.
- limit intake of saturated fats. If using margarine, choose one that has at least twice as much polyunsaturated fat as saturated and is low in trans-fatty acids.
- broil, bake, or boil foods instead of frying.

- cut back on fat-laden snack foods, e.g., potato chips, cookies, and pastries.
- switch as many fats as possible to the healthier monounsaturated oils such as olive oil and canola oil.

Cholesterol

Cholesterol is actually not a fat at all; it is an "alcohol wax" that at times behaves like a fat. It is a natural compound found in all animal tissues. It is essential for life, so much so that the human body manufactures all it needs without any help from dietary cholesterol. Cholesterol is also important as a structural component of cell membranes and blood lipids, and in the production of hormones and bile (aids in the digestion of fat). Eating cholesterol-rich foods is not the primary cause of high cholesterol; a high-fat diet, especially one high in saturated fats, is the major cause. Nevertheless, the AHA recommends that no more than 300 milligrams of cholesterol be eaten per day (American Heart Association, 2002).

Cholesterol is carried in the bloodstream in the form of lipoproteins, of which there are two main types.

- **High-density lipoproteins** (HDLs), "good" blood cholesterol, help to remove plaque from the arterial walls, returning it to the liver for eventual excretion from the body. Having a high serum HDL level of 60 mg/dl or more provides protection from heart disease. HDL cholesterol can be increased by exercising (cardiorespiratory exercise has the most beneficial effect), and by losing weight if overweight. Reducing total fat intake to less than 30% of daily calories, decreasing saturated fats, and stopping smoking are other key strategies.
- **Low-density lipoproteins** (LDLs), "bad" blood cholesterol, on the other hand, deliver plaque to the arterial walls, causing plaque build-up and increasing atherosclerosis and risk of heart disease. For optimal health, a blood LDL of < 100 mg/dl is best. To reduce LDLs, decrease all fats to less than 30% of daily calories, decrease high-cholesterol foods, cut back on trans-fatty acids, and substitute monounsaturated fats for saturated fats. Increasing soluble fiber, soy protein, and decreasing excess body weight are also helpful.

For clients with high cholesterol, the primary strategy is to lower LDL levels; the other important areas of focus are to decrease obesity and increase physical activity. If your client has high cholesterol, make certain he or she is working with a physician to manage this risk factor for CHD.

The National Cholesterol Education Program Expert Panel (2001) Cholesterol Guidelines				
(all values in mg/dl)	**Desirable**	**Borderline**	**High Risk**	**Very High Risk**
Total Cholesterol	< 200	200–239	≥ 240	
HDL Cholesterol	> 40			
LDL Cholesterol	< 130	130–159	160–189	≥ 190
Triglycerides	< 150	150–199	200–499	> 500

Vitamins

Vitamins are non-caloric, organic compounds that the human body cannot produce on its own. It is essential for optimal health that these substances be ingested in adequate quantities to support proper body function, growth, and repair. These nutrients fall into one of two groups: fat soluble and water soluble. The fat-soluble vitamins (A, D, E, and K) can be stored in the liver. The kidneys excrete excess water soluable vitamins, although toxicity has been reported with mega doses of vitamin C and vitamin B_6. Vitamins and minerals have no caloric value and cannot provide energy.

Minerals

Minerals are inorganic compounds that assist processes, such as regulating activity of many enzymes and maintaining acid-base balance, and are structural constituents of body tissues. Minerals are classed as either major (e.g., calcium, phosphorus) or minor (e.g., zinc, copper). For example, iron is part of red blood cells, and calcium is found abundantly in bone and teeth. The following minerals are of especial importance.

- Iron—The current DRI for iron is 8 mg per day for nonvegetarian men, 18 mg per day for menstruating women, and 8 mg per day for women over 50; iron can be found in liver, lean meat, dark green leafy vegetables, enriched whole grain cereals, and acidic foods (e.g., tomato sauce) cooked in iron skillets. Female athletes are at especial risk for iron-deficiency anemia due to iron lost during menstruation. Too much iron on the other hand can be harmful. It is a double-edged sword at times and can be harmful in people with iron overload conditions such as hemochromatosis. It is estimated that 1 in 300 Americans have undiagnosed hemochromatosis (Felitti, 1999).
- Calcium—The current DRI for calcium is 1,000 mg/day for adults under 50, and 1,200 mg/day for adults 50 and over. Sources include dairy products, kale, and broccoli.
- Potassium—Based on recent research, a new DRI for potassium of 4.7 grams (4,700 mg) per day has been established. This mineral has recently been shown to play a critical role in blood pressure regulation (Whelton et al., 1997). Potassium can be found in low-fat milk, yogurt, potatoes, and bananas. In people with renal insufficiency (kidney failure), potassium intake should be limited as it can build up to harmful levels.

Water

Water is the largest single component of the body. Muscle holds the highest concentration of water in the body while fat tissue holds some of the lowest amounts. Water has a variety of functions that are essential to life.

- Fluid in blood transports glucose to working muscles and carries away metabolic by-products.
- Fluid in urine eliminates metabolic waste products.
- Fluid in sweat dissipates heat through the skin.

Adequate hydration is important for everyone, but it is especially critical for regular exercisers to replace body fluids as dehydration is more likely during and after prolonged exercise and can have serious consequences. At the least, dehydration may cause decreased performance, headaches, and constant fatigue. More serious consequences can include muscle cramping, syncope (fainting), heat exhaustion, and heat stroke.

Although hyponatremia (a serious condition of over-hydration that can disrupt the body's sodium levels) is a potential concern for competitive endurance athletes, the ACSM states that dehydration is a far more common problem for most athletes and the general public, especially those unaccustomed to strenuous activity in hot environments.

Recommendations from *The ACSM's Position Stand on Exercise and Fluid Replacement* (1996) include the following.

- Drink approximately 500 ml (~17 oz.) of fluid about 2 hours before exercise to promote adequate hydration and allow time for excretion of excess ingested water.
- During exercise, start drinking early and at regular intervals in an attempt to consume fluids at rate to equal water lost through sweating.
- Fluids should be between 59–72° F and flavored to enhance palatability and promote fluid replacement.
- Sports drinks with proper amounts of carbohydrates and electrolytes are recommended for events longer than 1 hour (American College of Sports Medicine, 1996).

Additionally, check the color and quantity of your urine (it should be clear and copious). Weigh yourself before and after exercise. For every pound of weight lost, drink 2 cups of fluid. AFAA recommends drinking 1–2 cups of water 5–15 minutes before your workout, and a minimum of 3 ounces every 20 minutes of exercise. During hot and humid conditions and during prolonged and/or intense exercise, even more water is required—drink up to 8–10 ounces every 20 minutes. After exercise, continue to drink when thirsty, plus more. For exercise bouts lasting longer than 90 minutes, diluted juice and/or a sports drink will add beneficial electrolytes and help maintain blood sugar balance. After prolonged exercise, juice is preferable because of its higher levels of carbohydrates and electrolytes.

Alcohol

While the negative effects of excessive alcohol drinking are well known, the AHA suggests that moderate alcohol consumption (one drink per day for women and two drinks per day for men) may help reduce the risk of CHD (Kraus et al., 2000). This includes red wine (the phenolic compounds are thought to be especially beneficial), as well as other wines, beer, and spirits. However, alcohol may be problematic or even dangerous for those on certain medications, or for people with diabetes, hypertension, cancer risk, liver disease, and a family history of alcoholism. Recommendations state that those who do not currently consume alcohol should not be encouraged to begin. Note that 1 gram of alcohol equals 7 calories.

Antioxidants and Phytochemicals

The evidence is not yet clear on whether high dosages of **antioxidant vitamins** (C, E, and beta-carotene) significantly reduce the risk of heart disease, cataracts, and various cancers. Early reports (Reynolds, 1994) were encouraging, but recent studies have failed to find convincing results (Heart Protection Study Collaborative Group, 2002). Antioxidants are so-called because they appear to neutralize a class of atomic particles known as "free radicals" (unstable oxygen molecules created during normal cellular metabolism that can cause structural damage to the cells themselves). Most people can absorb enough vitamin C and beta-carotene from food if they eat plenty of citrus fruits and orange, red, yellow, and dark green fruits and vegetables. Those with low fat intakes (below 25%) may have trouble consuming enough vitamin E. It is recommended that vitamins and minerals come from food sources whenever possible. Remember that the fat-soluble vitamins A, D, E, and K are toxic when taken in high doses. Watch for the results of additional research in this area.

Phytochemicals, or phytonutrients, are neither vitamins nor minerals; they are substances that plants manufacture to protect themselves from viruses, bacteria, fungi, insects, drought, and the harmful effects of the sun. Research continues to try to identify beneficial effects of phytochemicals on human health; they may help prevent some cancers, heart disease, high blood pressure, cataracts, osteoporosis, and other conditions. Most fruits and vegetables contain phytochemicals; rich sources include leafy green vegetables, broccoli, strawberries, carrots, papayas, tomatoes, onions, whole grains, and tea.

Healthy Eating Guidelines

According to the Third National Health and Nutrition Examination Survey (McDowell et al., 1994), the average diet for adults in the United States consists of 49% carbohydrates, 15–16% protein, 34% fat, and 2–3% alcohol. In 2004, a study found that one third of the American diet comes from junk food and soft drinks (Block, 2004). Analysis revealed that two food groups, sweets/desserts and soft drinks/alcoholic beverages, comprised almost 25% of all calories consumed by Americans. Salty snacks and fruit-flavored drinks made up another 5%, bringing the total energy consumed by these nutrient-poor foods to at least 30% of total daily intake.

In an effort to promote increased health and wellness and reduce the high incidence of obesity, major organizations have developed healthy dietary guidelines. Personal fitness trainers should help promote healthy eating and need to be aware of the most recent government-issued guidelines for proper nutrition: the 2005 Food Guide Pyramid, called MyPyramid, (U.S. Department of Agriculture, 2005c) and the USDA Dietary Guidelines for Americans (U.S. Department of Agriculture and Health and Human Services, 2005). MyPyramid, shown below, is designed to be personalized for each individual; an interactive Web site (www.mypyramid.gov) is available with a number of helpful guides for consumers, including the following.

- An individualized eating plan based on a client's age, gender, and activity level
- Detailed explanations of the key food topic areas: grains, vegetables, fruits, milk, meat and beans, oils, and discretionary calories
- Personalized physical activity recommendations
- Sample menus and recipes for an entire week for a 2,000 calorie diet
- Tips for eating out
- Tips for health care professionals, including a PowerPoint presentation

Sample Menu for a 2,000 Calorie Day	
Breakfast	French toast *2 slices whole wheat French toast* *2 tsp. soft margarine* *2 tbsp. maple syrup*
	1/2 medium grapefruit
	1 cup fat-free milk
Lunch	Vegetarian chili on baked potato *1 cup kidney beans* *1/2 cup tomato sauce w/tomato tidbits* *3 tbsp. chopped onions* *1 oz. low-fat cheddar cheese* *1 tsp. vegetable oil* *1 medium baked potato*
	1/2 cup cantaloupe
	3/4 cup lemonade
Dinner	Hawaiian pizza *2 slices cheese pizza* *1 oz. Canadian bacon* *1/4 cup pineapple* *2 tbsp. mushrooms* *2 tbsp. chopped onions*
	Green salad *1 cup leafy greens* *3 tsp. sunflower oil and vinegar dressing*
	1 cup fat-free milk
Snacks	5 whole wheat crackers
	1/8 cup hummus
	1/2 cup fruit cocktail (in water or juice)

(U.S. Department of Agriculture, 2005b)

- Related links, including those for label reading and disease prevention
- MyPyramid Web site tracker—an interactive assessment tool that provides a step-by-step method for tracking personal progress in healthy eating and increased physical activity

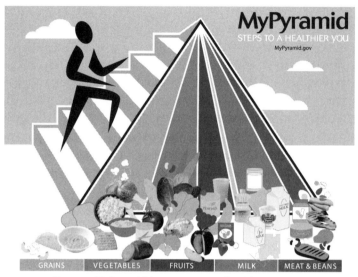

Fig. 12-1. MyPyramid (2005 USDA Food Guide Pyramid)

MyPyramid represents a major step forward in helping Americans adopt healthier physical activity and eating patterns. Unfortunately, it is not without controversy. Some of the weaknesses identified include the following.

- The implication that it is okay to acquire half your grains from refined starches
- The implication that red meat, poultry, fish, and beans are equivalent nutrient sources (e.g., that bologna is as good for you as beans)
- The controversy over the number of dairy servings per day (three)
- The choice of ounces, cups, and teaspoons as portion equivalents
- The visual illustration of the pyramid contains no text and may be confusing for those without computer access
- The inability of people without computer access to benefit from the personalized plans and information

Even so, the MyPyramid Web site (www.mypyramid.gov) contains a tremendous amount of advice that is important for consumers, and by all accounts, is a major improvement over the 1992 USDA Food Guide Pyramid. Key food messages from the MyPyramid Web site (U.S. Department of Agriculture, 2005c) include the following.

- Focus on fruits.
- Vary your vegetables.
- Eat calcium-rich foods.
- Make half your grains whole grains.
- Go lean with protein.
- Know the limits on fat, salt, and sugars.
- Find your balance between food and physical activity.

Below are the recommended daily intakes for a range of calorie levels according to the MyPyramid Web site (U.S. Department of Agriculture, 2005c).

Recommended Daily Intakes								
Calorie level	1,600	1,800	2,000	2,200	2,400	2,600	2,800	3,000
Grains	5 oz.	6 oz.	6 oz.	7 oz.	8 oz.	9 oz.	10 oz.	10 oz.
Vegetables	2 c.	2 1/2 c.	2 1/2 c.	3 c.	3 c.	3 1/2 c.	3 1/2 c.	4 c.
Fruits	1 1/2 c.	1 1/2 c.	2 c.	2 c.	2 c.	2 c.	2 1/2 c.	2 1/2 c.
Milk	3 c.	3 c.	3 c.	3 c.	3 c.	3 c.	3 c.	3 c.
Meat & Beans	5 oz.	5 oz.	5 1/2 oz	6 oz.	6 1/2 oz.	6 1/2 oz.	7 oz.	7 oz.
Oils	5 tsp.	5 tsp.	6 tsp.	6 tsp.	7 tsp.	8 tsp.	8 tsp.	10 tsp.
Discretionary Calories	132	195	267	290	362	410	426	512

These suggested food amounts are calculated to meet USDA recommended nutrient intakes. The contributions from each group are based on the "nutrient-dense" form of the food, without added fats or sugars (e.g., lean meats, fat-free dairy products, grains with no added sugars). DISCRETIONARY CALORIES are those remaining in the calorie total after all the food group portions and nutrients are consumed.

The 2005 USDA Dietary Guidelines were released along with MyPyramid; below are the key recommendations (U.S. Department of Health and Human Services and U.S. Department of Agriculture, 2005).

Dietary Guidelines for Americans 2005 Key Recommendations	
ADEQUATE NUTRIENTS WITHIN CALORIE NEEDS	• Consume a variety of nutrient-dense foods and beverages within and among the basic food groups while choosing foods that limit the intake of saturated and trans fats, cholesterol, added sugars, salt, and alcohol. • Meet recommended intakes within energy needs by adopting a balanced eating pattern, such as the USDA Food Guide or the Dietary Approaches to Stop Hypertension (DASH) Eating Plan.
WEIGHT MANAGEMENT	• To maintain body weight in a healthy range, balance calories from foods and beverages with calories expended. • To prevent gradual weight gain over time, make small decreases in food and beverage calories and increase physical activity.
PHYSICAL ACTIVITY	• Engage in regular physical activity and reduce sedentary activities to promote health, psychological well-being, and a healthy body weight. – To reduce the risk of chronic disease in adulthood: Engage in at least 30 minutes of moderate-intensity physical activity, above usual activity, at work or home on most days of the week. – For most people, greater health benefits can be obtained by engaging in physical activity of more vigorous intensity or longer duration. – To help manage body weight and prevent gradual, unhealthy body weight gain in adulthood: Engage in approximately 60 minutes of moderate- to vigorous-intensity activity on most days of the week while not exceeding caloric intake requirements. – To sustain weight loss in adulthood: Participate in at least 60–90 minutes of daily moderate-intensity physical activity while not exceeding caloric intake requirements. Some people may need to consult with a health care provider before participating in this level of activity. • Achieve physical fitness by including cardiovascular conditioning, stretching exercises for flexibility, and resistance exercises or calisthenics for muscle strength and endurance.
FOOD GROUPS TO ENCOURAGE	• Consume a sufficient amount of fruits and vegetables while staying within energy needs. Two cups of fruit and 2 1/2 cups of vegetables per day are recommended for a reference 2,000-calorie intake, with higher or lower amounts depending on the calorie level. • Choose a variety of fruits and vegetables each day. In particular, select from all five vegetable subgroups (dark green, orange, legumes, starchy vegetables, and other vegetables) several times a week. • Consume 3 or more ounce-equivalents of whole-grain products per day, with the rest of the recommended grains coming from enriched or whole-grain products. In general, at least half the grains should come from whole grains. • Consume 3 cups per day of fat-free or low-fat milk or equivalent milk products. *cont.*

cont.	Dietary Guidelines for Americans 2005 Key Recommendations
FATS	• Consume less than 10% of calories from saturated fatty acids and less than 300 mg/day of cholesterol, and keep trans fatty acid consumption as low as possible. • Keep total fat intake between 20–35% of calories, with most fats coming from sources of polyunsaturated and monounsaturated fatty acids, such as fish, nuts, and vegetable oils. • When selecting and preparing meat, poultry, dry beans, and milk or milk products, make choices that are lean, low-fat, or fat-free. • Limit intake of fats and oils high in saturated and/or trans-fatty acids, and choose products low in such fats and oils.
CARBOHYDRATES	• Choose fiber-rich fruits, vegetables, and whole grains often. • Choose and prepare foods and beverages with little added sugars or caloric sweeteners, such as amounts suggested by the USDA Food Guide and the DASH Eating Plan. • Reduce the incidence of dental caries by practicing good oral hygiene and consuming sugar- and starch-containing foods and beverages less frequently.
SODIUM AND POTASSIUM	• Consume less than 2,300 mg of sodium (approximately 1 teaspoon of salt) per day. • Choose and prepare foods with little salt. At the same time, consume potassium-rich foods, such as fruits and vegetables.
ALCOHOLIC BEVERAGES	• Those who choose to drink alcoholic beverages should do so sensibly and in moderation—defined as the consumption of up to one drink per day for women and up to two drinks per day for men. • Alcoholic beverages should not be consumed by some individuals, including those who cannot restrict their alcohol intake, women of childbearing age who may become pregnant, pregnant and lactating women, children and adolescents, individuals taking medications that can interact with alcohol, and those with specific medical conditions. • Alcoholic beverages should be avoided by individuals engaging in activities that require attention, skill, or coordination, such as driving or operating machinery.

FOOD SAFETY	• To avoid microbial food-borne illness:
	  – clean hands, food contact surfaces, and fruits and vegetables. Meat and poultry should not be washed or rinsed.
	  – separate raw, cooked, and ready-to-eat foods while shopping, preparing, or storing foods.
	  – cook foods to a safe temperature to kill microorganisms.
	  – chill (refrigerate) perishable food promptly and defrost foods properly.
	  – avoid raw (unpasteurized) milk or any products made from unpasteurized milk, raw or partially cooked eggs, foods containing raw eggs, raw or undercooked meat and poultry, unpasteurized juices, and raw sprouts

NOTE: The Dietary Guidelines for Americans 2005 contains additional recommendations for specific populations. The full document is available at www.healthierus.gov/dietaryguidelines.

Other Dietary Options

Other food guide pyramids have been proposed, presumably with less "political" influence. These include The New Healthy Eating Pyramid proposed by Dr. Walter Willett (2005) and the Harvard School of Public Health, and several pyramids suggested by Oldways Preservation & Exchange Trust (see Figures 12-2 and 12-3).

The New Healthy Eating Pyramid (Willett, 2005) emphasizes daily exercise and weight control, whole grains, healthy oils, vegetables, fruits, nuts, and legumes. The top of the pyramid identifies red meat, butter, white rice, white bread, white pasta, potatoes, soda, and sweets for sparse consumption only.

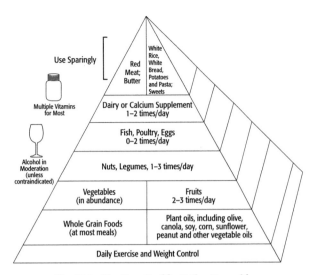

Fig. 12-2. The New Healthy Eating Pyramid
(Reprinted with the permission of Simon and Schuster Adult Publishing Group from *Eat, Drink and Be Healthy: The Harvard Medical School Guide to Healthy Eating* by Walter C. Willett, M.D. © 2001 by President and Fellows of Harvard College)

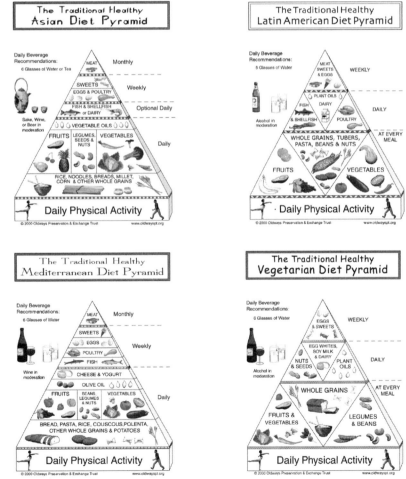

Fig. 12-3. Ethnic Pyramids

(Reprinted with permission. © 2000 Oldways Preservation & Exchange Trust, www.oldwayspt.org)

Nutrition Concepts

Nutrient Density

Nutrient density is the concept of eating foods that are very nutritious relative to the number of calories. Specifically, a high nutrient-dense food provides at least 5% of the RDA of one or more nutrients at a modest caloric cost (e.g., broccoli). At the other end of the spectrum, a food low in nutrient density provides a small amount of nutrition relative to the calories (e.g., potato chips). Usually, foods high in fat, sugar, refined carbohydrates, or alcohol are low in nutrient density. During certain phases of life and for some populations, eating nutrient-dense foods is especially important. Seniors, children, and people on weight-reduction-type diets, as well as pregnant or breast-feeding women, can't afford to waste many of their calories on low nutrient-dense (junk) foods. Examples of high nutrient-dense foods include: spinach, greens, bell peppers, cantaloupe, papaya, brown rice, wheat bran, whole wheat bread, nonfat plain yogurt, skim milk, water-packed tuna, and black beans.

Supplementation

More than half of American adults take dietary supplements (the incidence is even higher among the athletic population), making the supplement industry a $19 billion-per-year business (American Dietetic Association, 2005). Many believe dietary supplements (pills, powders, drinks, bars) provide nutritional "insurance"—that even if breakfast is skipped and a fast food lunch is eaten, supplements constitute a nutritional shortcut. Vitamins and minerals, however, work with other nutrients in food, and relying on supplements cannot compensate for a poor diet. No supplement will replace what a healthy diet can do for your body. Authorities are divided on whether most people really need a multi-vitamin supplement. However, the following people may need supplements and should seek the advice of a registered dietitian: pregnant women, seniors, those who take aspirin frequently, heavy drinkers, smokers, the chronically ill, vegetarians, those with food allergies, those on restricted calorie diets, and those who are unable or unwilling to consume a healthful diet. If clients are taking supplements because they question the adequacy of their diet, they should have a nutrition check-up with a registered dietitian who can teach them to obtain the nutrients they need from the foods they eat (see www.eatright.org to find a local registered dietitian.)

Megadosing (any dose greater than 10 times the RDA) is not only wasteful, but potentially dangerous. Note that the Food and Drug Administration (FDA) warns against the use of botanical supplements with the following ingredients because they may have serious, possibly even fatal, side effects: aristolochic acid (found in some Chinese herbals), chaparral, comfrey, ephedrine, ma huang, lobelia, germander, willow bark, wormwood, and yohimbe. For further information on nutritional supplementation, see Appendix D, "AFAA's Nutritional Supplement Policy."

Many people assume that vitamin and mineral products and other ergogenic aids (substances used to enhance performance) will affect their bodies as advertised. In fact, many distributors of supplements often promote their products with pseudoscience, utilizing questionable marketing techniques such as:

- relying on invalid or inappropriate research and taking advantage of consumers' ignorance about research methodology and applications.

- claiming that research is underway (in other words, there's no data to support the product).
- suggesting that there is a need for a particular product when in fact there is no need.
- claiming endorsement by professional organizations or groups without their full or informed consent.
- relying on testimonials instead of peer-reviewed, controlled studies.
- using a patent number as if it were a government endorsement (which it is not).
- misleading consumers by making advertisements appear to be news stories.
- promoting the myth that if a little is good, more is even better.

When evaluating claims, be sure they have been substantiated in a reputable, peer-reviewed scientific journal. Determine if the claim has been studied by other credible researchers and whether or not the same results were achieved. Look for research studies carried out by scientists using objective methods, without financial connections to the end result. (Who paid for the study?) If it was a long-term study, a control group should have been utilized. Finally, if the claim sounds too good to be true, it probably is!

The Glycemic Index and Glycemic Load

The **Glycemic Index** (GI) was developed by David Jenkins, MD, PhD, DSc to help assign values to carbohydrates based on their ability to release glucose into the bloodstream (Jenkins et al., 2002). This concept moves beyond the traditional simple-versus-complex definition of carbohydrates and instead evaluates them according to how much or little they elevate blood sugar in the body. The GI is a ranking that measures how much a given carbohydrate (50 grams worth) elevates blood sugar above normal. Several factors are involved in assigning GI values to carbohydrates, including: the food's rate of digestion, fiber content, type of fiber, cooking, ripeness, and presence of protein or fat, etc. (Ludwig, 2002). A related concept, developed by the Harvard School of Public Health, is the **Glycemic Load** (GL), which is calculated by multiplying the grams of carbohydrate by the GI. This is important, because both the amount of carbohydrate and its GI create the blood glucose and insulin level response in the body. See below for selected food values.

Glycemic Index and Glycemic Load Values for Commonly Eaten Foods				
The GI and GL offer information about how a food affects blood sugar and insulin. The lower the GI or GL, the less the food affects blood sugar and insulin levels. A GI below 55 and a GL below 10 are considered low.				
Foods	**Serving Size**	**Glycemic Index (%)**	**Grams of Carbs**	**Glycemic Load**
Pancakes	2–6"	67	58	39
Cornflakes	1 cup	81	26	21
Cranberry juice	1 cup	68	35	24
White rice	5 oz.	64	36	23
Jelly beans	1 oz.	78	28	22
Snickers bar	2 oz. bar	68	34	23
Spaghetti	1 cup	42	47	20
Oatmeal	1 cup	58	22	13
Banana	1 medium	51	25	13
Orange juice	1 cup	52	23	12
White bread	1 slice	70	14	10
Apple	1 medium	38	15	6
Skim milk	1 cup	32	13	4
Carrots	1/2 cup	47	6	3

(Adapted with permission by *The American Journal of Clinical Nutrition.* © Am J Clin Nutr. American Society for Nutrition.)

The most important benefits of managing GI and GL have to do with the reduction in blood sugar swings as well as insulin surges and declines. This may help prevent heart disease, diabetes, and obesity.

Pre- and Post-Exercise Eating

Eating appropriately prior to exercise helps boost carbohydrate energy and minimizes an insulin surge. (High insulin levels in the blood can contribute to low blood sugar and potential hypoglycemia when combined with exercise.) Foods low on the GI, such as lentils, apples, oranges, and raw carrots make good pre-exercise meals or snacks because they provide a prolonged, sustained entry of glucose into the bloodstream.

Conversely, foods high on the GI scale are released more quickly into the blood and are better for recovery and refueling after exercise.

It is recommended that you eat at least 50 grams (200 calories) of a high- or moderate-glycemic carbohydrate as soon after exercise as possible (Coyle & Coyle, 1993). Two hours later, eat another 50 grams or so of a high-glycemic carbohydrate. Bagels, pasta, raisins, and baked potatoes are good recovery foods (be sure to limit or omit fats such as butter or cream cheese on these carbohydrates as fat slows down the release of sugar into the bloodstream). These suggestions are particularly important for endurance athletes and those exercising twice a day. In addition, foods high in electrolytes (minerals such as potassium, calcium, and sodium) are important for recovery after prolonged exercise (2 or more hours). Good choices include potatoes, low-fat yogurt, bananas, and orange juice.

Carbohydrate loading is a pre-event practice used by endurance athletes to maximally load their muscles with stored glycogen. When preparing for marathons or other events lasting more than 90 minutes, it is recommended that atheltes: (1) cut back on exercise and rest their muscles prior to competition, and (2) continue to eat a high-carbohydrate diet (60–70%) for three days prior to the event in order to "super-saturate" the muscles with glycogen (Clark, 2003). Eating a diet high in carbohydrates can help prevent the problems known as "hitting the wall" or "bonking." Hitting the wall refers to having an inadequate supply of glycogen (carbohydrate) for muscular work, resulting in excessive fatigue and a desire to quit. Bonking is used to describe an inadequate supply of glucose to the brain, leading to light-headedness, lack of coordination, and weakness. Both phenomena can happen to endurance athletes during prolonged training or competition.

Label Reading

Food labels are mandated by the FDA for processed foods, while single-ingredient foods, such as fresh fruits, vegetables, meat, poultry, fish, and unprocessed grains are not required to have labels. Food labels must contain the following information under "Nutrition Facts":

total calories	calories from fat	total fat	saturated fat
cholesterol	dietary fiber	sodium	total carbohydrates
sugars	protein	vitamin A	vitamin C
calcium	iron		

Note that there are two parts to the Nutrition Facts label: (1) information that is specific to the item (serving size, calories, etc.), and (2) general information in the footnote on the bottom.

When reading labels, consider the following.

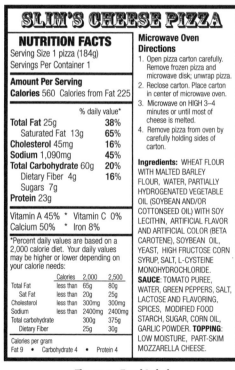

Fig. 12-4. Food Label

1. Look carefully at the serving size. If your normal serving size is more or less than the serving that is listed, you'll need to adjust when considering the amount of calories and nutrients in the product. Note that the serving size is often much smaller than what the average American actually eats.

2. To find out if a food is low fat, look at the number and percent of calories coming from fat. To figure the percent of calories coming from fat, divide the total calories per serving into the number of calories from fat. For example, to find the percent fat in a small, one-person-sized cheese pizza that contains a total of 560 calories with 230 calories from fat, divide 230 calories by 560 calories. You'll find that 41% of the calories are fat calories, hardly a low-fat choice! (Low fat is defined as less than 3 grams of fat per serving. In this example, there are more than 25 grams of fat.)

3. Look at the types of fat used in the product. Does it contain saturated fat and/or trans fats?

4. If the product contains grains, look for the word "whole", as in whole wheat flour, on the ingredient list. Oats, corn, and rye are healthy grains as well.

5. Look for foods high in fiber. Whole grains contain large amounts of fiber.

6. Minimize foods that are high in sugar; sugar is full of empty calories and lowers the nutrient density of any food.

7. The percentage (%) daily value can be confusing for some clients. It measures the amount of the particular nutrient in the food (e.g., fat) against the amount of that nutrient an average person is supposed to

have in one day. So, if you consume a 2,000-calorie-per-day diet, 30% fat is 600 calories from fat or about 65–66 grams of fat (see bottom of label in Figure 12-4). A serving of six cookies nets 4 grams of fat, which is 6% of the 66 total grams of fat you are allowed per day.

8. On the bottom of each label (the footnote) is a little nutrition lesson. Teach your clients what these numbers mean. For people consuming 2,000 or 2,500 calories per day, total fat, saturated fat, cholesterol, sodium, total carbohydrate, and dietary fiber recommendations are right there. In addition, calorie values per gram of fat, carbohydrates, and protein are on the labels for easy reference.

Eating Disorders

How do you know when food obsessions cross over into eating disorders? The American Psychiatric Association (APA) (1994) lists anorexia nervosa, bulimia nervosa, and binge-eating disorder as eating disorders. According to the *Diagnostic and Statistical Manual of Mental Disorders* (American Psychiatric Association, 1994), criteria for **anorexia nervosa** include the following.

- Intense fear of becoming obese, which does not diminish as weight loss progresses
- Disturbance of body image, e.g., claiming to "feel fat" even when emaciated
- Weight loss of at least 15% of original body weight
- Refusal to maintain body weight over a minimal normal weight for age and height
- No known physical illness that would account for the weight loss

Other symptoms of anorexia include: hyperactivity, compulsive exercising, loss of hair, amenorrhea (loss of menstrual periods), growth of fine body hair, extreme sensitivity to cold temperatures, feeling of being nervous at mealtime, denial, wearing clothing several sizes too large (due to the anorexic's perception that he or she is too large to fit into smaller sizes). Resulting health problems can include osteoporosis, muscle atrophy, electrolyte imbalances, cardiac arrhythmias, and occasionally even death.

Criteria for **bulimia nervosa** include the following.

- Recurrent episodes of binge eating
- Consumption of high-calorie, easily ingested food during a binge
- Inconspicuous eating during a binge
- Binge eating episodes terminating with abdominal pain, sleep, or self-induced vomiting
- Repeated attempts to lose weight with severely restrictive diets, self-induced vomiting, or use of diuretics
- Weight fluctuations of greater than 10 pounds due to alternating binges and fasts
- Depressed mood and self-deprecating thoughts following eating binges (American Psychiatric Association, 1994)

Other symptoms of bulimia include: frequent vomiting, damage to throat, bursting blood vessels in eyes, loss of tooth enamel, secretive behavior, excessive concern with physical appearance, and difficulty swallowing and retaining food. Note that a person with bulimia often appears to be of normal weight. Resulting health problems may include gastrointestinal difficulties, electrolyte imbalances, esophageal ruptures, pancreatitis, and tooth enamel erosion.

Binge-eating disorder is characterized by the following.

- Recurrent binge-eating episodes on at least 2 days per week over 6 months
- No purging-type behaviors are used to prevent weight gain
- Rapid eating
- Eating when not hungry
- Eating alone
- Feelings of guilt or disgust

This type of disordered eating results in rapid weight gain and loss of self-esteem, not to mention increased health risk due to obesity.

Research shows that these disorders are on the rise, especially among young, college-age women athletes. Over 2 million female Americans have a clinically relevant eating disorder (Mussell, Binford, & Fulkerson, 2000). Eating disorders and amenorrhea (cessation of the menstrual cycle) are part of the **female athlete triad**, along with osteoporosis. These three related problems can have serious, long-term repercussions for women. According to the ACSM, women with one component of the female athlete triad should be screened for the other components.

Internal and external pressures placed on girls and women to achieve or maintain an unrealistic body weight (in this case, an extremely low body weight) underlie the development of these disorders (American College of Sports Medicine, 1997). Fitness professionals should emphasize health and total well-being, not weight.

Helping clients who have eating disorders engage in fitness and exercise activities may be difficult. According to the ADA, nutrition education and intervention should be integrated into a team approach for individuals with anorexia, bulimia, and binge-eating (or compulsive overeating) disorder. If you suspect that a client has a disorder, be supportive and nonjudgmental. Try to build a bond of trust, which may help the person to be more receptive to your suggestions for help. Have available a referral to a health professional qualified to deal with eating disorders.

Help prevent eating disorders by giving your clients healthful messages. These can include the following.

- Avoid speaking disparagingly about your own body or anyone else's.
- Discourage thinking that equates thinness with happiness.
- Avoid promoting the idea that the best athlete is the thinnest athlete.
- Recognize that it is possible to be quite fit without being ultra-lean.
- Stay away from focusing on the "perfect" body.
- Emphasize feeling strong, fit, and healthy rather than thin or skinny.

Weight Management

Many personal fitness trainers will find that the primary reason clients come to them is for help with weight loss; clients often want to know what the best diet and exercise plans are to help them control problem areas and lose extra pounds. Now, more than ever, due to the increasing incidence of obesity, trainers need to be thoroughly familiar with the information contained in this chapter; accurate information about sound nutrition, appropriate referrals, and an understanding of obesity are critical.

Obesity Issues

Obesity is defined as a level of excess body fat that increases the risk of disease. More specifically, it is defined as a body mass index (BMI) of > 30 kg/m², or a waist girth > 102 cm for men and > 88 cm for women, or a waist/hip ratio of ≥ 0.95 for men and ≥ 0.86 for women.

According to recent data, approximately 65% of Americans are overweight and 31% are obese (Flegel, Carroll, Ogden, & Johnson, 2002). This represents a dramatic increase, considering that in 1960 obesity levels were at 13.4%. Obesity constitutes a significant health hazard; it is a contributing risk factor for heart disease, and influences the development of hypertension, diabetes, cholesterol abnormalities, and Metabolic Syndrome. It is a risk factor for certain kinds of cancer. It is associated with gall-stones, gout, respiratory insufficiency, sleep apnea, impaired heat tolerance, congestive heart failure, and increased risk from surgery, as well as musculoskeletal problems such as back and knee pain. Obesity also increases the likelihood of menstrual abnormalities, hemorrhoids, hernias, and varicose veins. These risks vary depending on genetic predisposition, other risk factors, degree of obesity, fitness level, and the location of body fat stores. Fat that is carried in the abdomen and upper body areas poses a greater health risk than that stored in the hips and thighs.

Several factors are responsible for obesity, including physical inactivity, poor nutrition, lack of nutrition education, genetics, socioeconomic factors, resting metabolic rate, number of fat cells (adipocytes), psychological factors, and ready availability of poor quality foods. Much research has been devoted to the study of fat cell development, number, and size. The body appears to increase its quantity of adipose tissue in two ways: (1) by increasing the size (hypertrophy) of existing fat cells (filling them with more fat), and (2) by increasing the number of fat cells (hyperplasia). Obese individuals typically have about twice as many fat cells as those who are not obese, with more fat per cell. This may partly account for the difficulty with weight loss and maintenance—when there is an elevated number of fat cells, they seem to resist shrinkage and do not disappear.

Researchers believe that the increase in obesity in the United States is due to an overabundance of food choices, large portion sizes, fast foods, and increasing technological and convenience devices that promote sedentary lifestyles. The 1996 U.S. Surgeon General's Report found that approximately 24% of Americans are completely sedentary, while another 54% spends only sporadic time in physical activity (U.S. Department of Health and Human Services, 1996).

Energy Balance

Energy balance is an important concept in weight management. Take in more calories than you expend and the excess will be stored as adipose tissue. Expend more calories than you consume and there will be a negative energy balance (weight loss). To maintain normal metabolic rate and provide energy for activities of daily living, the ADA recommends no less than 1,200 calories per day for women and no less than 1,400 calories per day for men. The ADA also states that energy intake should not exceed energy expenditure in order to prevent weight gain (American Dietetic Association, 2000). This message is key for clients: at the end of the day, the calories you've eaten need to equal the calories you've burned—if you want to maintain your weight.

Caloric expenditure has the following three components.
1.   Resting metabolic rate
2.   Energy expended with exertion (exercise and activities of daily living)
3.   The thermic effect of food

The **resting metabolic rate** (RMR) accounts for about 60–75% of daily caloric expenditure and is higher in individuals with a high percentage of lean body mass (fat-free mass). Resting (basal) metabolism refers to the amount of calories burned when the body is completely at rest; it is usually measured in laboratories first thing in the morning after the subject lies resting in a dark room for 30 minutes (prior to coffee, food, cigarettes, etc.) Because of the relationship between RMR and lean body mass, it is important to preserve lean body mass when losing weight (this helps maintain the metabolic rate). Several studies show that severely restricting calories lowers the RMR and may be appropriate only for the clinically treated and morbidly obese person (Wadden, Foster, & Letizia, 1994). Other factors affecting the RMR include: gender, age, height, air temperature, and physical activity.

Energy expended with exertion accounts for approximately 20–30% of daily caloric output, and is the easiest component to alter. There are at least three ingredients.
1.   Activities of daily living (e.g., washing, dressing, eating, driving)
2.   Bouts of exercise (may be as low-level as gardening or as intense as a 10-mile run)
3.   Recovery from exercise

The extra calories expended during recovery are often called EPOC (excess post-oxygen consumption). The amount of extra calories burned during EPOC appears to depend on both the duration and the intensity of the exercise bout, and is usually minor when compared to the amount of calories burned during the exercise itself (see Chapter 2, "Exercise Physiology"). Also, heavier people expend more calories with exertion than lighter people.

Many clients have misconceptions about the amount of calories they burn during exercise. They are usually surprised and discouraged to learn that a typical exercise session for the exerciser with average fitness burns only about 300 calories. An advantage to being fit is that the more fit you are, the longer, harder, and more often you can exercise, thus the more calories you'll burn.

Typical Calorie Expenditure Values for 30 Minutes of Exercise		
Activity (30 minutes)	130 lb. Body Weight	180 lb. Body Weight
Walking at 3.5 mph, 4% grade	173 cal.	241 cal.
Running at 6.0 mph, 0% grade	316 cal.	439 cal.
Cycling 10 mph on flat surface	177 cal.	243 cal.
Step aerobics, 6" step (124 bpm)	241 cal.	336 cal.
Swimming, fast crawl	276 cal.	378 cal.
Weight training (depends on length of rest periods between sets)	~150 cal.	~210 cal.

The **thermic effect of food** refers to the increase in RMR after eating and is roughly equivalent to 10% of the meal's total caloric value. For example, if you ate a 500 calorie meal, about 50 calories would be used for digestion and absorption.

Weight Loss Recommendations

The weight loss industry has traditionally focused on dietary changes and caloric restriction. In the past, few commercial diet centers had exercise facilities or offered exercise programming. This has resulted in temporary success for some; pounds were lost, but in most cases they were regained. Studies show that when exercise accompanies dietary changes, not only is lean body mass preserved, but the weight loss is much more likely to be maintained at 6 and 12 months after achieving goal weight than with individuals who dieted but didn't exercise (Skender et al., 1996). The presence of an exercise habit appears to prevent weight gain and predict success in the maintenance of lost weight (Jakicic et al., 2001). A combined program of dietary changes, exercise, and behavior modification is recommended for clients who want to lose weight. Several specific guidelines for counseling clients about weight reduction are listed below.

- Help clients focus on lifelong weight control strategies. Help them to choose diet modifications and exercise routines that they will adhere to over the long run. The exercise recommendation should be more concerned with adherence than with the specifics of frequency, intensity, and duration. With deconditioned and inactive clients it doesn't necessarily matter what exercise they do, as long as they do something. Brainstorm with your client about how to increase his/her physical activity level throughout the day in "non-exercise" endeavors (e.g., using stairs instead of elevators). Remember that high-intensity levels have been correlated with decreased adherence, especially for deconditioned exercisers.

- Teach clients that exercise is essential for lifelong weight control and good health. You rarely lose weight and keep it off without daily exercise. Remind clients of the other benefits of exercise, such as stronger bones, healthier heart, less stress and depression, and higher self-esteem. Have them work towards a balanced exercise program: cardiorespiratory exercise, resistance training, and stretching.

- Help clients to create an energy deficit of 500 calories per day or more. This can be accomplished by eating less (e.g., 250 calories less per day) and exercising more (e.g., 250 calories more burned per day). This can lead to a weight loss of about 1 pound per week. Some overweight individuals may need to gradually increase exercise to 200-300 minutes (3.3 to 5.0 hours) per week (Jakicic et al., 2001).

- Prepare clients for the possibility of a lapse or setback. This is very common when making a major behavior change and should not be interpreted as a failure or as a reason to quit. Teach them to persevere.

- Be careful when establishing an "ideal weight." This elusive number may be counterproductive and discouraging, and many clients may never actually achieve it. Instead, consider developing a "reasonable or healthy weight" based on: the lowest weight the client has been able to maintain in the past (for up to a year), loss and regain history, and/or medical history (at what weight, for instance, did high blood pressure develop). Look at the clients' abilities to control their eating habits, the extent of their social support, and their range of coping skills.

- Set short-term goals. For example, set a goal of a 5-pound weight loss, and when that has been achieved, then set a goal of maintaining the 5-pound weight loss for 1 month. When that has been achieved, then set another 5-pound weight loss goal, etc.

- Let clients know that losing even 10–15 pounds has positive benefits. Even a small weight loss can reduce blood pressure, lower LDLs, increase HDLs, and help with blood-sugar regulation. It's preferable to lose 10 pounds and keep it off than to lose 20 pounds and gain it back.

- Help clients realize that it's hard to eat a healthy diet if they're constantly exposed to poor food choices. As much as possible, eliminate high-calorie, high-fat, nutrient-poor food choices, as well as junk food stimuli (e.g., advertising on TV, as well as environments in which junk food is sold—malls, gas stations, convenience stores, etc.) from their environment. Help clients shop the perimeter of the grocery store (where produce, meat, poultry, fish, and dairy are usually placed) and bring home healthy, satisfying choices. Of course, teach label reading. Several excellent resources exist for clients who don't like to cook and who eat out frequently, as well as for those who enjoy cooking and spend a great deal of time in the kitchen (see the "Suggested Reading" and "Resources" at the end of this chapter). Eating well can be its own immediate reward. Healthy eating does not have to mean deprivation, self-pity, or "eating cardboard." People only believe this because they don't know any better. It's entirely possible to eat luxurious, delicious, beautiful meals that satisfy both mind and body, and are at the same time nutritious, wholesome, and low in fat.

- Teach portion control. Many people have become accustomed to overly large portions of food on their plates. Moderation is key.

- Have clients keep a food record: what and when they ate, as well as what mood they were in when eating. Do they skip meals? Do they consume large amounts of junk or processed food? Use the information at www.mypyramid.gov to help evaluate the number of calories in, and the quality of, their diet. Teach the concept of nutrient density.

- With your clients, develop a list of 10 non-food activities for them to do when they're bored, tired, lonely, etc. (e.g., take a bath, meditate, call a friend). Help them find substitute behaviors for eating (e.g., if they always eat snacks while watching TV, substitute exercise, sewing, or painting while watching TV).

- Remember that eating well isn't "all or nothing." It's what you do consistently (some say 80% of the time) that matters.

Gaining Weight

Gaining weight may be a priority for some clients. Nancy Clark, RD, offers the following six tips for healthful weight gain (Clark, 1991).

1. Consistently eat three hearty meals per day; make mealtime a priority.
2. Consistently eat larger than normal portions (e.g., instead of one sandwich at lunch, have two).

3. Eat an extra snack (e.g., a large peanut butter sandwich with a tall glass of milk) before bedtime. Pay attention to mid-morning and mid-afternoon snacks as well.
4. Select higher calorie foods (e.g., cranberry juice instead of orange juice, and split pea soup instead of vegetable soup).
5. Drink lots of juice and milk instead of water.
6. Perform resistance training exercises to build muscle.

Protein supplements and other "mass builders" are expensive and tend to promote misconceptions about muscle building. Increasing muscle mass results from the right kind of exercise and a healthy diet; the energy to exercise and fuel muscle activity is supplied by a diet high in carbohydrates. Extra, less expensive calories can easily come from juices and healthy foods.

Summary

In this chapter, fundamental concepts in nutrition were addressed, including: the 2005 USDA Food Guide Pyramid (MyPyramid), the U.S. Dietary Guidelines for Americans, and carbohydrate, protein, fat, cholesterol, vitamin and mineral, and hydration specifics. Nutrition and its impact on disease were covered. Label reading was reviewed step by step. Nutrient density, pre- and post-exercise eating, and supplementation were discussed. In addition, information was provided regarding eating disorders, gaining weight, and helping clients with weight loss/weight management.

References

American Cancer Society. (n.d.). *Food and fitness.* Retrieved November 16, 2005, from http://www.cancer.org/docroot/PED/ped_3.asp?sitearea=PED&level=1.

American College of Sports Medicine. (1996). The ACSM position stand on exercise and fluid replacement. *Medicine & Science in Sports & Exercise, 28*(1), i-vii.

American College of Sports Medicine. (ACSM). (1997). Position stand: The female athlete triad. *Medicine & Science in Sports & Exercise, 29*(5), i-ix.

American College of Sports Medicine, American Dietetic Association, and Dietitians of Canada. (2000). Joint position statement: Nutrition and athletic performance. *Medicine & Science in Sports & Exercise, 32*(12), 2130-2145.

American Diabetes Association. (2004). Nutrition principles and recommendations in diabetes. *Diabetes Care, 27,* S36-S46.

American Dietetic Association. (2000). Position of the American Dietetic Association: Weight management. *Journal of the American Dietetic Association, 102,* 1145-1155.

American Dietetic Association. (2005). *Dietary supplements: Practice paper.* Retrieved on February 13, 2006, from http://webdietitians.org/Public/GovernmentAffairs/index_21828.cfm.

American Heart Association. (1996). *Dietary guidelines for healthy American adults.* Retrieved November 16, 2005, from http://www.americanheart.org/presenter.jhtml?identifier=1466.

American Heart Association. (2002). Guidelines for primary prevention of cardiovascular disease and stroke: 2002 update. *Circulation, 106,* 388-391.

American Institute of Cancer Research. (1997). *Summary—Food nutrition and the prevention of cancer: A global perspective.* Retrieved November 16, 2005, from http://www.aicr.org/research/ report_summary.lasso.

American Psychiatric Association. (1994). *Diagnostic and statistical manual of mental disorders* (4th ed.). Washington, DC: American Psychiatric Association.

Block, G. (2004). Foods contributing to energy intake in the U.S.: Data from NHANES III and NHANES 1999-2000. *Journal of Food Composition and Analysis, 17,* 439-47.

Brower, M., & Leon, W. (1999). T*he consumer's guide to effective environmental choices.* New York: Three Rivers Press.

Calle, E.E., Rodriguez, C., Walker-Thurmond, K., Thun, M.J. (2003). Overweight, obesity, and mortality from cancer in a prospectively studied cohort of U.S. adults. *New England Journal of Medicine, 348*(17),1625-1638.

Centers for Disease Control and Prevention. (n.d.). *BMI-body mass index: BMI for adults.* Retrieved on November 16, 2005, from http://www.cdc.gov/nccdphp/dnpa/bmi/bmi-adult.htm.

Centers for Disease Control and Prevention Primary Prevention Working Group. (2004). Primary prevention of type 2 diabetes mellitus by lifestyle intervention: Implications for health policy. *Annals of Internal Medicine, 140,* 951-957.

Clark, N. (1991). Now to gain weight healthfully. *Physician and Sports Medicine, 19*(9), 53-54.

Clark, N. (2003). *Sports nutrition guidebook* (3rd ed.). Champaign, IL: Human Kinetics, Pub.

Coyle, E.F., & Coyle, E. (1993). Carbohydrates that speed recovery from training. *Physician and Sports Medicine, 21*(2), 111-123.

Felitti, V.J. (1999). A disease of too much iron. *Health News, 5*(1), 4-5.

Feskanich, D., Willett, W.C., & Colditz, G.A. (2003). Calcium, vitamin D, milk consumption, and hip fractures: A prospective study among post-menopausal women. *American Journal of Clinical Nutrition, 77,* 504-511.

Flegel, K.M., Carroll, M.D., Ogden, C.L, & Johnson, C.L. (2002). Prevalence and trends in obesity among U.S. adults, 1999-2000. *Journal of the American Medical Association, 288,* 1723-1727.

Foster-Powell, K., Holt, S.H., & Brand-Miller, J.D. (2002). International tables of glycemic index and glycemic-load values. *American Journal of Clinical Nutrition, 62,* 5-56.

Harper, C.R., & Jacobson, T.A. (2001). The fats of life: The role of omega-3 fatty acids in the prevention of coronary heart disease. *Archives of Internal Medicine, 161,* 2185-2192.

Heart Protection Study Collaborative Group. (2002). MRC/BHF heart protection study of antioxidant vitamin supplementation in 20,536 high risk individuals: A randomized placebo controlled trial. *Lancet, 360,* 23-33.

Institute of Medicine of the National Academies. (2002). Dietary reference intakes for energy, carbohydrate, fiber, fat, fatty acids, cholesterol, protein, and amino acids. Retrieved November 16, 2005, from http://www.iom.edu/report.asp?id=4340.

Jacobs, K.A., & Sherman, W.M. (1999). The efficacy of carbohydrate supplementation and chronic high-carbohydrate diets for improving endurance performance. *International Journal of Sport Nutrition, 9*, 92-115.

Jakicic, J.M., Clark, K., Coleman, E., Donnelly, J.E., Foreyt, J., Melanson, E., et al. (2001). American College of Sports Medicine position stand: Appropriate intervention strategies for weight loss and prevention of weight regain for adults. *Medicine & Science in Sports & Exercise, 33*, 2145-2156.

Jenkins, D.J., Kendall, C.W., Augustin, L.S., et al. (2002). Glycemic index: Overview of implications in health and disease. *American Journal of Clinical Nutrition, 76*(1), 266S-273S.

Kraus, R.M., Eckel, R.H., Howard, B., Appe, L.J., Daniels, S.R., Deckelbaum, R.J., et al. (2000). AHA dietary guidelines: Revision 2000: A statement for healthcare professionals from the Nutrition Committee of the American Heart Association. *Circulation, 102*, 2284-2299.

Lemon, P. (1995). Do athletes need more protein and amino acids? *International Journal of Sport Nutrition, 5* (Suppl.), S39-S61.

Ludwig, D.S. (2002). The Glycemic index: Physiological mechanisms relating to obesity, diabetes, and cardiovascular disease. *Journal of the American Medical Association, 287*, 2414-23.

McDowell, M.A., Briefel, R.R., Alaimo, K., Bischof, A.M., Caughman, C.R., Carroll, M.D., et al. (1994). *Energy and macronutrient intakes of persons ages 2 months and over in the United States: Third National Health and Nutrition Examination Survey, Phase I, 1988-1991.* Washington, D.C.: U.S. Government Printing Office.

Mussell, M.P., Binford, R.B., & Fulkerson, J.A. (2000). Eating disorders: Summary of risk factors, prevention programming, and prevention research. *The Counseling Psychologist, 28*(6), 764-796.

National Cholesterol Education Program Expert Panel. (2001). Executive summary of the third report of the National Cholesterol Education Program (NCEP) Expert Panel on detection, evaluation, and treatment of high blood cholesterol in adults (Adult Treatment Panel III). *Journal of the American Medical Association, 285*, 2486-2597.

National Institutes of Health Consensus Development Panel on Osteoporosis Prevention, Diagnosis and Therapy. (2001). Osteoporosis prevention, diagnosis, and therapy. *Journal of the American Medical Association, 285*, 785-795.

Pitsavos, C., Panagiotakos, D.B., Chrysohoou, C., Skoumas, J., Papaioannou, I., Stefanadis, C., et al. (2003). The effect of Mediterranean diet on the risk of the development of acute coronary syndromes in hypercholesterolemic people: A case control study (CARDIO2000). *Coronary Artery Disease, 13*, 295-300.

Reynolds, R.D. (1994). Vitamin supplements: Current controversies. *Journal of the American College of Nutrition, 13*, 118-126.

Shea, B., Wells, G., Cranney, A., Zytaruk, N., Robinson, V., Griffith, L., et al. (2004). Calcium supplementation on bone loss in postmenopausal women. *Cochrane Database of Systemataic Reviews*, Issue 1. Art. No: CD004526.pub2.DOI: 10.1002/14651858.CD004526.pub2.

Skender, M.L, Goodrick, K.G., Del Junco, D.J., Reeves, R.S., Darnell, L., Gotto, A.M., et al. (1996). Comparison of 2-year weight loss trends in behavioral treatments of obesity: Diet, exercise, and combination interventions. *Journal of the American Dietetic Association, 4*, 342-346.

U.S. Department of Agriculture. (2005a). *Dietary guidelines.* Retrieved November 16, 2005, from http://www.mypyramid.gov/guidelines/index.html.

U.S. Department of Agriculture. (2005b). *Dietary guidelines.* Retrieved November 16, 2005, from http://www.mypyramid.gov/downloads/sample_menu.pdf.

U.S. Department of Agriculture. (2005c). *Steps to a healthier you.* Retrieved September 1, 2005, from http://www.mypyramid.gov/index.html.

U.S. Department of Agriculture and Health and Human Services. (2005). *Nutrition and your health: Dietary guidelines for Americans* (6th ed.). Washington, DC: Government Printing Office.

U.S. Department of Health and Human Services. (1996). *Physical activity and health: A report of the Surgeon General.* Atlanta, GA: U.S. Department of Health and Human Services, Centers for Disease Control and Prevention, National Center for Chronic Disease Prevention and Health Promotion.

U.S. Department of Health and Human Services and U.S. Department of Agriculture. (2005). *Dietary Guidelines for Americans 2005.* Retrieved on February 13, 2006, from http://www.health.gov/dietaryguidelines/dga2005/document/pdf/DGA2005.pdf.

Wadden, T.A., Foster, G.D., & Letizia, K.A. (1994). One year behavioral treatment of obesity: Comparison of moderate and severe caloric restriction and the effects of weight maintenance therapy. *Journal of Consulting and Clinical Psychology, 62*, 165-171.

Whelton, P.K., He, J., Cutler, J.A., Brancati, F.L., Appel, L.J., Follmann, D., et al. (1997). Effects of oral potassium on blood pressure: Meta-analysis of randomized controlled clinical trials. *Journal of the American Medical Association, 277*, 1624-1632.

Whelton, S.P., He, J., Whelton, P.K., & Muntner, P. (2004). Meta-analysis of observational studies on fish intake and coronary heart disease. *American Journal of Cardiology, 93*, 1119-1123.

Willett, W.C. (2005). *Eat, Drink, and Be Healthy.* New York: Simon & Schuster, Inc.

Suggested Reading

Bernardot, D. (2000). *Nutrition for serious athletes.* Champaign, IL: Human Kinetics.

Berning, J.R., & Steen, S.N. (Eds). (1998). *Nutrition for sport and exercise* (2nd ed.). Gaithersberg, MD: Aspen Publishing.

Brownell, K.D., & Fairburn, C.G. (1995). *Eating disorders and obesity: A comprehensive handbook.* New York: Guilford Press.

Charney, P., & Malone, A. (2004). *Pocket guide to nutrition assessment.* Chicago, IL: American Dietetic Association.

Clark, N. (2003). *Sports nutrition guidebook* (3rd ed.). Champaign, IL: Human Kinetics.

Duyff, R.L. (2002). *The American Dietetic Association's complete food and nutrition guide* (2nd ed.). Hoboken, NJ: John Wiley & Sons, Inc..

Kleiner, S.M. (1998). *Power eating.* Champaign, IL: Human Kinetics.

Mahan, L.K., & Escott-Stump, S. (2003). *Krause's food, nutrition, & diet therapy* (11th ed.). Philadelphia: W.B. Saunders Company.

Ornish, D. (1993). *Eat more, weigh less.* New York: Harper Collins Publishers.

Ornish, D. (1998). *Love and survival.* New York: Harper Collins Publishers.

Rosenbloom, C. (Ed.). (2001). *Sports nutrition: A guide for the professional working with active people* (3rd ed.). Chicago, IL: American Dietetic Association.

Shils, M., Shike, M., Olson, J., & Ross, A.C. (1998). *Modern nutrition in health and disease* (9th ed.). Baltimore: Lippincott Williams & Wilkins.

Tribole, E. (1992). *Eating on the run.* Champaign, IL: Human Kinetics.

Willett, W.C. (2005). *Eat, drink, and be healthy.* New York: Simon & Schuster, Inc.

Resources

- www.aicr.org (American Institute for Cancer Research)
- www.americanheart.org
- www.anad.org (National Association of Anorexia Nervosa and Associated Disorders)
- www.cancer.org (American Cancer Society)
- www.cookinglight.com (*Cooking Light* Magazine)
- www.cspinet.org/nah/ (*Nutrition Action Health Letter*)
- www.diabetes.org
- www.eatingwell.com (*Eating Well* Magazine)
- www.eatright.org (find a registered dietitian)
- www.glycemicindex.com (click on GI database to access a search of a variety of foods)
- www.healthierus.gov/dietaryguidelines (2005 Dietary Guidelines)
- www.iom.edu (National Academy of Sciences Food and Nutrition Board, Institute of Medicine)
- www.mypyramid.gov (2005 USDA Food Guide Pyramid)
- www.nal.usda.gov/fnic/etext/000023.html (Food and Nutrition Information Center – food guide pyramids)
- www.nhlbi.gov/guidelines/hypertension
- www.nimh.gov/publicat/eatingdisorders.cfm (eating disorders)
- www.nof.org (National Osteoporosis Foundation)
- www.oldwayspt.org/pyramids (Mediterranean, vegetarian, Asian, and Latin American food guide pyramids)
- www.TheLifestyleCompany.com (includes the LEARN Program for Weight Management by Kelly Brownell, PhD)

Behavior Modification and Communication Skills

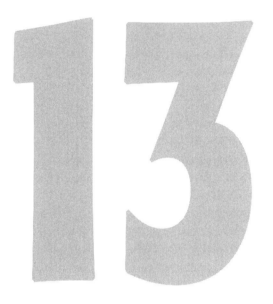

Outline

- Models for Behavior Change
- Barriers to Exercise
- Secrets of Goal Setting
- Fitness Motivation
- Supporting Behavior Change
- Communication Skills

We know that physical activity, exercise, healthy eating, and other positive lifestyle behaviors (such as not smoking) can prolong lives, prevent disease, and make life more enjoyable. Why then do so many people ignore these healthy behaviors that are widely known to be so beneficial? And an even more important question for personal fitness trainers is: how can you personally help people to modify their unhealthy behaviors in order to lead longer and happier lives? On a practical level, what can you actually do to affect change? Knowledge, of course, is critical; you must share the correct information. But many people have information about healthy living, yet they still do not change. In this chapter, behavior modification theories and practical tips for supporting change will be discussed. Additionally, communication skills will be addressed, and you will learn that honing these skills will enable you to help others more effectively and influence positive change.

Models For Behavior Change

Helping clients to modify their behavior to better maintain wellness is a continuing challenge for fitness professionals. Whether the lifestyle change is smoking cessation, alcohol abstinence, weight reduction and better eating habits, less stress, or the adoption of a regular exercise routine, clients who want to change share some common behavior patterns. Behavioral scientists have developed many models to explain these patterns and/or the motives behind change. Two of these models or theories, the Stages of Change model and the Social Cognitive Theory, may provide some insight into client behavior.

The Stages of Change Model

The Stages of Change model (also known as the readiness for change theory or the Transtheoretical Model) organizes people according to their level of motivation to change (Prochaska, 1979; Prochaska & DiClemente, 1983). This theory of behavior change, especially in regard to physical activity, has become increasingly popular and is widely accepted (Dunn et al., 1999). Some people have no intention to change whatsoever (at least right now), while others are quite motivated to make immediate changes, and may need help in maintaining their commitment. This model identifies the following five stages of change.

- **Stage One: Pre-Contemplation**—People in this stage are not even thinking about a new behavior pattern (such as exercising). They are usually unmotivated, resistant, and engaged in avoidance tactics (e.g., if exercise comes up in conversation, they change the subject). They are clearly not ready for change and may even deny the need for change. Typically, pre-contemplators tremendously underestimate the number of benefits of exercise, often citing only 1 or 2 when in actuality benefits number over 50. Instead, they may list many negatives (e.g., will get sweaty, have to buy new shoes, no time, might get injured, and will look silly). Since most American adults are sedentary (Schoenborn & Barnes, 2002) and appear to have little interest in exercising, a continuing challenge for fitness professionals lies in finding ways to move people out of this stage.
- **Stage Two: Contemplation**—During this stage individuals are seriously considering change. They are more aware of the benefits of change but

still are not ready to initiate new behavior. They may talk about losing weight or starting an exercise program, but have not yet taken any steps.

- **Stage Three: Preparation**—Individuals in this stage are "preparing" to change by initially making small changes. They may call a health club, buy an exercise video, or even buy a piece of home exercise equipment. They usually intend to take action within a month or so.

- **Stage Four: Action**—At this point, people are actively changing their behavior. Note that the first 6 weeks to 6 months is the most difficult period and the most common time to drop out (Dishman, 1994); 50% of new exercisers starting a fitness program drop out in the first 6 months. Many clients initiating change are not really prepared for a 6-month commitment; they think they'll achieve results much more quickly. Development of self-efficacy (the inner confidence a person has that he or she will be able to accomplish a given task) is critical, as is a supportive, motivating personal fitness trainer who provides realistic expectations.

- **Stage Five: Maintenance**—This is the stage that sustains long-term, ongoing consciousness of the new behavior and successful integration of it into the lifestyle.

Yet another way to define the five stages of change in regard to physical activity follows.

Stage One: the inactive and not thinking about becoming active stage

Stage Two: the inactive and thinking about becoming more active stage

Stage Three: the doing some physical activity stage (yet still not at the levels recommended by ACSM)

Stage Four: the doing enough physical activity stage (at the levels recommended by ACSM, but for less than six months)

Stage Five: the making physical activity a habit stage (longer than 6 months) (Marcus & Forsyth, 2003)

The Stages of Change model is a continuum and suggests that individuals often move back and forth cyclically between the stages, and do not necessarily progress through them in a linear fashion. Success, for some, may take many cycles or attempts. A sixth stage, termination, is sometimes added, but not in regard to physical activity, since vigilance seems to be constantly necessary to maintain the physical activity habit.

Studies have shown that once you have identified your client's level of motivation according to the Stages of Change model, it is important to match your response and information to his or her stage (Marcus, Rossi, Selby, Niaura, & Abrams, 1992). For example, giving an individual in stage one (pre-contemplation) information suited to stage five (maintenance) increases the likelihood of disinterest and/or refusal to participate. Following are some suggested strategies for each stage of change.

Stage of Change/ Level of Motivation	Strategy
Stage One: Pre-Contemplation	Encourage the person to begin thinking about the behavior change; discuss the pros and cons of the change; discuss the barriers to the change; have client set goals for reading about the new behavior
Stage Two: Contemplation	Encourage the person to begin taking steps towards the new behavior; have client read about starting; consider client's personal preferences; have client enlist the support of one or two others; build client's confidence by matching him or her with a successful role model
Stage Three: Preparation	Encourage the person to increase his or her sporadic attempts at the new behavior to consistent and recommended levels; identify barriers that prevent client from increasing the new behavior; use goal setting; use self-monitoring devices, logs, etc.; help client develop environmental cues for exercise.
Stage Four: Action	Continue to make the new behavior a part of the client's life; set short-term goals; try new activities; discuss relapse prevention; provide rewards.
Stage Five: Maintenance	Prepare for future setbacks; increase enjoyment of new activity; prevent boredom; use variety; have client reflect on achievements.

Social Cognitive Theory

Social Cognitive Theory states that there is a relationship between the environment, personal factors, and the behavior in question; the premise is that changing one of these variables influences the other variables. A key concept in Social Cognitive Theory is **self-efficacy**, which may be defined as the inner confidence that a person has that he or she will be able to accomplish a task. Personal fitness trainers should try to build a client's self-efficacy in relation to physical activity and healthy lifestyle choices. Four factors have been identified that may increase feelings of self-efficacy (Bandura, 1986).

1. Successful personal experiences—Set your client up for success with initial programs carefully matched to his or her level; as your client masters each small step, self-efficacy improves.

2. Vicarious experiences—Self-efficacy can be improved by observing others being successful, particularly if these individuals are similar to you.

3. Verbal persuasion—A positive and motivating personal fitness trainer can influence the development of self-efficacy. A cue such as, "I know you can do this!" is very powerful.

4. Measurable physiological responses—A client whose blood pressure decreases as a result of exercise usually experiences an increase in self-efficacy.

Another important concept in Social Cognitive Theory is known as outcome expectations. Helping your client understand that his or her exercise behavior will lead to fairly predictable results, in turn leads to realistic expectations, which, consequently, enhance continued behavior change. Often clients have an unrealistic perception of the results of exercise. They may think that exercising at a vigorous intensity for 5 days in a row will lead to a 20 lb. weight loss; when they fail to achieve this outcome, they may become discouraged and drop out. You can help your client have reasonable expectations by setting appropriate goals. Goal setting will be discussed later in this chapter. Remember, believing that physical activity has positive outcomes enhances motivation.

Barriers to Exercise

Many people aren't active because barriers, real or perceived, stand in their way (Rhodes et al, 1999). To find out what may stop your clients from achieving their goals, simply ask them about barriers, and then brainstorm with them for possible solutions. Common barriers include lack of time, effort required, and lack of interest. Exercise requires much more time and energy than other similar activities. Individuals who are time-pressed can be shown how to incorporate more activity into daily life. You can advise non-exercisers to use stairs instead of escalators, stretch during TV commercials, or walk that extra block to burn a few more calories. Exercising in short bouts, exercising earlier in the day, and riding an exercise bike while watching the nightly news are all possible solutions to a lack of time. Many clients aren't prepared for the effort required to achieve their goals, while some dislike being hot and sweaty. Making time for a post-exercise shower can be perceived as a barrier. And some people, particularly those in the pre-contemplation stage, simply aren't interested in exerting themselves, while others find exercise boring. Barriers exist inside the health fitness facility as well, including unavailable equipment, classes scheduled at inconvenient times, and poorly trained instructors.

Other common barriers have been identified (Dunlap & Barry, 1999) and include: lack of access to exercise, expense of exercise, depression and lethargy, multiple health problems, fear of injury, low fitness level, and a history of sedentary lifestyle. Lack of self-efficacy is also a barrier; people may not believe that they are physically able to exercise, or they may believe they're too heavy, too old, or too uncoordinated. In all these cases, your job is help identify the barriers, come up with solutions or small steps toward positive change, and support your clients in the process.

Secrets of Goal Setting

Helping clients set appropriate goals may be one of the most important things you can do to help them achieve change. There are two main types of goals: **approach goals** and **avoidance goals**. Of these two, approach goals appear to yield more positive results (Singer & Salovey, 1996) because positive outcomes are emphasized, often yielding happy memories. An example of an approach goal is to take a walk every day at sunset. An avoidance goal, on the other hand, may result in more anxiety, depression, and less enjoyment, even if the goal is achieved. An example of an avoidance goal is to deny yourself all sweets for a month.

The SMART system of goal setting has become a popular approach. SMART stands for the following: Specific, Measurable, Action-oriented, Realistic (or Relevant), and Timed.

- **Specific**—Defined, specific goals (e.g., "I want to lose 10 pounds" or "I want to see some definition on my arms and shoulders") are much easier to focus on than vague statements, such as, "I want to get in shape."
- **Measurable**—Help your client define measurable, tangible goals; then it will be clear when the goal has been achieved, and thus enhance motivation. Fitness assessments are ideal for establishing a base line and then giving proof of progress at later reevaluations. Structure at least one goal to allow you to measure progress during reassessment.
- **Action-oriented**—When you choose your goals, write out the details of the plan, including the days, times, duration, and intensity.
- **Realistic/relevant**—Choosing goals that are realistic and appropriate is critical for ensuring the success of your client; attainable goals set your client up for success.
- **Timed**—A timed goal is one with a target date for reassessment. Having a target date gives your client something to work toward and provides additional focus.

In general, for deconditioned and unmotivated clients, short-term goals of 2 weeks or less are more effective than long-term goals, as they can increase a person's sense of mastery and self-efficacy. Even though a client's long-term goal may be to lose 60 lb., focusing on what he or she can do this week, or today, is generally most helpful. For example, if your client's goal is to become more active in order to burn more calories, set a goal for this week only (e.g., "This week I'll walk on Monday, Wednesday, and Friday at 7:30 AM for 20 minutes."). When you see your client next, check to see whether this goal was accomplished and then set a new goal for the upcoming week. Additionally, goals that can be accomplished within a single session (process goals) are effective; examples include walking on the treadmill for 22 minutes instead of 20 minutes, doing just one more abdominal crunch than usual, or holding a stability exercise such as a plank for 5 more seconds than before. In this way, session by session and week by week, you help build steps to success.

A good goal is one that holds a challenge but is nevertheless attainable. The definition of a challenge will vary tremendously from client to client. Novice and deconditioned clients will appreciate only the gentlest challenge, whereas experienced and athletic clients may need rigorous challenges in order to stay motivated. Of course, it is extremely important to find out what your clients really want and why they want it. Use your best communication skills (discussed later in this chapter) to uncover your clients' feelings and thoughts about lifestyle change and what goals they think are effective.

Avoid setting unrealistic or hyper-inflated goals. Many clients may be initially attracted by marketing claims such as, "Get a new body in 4 weeks," but they will only be discouraged and possibly drop out when they discover that they are unable to meet such an unrealistic expectation. Finally, be sure to record your clients' goals and track their progress. It is very satisfying for clients to see how much they've improved and how successful they've been. For help with goal setting, please see the "Goal Setting Form" in Appendix C.

Fitness Motivation

The best motivation comes from within. **Intrinsic motivation** is the motivation that people have inside themselves to accomplish a goal, whereas **extrinsic motivation** is motivation that comes from something or someone else, such as a personal fitness trainer. Intrinsically motivated people are pursuing the "pleasure principle" and strive to be competent and self-determining. They enjoy mastering a task and being successful and take pride in their exercise and positive lifestyle experiences. Intrinsically motivated clients are more likely to maintain their positive lifestyle behaviors (Ryan, Frederick, Lepes, Rubio, & Sheldon, 1997). Knowledge, skill development, and social support can all help to foster intrinsic motivation.

Extrinsic motivation comes from outside, and the concern here is more with the outcome, not the process. For example, exercisers who are extrinsically motivated may have a certain body weight or percent body fat as their goal. They may work out—perhaps even in an addictive or compulsive way—to avoid the negative consequences of being overweight and out of shape. Personal fitness trainers need to find a way to turn extrinsic motivation into intrinsic motivation. This can be accomplished by emphasizing enjoyment, moderation, and variety; by creating a warm and supportive environment and the possibility of a positive experience; and by rewarding personal achievements, such as attitude changes, and ignoring negative behaviors.

How can you best motivate your clients? You'll find that different strategies may be needed for different clients. Beginners, for instance, typically need more support and encouragement than people who are already dedicated to exercise. The following is a list of possible strategies to inspire motivation.

- Empathize and connect with your client.
- Train clients in pairs or small groups; encourage your client to have a workout buddy.
- Encourage a sense of belonging.
- Use music that your client finds pleasurable.
- Provide choices when possible.
- Check up on your client regularly by phone or email.
- Encourage your client to increase his or her knowledge of fitness and health.
- Use rewards.
- Give specific positive feedback about your client's progress.
- Affirm your client's positive qualities and use motivational cues (see Chapter 8, "Applied Resistance Training Skills," for a discussion of affirmations and cueing).
- Help your clients believe that they will succeed.
- Be an enthusiastic role model.

Supporting Behavior Change

Additional strategies and techniques for supporting behavior change follow.

- **Emphasize benefits**—Educate clients about the 50+ benefits of exercise, the benefits of a heart-healthy diet, etc. Ask them what benefits they feel they're receiving. Remind them of their continued fitness progress, increased energy, and better sleep as they stick with their program. Most people feel much better at the end of an exercise session; help your clients to internalize this sense of well-being with a simple question, such as, "So, how do you feel now?" Help them develop an inner sense of satisfaction, and increase their intrinsic motivation for behavior change.

- **Ask the doctor**—Enlist the support and recommendations of your client's physician. Studies show that a personal physician's recommendation is one of the most important predictors of exercise participation and adherence (Petrella, Koval, Cunningham, & Patterson, 2003).

- **Avoid giving "too much, too soon"**—This is the major cause of injury and drop-out with new exercisers. When beginners exercise 5 or more days per week, and/or for longer than 45 minutes at a time, and/or at intensities greater than 85% of max VO_2, studies show increased injury rates and decreased compliance with the exercise program (Pollock & Wilmore, 1990). Instead, utilize the behavioral principle of shaping, or progression. This is the concept of slow, steady, gradual, one-step-at-a-time improvement. When applying the principle of overload, it's best to do so conservatively, especially with beginner exercisers.

- **Provide rewards and reinforcement**—This is said to be the most effective method for changing behavior. Let the client have a say in what type of reward works best for him/her, e.g., praise, certificates, headbands, and public recognition (as in an incentive contest, such as Travel Across America or Member of the Month). A fitness reassessment documenting positive change can also be a motivating reinforcer. The deposit-and-refund system of rewarding oneself has been shown to be effective (Jeffery, Gerber, Rosenthal, Lindquist, 1983). This system entails your client entrusting a friend with a certain dollar amount (e.g., $500), and then the friend "rewarding" your client a certain amount as each short-term goal is achieved (e.g., if a client wants to lose 10 lb., the friend refunds the client $50 as each pound is lost).

- **Give feedback**—This can be a formalized fitness reassessment or a simple day-to-day reminder of progress. Pointing out to your client that he or she is able to lift more weight or walk faster than was possible 2 weeks before provides continuing reassurance of progress. Documentation in the form of an exercise record or log is essential for tracking accomplishments.

- **Prepare your client for potential setbacks**—Find out what kinds of obstacles your client might face and discuss strategies for difficult times. Vacations, holidays, family obligations, and work pressures may all be cause for a temporary lapse. Help the client understand that this is normal; however, the goal is to persevere and not let the lapse turn into a "collapse" (relapse) or a cessation of the behavior.

- **Help the client use reminders**—Reminders are environmental cues or prompts that are used, for example, at home, in the car, and at the workplace, to help remind you, or provide a stimulus, to exercise (or continue the desired behavior). Examples include: setting out exercise clothes the night before, always carrying exercise shoes in the car, writing exercise times into an appointment book, setting a timer to go off when it's time to exercise, placing post-it notes on the refrigerator, and always exercising with a buddy.

- **Use behavioral contracts**—Contracts have been found to enhance success in 12-step programs. They help clients accept self-responsibility for their behavior as well as provide a time frame and focus for their goals. Many contracts include a reward for goal accomplishment and involve a significant other (as a witness). Be sure the goal is realistic and achievable (see "Behavior Contract" in Appendix C).

- **Help "generalize" behavior**—Encourage clients to practice the new behavior (e.g., exercise) on their own, when they're not with you. Provide them with alternatives for home exercise as well as exercise when traveling or on vacation. Develop your clients' confidence so they can continue the behavior independently. Help clients incorporate increased activity into their daily lives; exercise does not always have to be programmed and routine.

- **Prevent boredom**—Many people view exercise as boring and unpleasant. Devise strategies that work for each client that help make exercise fun, motivating, and interesting. This may mean adding variety with cross-training, taking indoor exercise outside and vice versa, or exercising with a friend. Recognize that the sheer repetitiveness of cardiorespiratory exercise (such as treadmill walking or stair-climbing) is boring for most. If possible, encourage reading, watching TV, listening to music, or some other distraction to help clients stick with it.

- **Minimize injuries**—Beginner and older exercisers, especially, often need a light to moderate program that keeps them free from injuries or other complications. A "twinge" that leads to an actual injury is a deterrent to all but the most dedicated exerciser.

- **Be a good role model**—Practicing what you preach, in terms of exercise, healthy eating habits, positive body image, not smoking, and through wellness practices, promotes and maintains a positive lifestyle (such as proper lifting to prevent future back problems). All of these tactics will provide an incentive for clients who see that a positive and fit lifestyle is possible.

Communication Skills

Good communication is vital for personal fitness trainers. For most clients, an ability to comfortably communicate with their trainer is an essential requirement; to many clients it may be more important than the trainer's level of fitness, experience, or knowledge. Being a good communicator is a key life skill as well; both personal and professional relationships are enhanced when you communicate openly, honestly, assertively, and with kindness. Clear communication reduces both personal stress and the stress felt by those around you. It helps you be a more effective, inspiring leader. It also helps you understand your client better and allows you to work together to create the best program for optimal results.

- Being empathetic means putting yourself in your clients' shoes and really seeing their point of view. It means being open and receptive to your clients.

- Being warm is exemplified by a spirit of friendliness and openness that is nonjudgmental. Giving clients your understanding and undivided attention helps them to open up, feel safe, and foster self-acceptance.

- Being genuine is simply letting your deep sense of caring come through. Think back to why you wanted to become a personal trainer. Let your spirit of earnestness and honesty be there for your clients.

Active, Conscious Listening

Giving full support to clients demands your full attention. When you utilize good listening skills, your clients feel valued, understood, and truly heard; listening well is key to skilled communication. You can practice **attending behaviors** to help your client feel that you are fully present and there for him or her; these behaviors can be verbal or nonverbal, as shown below. Following are several attending behaviors and steps toward active listening.

- Use open body language. Breathe deeply and allow your body to relax. Face your client and angle your body slightly toward him or her. Sit at the client's eye level and keep arms and legs uncrossed.
- Maintain eye contact; a relaxed focus on your client without constantly shifting your eyes helps him or her to feel safe.
- Remind yourself that your client is worthy of respect and attention.
- Take the time to really listen. Be patient.
- Drop expectations and fears about what you're going to do and how you'll respond to your client.
- Use encouraging phrases that tell the client you're really listening and want to hear more (e.g., "I see," "Really," "Mmm, hmm"). Note: this seems to work especially well with women (James & Clarke, 1993).
- Minimize distractions. Find a place where you won't be interrupted by other members, phone calls, etc.

Following are common roadblocks to active listening; these behaviors tend to inhibit clear communication.

- **Comparing, always assessing, always noticing who is more fit, smart, emotionally healthy, or who has suffered more, etc.**—You won't really hear or understand your client if your thoughts always come back to yourself.
- **Rehearsing**—If you're always busy planning what you'll say next, or what story you'll tell, you won't really hear your client.
- **Filtering, or listening to some things but not to others**–Letting your mind wander or avoiding hearing certain things (such as negative or critical statements) will prevent you from completely hearing what the client is saying.
- **Judging**—Labeling someone as stupid, crazy, or any other negative term means you've stopped listening and are having a "knee jerk" reaction.
- **Blaming or criticizing**—This tends to shame the client, creating a loss of self-confidence.
- **Being right**—If you always have to be right, you may go to any lengths to avoid being wrong (twisting the facts, making excuses, etc.).
- **Dreaming, half-listening**—If you tend to dream often when others are talking, you may be bored or anxious. Reconsider your commitment to really knowing your clients and valuing what they have to say.
- **Identifying**—Here again, the focus has more to do with you than with your client. In this case, everything the client says reminds you of something you've felt, done, or suffered. You're so busy thinking about your life that you don't really hear your client.
- **Advising**—Even though you are being paid to support, help, and advise, be sure you fully listen before jumping in with suggestions. Some

trainers only hear a sentence or two before they start trying to problem-solve, often missing what's really important in the process.

- **Derailing**—Suddenly changing the subject or "joking it off" causes you to avoid seriously listening to your client.
- **Placating**—Wanting to be liked, you simply go along with whatever is said. You agree without really hearing.
- **Minimizing**—Telling clients not to worry, or that their particular problem isn't so bad, lessens the importance of the message.
- **Denying**—Implying that clients don't have a problem when they feel they do, makes them feel as if they haven't been heard or understood.

Active Listening: Supporting through Verbal Responses

Giving appropriate verbal responses that encourage your client to keep talking is a form of active listening. Technique examples include the following.

- **Mirror**—Restate the client's message.
- **Paraphrase**—Put the core of the client's message into your own words for greater clarity.
- **Ask for clarification of a client's statements.**
- **Search for more information**—Use open-ended questions (see below).
- **Acknowledge**—Give the client direct feedback about what you hear the client saying. This is better accepted if your statements begin with "I" or another personal pronoun (e.g., "I hear that you're not feeling well today").
- **Summarize**—Recap what was said and never let a conversation end without being sure of what was said and why. Don't pretend to understand if you don't.

Using Open- and Closed-Ended Questions

The use of **open-ended questions** encourages more conversation and disclosure of information (Gavin & Gavin, 1995). This is ideal when you are trying to really understand a client. Examples of open-ended questions might include the following.

- Invite a free-flowing answer.
- Open up conversations.
- Usually start with words like how, what, why, could, or would.

Examples of open-ended questions are: "Would you tell me about your goals?" "What would you like to get out of our session today?" "How do you think you can best improve your well-being?"

On the other hand, **closed-ended questions** may be used to gain facts and narrow the discussion. Closed-ended questions:

- can be answered in a few words.
- close off discussion.
- give the questioner control of the conversation.
- direct the discussion.
- limit the kind of information obtained.

Examples of closed-ended questions are: "How old are you?" and "Do you like weight training?"

Clearer Communication through "I" Statements

Owning your thoughts and feelings helps you gain personal control of yourself, both in professional and personal interactions. Statements that use such words as "it," "you," "people," "they," and "we" place responsibility on someone or something else besides yourself. Examples include:

"It is strange talking to you" instead of "I feel strange talking to you."

"People feel nervous in new situations" instead of "I feel nervous in new situations." "We should end the session now" instead of "I think it's time to end the session."

It also helps to avoid the use of qualifiers and nullifiers. Qualifiers are ways of watering down the truth; nullifiers help avoid or escape the truth. Both decrease self-responsibility. Examples of qualifiers include: "I guess," "I suppose," "perhaps," "maybe," "kind of," "probably," "only," "just," and "sort of." Examples of nullifiers include: "I should" instead of "I could;" "I can't" instead of "I won't;" and "I don't know" instead of "I don't care to find out."

Communication Styles

Four basic styles of communication have been identified (Lange & Jakubowski, 1976): aggressive, passive-aggressive, passive, and assertive.

1. The **aggressive** communicator intimidates others and engages in verbal abuse. This leads to bad feelings on both sides, in addition to increased heart rates, higher blood pressure, and greater overall stress. The goal of aggression is domination and winning no matter what.

2. The **passive-aggressive** person tends to be indirect. Instead of saying what he or she means, this type of communicator remains silent, perhaps even with a forced air of politeness, yet later he or she will vent frustrations to or on someone else. Since problems are never resolved, increased stress results.

3. The **passive** person simply doesn't express feelings at all, holding everything in and avoiding conflict at all cost. He or she may have low self-esteem, believing that they do not have a right to their own opinion or that no one will listen anyway.

4. **Assertive** communication is the ideal. An assertive communicator is constantly trying to create a win/win situation. Opinions and feelings are clearly and respectfully expressed in such a way that the rights of others are supported and not infringed upon. An assertive person can stand up for him or herself without being intimidating or abusive. This communication style works to improve relationships, reduce stress, and promote a sense of well-being.

Personal fitness trainers are encouraged to become assertive communicators.

Roles You May Play

In the course of working with clients over time, you may find yourself in several different roles that involve behaving in a variety of ways. These roles may include the following.

- **The educator.** This role is especially suitable in the initial training sessions with a new client, but you will find yourself in "teaching" mode even with long-standing clients. As the educator, you answer your client's questions and teach them about a variety of topics, such as the components of fitness, how to assess exercise intensity, what muscles are being worked in a squat, how to avoid a sprained ankle, and how to access the USDA Food Guide Pyramid.

- **The nurturer.** Some clients want and need a great deal of support. Even dedicated clients may want empathy and a little hand-holding after a hard day or during a difficult time in their lives. Remember that not all clients want a vigorous, challenging, hard-core workout each and every time they see you (this is especially true for beginners, those with special conditions such as pregnancy, obesity, or diabetes, and older adults).
- **The conversationalist.** Occasionally, depending on the client, you may find yourself engaged in non-exercise-related conversation. Many clients are hungry for connection: with you, with other trainers or instructors, and with other club members. You can help facilitate this by introducing them to other clients and club members whenever possible. Obviously, most clients also want results and want to feel as if they're getting their money's worth; therefore, it is important to find a balance between guiding a client through a workout and engaging in some occasional playful banter and friendly conversation.
- **The motivator.** This is the "hat" you'll wear for clients wanting a tough and challenging workout. In this role, you may limit conversation and stay focused on directive and motivating cues as you lead your client from one exercise to the next. See Chapter 8, "Applied Resistance Training Skills," for a discussion of types of cues.

Personal fitness trainers need to find a balance between these and other roles. You may find that you are more comfortable in one of the above roles than another, or you may become adept at switching back and forth between them, depending on your client's needs. Of course, behaving professionally is key; make certain to keep all client conversation and information confidential, and avoid acting as a psychiatrist or therapist for your clients. Be friendly, warm, empathetic, generous, and kind, even while maintaining appropriate boundaries.

Perhaps the ultimate measure of success is to find that your clients have become so intrinsically motivated that they are maintaining a positive lifestyle simply because it feels good and because they want to. Their sense of inner satisfaction is the ongoing motivator; their good lifestyle habits are their own immediate reward. Once a client has reached this level of self-motivation, he or she may no longer need your professional support and guidance (although you can be sure you'll receive additional clients through word of mouth), and you'll know you have achieved the fulfilling reward of being an educator and a motivator of people.

Summary

In this chapter, two models for behavior change were discussed: the Stages of Change model and Social Cognitive Theory. Barriers to change, goal setting, motivation, and a number of practical strategies for helping clients with behavior change were outlined. Basic communication skills were introduced, including active listening, blocks to listening, supportive verbal responses, open-ended questions, and communication styles.

References

Bandura, A. (1986). *Social foundations of thought and action: A social cognitive theory.* Englewood Cliffs, NJ: Prentice-Hall.

Dishman, R.K. (1994). *Advances in exercise adherence.* Champaign, IL: Human Kinetics.

Dunlap, J., & Barry, H.C. (1999). Overcoming exercise barriers in older adults. *Physician and Sportsmedicine, 27*(11), 69-74.

Dunn, A.L., Marcus, B.H., Kampert, J.B., Garcia, M.E., Kohl, H.W., & Blair, S.N. (1999). Comparison of lifestyle and structured interventions to increase physical activity and cardiorespiratory fitness: A randomized trial. *Journal of the American Medical Association, 281*, 327-334.

Gavin, J., & Gavin, G. (1995). *Psychology for health fitness professionals.* Champaign, IL: Human Kinetics.

James, D., & Clarke, S. (1993). Women, men, and interruptions: A critical review. In D. Tannen (Ed.), *Gender and conversational interaction* (pp. 231-280). New York: Oxford University Press.

Jeffery, R.W., Gerber, W.M., Rosenthal, B.S., & Lindquist, R.A. (1983). Monetary contracts in weight control: Effectiveness of group and individual contracts of varying size. *Journal of Consulting and Clinical Psychology, 51*, 242-248.

Lange, A., & Jakubowski, P. (1976). *Responsible assertive behavior.* Champaign, IL: Research Press.

Marcus, B.H., & Forsyth, L.H. (2003). *Motivating people to be physically active.* Champaign, IL: Human Kinetics.

Marcus, B.H., Rossi, J.S., Selby, V.C., Niaura, R.S., & Abrams, D.B. (1992). The stages and processes of exercise adoption and maintenance in a worksite sample. *Health Psychology, 11*, 386-395.

Petrella, R.J., Koval, J.J., Cunningham, D.A., & Paterson, D.H. (2003). Can primary care doctors prescribe exercise to improve fitness? The step test exercise prescription (STEP) project. *American Journal of Preventive Medicine, 24*, 316-322.

Pollock, M.L., & Wilmore, J.H. (1990). *Exercise in health and disease: Evaluation and prescription for prevention and rehabilitation* (2nd ed.). Philadelphia: W.B. Saunders Co.

Prochaska, J.O. (1979). *Systems of psychotherapy: A transtheoretical analysis.* Homewood, IL: Dorsey Press.

Prochaska, J.O., & DiClemente, C.C. (1983). The stages and processes of self-change in smoking: Towards an integrative model of change. *Journal of Consulting and Clinical Psychology, 51*, 390-395.

Rhodes, R.E., Martin, A.D., Taunton, J.E., Rhodes, E.C., Donnelly, M., & Elliot, J. (1999). Factors associated with exercise adherence among older adults: An individual perspective. *Sports Medicine, 28*, 397-411.

Rogers, C.R., Gendlin, E.T., Keisler, D.J., & Truax, C.D. (1967). *The therapeutic relationship and its impact.* Madison, WI: University of Wisconsin Press.

Ryan, R.M., Frederick, C.M., Lepes, D., Rubio, N., & Sheldon, K.M. (1997). Intrinsic motivation and exercise adherence. *International Journal of Sport Psychology, 28*, 335-354.

Schoenborn, C.A. & Barnes, P.M. (2002, April 7). Leisure-time physical activity among adults: Advanced statistics. *Vital and Health Statistics*, No. 325. Retrieved on November 1, 2005, from http://www.cdc.gov/nchs/data/ad/ad325.pdf.

Singer, J.A., & Salovey, P. (1996). Motivated memory: Self-defining memories, goals and affect regulation. In L.L. Martin and A. Tesser (Eds.), *Striving and feeling: Interactions among goals, affect and self-regulation* (pp. 229-250). Mahwah, NJ: Lawrence Erlbaum Associates.

Suggested Reading

American College of Sports Medicine. (2003). *ACSM fitness book* (3rd ed.). Champaign, IL: Human Kinetics.

Annesi, J.J. (1996). *Enhancing exercise motivation.* Los Angeles: Fitness Management.

Bandura, A. (1997). *Self-efficacy: The exercise of control.* New York: W.H. Freeman and Company.

Blair, S.N., Dunn, A.L., Marcus, B.H., Carpenter, R.A., & Jaret, P. (2001). *Active living every day.* Champaign, IL: Human Kinetics.

Brehm, B.A. (2004). *Successful fitness motivation strategies.* Champaign, IL: Human Kinetics.

Gavin, J., & Gavin, G. (1995). *Psychology for health fitness professionals.* Champaign, IL: Human Kinetics.

Marcus, B.H., & Forsyth, L.H. (2003). *Motivating people to be physically active.* Champaign, IL: Human Kinetics.

Prochaska, J.O., Norcross, J.C., & DiClemente, C.C. (1994). *Changing for good.* New York: Avon Books.

Rejeski, W.J., & Kenney, E.A. (1988). *Fitness motivation.* Champaign, IL: Human Kinetics.

Rollnick, S., Mason, P., & Butler, C. (1999). *Health behavior change: A guide for practitioners.* New York: Churchill Livingstone.

Sallis, J.F., & Owen, N. (1998). *Physical activity and behavioral medicine.* Thousand Oaks, CA: Sage Publications.

Business Aspects, Legal Issues, and Professional Responsibilities

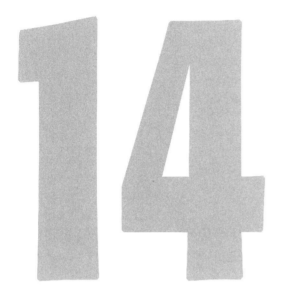

Outline

- Starting Your Business

- Marketing and Promoting Your Business

- Establishing Your Business Policies

- Managing and Expanding Your Business

- Legal Considerations

- Equipment Needs and Responsibilities

- Professional Responsibilities

Are you ready to be a personal fitness trainer? In the previous chapters of this book, the major areas of knowledge for personal trainers have been presented and addressed. Now it is up to you to integrate this information into your services and practice the skills and techniques that have been presented. There is, however, one final and important subject area remaining: the business side of personal fitness training. Any discussion of business and occupational matters also requires a discussion of legal and professional responsibilities. Whether you manage your own personal training business, or work as a trainer in a club, gym, or corporate setting, you will still need to understand certain legal issues and conduct yourself professionally. This chapter covers the basics of running a personal fitness training business, introduces and explains key legal concepts, and outlines major professional responsibilities for fitness professionals.

Starting Your Business

Writing Your Mission Statement

Whether you're starting your own business or you're in the business of personal training and working for someone else, it's helpful to think about the five questions listed below; these questions and concepts are fully explained by Kevin W. McCarthy in his motivating book, *The On-Purpose Person*. Articulating these ideas for yourself will help you to become more purposeful and clear about your life.

1. Answer the question, "Why am I here, or, what is my purpose in this life?"
2. Consider your **vision**, "Where am I going in my life; what do I want my future to look like?"
3. Formulate your **mission statement**, "How am I going to fulfill my purpose on a daily basis?"
4. Identify your **values**, "What is truly important to me and how will I act as I go about my mission?"
5. List your **commitments**, "In order to fulfill my purpose, vision, and mission, I commit to…".

As you can see, these are profound and important questions that will most likely require considerable thought. Yet thinking about what is most important to you and how you plan to show up in the world can make all the difference to your clients, friends, and family, not to mention your own sense of satisfaction and self-worth. The answers to these essential questions can be helpful to you in developing your mission statement as part of your overall business plan.

Many businesses develop such a mission statement; this statement is often featured on marketing and informational pieces, such as brochures, business cards, stationery, and Web sites. The mission statement defines your standards and intentions to your clients and may contain your vision statement as well.

Creating Your Advisory Board

If you are going into business for yourself, it makes sense to create an advisory board. Your advisory board should consist of outstanding professionals who are willing to support you with their knowledge, experience, and (occasionally) with their time. These are individuals to whom you can turn with technical questions and problems, and they can link your business to the real world. In return, they receive referrals from you, as well as publicity on your marketing materials and Web site. Consider including the following professionals on your board.

- Attorney
- Accountant
- Registered Dietitian
- Physical Therapist
- Chiropractor
- Orthopedist
- Obstetrician/Gynecologist
- Cardiologist
- Exercise Physiologist
- Professor specializing in Exercise Science Research
- Massage Therapist

Decide Where You'll Train

In deciding to become a personal fitness trainer, you have several options regarding the venue for personal training, including the following.

- Working as an employee of a commercial fitness facility, corporate fitness facility, or hospital-based facility
- Operating your own independent business, but renting training space in a commercial, corporate, or hospital-based facility
- Opening your own gym in either a commercial space or in your own home
- Training clients in the privacy of their own homes or offices

Each of these venues has advantages and disadvantages. Legal implications are associated with each venue and will be discussed later in this chapter.

Formulating a Business Plan

One of the most important aspects of managing a business is keeping your focus. This is why it's so helpful to find the answers to the questions posed at the beginning of this chapter, against which you can evaluate your daily decisions and the distribution of your time. Are you staying true to your purpose, vision, and mission? Are you continuing to uphold your values and commitments?

Where would you like your business to be in a year, five years, or ten years? How many clients would you like to have? How much money do you want or need to make? How much time and energy is needed to commit to making this happen? Do you want to eventually hire other trainers? Write down the steps you will need to take to meet your goals, and develop a timeline for completing those steps. A comprehensive business plan is particularly important if you are going to apply for a bank loan or solicit investors for your business.

To help you get started there are four aspects to effectively formulating your business plan, including the following.

1. Identify the personal trainer needs of your community. Is there a niche or target market for you as a personal trainer? It is important to determine this first. Do you prefer working with men or women? Are you interested in working with youth, young professionals, blue collar workers, executives, mid-life clients, or seniors? Perhaps your expertise is in working with special needs clients: those with disabilities, post-rehabilitation, pregnant, diabetic, or overweight (note that it's best that you

have specialty certifications and proper credentials for working with these types of clients). Do you prefer athletes, bodybuilders, dancers, or the deconditioned, harder-to-motivate client? Determining your target market will affect your marketing strategies.

2. Develop your business plan specific to this area of focus (plan includes vision, mission, goals, objectives, financial management, marketing and promotions, staffing, programs and services, in addition to other capital expenses, such as equipment, utilities, and insurance).

3. Implement your plan.

4. Evaluate your success. (Are you where you wanted to be after one year? If not, what changes need to be made?)

Marketing and Promoting Your Business

When starting out as a personal fitness trainer you'll need to find ways to let potential clients know about you and your services. To do this, you'll need to develop the marketing and promotion aspect of your business plan. Following are some strategies for business marketing and promotion.

1. Develop your marketing materials specifically for your target market. Choose professional-looking business cards, stationery, and resume. You may want to formulate a business name and/or logo; the services of a graphic designer can be valuable in helping to devise a business look and identity that is truly yours. Many trainers also develop an advertising brochure that lists their services and qualifications. Consider including your qualifications and the services you offer on your marketing materials, as well as solution-oriented points that identify your typical client's needs and how you can help. For instance, if you're working with a clientele primarily interested in weight loss, you might offer, "Interested in losing those last 10 pounds? Interested in feeling stronger and more fit? Here's what I (or your business name) can do for you." And then list the solutions to your potential client's problems that you offer.

2. Decide how you will attract your target market. For instance, if your target market consists of clients with special needs, networking with physicians (e.g., orthopedists, cardiologists, and rheumatologists) and physical therapists may help you gain referrals. In addition, ob-gyns may be willing to refer their pregnant or postnatal patients to you, if that is your specialty client focus. When approaching physicians, be organized and concise. Describe your credentials, explain what you can do for their patients, and ask if you may leave your cards, brochures, or flyers in the office waiting room. Consider what your target clients do for work and in their free time, what organizations they may belong to, what papers they read, what places they may frequent, and so on. Below are additional strategies for attracting clients.

   • Network with fitness-conscious health care professionals. Set up referral networks with massage therapists, dietitians, nutritionists, psychotherapists, social workers, registered nurses, and chiropractors. Ask for referrals. Tell them what you can do for their patients.

   • Network with exercise equipment stores. Small, independent, equipment-only stores are often open to developing relationships with trainers. This may include referrals for training sessions, free consultations for customers who spend a certain amount of money in the store, or allowing you to leave your brochures in a visible place.

- Speak for local organizations. Volunteer your expertise at the Rotary Club, National Association of Women Business Owners, church groups, social clubs, support groups, and other community associations. Look through the telephone book's yellow pages to see what organizations are nearby. Most groups appreciate a generalized presentation on such subjects as the benefits of exercise, how to incorporate exercise into your daily life, travel and exercise, and getting started with a walking program. This would not be the time to make a sales pitch, but if you speak in a professional manner and you are informative, people will listen and want to know more (have your brochures and business cards available).

- Write fitness and health promotion articles for newspapers and/or have a fitness message on the radio as part of a station's regular programming.

- Create a press release of your company's strengths. List all attributes, education, abilities, equipment, and experience in short, detailed sentences, succinctly answering the five W's: Who, What, When, Where, and Why. Emphasize your education, and highlight your Aerobics and Fitness Association of America (AFAA) certification (and other certifications, if appropriate) because it brings prestige and international credibility to your business. Examine the "bullet points" of your strengths and keep them readily available on your computer in order to make updating both continual and effortless. In the rapidly changing fitness environment today, information must be updated at least every 4 months to successfully promote yourself as current and credible. Continuously frequent the competition to see how you can better adapt your descriptions to include the evolving fitness market. You may wish to include the logo of your business on your press release. Use key bullets on business cards that correlate to your press release, and always keep these business cards handy. You can also write news releases on such noteworthy occasions as attending a major fitness conference, hiring a new trainer, or expanding to new locations. Send these releases to fitness and health writers at a variety of local papers and periodicals and follow up a week later.

- Use word of mouth. Offer your current clients a free session or two for every person they refer who starts a training program. You may also consider offering a free session to visible professionals, such as hairdressers, hotel concierges, and journalists, in exchange for referrals.

- Offer a complimentary consultation or session to potential new clients. Some individuals may not understand what is involved in personal training, and a no-cost initial session may be what they need in order to sign up as a client.

- Offer gift certificates to existing clients that they can use as gifts for friends (these can also be advertised in your flyers or brochures).

- Direct mail your flyers and/or distribute them in parking lots, stores, and health clubs. Direct mail can be expensive (figure the cost of a mailing list and stamps, plus the cost of your flyers), but may be a valuable source of clients.
- Use the Internet. Establish email addresses and perhaps a Web page. Costs can add up quickly, so investigate all alternatives before committing to an investment. Weigh the benefits of your company's exposure on the Web against your capital investment for online exposure. Having at least one electronic access in today's market speaks favorably about your company's success.
- Become involved in charity events. By helping others, you also help yourself. Have your name closely associated with worthwhile charities at least two to four times per year. Offer your services in warm-ups, sponsor activities, speaking engagements, and planning committee meetings associated with the events. To build a relationship over time you may choose to work with just one charity.
- Consider piggy-backing. This technique refers to two individuals or companies that come together, forming a symbiotic relationship. Each may offer a necessary skill without which the other would be rendered less effective, and thus more attention is drawn to the successful pairing. For example, if legally permissible, you may decide to go into business with a physical therapist, or open up a facility with a registered dietitian and share space, facilities, and associated costs.
- Explore sponsorships and references. Occasionally some products and services do well when backed by a sponsor; a new gym offering specialized equipment may do well to approach that equipment manufacturer with an inquiry regarding sponsorship, and thus profit from yet another source of publicity. Closely linked with sponsorships are references—if you have permission to cite a high-profile client linked in some capacity to your product, doing so on your promotional material can bolster your exposure.
- If you or your company's personnel can speak another language other than English, market this skill. Many fitness facilities in the United States and abroad continuously search for employees who may be multilingual. Stating "Spanish available" on promotional materials, for example, instantly doubles the accessibility of your product and makes you more marketable.
- Ask for feedback from professionals. After forming a relationship with a sponsor or the media, ask for input regarding the impact of your marketing materials. "How can I make this information even more stimulating for the public" is an excellent question for them.

Establishing Your Business Policies

Decide How Much You'll Charge

Rates for personal training vary according to where you live. In general, the closer you are to a metropolitan area, the higher the rate. The best way to determine how much you will charge is to find out what other trainers in the area are charging and decide on a similar fee. Rates should also be based on your education and experience; if you have a college degree in the health sciences and several certifications you should be able to charge (and receive) a higher rate than a trainer with only one certification. Also, it is fairly common for trainers to discount when several sessions are purchased in advance (e.g., a client can buy 10 sessions for the price of 8). Set clear policies regarding how and when your clients should pay for their personal training; it is helpful to create a billing agreement document and have clients sign it. Note that having clients pay in advance for a certain number of sessions may enhance their adherence. Also note that laws and even local ordinances may require you to comply with certain legal formalities for advance or pre-paid sessions. Individual legal representation in this regard is necessary.

Establish No-Show, Late, and Cancellation Policies

Many trainers and businesses require a 24-hour notice of cancellation; otherwise, the client is charged full price for missed, late, or cancelled sessions. Your time is valuable and you are a professional; it is perfectly legitimate for you to expect clients to fulfill their commitments to you. Note that your cancellation policies need to be clearly posted and explained to your clients in advance; some trainers have clients sign a document showing that they understand they will be billed for missed sessions. Legal advice for compliance with local ordinances is again required.

Establish Policies for Entry into Your Training Program

It is strongly recommended that you adhere to the guidelines established by American College of Sports Medicine (ACSM), the American Heart Association (AHA), and other respected standard-setting organizations for health screening (see Chapter 4, "Health Screening and Risk Appraisal") and fitness assessment (see Chapter 5, "Fitness Assessment"). Let your clients know that you follow these guidelines (in order to help protect them and yourself), and then take your clients through the proper steps for entry into personal training: initial interview, medical history form, analysis of risk factors, risk-factor stratification, physician's clearance form if necessary, informed consent, fitness assessment, goal setting, and finally, the exercise program itself, followed eventually by reassessment and more goal setting.

Once your business is up and running and you are busy training clients, you'll find there are a number of day-to-day duties. These can include: financial management (billing clients, paying bills, keeping track of expenses, tax preparation, etc.), maintenance of current client training records (updating workout logs and keeping careful notes on client needs, questions, and issues), communication with your clients' health-care providers (physicians, physical therapists, dietitians, etc.), facility maintenance, marketing material updates, and the continuation of your own education, fitness journal and text reading, or class attendance. Eventually, you may find your business expanding and you may need to hire employees.

Managing and Expanding Your Business

Business Expansion

Some personal fitness trainers find that after months or years of working 8 or more hours per day, training client after client, they are ready for a change and want to move towards managing other trainers and owning a larger business. Or, perhaps the number of clients wanting personal training exceeds the number of hours in the day. In this case, you can develop a waiting list, only taking clients when other clients move on, or you can hire, or go into business with, other trainers.

Becoming an employer requires a number of new skills, such as the ability to recruit, interview, and hire qualified trainers, manage conflict, delegate tasks and responsibilities, and motivate your staff. You'll need to establish fair policies for wages, benefits (if any), continuing education, and possible advancement within your company.

Other options for business expansion include selling products (such as exercise equipment or exercise clothing), or continuing your education and developing your skills so that you can work with specialty clients (e.g., athletes, dancers, seniors, children). Additionally, an exciting new area of training is wellness coaching or lifestyle consulting, often offered over the telephone or Internet (special training programs and certification programs exist for wellness coaching).

Reimbursement Issues

Of growing interest to personal fitness trainers is the possibility of third-party reimbursement, meaning payment from health insurance companies or HMOs, for personal training services. As the population grows steadily more overweight and obese, with resulting increases in disease, disability, and health care costs, some health insurance companies are becoming more open to providing reimbursement for fitness, wellness, and preventive types of services. Third-party reimbursement for trainers has advantages and disadvantages. On the one hand, it could greatly increase the number of people who are active and receive appropriate fitness and wellness advice. In addition, physicians would be more likely to refer sedentary and overweight patients to qualified trainers. And the credibility and perceived value of personal fitness training as a viable career path would improve.

However, there are some disadvantages, including the fact that insurance companies may be involved in cost reimbursement decisions. This involvement could have an impact on the price to be paid for personal training, which may well be considerably less than fees currently earned, especially in large metropolitan areas. Additionally, trainers would become much more involved in filling out necessary paperwork for reimbursement and may have to wait longer to receive payment. Insurance companies could be motivated in setting the standards for who qualifies as a personal fitness trainer, requiring degrees and certain certifications (this may be a positive benefit), as well as impacting what the trainer can and cannot do to remain within their permissible scope of practice. The additional insurance paperwork and regulations would probably drive up the cost of insurance premiums for all. At this point it is difficult to say whether or not the benefits of insurance coverage would outweigh the disadvantages. Personal fitness trainers should stay informed about the possible move towards insurance reimbursement in the fitness industry, and you would be wise to position yourself for the best opportunities by becoming (and staying) as educated and qualified as possible.

Legal Considerations

Choosing a Business Entity

If you work for a club, you may be either an employee or an independent contractor (in this case, self-employed).

An **employee**:

- must adhere to certain standards and methods specified by his or her employer.
- is often paid by the hour and not by the job.
- is usually hired for longer periods, such as months or years.
- is sometimes trained by the employer.
- generally provides services exclusively to the employer.
- provides work necessary to the employer's business on a consistent basis.
- may typically receive benefits such as health insurance and paid vacations.
- has his or her taxes deducted.

An **independent contractor**:

- is more likely to set his or her own hours and work agendas.
- typically must pay for his or her own benefits such as health insurance and vacation time.
- often receives a single payment for a specific job.
- is already skilled and may not require training by an employer.
- often provides services to several businesses.
- often provides his or her own equipment.
- is responsible for his or her own taxes.

If you are self-employed, you will need to make a number of business decisions, many of which were discussed earlier in this chapter. You will also need to decide what form of business or business entity you will have. Note that it is important to obtain the services of an attorney, as each state has differing legal requirements. There are three main business entity choices: (1) corporate, including so-called limited liability corporations, (2) partnership, or (3) sole proprietorship.

1. Technically, a **corporation** is a legal and distinct entity, having an independent existence separate of any owners, shareholders, or employees of that corporation. This fact may make it easier for you to protect your personal assets in the event of a lawsuit filed against your corporation, and this may be the most important potential benefit of becoming incorporated. This may be especially true with a somewhat newer form of corporate entity—a limited liability company, which provides even greater protection from personal liability. Keep in mind that incorporation can be somewhat more expensive than other entity forms and may be subject to many complicated legal regulations. However, more and more states have now streamlined the processes required for corporations, and the benefits of incorporating (such as personal liability limitation) may well offset any potential costs or formalities.

2. A **partnership** is a business owned by two or more individuals. This type of entity can offer some valuable advantages, such as access to the partner's assets and expertise, and less government regulation. Note that a successful partnership usually requires compatible partners; it helps if the partners share the same vision, mission, values, and commit-

ments. A major disadvantage is that partners can be held liable for each other's actions and debts.

3. The **sole proprietorship**, as its name implies, is owned and operated by one person. This individual is solely responsible for all debts and business issues, and is responsible for all liabilities connected to the business; on the plus side, he or she receives all the profit and may have more freedom in making business decisions. A sole proprietorship is the least costly way to start out in business.

After you have decided whether to run your business as a sole proprietorship, a partnership, or a corporation, you will need to obtain several licenses and permits, depending on where you live. At the county clerk's office inquire about: a business license, a state sales tax license, and registering your business name. You will probably also need to set up a business checking account, and you will find that the services of an attorney are invaluable. Lastly, always carry liability insurance (see discussion below).

Risk Management

Risk management refers to managing yourself and your business in such a way as to reduce your risk of being sued. Risk management emphasizes a process designed to identify and assess legal risks, provides a means to reduce, minimize, or eliminate those risks, and is a way to offset risks that cannot be entirely eliminated through processes, forms, and liability insurance. A related meaning is to take steps to reduce your client's risk of being injured or having any reason to initiate a lawsuit against you. In order to provide effective risk management for your business, you will need to understand the following concepts.

- **Standard of care**—When providing your personal fitness services, you must do so according to the industry-wide standard of care. Various health and fitness organizations have established standards of care, including: Aerobics and Fitness Association of America (AFAA), ACSM, the American Council on Exercise (ACE), the National Strength and Conditioning Association (NSCA), the International Health and Racquet Sports Association (IHRSA), and a number of other professional associations including the AHA. Fitness facility standards of care are presented in *ACSM's Health/Fitness Facility Standards and Guidelines* (1997). A new third edition of this work is due to be published in 2006. You will need to align your fitness services as closely as possible with these industry standards of care, and stay up to date with any changes as the fitness industry evolves. In the event of a claim and lawsuit against you, expert witnesses may be called who will compare your actions to the standards of care outlined by ACSM in the above mentioned text or by other similar organizations. For example, a failure to offer health screening (i.e., medical history form, risk factor analysis, risk factor stratification, physician's clearance if necessary) to your clients is deemed beneath the standard of care according to the standards of most major fitness organizations, and would increase your risk of liability in the event of a lawsuit.

- **Negligence**—This is a failure to conform your conduct to a generally accepted standard of care (Herbert, 2006, Chapter 5). A client may claim that a personal fitness trainer is negligent (leading to personal injury or harm) for a number of reasons, including the following.

- Screening was not performed or offered.
- An appropriate activity was not recommended.
- Proper supervision or instruction was not provided in the use of exercise equipment or in the recommendation of activities.
- Proper spotting was not performed when using free weights or other equipment.
- An exercise or exercise regimen was prescribed that was too rigorous or dangerous for the client.
- Equipment was not adjusted or maintained properly.
- Emergencies were not responded to appropriately and/or no emergency plan was in place or carried out in a proper and/or timely fashion.

- **Informed Consent/Assumption of Risk**—In the event of a lawsuit, a client's assumption of risk may become an issue, especially if you have had the client read and sign an express assumption of risk document or even a valid informed consent form (see Chapter 4, "Health Screening and Risk Appraisal"). The informed consent is an important document that should explain in reasonable detail the exercise test and/or program, outline potential risks, dangers, and discomforts, and describe the expected benefits of the test or program. The form should let the client know that he or she is free to stop the exercise test or program at any time. Clients should be advised of their responsibility to disclose all relevant information and ask any questions necessary to ensure a safe exercise experience. An assumption of risk document is written evidence of the client's assumption of the risks normally associated with a defined activity. The informed consent or similar express or written assumption of risk documents may offer you some degree of legal protection (although it is not a guarantee) if your client has voluntarily "assumed the risk" of the exercise test or program described. Of course, it is still your duty to uphold your professional standard of care to the best of your abilities, even if your client has signed an informed consent.

- **Releases/Waivers of Liability**—Aside from informed consent or express assumption of risk documents, written releases or waivers of liability signed by clients in advance of activity may well provide a very effective level of protection from claims and lawsuits in the event of client injury. Such documents, which are recognized in most states, specify that the client prospectively gives up or waives his or her right to sue for any injuries arising from participation in exercise and activity programs— even where a personal fitness trainer is negligent. So long as these documents are properly worded and executed they will frequently prevent the institution of a claim and/or suit. Moreover, even where a suit is filed, the litigation will often result in summary proceedings in favor of the fitness professional based upon the executed release documents. Examples of such a form can be found in Appendix C under "Agreement and Release of Liability" and "Alternative Form—Express Assumption of Risk/Prospective Waiver of Liability and Release Agreement." Remember that informed consents, waivers, and release documents must be properly written to be effective (and in some states these documents may not be recognized); therefore, consultation with an experienced and knowledgeable attorney is extremely important.

- **Liability Insurance**—It is strongly recommended that all personal fitness trainers carry appropriate professional liability insurance as a way to offset their personal risks associated with claims and/or lawsuits. Liability insurance protects you from potential serious financial loss in the event of a lawsuit and provides you with peace of mind. Reasonable group policies for health fitness professionals are offered through AFAA as well as other organizations. Such programs should be reviewed by all fitness professionals, as appropriate liability insurance is necessary and important.

Other steps you can take to manage your risk and protect your clients and yourself include the following.

- Regularly update your clients' medical history forms and be aware of changes in their health status. Refer to health care providers when and where indicated.
- Document everything. Keep clear, appropriate, and confidential records regarding your clients' health evaluations, fitness assessments, and session training logs. Document your clients' complaints, injuries, and successes, as well as your responses.
- Become, and stay, certified. Certification is a way for you to prove competency in the event of a lawsuit. Once certified, continue to educate yourself, including acquiring a college degree in a health-related field. Continuing education will be discussed later in this chapter.
- Stay up to date and follow exercise testing guidelines outlined by the ACSM. Do not attempt to administer maximal stress tests unless you have been specifically trained to do so. Refer specialized testing to physicians or exercise physiologists. When testing clients, always monitor the test properly and adhere to criteria for test termination as outlined by ACSM.
- Keep your instruction consistent with guidelines outlined by major organizations, such as ACSM, AFAA, ACE, NSCA, AHA, and the American Dietetic Association (ADA). Avoid contraindicated and controversial exercises; such exercises can put your clients in harm's way and increase your risk of a lawsuit.
- Be sure your clients' programs are appropriate for their health/fitness status, age, and ability to correctly carry out your instructions. This means selecting the appropriate intensity, frequency, duration, and mode, as well as carefully instructing your clients as to the safe performance of the program.
- Plan for emergencies. Rehearse for such emergencies on a regular basis—preferably quarterly or more frequently. Always know the location of the nearest telephone and how to activate the emergency medical system. Keep each client's emergency medical information with you for quick referencing during sessions. Always keep your CPR and first-aid certifications current. Learn how to use an automated, external defibrillator (AED); where required, purchase and keep an AED ready for use.
- Understand the limitations of your profession and stay within your scope of practice. This topic is discussed in more detail later in this chapter.

- Your ultimate responsibility is to the safety of your clients. Never leave a session unattended when you are being paid to work one-on-one. Be sure that your clients' exercise equipment and workout area are safe, clean, appropriate, and in repair. Be certain that you have instructed your clients in the proper use of all equipment. If you supervise and/or recommend exercise to be carried out offsite or in a client's home or office, make sure the exercise or activity is appropriate for that place and that emergency response can be carried out properly and timely if necessary.

Equipment Needs and Responsibilities

Most personal fitness trainers find they need several pieces of equipment, even if they are employed by a club, corporate fitness facility, or hospital-based program. Such business-related equipment includes a cell phone, answering machine (or service), pager, business or personal trainer software, and home computer or laptop. Additionally, even if you do not have your own training facility, you may want to purchase fitness assessment equipment, such as skinfold calipers, tape measures, heart rate monitors, and a step or sit-and-reach box. Trainers who work out of their own facility, or who travel to client's homes for training sessions, may invest in several versatile pieces of small equipment, including elastic tubing or bands, light handweights and ankle weights, medicine balls, a stability ball, BOSU, coreboard, slide, step, mat, jump rope, and pedometer.

Be aware that there are legal issues involved with the use of exercise equipment (both large and small) when training clients. It is your responsibility to make certain that equipment is maintained and is in good repair (and provide documentation upon request); you must also carefully explain to your clients the use of such equipment. Additionally, you must see that the training area or location is safe. If the equipment or training area is unsafe for any reason, it is your job to remove the equipment from service or at least to warn your client, even if the equipment and the space are in the client's own home. Failure to do so can be deemed negligent. If you recommend a particular area, for example, for your client to jog or run, you should determine that the area is relatively safe; if potential safety issues exist, you must tell your client about these issues, warning him or her of any concerns. If an area is unreasonably dangerous, you must recommend a different location.

Professional Responsibilities

Scope of Practice

An important professional responsibility is to stay within your scope of practice. In recent years, litigation has increased over scope of practice issues as lines have become somewhat blurred between certain health care professionals. Remember, you are not a physician, physical therapist, psychologist, or pharmacist. If you pretend to be one, you can be prosecuted for unlawfully practicing medicine or some other licensed health-care discipline, which is a criminal offense. If a death results from such unauthorized practices, you can be prosecuted for more serious crimes. Be careful about taking on clients with medical concerns; in some cases, the most prudent thing to do is refer them to a more clinically based program where they can have medical supervision. Advice that you give to clients must not be given nor construed as a diagnosis or a medical prescription. Additionally, avoid giving specific dietary advice unless qualified and/or using reliable software (see Appendix D, "AFAA's Nutritional Supplement Policy."). Dietitians, physicians, physical therapists, psychologists, and some other health care professionals have licenses; at present, personal fitness trainers do not. You must not cross over into the domains of licensed professionals. Follow codes of ethics. Determine if privacy laws apply. For applicability of federally enacted HIPAA see http://www.cms.hhs.gov/HIPAAGenInfo/06_AreYouaCoveredEntity.asp #TopOfPage. Consult a lawyer for interpretation of HIPAA and to examine the applicability of contracts and state laws.

Professionalism and Code of Ethics

How would you define professionalism? How would your clients define professionalism? Most clients want and appreciate a trainer who is a good role model and is professionally dressed (neat, clean, athletic-type clothes that are not too revealing, plus athletic shoes—no sandals or flip-flops) and practices good hygiene. A professional personal fitness trainer also conducts him or herself in a certain way—with appropriate, non-intimidating touch (always asking the client's permission), respectful listening skills, courteous, non-profane language, and a positive, upbeat demeanor. Professionalism means being punctual and honest. A professional trainer remembers that personal fitness training is a service business—you are there to help your client achieve his or her goals; you are not there to work out yourself or brag about your accomplishments. AFAA and other organizations, including the National Board of Fitness Examiners (NBFE), have established **codes of ethics** to help guide trainers toward professional behavior and an appropriate standard of care.

AFAA CERTIFIED FITNESS PROFESSIONALS' CODE OF ETHICS

- I do hereby attest to maintain the ethical and practical role of an AFAA Certified Instructor.

- I will uphold all of the standards and guidelines established by AFAA.

- I acknowledge the boundaries of my expertise as a fitness and exercise professional and will make referrals to other professionals as necessary.

- I will withhold personal judgment and be an unbiased advocate for lifestyle change.

- I will maintain responsibility and accountability to my clients while respecting their confidentiality.

- I accept the challenge of my professional growth and will update my practical and theoretical foundations through continuing education.

- My overall goal as an AFAA certified professional is to facilitate safe and effective exercise and instruction.

NATIONAL BOARD OF FITNESS EXAMINERS
PERSONAL FITNESS TRAINERS
CODE OF ETHICS

The NBFE Registered Personal Fitness Trainer should:

- Recognize that the principals of personal fitness training—improving physical strength, cardiovascular conditioning, flexibility, nutrition and overall wellness—are primary tools to improve public health in the United States.

- Regard client needs as the first responsibility in their practice. Recognize that client safety and health comes before all other fitness goals.

- Provide competent personal training instruction that fosters client dignity, self-worth, and confidentiality.

- Adhere to safe and recognized standards of practice and advocate healthy lifestyles for their clients.

- Practice within their knowledge and skill domain and refer clients to other fitness and health professionals as necessary.

- Actively maintain, upgrade and, where possible, add to the skills and knowledge domain of the fitness industry to increase their capacity to serve their clients.

- Observe and practice within all local, state, and national statutes and laws.

- Participate in a practice that is free of racial, cultural and gender bias and prejudice.

- Honestly and completely represent professional knowledge and skills, training, certifications to clients, employers, and colleagues.

- Involve clients in the decisions and determinations of all exercise programming.

- Follow the highest standards of business principals, integrity and professionalism.

(©2005 National Board of Fitness Examiners. Reprinted with permission.)

Continuing Education

Since the fitness industry interfaces with the scientific, research, and medical communities, it is a given that fitness guidelines and information are going to change over time. It is critical that you continue reading, attending seminars, workshops and conferences, and networking with health care professionals on a regular basis in order to remain professionally competent and be your best. Showing that you are serious about continuing your education and growing within the fitness industry is another mark of a professional (and can help in the event of a lawsuit). Below are some suggestions for educational growth.

- Return to school. The reality is, especially in the medical community, that degrees convey credibility and knowledge. Preparing for one (or even several) certifications can't possibly teach you as much as four years of college in a health-related field. Furthermore, in today's evolving fitness industry, the criteria for qualified fitness professionals is increasing. More and more health and fitness facilities are requiring degrees for employment. Go back to school now and grow with the industry!

- Attend higher level workshops and conferences. Most of the major fitness organizations, including AFAA, now provide appropriate seminars on a variety of topics.
- Go on for advanced certifications. Again, most major fitness organizations offer a "higher level" test of your competency.
- Prepare for, sit, and pass the national examination to be offered by the NBFE for personal trainers. It is believed that passing this examination and becoming registered with the NBFE will be a "gold standard" for personal trainers in the future. Study and prepare for the examination through an NBFE affiliate such as AFAA.
- Subscribe to (and read) as many professional journals as you can.
- Read textbooks. A large number of excellent textbook resources are provided at the end of each chapter in this book.
- Learn to read research. Reading research in quality, peer-reviewed journals will teach you to think scientifically. Critical, objective thinking is important in a field in which myths abound and naïve or misinformed clients are always trying to find a "magic pill, diet, or formula" to help them achieve their goals more easily.

Summary

Various aspects of developing a personal fitness training business, from marketing to insurance to pricing, were discussed in this chapter. Important legal issues, such as standard of care, negligence, and assumption of risk were introduced, and the importance of continuing education was emphasized.

References

American College of Sports Medicine. (1997). *ACSM's health/fitness facility standards and guidelines* (2nd ed.). Champaign, IL: Human Kinetics.

Herbert, D., & Herbert, W. (2006). Legal considerations. In *ACSM's resource manual for guidelines for exercise testing and prescription* (5th ed.), pp. 658-666. Baltimore: Lippincott Williams & Wilkins.

McCarthy, K.W. (1992). *The on-purpose person.* Colorado Springs, CO: Piñon Press.

Suggested Reading

Bangs, D.H. (1992). *The business planning guide.* Dover, NH: Upstart Publishing.

Brooks, D.S. (2004). *The complete book of personal training.* Champaign, IL: Human Kinetics.

Cotton, D.L., & Cotton, M.B. (1997). *Legal aspects of waivers in sport, recreation and fitness activities.* Canton, OH: PRC Publishing.

Durak, E.P. (1994). *The ins and outs of medical insurance billing.* Santa Barbara, CA: Medical Health and Fitness.

The Exercise Standard and Malpractice Reporter. (Journal). Canton, OH: PRC Publishing.

Gaut, E. (1995). *The personal trainer business handbook.* Gaithersburg, MD: Will Creek Publications.

Herbert, D., & Herbert, W. (2002). *Legal aspects of preventive, rehabilitative, and recreational exercise programs* (4th ed.). Canton, OH: PRC Publishing.

Kishel, G.F., & Kishel, P.G. (1993). *How to start, run, and stay in business.* New York: Wiley & Sons.

Koeberle, B.E. (1998). *Legal aspects of personal fitness training* (2nd ed.). Canton, OH: PRC Publishing.

Plummer, T. (1999). *Making money in the fitness business.* Monterey, CA: Healthy Learning.

Plummer, T. (2003). *The business of fitness: Understanding the financial side of owning a fitness business.* Monterey, CA: Healthy Learning.

Roberts, S.O. (1996). *The business of personal training.* Champaign, IL: Human Kinetics.

Emergency Protocol:
Standard First Aid, CPR, and AED

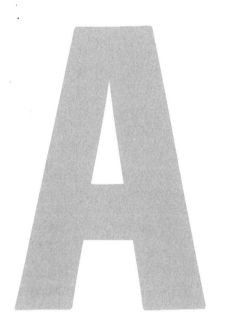

Outline

- Adult CPR, AED, and Airway Obstruction

- First Aid

Because emergency protocol techniques change often, the contents of this protocol are for reference and review purposes only. Reviewing and observing the following basic procedures will give you a jump start on any emergency situation.

- An emergency response plan should be developed and in writing for all to see.
- Post accurate telephone numbers for all available assistance. Make certain all staff members know where numbers are posted. Have a working telephone readily available at all times.
- Have a comprehensive first-aid kit on hand. Review contents regularly and ensure that used items are replaced immediately. Also ensure all staff members know where first-aid kit is stored. If automated external defibrillator (AED) is available, know location and how to operate.
- Train staff in emergency response procedures and rehearse regularly. Maintain records and document each rehearsal. Ensure all staff members know their responsibilities during an emergency.

In many emergencies, you will need to activate the Emergency Medical Services (EMS) system, including police, fire, and ambulance. In most areas, the emergency response contact number is 9-1-1. Verify and post the correct EMS contact number for your area.

In 2005, new cardiopulmonary resuscitation (CPR) guidelines were published by the American Heart Association (AHA). Additionally in 2005, the AHA joined with the American Red Cross (ARC) to release new guidelines for first aid. These guidelines are a culmination of ARC and AHA efforts, who together co-founded the National First Aid Science Advisory Board to review and evaluate current scientific information on first aid. All fitness professionals should remain current in CPR and first-aid procedures. And bear in mind that ARC and AHA are considered the gold standard for these certification trainings.

Brief reviews of CPR and first-aid procedures are provided in this appendix. However, please contact AHA and ARC for more comprehensive text and certification training programs in your area. The following bullet points are key considerations and steps to take when you are facing an emergency. Keep in mind that formal training and certification in these areas are essential.

Adult CPR, AED, and Airway Obstruction

- Check for unresponsiveness.
- Phone 9-1-1.
- Head-tilt/chin-lift method is to be used by all first responders (jaw-thrust method has been discontinued by first responders).
- Take 5–10 seconds to check for breathing in unresponsive victims.
- If no sign of breathing, attempt two breaths.
- If chest doesn't rise, perform abdominal thrusts (airway obstruction).
- If the chest rises, check for signs of a pulse. If there is no pulse, then immediately move to chest compressions.
- Provide 30 chest compressions and two ventilations (rate of 100 per minute).
- If using an AED, follow AED written protocols or AED machine prompts. If prompted, give one shock followed by immediate chest compressions.
- Check circulation every 2 minutes.

First Aid

Positioning the Body
- General rule—do not move victim unless in unsafe area.
- If face down, need to turn the victim over if CPR is required.
- If unresponsive but breathing and has a pulse, place on side.

Shock
If the victim goes into shock, he/she may be confused, have very fast or very slow heart and breathing rates, trembling and weakness in the arms and legs, cool and moist skin, pale or bluish skin, lips, and fingernails, or dilated pupils. Shock will lead to death if untreated.
- Activate the EMS system.
- If you do not suspect head injuries, spine injuries, or leg fractures, place victim on his or her back and elevate legs 9–12 inches. If you do suspect injuries, or specifically spine injuries or a leg fracture, do not move the victim.
- If the victim vomits, turn the victim on his or her side.
- If the victim is having trouble breathing, have him or her sit in a semi-reclining position.
- Maintain victim's body temperature by using blankets (cold victim) or providing shade and loosening clothing (hot victim).

Respiratory (Breathing) Emergencies
- If victim states he/she is having an asthma attack and has medication, assist victim in taking medication.
- If severe anaphylaxis and victim has auto-injector, assist victim in using device.
- If victim is unable to self-administer auto-injector, first responder can administer if previously prescribed by physician to victim.

Seizures
- Activate EMS system.
- Prevent injury to person.
- Ensure open airway.
- Ensure that airway remains open after seizure has ended (do not place anything in mouth).
- Place victim in recovery position—turn on his or her side.

Injury Emergencies
- External Bleeding
  - If severe, activate EMS.
  - Direct pressure on gauze or cloth until bleeding stops.
  - If bleeding doesn't stop, apply more pressure and use pressure bandage.
  - Do not use tourniquet.
- Wounds
  - If severe, activate EMS.
  - Irrigate wounds or abrasions with clean running water for at least 5 minutes.
  - Apply antibiotic ointment or cream if superficial wound.

- Burns
    - Superficial burns—cool with cold water to reduce pain.
    - Do not directly apply ice.
    - If blisters, cover with sterile dry bandage.
    - If electrocution, provide rescue breathing CPR/AED if necessary (do not put yourself in danger; ensure no electrical danger before approaching and assisting victim).
- Spine Stabilization

  You should suspect a spinal injury with anyone who has been involved in a motor vehicle, motorized cycle, or bicycle accident, whether he or she is the driver, a passenger, or an involved pedestrian. In addition, you should also suspect a spinal injury with anyone who has had a fall from greater than standing, complains of neck or back pain, has tingling in extremities, is not fully alert or is confused, and/or has a visible head or neck injury.
    - Activate EMS system.
    - Manually stabilize head, neck, and spine—do not move or use any external device to stabilize the victim.
    - Keep victim in line/keep in original position until EMS arrives.
    - If helmet is in place on victim, do not attempt to remove.

Musculoskeletal Injuries

- RICE (Rest, Ice, Compression, Elevation)
- Apply ice to the injured area (but not directly on the skin) for no longer than 20 minutes at a time.
- If open fracture, cover open wound with sterile bandage.
- Do not straighten an injured extremity.
- If extremity is blue or pale, activate EMS.

Medical Emergencies

- Nosebleeds
    - Nosebleeds may be an indication of head injury. Refer to the information on spinal stabilization.
    - Have this individual stop activity and rest.
    - To prevent re-bleeding in more severe nosebleeds, an icepack may be applied. Also, applying pressure by gently pinching nostrils together and tilting head downward slightly may be helpful (do not lean individual's head backward).
    - If bleeding persists, despite the pressure, for a prolonged period of time (15 minutes), call 9-1-1 or the emergency response number in your area.
- Diabetic Emergencies (Hypoglycemia)
    - Activate EMS system.
    - If the individual can drink and swallow, offer fruit juices or non-diet soda.
    - If person refuses juice or soda, rub cake icing or contents of a sugar packet in the gum area of the victim's mouth.
    - If the individual is becoming unresponsive, put him or her in shock position (on back with legs elevated).
    - Monitor person's condition.

- Stroke
  - Activate EMS system.
  - Keep a stroke victim lying down and protected.
  - Attempt to maintain normal body temperature.
  - Do not give the victim anything to eat or drink.
  - If victim begins to vomit, lay victim on his or her side.
  - Monitor person's condition

Environmental Emergencies

- Heat Exhaustion
  - Activate EMS system.
  - Move the victim out of direct sun and preferably into a cooler environment.
  - Reduce body temperature with cool, wet cloths or towels.
  - Loosen all tight clothing.
  - If the victim is able to swallow, give cool water to drink (slowly).
  - Minimize shock (see above).
  - Monitor the victim until EMS arrives.
- Heat Stroke
  This is the least common heat emergency, but it is the most severe. It usually occurs if heat exhaustion is left unchecked. With heat stroke, a dangerously elevated internal body temperature can cause vital body systems to fail.
  - Activate EMS system.
  - Move the victim out of direct sun and preferably into a cooler environment.
  - Reduce body temperature with cool, wet cloths or towels.
  - Loosen all tight clothing.
  - Do not give anything by mouth.
  - Minimize shock (see above).
  - Monitor victim until EMS arrives.
- Hypothermia
  - Activate EMS system.
  - Remove wet clothing and dry the victim.
  - Have victim put on dry clothing and gradually warm up the body with blankets.
  - Move to a dry, warmer environment.
  - Do not warm victim too quickly as this could lead to heart problems.
  - Monitor vital signs until EMS arrives.
- Frostbite
  - Handle the area gently and with extreme care.
  - Never rub the affected area as that could cause further damage.
  - Gradually warm the affected area in 100-105°F water.
  - Affected area should not touch side or bottom of tub or container.
  - Keep in water until area is red and warm to the touch.
  - Bandage area in dry, sterile dressing.
  - If the affected area is a toe or finger, place gauze between digits.
  - Get medical attention as soon as possible.

Summary

Review these protocols frequently and keep your CPR/AED and first-aid certifications current. You must be prepared for emergencies in order to react quickly and appropriately when necessary. Remember that the American Heart Association and the American Red Cross are the gold standard in these certifications.

References

American Heart Association. (2005). *2005 American Heart Association Association guidelines for cardiopulmonary resuscitation and emergency cardiovascular care.* Retrieved December 3, 2005, from http://www.americanheart.org/eccguidelines.

American Heart Association and American Red Cross. (2005). Guidelines for first aid. *Circulation, 112*, IV-196-IV-203. Retrieved December 3, 2005, from http://www.circulationaha.org.

Effects of Medications

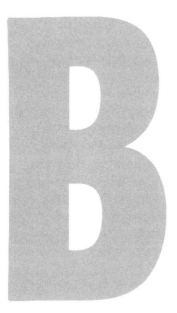

Caveat

"The following information is provided for educational purposes only and is based upon available source materials that are believed to be accurate and are reprinted with permission. However, any decisions that are made as to the appropriateness of recommending or supervising specific client activity while a client is taking medications, or as to the intensity/duration of such activity while clients are taking medications, or as to the use of medications or the interactions of medications with other medications or substances must be made by the client's health care provider."

Effects of Medications on Heart Rate, Blood Pressure, the Electrocardiogram (ECG), and Exercise Capacity

Medications	Heart Rate	Blood Pressure	ECG	Exercise Capacity
I. ß-Blockers (including carvedilol and labetalol).	↓* (R and E)	↓ (R and E)	↓ HR* (R) ↓ ischemia** (E)	↑ in patients with angina; ↓ or ↔ in patients without angina
II. Nitrates	↑ (R) ↑ or ↔ (E)	↓ (R) ↓ or ↔ (E)	↑ HR (R) ↑ or ↔ HR (E) ↓ ischemia** (E)	↑ in patients with angina; ↔ in patients without angina; ↑ or ↔ in patients with congestive heart failure (CHF)
III. Calcium channel blockers Amlodipine Felodipine Isradipine Nicardipine Nifedipine Nimodipine Nisoldipine	↑ or ↔ (R and E)	↓ (R and E)	↑ or ↔ HR (R and E) ↓ ischemia** (E)	↑ in patients with angina; ↔ in patients without angina
Diltiazem Verapamil	↓ (R and E)		↓ HR (R and E) ↓ ischemia** (E)	
IV. Digitalis	↓ in patients with atrial fibrillation and possibly CHF Not significantly altered in patients with sinus rhythm	↔ (R and E)	May produce non-specific ST-Twave changes (R) May produce ST segment depression (E)	Improved only in patients with atrial fibrillation or in patients with CHF
V. Diuretics	↔ (R and E)	↔ or ↓ (R and E)	↔ or PVCs (R) May cause PVCs and "false-positive" test results if hypokalemia occurs May cause PVCs if hypomagnesemia occurs (E)	↔, except possibly in patients with CHF
VI. Vasodilators, nonadrenergic	↑ or ↔ (R and E)	↓ (R and E)	↑ or ↔ HR (R and E)	↔, except ↑ or ↔ in patients with CHF
ACE inhibitors and Angiotensin II receptor blockers	↔ (R and E)	↓ (R and E)	↔ (R and E)	↔, except ↑ or ↔ in patients with CHF
a-Adrenergic blockers	↔ (R and E)	↓ (R and E)	↔ (R and E)	↔
Antiadrenergic agents without selective blockade	↓ or ↔ (R and E)	↓ (R and E)	↓ or ↔ HR (R and E)	↔
VII. Antiarrhythmic agents	All antiarrhythmic agents may cause new or worsened arrhythmias (proarrhythmic effect)			
Class I Quinidine Disopyramide	↑ or ↔ (R and E)	↓ or ↔ (R) ↔ (E)	↑ or ↔ HR (R) May prolong QRS and QT intervals (R) Quinidine may result in "false-negative" test results (E)	↔
Procainamide	↔ (R and E)	↔ (R and E)	May prolong QRS and QT intervals (R) May result in "false-positive" test results (E)	↔
Phenytoin Tocainide Mexiletine	↔ (R and E)	↔ (R and E)	↔ (R and E)	↔
Moricizine	↔ (R and E)	↔ (R and E)	May prolong QRS and QT intervals (R) ↔ (E)	↔

Medications	Heart Rate	Blood Pressure	ECG	Exercise Capacity
Propafenone	↓ (R) ↓ or ↔ (E)	↔ (R and E)	↓ HR (R) ↓ or ↔ HR (E)	↔
Class II ß-Blockers (see I.) *Class III* Amiodarone Sotalol *Class IV* Calcium channel blockers (see III.)	↓ (R and E)	↔ (R and E)	↓ HR (R) ↔ (E)	↔
VIII. Bronchodilators	↔ (R and E)	↔ (R and E)	↔ (R and E)	Bronchodilators ↑ exercise capacity In patients limited by bronchospasm
Anticholinergic agents Xanthine derivatives	↑ or ↔ (R and E)	↔	↑ or ↔ HR May produce PVCs (R and E)	
Sympathomimetic agents	↑ or ↔ (R and E)	↑, ↔, or ↓ (R and E)	↑ or ↔ HR (R and E)	↔
Cromolyn sodium	↔ (R and E)	↔ (R and E)	↔ (R and E)	↔
Steroidal anti-inflamatory agents	↔ (R and E)	↔ (R and E)	↔ (R and E)	↔
IX. Antilipemic agents	Clofibrate may provoke arrythymias, angina in patients with prior myocardial infarction Nicotinic acid may ↓ BP All other hyperlipidemic agents have no effect on HR, BP, and ECG			↔
X. Psychotropic medications				
Minor tranquilizers	May ↓ HR and BP by controlling anxiety; no other effects			
Antidepressants	↑ or ↔ (R and E)	↓ or ↔ (R and E)	Variable (R) May result in "false positive" test results (E)	
Major tranquilizers	↑ or ↔ (R and E)	↓ or ↔ (R and E)	Variable (R) May result in "false positive" or "false negative" test results (E)	
Lithium	↔ (R and E)	↔ (R and E)	May result in T wave changes and arrythmias (R and E)	
XI. Nicotine	↑ or ↔ (R and E)	↑ (R and E)	↑ or ↔ HR May provoke ischemia, arrythmias (R and E)	↔, except ↓ or ↔ in patients with angina
XII. Antihistamines	↔ (R and E)	↔ (R and E)	↔ (R and E)	↔
XIII. Cold medications with sympathomimetic agents	Effects similar to those described in sympathomimetic agents, although magnitude of effects is usually smaller			↔
XIV. Thyroid medications Only levothyroxine	↑ (R and E)	↑ (R and E)	↑ HR May provoke arrhythmias ↑ ischemia (R and E)	↔, unless angina is worsened

Medications	Heart Rate	Blood Pressure	ECG	Exercise Capacity
XV. Alcohol	↔ (R and E)	Chronic use may have role in ↑ BP (R and E)	May provoke arrhythmias (R and E)	↔
XVI. Hypoglycemic agents Insulin and oral agents	↔ (R and E)	↔ (R and E)	↔ (R and E)	↔
XVII. Blood Modifiers (Anticoagulants and antiplatelets)	↔ (R and E)	↔ (R and E)	↔ (R and E)	↔
XVIII. Pentoxifylline	↔ (R and E)	↔ (R and E)	↔ (R and E)	↑ or ↔ in patients limited by intermittent claudication
XIX. Antigout medications	↔ (R and E)	↔ (R and E)	↔ (R and E)	↔
XX. Caffeine	Variable effects depending on previous use Variable effects on exercise capacity May provoke arrhythmias			
XXI. Anorexiants/diet pills	↑ or ↔ (R and E)	↑ or ↔ (R and E)	↑ or ↔ HR (R and E)	

*ß Blockers with ISA lower resting HR only slightly.
** May prevent or delay myocardial ischemia.
Abbreviations: PVCs = premature ventricular contractions; ↑ = increase; ↔ = no effect; ↓ = decrease; R = rest; E = exercise; HR = heart rate.

(American College of Sports Medicine. [2006]. *ACSM's guidelines for exercise testing and prescription* [7th ed.]. Baltimore: Lippincott Williams & Wilkins. Reprinted with permission.)

Personal Fitness Trainer Forms, Questionnaires, and Assessment Norms

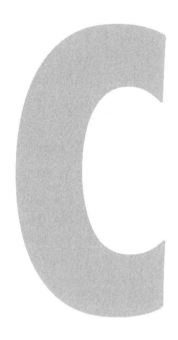

Outline

- AHA/ACSM Health/Fitness Facility Preparticipation Screening Questionnaire (Medical History Form)
- Physician's Clearance Form
- PAR-Q & You
- Informed Consent Forms
- Agreement and Release of Liability
- Express Assumption of Risk Forms
- Exercise and Activity Quiz
- Nutrition and Weight Profile
- Self-Assessment Quiz
- Fitness Assessment Data Sheet
- Percent Fat Estimations for Men and Women
- Classification of Disease Risk Based on Body Mass Index (BMI) and Waist Circumference
- Body Mass Index Nomogram
- Step Test Norms for Men and Women
- Rockport Walking Test Norms
- Rockport Walking Treadmill Test Norms
- Upper Body Strength Norms
- Standard Values for Push-Up Endurance
- Fitness Categories by Age Groups and Gender for Partial Curl-Up
- Standard Values for Trunk Flexion in Inches (Sit and Reach Norms)
- Postural Analysis Guide
- Exercise Session Recording Form
- Example of Hands-On Technique Consent Form
- Goal Setting Form
- Behavior Contract

Legal Forms

The following materials, written by David L. Herbert, J.D. and William G. Herbert, Ph.D. and taken from the book *Legal Aspects of Preventive Rehabilitative and Recreational Exercise Programs*, fourth edition, are being reproduced with permission from PRC Publishing, Inc., Canton, OH 1-800-336-0083 ©2002 PRC Publishing, Inc. all other rights reserved.

- Informed Consent for Exercise Testing of Apparently Healthy Adults
- Alternative Form for Informed Consent for Exercise Testing Procedures of Apparently Healthy Adults
- Informed Consent for Participation in an Exercise Program for Apparently Healthy Adults
- Agreement and Release of Liability
- Alternative Form—Express Assumption of Risk/Prospective Waiver of Liability and Release Agreement
- Express Assumption of Risk for Participation in Specified Activity

Caveat

"No form should be adopted by any program until it has first been reviewed by legal counsel and other advisors to the program. Each such form must be written in accordance with prevailing state laws by knowledgeable legal counsel and should state to the participant the reasons for the procedures, the risks and benefits of the procedure, etc. in a manner specific to the program activities for which consent or other form or contractual document is being obtained."

AHA/ACSM Health/Fitness Facility Preparticipation Screening Questionnaire* (Medical History Form)

Assess your health status by marking all true statements

History

You have had:

_____ a heart attack	_____ heart valve disease
_____ heart surgery	_____ heart failure
_____ cardiac catheterization	_____ heart transplantation
_____ coronary angioplasty (PTCA)	_____ congenital heart disease
_____ pacemaker/implantable cardiac defibrillator, or rhythm disturbance	

Symptoms

_____ You experience chest discomfort with exertion.

_____ You experience unreasonable breathlessness.

_____ You experience dizziness, fainting, or blackouts.

_____ You take heart medications.

> If you marked any of these statements in this section, consult your physician or other appropriate health care provider before engaging in exercise. You may need to use a facility with a **medically qualified staff**.

Other Health Issues

_____ You have diabetes.

_____ You have asthma or other lung disease.

_____ You have burning or cramping sensation in your lower legs when walking short distances.

_____ You have musculoskeletal problems that limit your physical activity.

_____ You have concerns about the safety of exercise.

_____ You take prescription medication(s).

_____ You are pregnant.

Cardiovascular Risk Factors

_____ You are a man older than of 45 years.

_____ You are a woman older than 55 years, have had a hysterectomy, or are postmenopausal.

_____ You smoke, or quit smoking within the previous 6 months.

_____ Your blood pressure is > 140/90 mmHg.

_____ You do not know your blood pressure.

_____ You take blood pressure medication.

_____ Your blood cholesterol level is > 200 mg/dl.

_____ You do not know your cholesterol level.

_____ You have a close blood relative who had a heart attack or heart surgery before age 55 (father or brother) or age 65 (mother or sister).

_____ You are physically inactive (i.e., you get < 30 minutes of physical activity on at least 3 days per week.)

_____ You are > 20 pounds overweight.

> If you marked two or more of the statements in this section you should consult your physician or other appropriate health care provider before engaging in exercise. You might benefit from using a facility with a **professionally qualified exercise staff+** to guide your exercise program.

_____ None of the above

> You should be able to exercise safely without consulting your physician or other appropriate health care provider in a self-guided program or almost any facility that meets your exercise program needs.

+Professionally qualified exercise staff refers to appropriately trained individuals who possess academic training, practical and clinical knowledge, skills, and abilities commensurate with the credentials defined in Appendix F of the ACSM Guidelines 2006.

*Modified from American College of Sports Medicine and American Heart Association. (1998). ACSM/AHA joint position statement: Recommendations for cardiovascular screening, staffing, and emergency policies at health/fitness facilities. *Medicine & Science in Sports & Exercise*: 1018. Reprinted with permission.

Physician's Clearance Form

Please return this form to: _____
(Personal Fitness Trainer's Name)

Address: _____

Phone: _____

Date: _____

Patient's name: _____ Age: _____

Date of last physical examination: _____

_____ This patient may/may not participate fully in a physical activity program consisting of cardiovascular, strength, and flexibility training without limitation.

_____ This patient may participate in a physical activity program with the following limitations and/or recommendations: _____

_____

_____

Please include a brief description of any medical condition that might affect his/her physical activity program: _____

_____

If this patient is on any medication that may affect the heart rate or the blood pressure response to exercise (elevating or suppressing), please indicate: _____

I consider the above individual to be: _____ normal

                                       _____ cardiac patient

                                       _____ prone to coronary heart disease

                                       _____ other (explain): _____

Please fill in the following information if available:

      result of last GXT   _____

      blood pressure _____

      glucose_____

      total serum cholesterol   _____

      HDL-C _____ LDL-C _____

      triglycerides_____

Physician's Signature _____ Date _____

Please Note: This record must be signed by the physician or at least stamped by the physician and verified if stamped by a typed letter on the provider's letterhead. THE PHYSICIAN'S CLEARANCE FORM WILL NOT BE ACCEPTED WITHOUT SUCH PROPER VERIFICATION.

PAR-Q & You

A questionnaire for people age 15–69

Regular physical activity is fun and healthy, and increasingly more people are starting to become more active every day. Being more active is very safe for most people. However, some people should check with their doctor before they start becoming much more physically active.

If you are planning to become much more physically active than you are now, start by answering the seven questions in the box below. If you are between the ages of 15–69, the PAR-Q will tell you if you should check with your doctor before you start. If you are over 69 years of age, and you are not used to being very active, check with your doctor.

Common sense is your best guide when you answer these questions. Please read the questions carefully and answer each one honestly. Check YES or NO.

YES	NO	
❏	❏	1. Has your doctor ever said that you have a heart condition <u>and</u> that you should only do physical activity recommended by a doctor?
❏	❏	2. Do you feel pain in your chest when you do physical activity?
❏	❏	3. In the past month, have you had chest pain when you were not doing physical activity?
❏	❏	4. Do you lose your balance because of dizziness or do you ever lose consciousness?
❏	❏	5. Do you have a bone or joint problem (for example, back ,knee, or hip) that could be made worse by physical activity?
❏	❏	6. Is your doctor currently prescribing drugs (for example, water pills) for your blood pressure or heart condition?
❏	❏	7. Do you know of <u>any other reason</u> why you should not do physical activity?

If you answered

YES to one or more questions:

Talk with your doctor by phone or in person BEFORE you start becoming much more physically active or BEFORE you have a fitness appraisal. Tell your doctor about the PAR-Q and which questions you answered YES.

- You may be able to do any activity you want—as long as you start slowly and build up gradually. Or, you may need to restrict your activities to those which are safe for you. Talk with your doctor about the kinds of activities you wish to participate in and follow his/her advice.

- Find out which community programs are safe and helpful for you.

NO to all questions:

If you answered NO honestly to <u>all</u> PAR-Q questions, you can be reasonably sure that you can:

- start becoming much more physically active—begin slowly and build up gradually. This is the safest and easiest way to go.

- take part in a fitness appraisal-this is an excellent way to determine your basic fitness so that you can plan the best way for you to live actively. It is also highly recommended that you have your blood pressure evaluated. If your reading is over 144/94, talk with your doctor before you start becoming much more physically active.

Delay Becoming Much More Active:

- if you are not feeling well because of temporary illness such as a cold or a fever—wait until you feel better; or

- if you are or may be pregnant—talk to your doctor before you start becoming more active.

PLEASE NOTE: If your health changes so that you then answer YES to any of the above questions, tell your fitness or health professional. Ask whether you should change your physical activity plan.

<u>Informed Use of the PAR-Q</u>: The Canadian Society for Exercise Physiology, Health Canada, and their agents assume no liability for persons who undertake physical activity, and if in doubt after completing this questionnaire, consult your doctor prior to physical activity.

No changes permitted. You are encouraged to photocopy the PAR-Q but only if you use the entire form.

NOTE: If the PAR-Q is being given to a person before he or she participates in a physical activity program or a fitness appraisal, this section may be used for legal or administrative purposes.

"I have read, understood and completed this questionnaire. Any questions I had were answered to my full satisfaction."

Name _____

Signature _____   Date _____

Signature of Parent _____   Witness _____
or Guardian (for participants under the age of majority)

Note: This physical activity clearance is valid for a maximum of 12 months from the date it is completed and becomes invalid if your condition changes so that you would answer YES to any of the seven questions.

(Source: Physical Activity Readiness Questionnaire (PAR-Q) ©2002. Reprinted with permission from the Canadian Society for Exercise Physiology. http://www.csep.ca/forms.asp.)

Informed Consent for Exercise Testing of Apparently Healthy Adults
(without known heart disease)

Name: _____

1. Purpose and Explanation of Test

I hereby consent to voluntarily engage in an exercise test to determine my circulatory and respiratory fitness. I also consent to the taking of samples of my exhaled air during exercise to properly measure my oxygen consumption. I also consent, if necessary, to have a small blood sample drawn by needle from my arm for blood chemistry analysis and to the performance of lung function and body fat (skinfold pinch) tests. It is my understanding that the information obtained will help me evaluate future physical activities and sports activities in which I may engage.

Before I undergo the test, I certify to the program that I am in good health and have had a physical examination conducted by a licensed medical physician within the last _____ months. Further, I hereby represent and inform the program that I have accurately completed the pre-test history interview presented to me by the program staff and have provided correct responses to the questions as indicated on the history form or as supplied to the interviewer. It is my understanding that I will be interviewed by a physician or other person prior to my undergoing the test who will in the course of interviewing me determine if there are any reasons which would make it undesirable or unsafe for me to take the test. Consequently, I understand that it is important that I provide complete and accurate responses to the interviewer and recognize that my failure to do so could lead to possible unnecessary injury to myself during the test.

The test which I will undergo will be performed on a motor driven treadmill or bicycle ergometer with the amount of effort gradually increasing. As I understand it, this increase in effort will continue until I feel and verbally report to the operator any symptoms such as fatigue, shortness of breath or chest discomfort which may appear. It is my understanding and I have been clearly advised that it is my right to request that a test be stopped at any point if I feel unusual discomfort or fatigue. I have been advised that I should, immediately upon experiencing any such symptoms or if I so choose, inform the operator that I wish to stop the test at that or any other point. My wishes in this regard shall be absolutely carried out.

It is further my understanding that prior to beginning the test, I will be connected by electrodes and cables to an electrocardiographic recorder which will enable the program personnel to monitor my cardiac (heart) activity. During the test itself, it is my understanding that a trained observer will monitor my responses continuously and take frequent readings of blood pressure, the electrocardiogram, and my expressed feelings of effort. I realize that a true determination of my exercise capacity depends on progressing the test to the point of my fatigue.

Once the test has been completed, but before I am released from the test area, I will be given special instructions about showering and recognition of certain symptoms which may appear within the first 24 hours after the test. I agree to follow these instructions and promptly contact the program personnel or medical providers if such symptoms develop.

2. Risks

It is my understanding and I have been informed that there exists the possibility of adverse changes during the actual test. I have been informed that these changes could include abnormal blood pressure, fainting, disorders of heart rhythm, stroke and very rare instances of heart attack or even death. Every effort, I have been told, will be made to minimize these occurrences by preliminary examination and by precautions and observations taken during the test. I have also been informed that emergency equipment and personnel are readily available to deal with these unusual situations should they occur. I understand that there is a risk of injury, heart attack, stroke or even death as a result of my performance of this test, but knowing those risks, it is my desire to proceed to take the test as herein indicated.

3.   Benefits to be Expected and Alternatives Available to the Exercise Testing Procedure

The results of this test may or may not benefit me. Potential benefits relate mainly to my personal motives for taking the test, i.e., knowing my exercise capacity in relation to the general population, understanding my fitness for certain sports and recreational activities, planning my physical conditioning program or evaluating the effects of my recent physical activity habits. Although my fitness might also be evaluated by alternative means, e.g., a bench step test or an outdoor running test, such tests do not provide as accurate a fitness assessment as the treadmill or bike test nor do those options allow equally effective monitoring of my responses.

4.   Confidentiality and Use of Information

I have been informed that the information which is obtained from this exercise test will be treated as privileged and confidential and will consequently not be released or revealed to any person without my express written consent or as required by law. I do, however, agree to the use of any information for research or statistical purposes so long as same does not provide facts which could lead to the identification of my person. Any other information obtained, however, will be used only by the program staff to evaluate my exercise status or needs.

5.   Inquiries and Freedom of Consent

I have been given an opportunity to ask questions as to the procedure. Generally these requests, which have been noted by the testing staff, and their responses are as follows:

_____

_____

_____

I further understand that there are also other remote risks that may be associated with this procedure. Despite the fact that a complete accounting of all remote risks is not entirely possible, I am satisfied with the review of these risks which was provided to me and it is still my desire to proceed with the test.

I acknowledge that I have read this document in its entirety or that it has been read to me if I have been unable to read same.

I consent to the rendition of all services and procedures as explained herein by all program personnel and to the provision of emergency care response and CPR if necessary.

Date _____   _____

                                                                    Participant's Signature

_____

    Witness's Signature

_____

    Test Supervisor's Signature

Alternative Form for Informed Consent for
Exercise Testing Procedures of Apparently Healthy Adults

Name: _____

1. Purpose and Explanation of Test

It is my understanding that I will undergo a test to be performed on a motor driven treadmill or bicycle ergometer with the amount of effort gradually increasing. As I understand it, this increase in effort will continue until I feel and verbally report to the operator any symptoms such as fatigue, shortness of breath or chest discomfort which may appear or until the test is completed or otherwise terminated. It is my understanding and I have been clearly advised that it is my right to request that a test be stopped at any point if I feel unusual discomfort or fatigue. I have been advised that I should, immediately upon experiencing any such symptoms or if I so choose, inform the operator that I wish to stop the test at that or any other point. My stated wishes in this regard shall be carried out. **IF CORRECT AND YOU AGREE AND UNDERSTAND, INITIAL HERE** _____.

It is further my understanding that prior to beginning the test, I will be connected by electrodes and cables to an electrocardiographic recorder which will enable the program personnel to monitor my cardiac (heart) activity. During the test itself, it is my understanding that a trained observer will monitor my responses continuously and take frequent readings of blood pressure, the electrocardiogram and my expressed feelings of effort. I realize that a true determination of my exercise capacity depends on progressing the test to a point of my fatigue. Once the test has been completed, but before I am released from the test area, I will be given special instructions about showering and recognition of certain symptoms which may appear within the first 24 hours after the test. I agree to follow these instructions and promptly contact the program personnel or medical providers if such symptoms develop. **IF CORRECT AND YOU AGREE AND UNDERSTAND, INITIAL HERE** _____.

Before I undergo the test, I certify to the program that I am in good health and have had a physical examination conducted by a licensed medical physician within the last _____ months. Further, I hereby represent and inform the program that I have accurately completed the pre-test history interview presented to me by the program staff and have provided correct responses to the questions as indicated on the history form or as supplied to the interviewer. It is my understanding that I will be interviewed by a physician or other person prior to my undergoing the test who will, in the course of interviewing me, determine if there are any reasons which would make it undesirable or unsafe for me to take the test. Consequently, I understand that it is important that I provide complete and accurate responses to the interviewer and recognize that my failure to do so could lead to possible unnecessary injury to myself during the test. **IF CORRECT AND YOU AGREE, INITIAL HERE** _____.

2. Risks

It is my understanding, and I have been informed, that there exists the possibility of adverse changes during the actual test. I have been informed that these changes could include abnormal blood pressure, fainting, disorders of heart rhythm, stroke and very rare instances of heart attack or even death. I have also been informed that aside from the foregoing other risks exist. These risks include, but are not necessarily limited to the possibility of stroke, or other cerebrovascular or cardiovascular incident or occurrence, mental, physiological, motor, visual or hearing injuries, deficiencies, difficulties or disturbances, partial or total paralysis, slips, falls, or other unintended loss of balance or bodily movement related to the exercise treadmill (or bicycle ergometer) which may cause muscular, neurological, orthopedic or other bodily injury as well as a variety of other possible occurrences, any one of which could conceivably, however remotely, cause bodily injury, impairment, disability or death. Any procedure such as this one carries with it some risk however unlikely or remote. THERE ARE ALSO OTHER RISKS OF INJURY, IMPAIRMENT, DISABILITY, DISFIGUREMENT, AND EVEN DEATH. I ACKNOWLEDGE AND AGREE TO ASSUME ALL RISKS. **IF YOU UNDERSTAND AND AGREE, INITIAL HERE** _____.

Every effort, I have been told, will be made to minimize these occurrences by preliminary examination and by precautions and observations taken during the test. I have also been informed that emergency equipment and personnel are readily available to deal with these unusual situations should they occur.

Knowing and understanding all risks, it is my desire to proceed to take the test as herein described. **IF CORRECT AND YOU AGREE AND UNDERSTAND, INITIAL HERE _____.**

3. Benefits to be Expected and Alternatives Available to the Exercise Testing Procedure

I understand and have been told that the results of this test may or may not benefit me. Potential benefits relate mainly to my personal motives for taking the test, i.e., knowing my exercise capacity in relation to the general population, understanding my fitness for certain sports and recreational activities, planning my physical conditioning program or evaluating the effects of my recent physical activity habits. Although my fitness might also be evaluated by alternative means, e.g., a bench step test or an outdoor running test, such tests do not provide as accurate a fitness assessment as the treadmill or bike test nor do those options allow equally effective monitoring of my responses. **IF YOU UNDERSTAND, INITIAL HERE _____.**

4. Consent

I hereby consent to voluntarily engage in an exercise test to determine my circulatory and respiratory fitness. I also consent to the taking of samples of my exhaled air during exercise to properly measure my oxygen consumption. I also consent, if necessary, to have a small blood sample drawn by needle from my arm for blood chemistry analysis and to the performance of lung function and body fat (skinfold pinch) tests. It is my understanding that the information obtained will help me evaluate future physical fitness and sports activities in which I may engage. **IF CORRECT AND YOU AGREE, INITIAL HERE _____.**

5. Confidentiality and Use of Information

I have been informed that the information which is obtained in this exercise test will be treated as privileged and confidential and will consequently not be released or revealed to any person without my express written consent or as required by law. I do, however, agree to the use of any information for research or statistical purposes, so long as same does not provide facts which could lead to the identification of my person. Any other information obtained, however, will be used only by the program staff to evaluate my exercise status or needs. **IF YOU AGREE, INITIAL HERE _____.**

6. Inquiries and Freedom of Consent

I have been given an opportunity to ask questions as to the procedures. Generally these requests, which have been noted by the testing staff, and their responses are as follows:

_____

IF THIS NOTATION IS COMPLETE AND CORRECT, INITIAL HERE _____.

I acknowledge that I have read this document in its entirety or that it has been read to me if I have been unable to read same.

I consent to the rendition of all services and procedures as explained herein by all program personnel and to the provision of emergency care response and CPR if necessary.

I consent to the rendition of all services and procedures as explained herein by all program personnel and to the provision of emergency care response and CPR if necessary.

Date _____

_____ _____
Witness's Signature   Participant's Signature

_____ _____
Witness's Signature   Spouse's Consent

                                 _____
                                 Test Supervisor's Signature

Informed Consent for Participation in an Exercise Program for Apparently Healthy Adults
(without known or suspected heart disease)

Name: _____

1. Purpose and Explanation of Procedure

I hereby consent to voluntarily engage in a program of exercise conditioning. I also give consent to be placed in program activities which are recommended to me for improvement of my general health and well-being. These may include dietary counseling, stress reduction, and health education activities. The levels of exercise which I will perform will be based upon my cardiorespiratory (heart and lungs) fitness as determined through my recent laboratory graded exercise evaluation. I will be given exact instructions regarding the amount and kind of exercise I should do. I agree to participate three times per week in the formal program sessions. Professionally trained personnel will provide leadership to direct my activities, monitor my performance, and otherwise evaluate my effort. Depending upon my health status, I may or may not be required to have my blood pressure and heart rate evaluated during these sessions to regulate my exercise within desired limits. I understand that I am expected to attend every session and to follow staff instructions with regard to exercise, diet, stress management, and smoking cessation. If I am taking prescribed medications, I have already so informed the program staff and further agree to so inform them promptly of any changes which my doctor or I have made with regard to use of these. I will be given the opportunity for periodic assessment with laboratory evaluations at 6 months after the start of my program. Should I remain in the program thereafter, additional evaluations will generally be given at 12 month intervals. The program may change the foregoing schedule of evaluations if this is considered desirable for health reasons.

I have been informed that during my participation in exercise, I will be asked to complete the physical activities unless symptoms such as fatigue, shortness of breath, chest discomfort or similar occurrences appear. At that point, I have been advised it is my complete right to decrease or stop exercise and that it is my obligation to inform the program personnel of my symptoms. I hereby state that I have been so advised and agree to inform the program personnel of my symptoms, should any develop.

I understand that during the performance of exercise, a trained observer will periodically monitor my performance and perhaps measure my pulse, blood pressure, or assess my feelings of effort for the purposes of monitoring my progress. I also understand that the observer may reduce or stop my exercise program when any of these findings so indicate that this should be done for my safety and benefit.

2. Risks

It is my understanding, and I have been informed, that there exists the remote possibility during exercise of adverse changes, including abnormal blood pressure, fainting, disorders of heart rhythm, and very rare instances of heart attack, stroke or even death, as well as other risks of injury or impairment, due to my participation in activity. Often injuries to bones, muscles, tendons, ligaments, and other parts of my body may also occur. Every effort, I have been told, will be made to minimize these occurrences by proper staff assessment of my condition before each exercise session, through staff supervision during exercise and by my own careful control of exercise efforts. I have also been informed that emergency equipment and personnel are readily available to deal with unusual situations should these occur. I understand that there is a risk of injury, heart attack or even death as a result of my exercise, but knowing those risks, it is my desire to participate as herein indicated.

3. Benefits to be Expected and Alternatives Available to Exercise

I understand that this program may or may not benefit my physical fitness or general health. I recognize that involvement in the exercise sessions will allow me to learn proper ways to perform conditioning exercises, use fitness equipment, and regulate physical effort. These experiences should benefit me by indicating how my physical limitations may affect my ability to perform various physical activities. I further understand that if I closely follow the program instructions, that I will likely improve my exercise capacity after a period of three (3) to six (6) months.

4. Confidentiality and Use of Information

I have been informed that the information which is obtained in this exercise program will be treated as privileged and confidential and will consequently not be released or revealed to any person without my express written consent or as required by law. I do, however, agree to the use of any information which is not personally identifiable with me for research and statistical purposes so long as same does not identify my person or provide facts which could lead to my identification. Any other information obtained, however, will be used only by the program staff in the course of prescribing exercise for me and evaluating my progress in the program.

5. Inquiries and Freedom of Consent

I have been given an opportunity to ask certain questions as to the procedures of this program. Generally speaking, the questions I have asked, which have been noted by the interviewing staff member, and the responses I have received from that staff member are as follows:

_____

_____

_____

I further understand that there are also other remote risks that may be associated with this program. Despite the fact that a complete accounting of all these remote risks is not entirely possible, I am satisfied with the review of these risks which was provided to me and it is still my desire to participate.

I acknowledge that I have read this document in its entirety or that it has been read to me if I have been unable to read same.

I consent to the rendition of all services and procedures as explained herein by all program personnel and to the provision of emergency care response and CPR if necessary.

Date _____   _____
                                                    Participant's Signature

_____
        Witness's Signature

_____
        Test Supervisor's Signature

Agreement and Release of Liability

1. In consideration of being allowed to participate in the activities and programs of _____ _____ and to use its facilities, equipment and machinery, in addition to the payment of any fee or charge, I do hereby waive, release and forever discharge _____ and its directors, officers, agents, employees, representatives, successors and assigns, administrators, executors, and all others from any and all responsibilities or liability from injuries or damages resulting from my participation in any activities or my use of facilities, equipment or machinery in the above mentioned activities. I do also hereby release all of those mentioned and any others acting upon their behalf from any responsibility or liability for any injury or damage to myself, including those caused by the ordinary negligence of the program or any of its agents due to any such ordinary negligent act or omission of any of those mentioned or others acting on their behalf or in any way arising out of or connected with my participation in any activities of _____ or the use of any facilities/equipment or machinery at _____. I acknowledge and understand that this release is given in advance of any injury or damage to me and that it includes injury or damage to me caused by the ordinary negligence of those released hereby but not from any claims related to gross negligence or willful/wanton/criminal/intentional conduct or acts of those who are otherwise released hereby.

   IF YOU UNDERSTAND AND AGREE, PLEASE INITIAL _____.

2. I understand and am aware that strength, flexibility and aerobic exercise, including the use of equipment, is a potentially hazardous activity. I also understand that fitness activities involve the risk of injury and even death, and that I am voluntarily participating in these activities and using facilities, equipment and machinery with knowledge of the dangers involved. I hereby agree to expressly assume and accept any and all risks of injury or death.

   IF YOU UNDERSTAND AND AGREE, PLEASE INITIAL _____.

3. I do hereby further declare myself to be physically sound and suffering from no condition, impairment, disease, infirmity or other illness that would prevent my participation or use of equipment or machinery except as hereinafter stated. I do hereby acknowledge that I have been informed of the need for a physician's approval for my participation in an exercise/fitness activity or in the use of exercise equipment and machinery. I also acknowledge that it has been recommended that I have a yearly or more frequent physical examination and consultation with my physician as to physical activity, exercise and use of exercise and training equipment so that I might have his recommendations concerning these fitness activities and equipment use. I acknowledge that I have either had a physical examination and have been given my physician's permission to participate, or that I have decided to participate in activity and use of equipment and machinery without the approval of my physician and do hereby assume all responsibility for my participation and activities, and utilization of equipment and machinery in my activities.

   IF YOU UNDERSTAND AND AGREE, PLEASE INITIAL _____.

   This Agreement shall be binding upon the undersigned, his/her heirs, executors, administrators and assigns.

Date _____   _____
                                              Signature

Alternative Form–Express Assumption of Risk/Prospective Waiver of Liability and Release Agreement

I, the undersigned, hereby expressly and affirmatively state that I wish to participate in fitness assessments, activities and programs and in the use of exercise equipment at various sites, including home, club or worksite, that may be provided or recommended by (_____) (hereinafter "Facility"). I realize that my participation in these activities or in the use of equipment involves various risks of injury including, but not limited to (list) _____

_____

and even the possibility of death. I also recognize that there are many other risks of injury, including serious disabling injuries, that may arise due to my participation in these activities or in the use of equipment and that such risks, including remote ones, have been reviewed with me. I also understand that under some circumstances I may choose to engage in activity in a non-supervised setting under circumstances where there is no one to respond to any emergency that may arise as a result of my participation or use of equipment on an individual basis, in an unsupervised setting. Despite the fact that I have been duly cautioned as to such unsupervised and unattended activity or equipment use, and despite the fact that I have been advised against such activity and equipment use in an unsupervised and unattended setting, I, knowing the material risks and appreciating, knowing and reasonably anticipating that other injuries and even death are a possibility as a result of my participation in fitness assessments, activities or programs, or in the use of equipment in supervised/attended and unsupervised/unattended settings (within which settings I acknowledge that the risks of injury or death may be greater than in other settings), I hereby expressly assume all of the delineated risks of injury, all other possible risks of injury and even the risk of death which could occur by reason of my participation in any of the assessments, activities or programs or in the use of equipment in any or all settings. **IF YOU UNDERSTAND AND AGREE, PLEASE INITIAL _____.**

I have had an opportunity to ask questions regarding my participation in various activities and in the use of exercise equipment. Any questions I have asked have been answered to my complete satisfaction. I subjectively understand the risks of my participation in various activities or in the use of equipment and knowing and appreciating these risks, I voluntarily choose to participate, assuming all risks of injury and death which may arise due to my participation. **IF YOU UNDERSTAND AND AGREE, PLEASE INITIAL _____.**

I further acknowledge that my participation in the activities and use of equipment is completely voluntary and that it is my choice to participate and/or reuse equipment or not to participate as I see fit. **IF YOU UNDERSTAND AND AGREE, PLEASE INITIAL _____.**

In consideration of being allowed to participate in the activities and programs provided through Facility and/or in the use of its facilities, equipment and machinery, I do hereby waive, release and forever discharge Facility, and all of its directors, officers, agents, employees, representatives, successors and assigns, and all others from any and all responsibility or liability for injuries or damages resulting from my participation in any activities at Facility or elsewhere. I do also hereby release all of those mentioned and any others acting on their behalf from any responsibility or liability for any injury or damage to myself, including those caused by the ordinary negligence of the program or any of its agents due to any such ordinary negligent act or omission of any of those mentioned or others acting on their behalf or in any way arising out of or connected with my participation in any of the contemplated activities or in the use of equipment through Facility or otherwise. I acknowl edge that this release is given in advance of any injury or damage to me and that it includes injury or damage to me caused by the ordinary negligence of those released hereby but shall not apply to any claims related to gross negligence, or willful/wanton/criminal/intentional conduct or acts of those who are otherwise released hereby. **IF YOU UNDERSTAND AND AGREE, PLEASE INITIAL _____.**

I understand and am aware that strength, flexibility and aerobic exercise, including the use of equipment, is a potentially hazardous activity. I also understand that fitness activities involve a risk of injury and even death and that I am voluntarily participating in these activities and using equipment with knowledge of the dangers involved. **IF YOU UNDERSTAND AND AGREE, PLEASE INITIAL _____.**

I do further declare myself to be physically sound and suffering from no condition, impairment, disease, infirmity or other illness that would prevent my participation in any of the activities and programs provided through Facility or in the use of equipment and machinery except as hereinafter stated: _____ _____. I do hereby acknowledge that I have been informed of the need or desirability for a physician's approval for my participation in exercise/fitness activity or in the use of exercise equipment. I also acknowledge that it has been recommended that I have a yearly or more frequent physical examination and consultation with my physician as to physical activities and exercise, and as to the use of exercise equipment, so that I might have recommendations concerning these physical activities and equipment use. I acknowledge that I have either had a physical examination and have been given my physician's permission to participate or that I have decided to participate in activity and/or use of equipment without the approval of my physician and do hereby assume all responsibility for my participation and activities or in the utilization of equipment without that approval. **IF YOU UNDERSTAND AND AGREE, PLEASE INITIAL _____.**

I, the undersigned spouse of the participant, do hereby further acknowledge that my spouse (participant) wishes to engage in certain activities and programs provided by Facility including the use of various facilities and equipment. In consideration of my spouse's (participant's) voluntary decision to engage in such activities, and in consideration of the provision of such activities and equipment to spouse by Facility, I, the undersigned, do hereby waive, release and forever discharge Facility and its directors, officers, agents, employees, representatives, successors and assigns, and all others from any and all responsibility or liability for any injuries or damages resulting from my spouse's participation in any activities or in my spouse's use of equipment as a result of participation in any such activities or otherwise arising out of that participation. I do further release all of those above mentioned and any others acting upon their behalf from any responsibility or liability for any injury to, or even death of, my spouse, including that caused by the ordinary negligent act or omission of any of those mentioned or others acting upon their behalf, or in any way arising out of or connected with my spouse's participation in any of the activities provided by Facility or in the use of any equipment at any location, but shall not apply to any claims related to gross negligence or willfull/wanton/criminal/intentional conduct or acts. I specifically acknowledge that my execution of this prospective Waiver and Release relinquishes any cause of action that I may have either directly through my spouse or independently by way of a loss of consortium or other type of action of any kind or nature whatsoever and I do hereby further agree to my spouse's participation in the activities as above mentioned and in the use of any equipment at any location. **IF SPOUSE UNDERSTANDS AND AGREES, SPOUSE TO INITIAL HERE _____.**

IN WITNESS WHEREOF, the participant and the participant's spouse, if any, have executed this Express Assumption of Risk/Prospective Waiver of Liability and Release Agreement this _____ day of_____, 20___, which shall be binding upon each of them and their respective heirs, executors, administrators and assigns. Each does hereby further agree to indemnify and hold Facility and all those identified or named herein absolutely harmless in the event that anyone claiming any cause of action as a result of any injury and/or death to participant or spouse attempts at any time to institute any claim or suit against the Facility arising out of any of the activities or programs herein or in the use of any equipment.

Signed in the presence of:

_____   _____
                                                    Participant

_____   _____
                                                Participant's Spouse

Express Assumption of Risk for Participation in Specified Activity

I, the undersigned, hereby expressly and affirmatively state that I wish to participate in _____. I realize that my participation in this activity involves risks of injury, including but not to limited to (list) _____ _____ and even the possibility of death. I also recognize that there are many other risks of injury, including serious disabling injuries, which may arise due to my participation in this activity and that it is not possible to specifically list each and every individual injury risk. However, knowing the material risks and appreciating them, and knowing and reasonably anticipating that other injuries and even death are a possibility, I hereby expressly assume all of the delineated risks of injury, all other possible risks of injury and even death which could occur by reason of my participation.

I have had an opportunity to ask questions. Any questions which I have asked have been answered to my complete satisfaction. I subjectively understand the risks of my participation in this activity, and knowing and appreciating these risks I voluntarily choose to participate, assuming all risks of injury or even death due to my participation.

_____   _____
            Witness   Participant

Date _____

NOTES OF QUESTIONS AND ANSWERS

_____

_____

_____

_____

_____

This is as stated, a true and accurate record of what was asked and answered.

                              _____
                                        Participant

Exercise and Activity Quiz

Name:_____ Date: _____

How fit do you feel now? _____
(assign #1-5 with 1 being poor and 5 being excellent)

Exercise/activity habits:

In an average day, I climb _____ flights of stairs (~12 stairs/flight).

My job requires that I be on my feet and moving _____ hours a day (example: waitress, industrial inspector, nurse). Count actual time moving only.

My job requires that I be on my feet _____ hours a day, but I move around very little (example: sales clerk).

In an average day I walk _____ miles (walking at least one mile at a time without stopping).

I spend about _____ hours a week tending a garden or lawn.

I am a parent who assumes primary responsibility for a preschool child ____.

— child and parent at home all day

— child spends half day in day care

— child spends full day in day care

My job is physically demanding (lifting, carrying, shoveling, climbing) for _____ hours a day (consider only the time you are actually involved in vigorous activity).

I perform household chores (laundry, cleaning, cooking) an average of _____ hours a week.

I have a desk job, but leave my desk regularly to run errands, greet visitors, attend meetings, etc. at least _____ times an hour.

I engage in light sports activities (doubles tennis, softball, volleyball, social dancing) _____ hours a week.

I engage in vigorous exercise ____ times a week for _____ minutes each time.

Please list your fitness goals: _____

Why are these goals important to you? _____

_____

How long do you think it will take to achieve these goals?_____

How committed are you to improving your fitness at this time? _____

What are your favorite exercise activities? _____

_____

What types of exercise have you tried in the past? _____

Have you had any negative exercise experiences? _____

Nutrition and Weight Profile

Name: _____ Date: _____

What is your current weight? _____ What would you like to weigh? _____

If you are trying to lose weight:

What is the most you have weighed as an adult? _____

What is the least you have weighed as an adult? _____

How long did you maintain this weight? _____

What is the lowest weight you have maintained for a year? _____

How many times have you lost and regained weight? _____

What types of diets have you tried? _____

If you have high blood pressure or high cholesterol,
at what weight did these problems develop? _____

Do you have parents or siblings who are overweight?   Yes ❏   No ❏

Is this a good time in your life to commit to a weight loss program (think about possible pressing responsibilities, unusual stressors or distractions, etc.)?   Yes ❏   No ❏

What obstacles are in the way of achieving your goal? _____

_____

Which do you eat regularly (check all that apply):
❏ Breakfast   ❏ Lunch   ❏ Dinner
❏ Midmorning snack   ❏ Midafternoon snack ❏ After-dinner snack

How often do you eat out each week? _____ times

What size portions do you normally have?
❏ Small   ❏ Moderate   ❏ Large   ❏ Extra-large   ❏ Uncertain

How often do you eat more than one serving?
❏ Always   ❏ Usually   ❏ Sometimes   ❏ Never

How long does it usually take you to eat a meal? _____ minutes

Do you eat while doing other activities (e.g., watching TV, reading, working)?   Yes ❏   No ❏

How many times a week do you eat or drink the following?

_____ cookies, cake, pie

_____ candy

_____ doughnuts

_____ ice cream

_____ commercial muffins

_____   soft drinks

_____   potato chips, corn chips, etc.

_____   fried foods

_____   peanut butter, nuts or seeds

_____   crackers

_____   fast food (McDonald's, Taco Bell, etc.)

_____   cheese

_____   whole milk, cream, non-dairy creamer

_____   red meat (beef, pork, lamb)

_____   butter, margarine, mayonnaise

_____   breakfast meat or luncheon meat (bacon, sausage, hot dogs, salami)

_____   convenience items (frozen foods, instant products, canned soup, etc.)

_____   refined grains (e.g., white rice & breads) vs. whole grain

_____   more than one serving of alcohol daily (4 oz. wine, 1.5 oz. liquor, 12 oz. beer)

_____   more than two servings of a caffeinated beverage in a day

How many servings of the following foods do you eat each day:

_____   fruit (1 small whole, or ½ cup)

_____   vegetables (½ cup)

_____   bread (1 slice)

_____   cereal (½ cup)

_____   pasta, rice, other grain (½ cup)

_____   dairy product (½ cup)

_____   meat (3 oz.)

_____   dried beans, peas, tofu, etc. (½ cup)

Self-Assessment Quiz

The following questionnaire is designed to increase your knowledge and awareness of your overall health, and to highlight potential areas of concern. It doesn't pinpoint how you compare to the rest of the population, but the scoring chart at the end will show you areas where you are making healthy choices and where there is room for improvement. Keep in mind that although health risks associated with age, gender, and heredity are beyond your control, you can modify a range of other factors, such as blood pressure, smoking, blood cholesterol levels, exercise, diet, stress, and excess body weight.

Section A: PHYSICAL FITNESS

1. Do you exercise or play a sport for at least thirty minutes three or more times a week? — Yes ❑ No ❑

2. Do you warm up and cool down by stretching before and after exercising? — Yes ❑ No ❑

3. Do you fall into the appropriate weight category for someone your height and gender? — Yes ❑ No ❑

4. In general, are you pleased with the condition of your body? — Yes ❑ No ❑

5. Are you satisfied with your current level of energy? — Yes ❑ No ❑

6. Do you use stairs rather than escalators or elevators whenever possible? — Yes ❑ No ❑

NUMBER OF ANSWERS EACH COLUMN ____ ____

Section B: FAMILY HISTORY

Do you have a grandparent, parent, aunt, uncle, brother, or sister who:

1. Had a heart attack before age forty? — No ❑ Yes ❑

2. Had high blood pressure requiring treatment? — No ❑ Yes ❑

3. Developed diabetes? — No ❑ Yes ❑

4. Developed glaucoma? — No ❑ Yes ❑

5. Developed gout? — No ❑ Yes ❑

6. Developed breast cancer? — No ❑ Yes ❑

NUMBER OF ANSWERS EACH COLUMN ____ ____

Section C: SELF-CARE AND MEDICAL CARE

1. Do you floss your teeth daily? — Yes ❑ No ❑

2. Do you have a dental checkup at least one a year? — Yes ❑ No ❑

3. Do you use sunscreen regularly and avoid extensive exposure to the sun? — Yes ❑ No ❑

4. For women: do you examine your breasts for unusual changes or lumps at least once a month? — Yes ❑ No ❑

5. For men: do you examine your testicles for unusual changes or lumps at least once every three months? — Yes ❑ No ❑

6. Do you usually know what to do in case of illness or injury? — Yes ❑ No ❑

7. Do you avoid unnecessary X-rays? — Yes ❑ No ❑

8. Do you normally get an adequate amount of sleep? — Yes ❑ No ❑

9. Have you had your blood pressure checked in the past year?   Yes ❑   No ❑

10. For women: have you had a Pap smear within the last two years?   Yes ❑   No ❑

11. If you are over forty: have you had a test for glaucoma within the last four years?   Yes ❑   No ❑

12. If you are over forty: have you had a test for hidden blood in your stool
    within the last two years? If you are over fifty: within the last year?   Yes ❑   No ❑

13. If you are over fifty: have you had a least one endoscopic exam of the lower bowel?   Yes ❑   No ❑

NUMBER OF ANSWERS EACH COLUMN   ____   ____

Section D: EATING HABITS

1. Do you drink enough fluids so that your urine is a pale yellow color?   Yes ❑   No ❑

2. Do you try special or fad diets?   No ❑   Yes ❑

3. Do you add salt to foods during cooking and at the table?   No ❑   Yes ❑

4. Do you minimize your intake of sweets, especially candy and soft drinks,
    and avoid adding sugar to foods?   Yes ❑   No ❑

5. Is your diet well-balanced (including vegetables, fruits, breads, cereals,
    dairy products, and adequate sources of protein)?   Yes ❑   No ❑

6. Do you limit your intake of saturated fats (butter, cheese, cream, fatty meats)?   Yes ❑   No ❑

7. Do you limit your intake of cholesterol (eggs, liver, meats)?   Yes ❑   No ❑

8. Do you eat fish and poultry more often than red meats?   Yes ❑   No ❑

9. Do you eat high-fiber foods (vegetables, fruits, whole grains) several times a day?   Yes ❑   No ❑

NUMBER OF ANSWERS EACH COLUMN   ____   ____

Section E: ALCOHOL, NICOTINE, AND OTHER DRUG USE

1. Do you smoke cigarettes, cigars, or a pipe, chew tobacco, or use other drugs?   No ❑   Yes ❑

2. Do you limit yourself to no more than two drinks a day?   Yes ❑   No ❑

3. Have family members or friends ever commented on or complained
    about your drinking or your use of other drugs?   No ❑   Yes ❑

4. Have you been unable to recall things you did when you are drinking or
    using other drugs?   No ❑   Yes ❑

5. Do you use alcohol or other drugs as a way of handling stressful
    situations or problems in your life?   No ❑   Yes ❑

6. Do you read and follow the label directions when using prescribed
    and over-the-counter drugs?   Yes ❑   No ❑

NUMBER OF ANSWERS EACH COLUMN   ____   ____

Section F: ACCIDENTS

1. Do you drive after drinking alcohol or using other drugs, or ride with
    drivers who have been drinking or using other drugs?   No ❑   Yes ❑

2. Do you obey traffic rules and stay within the speed limit when you drive?   Yes ❑   No ❑

3. As a driver and passenger, do you wear a seat belt at all times?   Yes ❑   No ❑

4. Are the vehicles you drive well-maintained?   Yes ❑   No ❑

5. Do you smoke in bed?   No ❑   Yes ❑

6. Are you informed and careful when using potentially harmful products or substances, such as household cleaners, poisons, flammables, solvents, and electrical devices?   Yes ❑   No ❑

7. Do you own a gun?   No ❑   Yes ❑

NUMBER OF ANSWERS EACH COLUMN   ____   ____

Section G: INTELLECTUAL LIFE, VALUES, AND SPIRITUALITY

1. Are you interested in, and do you keep up to date on, social and political issues?   Yes ❑   No ❑

2. Are you satisfied with what you do for entertainment?   Yes ❑   No ❑

3. Do you engage in creative and stimulating activities as often as you would like?   Yes ❑   No ❑

4. Are you satisfied with the degree to which your work is consistent with your values?   Yes ❑   No ❑

5. Are you satisfied with the degree to which your leisure activities are consistent with your values?   Yes ❑   No ❑

6. Is it difficult for you to accept the values and life-styles of others when they are different from your own?   No ❑   Yes ❑

7. Are you satisfied with your spiritual life?   Yes ❑   No ❑

NUMBER OF ANSWERS EACH COLUMN   ____   ____

Section H: STRESS AND SOCIAL SUPPORT

1. Are you satisfied with the amount of excitement in your life?   Yes ❑   No ❑

2. Do you find it easy to laugh?   Yes ❑   No ❑

3. Do you hold in your angry feelings without expressing them?   No ❑   Yes ❑

4. Do you make decisions with minimum stress and worry?   Yes ❑   No ❑

5. Do you include relaxation time as part of your daily routine?   Yes ❑   No ❑

6. Do you anticipate and prepare for events or situations likely to be stressful?   Yes ❑   No ❑

7. Have you had to make difficult readjustments at home or work in the past year?   Yes ❑   No ❑

8. Has a family member or close friend died, been seriously ill, or been injured within the past year?   No ❑   Yes ❑

9. Are you a chronic worrier, subject to guilt feelings or self-punishment?   No ❑   Yes ❑

10. Have your health, eating, or sleeping habits changed as a result of a stressful incident or situation during the past year?   No ❑   Yes ❑

11. Are you able to fall asleep when you are ready and to sleep through the night uninterrupted?   Yes ❑   No ❑

12. Do you wake up feeling rested?   Yes ❑   No ❑

13. Do you have one or more persons with whom you can discuss personal concerns, worries, or problems?   Yes ❑   No ❑

14. Do they make you feel respected and/or admired?   Yes ❏ No ❏

15. Is there someone to whom you can turn if you need help, such as
    to lend you money?   Yes ❏ No ❏

16. Are you satisfied with the support you provide to others?   Yes ❏ No ❏

NUMBER OF ANSWERS EACH COLUMN ____ ____

Section I: **ENVIRONMENT**

1. Are you often in an environment that has significant air and/or noise pollution?   No ❏ Yes ❏

2. Are you often exposed to asbestos, vinyl chloride, formaldehyde, or other toxins?   No ❏ Yes ❏

3. Do you miss many days at work due to illness or just not feeling up to it?
   ("Work" refers to daily activities, including school or work in the home.)   No ❏ Yes ❏

4. Do you often sit for periods of an hour or more at a time?   No ❏ Yes ❏

5. Are you satisfied with your ability to plan your workload?   Yes ❏ No ❏

6. Do you receive adequate feedback to judge your performance?   Yes ❏ No ❏

7. Are you satisfied with your balance between work and leisure time?   Yes ❏ No ❏

NUMBER OF ANSWERS EACH COLUMN ____ ____

Section J: **SEXUALITY**

1. Are you satisfied with your level of sexual activity?   Yes ❏ No ❏

2. Are you satisfied with your sexual relationship?   Yes ❏ No ❏

3. Are you satisfied with your use (or nonuse) of contraceptives?   Yes ❏ No ❏

4. Are you satisfied with your use (or nonuse) of "safer sex" practices?   Yes ❏ No ❏

NUMBER OF ANSWERS EACH COLUMN ____ ____

Scoring the Self-Assessment Quiz

For each section of the quiz, write the number of answers you marked in the left-hand column in the blanks below.

Sections: A____   B____   C____   D____   E____   F____   G____   H____   I____   J____

In the circle graph below, shade in the number of subsections to correspond with the numbers you wrote above. Start with the innermost section. For example, if there are four answers marked in the left-hand answer column of Section D, that portion of the circle graph will look like this:

Sections that are completely shaded: you are making healthy behavior and life-style choices in these areas. Keep up the good work.

Sections that are partially shaded: with a little more awareness and effort in these areas, you could improve the quality of your life—and live longer.

Sections that are barely shaded or not shaded at all: there is significant room for increasing your health and satisfaction in these areas. Work first on those areas where you are most likely to be successful, then tackle the tougher sections.

Note: This grading system doesn't apply to section B since you have no control over your family history. If you answered "yes" to several questions about family history, try to compensate by concentrating on the other areas over which you do have control.

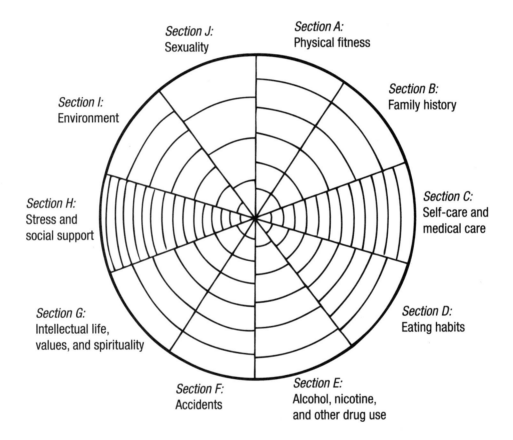

Fitness Assessment Data Sheet

Name _____ Date _____

Age _____ Wt. _____ Ht. _____ _____ Medications _____

Risk Factor Status _____

Resting HR _____   Resting BP   (1) _____   (2) _____

Skinfolds: WOMEN   MEN

             Triceps   ___ ___ ___   Pectoral   ___ ___ ___

             Suprailiac   ___ ___ ___   Abdomen   ___ ___ ___

             Thigh   ___ ___ ___   Thigh   ___ ___ ___

Estimated % Body Fat _____

Waist-to-Hip Ratio (divide waist by hip)   _____

BMI   _____

Circumferences:

Waist _____ Hip _____ Thigh _____

Calf _____ Upper arms _____ Forearm _____

Step Test (60 sec. HR) _____ Rockport Walking Test (60 sec. HR) _____

Comments   _____

_____

Bench Press 1 RM _____ /Wt. in lb. _____ = _____

Crunch Test (#/min.)   _____

Push-up Test (total #)   _____

Sit and Reach Test (inches) _____

Muscle-Specific Flexibility Tests

	Adequate	Needs improvement
Hamstrings	_____	_____
Iliopsoas	_____	_____
Quadriceps	_____	_____
Calves	_____	_____
Shoulders	_____	_____

Posture Assessments (visual)

	Yes	No
Lordosis	_____	_____
Kyphosis	_____	_____
Forward head	_____	_____
Hip height discrepancy	_____	_____
Shoulder height	_____	_____

Percent Fat Estimations For Men

Sum of Three Skinfolds	Age (years)								
	18–22	23–27	28–32	33–37	38–42	43–47	48–52	53–57	> 57
8–12	1.8	2.6	3.4	4.2	4.9	5.7	6.5	7.3	8.1
13–17	3.6	4.4	5.2	6.0	6.8	7.6	8.4	9.1	9.9
18–22	5.4	6.2	7.0	7.8	8.6	9.3	10.1	10.9	11.7
23–27	7.1	7.9	8.7	9.5	10.3	11.1	11.9	12.6	13.4
28–32	8.8	9.6	10.4	11.2	12.0	12.8	13.5	14.3	15.1
33–37	10.4	11.2	12.0	12.8	13.6	14.4	15.2	15.9	16.7
38–42	12.0	12.8	13.6	14.4	15.2	15.9	16.7	17.5	18.3
43–47	13.5	14.3	15.1	15.9	16.7	17.5	18.3	19.0	19.8
48–52	15.0	15.8	16.6	17.4	18.1	18.9	19.8	20.5	21.3
53–57	17.8	18.5	19.3	20.1	20.9	21.7	22.5	23.3	24.1
58–62	19.1	19.9	20.6	21.4	22.2	23.0	23.8	24.5	25.4
63–67	20.3	21.1	21.9	22.7	23.5	23.8	25.1	25.8	26.6
68–72	21.5	22.3	23.1	23.9	24.7	25.5	26.3	27.0	27.8
73–77	22.7	23.5	24.3	25.0	25.8	26.6	27.4	28.2	29.0
78–82	23.8	24.6	26.4	27.2	28.0	28.8	29.6	30.3	31.1
83–87	24.8	25.6	26.4	27.2	28.0	28.8	29.6	30.3	31.1
88–92	25.8	26.6	27.4	28.2	29.0	29.8	30.5	31.3	32.3
93–97	26.7	27.5	28.3	29.1	29.9	30.7	31.5	32.3	33.4
98–102	27.6	28.0	29.2	30.0	30.8	31.6	32.4	33.2	33.9
103–107	28.5	29.3	30.1	30.8	31.6	32.4	33.2	34.0	34.8
108–112	29.3	30.0	30.8	31.6	32.4	33.2	32.0	34.8	35.6
113–117	30.0	30.8	31.6	32.4	33.1	33.9	34.7	35.5	36.3
118–122	30.7	31.5	32.3	33.0	33.8	34.6	35.4	36.2	37.0
123–127	31.3	32.1	32.9	33.7	34.4	35.2	36.0	36.8	37.6
133–137	31.9	32.7	33.4	42.2	45.0	35.8	36.6	37.4	38.2
138–142	32.4	33.6	34.4	35.2	36.0	36.8	37.6	38.4	39.2
143–147	32.9	33.6	34.4	25.2	36.0	36.8	37.6	38.4	39.2
148–152	33.3	34.1	34.8	35.6	36.4	37.2	38.0	38.8	39.6
153–157	33.6	34.4	35.2	36.0	36.8	37.6	38.4	39.2	39.9
158–162	33.9	34.7	35.5	36.3	37.1	37.9	38.7	39.5	40.3
163–167	34.2	35.0	35.8	36.3	37.4	38.1	38.9	39.7	40.5
168–172	34.4	35.2	36.0	36.8	37.6	38.4	39.1	39.9	40.7
173–177	34.6	35.3	36.1	36.9	37.8	38.5	39.2	40.1	40.9
178–182	34.7	35.4	36.2	37.0	37.8	38.6	39.4	40.2	42.1

(Source: Jackson, A.S., & Pollock, M.L. [1985]. Tables determining relative body fat percent for men & women. *The Physician and Sportsmedicine, 13*[5], 76-90.)

Percent Fat Estimations For Women

Sum of Three Skinfolds	Age (years)								
	18–22	23–27	28–32	33–37	38–42	43–47	48–52	53–57	> 57
8–12	8.0	9.0	9.2	9.4	9.5	9.7	9.9	10.1	10.3
13–17	10.8	10.9	11.1	11.3	11.5	11.7	11.8	12.0	12.2
18–22	12.6	12.8	13.0	13.2	13.4	13.5	13.7	13.9	14.1
23–27	14.5	14.6	14.8	15.0	15.2	15.4	15.6	15.7	15.9
28–32	16.2	16.4	16.6	16.8	17.0	17.1	17.3	17.5	17.7
33–37	17.9	18.1	18.3	18.5	18.7	18.9	19.0	19.2	19.4
38–42	19.6	19.8	20.0	20.2	20.3	20.5	20.7	20.9	21.1
43–47	21.2	21.4	21.6	21.8	21.9	22.1	22.3	22.5	22.7
48–52	22.8	22.9	23.1	23.3	23.5	23.7	23.8	24.0	24.2
53–57	24.4	24.4	24.6	24.8	25.0	25.2	25.3	25.5	25.7
58–62	25.7	25.9	26.0	26.2	26.4	26.6	26.8	27.0	27.1
63–67	27.1	27.2	27.4	27.6	27.8	28.0	28.2	28.3	28.5
68–72	28.4	28.6	28.7	28.9	29.1	29.3	29.5	29.7	29.8
73–77	29.6	29.8	30.0	30.2	30.4	30.6	30.7	30.9	31.3
78–82	30.9	31.0	31.2	31.4	31.6	31.8	31.9	32.1	32.3
83–87	30.0	32.2	32.4	32.6	32.7	32.9	33.1	33.3	33.5
88–92	33.1	33.3	33.5	33.7	33.8	34.0	34.2	34.4	34.6
93–97	34.2	34.4	34.5	34.7	34.9	35.1	35.2	35.4	35.6
98–102	35.1	35.3	35.5	35.7	35.9	36.0	36.2	36.6	36.7
103–107	36.1	36.2	36.4	36.6	36.8	37.0	37.2	37.3	37.5
108–112	36.9	37.1	37.3	37.5	37.7	37.9	38.0	38.2	38.4
113–117	37.9	38.9	38.1	38.3	39.2	39.4	39.6	39.8	39.5
118–122	38.5	38.7	38.9	39.1	39.4	39.6	39.8	40.0	40.0
123–127	39.2	39.4	49.6	39.8	40.0	40.2	40.3	40.5	40.7
133–137	40.5	40.7	40.8	41.0	41.2	41.4	41.6	41.7	41.9
138–142	41.0	41.2	41.4	41.6	41.7	41.9	42.1	42.3	42.5
143–147	41.5	41.7	41.9	42.0	42.2	42.4	42.6	42.8	43.0
153–157	42.3	42.5	42.6	42.8	43.0	43.2	43.4	43.6	43.4
158–162	42.6	42.8	42.0	43.1	43.4	43.5	43.7	43.9	44.1
163–167	42.9	43.0	43.2	43.4	43.6	43.8	44.0	44.1	44.3
168–172	43.1	43.2	43.4	43.6	43.8	44.0	44.2	44.3	44.5
173–177	43.2	43.4	43.6	43.8	43.9	44.1	44.3	44.5	44.7
178–182	43.3	43.5	43.7	43.8	44.0	44.2	44.4	44.6	44.8

(Source: Jackson, A.S., & Pollock, M.L. [1985]. Tables determining relative body fat percent for men & women. *The Physician and Sportsmedicine, 13*[5], 76-90.)

Classification of Disease Risk Based on
Body Mass Index (BMI) and Waist Circumference

		Disease risk* relative to normal weight and waist circumference	
	BMI (kg/m²)	**Men, < 102 cm**	**Men, > 102 cm**
		Women, ≤ 88 cm	**Women, > 88 cm**
Underweight	< 18.5	–	–
Normal	18.5–24.9	–	–
Overweight	25.0–29.9	Increased	High
Obesity, class			
I	30.0–34.9	High	Very high
II	35.0–39.9	Very high	Very high
III	≥ 40	Extremely high	Extremely high

*Disease risk for type 2 diabetes, hypertension, and cardiovascular disease. Dashes (–) indicate that no additional risk at these levels of BMI was assigned. Increased waist circumference can also be a marker for increased risk even in persons of normal weight.

(Modified from Expert Panel: Executive summary of the clinical guidelines on the identification, evaluation, and treatment of overweight and obesity in adults. *Archives of Internal Medicine* [1998] *158*: 1855-1867.)

Body Mass Index Nomogram

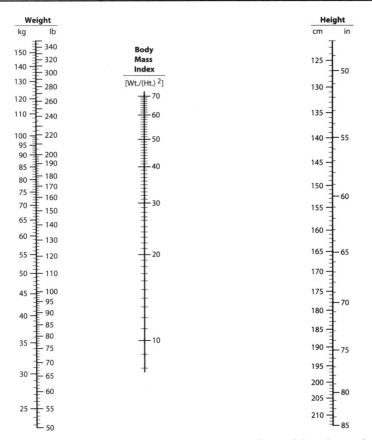

NOTE: Body mass index is determined by connecting your weight and height with a straight edge and reading your body mass index where the edge intersects the central scale.

(Adapted from Positively Aging® & M.O.R.E. Curricular Programs. [2006]. *Teacher enrichment initiatives: Multidisciplinary health science curriculum, nomogram for body mass index*. Retrieved May 5, 2006, from University of Texas, San Antonio Web site: http://teachhealthk-12.uthscsa.edu/curriculum/nutrition-aging/pa08pdf/0804B-SHO.pdf)

Norms for 3-Minute Step Test (Men)

Fitness Category	Age					
	18–25	**26–35**	**36–45**	**46–55**	**56–65**	**65+**
Excellent	< 79	< 81	< 83	< 87	< 86	< 88
Good	79–89	81–89	83–96	87–97	86–97	88–96
Above average	90–99	90–99	97–103	98–105	98–103	97–103
Average	100–105	100–107	104–112	106–116	104–112	104–113
Below average	106–116	108–117	113–119	117–122	113–120	114–120
Poor	117–128	118–128	120–130	123–132	121–129	121–130
Very poor	> 128	> 128	> 130	> 132	> 129	> 130

(Reprinted from *YMCA Fitness Testing and Assessment Manual*, 4th edition, 2000 with permission of YMCA of the USA, 101 N. Wacker Drive, Chicago, IL 60606)

Norms for 3-Minute Step Test (Women)

Fitness Category	Age					
	18–25	**26–35**	**36–45**	**46–55**	**56–65**	**65+**
Excellent	< 85	< 88	< 90	< 94	< 95	< 90
Good	85–98	88–99	90–102	94–104	95–104	90–102
Above average	99–108	100–111	103–110	105–115	105–112	103–115
Average	109–117	112–119	111–118	116–120	113–118	116–122
Below average	118–126	120–126	119–128	121–126	119–128	123–128
Poor	127–140	127–138	129–140	127–135	129–139	129–134
Very poor	> 140	> 138	> 140	> 135	> 139	> 134

(Reprinted from *YMCA Fitness Testing and Assessment Manual*, 4th edition, 2000 with permission of YMCA of the USA, 101 N. Wacker Drive, Chicago, IL 60606)

Rockport Walking Test Norms

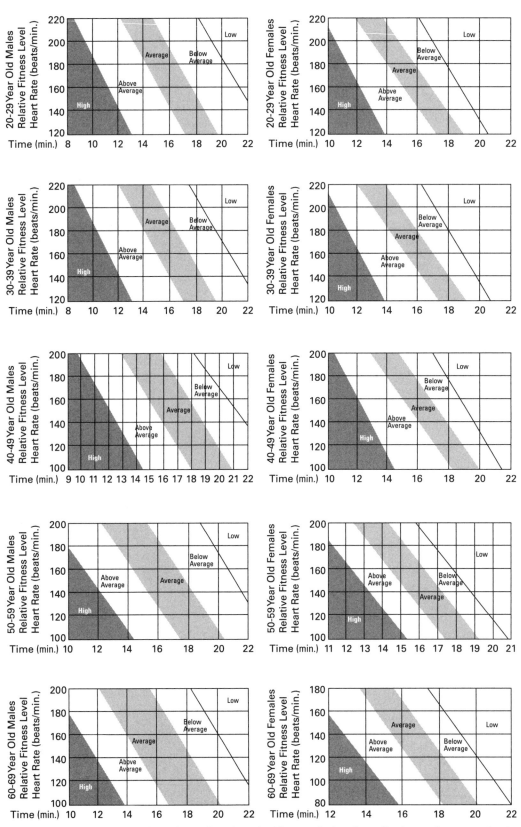

Rockport Fitness Walking Test charts (reprinted with permission from Rockport Company, Inc.)

Rockport Walking Treadmill Test Norms

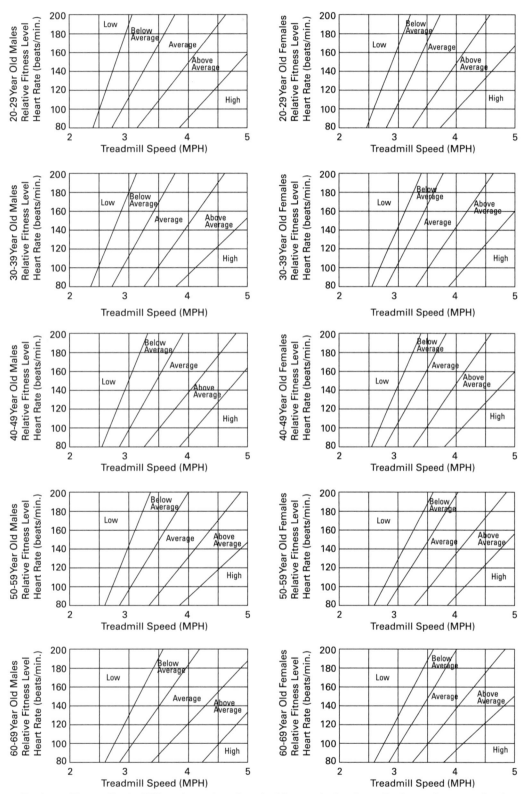

Rockport Fitness Tredmill Test charts (reprinted with permission from Rockport Company, Inc.)

Upper Body Strength Norms*†

Percentile	20–29	30–39	40–49	50–59	60+
Men					
90	1.48	1.24	1.10	0.97	0.89
80	1.32	1.12	1.00	0.90	0.82
70	1.22	1.04	0.93	0.84	0.77
60	1.14	0.98	0.88	0.79	0.72
50	1.06	0.93	0.84	0.75	0.68
40	0.99	0.88	0.80	0.71	0.66
30	0.93	0.83	0.76	0.68	0.63
20	0.88	0.78	0.72	0.63	0.57
10	0.80	0.71	0.65	0.57	0.53
Women					
90	0.90	0.76	0.71	0.61	0.64
80	0.80	0.70	0.62	0.55	0.54
70	0.74	0.63	0.57	0.52	0.51
60	0.70	0.60	0.54	0.48	0.47
50	0.65	0.57	0.52	0.46	0.45
40	0.59	0.53	0.50	0.44	0.43
30	0.56	0.51	0.47	0.42	0.40
20	0.51	0.47	0.43	0.39	0.38
10	0.48	0.42	0.38	0.37	0.33

*One repetition maximum bench press, with bench press weight ratio= weight pushed/body weight.
†Adapted From Institute for Aerobics Research, Dallas, 1994. Study population for the data set was predominantly White and college educated. A Universal DVR machine was used to measure the 1-RM. The following may be used as descriptors for the percentile rankings: well above average (90), above average (70), average (50), below average (30), and well below average (10).

(Fitness norms used with permission of the Cooper Institute, Dallas, TX)

Standard Values for Push-Up Endurance

Rating	Age				
	20–29	30–39	40–49	50–59	60+
Men					
Excellent	> 55	> 45	> 40	> 35	> 30
Good	45–54	35–44	30–39	25–34	20–29
Average	35–44	25–34	20–29	15–24	10–19
Fair	20–34	15–24	12–19	8–14	5–9
Poor	< 19	< 14	< 11	< 7	< 4
Women					
Excellent	> 49	> 40	> 35	> 30	> 20
Good	34–48	25–39	20–34	15–29	5–19
Average	17–33	12–24	8–19	6–14	3–4
Fair	6–16	4–11	3–7	2–5	1–2
Poor	< 5	< 3	< 2	< 1	< 0

(Adaptation of Table 3.11, p. 109 from *Health and Fitness through Physical Activity* by Michael L. Pollock, Jack H. Wilmore and Samuel M. Fox III. Copyright © 1985 by Macmillan Publishing Co. Reprinted by permission of Pearson Education, Inc.)

Fitness Categories by Age Groups and Gender for Partial Curl-Up

Category	Age									
	20–29		30–39		40–49		50–59		60–69	
Gender	M	F	M	F	M	F	M	F	M	F
Excellent	25	25	25	25	25	25	25	25	25	25
Very Good	24	24	24	24	24	24	24	24	24	24
	21	18	18	19	18	19	17	19	16	17
Good	20	17	17	18	17	18	16	18	15	16
	16	14	15	10	13	11	11	10	11	8
Fair	15	13	14	9	12	10	10	9	10	7
	11	5	11	6	6	4	8	6	6	3
Needs Improvement	10	4	10	5	5	3	7	5	5	2

(*The Canadian Physical Activity, Fitness & Lifestyle Approach: CSEP-Health & Fitness Program's Health-Related Appraisal and Counseling Strategy.* 3rd ed. Reprinted with permission from the Canadian Society for Exercise Physiology, 2003.)

Standard Values for Trunk Flexion in Inches (Sit and Reach Norms)

Rating	Age				
	20–29	30–39	40–49	50–59	60+
Men					
Excellent	> 22	> 21	> 20	> 19	> 18
Good	19–21	18–20	17–19	16–18	15–17
Average	13–18	12–17	11–16	10–15	9–14
Fair	10–12	9–11	8–10	7–9	6–8
Poor	< 9	< 8	< 7	< 6	< 5
Women					
Excellent	> 24	> 23	> 22	> 21	> 20
Good	22–23	21–22	20–21	19–20	18–19
Average	16–21	15–20	14–19	13–18	12–17
Fair	13–15	12–14	11–13	10–12	9–11
Poor	< 12	< 11	< 10	< 9	< 8

(Reprinted from *YMCA Fitness Testing and Assessment Manual*, 4th edition, 2000 with permission of YMCA of the USA, 101 N. Wacker Drive, Chicago, IL 60606)

Postural Analysis Guide

I. Side View

Head	___ neutral
	___ forward
Cervical spine	___ normal extension
	___ excessive extension
	___ flat
Thoracic spine	___ normal flexion
	___ excessive kyphosis
	___ flat
Lumbar spine	___ normal extension
	___ excessive lordosis
	___ flat
Pelvis	___ neutral pelvis
	___ anterior pelvic tilt
	___ posterior pelvic tilt
Hips	___ neutral
	___ flexed
	___ extended
Knees	___ neutral
	___ flexed
	___ extended
Ankle	___ neutral
	___ plantar flexed
	___ dorsiflexed

II. Front View

Head	___ straight
	___ tilted R L
	___ shifted R L
Shoulders	___ level
	___ right high
	___ left high
Pelvis	___ level
	___ right high
	___ left high
	___ rotated R L
Knees	___ normal
	___ knock-kneed
	___ bow-legged
Feet	___ inverted
	___ everted

III. Back View

Scapulae	___ normal
	___ protracted R L
	___ retracted R L
	___ elevated R L
	___ winged R L
Spine	___ scoliosis

Exercise Session Recording Form

Client Name _____ Date _____

Location _____ Time _____

Pre-exercise Client Affect

How do you feel? _____

How did you feel after last session? _____

_____

— Exercise Session —

I. **Warm-up Component (Summary)**

_____

_____

II. **Cardiovascular Component**

Target Heart Rate _____

Type of Exercise	Intensity	HR Response	Time	Client Response
_____	_____	_____	_____	_____
_____	_____	_____	_____	_____

III. **Strength Component**

	Type of Exercise	Set	Reps	Weight	Client Response
1.	_____	____	____	_____	_____
		____	____	_____	_____
		____	____	_____	_____
2.	_____	____	____	_____	_____
		____	____	_____	_____
		____	____	_____	_____
3.	_____	____	____	_____	_____
		____	____	_____	_____
		____	____	_____	_____

4. _____   _____ _____ _____ _____

    _____ _____ _____ _____

    _____ _____ _____ _____

5. _____   _____ _____ _____ _____

    _____ _____ _____ _____

    _____ _____ _____ _____

6. _____   _____ _____ _____ _____

    _____ _____ _____ _____

    _____ _____ _____ _____

7. _____   _____ _____ _____ _____

    _____ _____ _____ _____

    _____ _____ _____ _____

8. _____   _____ _____ _____ _____

    _____ _____ _____ _____

    _____ _____ _____ _____

IV. Cool-down Component (Summary of Cool-down Exercises and Client's Response)

_____

_____

_____

General Summary of Session

_____

_____

_____

_____

Example of Hands-On Technique Consent Form

Consent to the Use of Systematic T.O.U.C.H. Training℠ (STT) As Part of My Regular Physical Fitness Program and Exercise Activities

I understand that the exercise activities and physical fitness program conducted by John Doe and XYZ Personal Fitness Trainers may include the use of Systematic T.O.U.C.H. Training also known as STT.

STT is a method in which the trainer attempts to enhance muscle strength and function by stimulating the central nervous system of the exerciser through the use of specific and repetitive patterns of touch. STT is based upon the theory that the receptors of the skin are able to transmit precise information to the central nervous system when stimulated through touch. STT is not medical treatment, nor is it any form of massage, acupressure, or other similar body work. I understand that STT will be used in conjunction with my regular exercise program and that it may provide the following potential benefits. 1) It may help direct the focus of my attention on the muscle I am working. 2) It may help to provide information to both me and my trainer about which muscles are involved in the exercise and how much tension they are producing. 3) It may help to increase the tension of my muscle contractions. 4) It may help my trainer evaluate the tension in my muscles and detect any muscle imbalances. 5) It may help to eliminate tension in those muscles that should not be involved during a particular exercise.

STT does not require that my trainer touch my bare skin. The method works equally well over light clothing, such as leggings., light sweat shirts, and sweat pants. I have been informed that the aim of STT is to stimulate the receptors of the skin over my muscles and that there is no reason to touch any intimate part of my body, such as the face, mouth, breasts, genitals, or any body orifice. STT is totally non-sexual. I have been advised that attitudes toward touching and being touched by others are sometimes influenced by culture, religious upbringing, individual preferences, and gender differences. In addition, I understand that every person has different hypersensitivities. It is therefore important for me to advise my trainer in advance if there is /are any part(s) of my body that I would prefer he/she not touch. I have been informed that this is perfectly acceptable to my trainer, and he/she will refrain from touching those areas without any comment or further discussion. On the attached drawing I will mark an X on those locations (if any) that the trainer should avoid touching. I have been informed that I am free to decline the use of STT, or any portion thereof, in my training program. I may also verbally withdraw my consent at any time and for any reason, either before or after we begin using the STT method, without prejudice and without fear of offending my trainer. By the same token, I understand that my trainer reserves the right to discontinue using STT if for any reason he/she decides that it will be of no further benefit to me.

STT produces no pain and is non-invasive. However, each exerciser's sensitivities, tactile thresholds, and sensations determine how much pressure the trainer will use. Therefore, my trainer will test me in advance for the particular scale of pressure with his/her forefinger to the underside of my forearm. I may experience momentary pain in that area because of the pressure applied. I understand that my trainer will make every effort to avoid causing a bruise to the forearm, but there is a potential risk that I may develop a bruise.

The trainer will begin using STT by demonstrating on his/her body where he/she intends to touch me, and provide a brief explanation of the reason. Once I have become comfortable and familiar with the technique, this practice will be discontinued, as it is time-consuming.

Unless I instruct otherwise, my trainer may sometimes demonstrate an exercise by asking me to touch his/her muscles, so that I will understand how a properly executed muscle should feel through its full range of motion.

While there is substantial experimental evidence from personal trainers and strength coaches on the value and effectiveness of this technique, there is presently no scientific explanation as to why STT works. However, there is growing evidence from scientific research that cutaneous receptors play an important role in muscle control. Together with the known effectiveness of touch as a means of communicating, there is reason to believe that touch can be used effectively by strength trainers and coaches to improve strength and function, and to teach exercise techniques. However, I understand that STT may or may not benefit my physical fitness, general health, exercise techniques, or sports ability.

I have been informed by my trainer that the information about me obtained as a consequence of using the STT technique will be treated as privileged and confidential, and that he/she will make every effort, to the extent permitted by law, not to release or reveal said information to any person without my express written consent.

I have been given the opportunity to ask any questions about the scientific basis of STT, its techniques and procedures, and they have all been answered to my satisfaction. I acknowledge that I have carefully read and understood this document in its entirety. I consent to the use of STT by my trainer in conjunction with my regular exercise program.

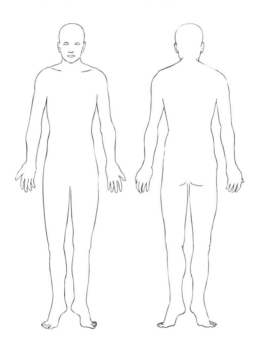

_____   _____
CLIENT SIGNATURE   TRAINER SIGNATURE

_____   _____
DATE   DATE

Cautionary Note: This form is illustrative only. No form that may have legal implication should ever be adopted for use or used without individualized legal advice.

(© PRC Publishing, 1995. From Rothenberg, O. (1995). Professional and legal concerns related to the use of Systematic T.O.U.C.H. Training^sm. _The Exercise Standards and Malpractice Reporter, 9_(1), 8-11. Reprinted by permission.)

Goal Setting Form

1. Please list your long-term health and fitness goals in order of importance.

    #1. _____

    Why is this goal important to you? _____

    #2. _____

    Why is this goal important to you? _____

    #3. _____

    Why is this goal important to you? _____

2. How do you plan to achieve these goals? (Consider frequency [list specific days and times], intensity, duration, mode, etc.)

    Goal #1 _____

    Goal #2 _____

    Goal #3 _____

3. How and when will these goals be measured? _____

    _____

4. What barriers or obstacles might keep you from reaching these goals?

Barriers	Strategies for overcoming barriers
_____	_____
_____	_____
_____	_____
_____	_____

5. What short-term goals can you set for yourself this week? _____

    _____

6. How will you reward yourself when your goal is achieved? _____

    _____

Behavior Contract

I, _____, am making a commitment to myself to change the following behavior(s):

_____.

I agree to adhere to an exercise program for _____ weeks. I commit to exercising _____ times per

week and to increasing my overall level of physical activity. I am doing this so that _____

_____.

I will reward myself by _____

_____.

Signed _____ Date_____

Witness_____ Date_____

AFAA's Nutritional Supplement Policy

Policy Statement on the Sale, Provision, or Recommendation of Nutritional Supplements by AFAA Certified Fitness Professionals to Clients

Aerobics and Fitness Association of America
Policy Statement on the Sale, Provision, or Recommendation of Nutritional Supplements by AFAA Certified Fitness Professionals to Clients
Copyright © 1999, 2006, 2007 by AFAA, Sherman Oaks, California

As part of its mission, the Aerobics and Fitness Association of America (AFAA) is committed to assisting AFAA certified fitness professionals in their provision of exceptional fitness-related services to clients. In so doing, AFAA gathers and publishes information on a wide variety of topics to inform such professionals and help them to provide the best possible services to their clients.

In 1999, AFAA originally developed this Policy Statement regarding the recommendation, provision, and/or sale of nutritional supplements to consumers. In 2006/2007, AFAA determined to review and update the statement. As with its first work on this subject, this revised Policy Statement is intended to assist professionals in determining how they might, in the exercise of independent professional judgment, provide relevant services or products to their clients. However, this statement is not intended to limit the recommendation or sale of nutritional supplement products by knowledgeable entities which use computerized programs or algorithms to recommend the use of nutritional products to individual clients, nor to limit the provision of relevant service by those who are qualified by reason of education, training, licensure or other form of regulation to provide nutritional supplement advice. By reason of the development and publication of this Policy Statement, neither the authors nor AFAA shall be deemed to be engaged in the practice of any form of health care or law; nor do they assume any duty toward clients of fitness professionals or fitness professionals themselves who consider the materials within this Policy Statement for adaptation to their professional practices. Fitness professionals considering these issues should consult with their individual medical and legal advisors for guidance.

As a starting point, fitness professionals must acknowledge that some manufacturers of nutritional supplements as well as others often encourage health and fitness facilities and fitness professionals to sell a wide range of nutritional products to their employees and customers. Many facilities and professionals have undertaken to do so for a variety of reasons. However, AFAA believes that the recommendation, sale, or provision of such products must be based upon a number of factors.

The sale of nutritional supplements in the United States involves literally hundreds, if not thousands, of products sold to most adult Americans through a variety of retail and service establishments as well as over the Internet. The range of nutritional supplement products is extremely diverse. As of 2005, the industry has been reported to be in excess of $20 billion in the United States and perhaps as large as $182 billion worldwide.

Nutritional supplements include vitamins, minerals, herbs, and even hormones. There are 13 vitamins, 15 minerals, and untold numbers of herbal and other similar products available for sale in this market. While vitamins and minerals may be the most studied, and perhaps the best understood, of all nutritional supplements, controversy continues to surround all such products.

As a general rule, vitamin and mineral supplements are not harmful unless taken in excessive doses, in which case, actual damage can result. Several herb products, such as aspirin, have proven medicinal properties, while many other herbs and even hormones can be clearly harmful, or are not yet well understood. Moreover, some nutritional products can be harmful when ingested along with other such products, prescriptions, over-the-counter medications, or even foods or beverages. Those with certain health conditions should not ingest some nutritional products. In addition, those who ingest certain nutritional products may have increased surgical- and anesthesia-related risks. Consequently, it is necessary to obtain health-care provider advice, approval, and monitoring of product use.

Generally, there is no legal requirement in the United States for nutritional supplements (as opposed to drug products) to be tested and/or approved for use by any governmental agency prior to their sale to consumers. While the Food and Drug Administration (FDA) does have some regulatory authority and responsibility as to nutritional products, such supplements are only subject to regulation after such products are determined to be dangerous or to the extent that claims are made that such products cure, mitigate, or treat various diseases.

Due to the present lack of pre-sale regulation of these products, some such products may not be "pure," or in other words, of a certain formula or strength; and some, potentially, may not contain what is actually on the product label. Since nutritional products are not sold as prescriptions by health-care providers, the legal doctrine applicable in some states and known as the "learned intermediary doctrine" does not limit the duty of producers and manufactures to warn consumers of adverse consequences associated with such products. Moreover, those who sell, provide, or recommend such products necessarily do so with only limited information, as compared to the information that is available for prescription drug products, which are subject to extensive testing and research before being approved by the FDA for sale to consumers.

Due to all of the foregoing, those recommending nutritional supplement products to consumers, and those actually involved in providing or selling such products to consumers, may well have increased ethical, professional, and legal duties and responsibilities to ensure that the products they recommend, sell, or provide are relatively safe for consumption and/or are beneficial to the user. This conclusion is due in part to the fact that such products are not "sanctioned" by any government agency and that there is often only limited information and research findings available from non-manufacturer sources as to the safety and efficacy of many of these products.

Since some nutritional supplements have been deemed by the FDA to be associated with certain adverse health effects, AFAA strongly discourages professionals from making any favorable recommendations to clients related to these specific products or from providing or selling same. A current listing of these nutritional products can be obtained from the FDA's Internet site at http://vm.cfsan.fda.gov/~dms/fdsuppch.html. AFAA also discourages professionals from making favorable product recommendations or from selling or providing products to clients when the available scientific evidence and research findings from sources other than manufacturers are insufficient to provide clear guidance as to whether such products are beneficial.

AFAA recognizes that some health/fitness facilities and professionals do not, as a matter of policy, sell or provide supplements or advice to others concerning nutritional products. Many believe it to be inappropriate and even unethical to do so. Others do not do so for fear of incurring additional legal exposure in the situation in which an untoward event occurs related to such products. These concerns are valid and must be given some deference by professionals.

In the event that any of these products are sold, provided, or recommended by professionals to consumers to treat, cure, or beneficially impact a disease process or infirmity, or perhaps even for preventive purposes, such professionals could be exposed to criminal and/or civil claims related to the unauthorized practice of medicine or other similar licensed health-care provider practices such as those reserved for provision by dietitians. If an untoward event occurred associated with a practice violating any of the foregoing kinds of statutes, a fitness professional who recommends, provides, or sells nutritional substances in the course of providing unauthorized advice could be exposed to rather substantial claims.

To illustrate what can happen in regard to advice given to a fitness client about nutritional supplements readers should consider what was alleged in a lawsuit that was filed in the state of New York. The suit arose from the 1998 death of a 37-year-old facility patron who allegedly took five nutritional supplements at the claimed, written recommendation of a personal trainer employed by a health and fitness facility. The suit sought $320 million in damages against the trainer, the facility, the named retail seller of the supplements, and five nutritional supplement manufacturers. The suit was based upon negligence, willful, wanton, malicious, and reckless conduct, improper and dangerous product use instructions, failure to warn, and the sale of unreasonably dangerous products. The action was recently resolved for an undisclosed, confidential settlement.

Based upon the foregoing concerns the following basic principles should be considered by professionals as to the sale, recommendation, or provision of nutritional supplement products to clients.

1. Health and fitness facilities and fitness professionals should not sell, recommend, or provide ("provide") nutritional supplement products, including vitamins, minerals, herbs, and/or hormones ("nutritional supplements") to their employees and/or members/guests/clients unless the sale, recommendation, or provision of such products is justified by existing scientific and medical research, which is derived independently from those who manufacture such products and which demonstrates some benefit or potential benefit to consumers who ingest such products.

2. Such facilities and personnel should not provide nutritional supplements unless there is adequate, independent, scientifically-based information other than manufacturer information available as to the use of such supplements to indicate that use is preferably beneficial or at least reasonably safe when taken in proper quantities and subject to health-care provider approval, review, and monitoring.

3. Nutritional supplements that have been determined by the FDA to be harmful or those that have been associated with certain adverse health effects should not be provided by fitness professionals to clients. A listing of such nutritional supplements that have been associated with certain adverse health effects can be obtained from the following FDA Internet site: http://vm.cfsan.fda.gov/~dms/fdsuppch.html.

4. If the provision of nutritional supplements is deemed by health/fitness facilities or fitness professionals to be appropriate based upon the foregoing principles, consumers of such products should be provided with certain information. This information should be specific and individual warnings and/or disclaimers advising the consumer of the potential adverse consequences associated with certain supplements should be included. Provided information should also include a statement about the limitations of present knowledge as to some products, and the unknown risks or adverse potential reactions or consequences that might be associated with the use of some products, either when ingested alone or in conjunction with other similar products, drugs, other substances, some foods or beverages, or when some such products are used prior to surgical procedures. Those products that may not provide anticipated or advertised benefits should also be identified for consumers. Products that may be inadequately labeled or those whose quality or purity cannot be verified independently should not be recommended, provided, or sold to consumers.

5. In conjunction with the provision of any nutritional supplement, scientifically formulated and derived information should be provided in writing to the consumer/purchaser of such supplements that is based upon information obtained from scientifically/medically reliable sources apart from the manufacturers or wholesalers of such products. These authoritative sources might include the FDA or organizations such as the American Medical Association (AMA) or the American Dietetic Association. Fitness professionals must stay current as to developments in this area and provide reasonably current information to clients, including manufacturer information.

Fitness professionals who decide to provide nutritional supplement products to clients while also providing information related to those products must be aware of and fully comply with applicable requirements related to such practices as provided by regulations issued under the Dietary Supplement Health and Education Act of 1994 (DSHEA) and the DSHEA, as those regulations and statutes may be amended or changed from time to time. Under the latest revisions to the regulations promulgated pursuant to the DSHEA, the FDA has established new rules as to what kinds of information may be supplied (and how and in what context) to consumers associated with the sale of dietary supplement products. As a consequence, fitness professionals providing products and information must review the Act and the regulations promulgated there under as same may be amended or changed from time to time to determine what is permissible and what is not permissible in that regard. It may also be helpful for such professionals to review Federal Trade Commission (FTC) requirements dealing with claims in advertising (including direct marketing materials) and even state/local law/regulations that may impact the provision of such products and information. Consequently, based upon all of the foregoing, professionals must independently determine how, when, and in what manner and context relevant information may be provided to consumers about nutritional supplement products.

6. The provision of nutritional supplements by health/fitness facilities/professionals should not under any circumstances be used to treat, cure, mitigate, or otherwise attempt to beneficially impact any condition, disease, or infirmity with which an individual is afflicted in violation of state health-care provider licensing and/or practice statutes, or be used in any way on the recommendation of a fitness professional, which would violate state practice of medicine acts or other similar statutes or laws. No exercise or fitness professional should ever recommend any supplement or even any activity under circumstances where the practice could be deemed to be the unauthorized practice of medicine or some other health-care discipline including those services reserved for provision by licensed nutritionists or dietitians.

7. Nutritional supplements must have appropriate and accurate labeling information that properly describes product purity, weight/size, quantity, and recommended dosages. Product information as required by law must be provided. Health claims associated with nutritional products must not be made unless specifically allowed by law.

8. The provision of nutritional supplements by health and fitness facilities/professionals should not be made for the purposes of enhancing or attempting to enhance athletic performance or the athletic condition of those clients participating in such activities.

9. Before a consumer begins using or ingesting a nutritional supplement that is provided by a fitness facility or professional, that individual's use of any nutritional supplement should be reviewed and approved by the consumer's health-care provider, especially when such supplements are provided to individuals who are taking other forms of prescription or over-the-counter medications or supplements. Moreover, an individual's use of such supplements should be monitored by his/her health-care provider. Due to the foregoing, fitness facilities and professionals must make such a recommendation to their members/guests/clients in writing before the provision of such a supplement product to seek such clearance, advice, guidance, and monitoring. Written documentation as to the client's receipt of such advice, and preferably the written acknowledgement of same by the recipient, should be secured if possible.

10. Health and fitness facilities and exercise professionals should document all of the foregoing in their written records. Such records should be maintained for a period of time coexistent with advice provided by their independent legal/professional advisors. The use of waivers, releases, or assumption-of-risk documents by fitness professionals to be executed by clients who are provided with nutritional supplements should be considered where warranted and as fitness personnel are advised by their individual professional/legal advisors.

C

cancer, 4-7, 10-12, 14-16, 18, 309, 334-337, 344-345, 348-349, 354, 366
    risk factors, 5-6
carbohydrate loading, 362
carbohydrates, 6, 345-347, 349, 354-355, 358, 360-364
cardiac
    cycle, 25
    muscle, 25, 39
    output, 24-25
cardiorespiratory, 24, 37-38, 41
    fitness, 81, 83, 93, 95, 108-109, 113-115, 117, 123, 126, 326
    system, 23-24, 37, 41
cardiovascular disease, signs and symptoms of, 74
carotid artery, 84
carpal tunnel syndrome, 219, 225-226, 306
cartilage, 27, 46, 49-50
case study, 72, 78-79
central nervous system, 38
cervical, 148, 239, 306-307
    See also spine
CHD, *See* coronary heart disease
children, 7, 329-330, 334, 337
cholesterol, 4, 7, 11-16, 18, 344-345, 348-352, 357-358, 363-364, 366
chronic obstructive pulmonary disease (COPD), 7, 18, 334, 337
claudication, 332
closed
    -ended questions, 385
    kinetic chain, 134, 315
coccygeal, 306
    See also spine
code of ethics, 404-405
communication styles, 386-387
concentric, 63
congestive heart failure, 12, 330, 344, 366
continuing education, 398, 402, 404-405
contractures, 300
contusion, 299
cool-down, 121-123, 326
COPD, *See* chronic obstructive pulmonary disease
core
    exercises, 136, 144
        See also resistance training
    training, 144
        See also resistance training
coronary heart disease (CHD), 3, 73-75, 77-79, 114, 117, 119, 325, 344, 349-350, 352, 354
    risk factors, 4, 73-75, 77, 117, 344
cross
    -country skiing, 116, 124, 126
    -training, 122-124

cues, types of, 165
cueing, 162, 165-166, 168
cycling, 116, 120, 124-125, 326, 332, 337

D

delayed onset muscle soreness (DOMS), *See* muscle
demo-detail-demo, 167
detraining, 129, 152-153
DEXA (dual-energy X-ray absorptiometry), 87
diabetes, 4, 6-7, 10, 12, 14-18, 321-322, 329, 332-334, 337, 344-345, 347, 349, 354, 362, 366, 420, 436, 444
diaphragm, 29
diarthrodial joints, 49
diastole, 25
dietary
    guidelines, 11, 347, 349-351, 355, 357-358
    supplements, *See* supplementation
Dietary Reference Intake (DRI), 346, 353
disk herniation, 310
dislocation, 299, 303-304
dual-energy X-ray absorptiometry, *See* DEXA
duration (time), 114, 116-117, 121-122, 124, 126
dynamic
    constant resistance, 141
        See also resistance training
    variable resistance, 141
        See also resistance training

E

eating disorders, 364-365
    See also anorexia nervosa, bulimia nervosa, binge-eating disorder
eccentric, 63
elbow joint, 55, 210, 217
    See also tennis elbow
energy balance, 366
epicondylitis, 305
EPOC (excess post-exercise oxygen consumption), 38
equipment, 130, 133, 135, 140-143, 149, 394-396, 398-399, 401, 403
    See also resistance training
ergometer, upper body, 126
excess post-exercise oxygen consumption, *See* EPOC
exercise
    barriers to, 379
    continuum, 168
    during pregnancy, 320-323, 337-338
    functional, 134, 159, 326, 329, 337
    variety of, 133-141
    waiver, 77, 79
exercises, order of, 133

Index

K

Karvonen formula, 117-118, 128
ketosis, 346
knee joint, 45, 60-61, 68, 247, 252
Krebs cycle, 34-36
kyphosis, 105, 306-308

L

label reading, 356, 363, 369
lactate, 24, 33, 38
lactic acid, 24, 33-35, 37-38
    system, *See* anaerobic glycolytic system
larynx, 27-28
learning styles, 165, 168
levers, 46, 63-64
liability insurance, 400, 402
lifting technique, 167
ligament
    injuries, 313-314
    laxity, 274
ligaments, 46, 50, 61, 273-274
listening, *See* active listening
lordosis, 105, 306, 308, 311
low
    -back pain, 8, 86, 98, 100-102, 105, 135, 144
    -density lipoproteins (LDLs), 73, 352
lumbar, 148, 239, 306
    See also spine

M

macronutrients, 29
marketing strategies, 394
maximal
    exercise test, 93
    oxygen uptake, 38
        See also VO$_2$ max
McKenzie, 311, 317
medical history form, 72-73, 76, 79, 418, 420
medications, 72, 76, 415-417
meniscus tears, 314
MET (metabolic equivalent), 120-121
Metabolic
    disease, 74
    Syndrome, 6-7, 345, 366
metatarsalgia, 316-317
minerals, 149, 346-348, 353, 355, 360, 362
    See also supplementation
mission statement, 392
mitochondria, 35, 40
mitral valve, 24
mode, 116-117, 119, 122, 126
motivation, 376-382, 387
multiple sclerosis, 336-337

muscle
    endurance, 98-100, 132, 135
    fiber types, *See* slow twitch fibers and fast twitch fibers
    groups, opposing, 43, 64, 135, 138
    imbalances, 271, 301, 307, 313, 317
    power, 131, 137
    soreness
        acute, 148
        delayed onset (DOMS), 141, 148
    spindles, 41, 271-272
    stability, 131
    strength, 83, 98, 102, 108, 130-156, 170, 181, 183, 185-188, 190, 192, 194, 196, 270
    See also agonist, antagonist, cardiac, skeletal, smooth, stabilizer
muscles, commonly tight, 271
muscular
    endurance, 131
    fitness, 83, 98, 101
        benefits of, 130
    strength, 130-156
        See also muscle strength
myocardial infarction, 4, 24
myocardium, 24-25
myofascial release, 273, 275
myosin, 39

N

near-infrared interactance, 88
negligence, 400
nervous system, 38, 41, 150
neutral spine, 171, 215, 220, 228, 239, 258, 309, 311
nonsynovial joints, 49
nutrient density, 360, 363, 369

O

obesity, 4-8, 12, 73-74, 344-345, 349, 352, 355, 362, 365-366
older adults, 320, 324-327, 337
omega-3 fatty acids, 344, 350
open
    -ended questions, 385, 387
    kinetic chain, 134, 315
opposing muscle groups, *See* muscle
osteoarthritis, 8, 18, 309, 311-315, 325, 327-328
osteopenia, 328
osteoporosis, 8, 15, 18, 308, 325, 328-329, 337, 344-346, 355, 364-365
overhead press, 172, 194-195, 197, 213, 251, 254, 264
overload, 116, 122-123, 131, 137, 139
    principle, 131
overtraining, 129, 138, 152
    syndrome, 299

Baltimore
CHARM CITY

By DAN RODRICKS *and* ROGER MILLER

❧

Profiles in Excellence and Captions by CAROLYN SPENCER BROWN

❧

Art Direction by BRIAN GROPPE

ENJOY BALTIMORE!

Dan Rodricks

URBAN
TAPESTRY
SERIES
TOWERY
PUBLISHING, INC.

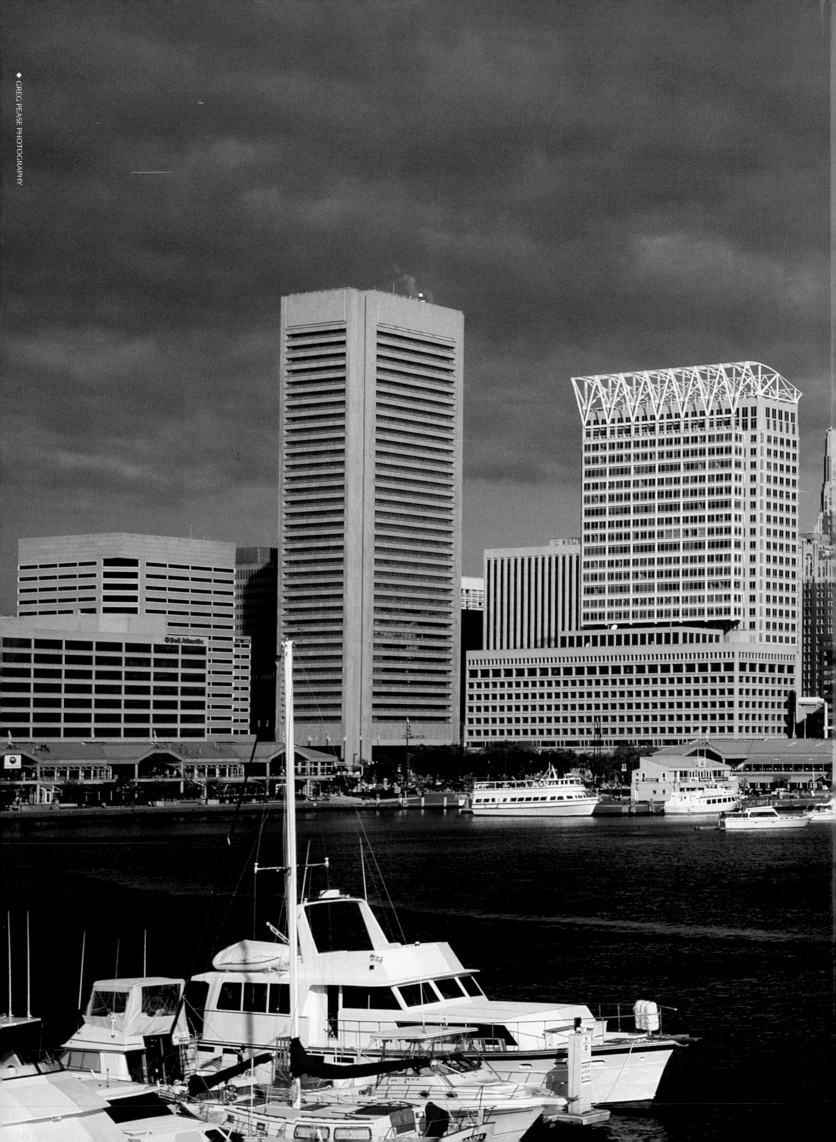

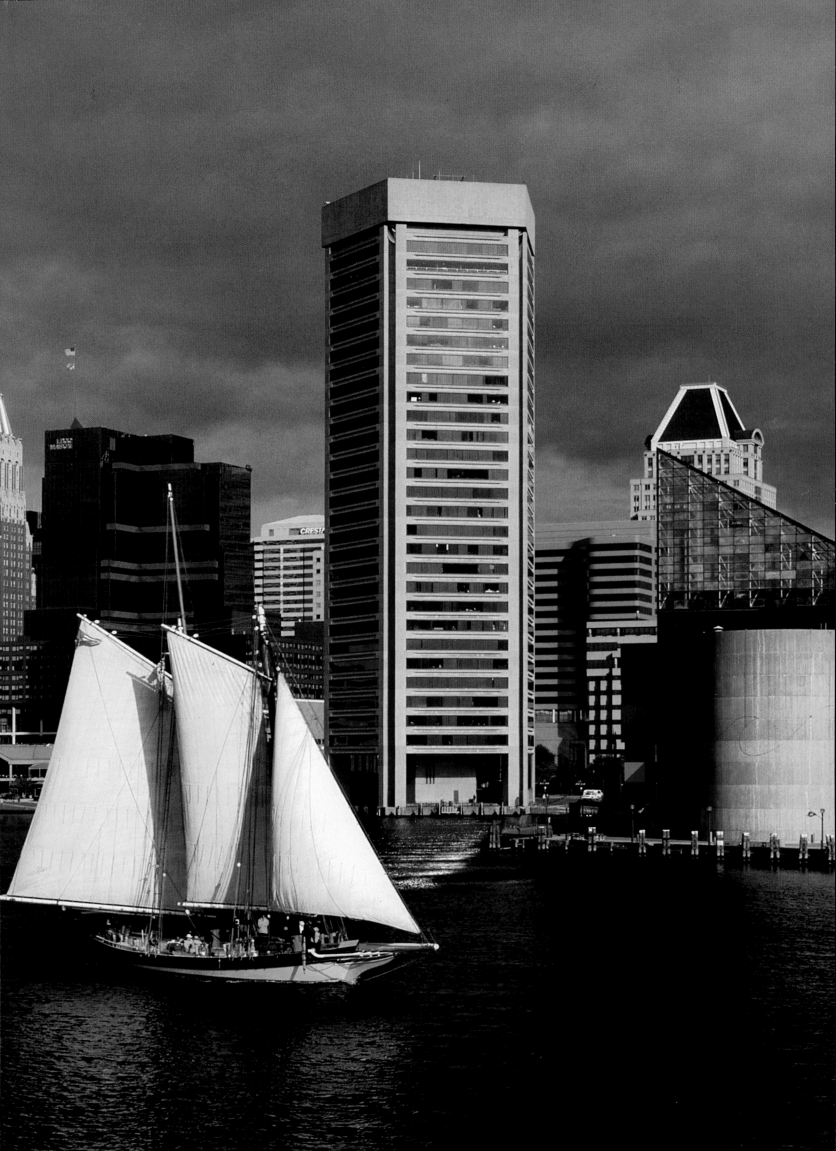

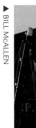
▲ BILL McALLEN

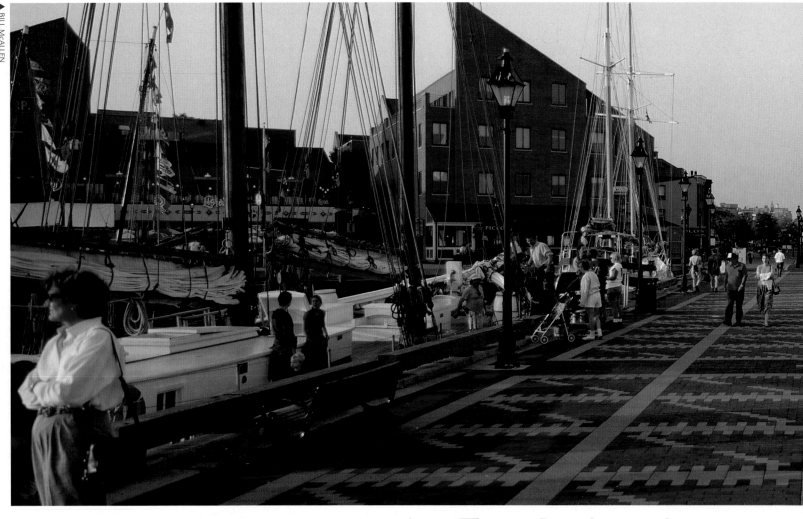

LIBRARY OF CONGRESS CATALOGING-IN-PUBLICATION DATA

Rodricks, Dan, 1954-

    Baltimore : charm city / by Dan Rodricks and Roger Miller ;
profiles in excellence and captions by Carolyn Spencer Brown ; art
direction by Brian Groppe.

      p. cm. – (Urban tapestry series)

    Includes index.

    ISBN 1-881096-50-5 (alk. paper)

    1. Baltimore (Md.)–Civilization. 2. Baltimore (Md.)–Pictorial
works. 3. Business enterprises–Maryland–Baltimore. 4. Baltimore
(Md.)–Economic conditions. I. Miller, Roger, 1946- .
II. Brown, Carolyn Spencer, 1962- . III. Title. IV. Series.

F189.B15R625 1997

975.2'6-dc21

                           97-40374

                             CIP

TOWERY PUBLISHING, INC., 1835 UNION AVENUE, MEMPHIS, TN 38104

Publisher:	J. Robert Towery
Executive Publisher:	Jenny McDowell
National Sales Manager:	Stephen Hung
Regional Sales Manager:	Dawn E. Park-Donegan
Marketing Director:	Carol Culpepper
Project Directors:	Aphrodite Corsi, Susan Kollet-Harris
Executive Editor:	David B. Dawson
Managing Editor:	Michael C. James
Senior Editors:	Lynn Conlee, Carlisle Hacker
Editor/Project Manager:	Lori Bond
Staff Editors:	Mary Jane Adams, Jana Files, Susan Hesson, Brian Johnston
Assistant Editors:	Pat McRaven, Jennifer C. Pyron, Allison Ring
Editorial Contributor:	Laura Reiley
Profile Designers:	Laurie Beck, Kelley Pratt, Ann Ward
Digital Color Supervisor:	Brenda Pattat
Digital Color Technicians:	Jack Griffith, Darin Ipema, Jason Moak
Production Resources Manager:	Dave Dunlap Jr.
Production Assistants:	Geoffrey Ellis, Enrique Espinosa, Robin McGehee
Print Coordinator:	Beverly Thompson

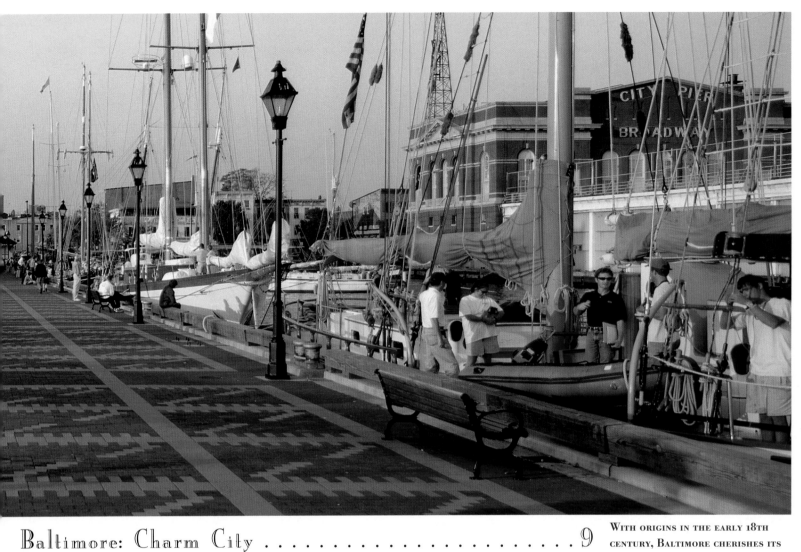

With origins in the early 18th century, Baltimore cherishes its colorful heritage, and former residents have long returned to their roots during Old Home Week (pages 6 and 7). The city's historic harbor-front neighborhood, Fells Point, dates back to 1730, when William Fell purchased the land. In 1763, his brother and fellow shipbuilder, Edward Fell, divided the urban port into 200 lots on which rowhouses, shops, and shipyards were built (above).

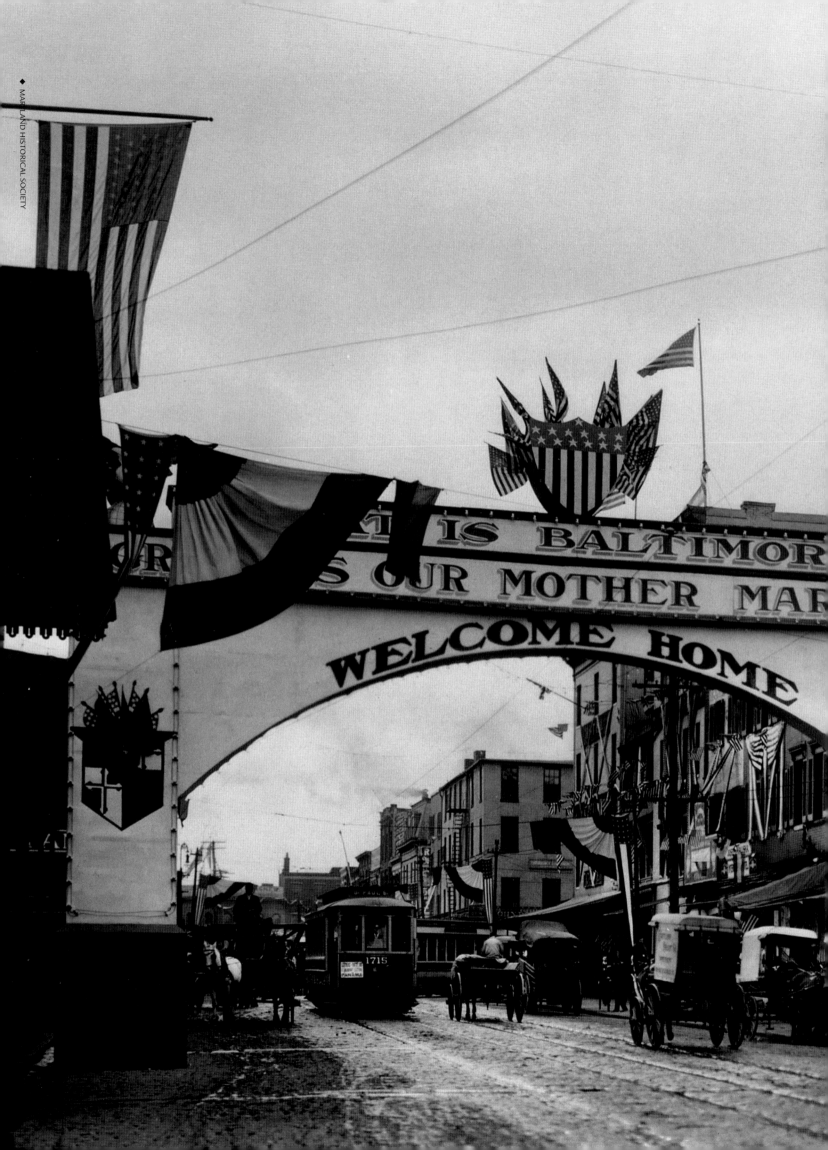

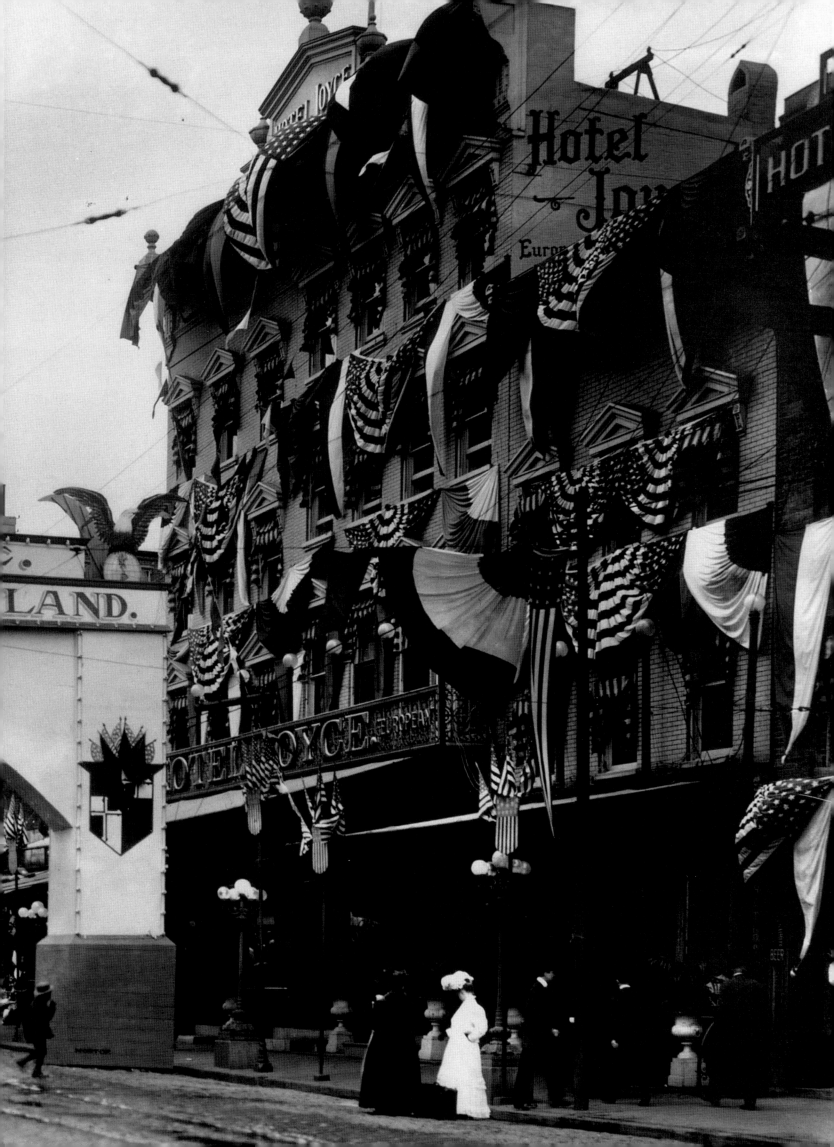

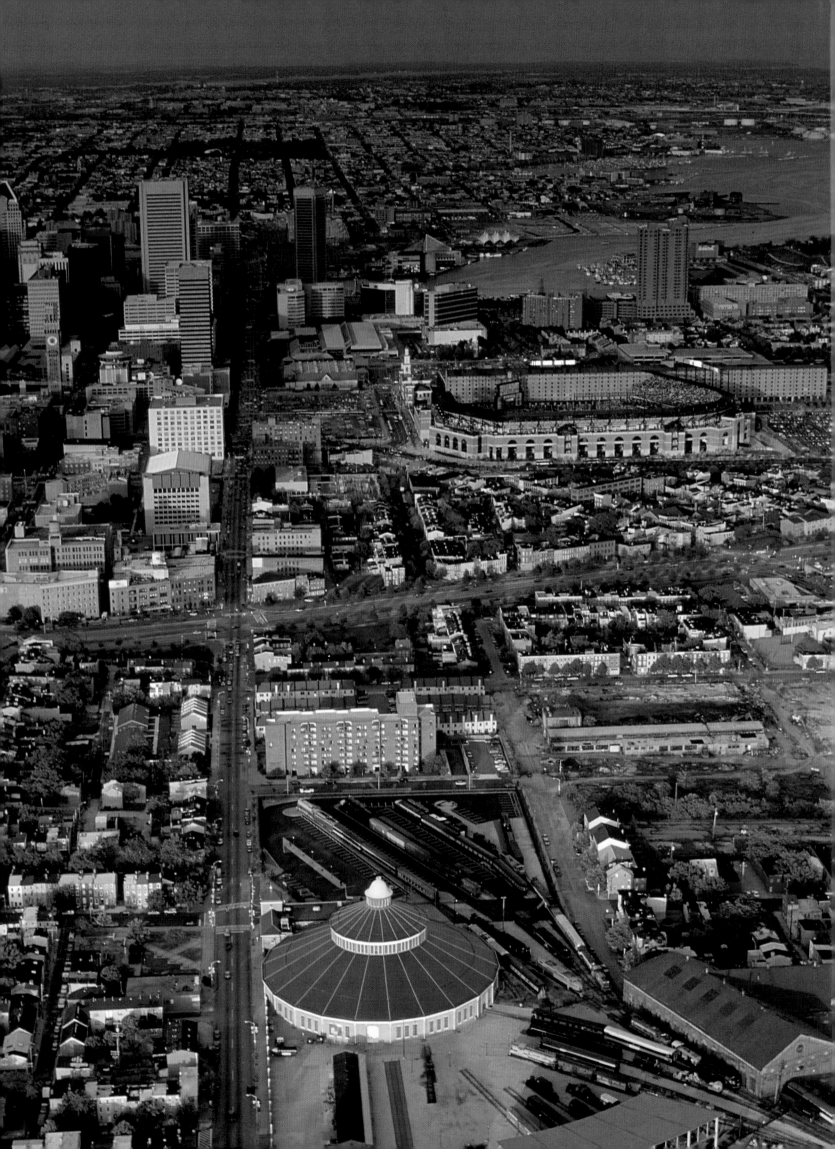

By Dan Rodricks

A FEW YEARS AGO, SOME WISE GUY SPRAY PAINTED "HON" ON THE WELCOME-TO-BALTIMORE sign at the city's south entrance—the one Washingtonians see during their drive to Orioles games—and never was one word of graffiti so appreciated. "Welcome to Baltimore, Hon!" Of course. It's the city's unofficial greeting. "Hon" is an old Baltimore tag, a verbal wink, a nostalgic nod. Newcomers might hear it when ordering lunch in a small restaurant and not know what to make of it. Don't worry: It's a term of endearment. It's not in everyone's greeting, but it settled on the Baltimore tongue long ago, and, though some people find it a cornball anachronism, it survives as a genuine provincialism.

"You want fries with that?" can be heard in every community in America by now.

But in Baltimore you'll be asked, "You want fries with that, hon?"

Correct answer: "Yeah, and with gravy please."

We eat them with the brown, gloppy stuff on top. Fries-and-gravy showed up in film director Barry Levinson's homage to his youth and his hometown, *Diner*, and he wasn't making it up.

The thing you discover about Baltimore is that you don't have to make it up. The city's full of peculiar, unpredictable, unpretentious delights—a million little roadside attractions.

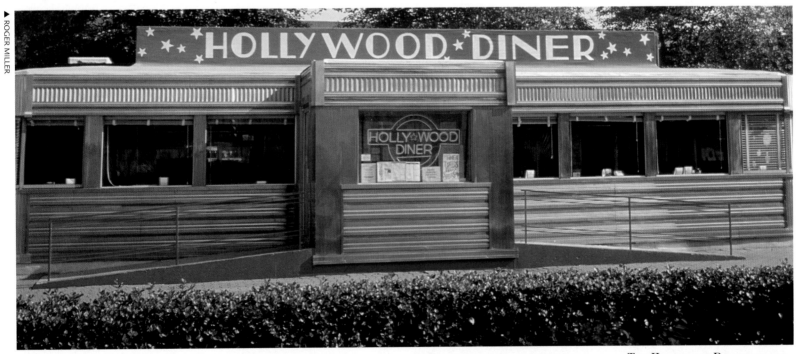

IN BALTIMORE, THE MORE THINGS CHANGE, THE MORE THEY STAY THE SAME. AN EASTWARD GLANCE TOWARD THE GLITTER OF THE INNER HARBOR IS MET BY A MIX OF OLD AND NEW, FROM THE ANCIENT B&O RAILROAD MUSEUM TO RETRO-NOUVEAU ORIOLE PARK AT CAMDEN YARDS (OPPOSITE).

THE HOLLYWOOD DINER WAS THE SETTING FOR BARRY LEVINSON'S AUTO-BIOGRAPHICAL FILM ABOUT A CLOSE-KNIT BUNCH OF GUYS WHOSE LIVES REVOLVED AROUND A LOCAL CAFÉ. TODAY, AT-RISK KIDS ARE GIVEN THE OPPORTUNITY TO LEARN THE RESTAU-RANT TRADE AT THE FAMOUS LOCALE (ABOVE).

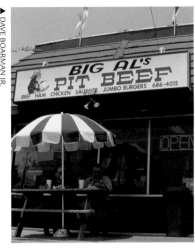

One of our downtown architectural wonders is a tribute to man's battle against indigestion—the Bromo Seltzer Tower.

We have a neighborhood called Pigtown, and one called Beverly Hills.

In West Baltimore, some streets are lined with flower urns made from old tires. They're filled with petunias and impatiens in the summer.

Locals actually have heated arguments over which restaurant serves the best crab cakes.

The man who operated Big Al's Pit Beef on Pulaski Highway—directly across from the Rosedale Loudmouths Club—was just barely five feet tall.

We have a fellow here named Abu. He makes musical wind instruments out of junk and can play a Rodgers and Hammerstein number on a chair leg.

We have a professional football team named after a roadkill-eating bird memorialized in a macabre poem by Edgar Allan Poe, who was not born in Baltimore but died a miserable death here (a local physician thinks it was rabies that killed him).

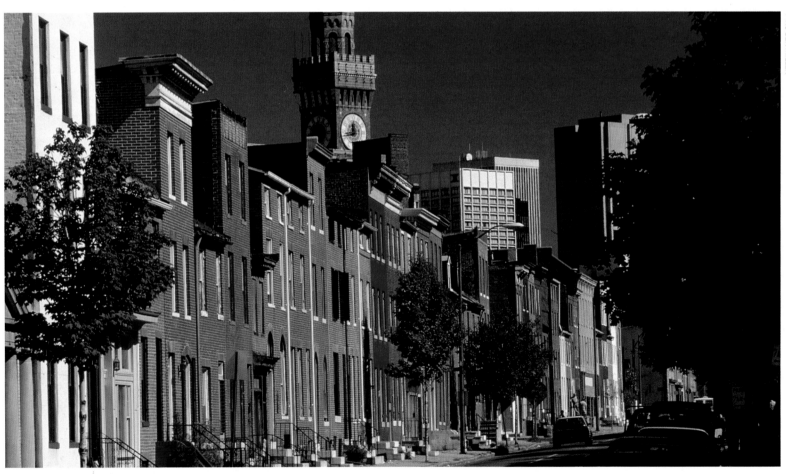

BALTIMORE IS A CITY OF NEIGHBOR-HOODS, WITH MORE THAN 1,000 OF THEM BY SOME RECKONINGS. EACH HAS ITS OWN INTRIGUING, AND OFTEN ECCENTRIC, CHARACTERISTICS. THE STEREOTYPICAL ROWHOUSE IS

BALTIMORE'S MOST COMMON RESI-DENCE, BUT STATELY VICTORIAN HOMES, MODERN CONDOMINIUM TOWERS, AND COZY, TREE-SHADED BUNGALOWS ALSO ABOUND.

PIT BEEF STANDS, SCATTERED ALL OVER THE CITY, ARE A POPULAR CHOICE FOR AN EASY, PICK-ME-UP MEAL (TOP).

The man who assassinated Abraham Lincoln is buried here, too.

We have a laundromat called the Up-To-Date. You can still buy a Polock Johnny's hot dog in Lexington Market. We have secondhand stores called Fat Elvis and Killer Trash. We have Rowley's, a tavern that serves beer on doilies, where you can tell if the place is open by the traffic light fixed to its exterior. If it's green, you go. Simple.

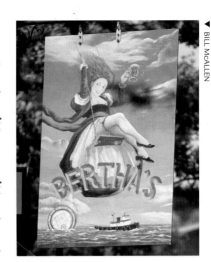

We have acres of Formstone, a gray masonry appliqué that a small army of mid-century salesmen convinced the owners of thousands of brick rowhouses they absolutely had to have. A lot of it disappeared in the 1970s and 1980s, when a new generation of home owners opted for the exposed brick look. But there's still plenty of the F stuff around.

Tube socks are big here. Our flea markets and discount stores sell them by the pile.

Our most popular bumper sticker has been seen all over the world by now. It advises all who see it to "Eat Bertha's Mussels."

If you want a fabulous dinner at Martick's, you might have to ask someone where it is. Then you have to ring the doorbell and hope Morris, the owner, feels like cooking. If he does, you're in for a treat. ☞

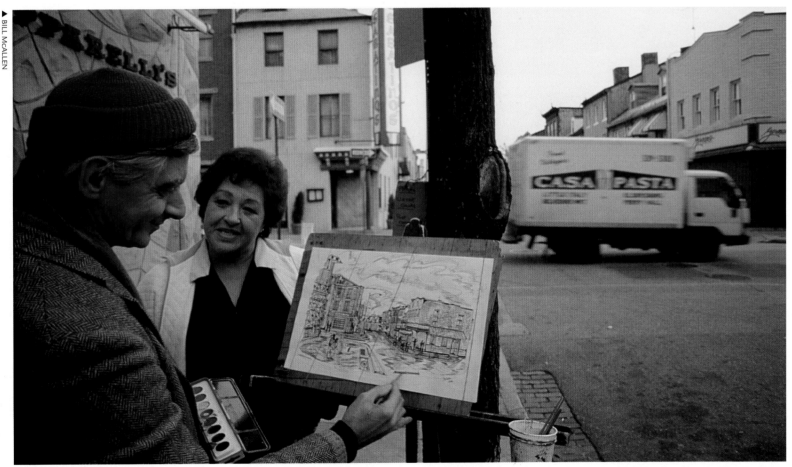

LOCATED JUST EAST OF THE INNER HARBOR, LITTLE ITALY HAS BEEN THE CENTER OF BALTIMORE'S ITALIAN POPULATION FOR MORE THAN A CENTURY. THE FRIENDLY NEIGHBORHOOD, KNOWN FOR ITS BOCCIE TOURNAMENTS AND AUTHENTIC ITALIAN RESTAURANTS, IS A FAVORITE SUBJECT OF LOCAL WATERCOLORIST TONY DeSALES, WHO PAINTS THE TOWN AT THE CORNER OF FAWN AND SOUTH HIGH. SINCE THE FOLKS AT BERTHA'S IN FELLS POINT PLASTERED "EAT BERTHA'S MUSSELS" ON THOUSANDS OF BUMPER STICKERS, THEIR WACKY MARKETING SLOGAN HAS BEEN SPOTTED ACROSS THE GLOBE FROM HONG KONG TO EDINBURGH (TOP).

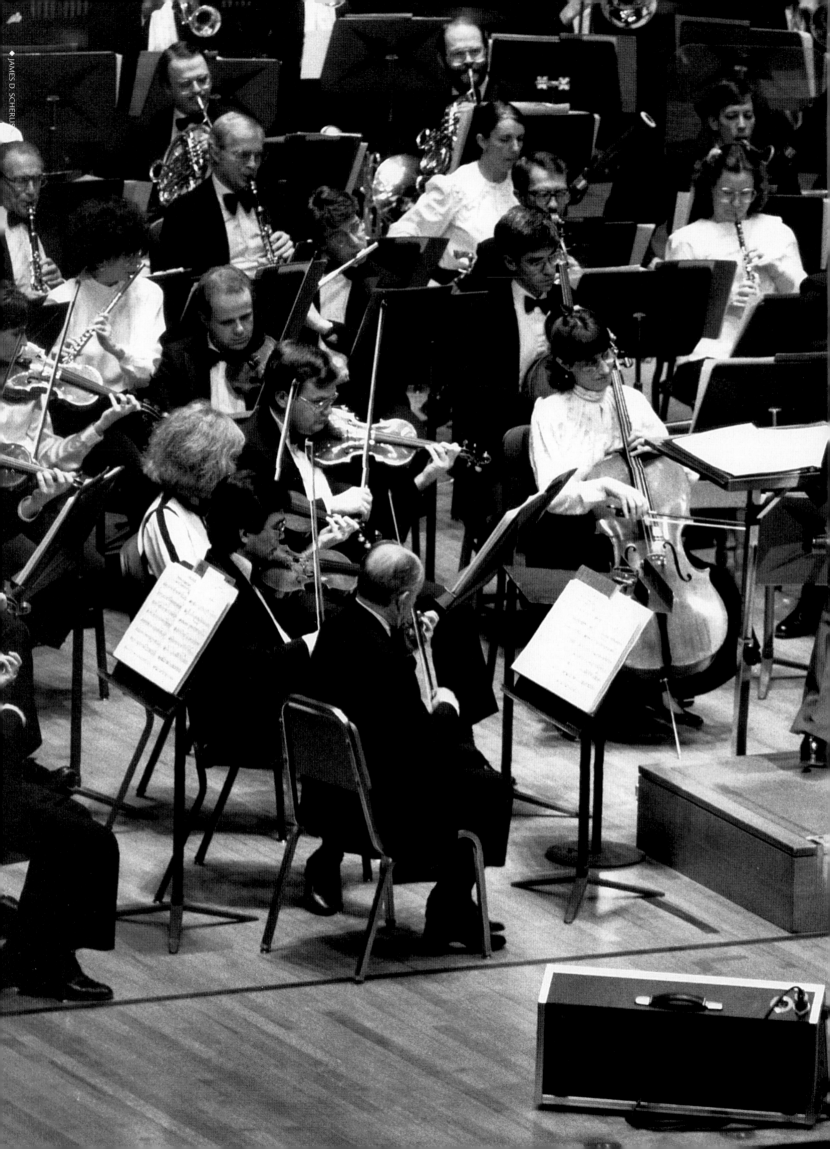

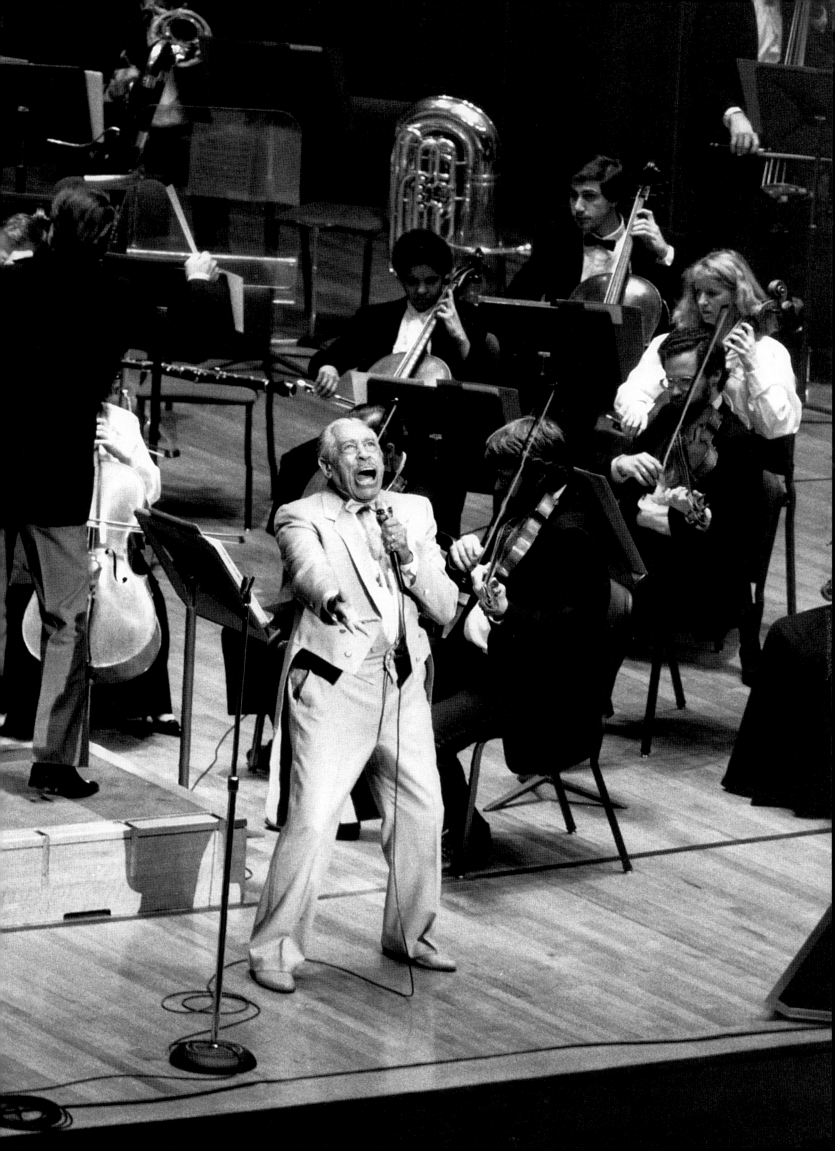

W E CHERISH THE FEW TRUE CELEBRITIES, NATIVE AND IMPORTED, WHO LIVE AROUND here—Kweisi Mfume, Artie Donovan, Cal Ripken Jr., Frank Robinson, Brooks Robinson, Boog Powell, Jim Palmer, Johnny Unitas, Tom Clancy, Pam Shriver, Roberto Alomar, Brady Anderson, Jim McKay, David Zinman, Anne Tyler, John Waters, Ethel Ennis, Barbara Mikulski. We take pride in those who came and went—Oprah Winfrey, Louis Rukeyser, Kathleen Turner, Robin Quivers. We even take pride in the ones who are dead—F. Scott Fitzgerald, Poe, H.L. Mencken, Wallis Warfield Simpson (the former Duchess of Windsor), Eubie Blake, Thurgood Marshall, Ogden Nash, Harold Rollins—not to mention Edith the Egg Lady and Divine, both stars of Waters' hilarious films.

Waters keeps making movies here, bless his heart. He's the bad boy who dubbed Baltimore the "hairdo capital of the world," a term that hasn't lost much of its relevance in the quarter-century since the director of *Hairspray*, *Polyester*, and *Pink Flamingos* came up with it. We have some amazing hair days here. The Cafe Hon even has an annual big-hair contest.

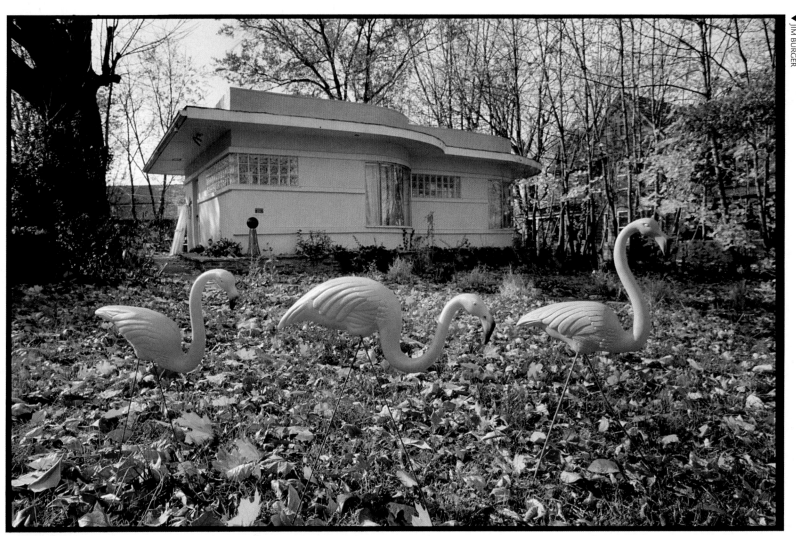

JIM BURGER

THE WORLD-RENOWNED BALTIMORE SYMPHONY ORCHESTRA ALWAYS DE-LIVERS MUSIC TO NURTURE THE SOUL, BUT NEVER SO MUCH AS IN THE FALL OF 1990, WHEN THE ENSEMBLE WAS FRONTED BY CAB CALLOWAY, A LEG-ENDARY JAZZMAN WHO HAILED FROM CHARM CITY (PAGES 12 AND 13).

Baltimore has also been called Mob Town—because of what rowdies did to Union troops as they passed through Pratt Street on their way to the Civil War. And I've heard it called the Renaissance City. Kurt Schmoke, who was elected mayor in 1987 and two more times after that, dubbed it The City That Reads. Some of us like to call it the Queen City of the Patapsco Drainage Basin.

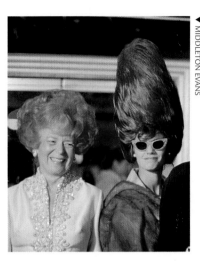

But Charm City seems to have stuck.

Baltimore might also be the Snow Panic Capital of the East. We are snowanoid. Baltimoreans have a habit of buying a month's supply of toilet paper and milk at the mere rumor of snow. Honest. You can see this demonstrated on the 11 o'clock news before every snowfall, year in and year out. We don't handle winters well, and that's probably because, until recent years, we haven't had all that much experience with bad ones. We have an in-between climate. It's not northeasterly, it's not southern—except in summer, when the place can feel like a swamp. The city in summer no longer smells "like 10,000 pole cats," as Mencken put it. But in July and August, Baltimore *does* belong to the 3-H Society—hazy, hot, and humid. ☛

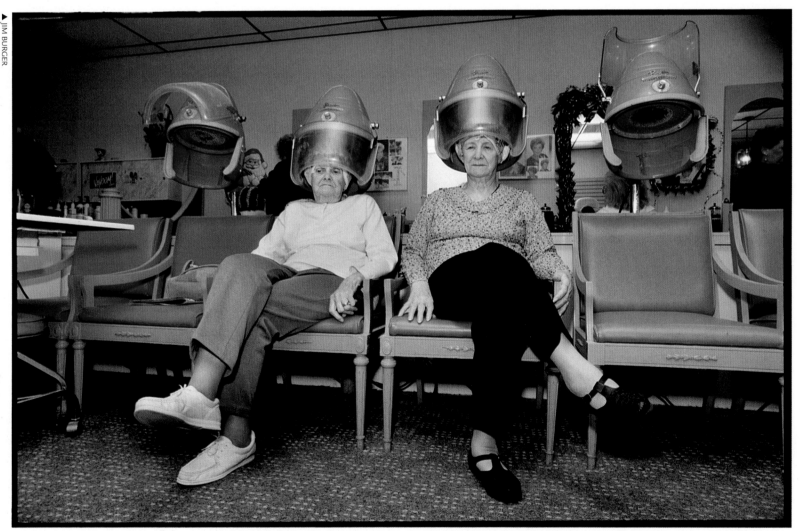

"TO ME, BAD TASTE IS WHAT ENTERTAINMENT IS ALL ABOUT. BUT ONE MUST REMEMBER THAT THERE IS SUCH A THING AS GOOD BAD TASTE AND BAD BAD TASTE." SO SAYS JOHN WATERS, A B-FILM AUTEUR WHO CREATED SUCH UNFORGETTABLE CLASSICS AS *Hairspray, Pink Flamingos, Polyester,* AND *Cry-Baby.* A NATIVE BALTIMOREAN, WATERS FOUND PLENTY OF INSPIRATION RIGHT HERE AT HOME.

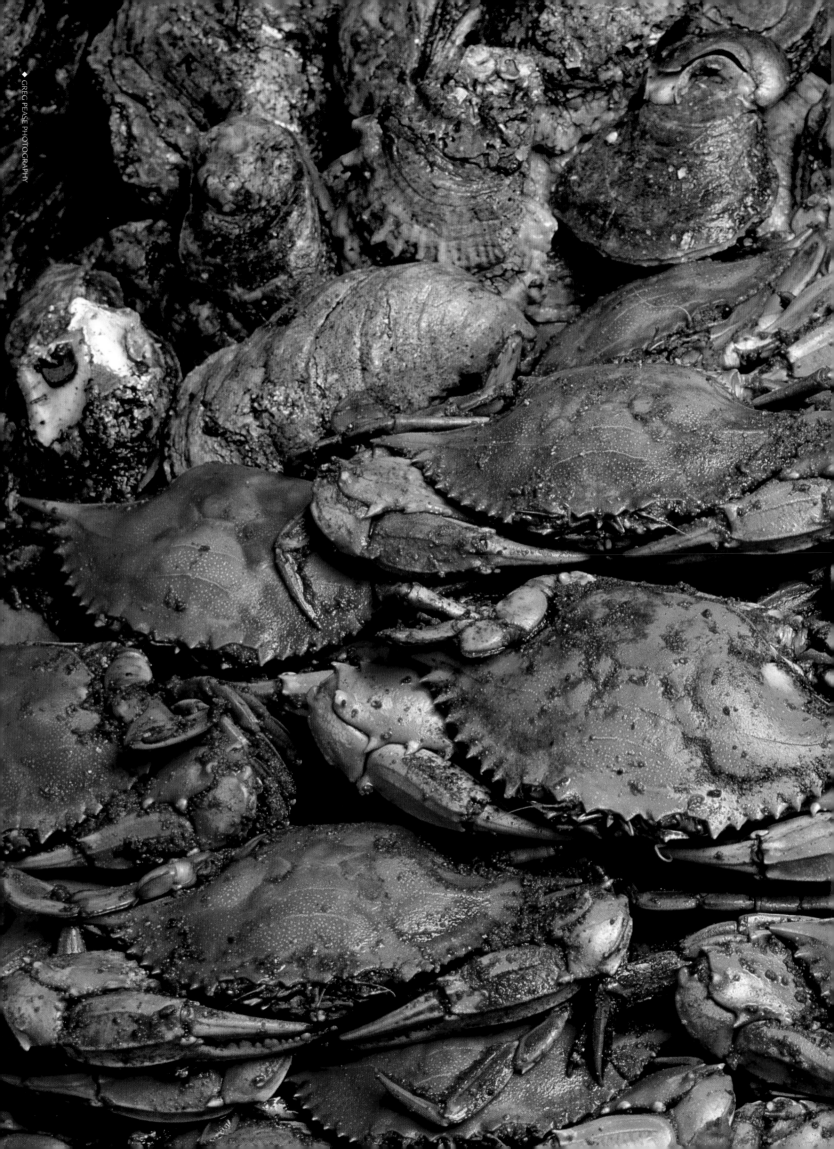

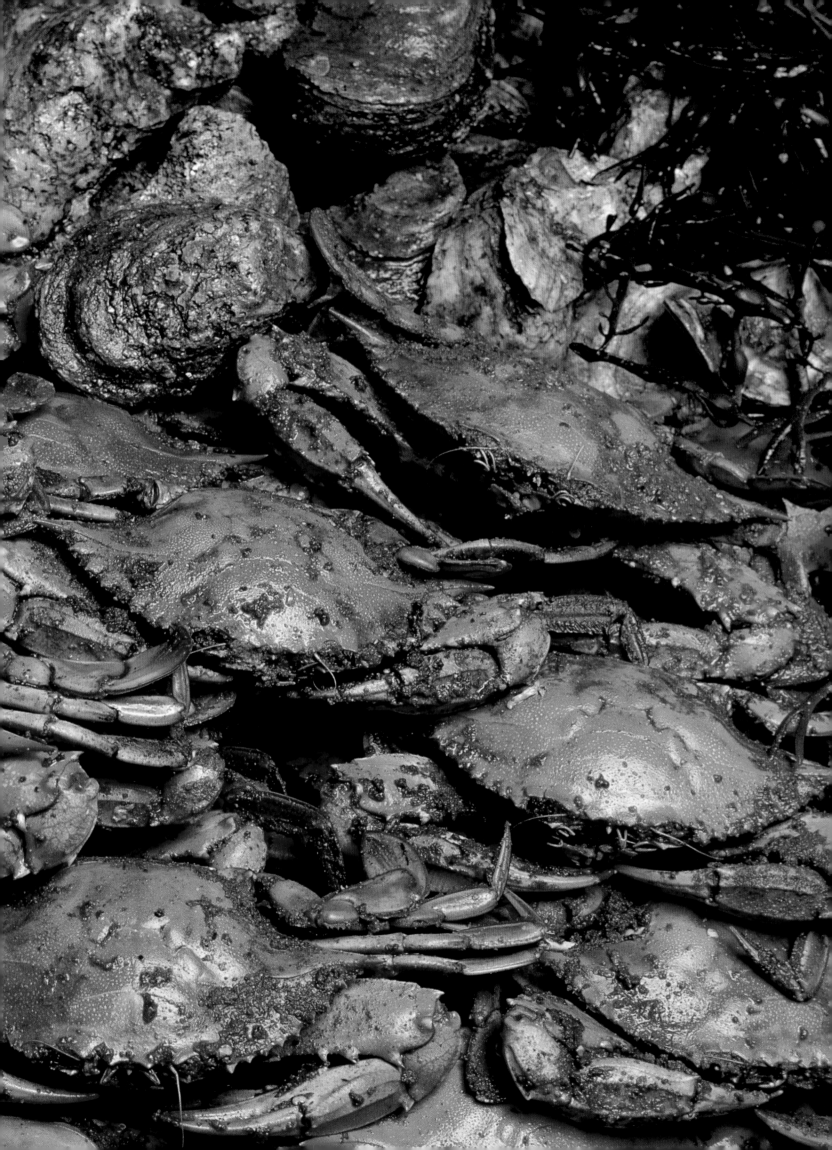

WE DON'T KNOW THE NAME OF THE FIRST MAN OR WOMAN WHO LOOKED AT A CHESAPEAKE blue crab and decided it would be good to eat. Whoever, he or she was a brave and/or hungry person, and we are forever indebted to such a pioneering palate. Crabs are, indeed, a local delicacy. You catch them by using chicken necks tied to butcher string. You drop the bait into a bay or creek, right off a bridge or a boat. When the crab grabs, you give the line a gentle tug, then hand-over-hand it. As the crab reaches the surface, still clutching the chicken neck, you snatch it with a net. Men line the Poteet Street bridge in South Baltimore all summer to do this.

Of course, you can buy live crabs by the bushel. Sometimes you'll find them for sale on the roadside, out of the back of a pickup. There are seafood shops that specialize in crabs all over town; in West Baltimore, there are even four at one intersection. When you see a sign for Steamed Females, it's crabs they're selling.

Order them in a crab house and the waitress will spread newspaper over your table and hand you a wooden mallet and maybe a nutcracker. (She might call you "hon," too.) Then, she'll pile heavily seasoned, steamed

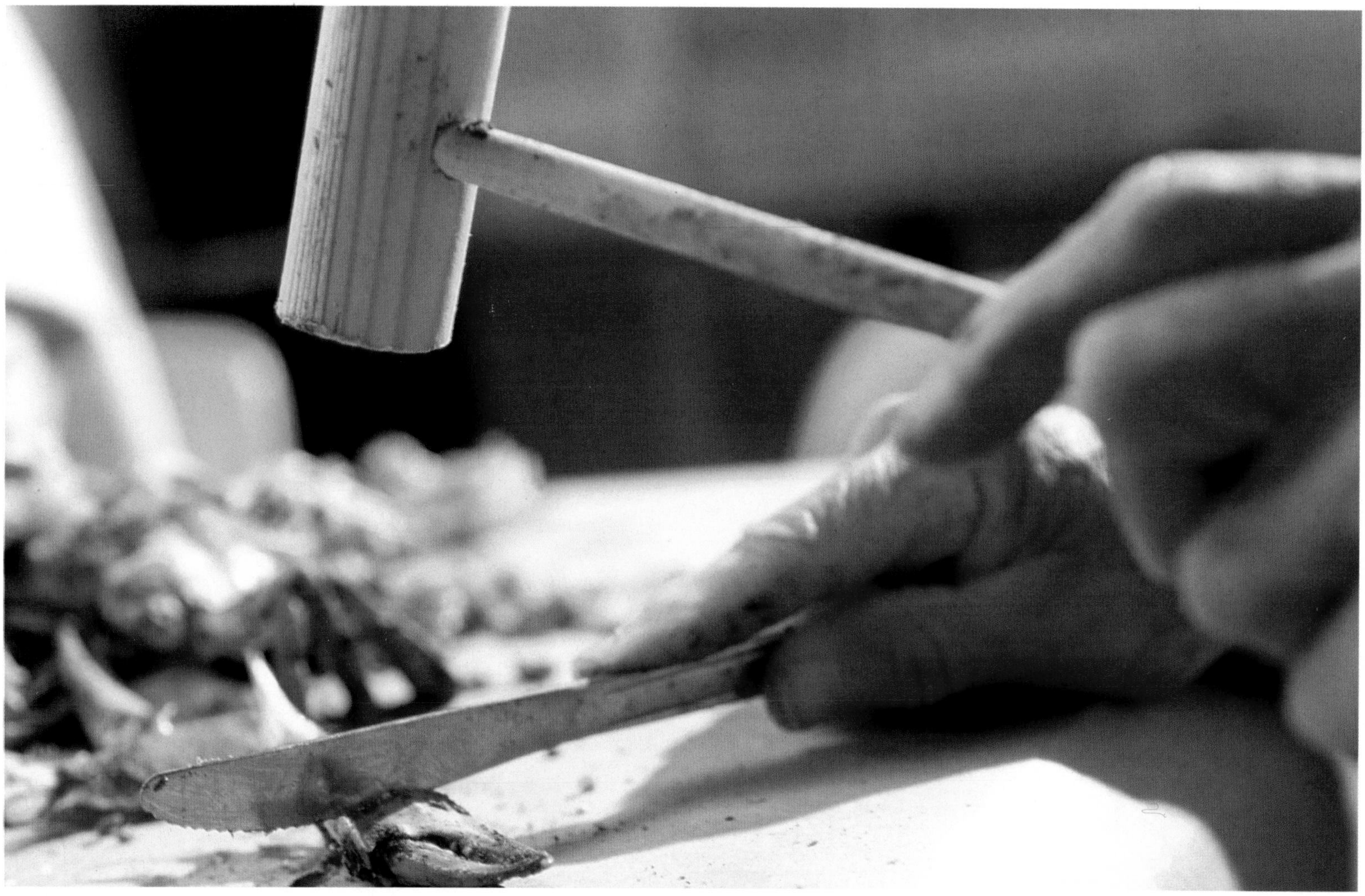

▶ GREG PEASE PHOTOGRAPHY

WROTE AUTHOR JAMES MICHENER IN *Chesapeake*: "A CRAB PROVIDES LITTLE FOOD, SO HE IS NOT EASY TO EAT. BUT THE LITTLE HE DOES OFFER IS THE BEST FOOD UNDER THE SKY. TO EAT CRAB YOU MUST WORK, WHICH MAKES YOU APPRECIATE HIM MORE." THE TRADITIONAL CRAB FEAST IS AN ALL-YOU-CAN-EAT AFFAIR WITH CRITTERS RANGING IN SIZE FROM SMALL TO JUMBO. THE MEAL IS USUALLY SERVED WITH HUSH PUPPIES, FRIED CHICKEN, FRESH CORN ON THE COB, COLESLAW, AND PITCHERS OF LOCALLY BREWED BEER.

crabs a dozen at a time on the table, and you attack the hard shells. A good crab feast can take hours. It's a social event.

So are bull roasts, or bull-and-oyster roasts. When someone needs money to campaign for public office or funds for a local booster club, they rent an American Legion post, volunteer fire company, or catering hall and sell tickets to an eat-a-thon. You get beer and setups; beef roasted on outdoor pits cut from steel tanks; oysters and clams on the half shell; maybe some steamed shrimp, potato salad, and coleslaw; and usually crab soup—although not necessarily in that order. Bull roasts are big in the winter and spring.

We have upscale restaurants—some truly fabulous places—that year after year make every list maker's top 10. But then there are all those diners and other little places—the Double T Diner, the Bel Loc, Rollo's, the Sip & Bite, Jimmy's, the Yellow Bowl, Werner's, and the House of Welsh—as well as numerous ethnic restaurants and a whole new generation of hip restaurants run by young, innovative chefs. ☛

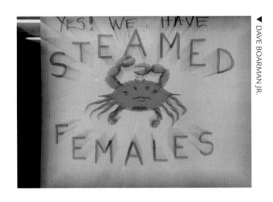

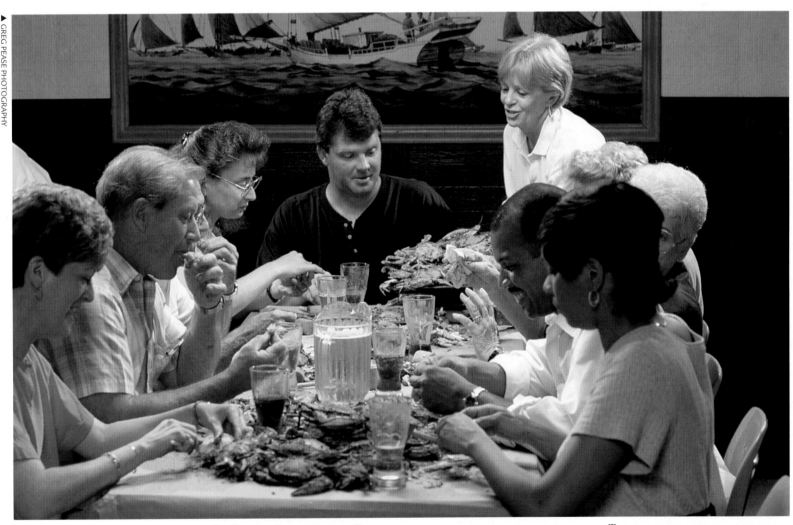

BO BROOKS CRABHOUSE AND RESTAU-RANT IS JUST ONE OF BALTIMORE'S SHRINES TO CLASSIC CRAB CONSUMP-TION, COMPLETE WITH BRASH WAIT-RESSES, PAPER-COVERED TABLES, AND LONG LINES OF HUNGRY DINERS WAIT-ING TO GET INSIDE (ABOVE). FAIDLEY'S SEAFOOD (PAGES 20 AND 21) SERVES UP SOME OF THE BEST CRAB CAKES IN THE CITY, ACCORDING TO LOCAL POLLS. THE FAMILY-RUN SHOP IS PART OF LEXINGTON MARKET, WHICH HAS BEEN A CENTRAL RESOURCE FOR FOODSTUFFS GROWN AND CAUGHT ON CHESAPEAKE BAY SINCE 1782.

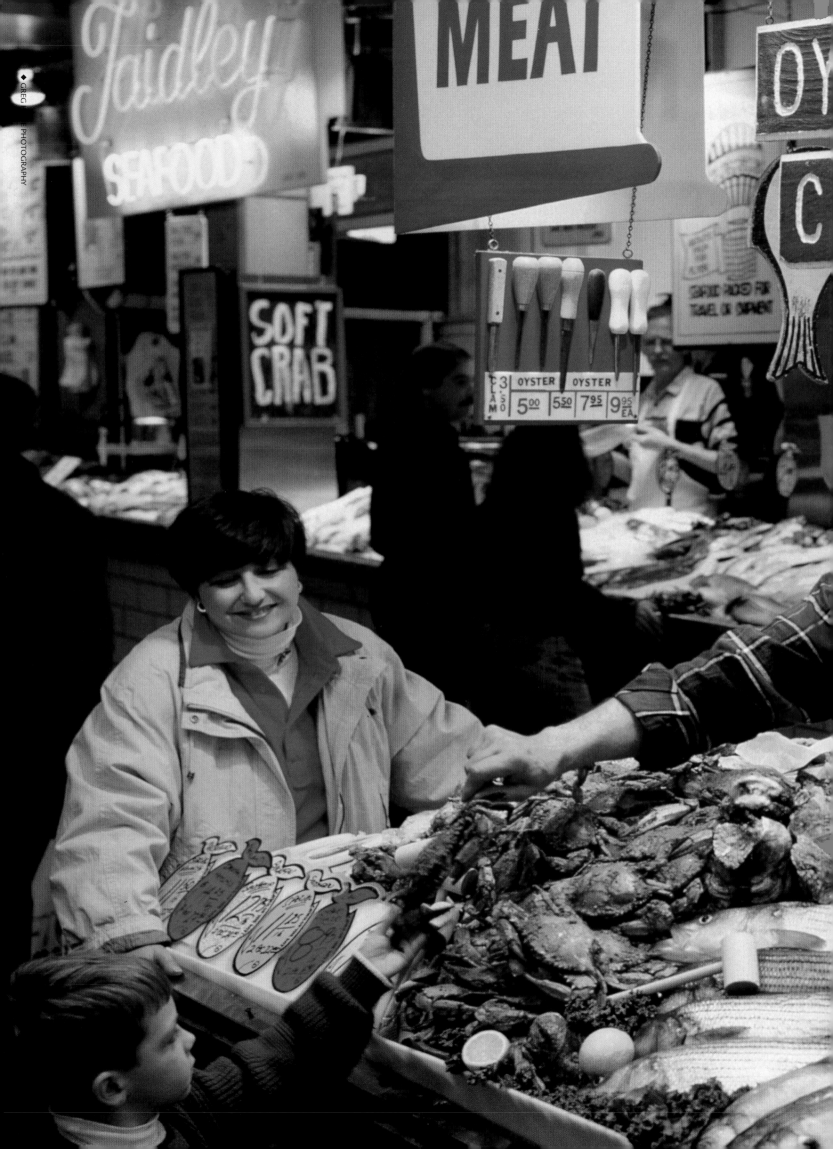

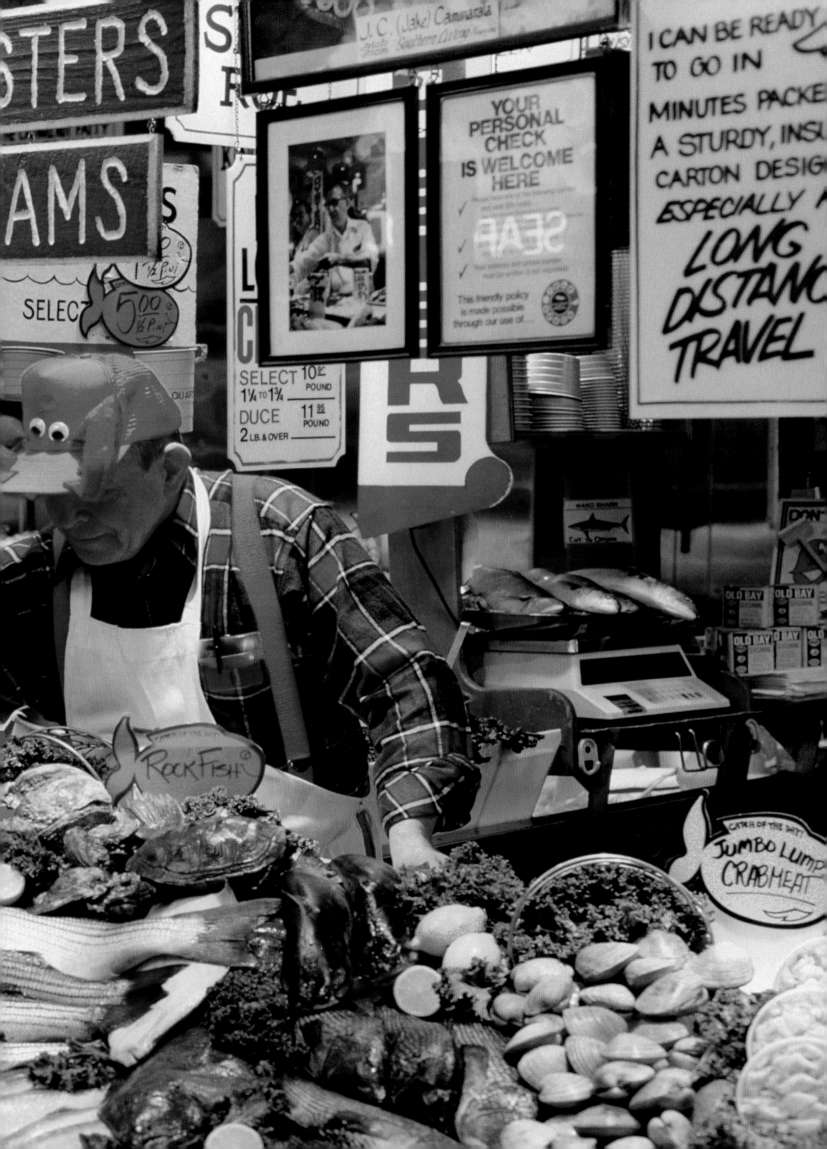

T

ELL YOU WHAT'S GOOD: LEXINGTON MARKET. YOU CAN GET JUST ABOUT ANYTHING THERE. It's full of butchers, bakers, produce vendors, and hundreds of shoppers at a time. It does a big weekday lunch business, and there might not be a better example of the "great good place" in Baltimore. The city is at its best when it gets together to chow down like that. Cross Street Market, in South Baltimore, is another great gathering place—black and white, young and old, longtime resident and sushi-eating yuppie, all moving, shopping, standing, drinking, eating, cruising, flirting, and talking under one long roof. There are eight public markets in the city, and they remain a focal point of neighborhood life.

Another thing about Baltimore: It actually begins before you get here, before you pass the welcome sign with the faded "Hon" graffiti. You feel the place before you're in the place.

From almost every approach—along the big waterfront and industrial ramparts on the south and east, the commercial corridors and rowhouse neighborhoods to the west, the spreading suburbs and big valleys to the north—you can sense a sympathetic force that pulls everyone, no matter how spiritually and physically scattered

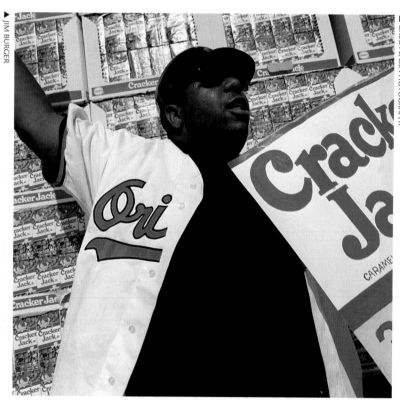

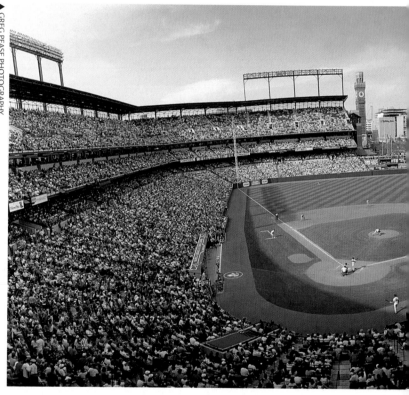

ORIOLE PARK AT CAMDEN YARDS SPARKED A REVOLUTION IN STADIUM DESIGN, THANKS TO A BACK-TO-THE-FUTURE APPROACH THAT MERGES OLD-FASHIONED TRADITION WITH NEW-FANGLED CONVENIENCE. ALTHOUGH REPLICAS OF THE BALLPARK HAVE SPROUTED UP IN CITIES LIKE DENVER AND CLEVELAND, NOTHING CAN BEAT BALTIMORE'S DIE-HARD FANS, SOME OF WHOM HAVE SPENT A LIFETIME CHEER-ING ON THEIR BELOVED BIRDS.

they might be, toward Baltimore. Or back to it. There's a Baltimore diaspora throughout the surrounding counties.

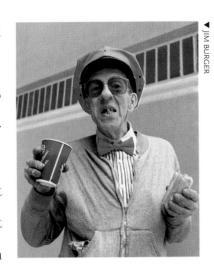

A man might say he lives in Linthicum; a woman might say Randallstown. But to someone from out of town, they simply say, "I'm from Baltimore." Not "the Baltimore area." Just "Baltimore."

And if it's someone who has spent an entire lifetime here, you're likely to hear it pronounced "Bawlmer," as in "Bawlmer, Merlin." Some people believe the accent is dying off as the old palatinate becomes more and more homogenized. But you can still hear "Bawlmerese" spoken here. You hear it in Highlandtown and Essex. You hear it in Parkville. You hear it whenever William Donald Schaefer, the mayor during the Baltimore Renaissance, gives a speech at a downtown business luncheon. When the Orioles still played in Memorial Stadium, you could hear a cheer in Section 34 for the great Cal Ripken Jr. (a native of Aberdeen, but a Baltimorean at heart) that went: "Come owen, Cal, put it in the bull pen now." (In Bawlmerese, "now" comes out "nal," and just about rhymes with Cal.) ☛

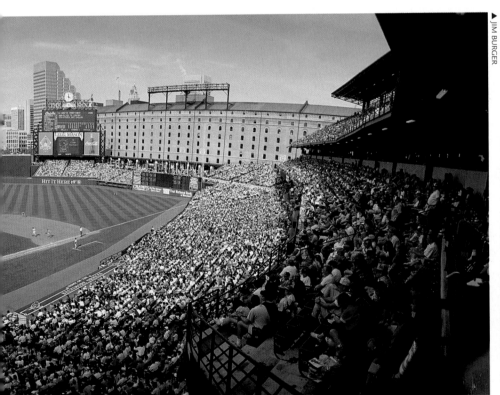

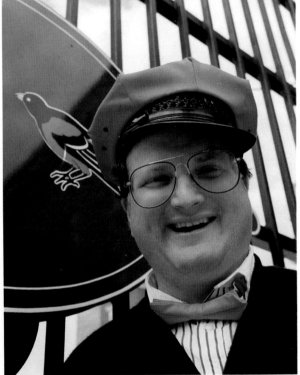

BALTIMORE'S BASEBALL HEROES—BOTH PAST AND PRESENT—ARE IMMORTAL IN THE MINDS OF LOCAL FANS: IN 1996, LONGTIME ORIOLE CAL RIPKEN JR. SURPASSED LOU GEHRIG'S RECORD FOR CONSECUTIVE GAMES PLAYED (PAGE 24). DESPITE DEVOTING MOST OF HIS CAREER TO THE NEW YORK YANKEES, NATIVE SON BABE RUTH IS AS BELOVED AS ANY ORIOLE (PAGE 25).

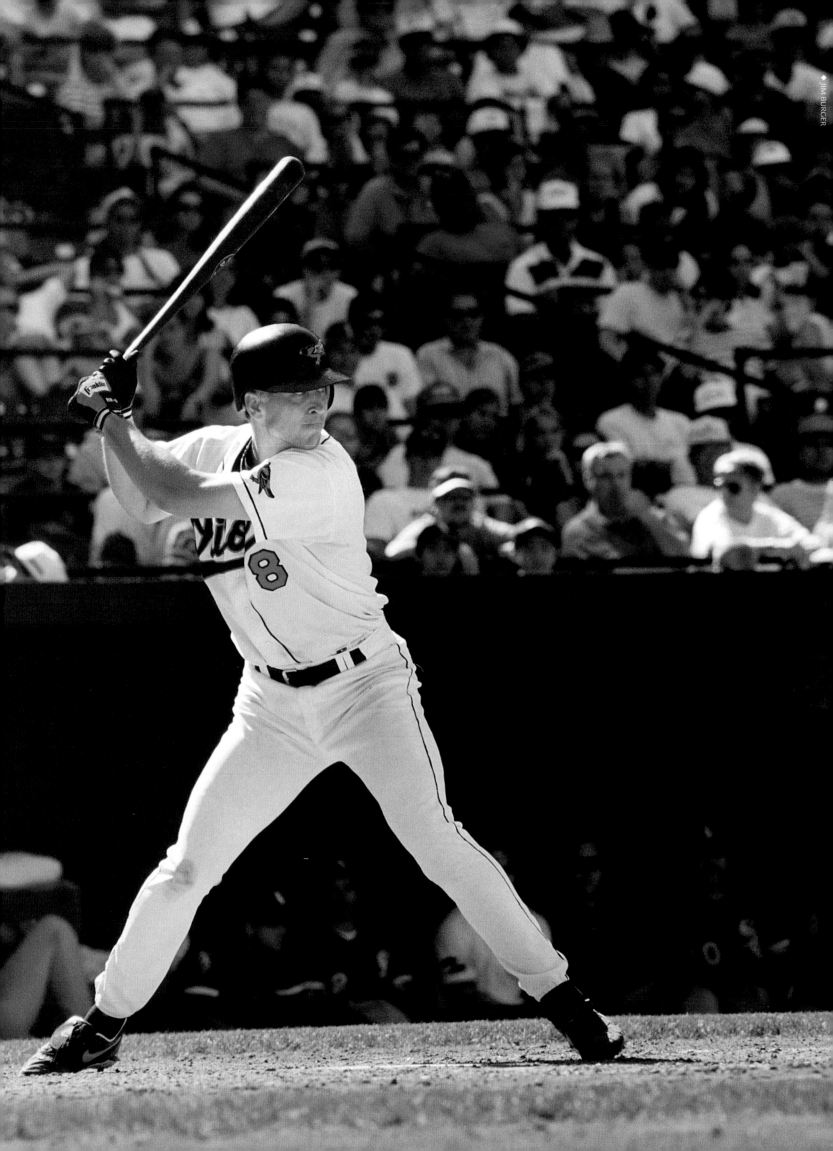

EUTAW STREET

Baltimore is a big place. Not dense. But big, wide, flat, sprawling. Someone drew a huge, curving, crooked line around it and built a beltway in 1962. It's 51.7 miles, with eight lanes in two loops—an inner loop and an outer loop—and helpful signs to tell you which one you're driving on at any given moment. ✺ As vast as Baltimore is, it's almost impossible to get lost around here—unless, of course, you go looking for Eutaw Street, and your brain locks on the conventional spelling, "Utah." All roads lead downtown, and the city traffic patterns have few surprises. The streets are basically a grid that never locks (except when we get snow). You can always find your way to the heart of the city, and you can do it the old-fashioned way if you have to: You can look up. The city emits a haze most days. The sky glows at night.

In Catonsville, a dozen miles to the southwest, you can stand on a front porch and see, from a surprising rise in the landscape, the tantalizing glitter of downtown, the lights at Oriole Park, and a few artistically illuminated

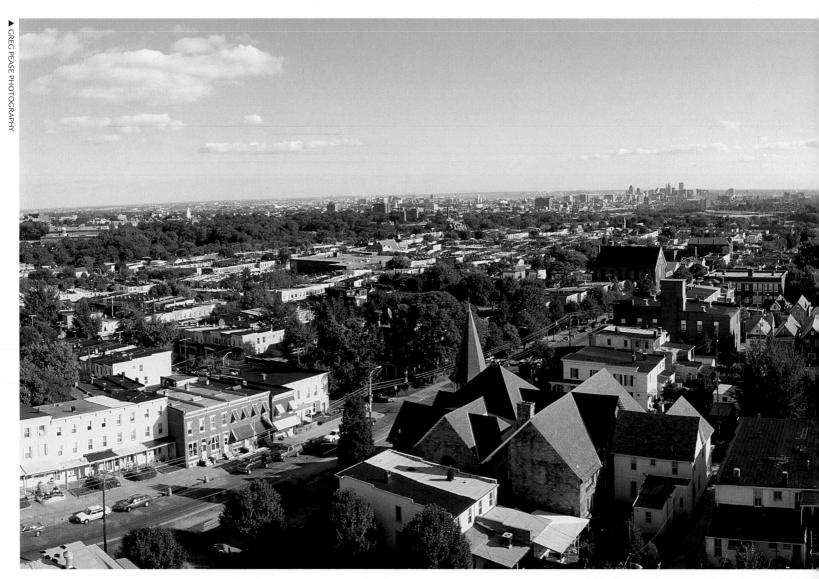

▲ GREG PEASE PHOTOGRAPHY

BALTIMORE'S METROPOLITAN SPRAWL IS KEPT IN CHECK BY ITS OMNIPRESENT NEIGHBORHOODS, KNOWN BY SUCH QUAINT NAMES AS RIDGELY'S DELIGHT, TUSCANY-CANTERBURY, PIGTOWN, AND MOUNT VERNON.

office towers. It makes the city seem more cosmopolitan than anyone here would claim it to be.

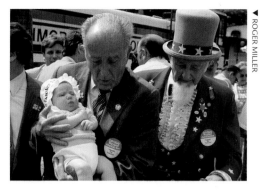

ROGER MILLER

On many nights, 30 miles away in the north woods of Baltimore County, near the vast reservoir that provides the metropolitan area with water, you can see the city's orange glimmer, like the campfires of a distant village.

Out on the Chesapeake Bay, aboard a tug or pleasure boat, there is no mistaking where you are headed or where you just came from—the Port of Baltimore. In this harbor, once upon a time, Francis Scott Key got the inspiration for the national anthem, hundreds of thousands of immigrants arrived from Europe, Bethlehem Steel created a small city within a city, and the Rouse Company built the centerpiece of our urban renewal efforts—Harborplace.

Baltimore is the glow at the top of the bay. ☞

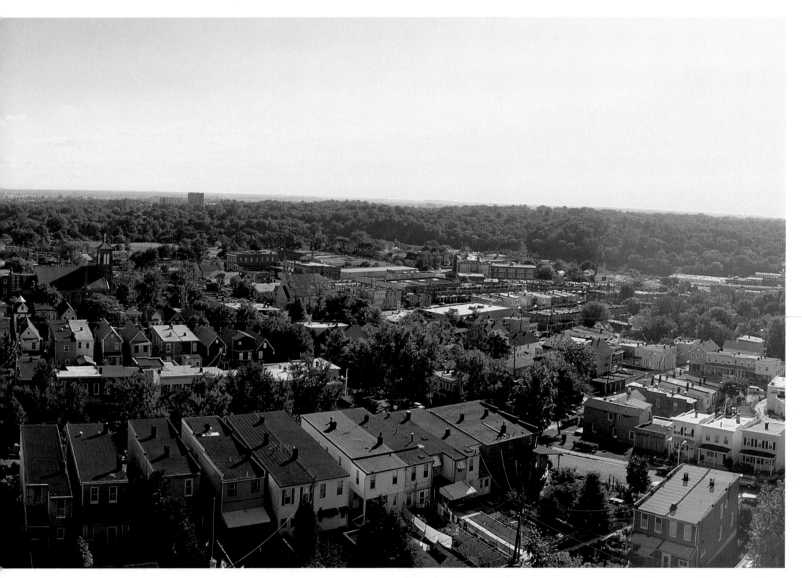

WILLIAM DONALD SCHAEFER IS A FAMILIAR FIGURE TO BALTIMOREANS YOUNG AND OLD (TOP). THE TWO-TERM STATE GOVERNOR WAS ALSO CITY MAYOR DURING THE BALTIMORE RENAISSANCE, WHICH RECEIVED NATIONAL ATTENTION IN THE 1970S.

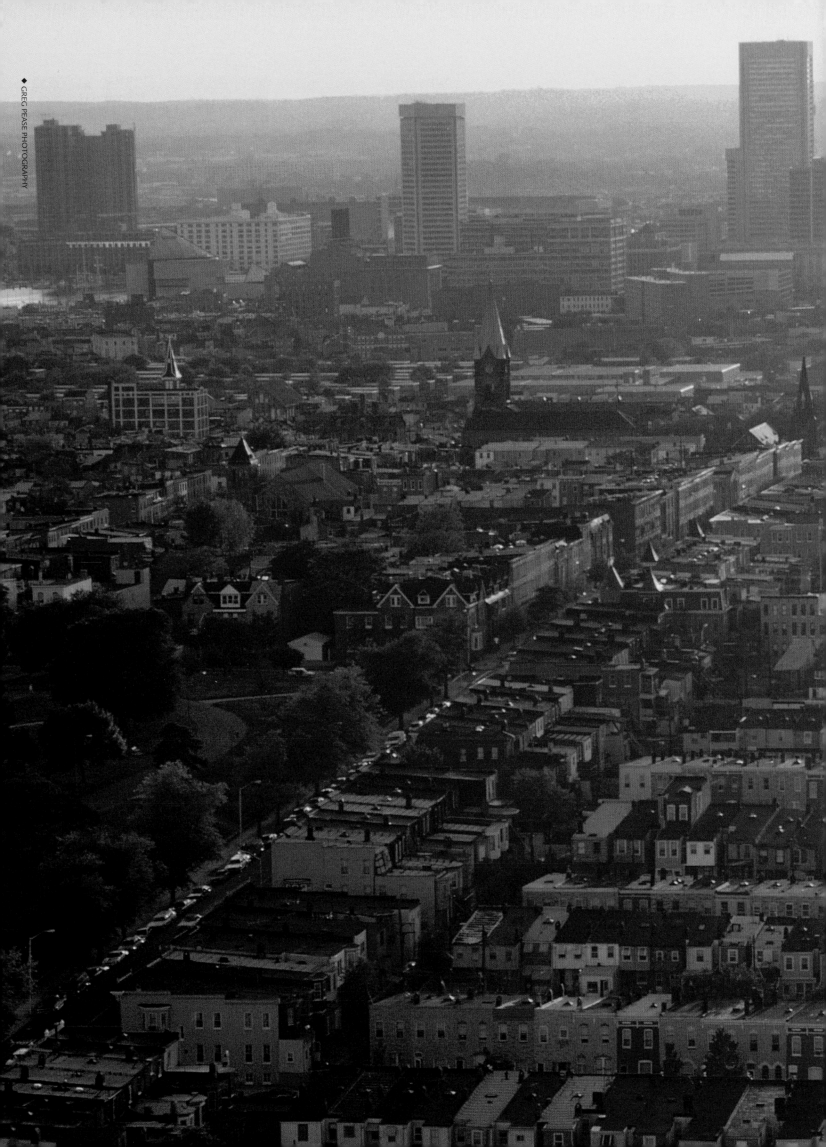

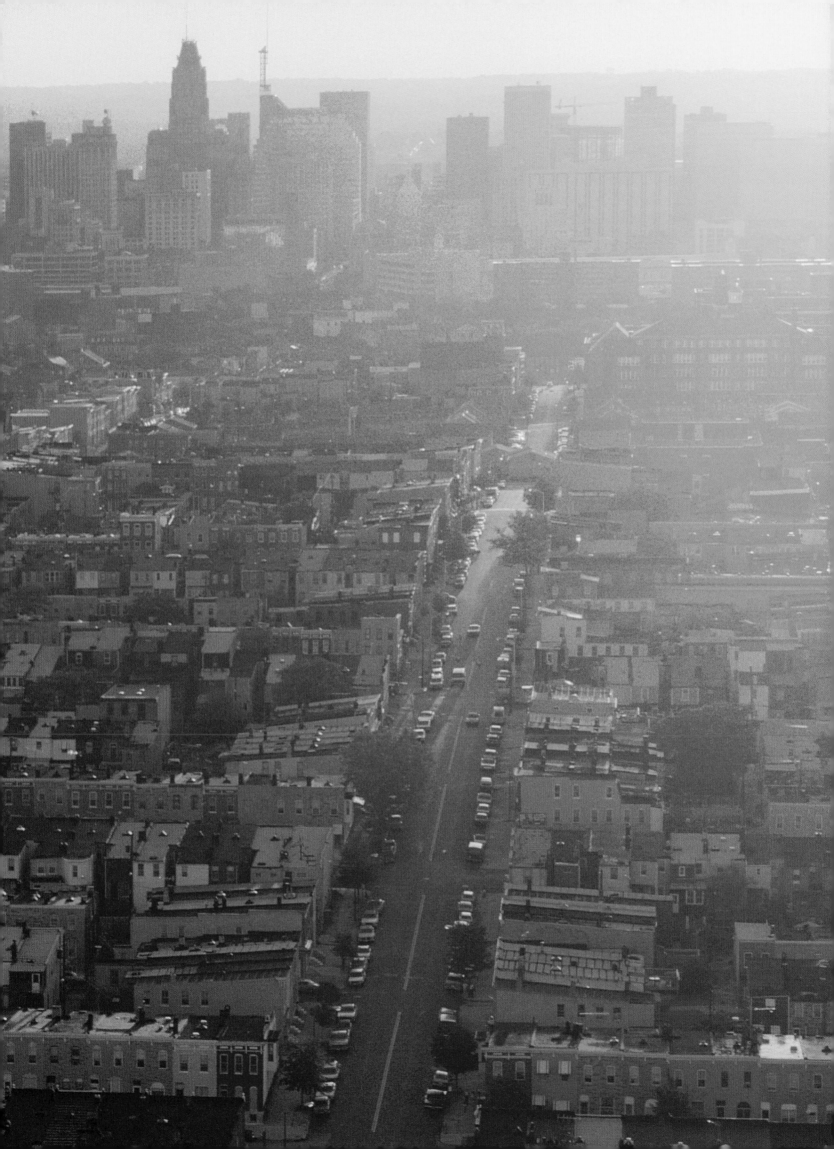

IN RECENT YEARS, MUCH HAS BEEN MADE OF THE SCHISM BETWEEN THE CITY AND ITS WEALTHIER, independent suburbs. But an alluring force remains in the atmosphere—a sense of center, anchored on the upper bay, home to people who no longer get their mail here. Suburbanites still connect to the rituals and traditions of Baltimore. They still take pride in its progress, still complain about its politics and its social problems, and still indulge themselves in its many charms.

The charms begin before you get here, too.

There are still valleys for the horse set—from the hard-sweat Thoroughbred farmers to the old-money foxhunters—to the north of the city. Though housing and commercial development continue to spread farther and farther away from the edges of Baltimore and its older suburbs, your approach from the north and east takes you through bucolic settings, with pastures and miles of four-board fence. The big, brawny Susquehanna River runs through Harford County and pours into the Chesapeake near Havre de Grace. The Gunpowder River, a blue-ribbon trout stream in Baltimore County, is a 35-minute drive from downtown, as is the popular hike-and-bike trail that runs high above its wooded banks. Just north of the city, the Baltimore County seat of Towson, once a dullsville of politicians and bureaucrats in polyester suits, now boasts the kind of nightlife amenities that had once only been found in the city.

Driving west from downtown, you hit Leakin Park, one of the largest city parks in America and site of the Baltimore Herb Festival, an annual earth-mother celebration; a little farther, and there's Dickeyville, a charming

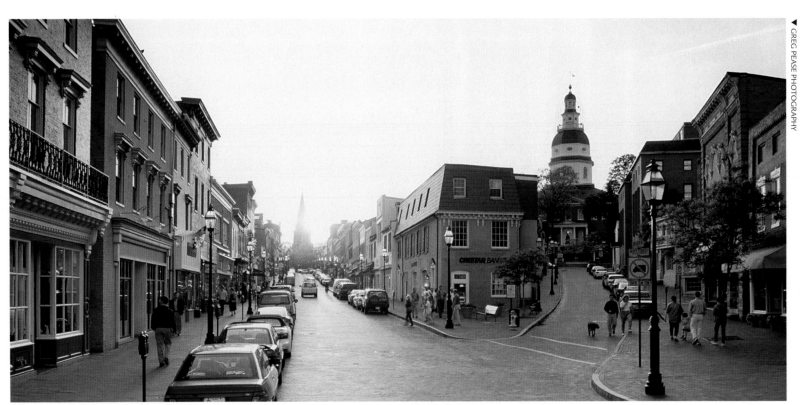

THE BRILLIANT SUN CASTS ITS DRA-MATIC GLOW ON SCENES THROUGHOUT MARYLAND, FROM AN EASTWARD VIEW OF DOWNTOWN BALTIMORE (PAGES 28 AND 29) TO THE INTERSECTION OF MAIN AND FRANCIS STREETS IN ANNAPOLIS (ABOVE), AND FROM A BUCOLIC HORSE FARM IN BALTIMORE COUNTY (OPPOSITE BOTTOM) TO A LONE FISHERMAN ENJOYING THE LAST MOMENTS OF DAYLIGHT (OPPOSITE TOP).

old mill village within the city limits; a little farther, and you're into a state park that runs along the Patapsco River.

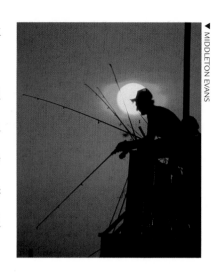

That puts you in Howard County, with its farmland and spreading suburbs, the old hospitable county seat of Ellicott City, and the planned community of Columbia (population 150,000). A little farther still, and Interstate 70 connects you to the western part of Maryland—Frederick, Hagerstown, Cumberland, the upper Potomac River, and the mountains of Garrett County. Someone once declared Maryland "America in Miniature." From Baltimore, you can get to America easily.

To the east of the city, there are hundreds of miles of nooks and crannies along dozens of coves and creeks—Frog Mortar, Turkey Neck, Booby Point—and rivers that feed the Chesapeake. And to the south, Annapolis, one of the nation's truly quaint state capitals, is a mere zip-trip now. You can be on the Bay Bridge, headed to Maryland's eastern shore and the Atlantic Ocean, in less than an hour. (The ocean, though, is still another two hours from there.)

The miracle miles—Ritchie Highway, Route 40, Reisterstown Road, Liberty Road, and Security Boulevard—provide the long, dense commercial strips in still-growing suburbs that have become economically strong jurisdictions independent of Baltimore.

But the city remains the centerpiece of this little universe. ☛

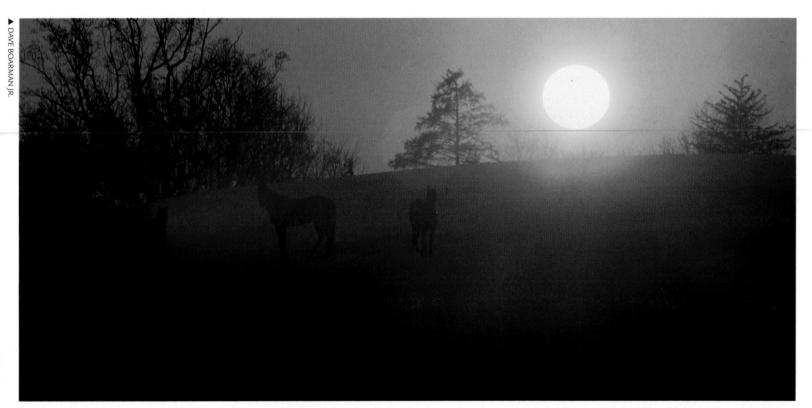

ALTHOUGH THE CITY IS BEST KNOWN FOR ITS RELATIONSHIP WITH THE CHESAPEAKE, LOCALS FIND PLENTY OF WAYS TO ENJOY THE AREA'S OTHER WATERWAYS. NESTLED IN A FORESTED WILDERNESS NORTH OF BALTIMORE, THE GUNPOWDER RIVER MAY BE FAMOUS FOR ITS TROUT AND FLY-FISHING, BUT IT'S ALSO A GREAT DESTINATION FOR AN AFTERNOON OF TUBING (PAGE 33). THOSE WHO PREFER THE RUSH OF KAYAKING THROUGH RAPIDS, HOWEVER, CAN GET THEIR FILL IN THE NEARBY POTOMAC RIVER (PAGE 32).

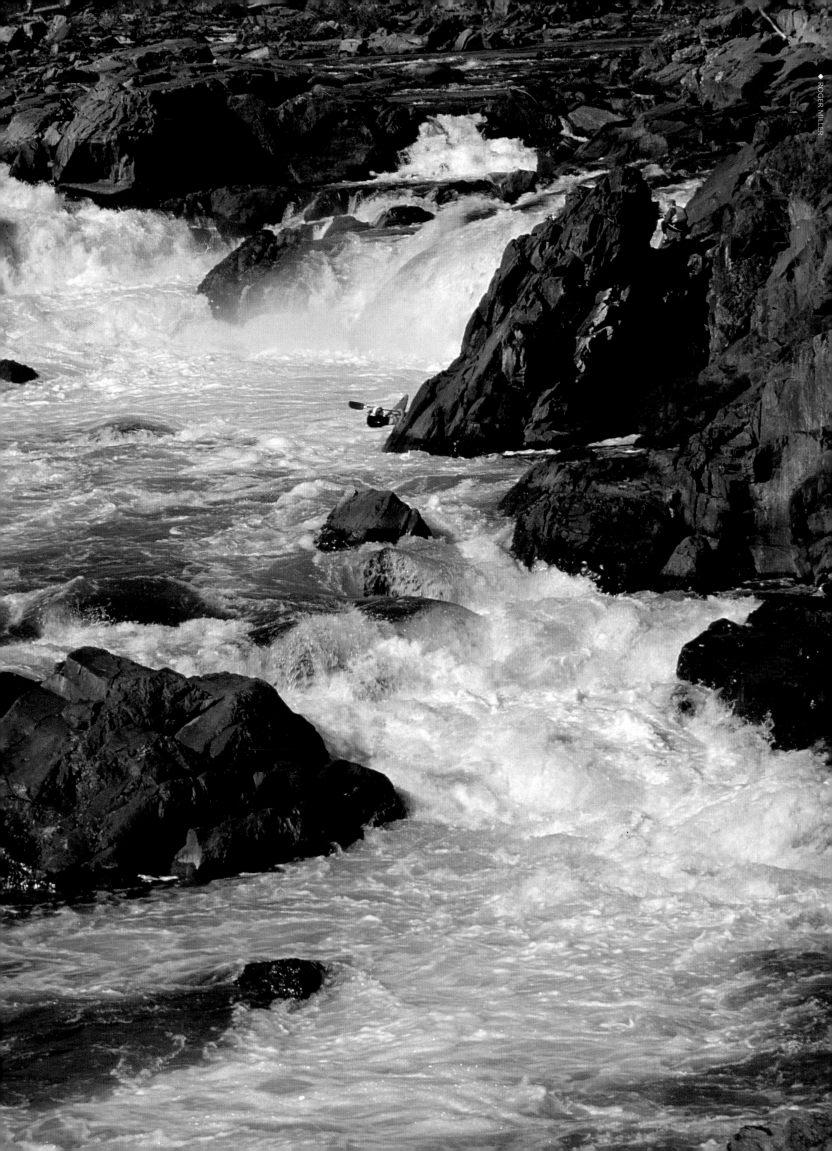

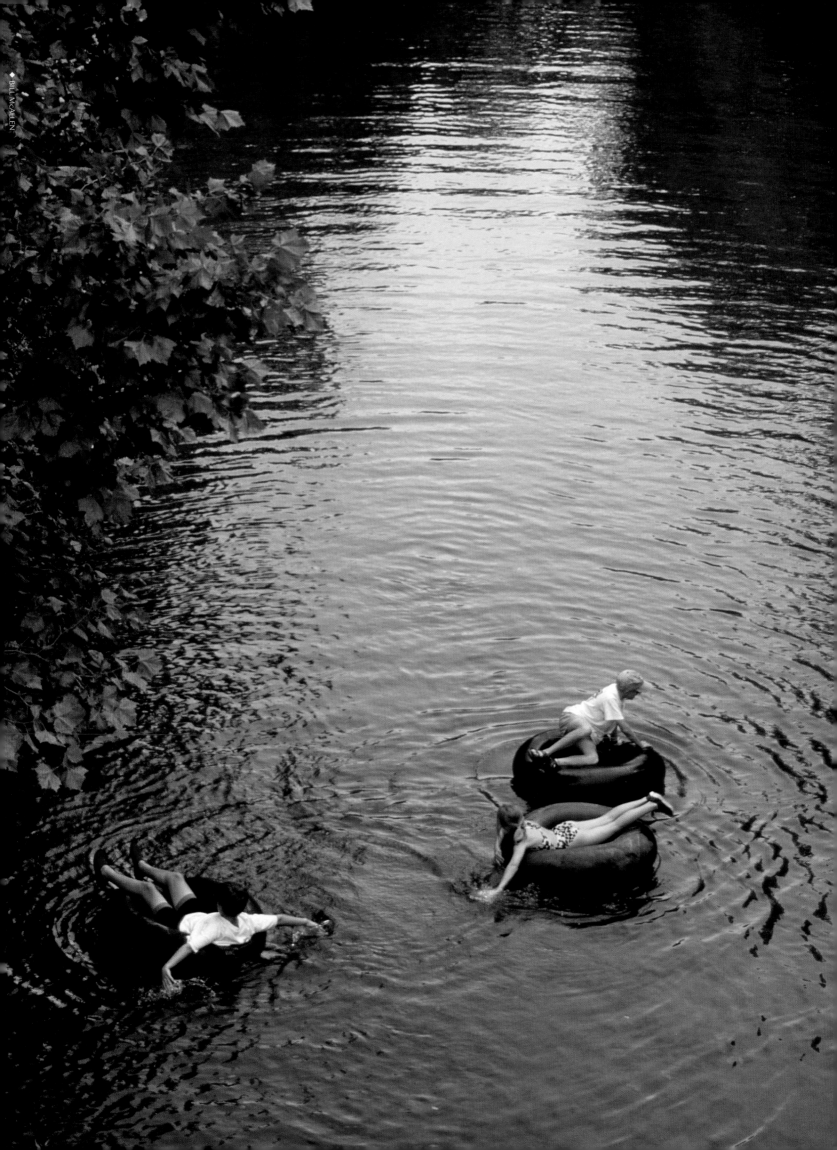

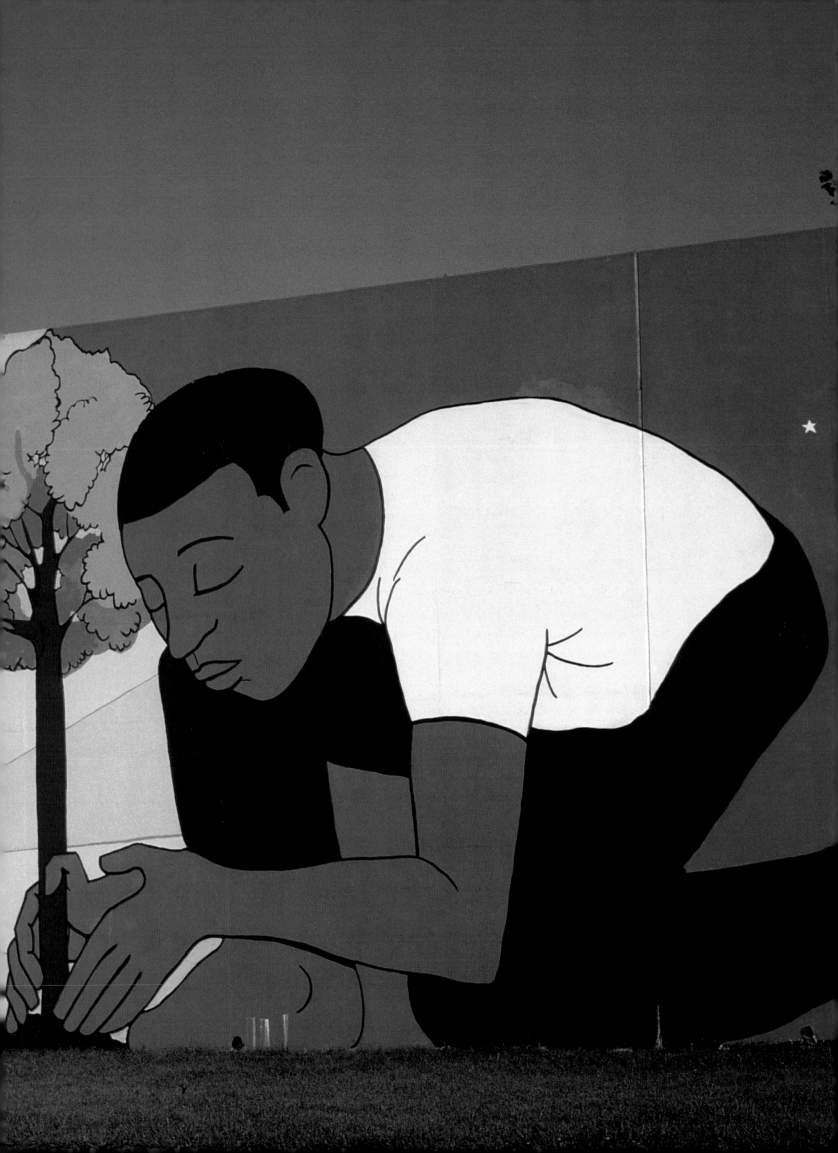

A ND IT'S THE CITY THAT, FOR ALL ITS SOCIAL ILLS, STILL OFFERS THE THINGS THAT, NO MATTER how hard the suburbs try to import them, can't be found anywhere else. One of the many travel writers who have come this way noted how, for years, all he ever knew of Baltimore was the industrial vista apparent from the Harbor Tunnel Thruway on his trips between New York and Washington. Once he got inside, he realized that this industrial facade was just the "tattered overcoat" of a busy northern city laced with old southern charm. That's a common description of Baltimore—we are, after all, south of the Mason-Dixon line—but you also hear this: big city/small town.

Actually, you could describe Baltimore as a series of small towns cobbled together and forming a sprawling metropolis.

That's because of the neighborhoods. Most of them still hold strong, while some have tottered under the weight of crime and poverty. Baltimore has the highest concentration of Maryland's poor, and its population has been in decline. That makes it a city of paradoxes—strong neighborhoods a few blocks from decaying pockets, enclaves of energy and civic health sometimes just a short stroll from abandoned rowhouses and corner stores, panhandlers

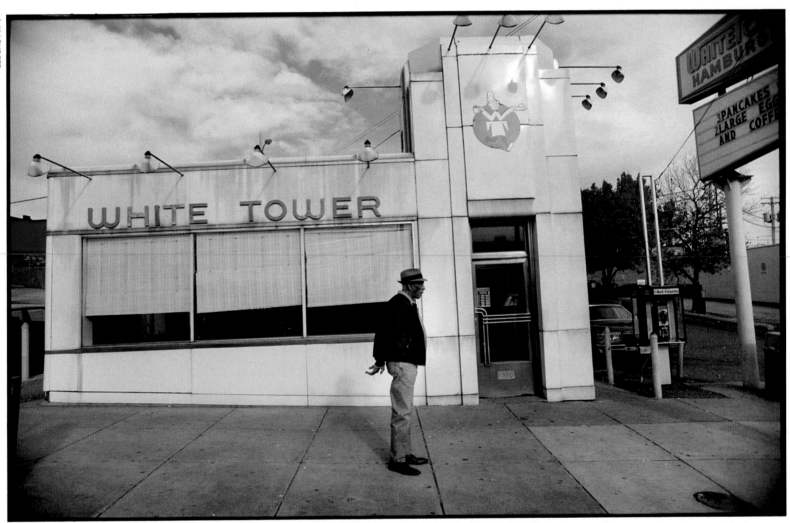

▲ JIM BURGER

BALTIMORE HAS A CHARM ALL ITS OWN, FROM OVERSIZED MURALS WITH AN ENVIRONMENTALLY FRIENDLY THEME TO THE WHITE TOWER COFFEE SHOP CHAIN, WHICH REMAINED A LOCAL ICON FOR DECADES. WHILE ALL WHITE TOWER LOCATIONS HAVE NOW CLOSED, THE 1940S-STYLE CAFÉ LIVES ON AT THE BLAUSTEIN CITY LIFE EXHIBITION CENTER, WHERE THE SHELL OF THE HOWARD STREET SITE WAS PRESERVED AND TURNED BACK INTO A WORKING DINER.

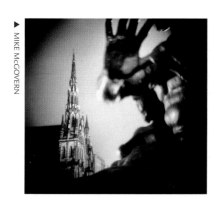

hovering outside the city's toniest restaurants. This is no secret here; the people who live and work in Baltimore are well aware of it.

But we go on, and look for what's good.

And there's a lot that's good—a strong religious life centered in churches and synagogues, diligent community associations that keep public officials on their toes, pride in the progress of the city over the last three decades, and the sense that Baltimore is the center around which life revolves.

Starting in the 1960s—and set to continue for the remainder of the century—Baltimore has benefited from a vigorous, federally funded urban renewal effort that shifted into high gear when Mayor Schaefer and the business leaders he constantly prodded pointed to the Inner Harbor and declared it ground zero for the Baltimore Renaissance. It happened. Harborplace, a modern, urban market at the corner of Light and Pratt streets, became a reality in 1980. The National Aquarium opened in 1981, with Schaefer, the city's greatest cheerleader, donning a Victorian bathing suit and, with a rubber duckie under his arm, plunging into the seal pool. Millions of tourists have been there since. It's been a boon to the city. Natives love to show it off to visitors.

We also love to show off other good stuff—Johns

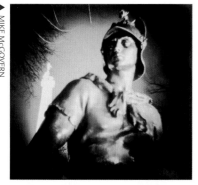

IN MOUNT VERNON SQUARE, IMPRESSIVE STATUES COMPLEMENT SUCH HISTORIC LANDMARKS AS THE ORIGINAL WASHINGTON MONUMENT, ERECTED IN 1829 (BOTTOM), AND MOUNT VERNON METHODIST CHURCH, COMPLETED IN 1872 (TOP).

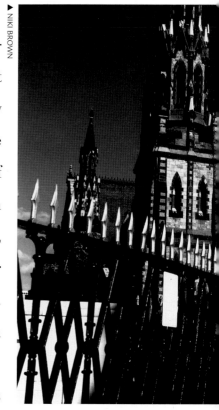

THE VICTORIAN GOTHIC MOUNT VERNON METHODIST CHURCH (ABOVE) STANDS ON THE SITE WHERE FRANCIS SCOTT KEY, WHO SCRIBED *The Star-Spangled Banner*, LIVED AND DIED.

Hopkins University, the world-renowned hospital and extensive medical system; the Walters Art Gallery; the Baltimore Museum of Art; Fort McHenry; the Basilica of the Assumption; the Enoch Pratt Free Library; Charles Street (especially in April, when the Bradford pear trees are in bloom); the Morgan University Choir; the Peabody Conservatory of Music; the Baltimore Symphony Orchestra; the Lyric Opera House, home of the Baltimore Opera; the historic Orchard Street Church;

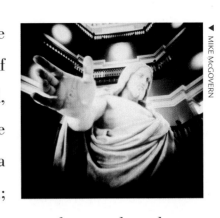

"A-rabbers" selling produce off their pony-drawn wagons; the grand rowhouses of Bolton and Reservoir hills; the redeveloped neighborhoods of Otterbein and Ridgely's Delight; Parks Sausages or Haussner's Restaurant, packed with Dutch and Flemish art; the Women's Industrial Exchange; Union Square and Mencken's home; the Babe Ruth birthplace and museum; boccie games on summer evenings in Little Italy; Mary Sue Easter Eggs; Ostrowski's Polish sausage; the Friday line for homemade pierogi at St. Michael's Ukrainian Catholic Church; the view from Federal Hill; the European look and feel of Mount Vernon on the approach from Charles Street; Druid Hill Park and the zoo. These are all points of great civic pride. We love to savor visitors' reactions to the discovery that there's really something to Baltimore besides the Harbor Tunnel, besides Harborplace. ☛

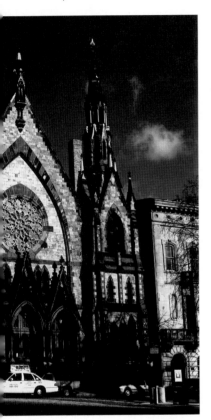

STATELY SCULPTURE IS SCATTERED THROUGHOUT THE CITY'S MUSEUMS AND INSTITUTIONS, INCLUDING JOHNS HOPKINS HOSPITAL (TOP RIGHT) AND THE WALTERS ART GALLERY (BOTTOM RIGHT).

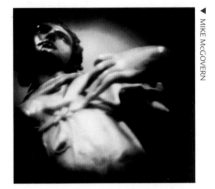

ONE OF THE INNER HARBOR'S BEST-KEPT SECRETS IS THE PEACEFUL PLAZA ATOP THE RENAISSANCE HARBORPLACE HOTEL'S FIVE-STORY ATRIUM (PAGES 38 AND 39).

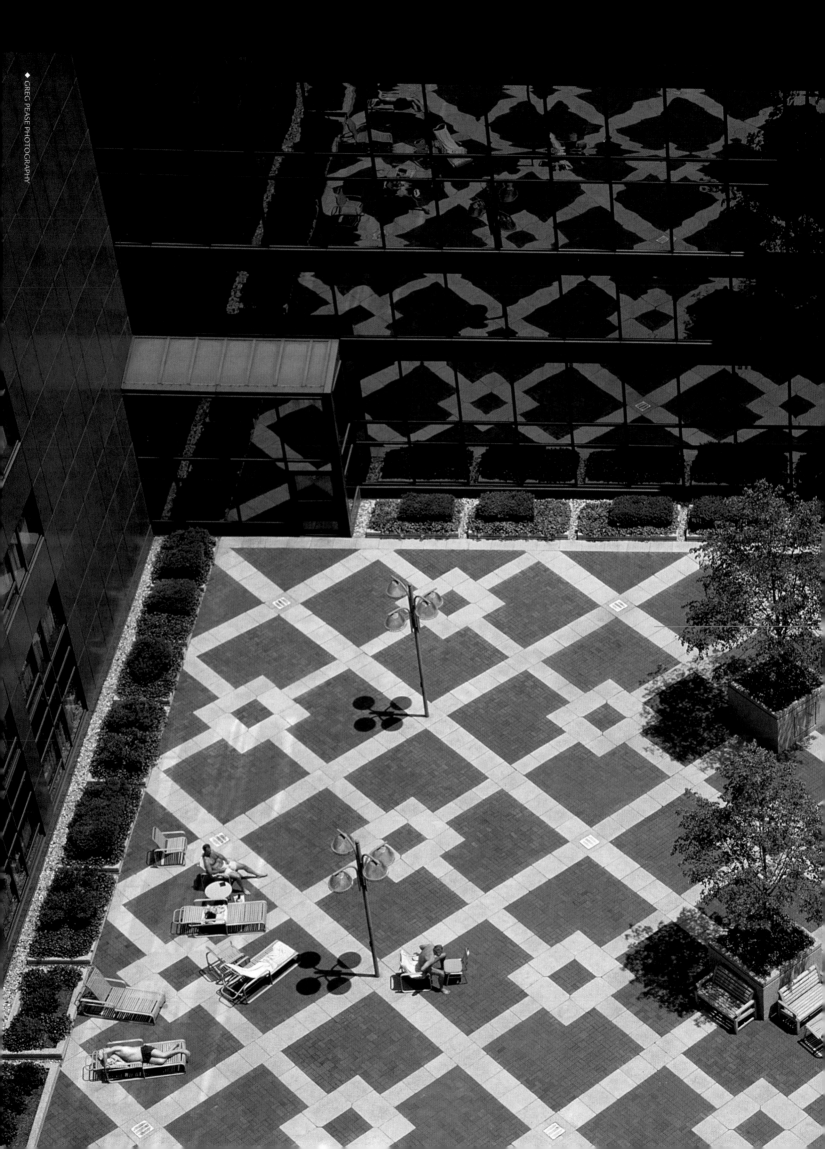

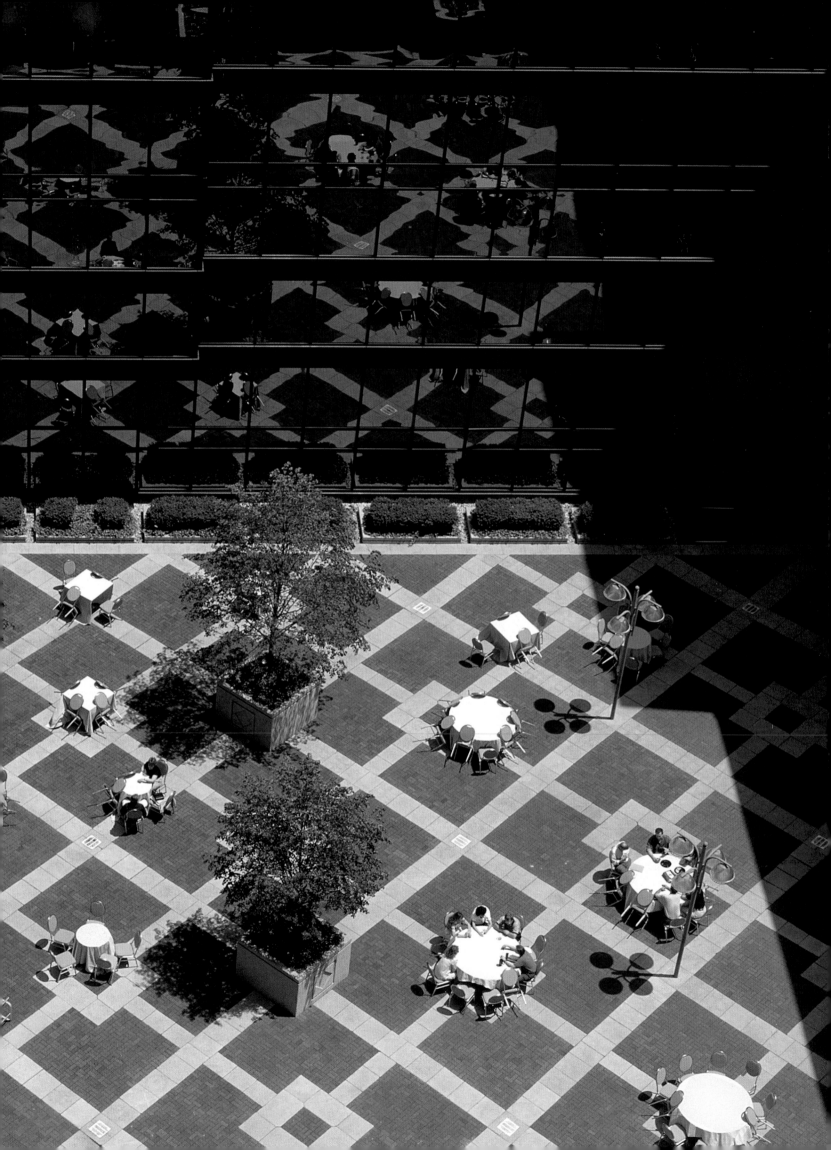

T HE CITY DECIDED TO TRY BECOMING A CONVENTION TOWN, AND IT SUCCEEDED. THE BALTIMORE Convention Center opened in 1979, and a new addition opened in 1996. Major hotels have been built downtown. Oriole Park opened in 1991 at Camden Yards, in the shadow of the old B&O Railroad Museum, bringing new life to what had been a gritty, industrial corner of the city. When the Birds play at home, the west end of downtown hops; it becomes festive and full of people again. A football stadium, home of the city's new National Football League franchise, the Ravens, is scheduled to open in 1998, just south of Oriole Park.

"I believe we're on the verge of a second renaissance," Schaefer said a decade after he'd left office. And that time he was looking east, beyond the aquarium, to the new Columbus Center, established in 1994 as a marine research center, and Inner Harbor East, one of the most ambitious residential and commercial ventures ever. Its promise to deliver new property owners and taxpayers to the city is huge. The old Power Plant at the Inner Harbor is on track to become another popular spot, with a new Hard Rock Cafe and a Barnes & Noble bookstore.

While all that is happening downtown, along the harbor, there are signs of mini-renaissances scattered

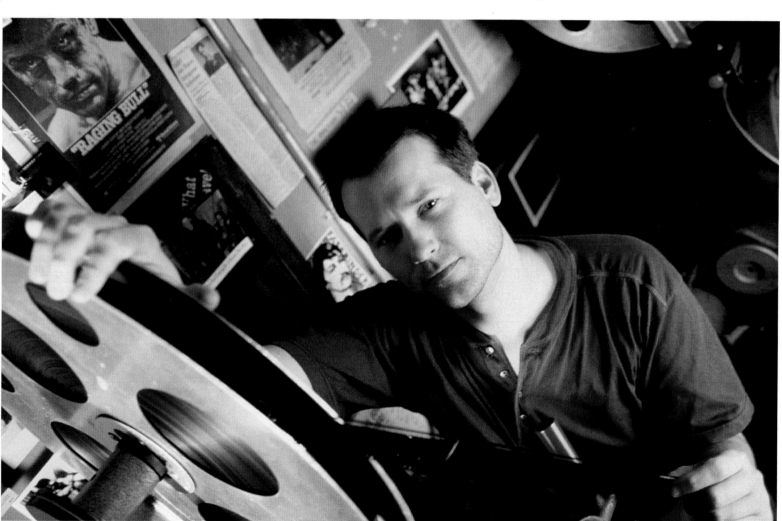

IN ADDITION TO A NUMBER OF MOTION PICTURES THAT HAVE BEEN FILMED IN BALTIMORE, TELEVISION'S *Homicide: Life on the Street* IS SHOT ON LOCA- TION HERE. IN FACT, THE ONGOING PRESENCE OF CAST AND CREW HAS EVEN EARNED THE CITY A NEW NICK- NAME: HOLLYWOOD ON THE HARBOR.

throughout the city. You see it in the neighborhoods. In Hampden, along 36th Street—known to long-timers as "The Avenue"—new restaurants and shops have opened. Artists and artisans have moved into old, industrial buildings in the city's Mill Valley.

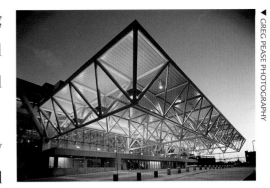

Fells Point, on the southeastern rim of the city's waterfront, remains very popular, with dozens of bars, restaurants, and stores. It's also the central location for NBC-TV's *Homicide: Life on the Street*. (Locals sometimes refer to it as "life without parking" because of the amount of space location shots take.) The old Rec Pier was turned into police headquarters for the TV cops. You're likely to bump into a cast member having a cup of coffee across the street at the Daily Grind or in the Waterfront Hotel, the bar/restaurant frequently featured on the show. It was Barry Levinson, the Academy Award-winning director, who made the decision to produce the show on location in his old hometown. It's estimated that *Homicide* puts about $23 million a year into the local economy.

Fells Point never seems to sleep. On Halloween, the streets fill with party animals in fantastic costumes, many

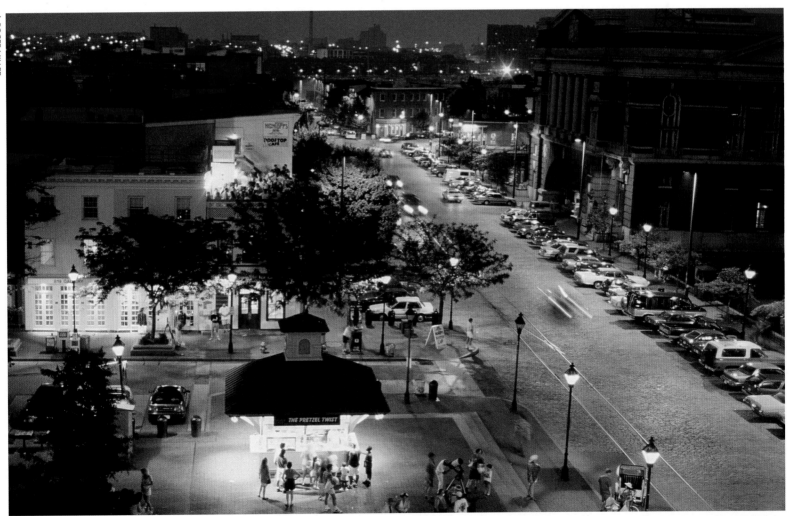

WITH A TOTAL OF 60,000 SQUARE FEET OF GLASS, THE BALTIMORE CONVENTION CENTER'S ORIGINAL BUILDING BOASTS THE LARGEST SUSPENDED GLASS SYSTEM IN THE WORLD (TOP).

HOME TO ONE OF AMERICA'S DENSEST ASSEMBLIES OF DRINKING ESTABLISHMENTS AND ENTERTAINMENT OPTIONS, FELLS POINT IS THE BELLE OF THE BALL ON ANY EVENING,

WHETHER IT'S NEW YEAR'S EVE, HALLOWEEN, ST. PATRICK'S DAY, OR JUST AN ORDINARY NIGHT ON THE TOWN (BOTTOM).

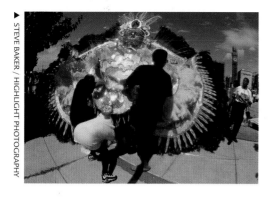

of them the creations of students from the Maryland Institute-College of Art. It's about as close to Mardi Gras as Baltimore gets. Each September, the Fells Point Fun Festival draws countless revelers over two days.

From Fells Point, the city's "gold coast" reaches along Boston Street, past the 24-hour-a-day Sip & Bite and Le Bistro Midi, to the new rowhouse community in Canton and resurgent O'Donnell Street. Farther to the east, you're in Highlandtown—pronounced "Hollandtown"—and acres of Baltimore rowhouses with their famous white marble steps and ceramic figurines in front windows. Still farther, and you're in Greektown, with its restaurants and ethnic groceries, more rowhouses, and a coffee shop where men from the old country sit, smoke, read Greek newspapers, and speak their native language.

I hear the same kind of kibitzing—but in English, with a little Yiddish thrown in here and there—at Attman's Deli on Corned Beef Row, just east of downtown. I feel part of a community in places like that, where people get to know your name. I feel happy to be part of a scene like Wednesday nights at the New Haven Lounge, with blues and barbecue, a happy crowd, and a singer named Big Jesse. I like to watch young men washing their cars under

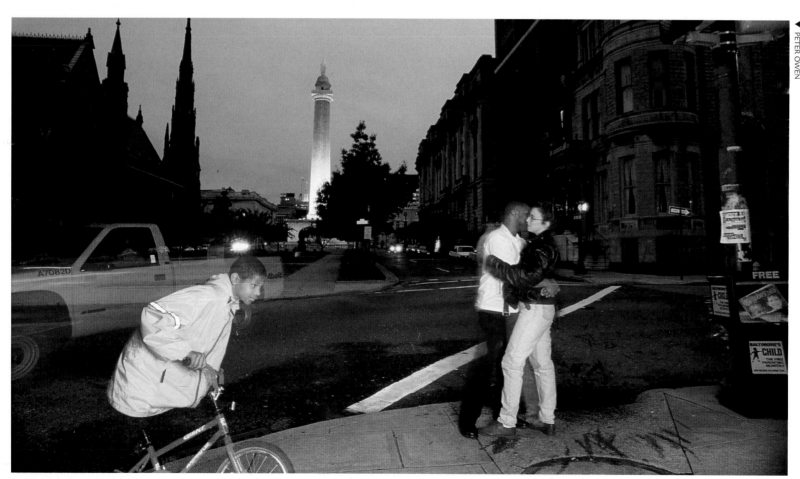

FOR JUST A BUCK, YOU CAN CLIMB THE 228 STEPS OF MOUNT VERNON SQUARE'S WASHINGTON MONUMENT (BOTTOM). THE LANDMARK WAS DESIGNED BY ROBERT MILLS, WHO CRAFTED A SIMILAR MEMORIAL TO THE NATION'S FIRST PRESIDENT IN WASHINGTON, D.C. THE MONUMENT ISN'T CHARM CITY'S ONLY NOTEWORTHY SIGHT, BY ANY STRETCH. HERE, A FESTIVE CHARACTER PUTS ON A SHOW OUTSIDE ORIOLE PARK (TOP).

the big trees in Druid Hill Park. I like buying fresh corn at the farmer's market in Waverly on Saturday, or under the Jones Falls Expressway on Sunday.

I savor the good feelings that come up Mount Royal Avenue like a summer breeze when ARTSCAPE opens for another big weekend. I like the way October sunlight filters through the tall sycamore trees in Cedarcroft, giving everything a soft edge. I like the stunning sight of a million tulips in Sherwood Gardens every spring. I like that I can never stop staring at all the elaborate Christmas decorations on the houses along 34th Street in Hampden.

I like the way the Senator Theater, a classic art deco movie house, shines when it's all lit up at night. I like the fresh look of children going to church on Easter morning, colorful as confetti and sprinkled through the streets of West Baltimore. I like to watch newlyweds emerging from the courthouse on Calvert Street. I think it's amusing to see men and women flirting around Harborplace in the summer.

I like the aroma of sausage frying in Mugs' sandwich shop in Little Italy. I like the smell of bread baking on the north end of Fells Point. And the smell of peanuts roasting outside Lexington Market. I like the smoky smell of Boog's Barbecue at Camden Yards. I even like the smell of Fleischmann's vinegar plant located along the Jones Falls Expressway near Cold Spring Lane. That tells me I'm close to home. 🖋

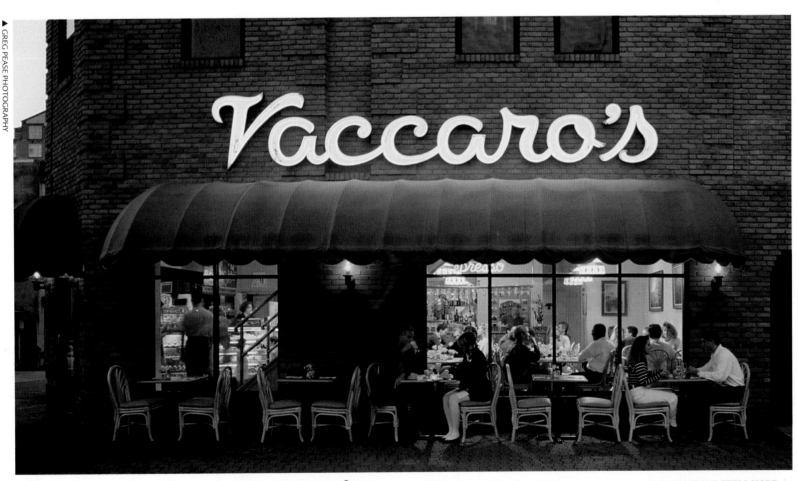

LOCATED IN THE HEART OF LITTLE ITALY, VACCARO'S PASTICCERIA PORTRAYS BALTIMORE AT ITS MOST EXOTIC. THANKS TO AN APPETIZING COMBINATION OF DECADENT PASTRIES, STRONG COFFEE, SMALL TABLES, AND PATRONS ENGAGED IN GOOD CONVERSATION, THE RESTAURANT FEELS MORE LIKE A CLASSIC VIENNESE COFFEE HOUSE THAN A MOB TOWN BAKERY.

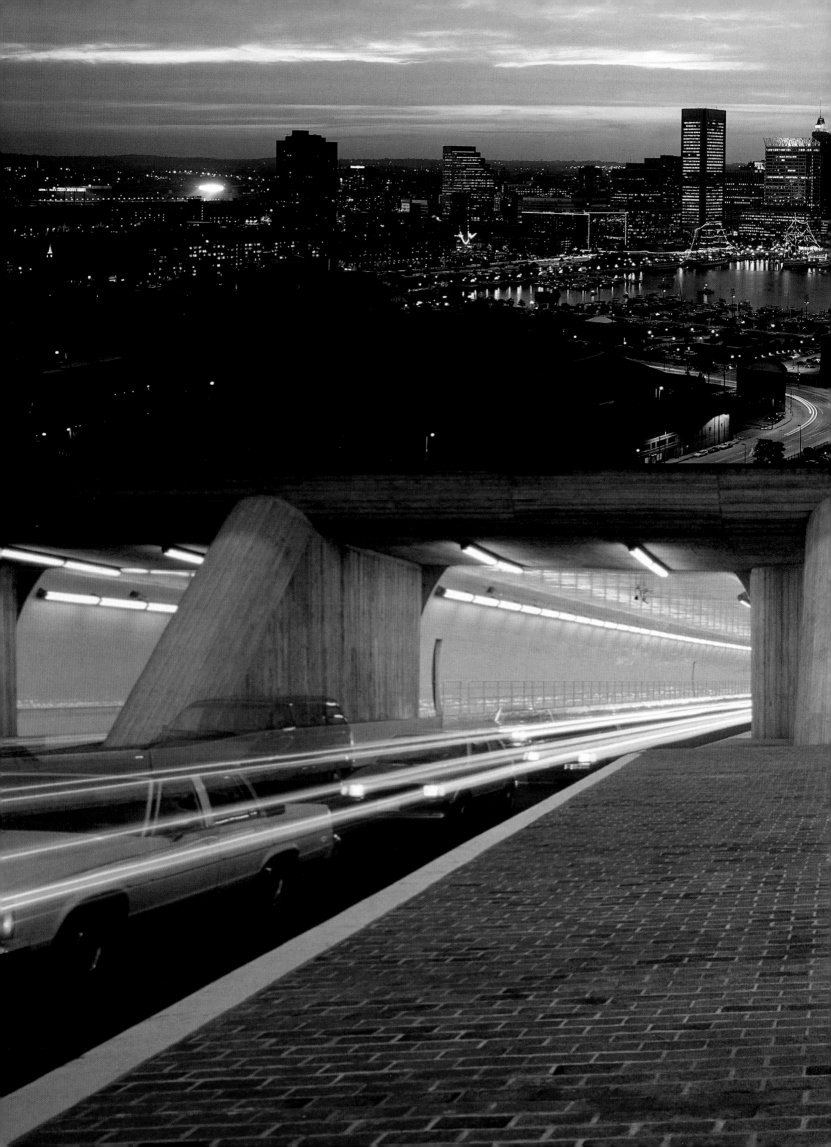

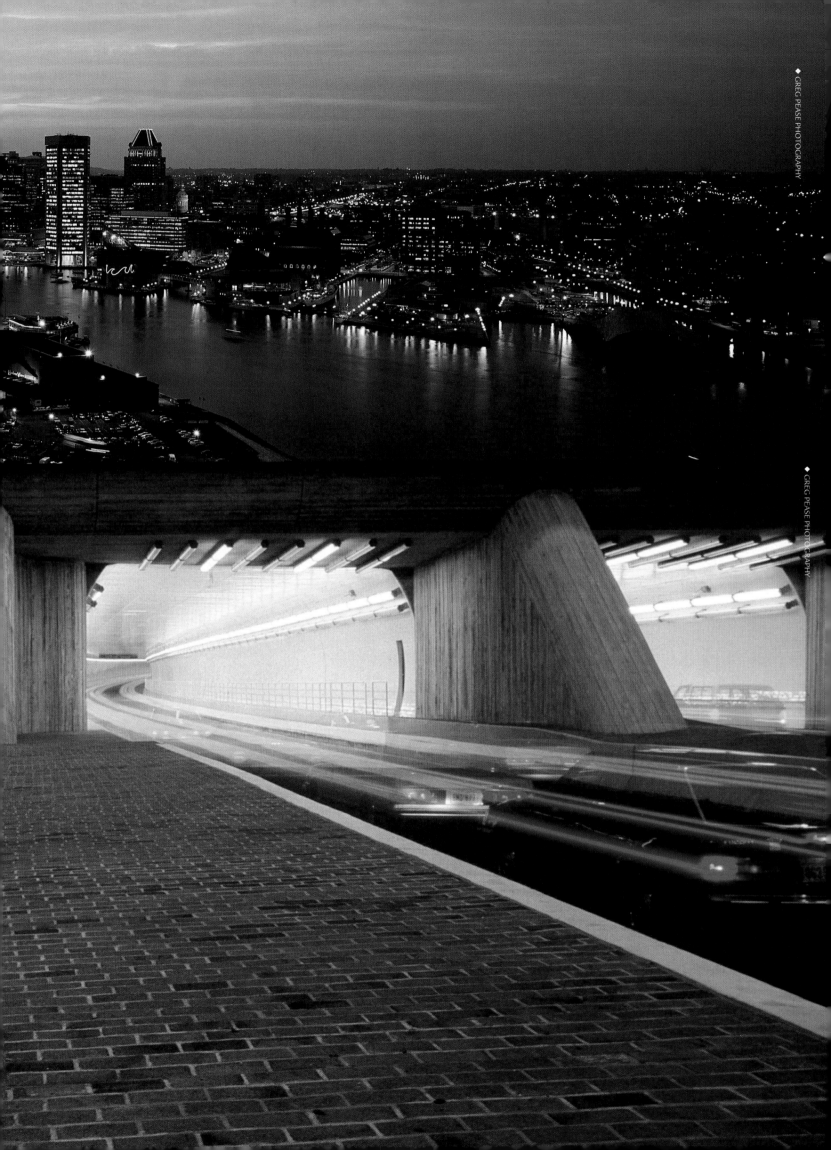

Once upon a time, Baltimore was considered merely a dot on the map between Philadelphia and Washington, D.C., and many people's knowledge of this seaport city did not go beyond the Harbor Tunnel. But a renaissance during the 1980s that replaced the Inner Harbor's dilapidated warehouses and old shipyards helped transform Baltimore into a dynamic, progressive metropolis (PAGES 44 AND 45).

Presiding over rush hour in the city is the giant clock at Penn Station, the terminus for Amtrak and the Maryland Rail Commuter system (OPPOSITE). A similar timepiece at the 15-story Bromo Seltzer Tower, located at Eutaw and Lombard streets, was completed in 1911; its hour hand weighs some 145 pounds (RIGHT).

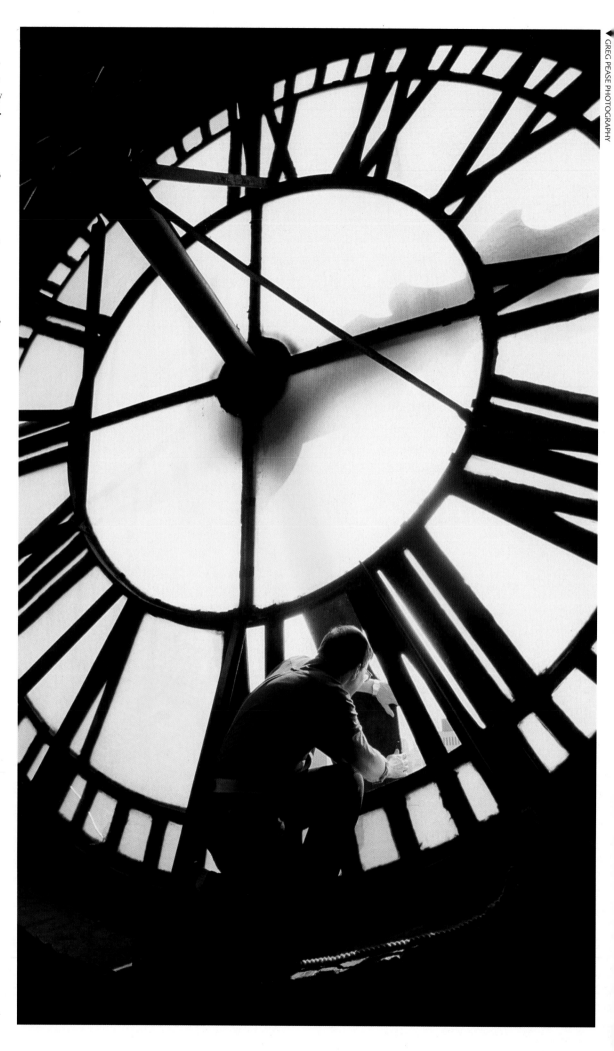

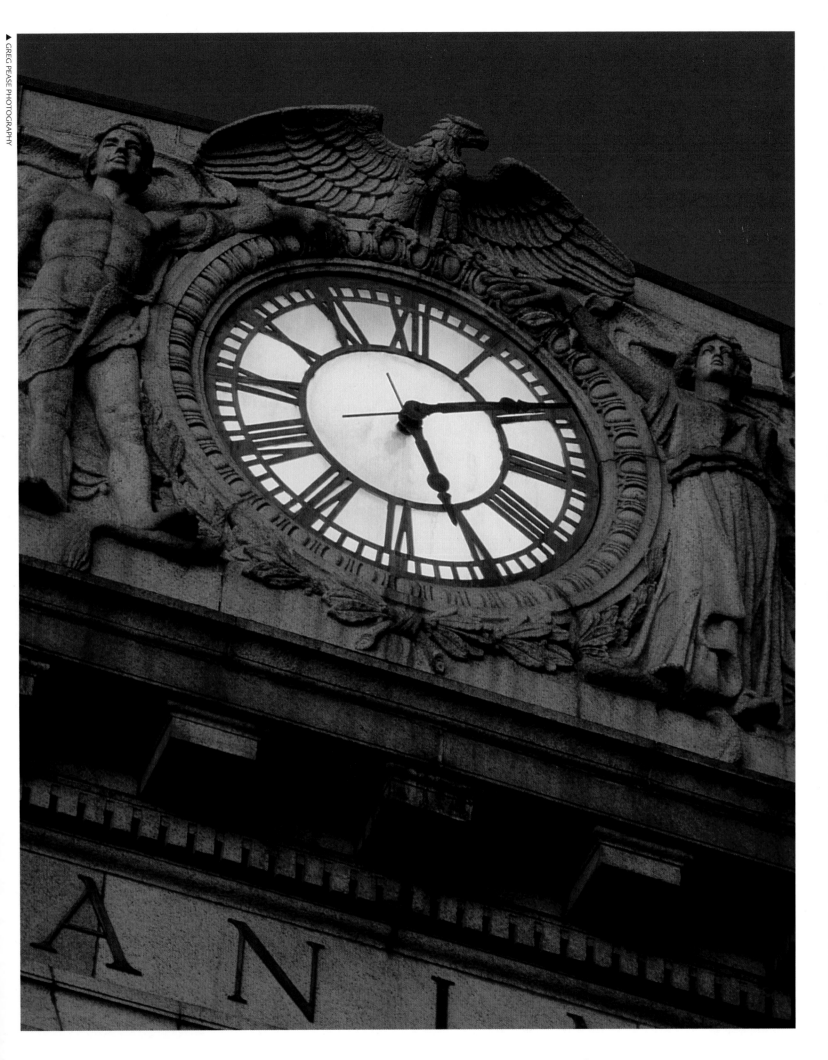

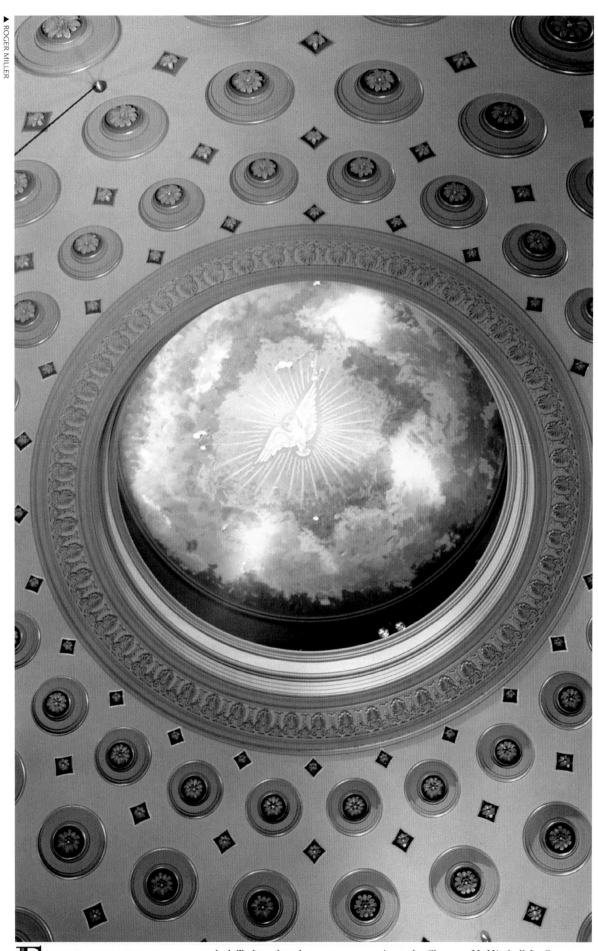

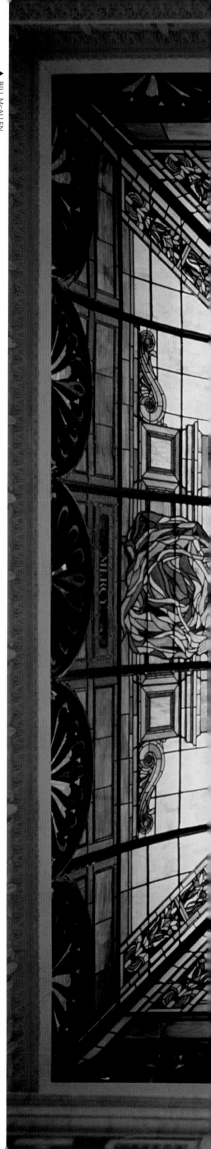

Eras ago, sailors knew they were approaching Baltimore when they saw the dome of the Basilica of the Assumption, the nation's first Roman Catholic cathedral. Today, churchgoers can appreciate the "heavenly" view from inside (ABOVE). Built in 1900 and known for its classical ornaments, stained-glass windows, and Beaux Arts architecture, the Clarence M. Mitchell Jr. Courthouse (OPPOSITE) was featured in the film . . . *And Justice for All*, starring Al Pacino.

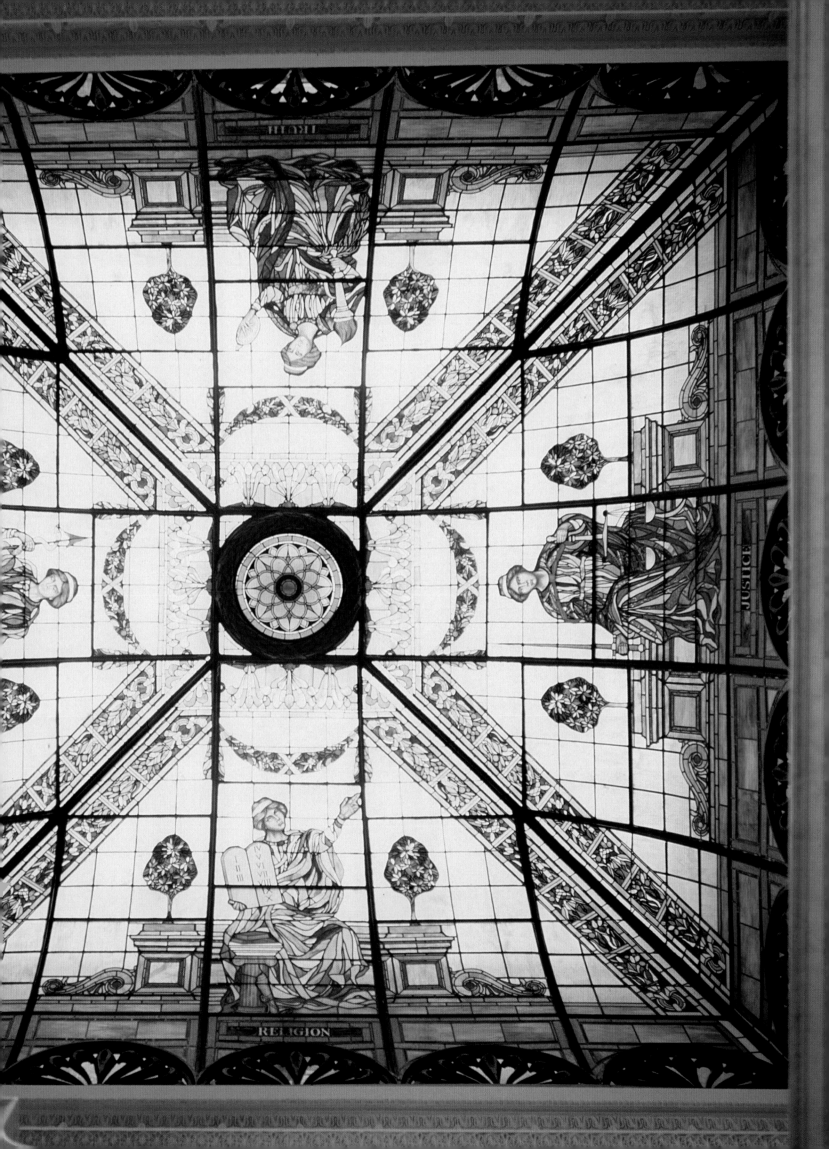

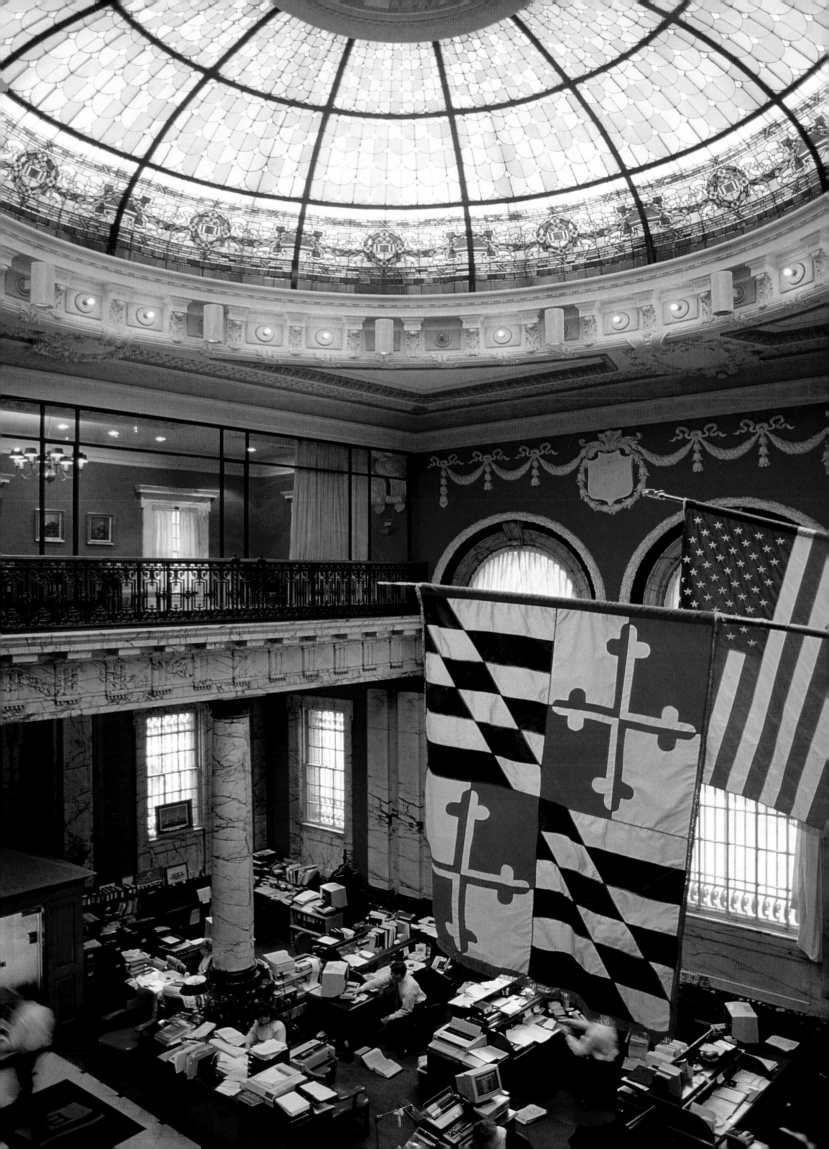

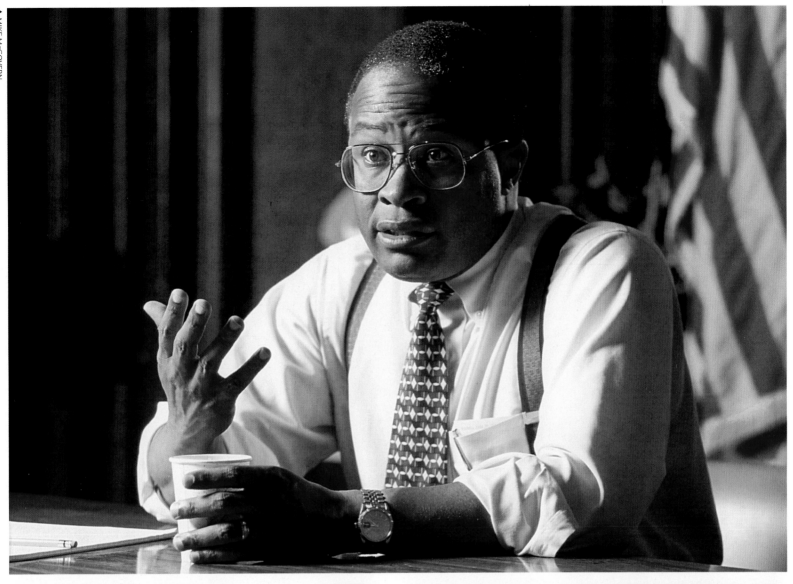

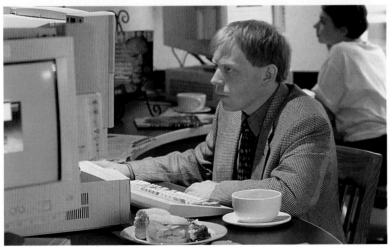

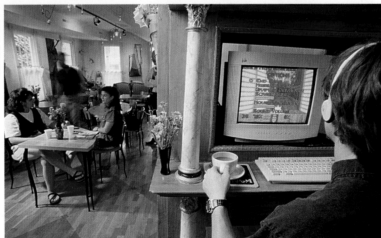

Tʜᴇ Bʀᴏᴡɴ ɴᴀᴍᴇ ʜᴀs ʙᴇᴇɴ important in Baltimore ever since Alexander Brown emi-grated from Northern Ireland and made money as an importer. Today, the company he started is one of the city's most prestigious brokerage houses (ᴏᴘᴘᴏsɪᴛᴇ). Whatever your line of business, however, nothing gets you through a hectic day better than a strong cup of coffee. Mayor Kurt Schmoke (ᴛᴏᴘ), who is presiding over the city's second renaissance, knows the value of the bean, as do Strand Cybercafe (ʙᴏᴛᴛᴏᴍ ʟᴇꜰᴛ) and Café Pangea (ʙᴏᴛᴛᴏᴍ ʀɪɢʜᴛ), both of which have merged the computer age with cappuccino to create the ultimate "surfer's" paradise.

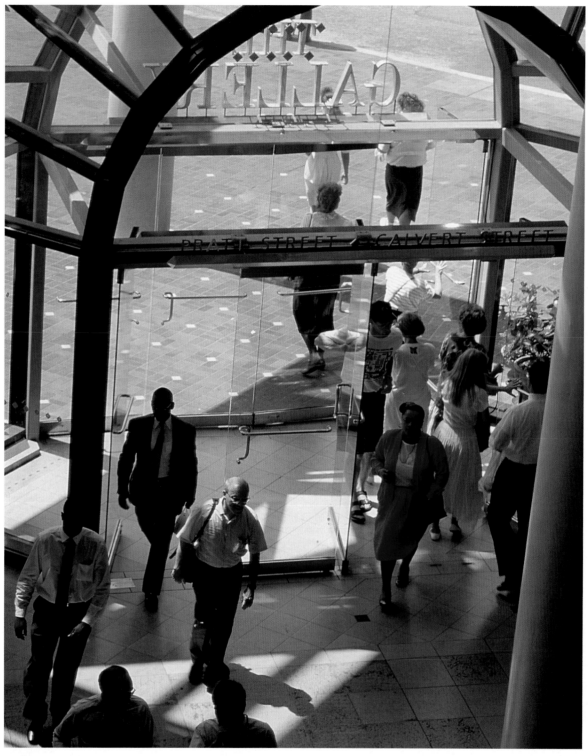

▲ GREG PEASE PHOTOGRAPHY ▲ PETER OWEN

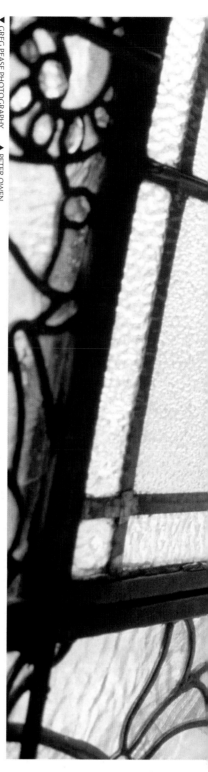

AN URBAN SHOPPING MALL OFFER-
ing the area's finest selection
of popular retailers, the Gallery at Harborplace is a magnet for
tourists and office workers alike.

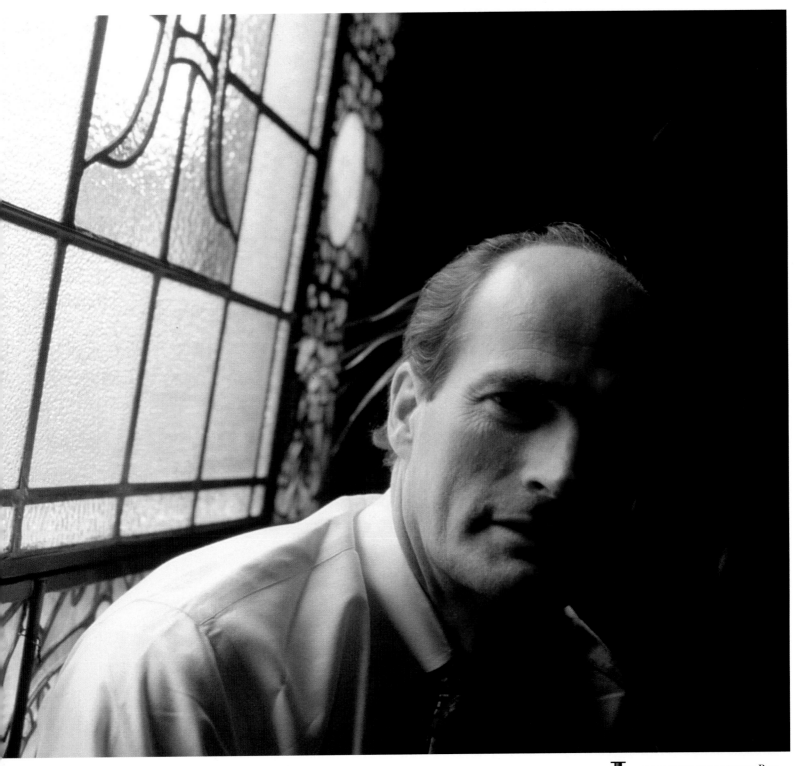

L OCAL PUBLISHING MAGNATE BILL Bonner has transformed a number of Mount Vernon's Victorian mansions into modern-day office buildings that merge two key functions: relevance and beauty.

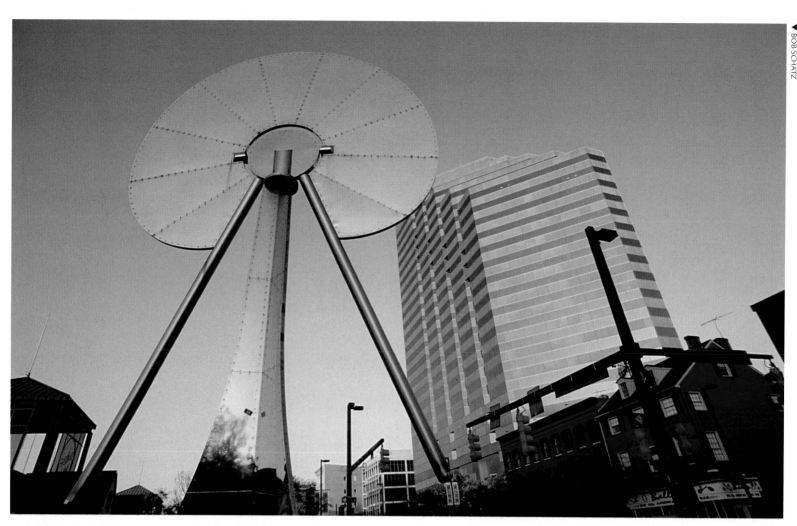

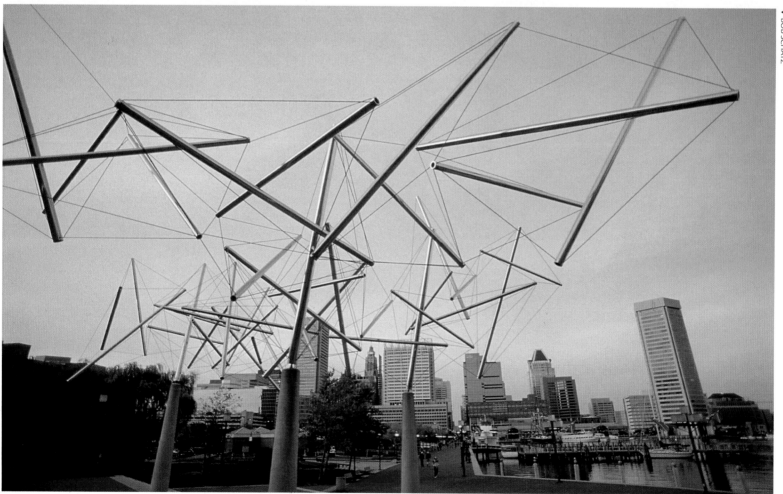

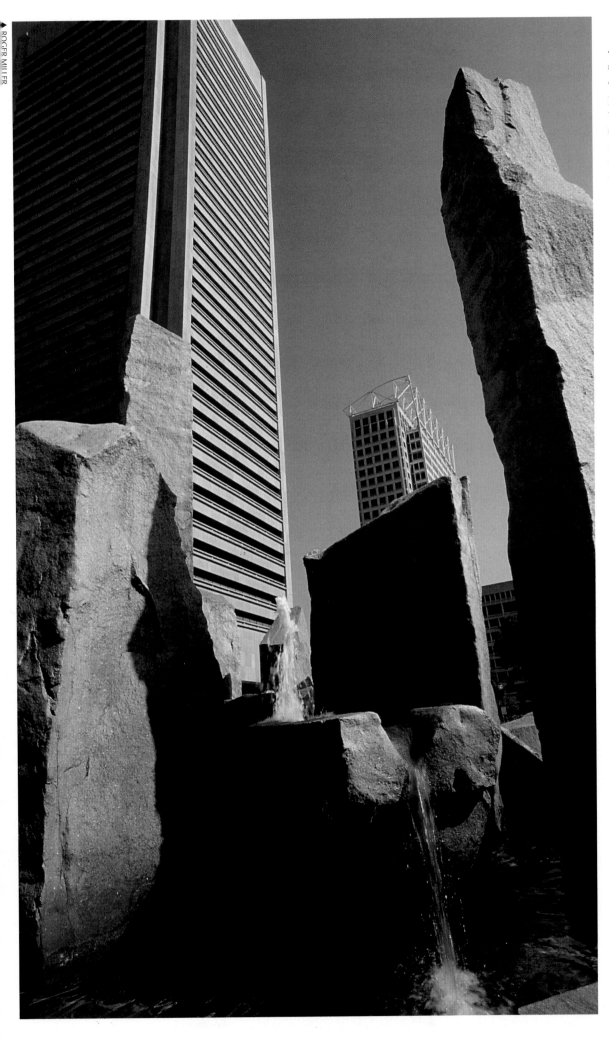

As downtown Baltimore has grown taller over the years, adding sleek contemporary skyscrapers to the "grandes dames" of yesteryear (PAGES 56 AND 57), city planners and corporations have strived to harmonize construction with public sculpture. From Thomas A. Todd's Stonehenge-like fountain in front of NationsBank's Bank Center (LEFT) to Greg Moring's *Fan Figure* on West Pratt (OPPOSITE TOP) to Kenneth Snelson's 1978 *Easy Landing* at the Maryland Science Center (OPPOSITE BOTTOM), Baltimore has worked to maintain and enhance its beautiful seaport setting.

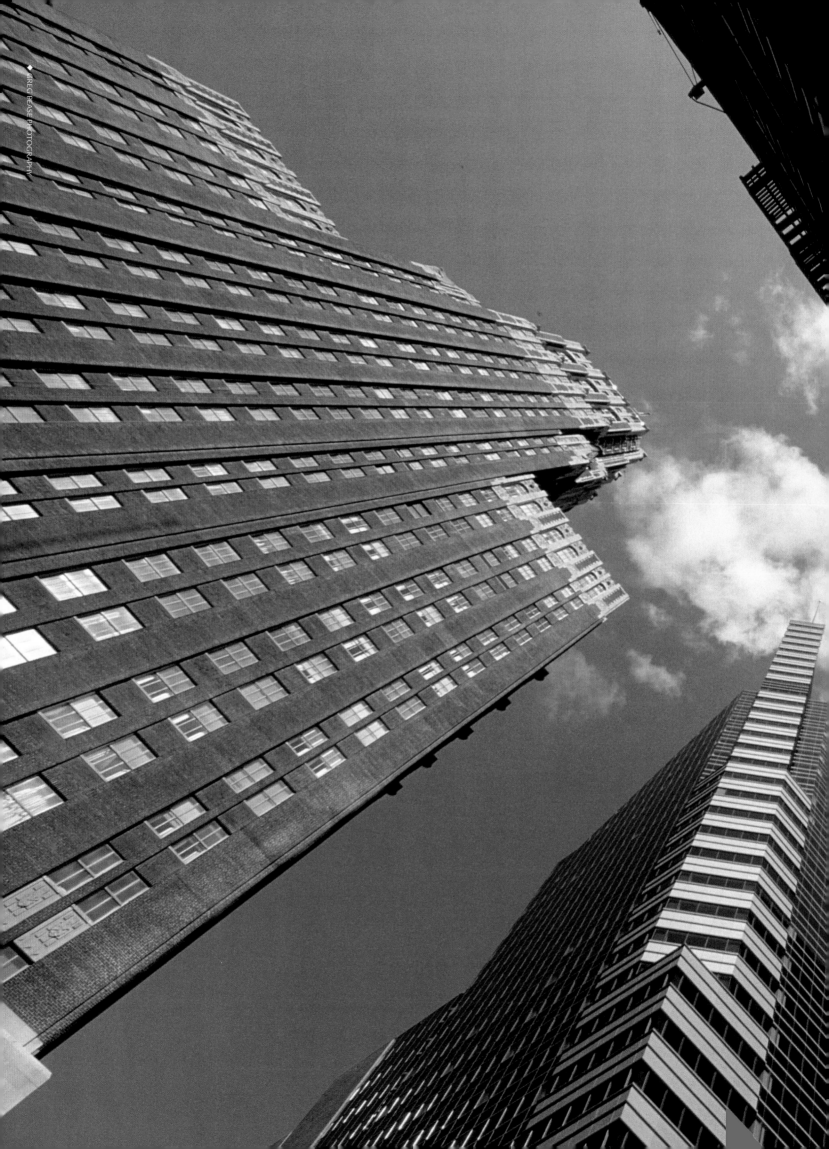

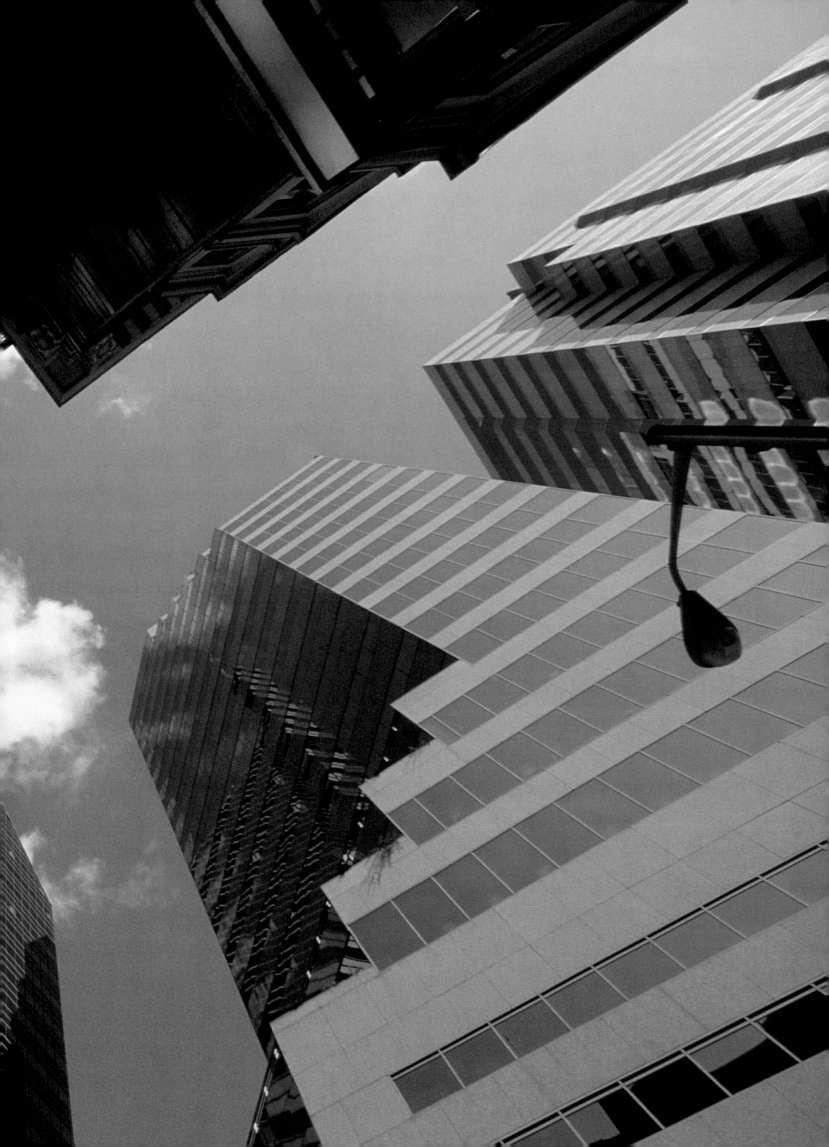

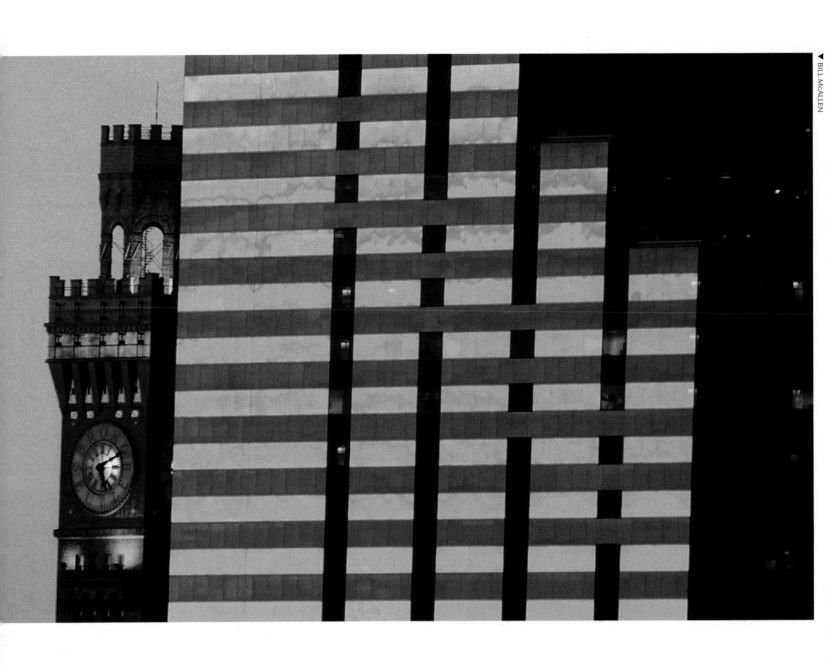

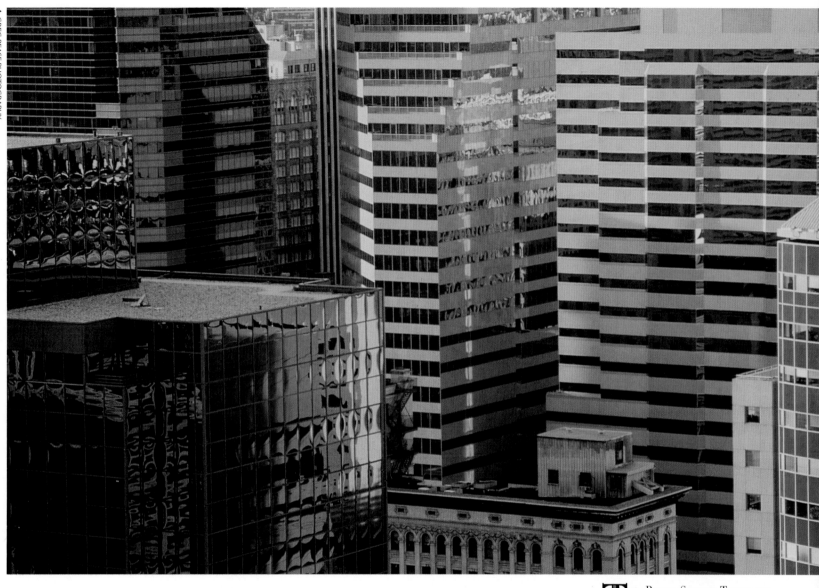

Tʜᴇ Bʀᴏᴍᴏ Sᴇʟᴛᴢᴇʀ Tᴏᴡᴇʀ ᴀɴᴅ 250 West Pratt (ᴏᴘᴘᴏsɪᴛᴇ) bask radiantly at sundown, while the waning light of another workday illuminates downtown's corporate canyons (ᴀʙᴏᴠᴇ).

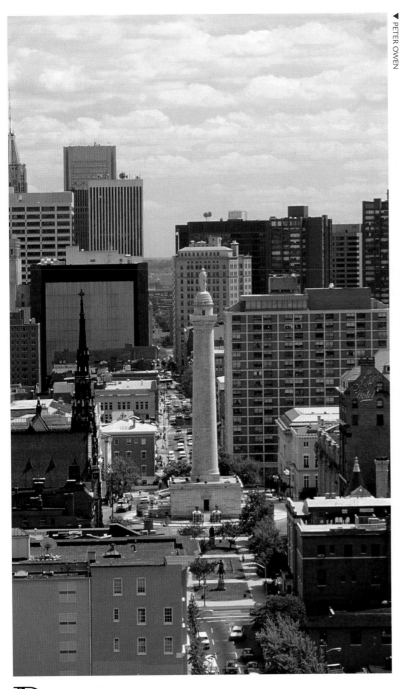

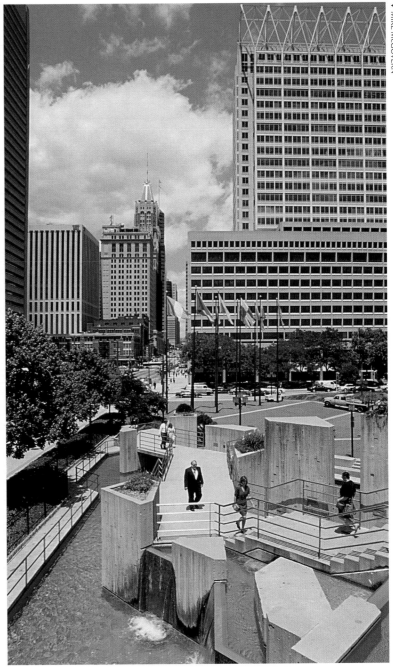

Downtown Baltimore offers a number of sanctuaries from the daily hustle and bustle, including the beautiful green spaces of Mount Vernon Square and a fountain oasis in the heart of the business district.

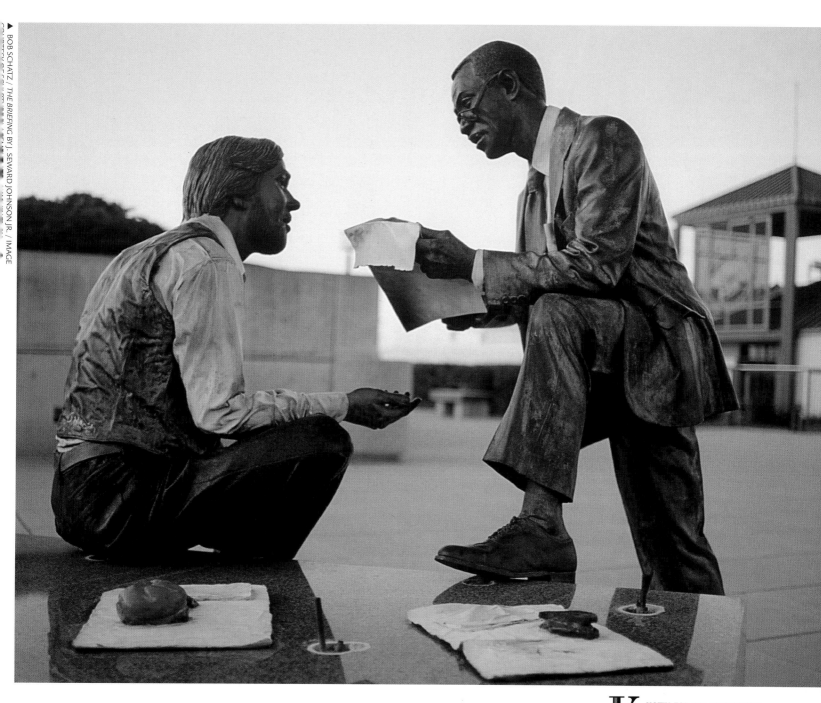

K NOWN FOR HIS INCREDIBLY realistic, life-size figures, J. Seward Johnson Jr. sculpted this pair of businessmen discussing the workday ahead. Titled *The Briefing*, the piece is located outside Baltimore's Convention Center.

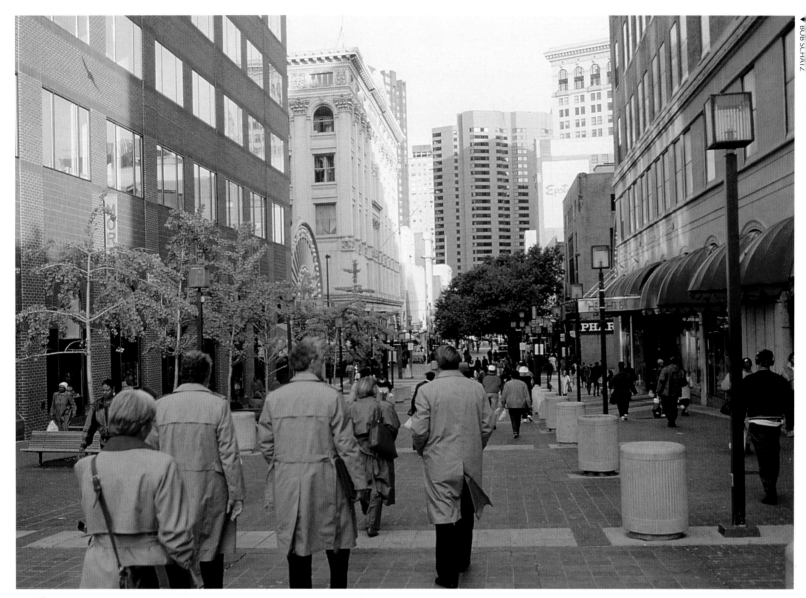

C HARLES CENTER, A 33-ACRE
business, hotel, and cultural
complex, sparked Baltimore's
first successful effort at urban revitalization when it was created in the
early 1960s.

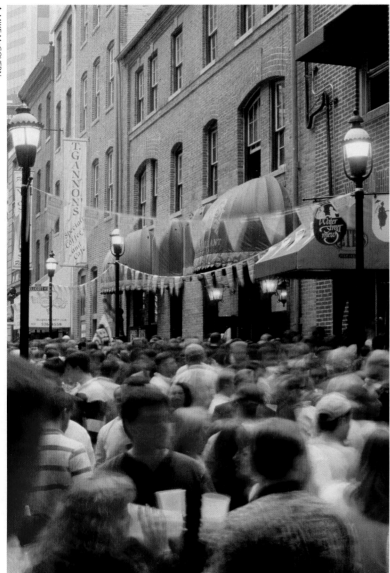

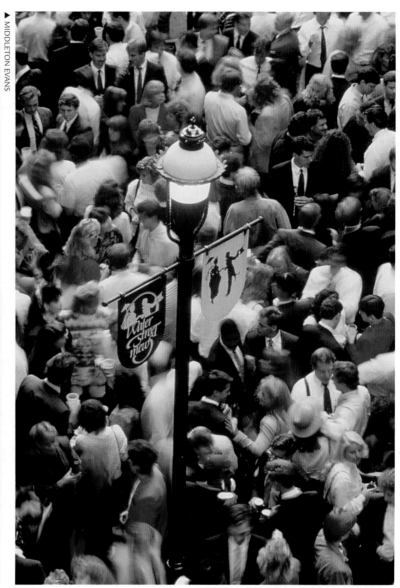

T HE PLACE TO MEET AND GREET IS
Water Street, a one-block sliver
of downtown where happy
hour—complete with live bands
and crowds of well-dressed young
professionals—is an institution for
the office worker set.

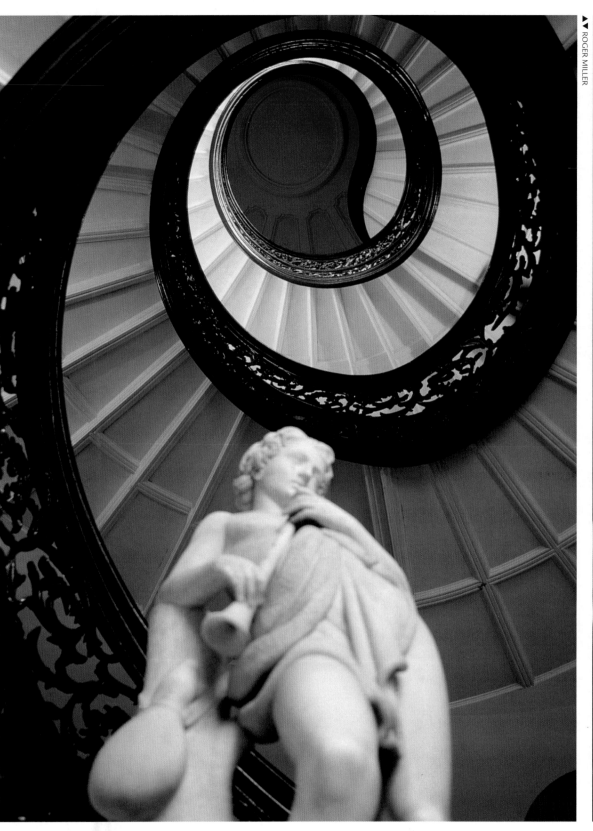
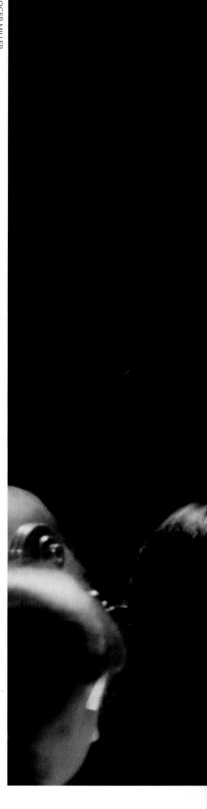

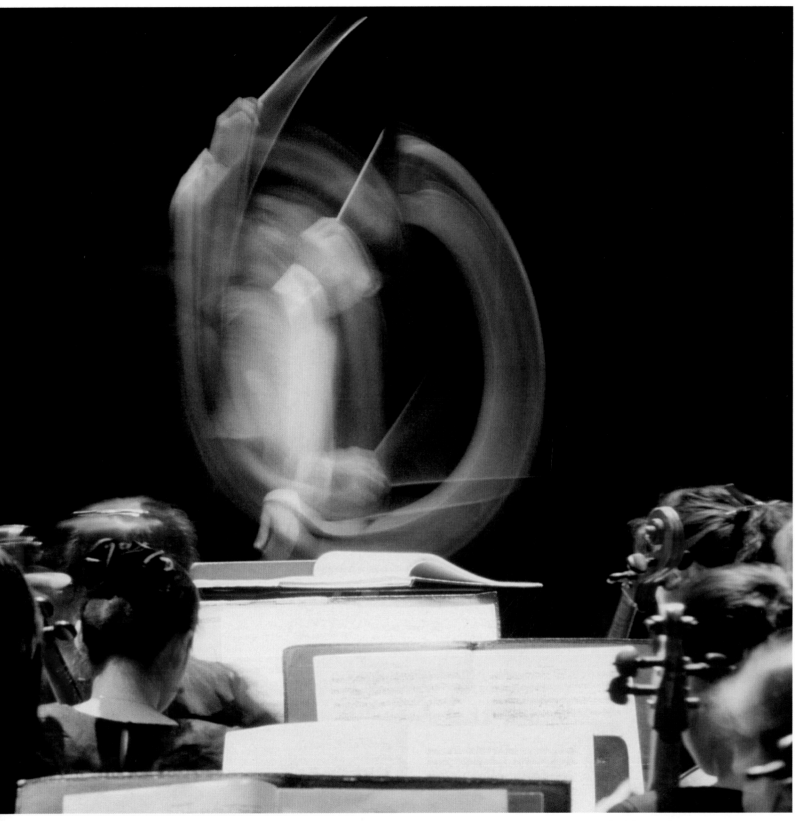

THE PEABODY CONSERVATORY
of Music, created in 1857 by
philanthropist George Peabody,
was designed as a temple of arts.
Today, it houses one of the nation's
most prestigious schools of music.

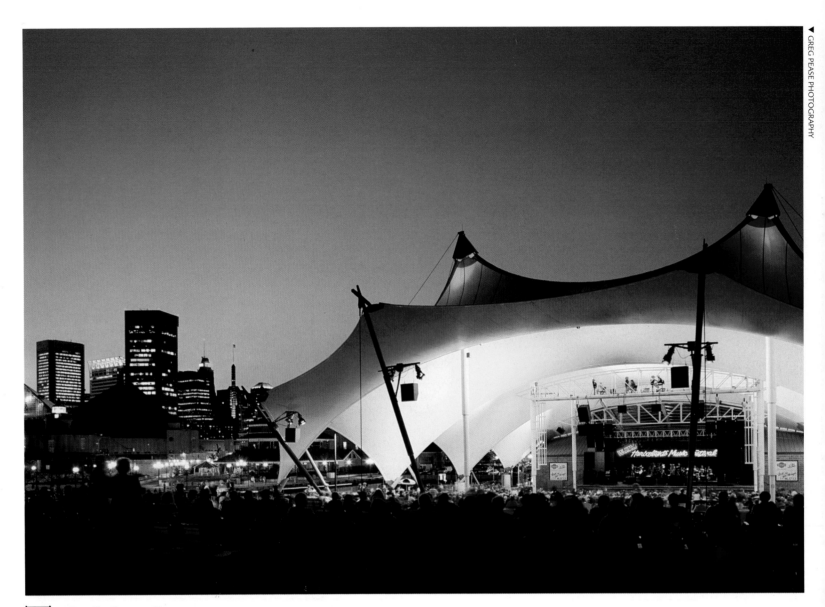

THE PIER SIX CONCERT PAVILION boasts the summer's most popular performers, along with a great moonlit view of the Inner Harbor.

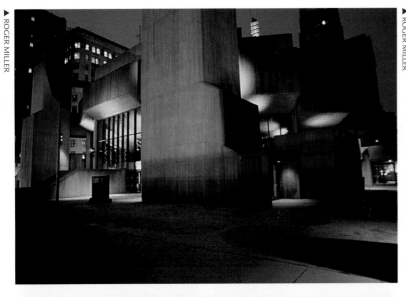

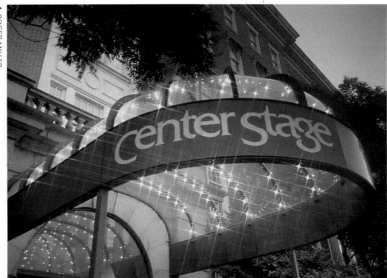

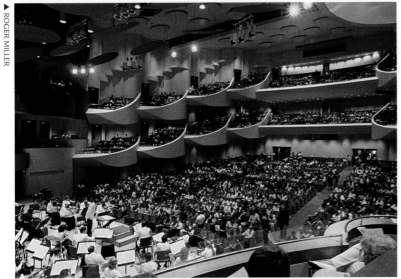

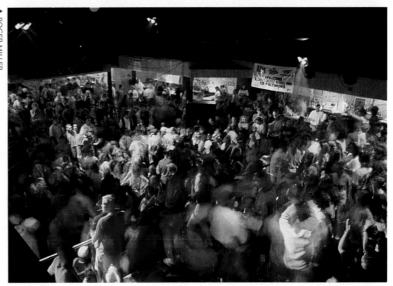

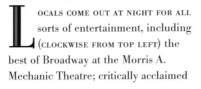

Locals come out at night for all sorts of entertainment, including (clockwise from top left) the best of Broadway at the Morris A. Mechanic Theatre; critically acclaimed productions, ranging from Shakespeare to avant-garde, at Center Stage; hip, funky dance music at Hammerjacks Concert Hall, which was recently razed to make room for the Ravens' new football stadium; and uplifting performances by the Baltimore Symphony Orchestra at the Meyerhoff Symphony Hall.

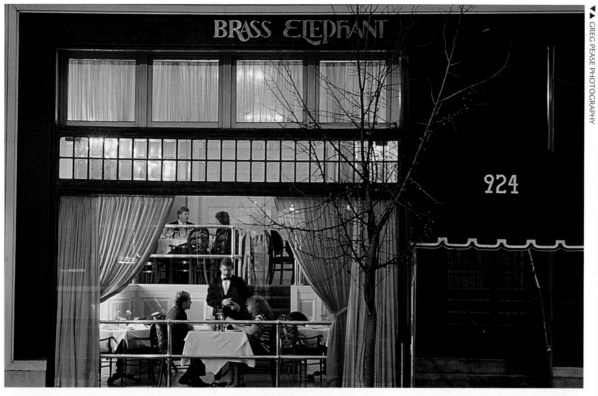

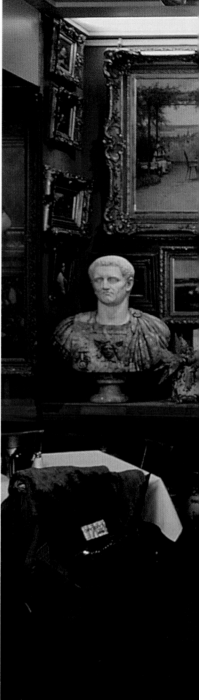

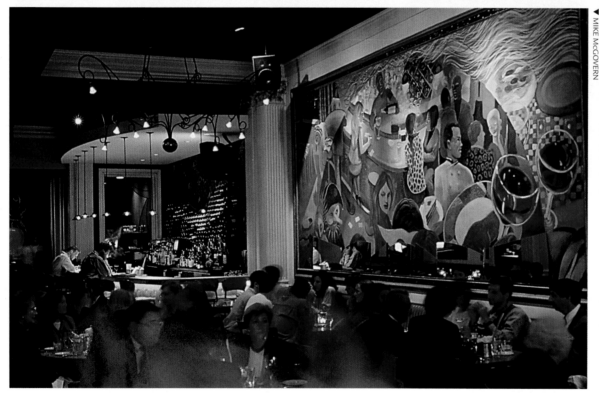

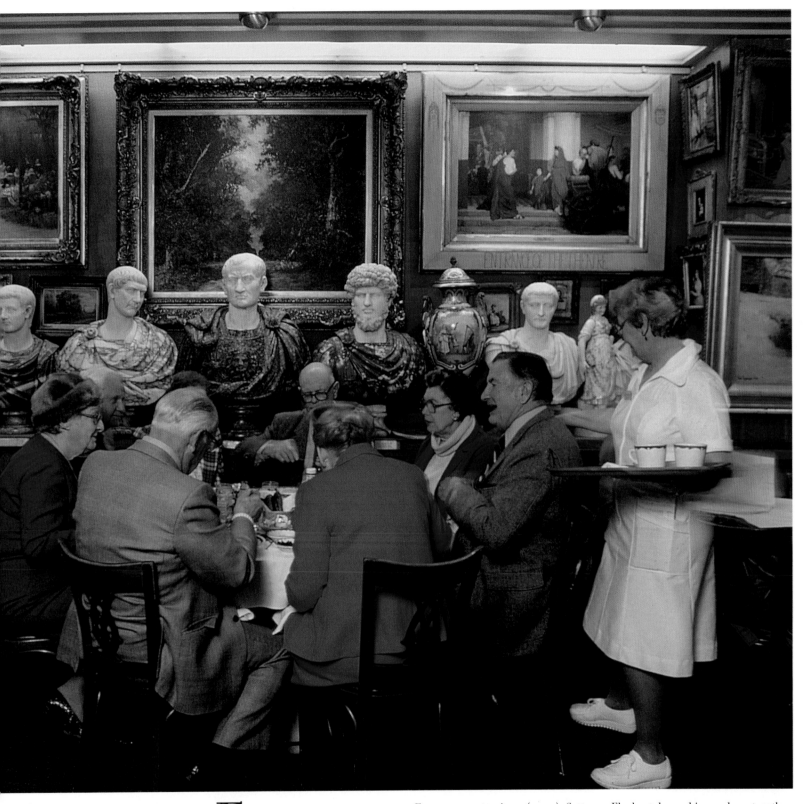

F INE ART AND CULINARY ARTISTRY
are de rigueur at several local
restaurants: Haussner's fine
German-style cuisine is matched
only by its 800-piece collection of
European masterpieces (ABOVE); Sotta
Sopra is sleek and urbane, with wall
murals that evoke festive scenes
(OPPOSITE BOTTOM); and the Brass
Elephant, housed in an elegant, 19th-
century Victorian mansion, is considered by many to be Baltimore's most
romantic café (OPPOSITE TOP).

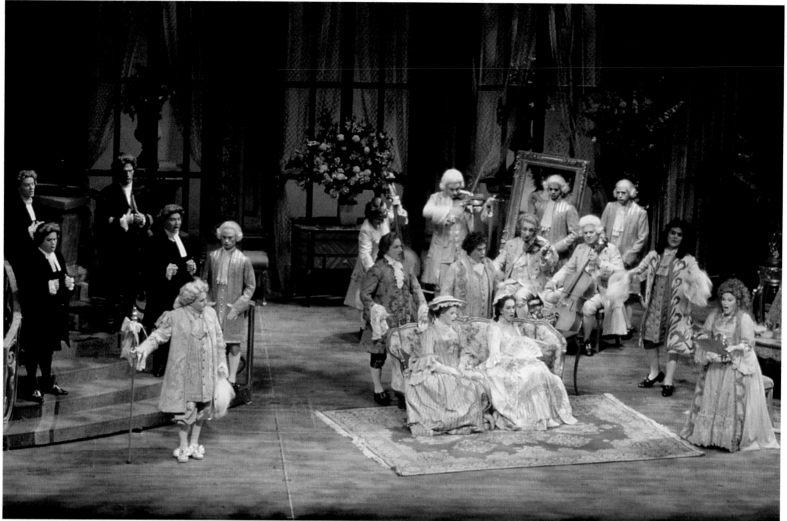

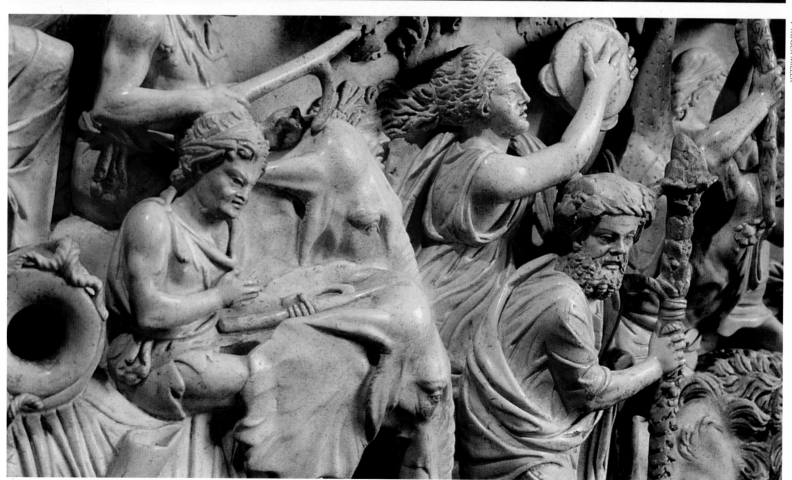

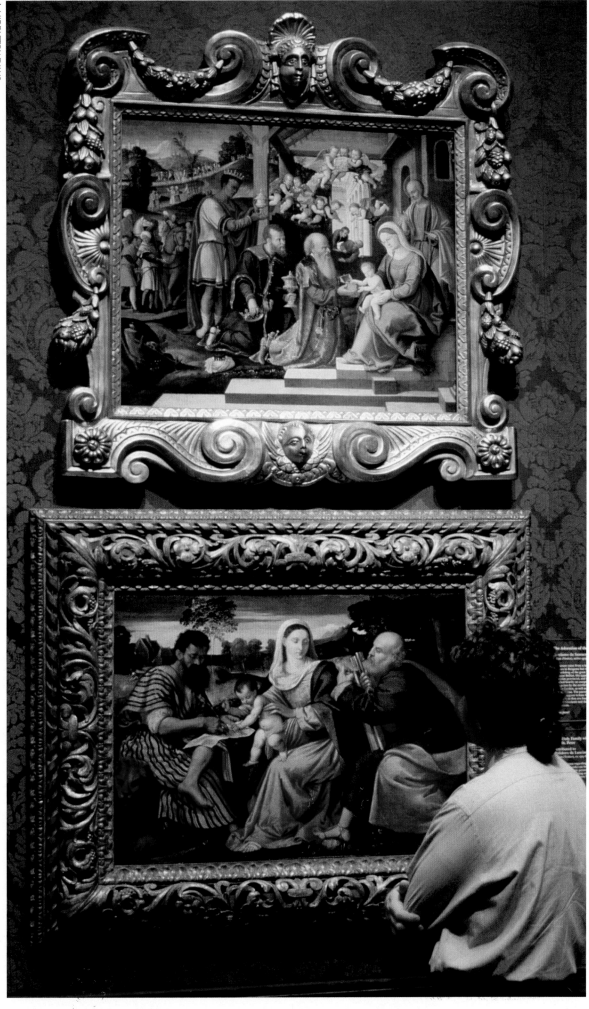

J UST BECAUSE OPERA IS HIGH ART, that doesn't mean we can't have a good time," teases an award-winning ad campaign for the Baltimore Opera (OPPOSITE TOP), which promises an evening of "bigamy, double-crossing, foul play, cheating, and all kinds of assorted depraved behavior." The Walters Art Gallery (LEFT AND OPPOSITE BOTTOM) offers an equally unforgettable experience, including a stunning array of paintings, ceramics, illuminated manuscripts, tapestries, stained glass, sculptures, and jeweled Fabergé eggs.

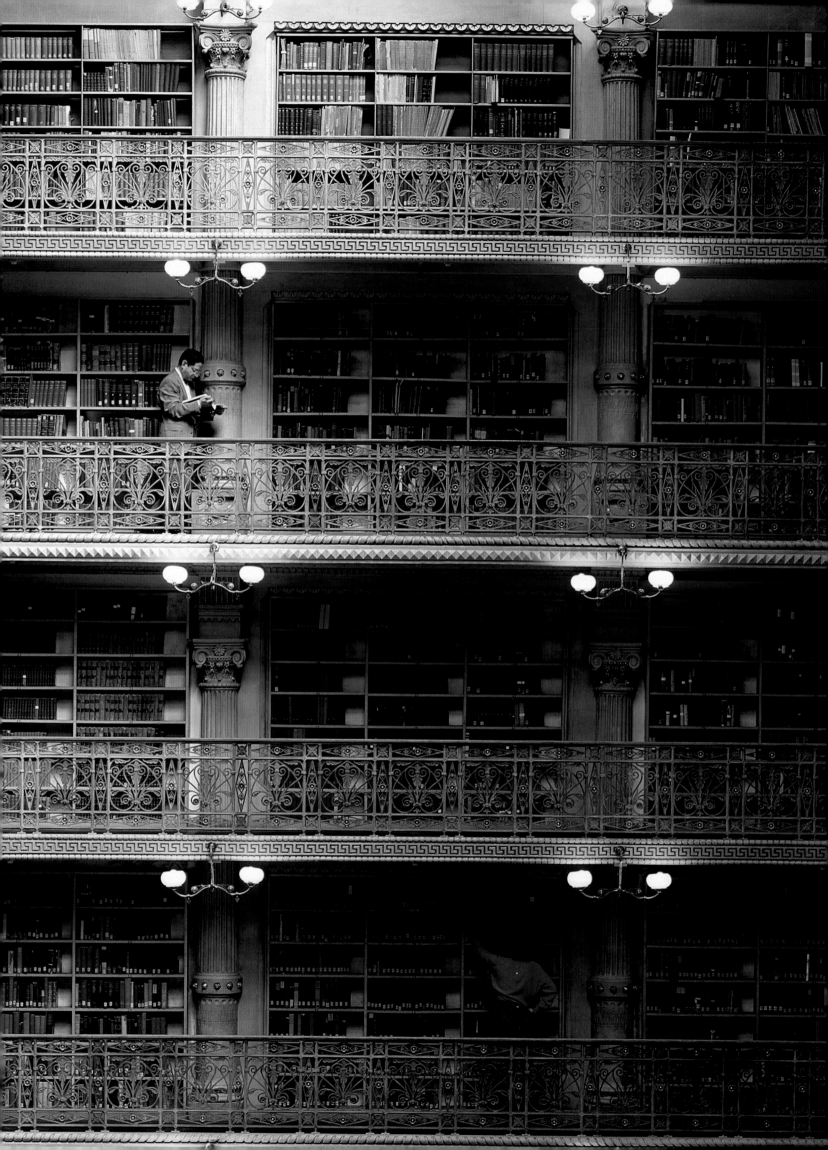

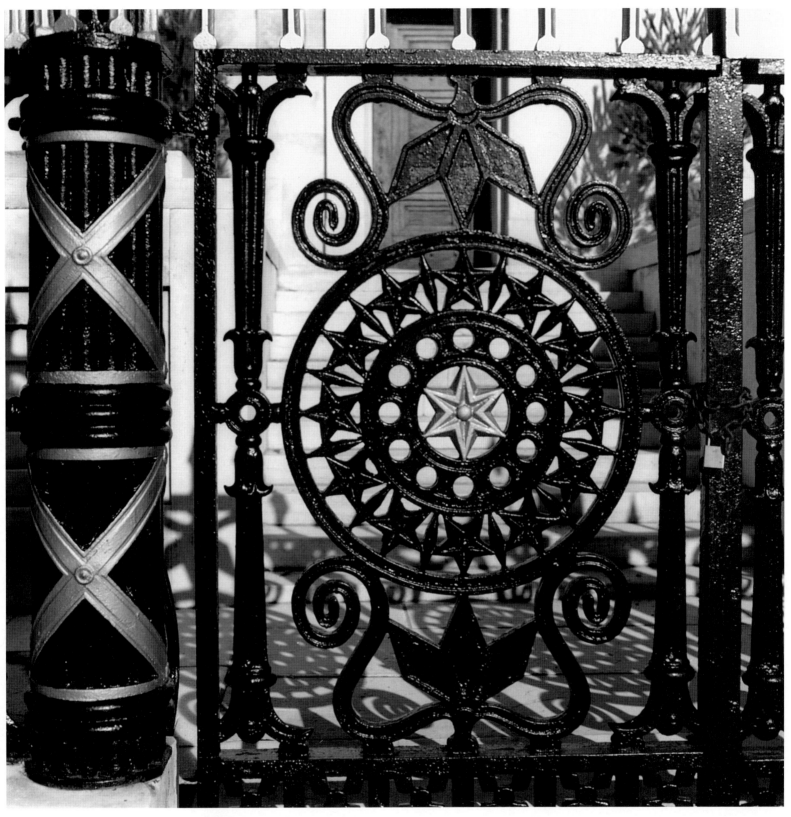

THE ORNATE IRONWORK THAT encircles the base of the Washington Monument in Mount Vernon Square competes for attention with the cast-iron balconies of the Peabody Library at the Peabody Conservatory of Music. Considered by many to be the most beautiful facility of its kind in the world, the 250,000-volume library also features a large skylight and a marble court.

A marriage of old and new: downtown's office buildings demonstrate the dramatic changes in architectural styles and materials over the decades (PAGES 74 AND 75).

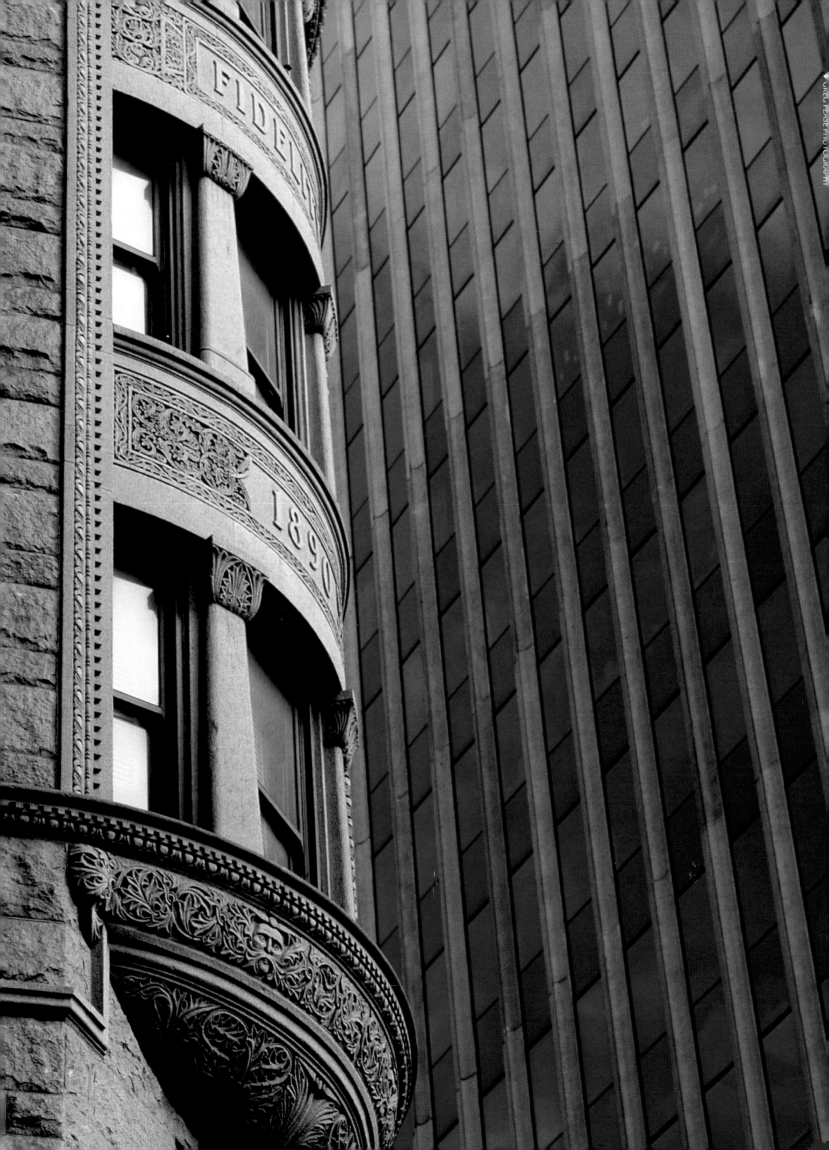

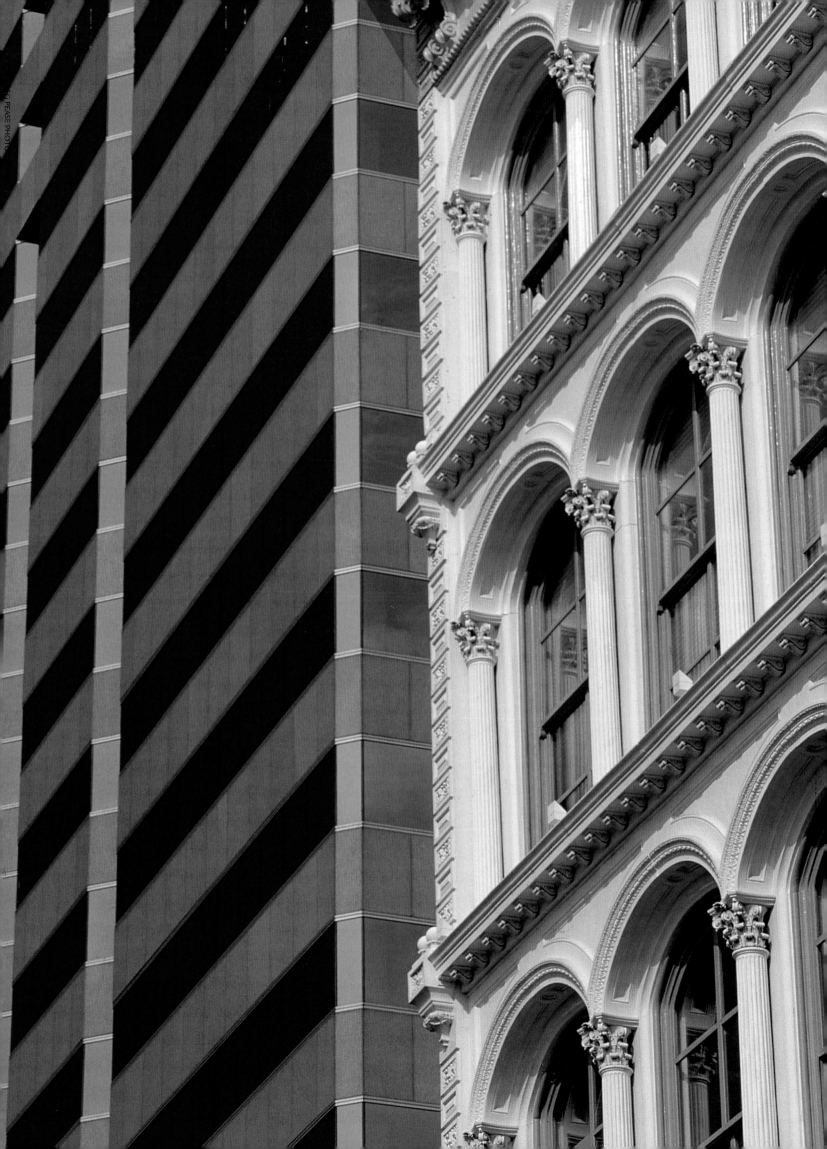

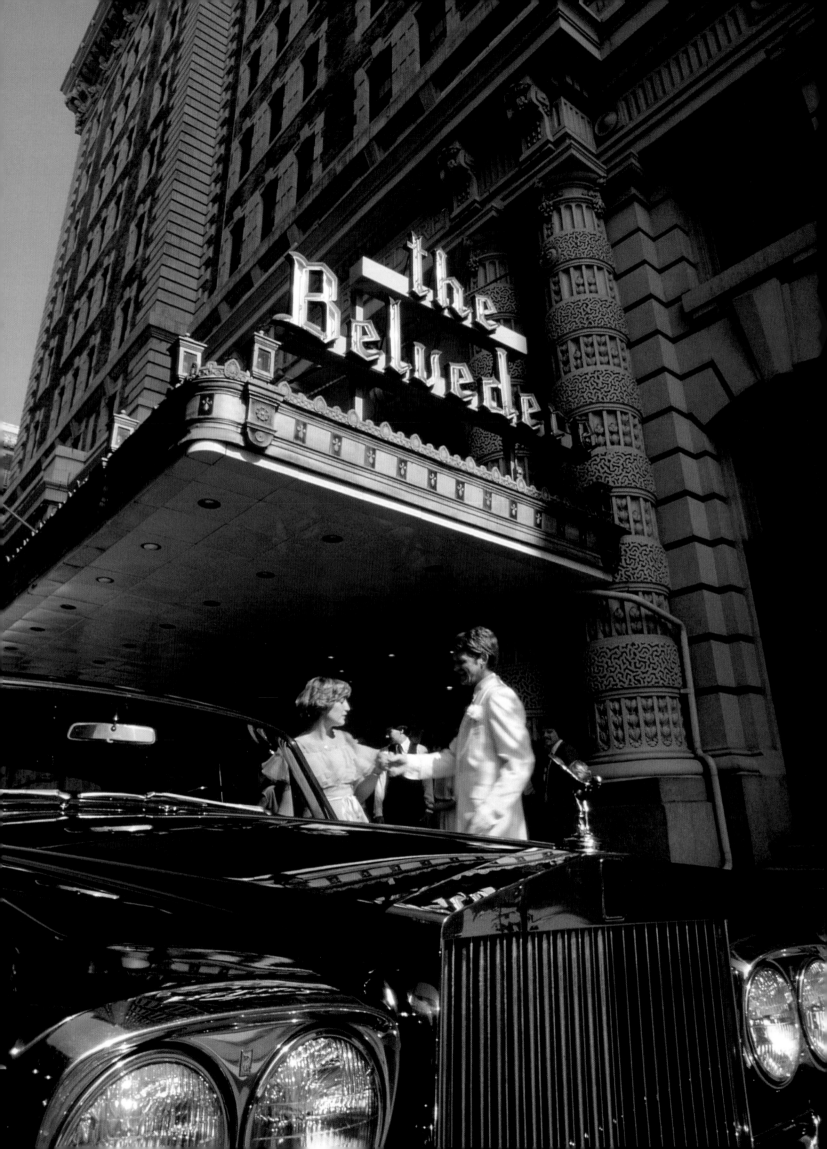

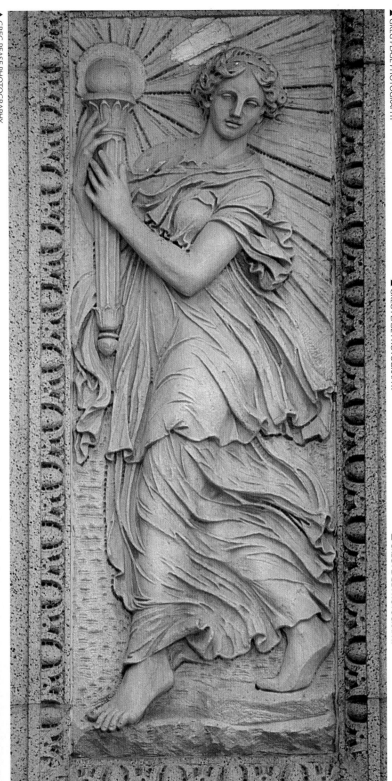

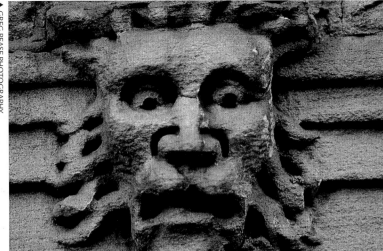

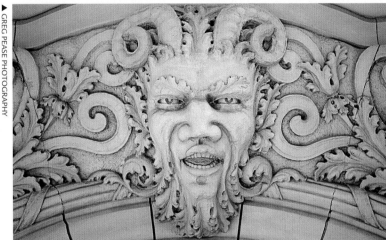

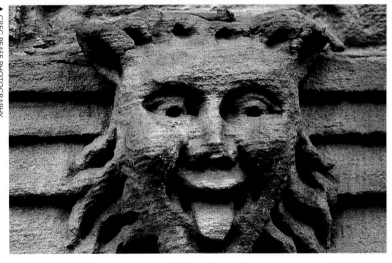

BUILT IN 1903 AS A LUXURY hotel, the Belvedere was—for generations—Baltimore society's favorite spot for elegant tea dances (OPPOSITE), and F. Scott Fitzgerald once threw a party here for his beloved daughter, Scottie. Today, the high French Renaissance/Second Empire-style chateau has been converted to condominiums, but thanks to its retro funky Owl Bar, it's still a popular gathering place.

In the 19th century, local office buildings and residences featured plenty of architectural flourishes.

A bas-relief adorns downtown's Baltimore Gas and Electric Building (LEFT), while expressive faces enliven the facades of area town houses (RIGHT).

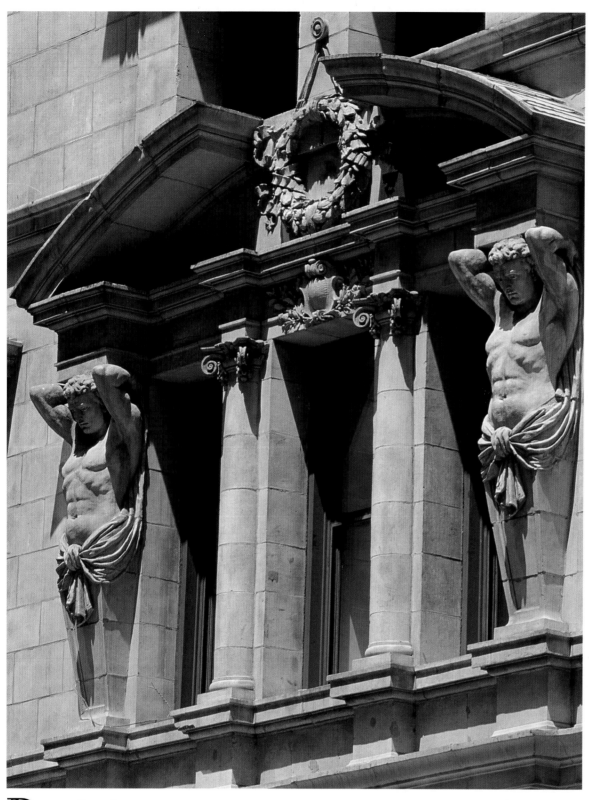

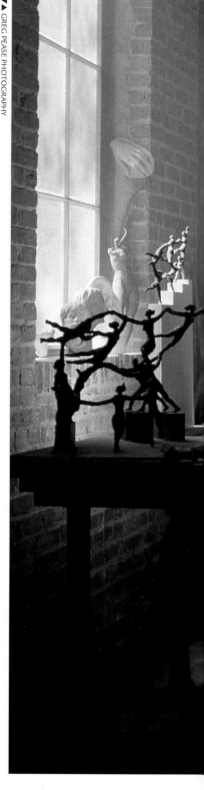

Built by Frank Junker, the former Junker Hotel was long a favorite resting spot for traveling salesmen. The structure's eye-catching architectural details have given passersby pause for nearly a century.

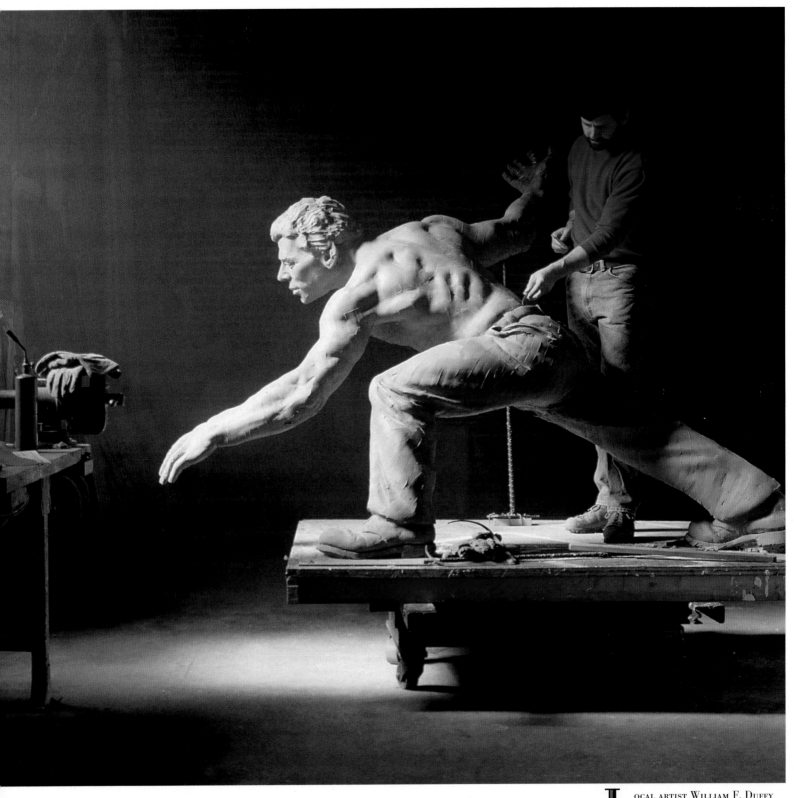

L OCAL ARTIST WILLIAM F. DUFFY
works on his sculptural tribute
to Baltimore's economic
heritage—*Monument to Labor.*

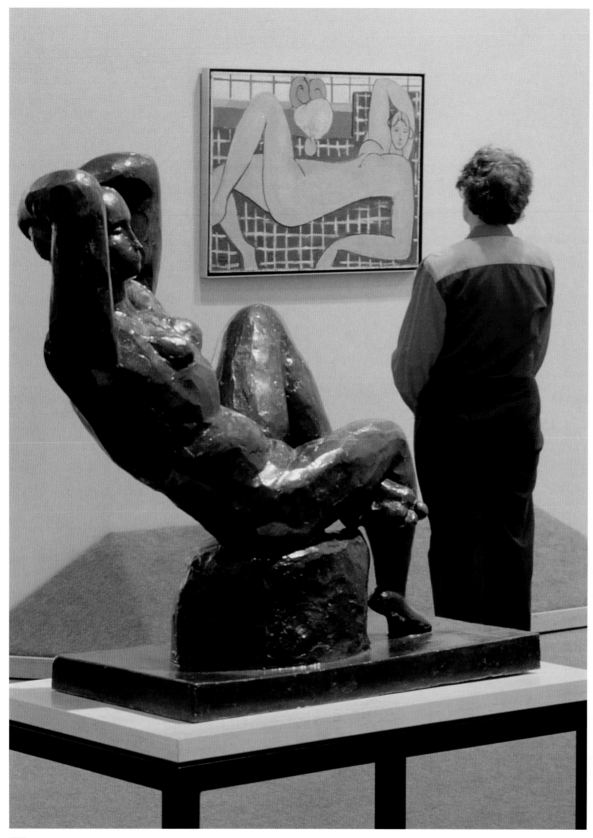

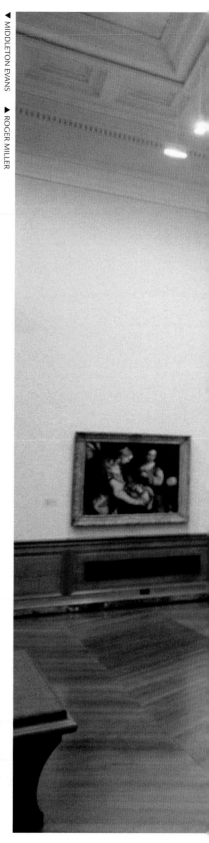

MIDDLETON EVANS ▲ ROGER MILLER ▲

I N THE EARLY 20TH CENTURY, DR. Claribel Cone and Miss Etta Cone, a pair of globe-trotting Baltimore sisters, amassed art by such masters as Picasso, van Gogh, Gauguin, and Matisse. Their prized acquisitions today comprise the Baltimore Museum of Art's Cone Collection, which also features notable works by Rodin, Cézanne, Renoir, and Degas.

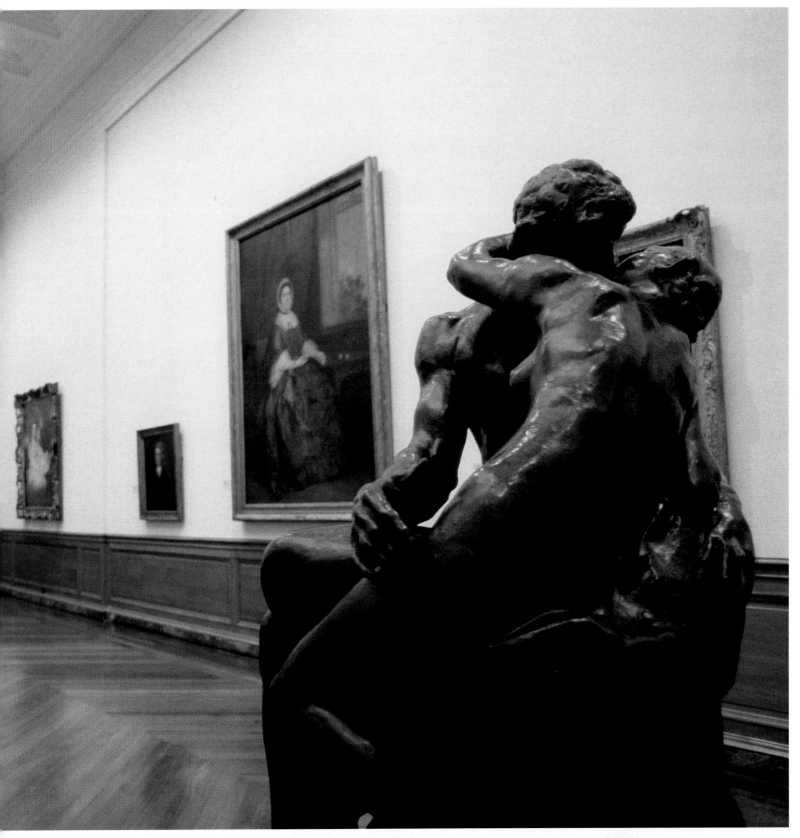

THEY MAY NOT BE THE FOUNTAIN OF youth, but the dramatic water sprays at the H.L. Mencken House (PAGE 82) and in Mount Vernon Square (PAGE 83) have a soothing power all their own.

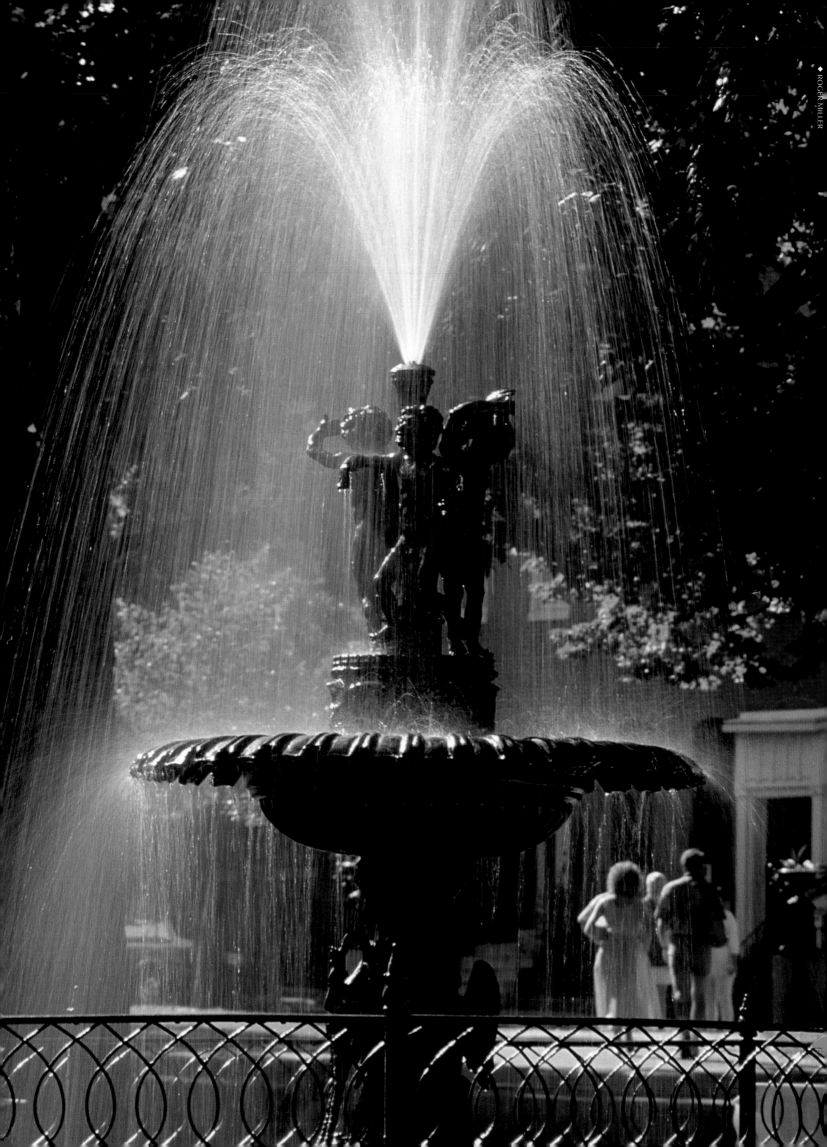

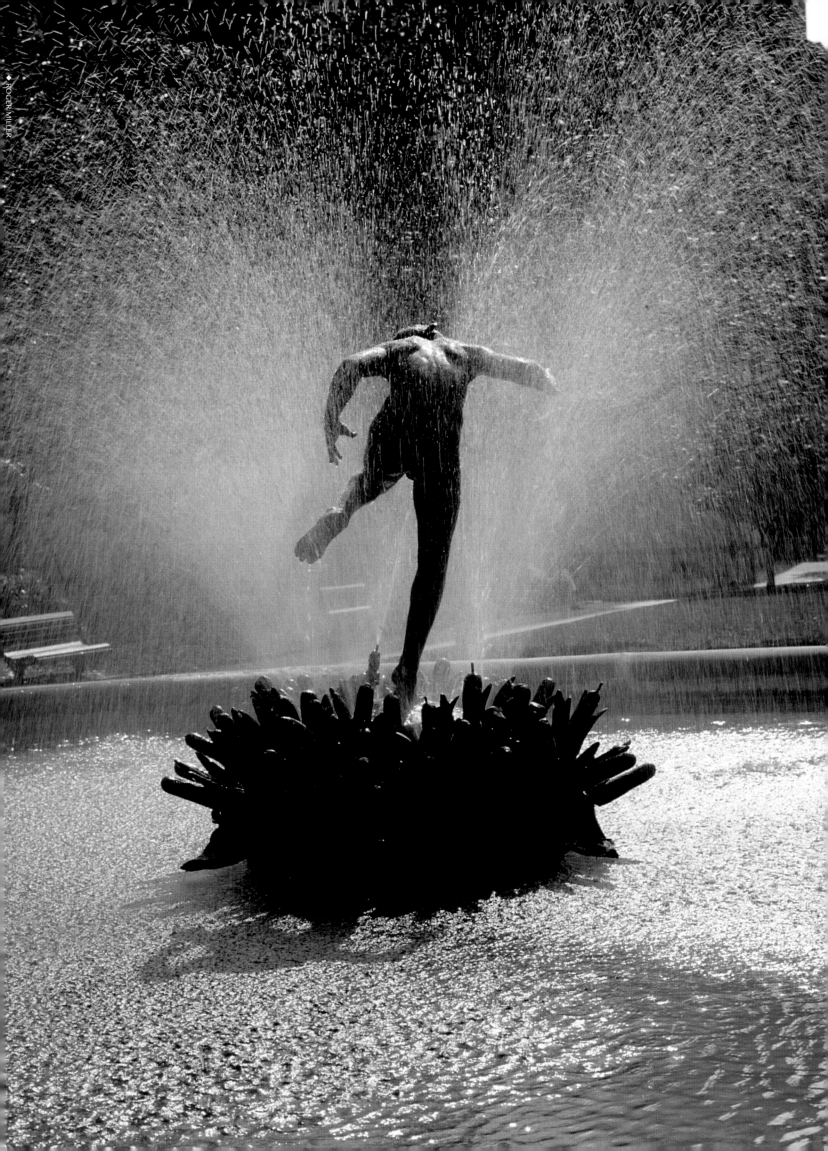

THE BALTIMORE MUSEUM OF ART (BMA) takes seriously its role as a premier showcase for post-1945 works, as evidenced by the West Wing for Contemporary Art, which opened in October 1994 (RIGHT). Housing some 16 galleries, the new space is devoted primarily to the works of Andy Warhol, making the BMA home to the world's second-largest collection of paintings by the artist on regular public display (OPPOSITE TOP).

Across town at the Walters Art Gallery, the Italianate sculpture court offers patrons an up close look at a number of Renaissance and baroque pieces (OPPOSITE BOTTOM). The benefactors of the museum were William Walters and his son, Henry, who believed that culture should be made available to the masses.

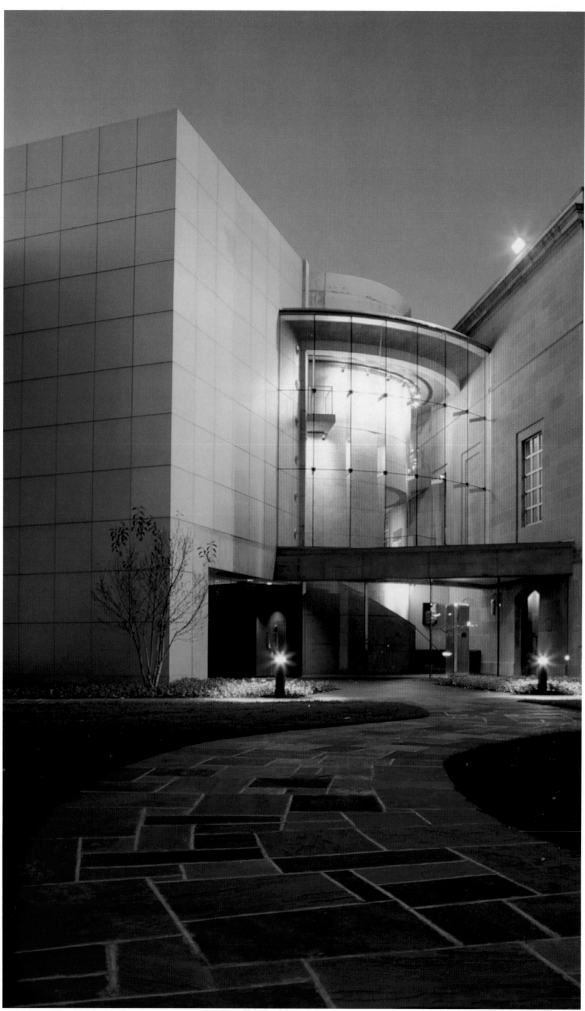

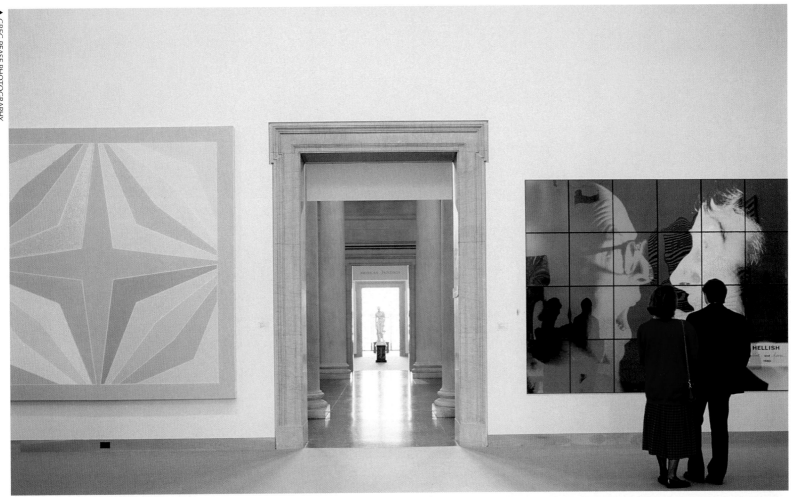

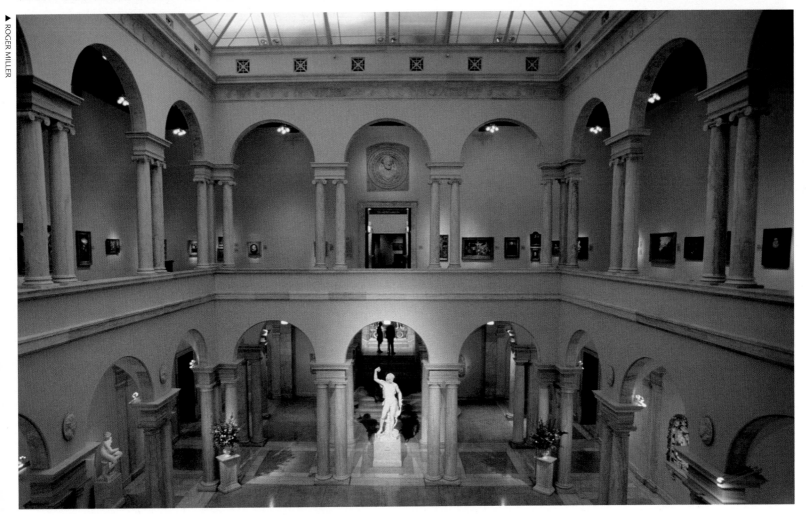

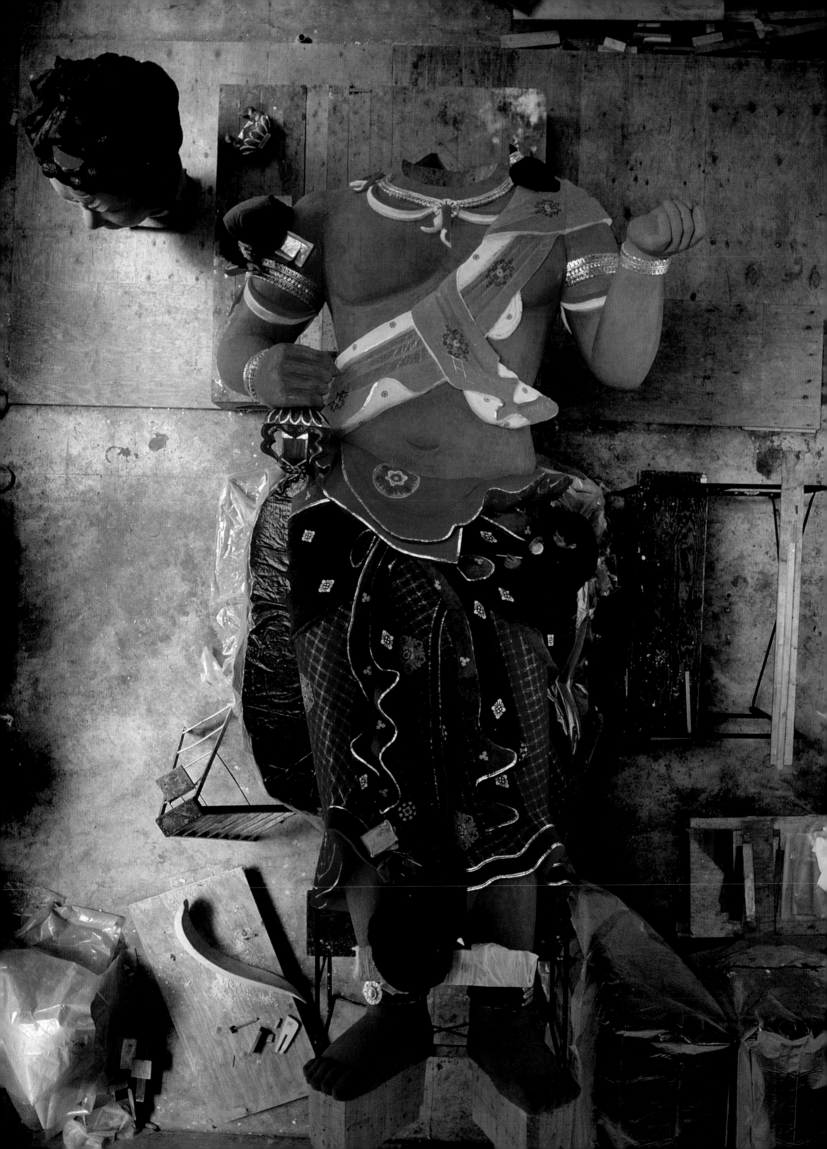

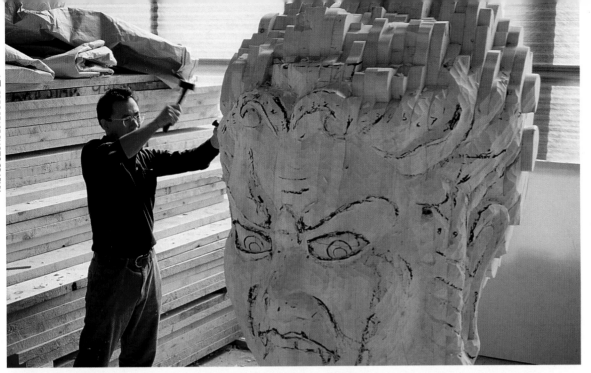

THE MARYLAND INSTITUTE-College of Art, which offers graduate and undergraduate degrees in a variety of artistic pursuits, is a cornerstone of historic Bolton Hill. One of the school's best-known projects was the construction of *Fudo Myoh-oh*, an incarnation of Buddha, led by Japanese sculptor Yasuhiko Hashimoto. The 33-foot-tall cedar statue took two and a half years to complete, and its fierce expression is said to scare people away from their egos on the way to enlightenment.

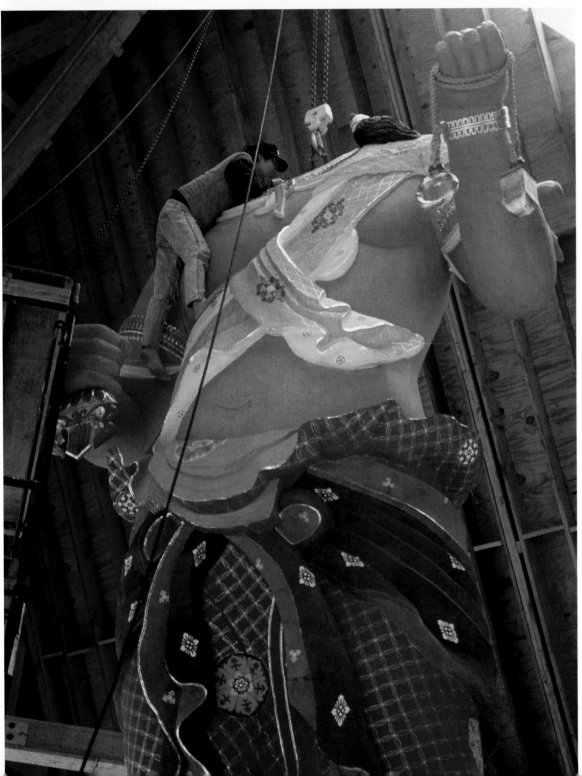

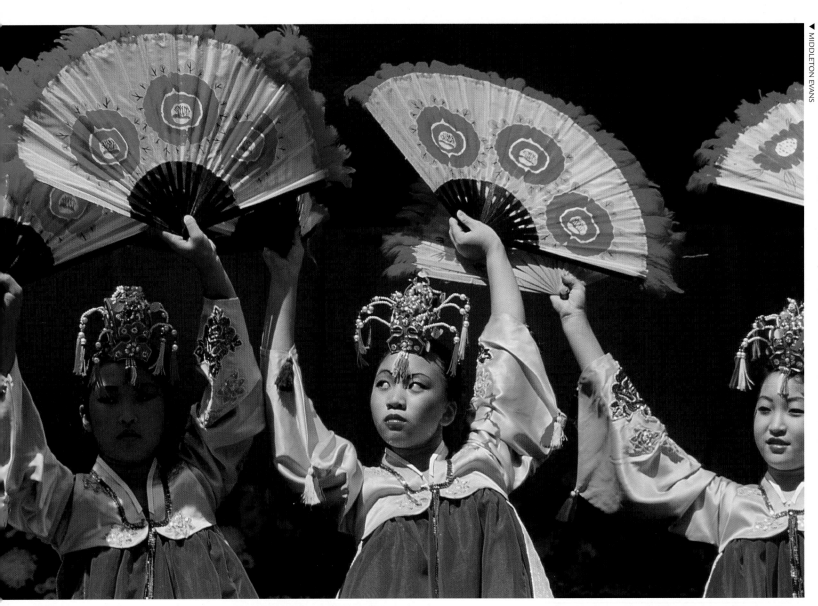

THE KOREAN FESTIVAL IS JUST one of many ethnic celebrations that honor Baltimore's diversity. This and other events—like those hosted by the Italian, Greek, and African-American communities—were spawned by the tremendous success of the first City Fair in 1970, which is often given credit for fueling Baltimore's modern renaissance.

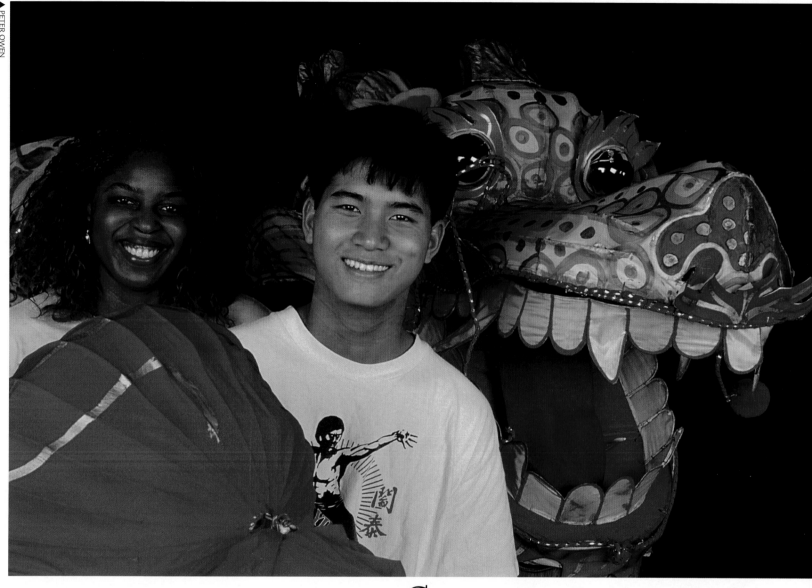

S TARTED IN THE EARLY 1980S, THE
annual ARTSCAPE celebration
features live music, exhibits,
international dance, theater, and a

crafts market. Opening the 1997 festivities was a traditional Chinese
dragon dance, complete with a
colorful, 100-foot-long beast.

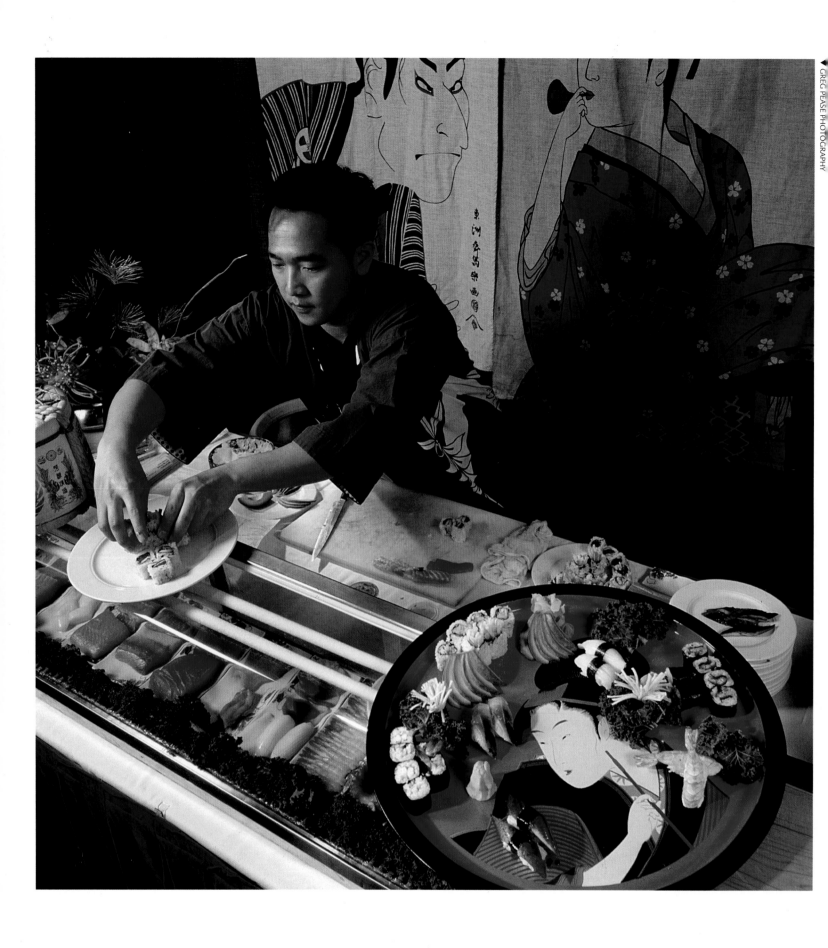

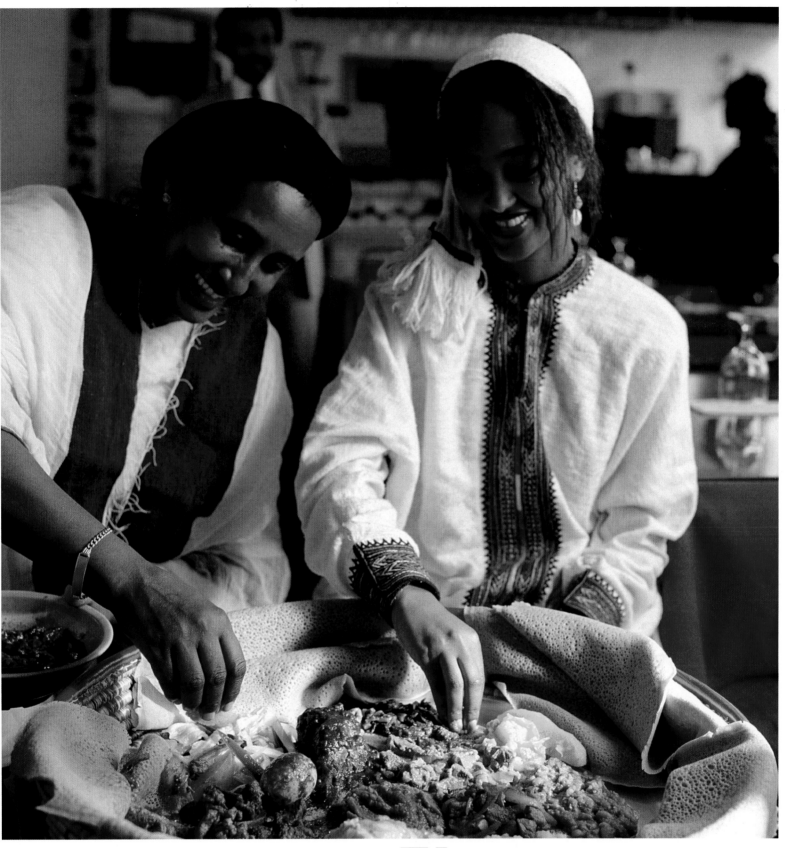

W HILE BALTIMOREANS HAVE long enjoyed the ethnic restaurants in such enclaves as Greektown and Little Italy, more recent newcomers to downtown reflect Asian, African, and Indian traditions.

As Jack Chang prepares the sushi buffet at the Omni Inner Harbor hotel (OPPOSITE), a couple of hungry customers enjoy the unusual Ethiopian fare at the Blue Nile (ABOVE).

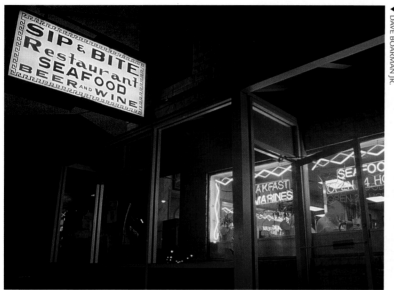

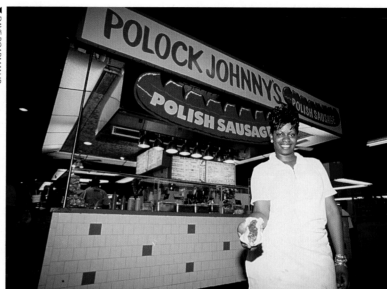

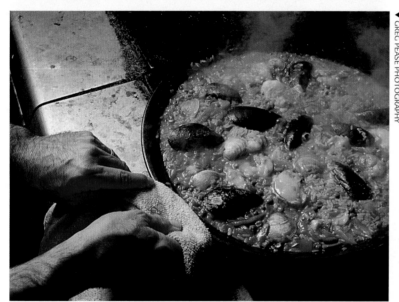

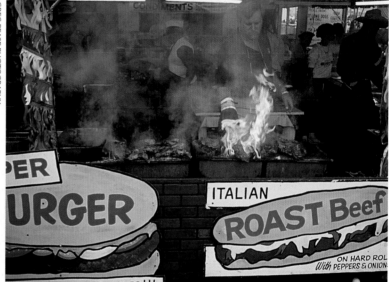

Dining options in Baltimore run the gamut, from a seafood feast at the Sip & Bite to a meaty dog at Polock Johnny's, paella à la Valenciana at Tio Pepe, and a choice of burgers, roast beef, and countless other treats at the Maryland State Fair.

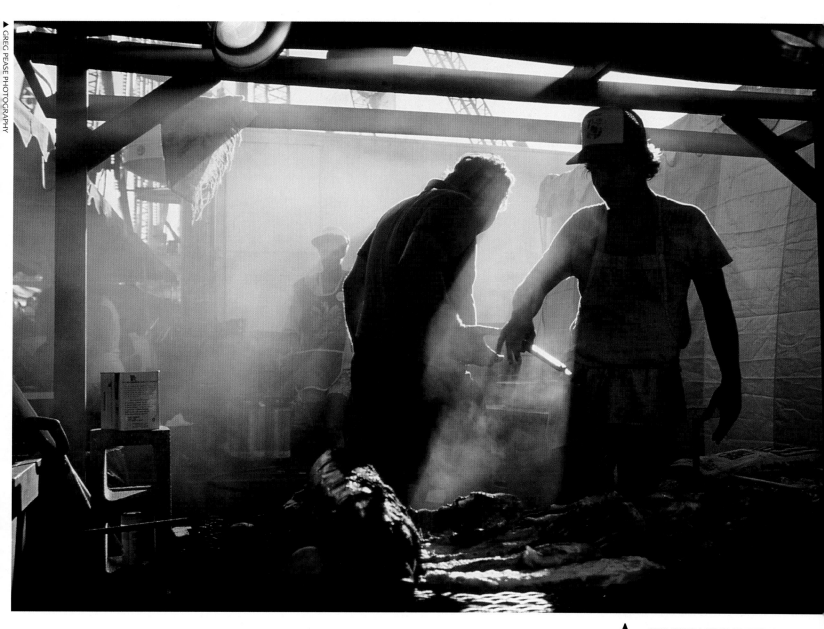

ASIDE FROM A HOST OF ATTRAC-
tions that range from live-
stock shows to Ferris wheel
rides, the 10-day Maryland State Fair
is famous for its barbecued ribs.

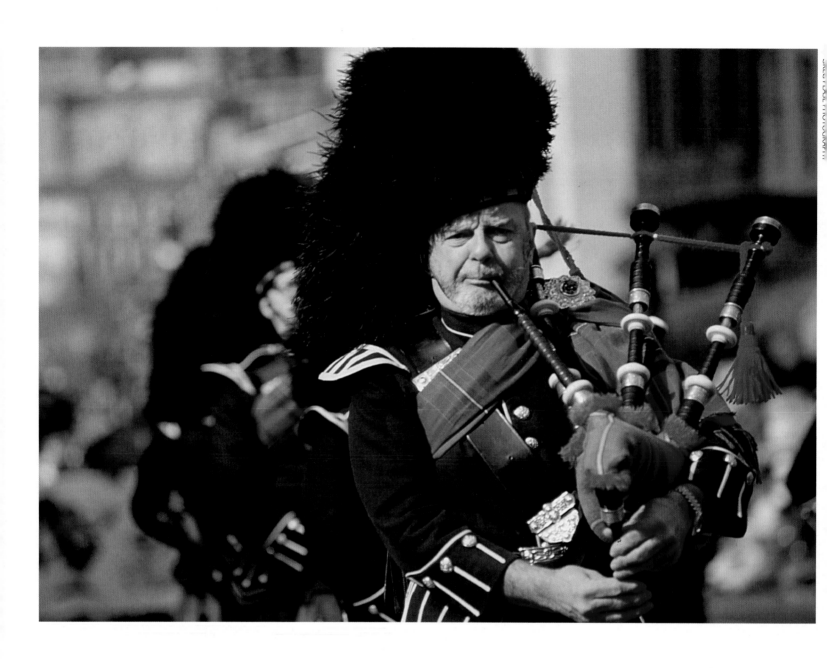

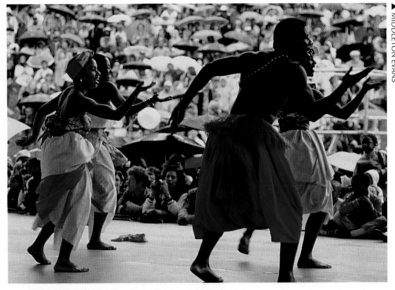

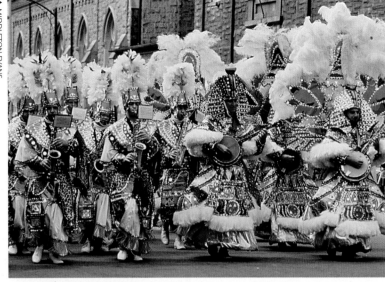

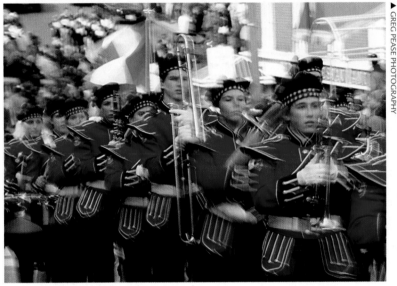

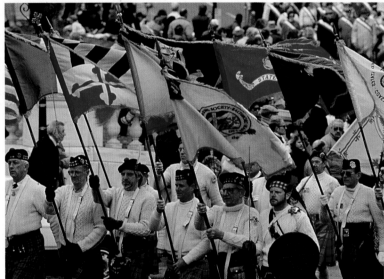

Y EAR-ROUND, LOCALS PROVE THEY
know how to throw a party at
such events as the annual St.
Patrick's Day Parade (BOTTOM AND
OPPOSITE), a colorful Shriners Parade
(TOP RIGHT), and a traditional African
performance at ARTSCAPE (TOP LEFT).

Young Baltimoreans of every stripe are reminded of their roots at numerous celebrations. Whether it's August's AFRAM Festival (TOP), the International Festival in War Memorial Plaza (CENTER), the Korean Festival at Hopkins Plaza (BOTTOM), or the St. Anthony Festival in Little Italy (OPPOSITE), youngsters get a chance to show the grown-ups what fun is really all about.

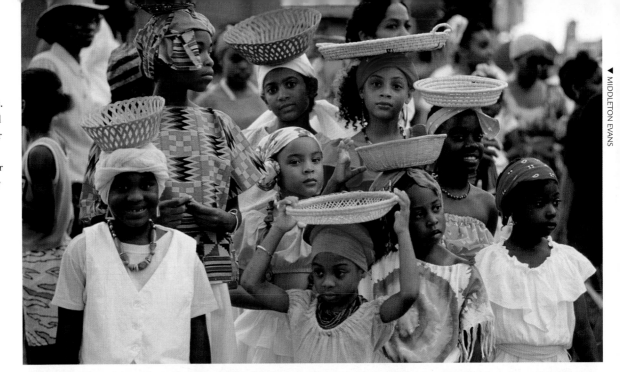

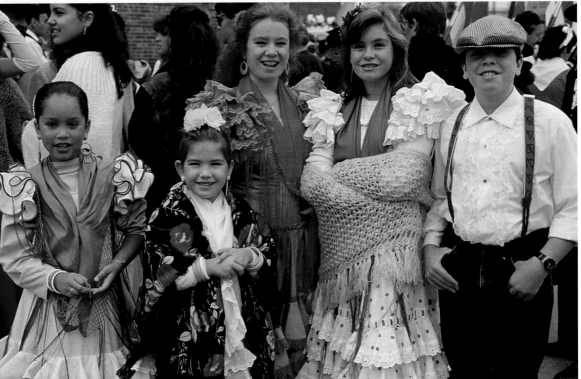

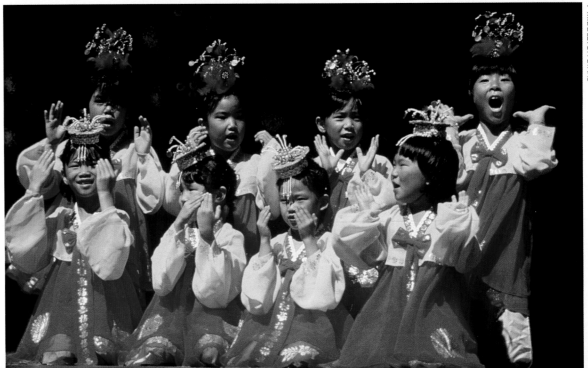

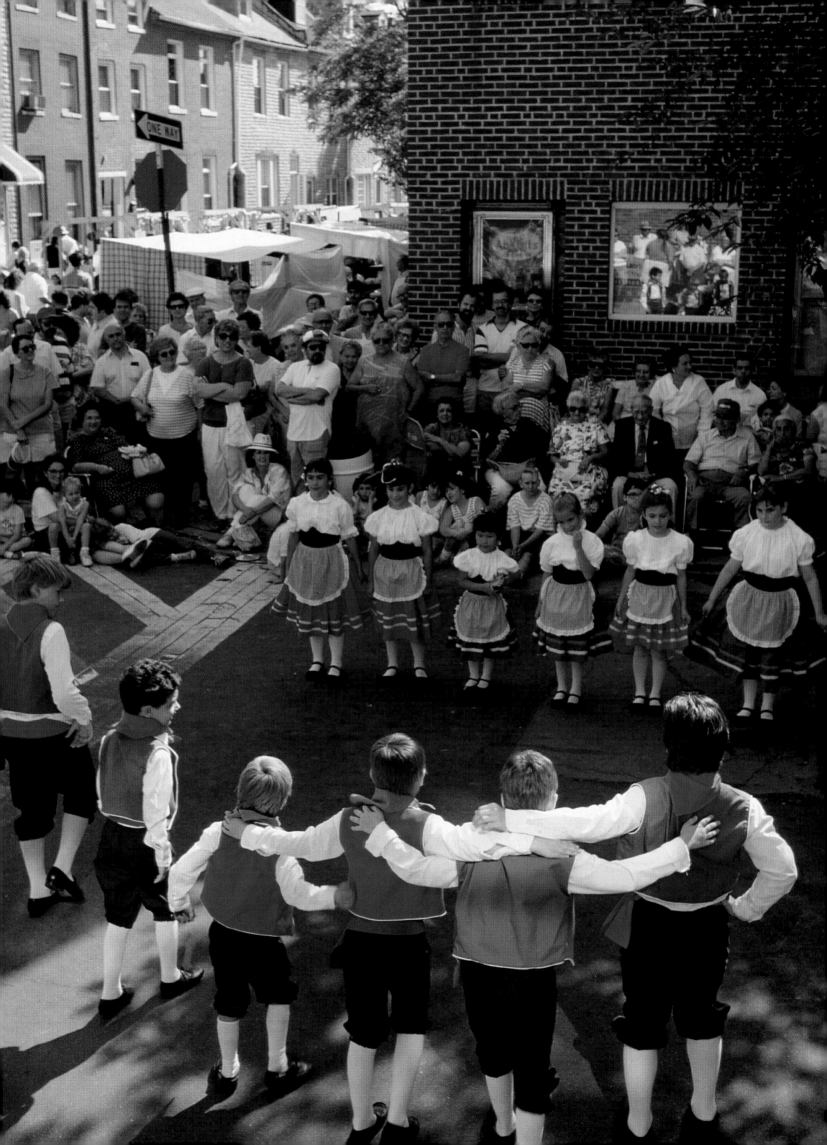

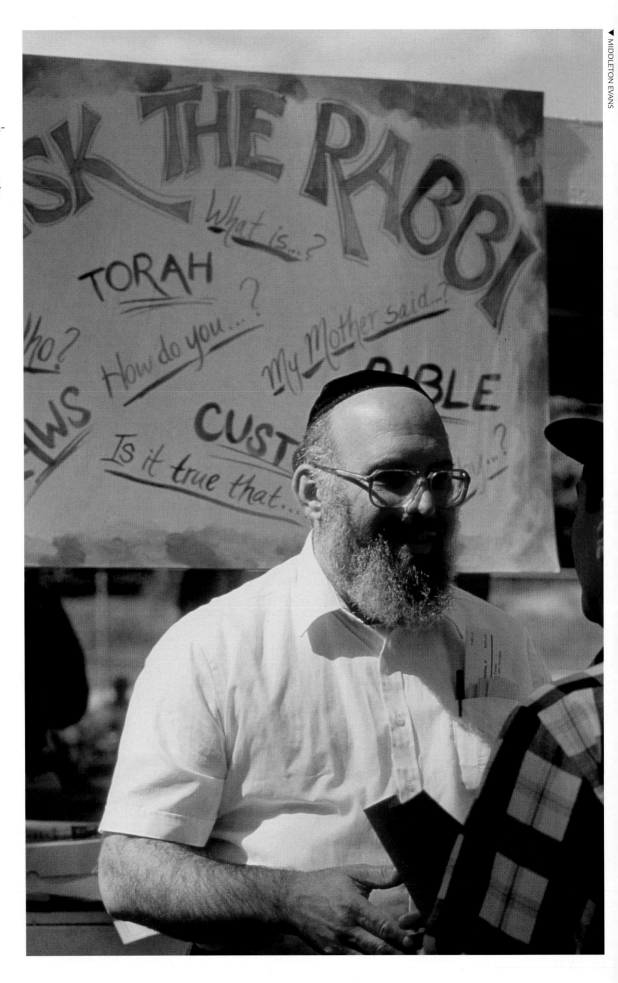

GREATER BALTIMORE'S LARGE Jewish population comes together to celebrate each May at the Jewish Festival, which features the popular Ask the Rabbi booth (RIGHT). Plenty of kibitzing can also be overheard at Attman's Authentic New York Delicatessen on East Lombard Street (OPPOSITE, TOP LEFT). Since 1915, folks have frequented the popular eatery for its hot corned beef and kosher hot dogs.

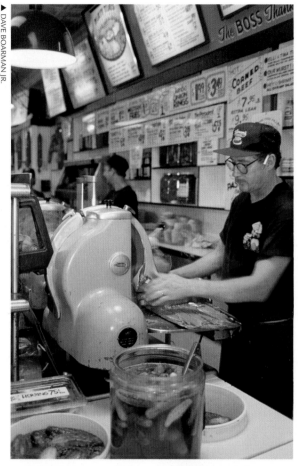

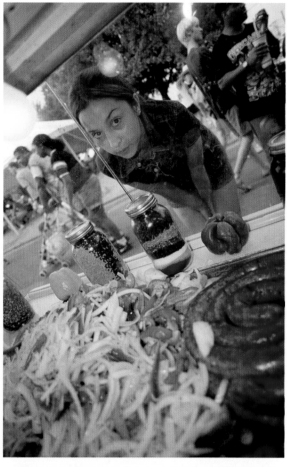

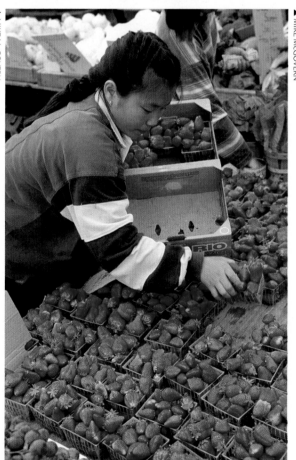

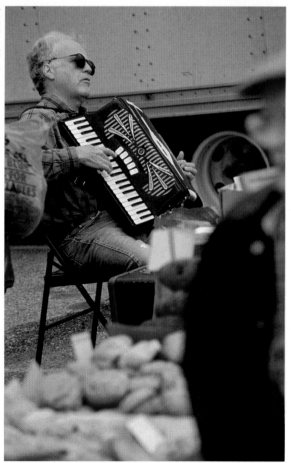

F OR MORE THAN 200 YEARS, Baltimoreans have bought their groceries—handpicked and fresh from the sea—at such local venues as the venerable Lexington Market on Eutaw Street and the Waverly Market in North Baltimore.

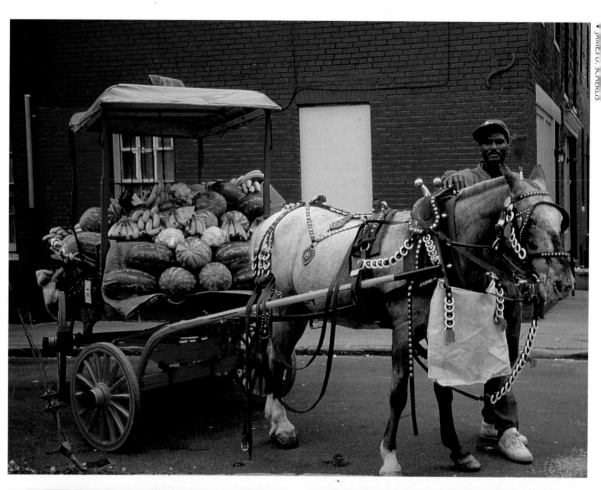

JAMES D. SCHERL

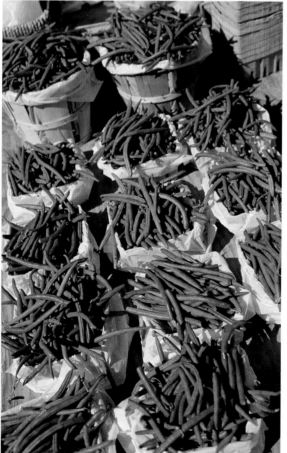

MIKE McGOVERN

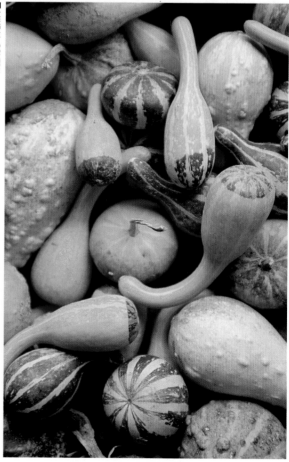

MIKE McGOVERN

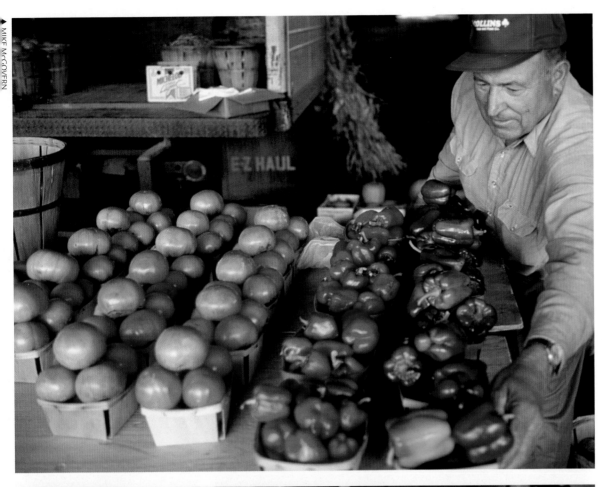

THERE'S NO SHORTAGE OF FRESH food in Charm City, where local markets offer everything from watermelons and green beans to squash, peppers, and juicy tomatoes. A familiar sight throughout downtown's rowhouse neighborhoods, Baltimore's street merchants, known as "A-rabbers," sell produce and oysters from horse-drawn carts (OPPOSITE TOP).

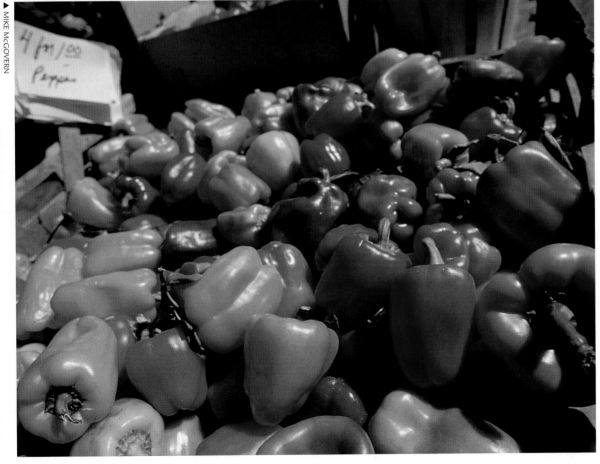

CHARM CITY

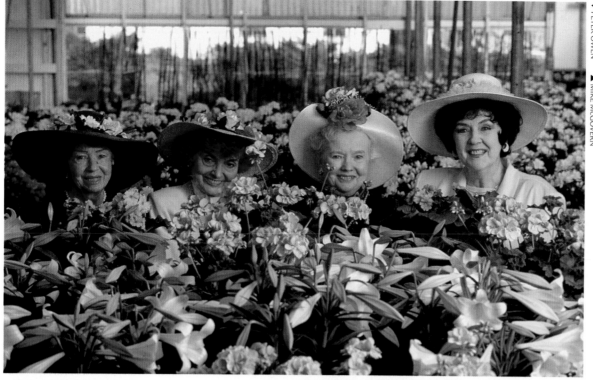

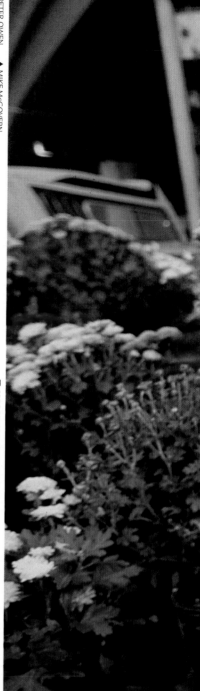

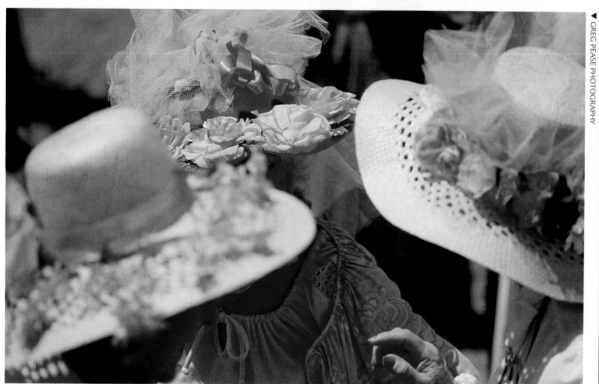

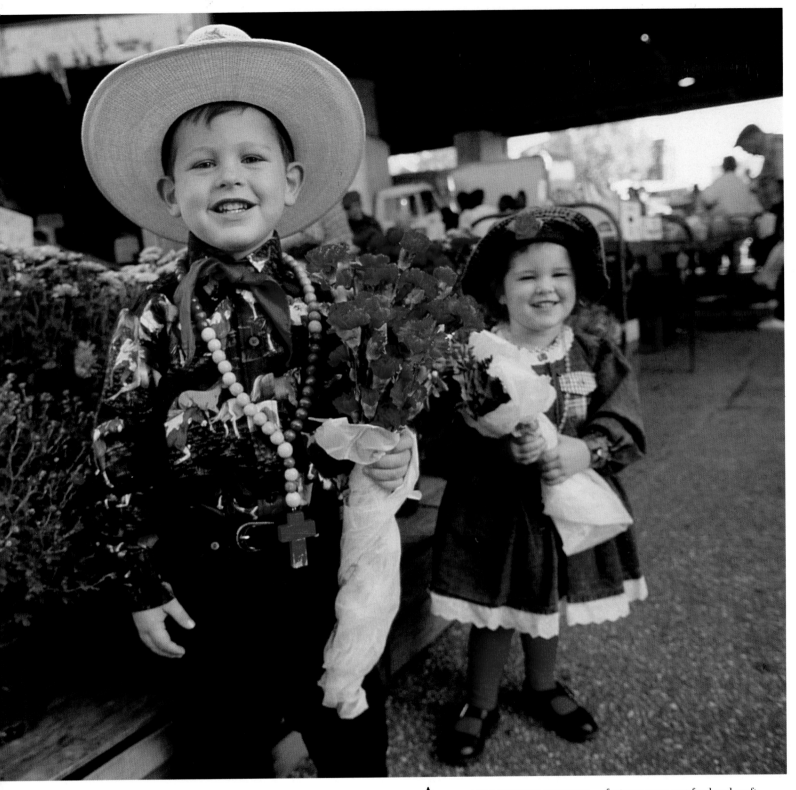

AN APPRECIATION FOR BEAUTIFUL blossoms begins early in Baltimore, thanks in part to the Women's Civic League's Flower Mart fund-raiser. Started in 1911, the Mount Vernon Square event today offers more than just flowers; it also features some 150 food and craft booths, where you'll find everything from chocolate-filled French pastries to personalized coat hangers to the Flower Mart's trademark lemon-with-peppermint sticks.

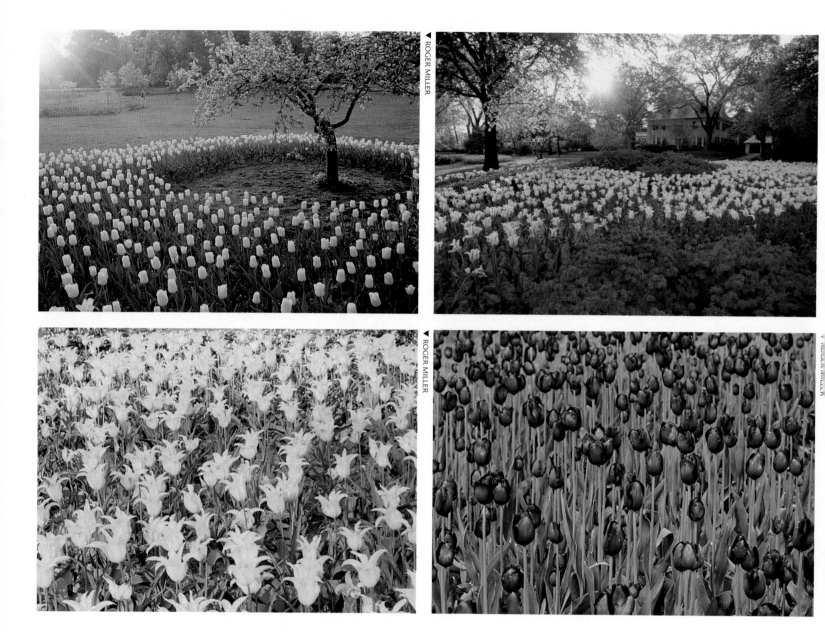

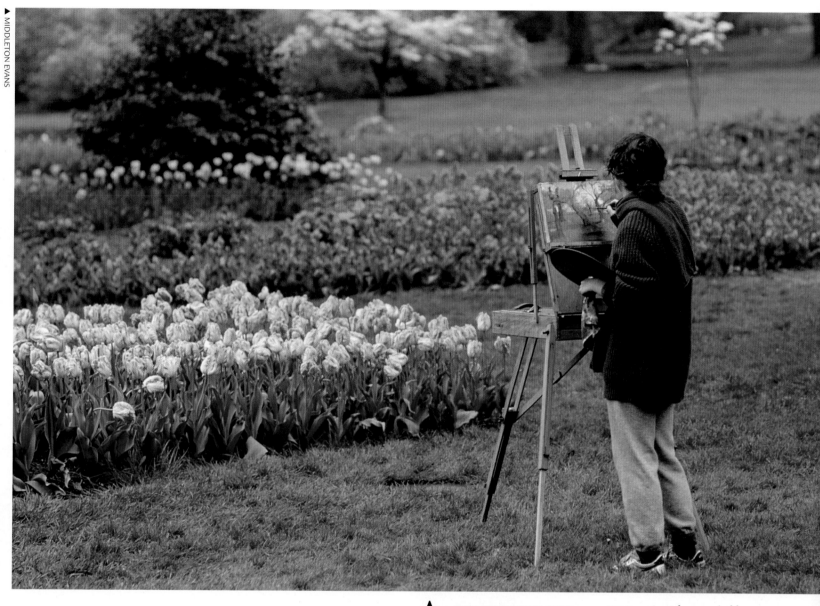

A T THE HEIGHT OF ITS GLORY between Easter and the end of May, Sherwood Gardens pays homage to spring with an explosion of more than 100,000 tulips. The seven-acre gardens are in bloom nearly year-round, with a seasonal array of daffodils, pansies, azaleas, and other colorful flora.

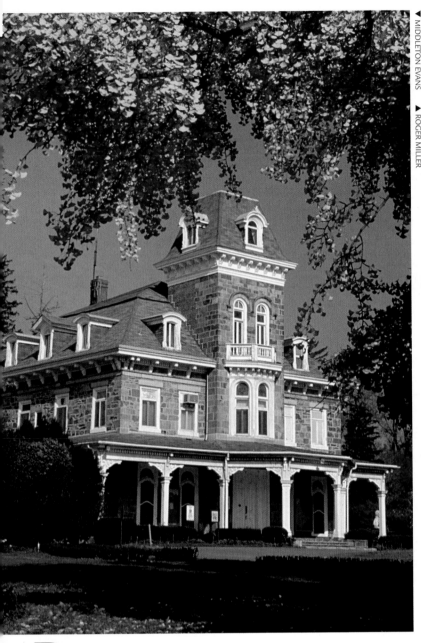

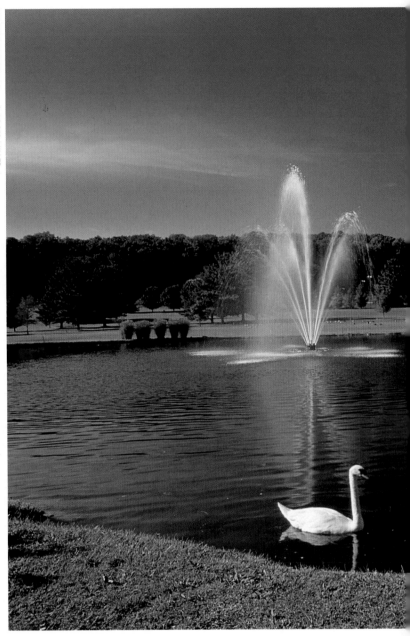

DURING THE CIVIL WAR, CYLBURN was one of Baltimore's grandest estates, complete with its own railroad station, a Louis XV drawing room, and a dozen servants. Today, the historic site is a wildflower and horticultural sanctuary (LEFT).

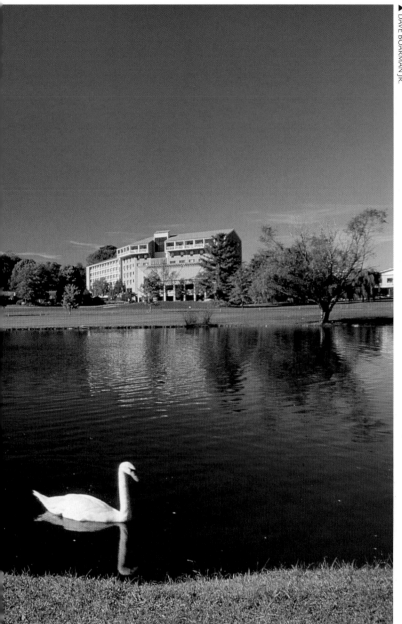

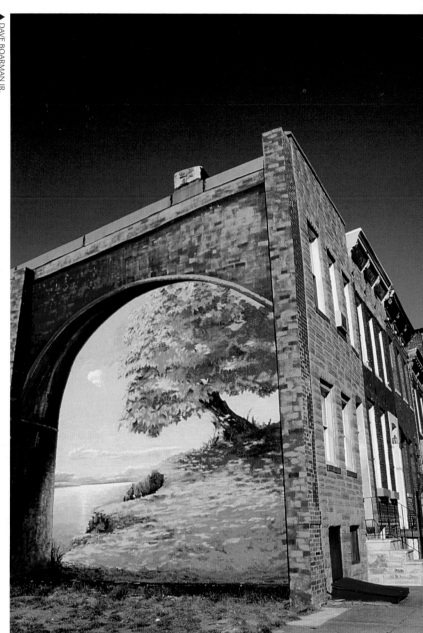

I N TOWN OR OUT, LOCALS KNOW HOW to appreciate Mother Nature. The Turf Valley Golf Club in nearby Howard County (CENTER) offers members and guests a picture-perfect setting, while back in the city, a building facade becomes an unexpected canvas for an enterprising craftsman (RIGHT).

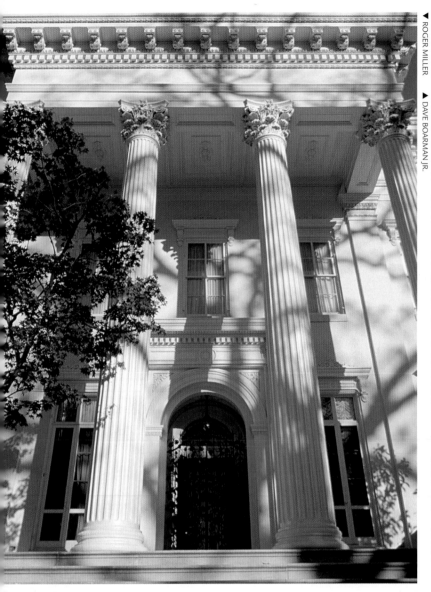

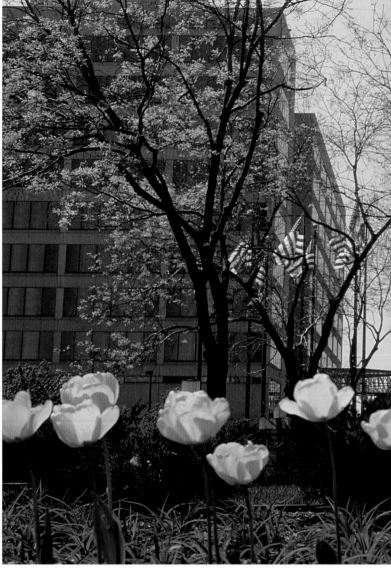

Tʜᴇ ᴍᴀɢɴɪꜰɪᴄᴇɴᴛ Cᴏʀɪɴᴛʜɪᴀɴ portico is just one distinguishing feature of Evergreen House (ʟᴇꜰᴛ), built circa 1855 by Baltimore's Garrett family. Today owned by Johns Hopkins University, the homestead has been transformed into a museum to showcase the Garretts' eclectic art collection, which ranges from Tiffany to Picasso.

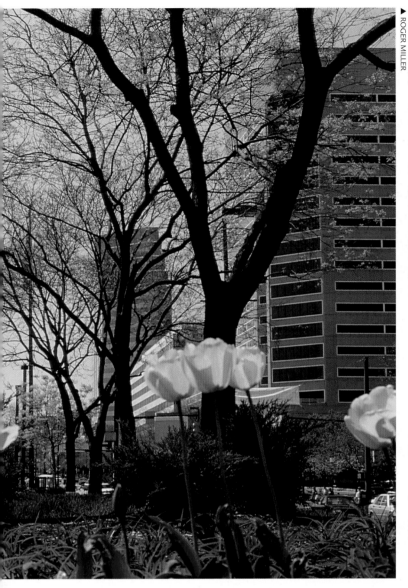

ROGER MILLER

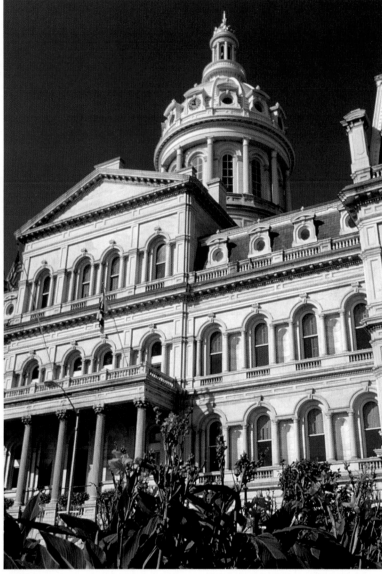

I N AN EFFORT TO ADD NATURAL
beauty to man-made facades, city
planners have landscaped portions
of downtown, including Metro Center,
a complex of office buildings north of
the Inner Harbor (CENTER).

Opened in 1875, City Hall and its
110-foot rotunda still stand tall today
(RIGHT). The building was one of the
few structures downtown that survived
the Great Fire of 1904.

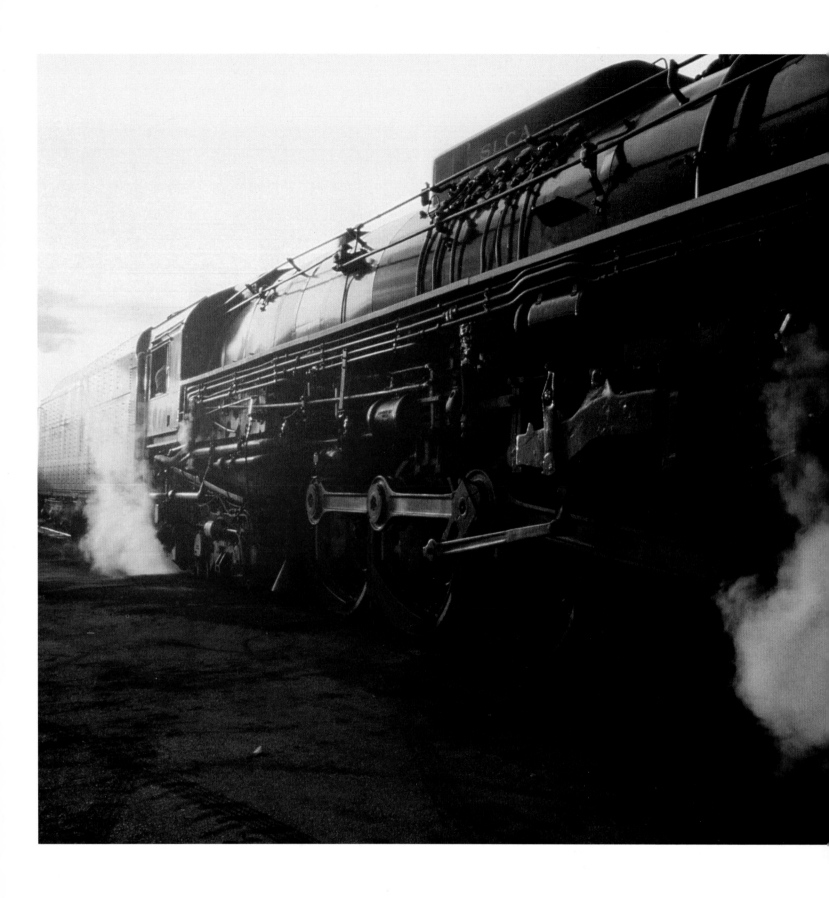

110

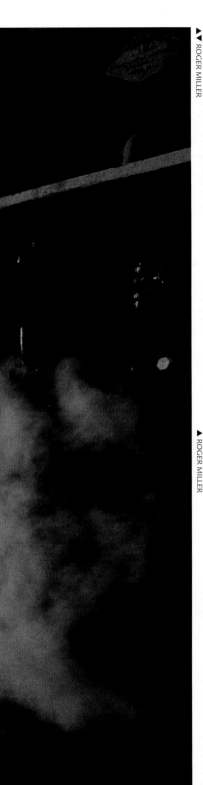

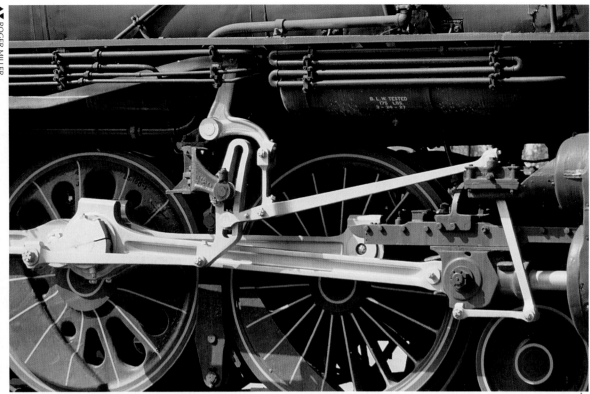

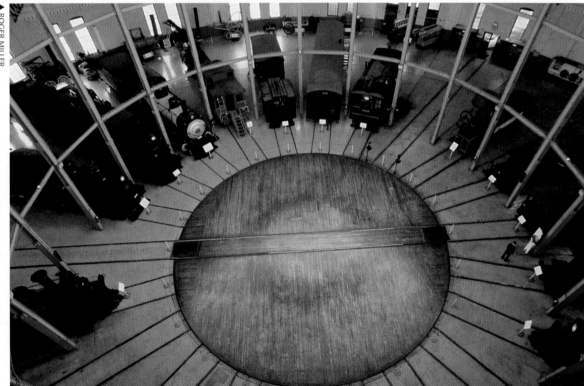

THE LARGEST FACILITY OF ITS KIND in the United States, the B&O Railroad Museum features a stunning collection of train engines, as well as a replica of the Tom Thumb, America's first steam locomotive. The museum's entrance is at the Mount Clare Station, a glorious roundhouse built in 1884.

IMAGES OF HISTORIC BALTIMORE: A funnel of smoke gracefully rises from a locomotive as it passes through Pennsylvania Train Yard in 1945.

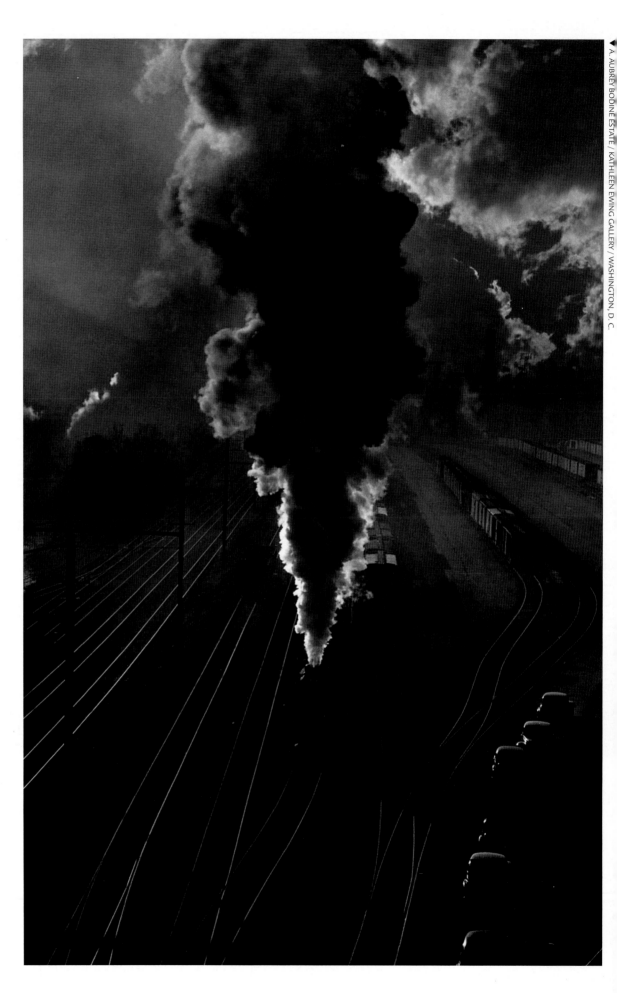

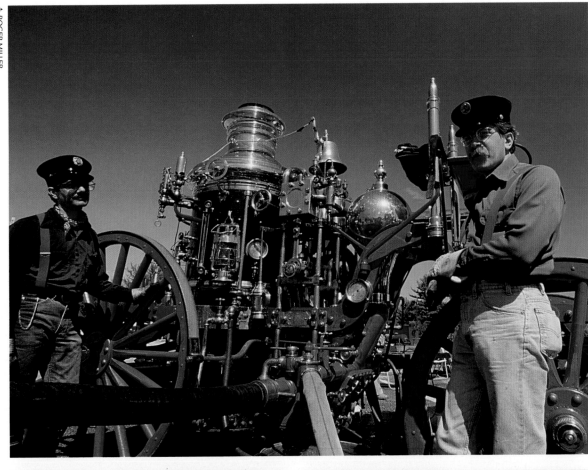

ROGER MILLER

B ALTIMORE COMMEMORATES ITS past in countless ways, including (CLOCKWISE FROM TOP) the Fire Museum of Maryland, which houses examples of antique fire fighting equipment, some of which are nearly 200 years old; the Baltimore Museum of Industry, a former oyster cannery on the Inner Harbor that celebrates the city's industrial and labor history; and the *Pride of Baltimore II*, shown here during its construction in 1987.

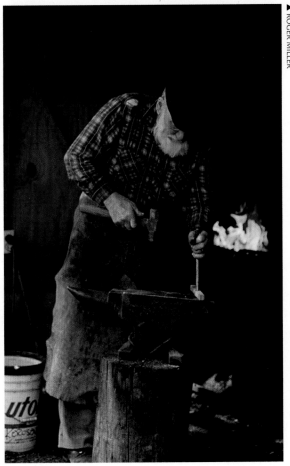

GREG PEASE PHOTOGRAPHY

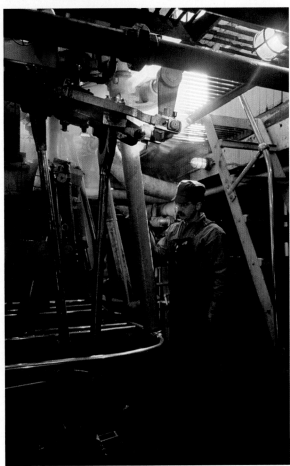

ROGER MILLER

THE GREAT FIRE OF 1904, THE cause of which was never determined, demolished more than 70 prime downtown blocks and the city's tallest buildings (OPPOSITE TOP). Today's firefighters work hard to prevent similar destruction.

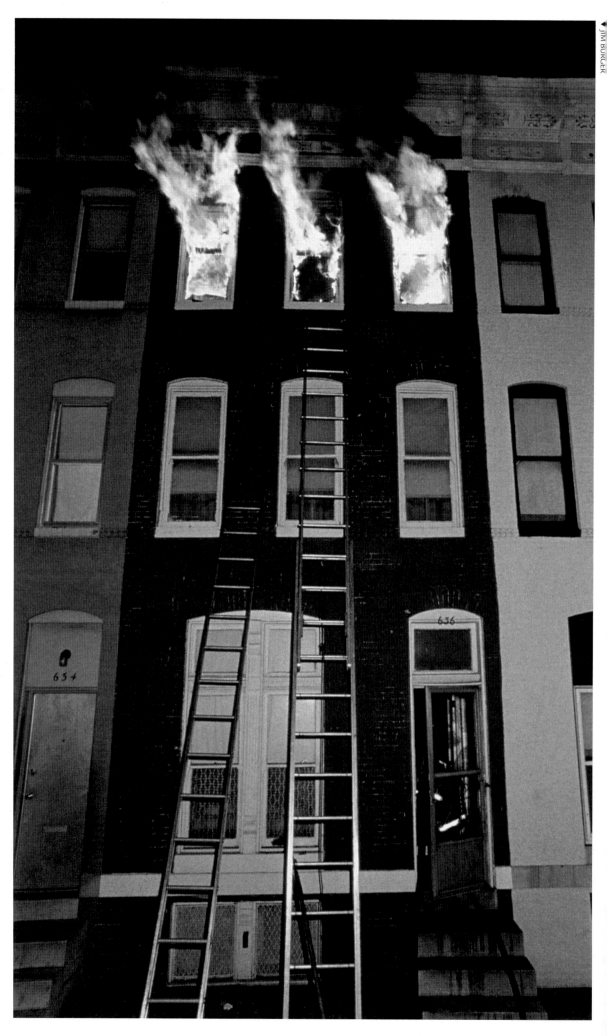

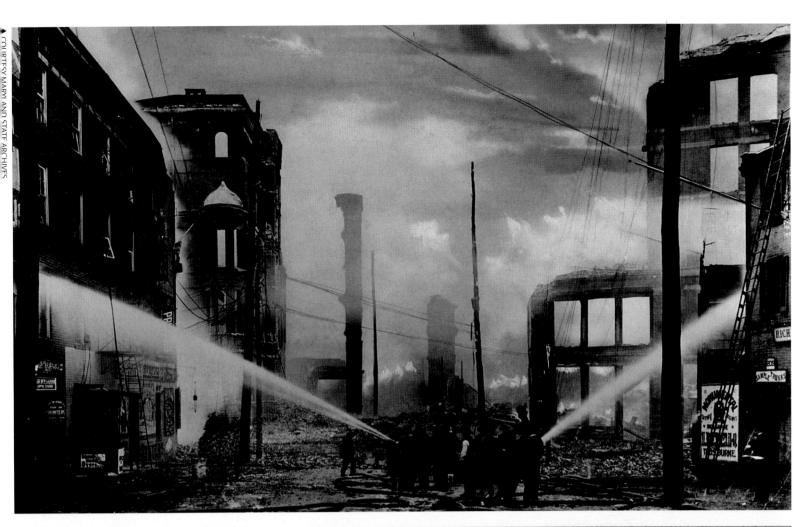

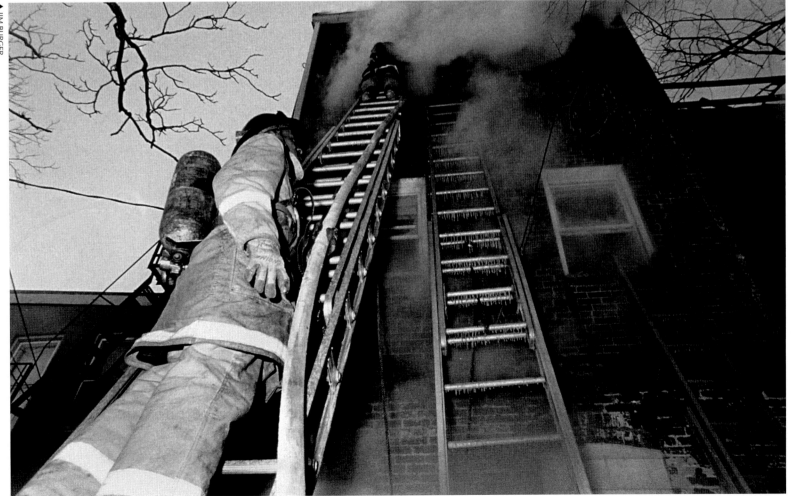

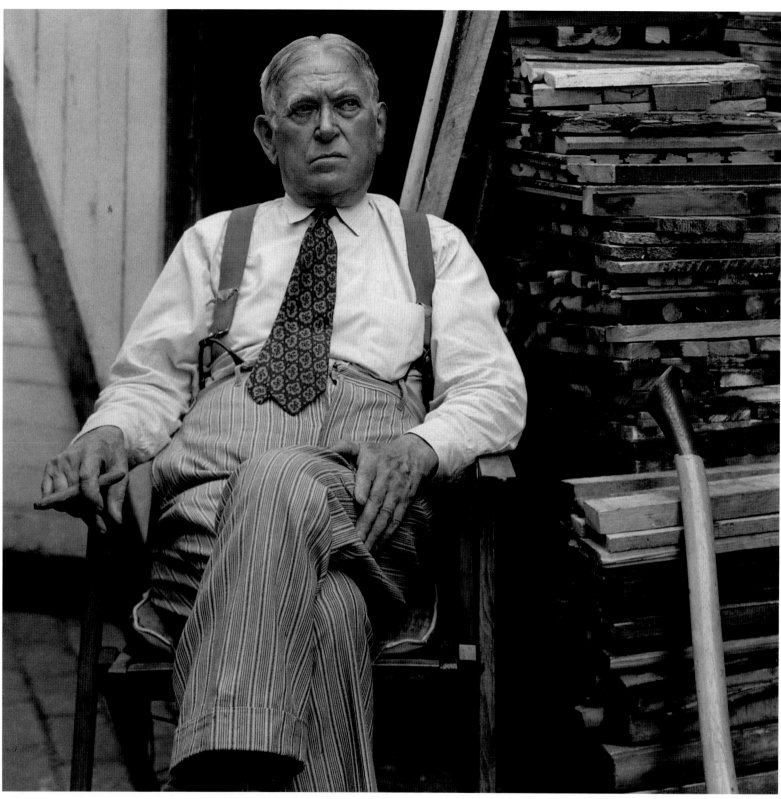

THE LATE H.L. MENCKEN, A PRO-
lific and powerful 20th-century
essayist and critic, was known
as the "sage of Baltimore," having
spent most of his life in the family
rowhouse on Union Square. His
sitting room, dining room, garden,
and second-floor study have been
preserved, and now are part of the
Mencken House museum.

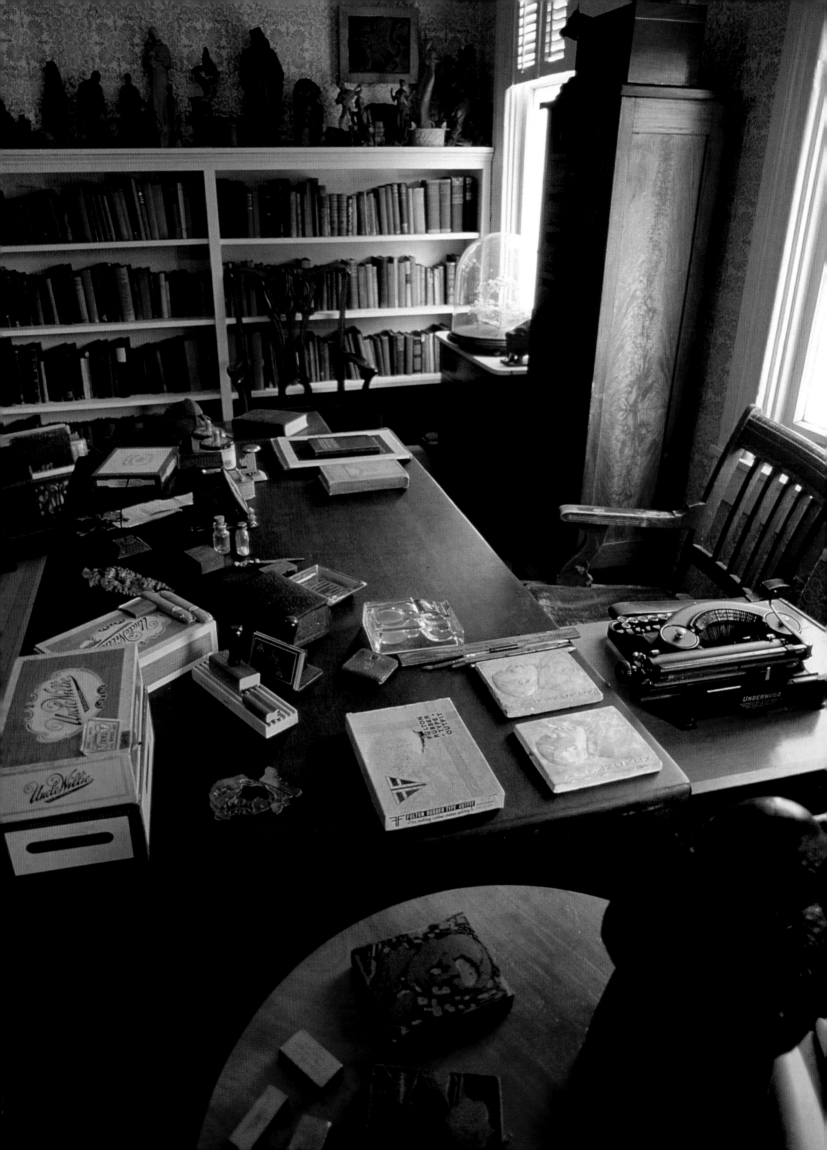

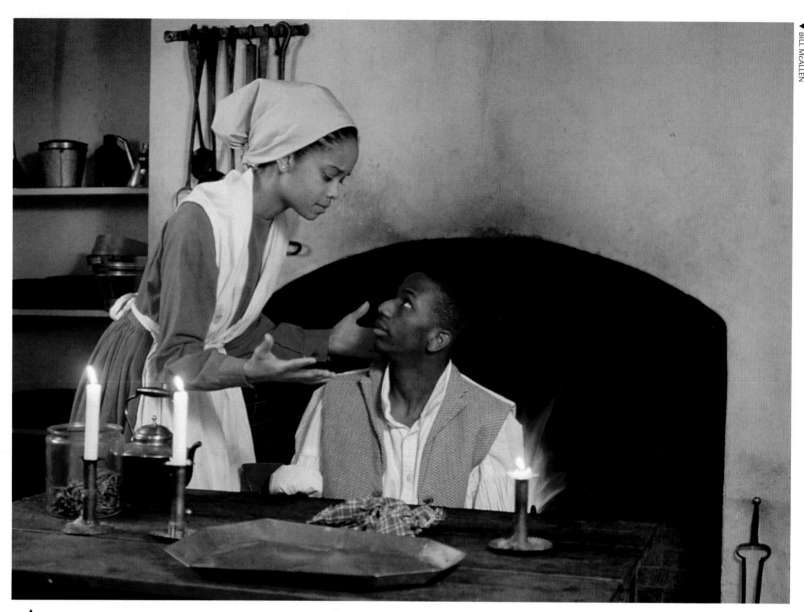

A RECONSTRUCTED ROWHOUSE that belonged to a wheelwright and his family, the 1840 House in Little Italy features a troupe of actors who re-create life as it existed in the 19th century.

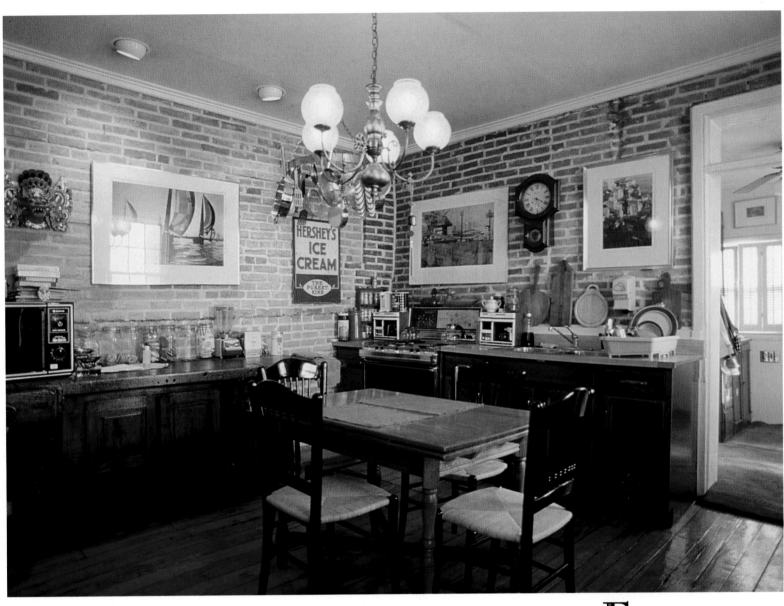

EVERYTHING OLD IS NEW AGAIN IN Baltimore. A contemporary kitchen belies the age of this homestead in historic Union Square.

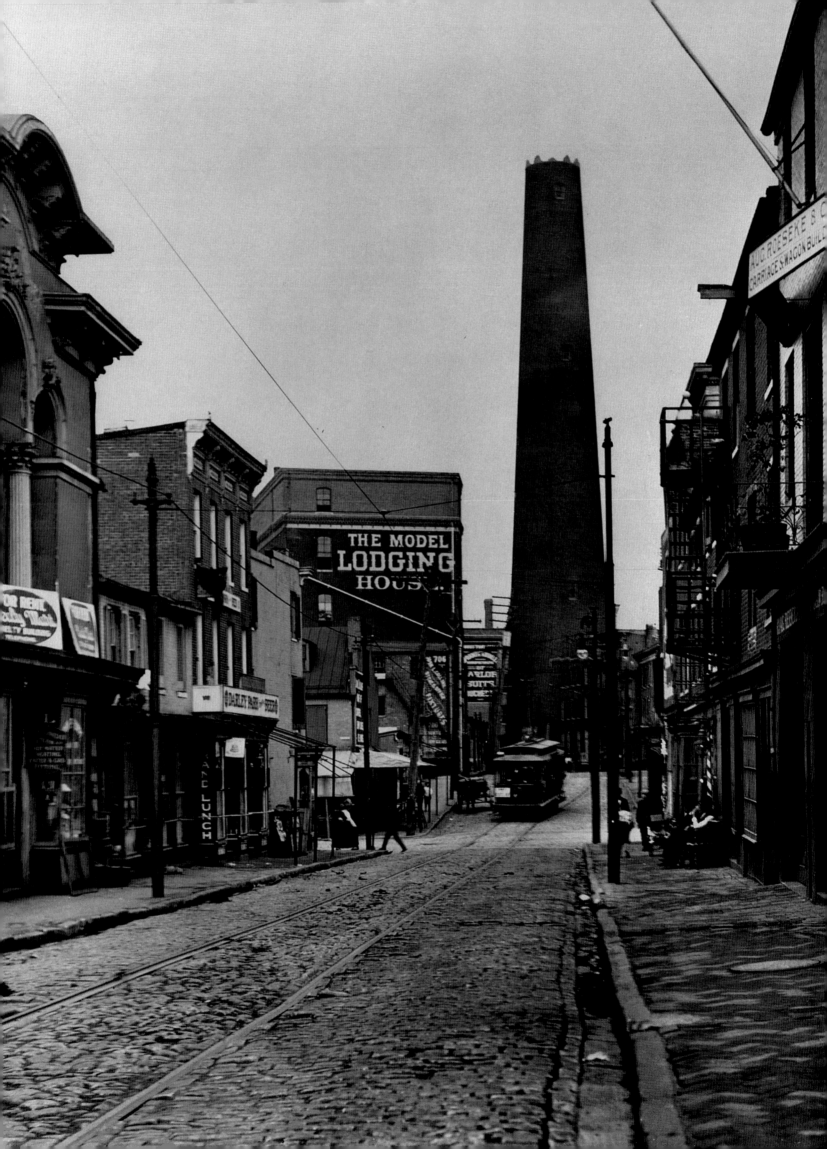

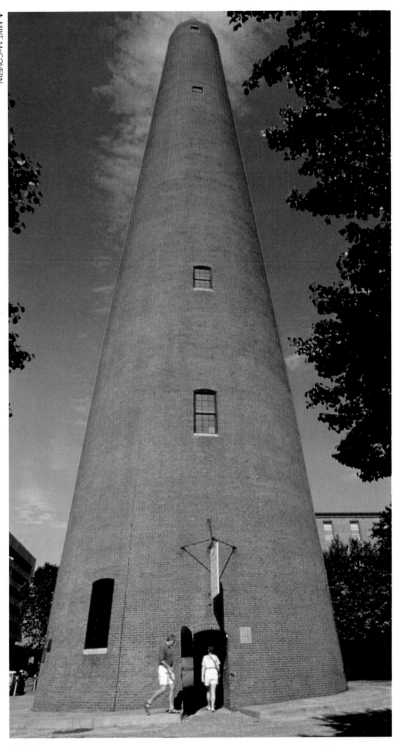

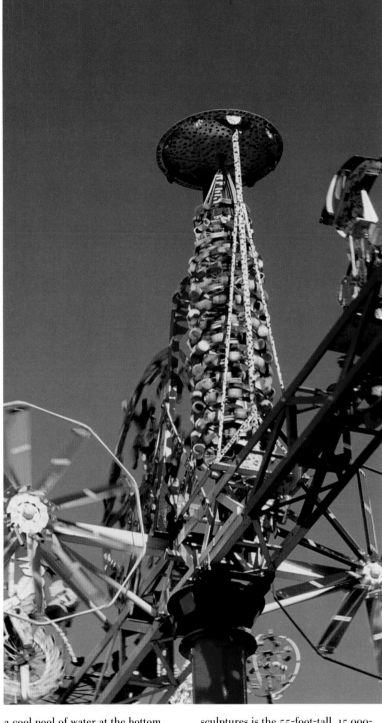

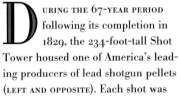URING THE 67-YEAR PERIOD following its completion in 1829, the 234-foot-tall Shot Tower housed one of America's leading producers of lead shotgun pellets (LEFT AND OPPOSITE). Each shot was formed by dropping tiny balls of molten lead through a sieve at the top of the structure. As they fell through the tower, the lead balls would form spheres that were then hardened by a cool pool of water at the bottom.

The American Visionary Art Museum is uniquely dedicated to showcasing the creations of untrained artists. One of its most distinctive sculptures is the 55-foot-tall, 15,000-pound *Whirligig* (RIGHT). The multicolored, wind-powered piece was created by Vollis Simpson, a mechanic, farmer, and visionary artist born in 1919.

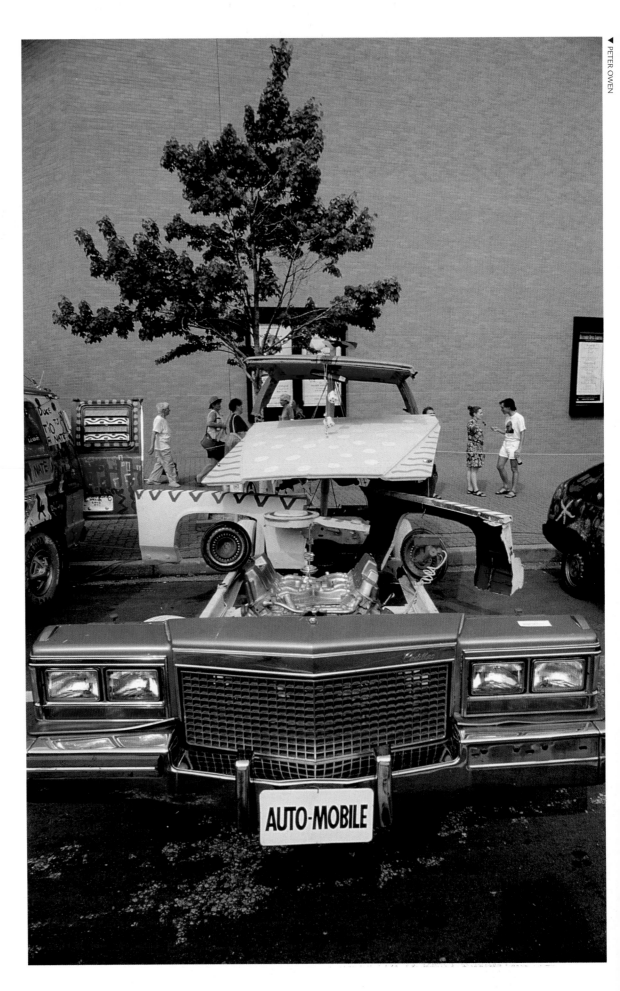

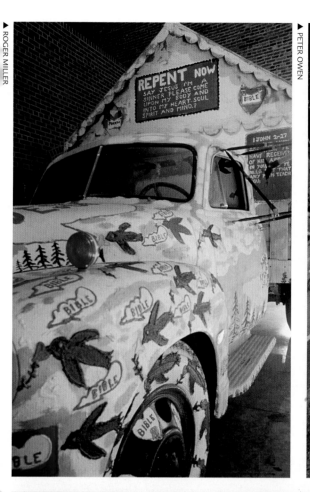

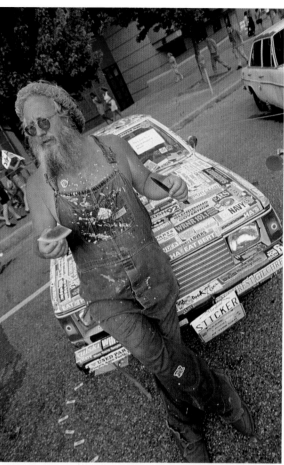

ARS AND CHARACTERS: An unmistakable love for the automobile, in all its incarnations, has created many a unique opportunity for self-expression in Baltimore.

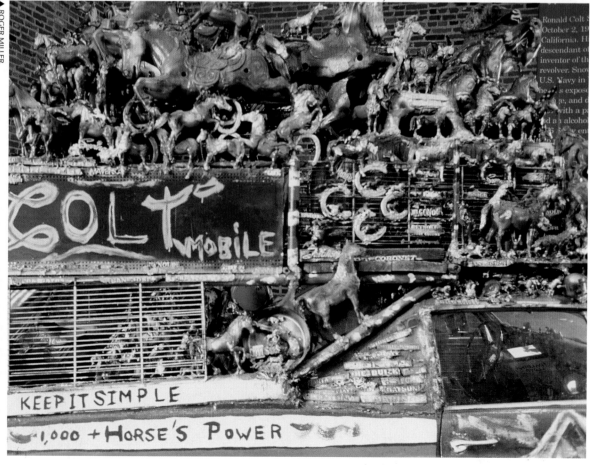

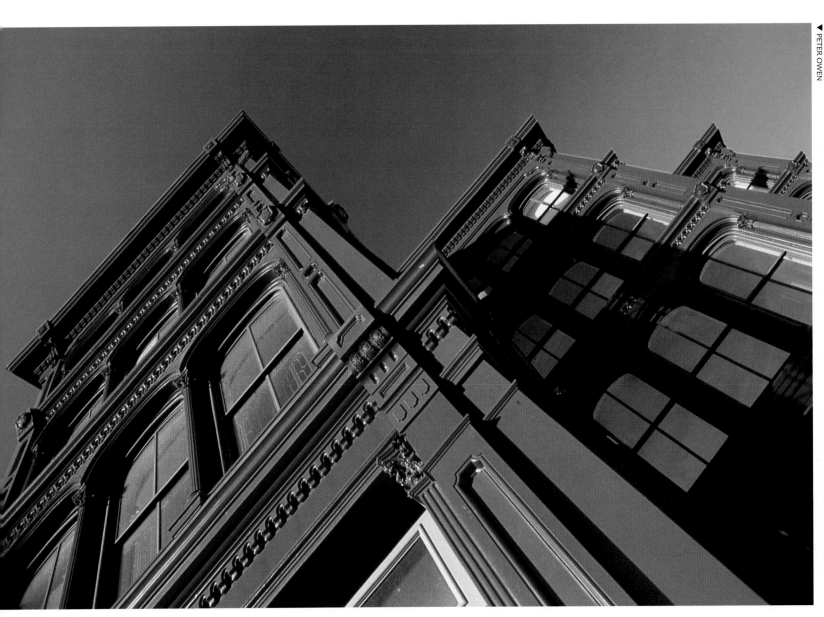

WITH ITS TIERED, MAROON facade of cast iron that has been salvaged and remolded, the Morton K. Blaustein City Life Ex- hibition Center is the newest addition to the Baltimore City Life Museums, a collection of eight landmarks dedi- cated to commemorating local history.

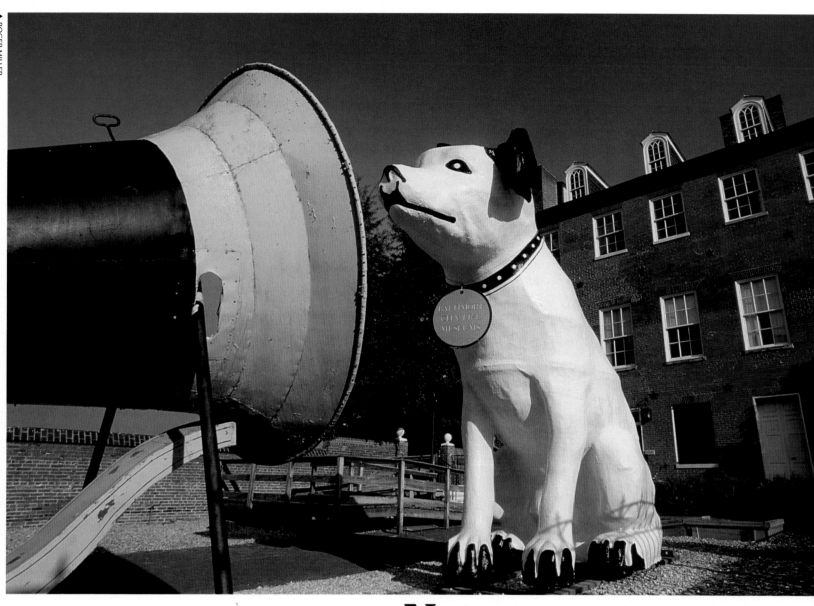

IPPER THE DOG—THE CITY'S beloved mascot—long presided over South Baltimore from the roof of the D&H Distribution Company warehouse. The 1,400-pound pooch, who was exiled for a time to Virginia, has recently returned to his hometown and now stands watch over the courtyard at the Baltimore City Life Museums.

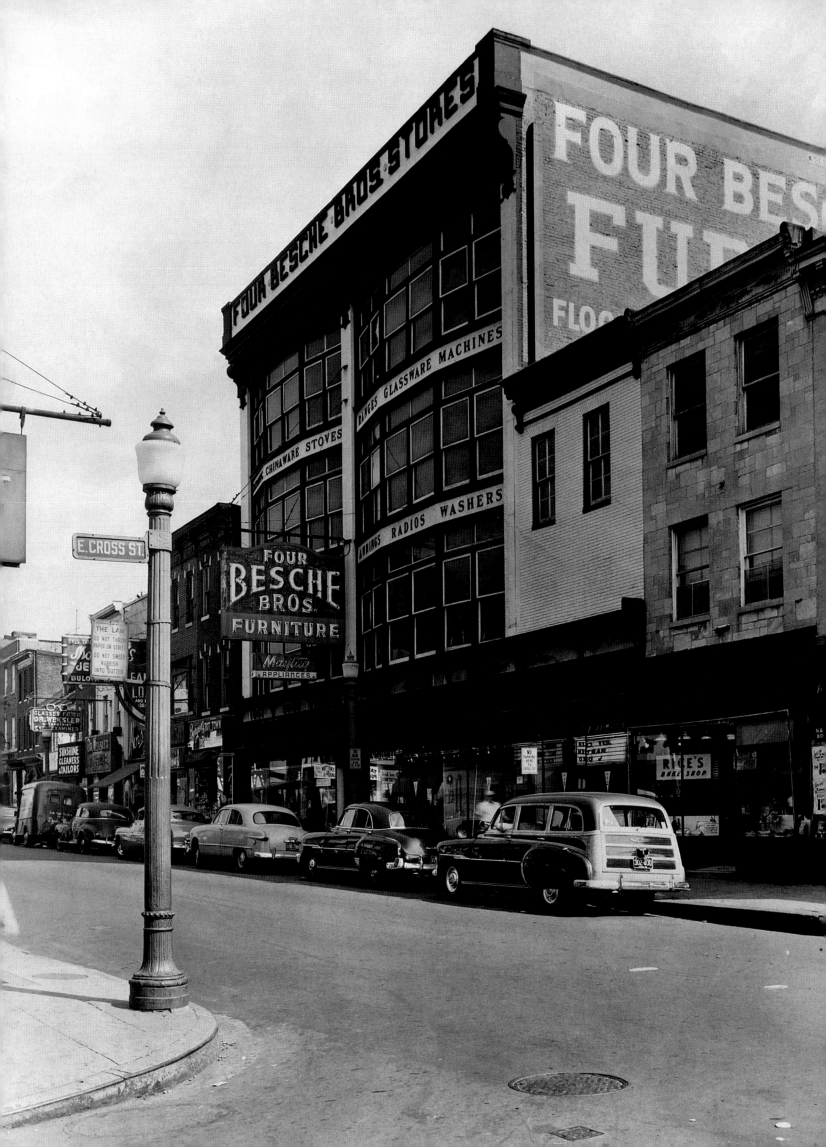

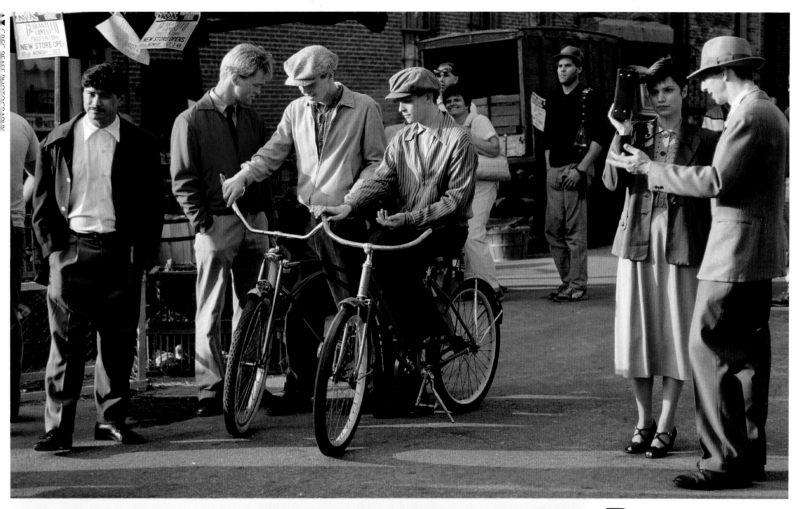

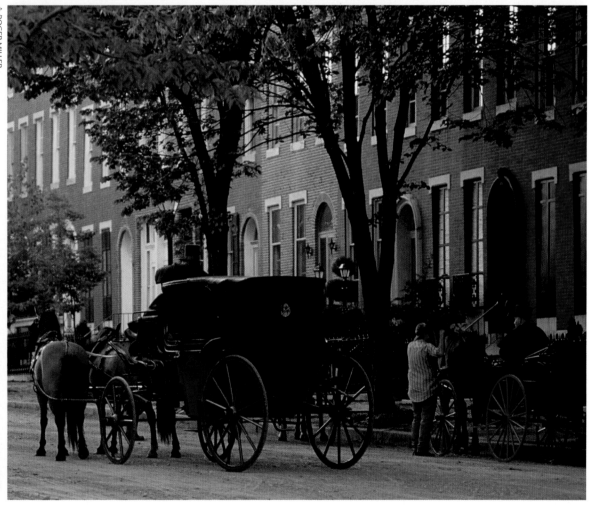

B ALTIMORE'S HISTORIC NEIGHBOR-
hoods have become a favorite
of Hollywood moviemakers,
who've traveled here to film scenes
from such period flicks as *Avalon*
(TOP) and *Washington Square* (BOTTOM).

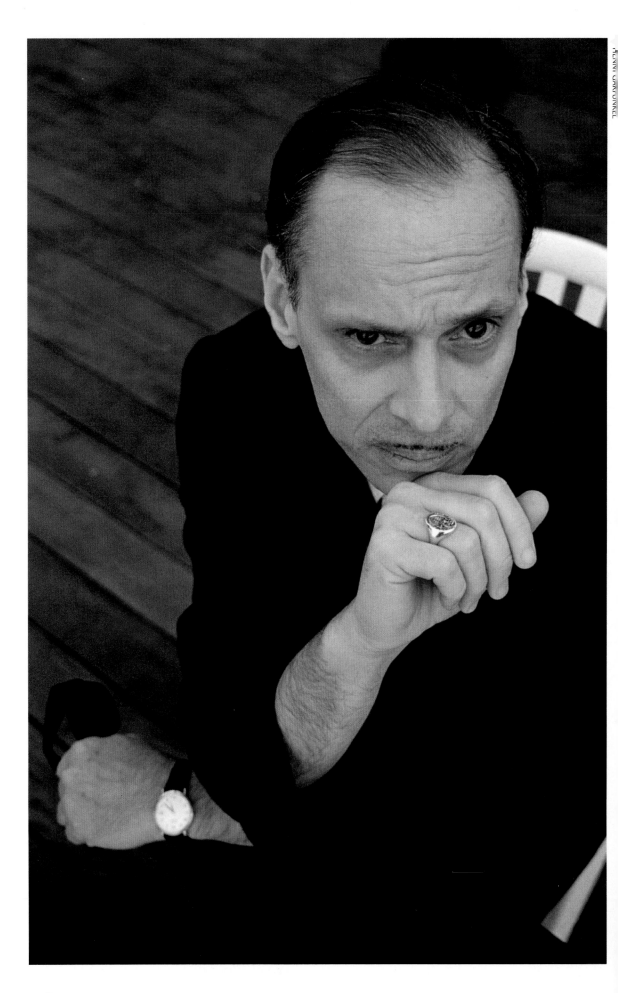

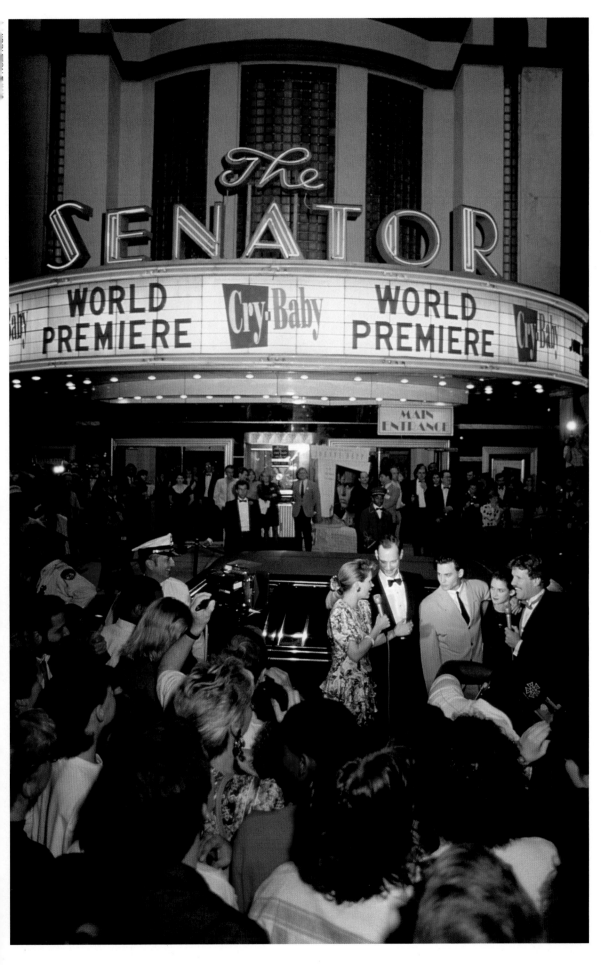

F ILM DIRECTOR AND BALTIMORE native John Waters (OPPOSITE) has set a good many of his movies in Charm City. The world premiere of *Cry-Baby*, held at Baltimore's historic Senator Theater, drew plenty of celebrities to the 900-seat movie house, including Waters himself and *Cry-Baby* star Johnny Depp.

A FELLS POINT INSTITUTION, THE Killer Trash vintage clothing store is a psychedelic version of the world's best yard sale.

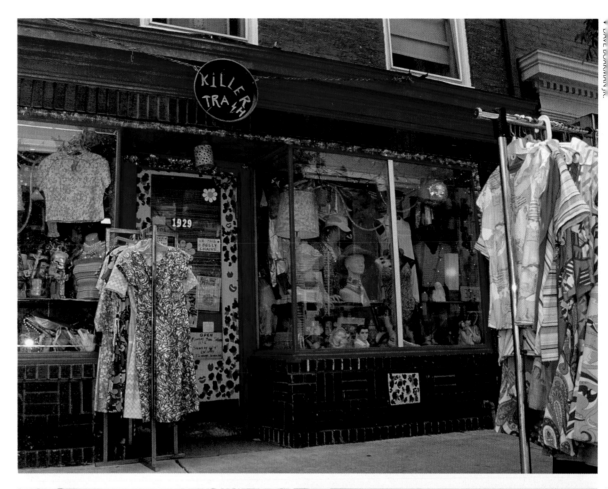

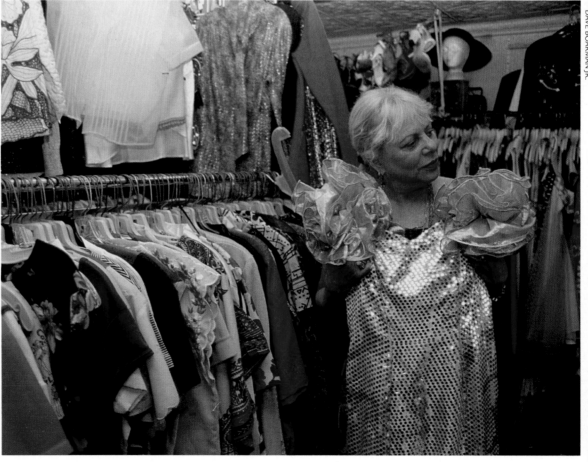

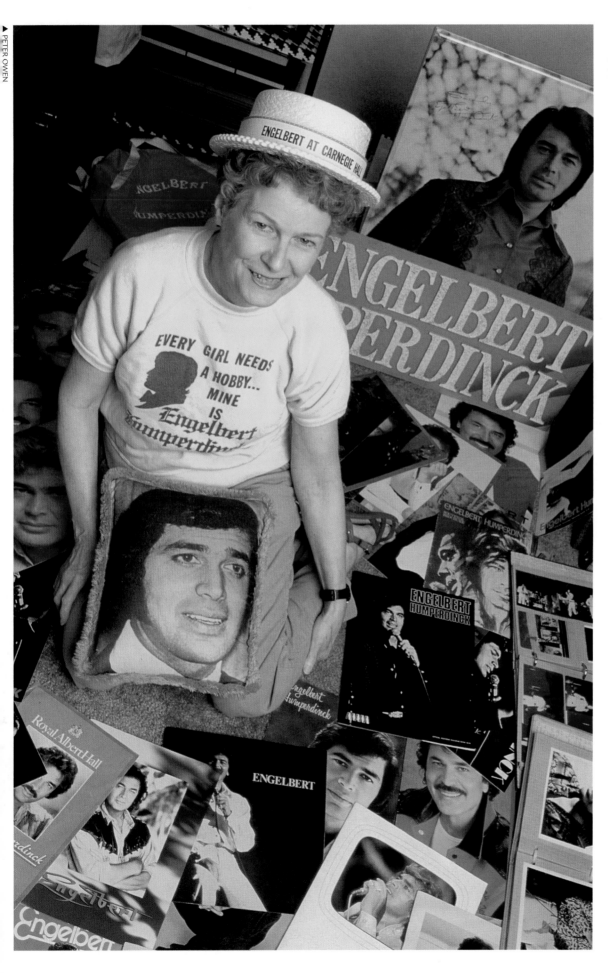

A FANATIC BALTIMOREAN SHOWS off her shrine to India-born balladeer Engelbert Humperdinck.

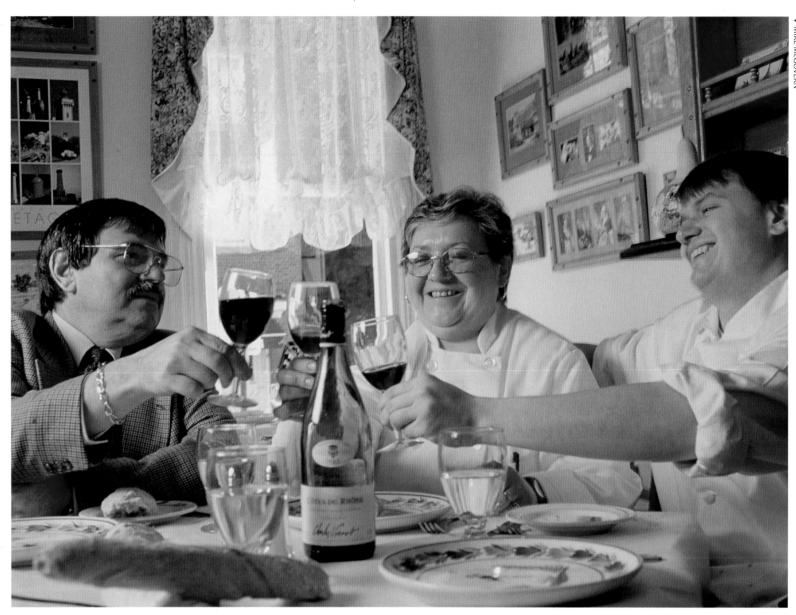

BALTIMORE MAY BE KNOWN AS Crab Town in many culinary circles, but French restaurants like Tersiguel's in Howard County speak to a sophisticate's sensibility and palate.

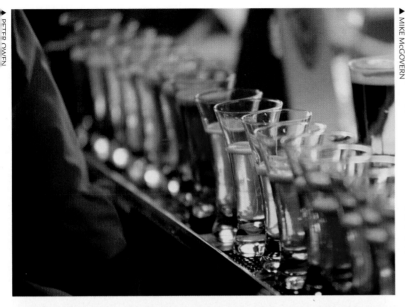

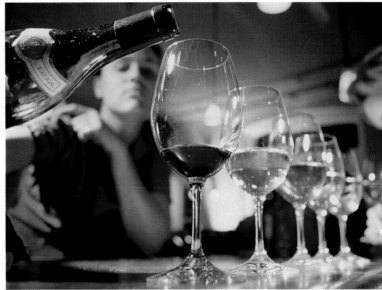

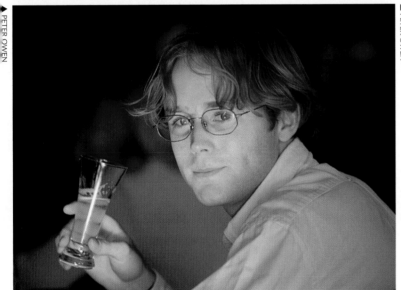

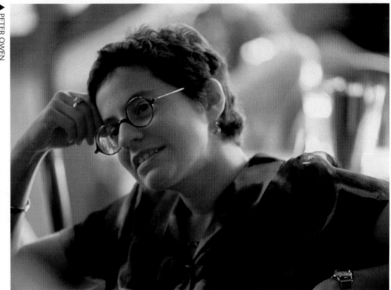

C ATERING TO LOCALS' THIRST FOR new and interesting beers and wines, joints like the Oxford Brewing Company and Spike & Charlie's Restaurant and Wine Bar invite folks to raise a glass or two.

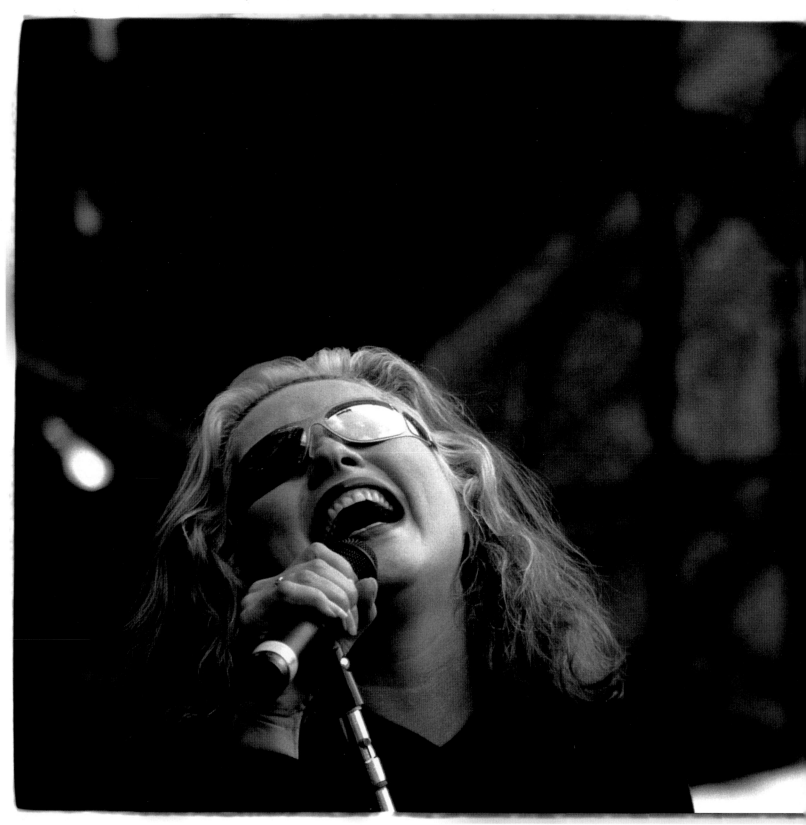

S HE MAY BE BEST KNOWN FOR HER
tenure as the lead singer of
Blondie, but many Baltimoreans
remember Deborah Harry for her
screen role in John Waters' *Hairspray*.

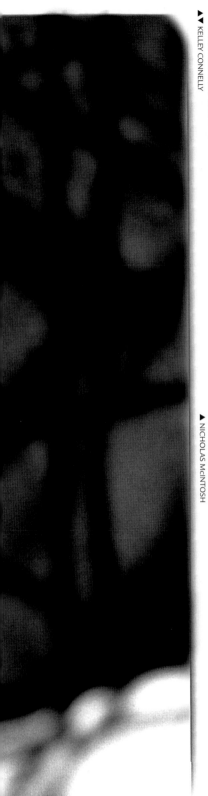

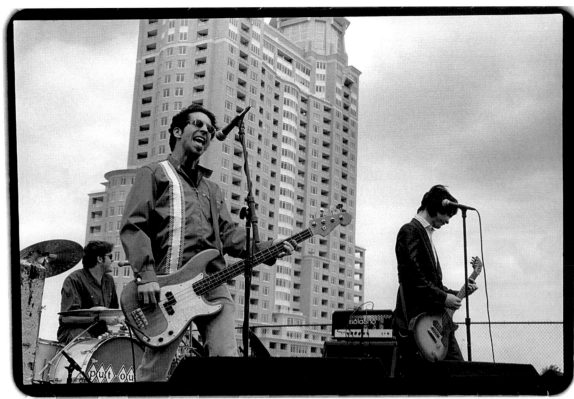

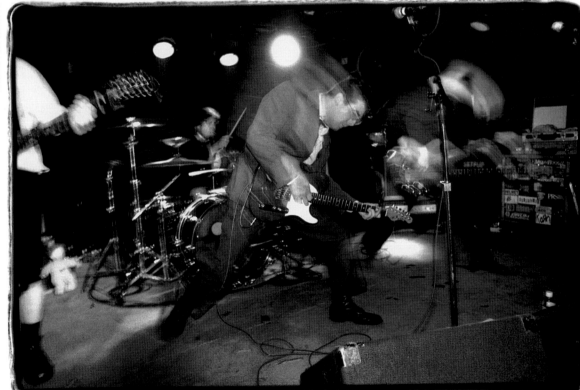

Music lovers have plenty to shout about in Charm City, thanks to such talented local groups as The Put-Outs (TOP) and the Lee Harvey Keitel Band (BOTTOM).

IN BALTIMORE, THERE'S NO SHORTAGE of musical talent, from gifted performers to the hardworking folks who make things happen behind the scenes. Popular guitarist Paul Bollenback has performed on a number of nationally released albums (RIGHT), while Jimmie's Chicken Shack made local history by becoming one of the first groups to sign with Elton John's new label, Rocket Records (OPPOSITE TOP). Joe Goldsborough and David Koslowski of Merkin Records spend their days making dreams come true for many area bands (OPPOSITE BOTTOM).

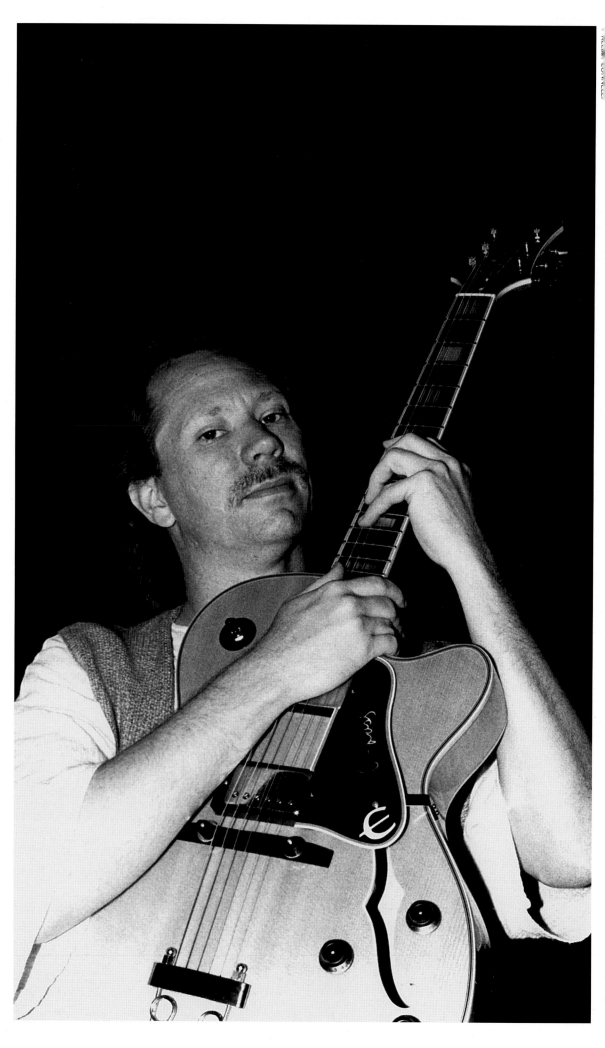

136

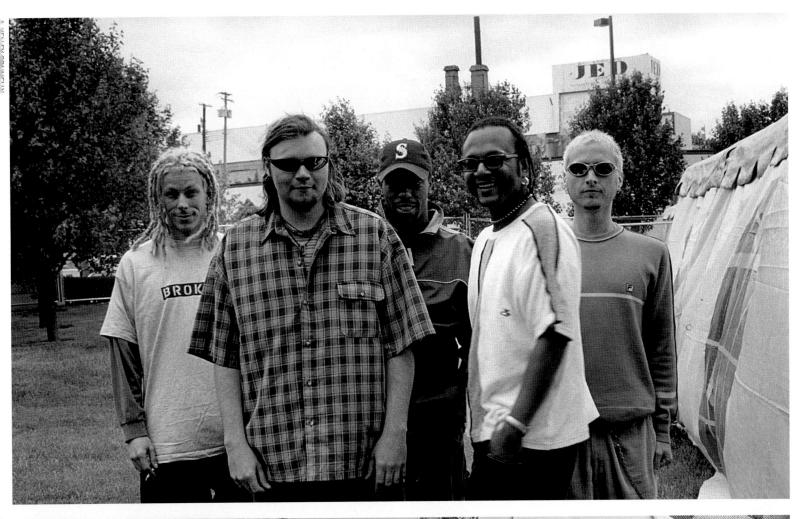

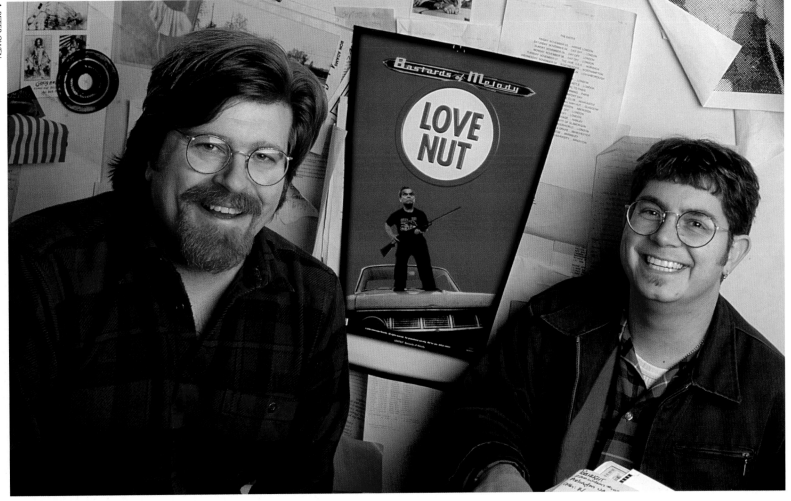

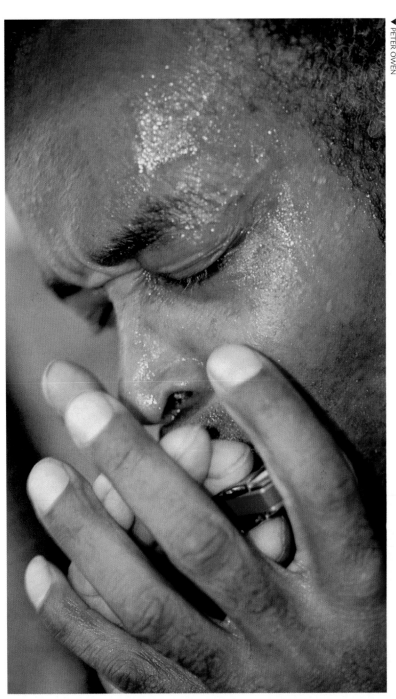

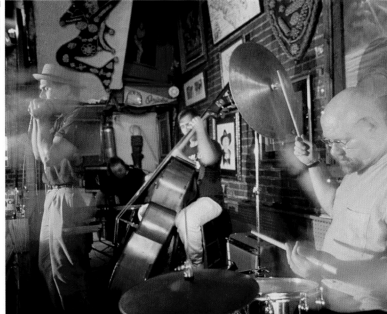

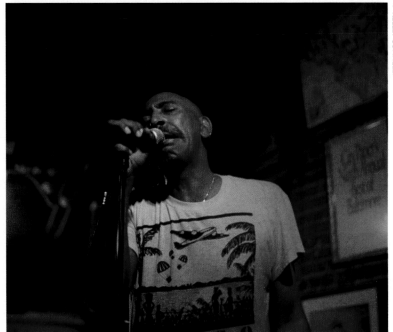

S INCE THE 1920S, WHEN THE Harlem Renaissance came to town, Baltimore has hosted big-name blues and jazz musicians like Eubie Blake, Cab Calloway, Duke Ellington, and Ella Fitzgerald. Known for one of the best blues jams around, the Cat's Eye Pub in Fells Point also offers a mix of live jazz, zydeco, and Irish music nightly.

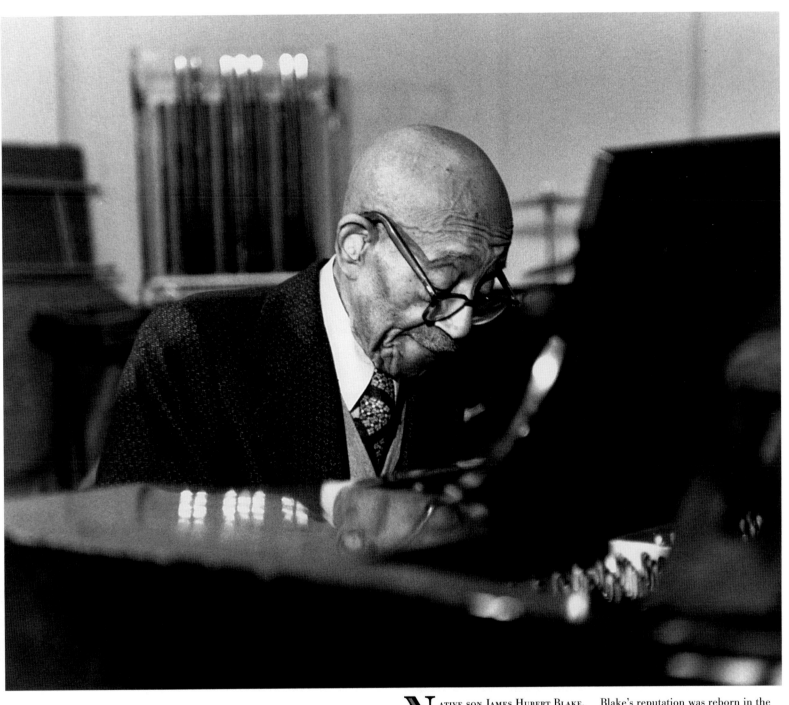

Nᴀᴛɪᴠᴇ ꜱᴏɴ Jᴀᴍᴇꜱ Hᴜʙᴇʀᴛ Bʟᴀᴋᴇ, better known as Eubie, was one of America's foremost composers of ragtime and stage music. The son of former slaves, he worked in vaudeville until its eventual demise. Blake's reputation was reborn in the 1980s when *The Sting* became a hit movie, bringing about a resurgence of ragtime and, thus, pulling the musician out of retirement.

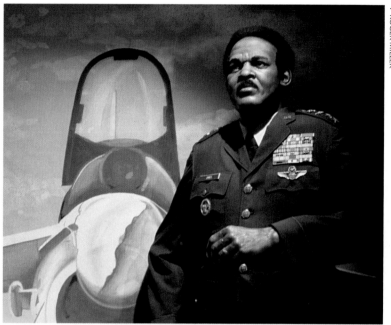

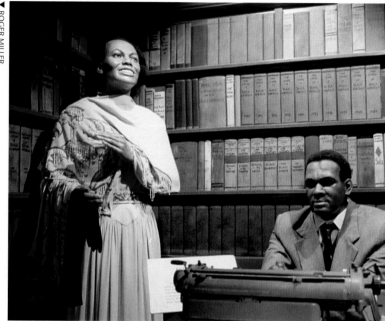

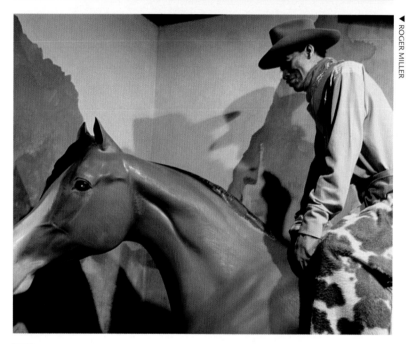

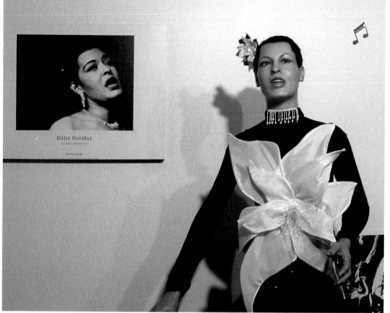

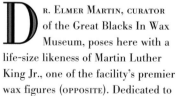

Dr. Elmer Martin, curator of the Great Blacks In Wax Museum, poses here with a life-size likeness of Martin Luther King Jr., one of the facility's premier wax figures (opposite). Dedicated to providing African-Americans with a glimpse at their ancestors and heroes, the museum includes displays featuring such notables as (clockwise from top left) Daniel "Chappie" James Jr., the first African-American four-star general; novelists Zora Neale Hurston and Richard Wright; jazz singer Billie Holiday; and Bill Pickett, the first African-American to be inducted into the Rodeo Hall of Fame.

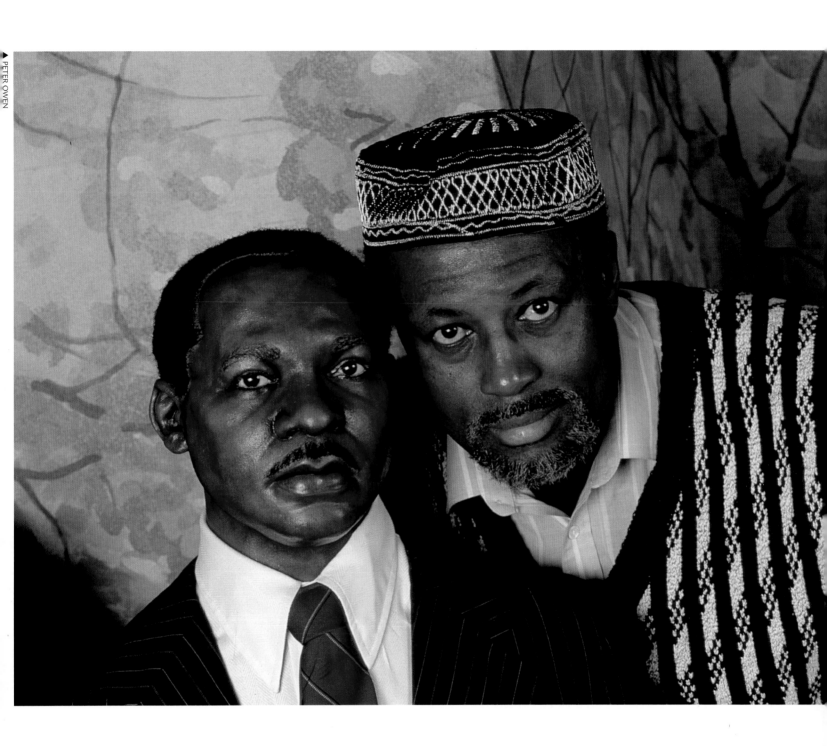

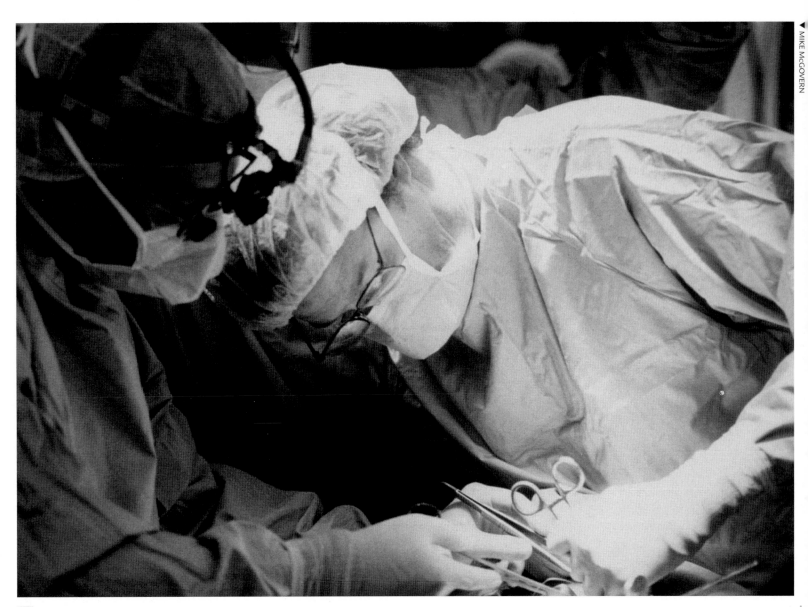

I T'S JUST ANOTHER DAY ON THE JOB for Dr. Levi Watkins Jr., a famous heart surgeon at Johns Hopkins Hospital. In 1980, Watkins became the first to implant an automatic defibrillator in a human heart.

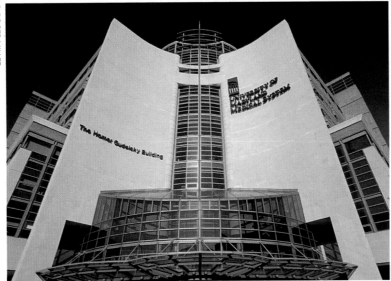

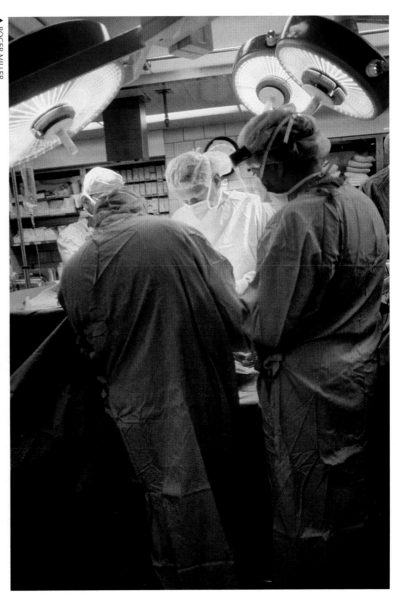

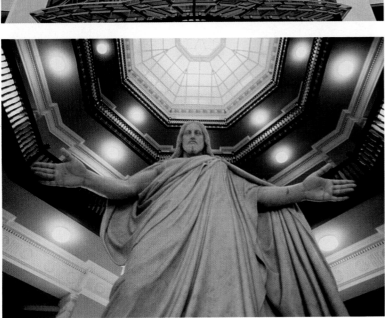

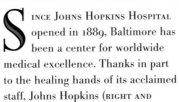

Since Johns Hopkins Hospital opened in 1889, Baltimore has been a center for worldwide medical excellence. Thanks in part to the healing hands of its acclaimed staff, Johns Hopkins (RIGHT AND BOTTOM LEFT) has been named by *U.S. News & World Report* as the top hospital in the country for seven consecutive years. The University of Maryland Medical System is also known for pioneering its share of medical techniques; the Homer Gudelsky Building, which opened downtown in 1994, houses state-of-the-art cancer, cardiological, and neurological care, as well as transplantation facilities (TOP LEFT).

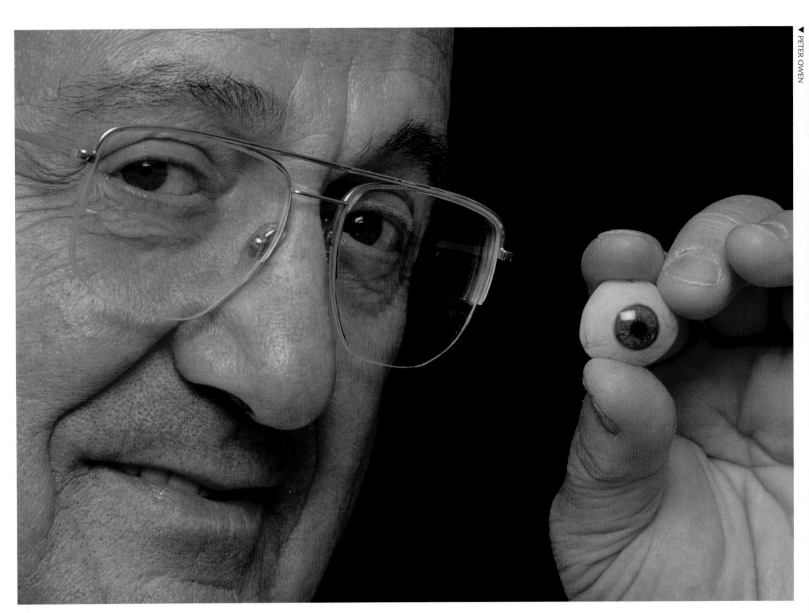

FOR MORE THAN 50 YEARS, Raymond Elia Peters has improved people's lives and appearances by crafting state-of-the-art ocular prosthetics. "The secret of this business," he says, "is to do your work so well that nobody notices it."

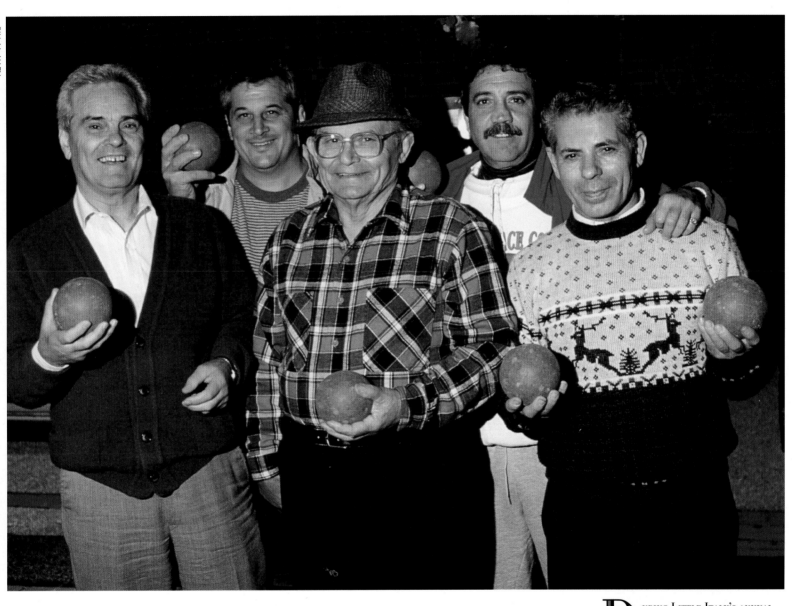

DURING LITTLE ITALY'S ANNUAL St. Leo's Festival, boccie—a game described as "rolling horseshoes"—takes on World Series-like intensity.

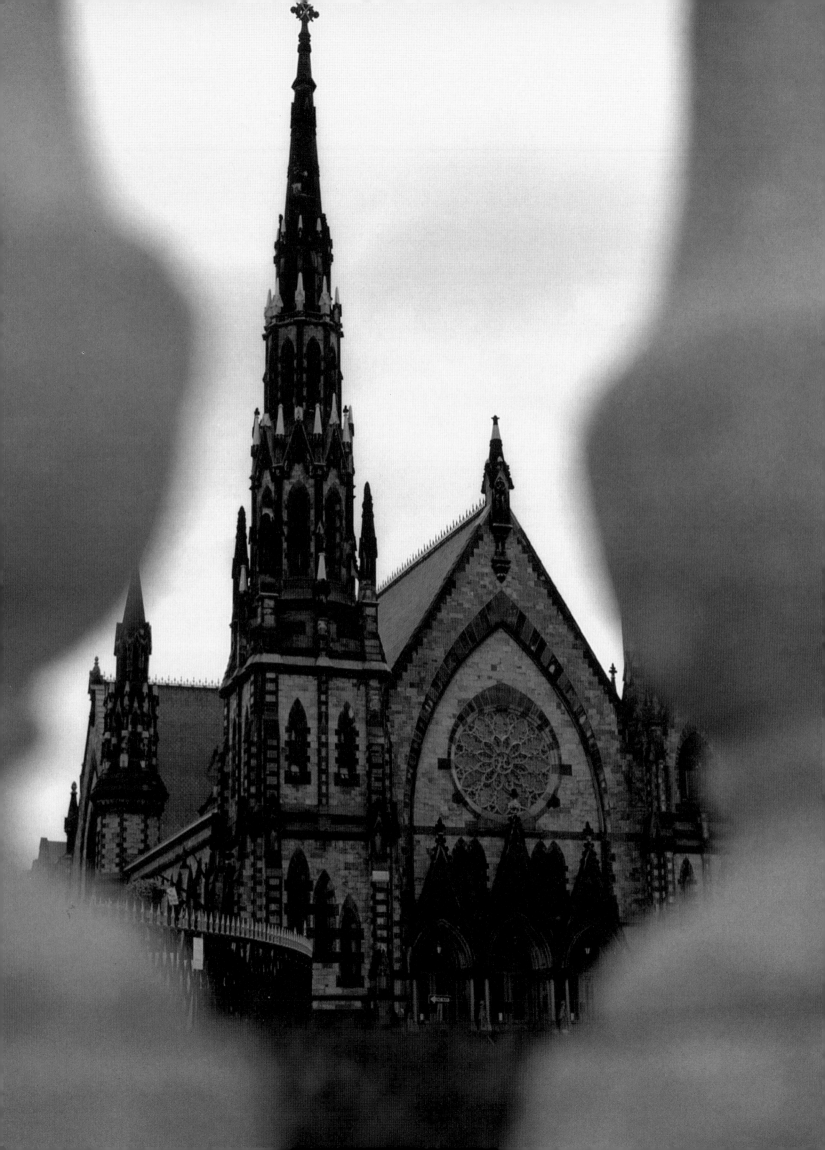

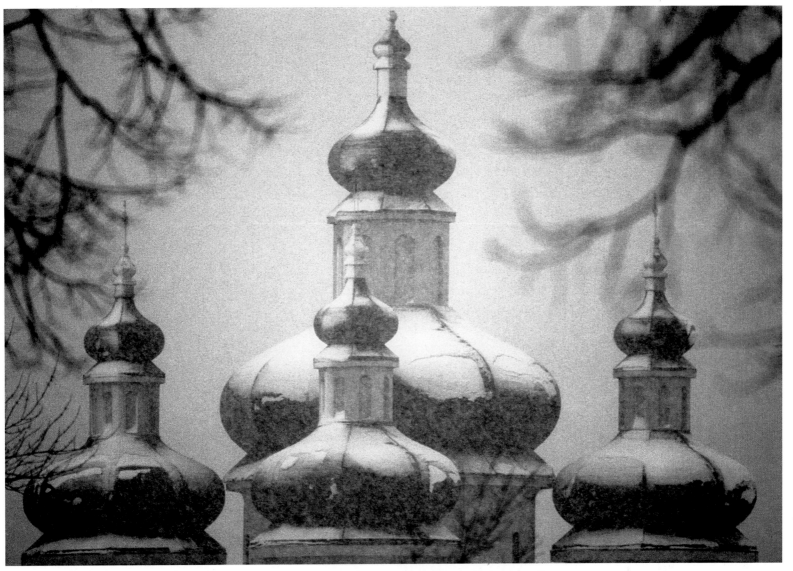

MOUNT VERNON METHODIST
Church—along with Balti-
more's stately Washington
Monument—forms the cornerstone of
Mount Vernon Square. The structure's
green serpentine marble, buff and red
sandstone trim, and tall spires are well
known throughout the city (OPPOSITE).

Even covered with snow, the
golden domes of St. Michael's Ukrainian Catholic Church accentuate the
landscape in Patterson Park (ABOVE).

COMPLETED IN 1959, THE CATHE-
dral of Mary Our Queen was
intended to combine Gothic
principles with modern expression.
Each Sunday, the church is filled with
the haunting strains of organ music
and natural light filtered through
magnificent stained-glass windows.

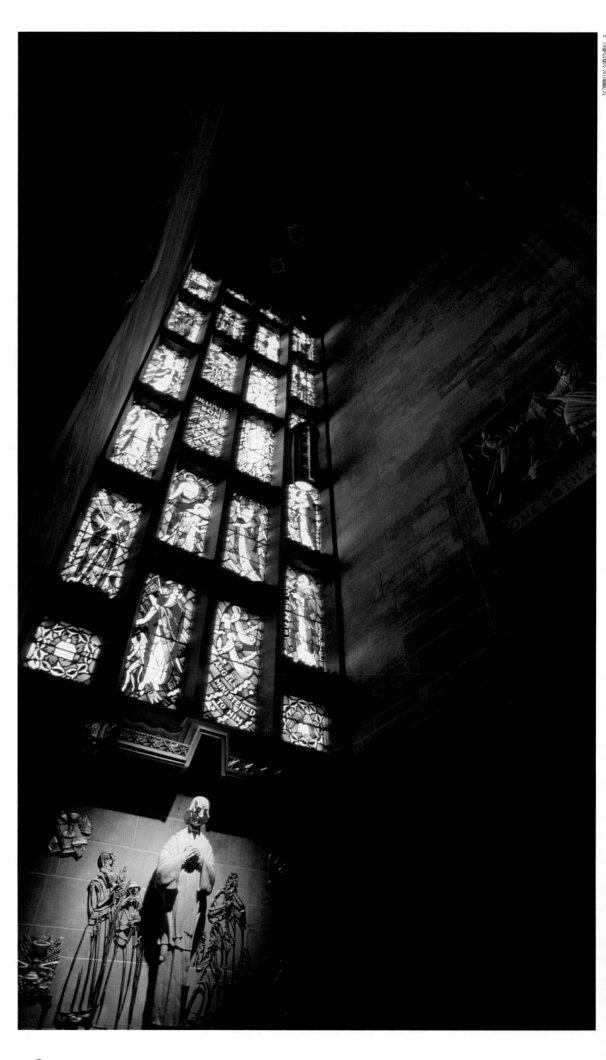

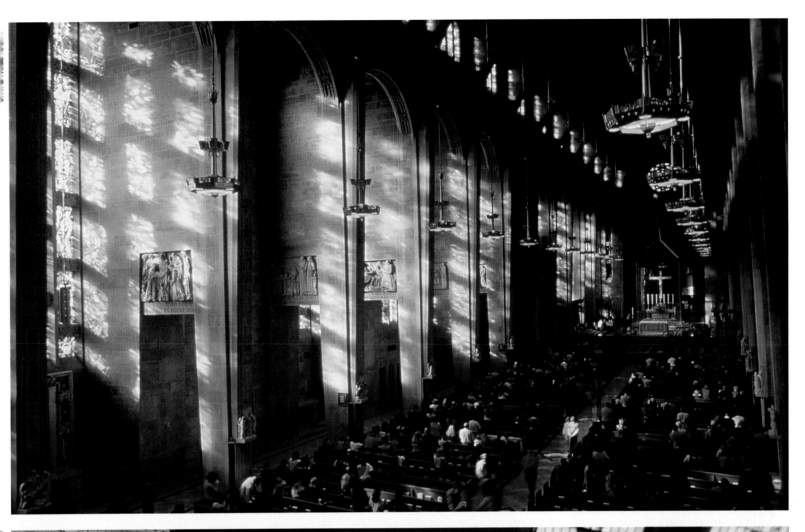

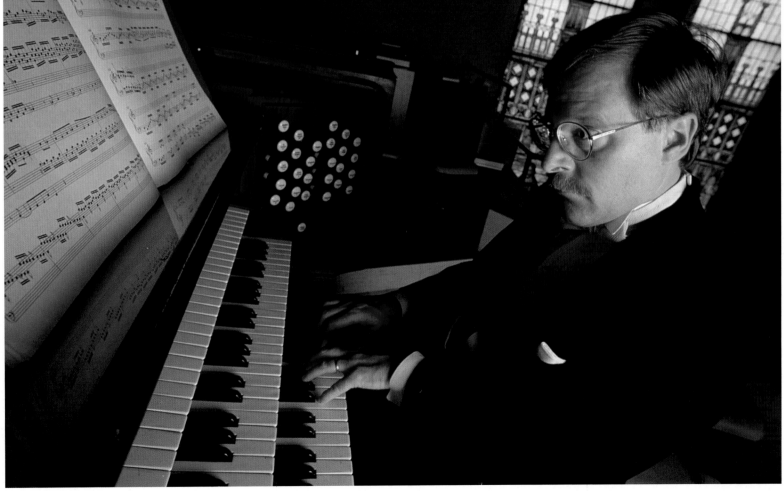

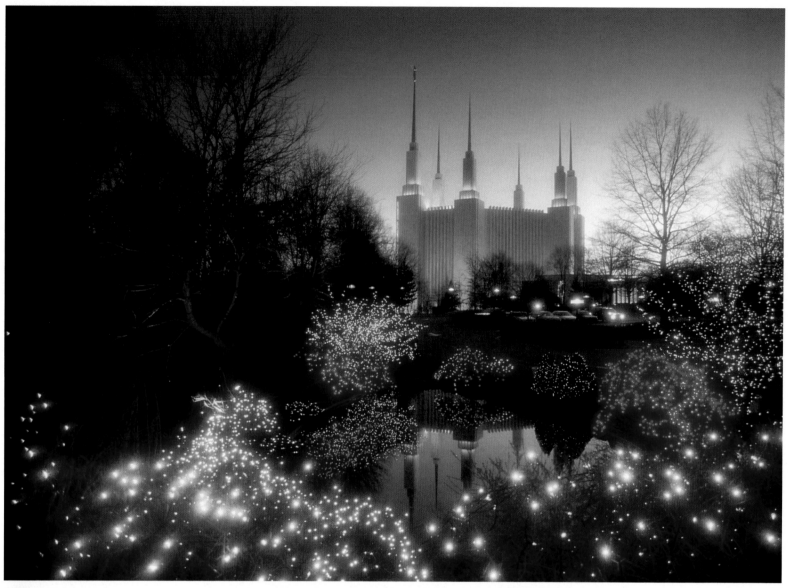

B**altimore's own "Miracle on 34th Street"** is a block-long stretch that has been dubbed the "House of Gawd" for its mind-boggling holiday light displays (opposite). Each house tries to outdo the others, and the brightly lit tributes to Santa, the baby Jesus, and countless other icons of the season draw people from all the over the world. Offering a contrasting image, the mormon temple in Kensington in Montgomery County creates a subtle backdrop for a festive holiday display (above).

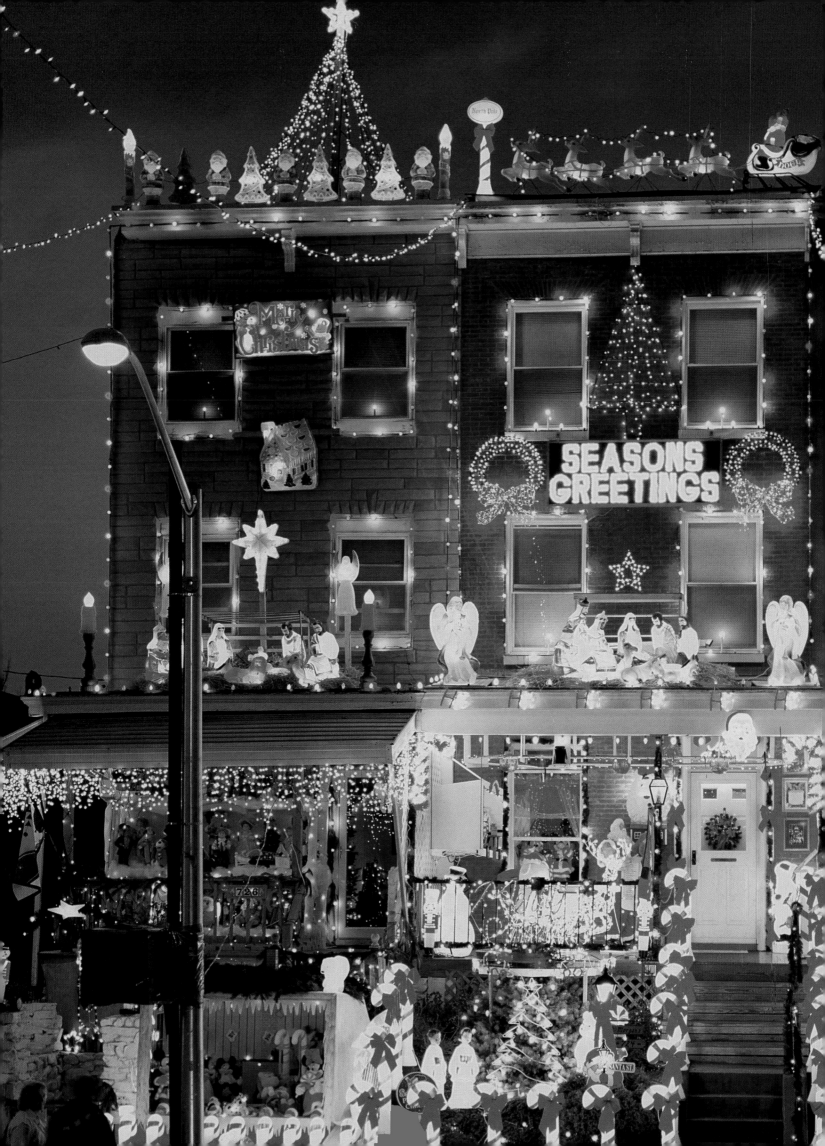

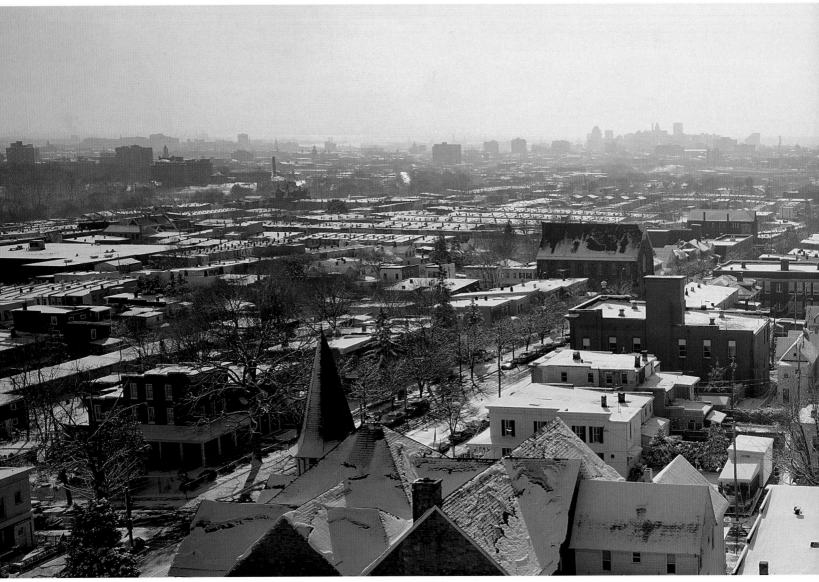

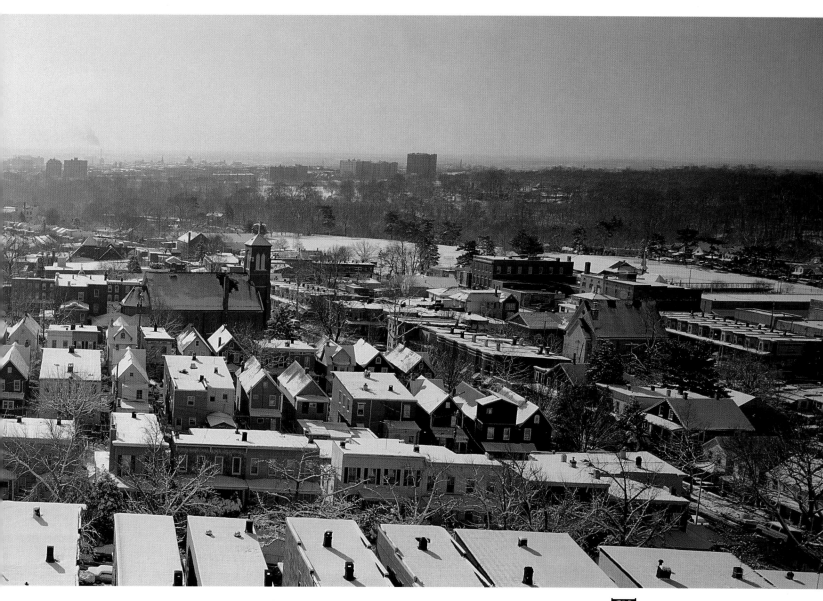

T HE OMNIPRESENT HUM OF THE city is muffled—for a time, at least—by a quieting snowfall.

THOUGHTS OF THE AMERICAN DREAM, complete with a cottage house and a white picket fence, start early in Baltimore. But in at least one town, the dream has been realized. A one-time mill town whose decline led to its sale at auction for $42,000 in 1934, Dickeyville is now one of the area's most bucolic neighborhoods (TOP). The efforts of its residents to rehabilitate the old mill houses have been so successful that Dickeyville is arguably lovelier today than ever before.

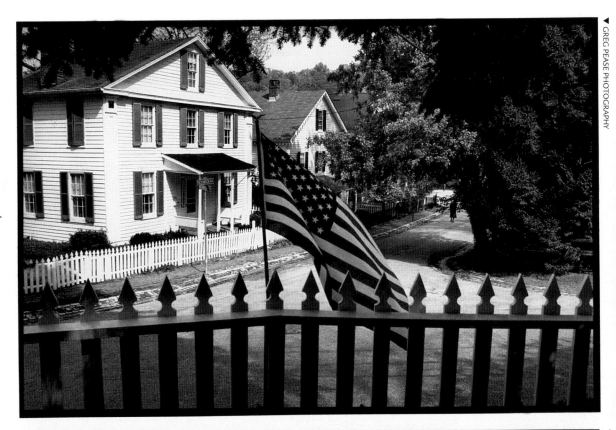

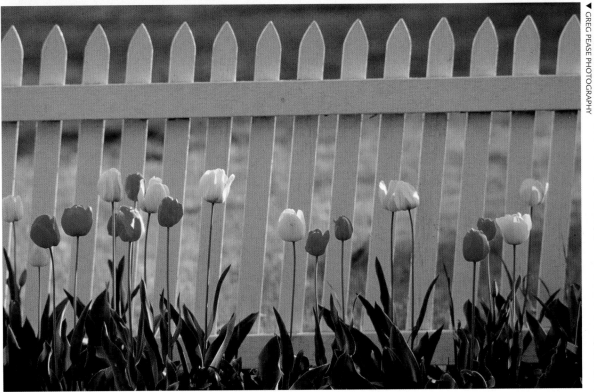

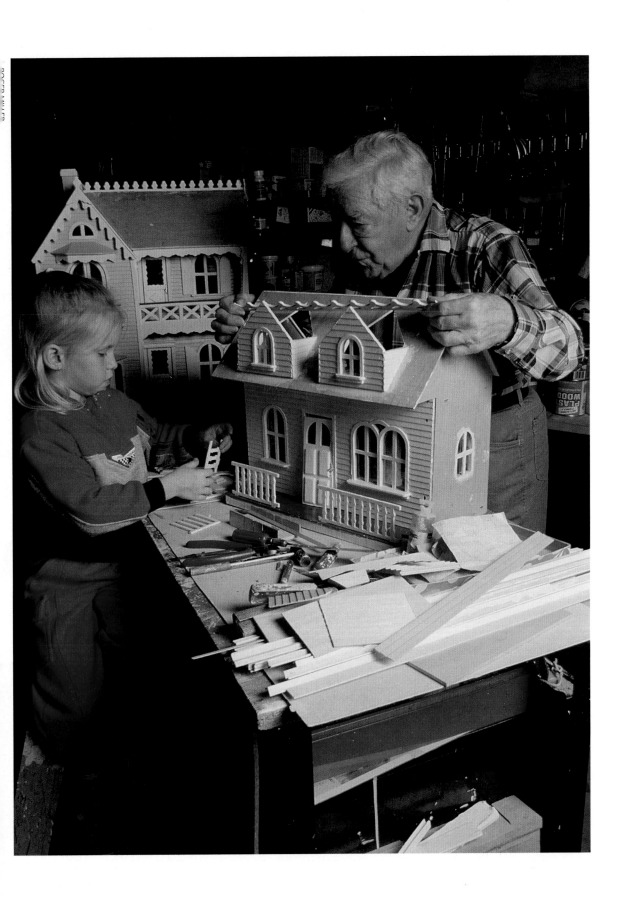

RIDGELEY'S DELIGHT, LOCATED near the University of Maryland Medical System complex, has undergone extensive renewal in recent years. Today, the historic neighborhood boasts a charming mix of apartments and rowhouses.

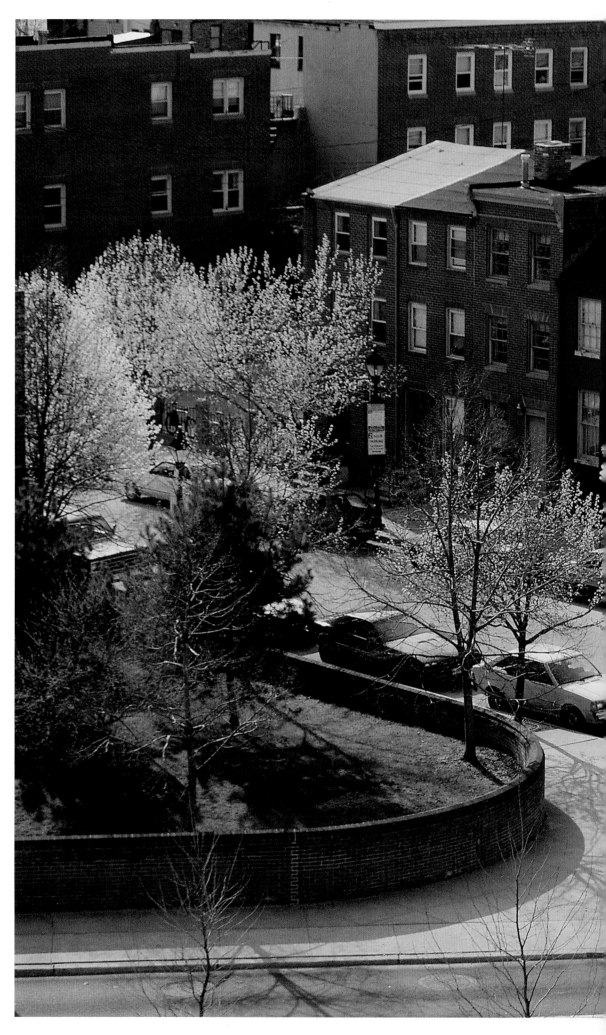

156

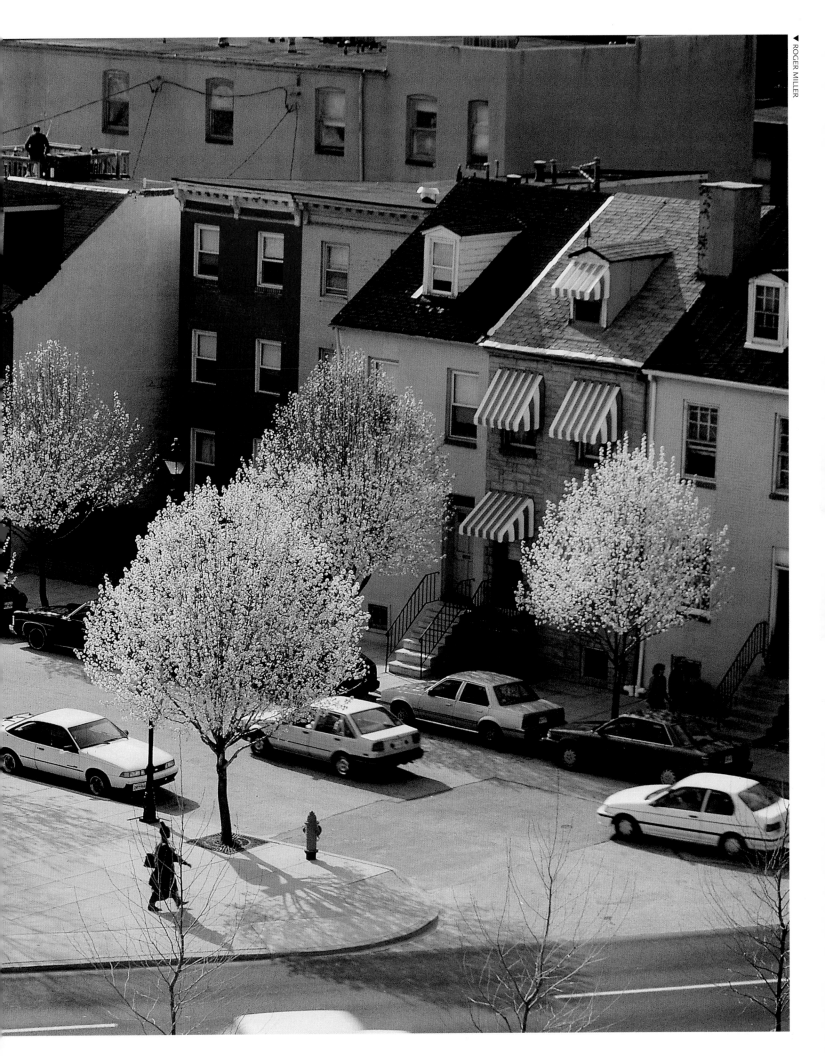

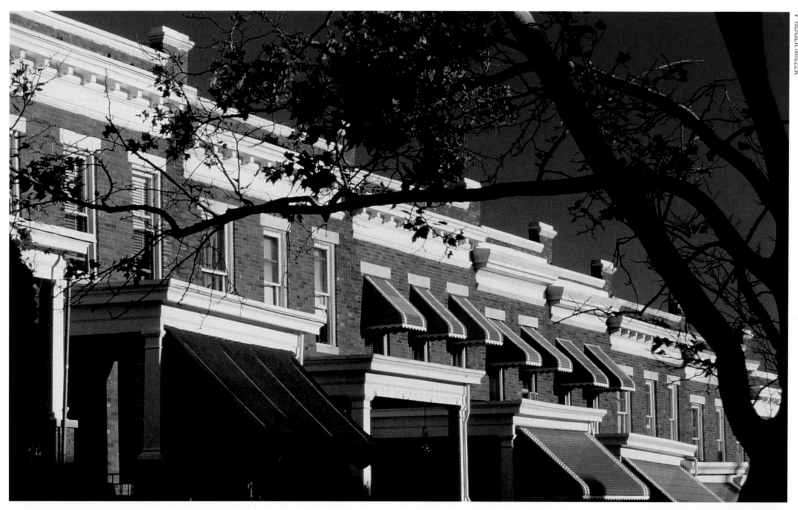

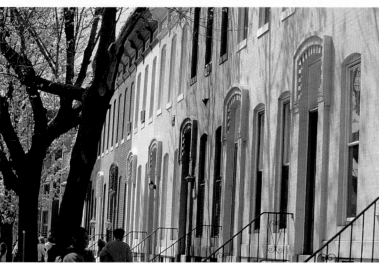

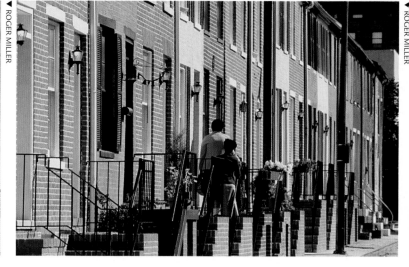

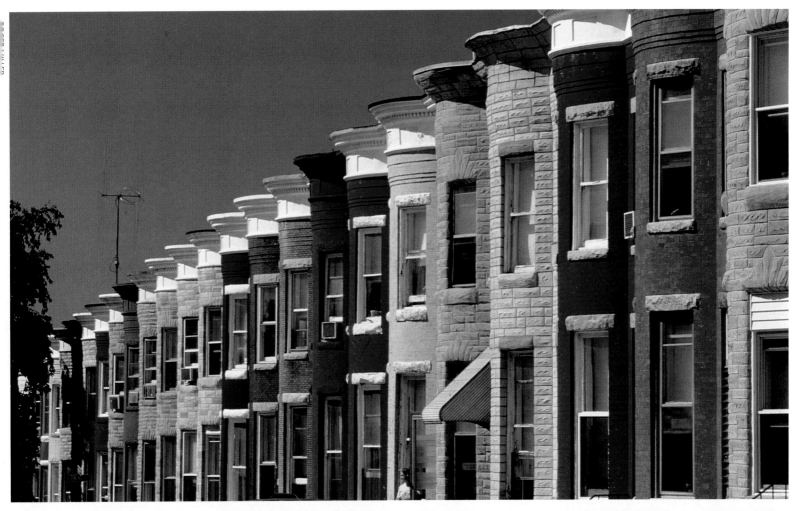

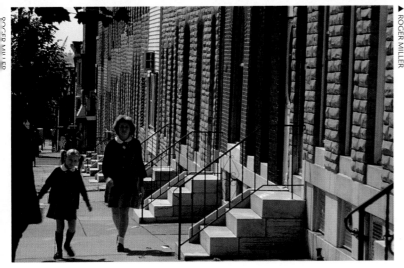

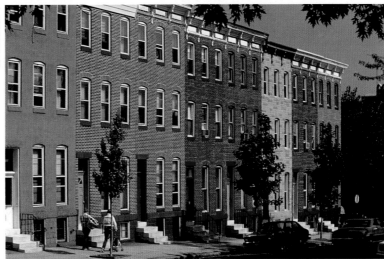

BROWNSTONE FACADES OR Form-stone? Brick steps or marble ones? Porch or stoop? So many choices, yet Baltimore's rowhouses were actually designed for economy rather than beauty. Today, their enduring charm provides the city's distinctive architectural ambience.

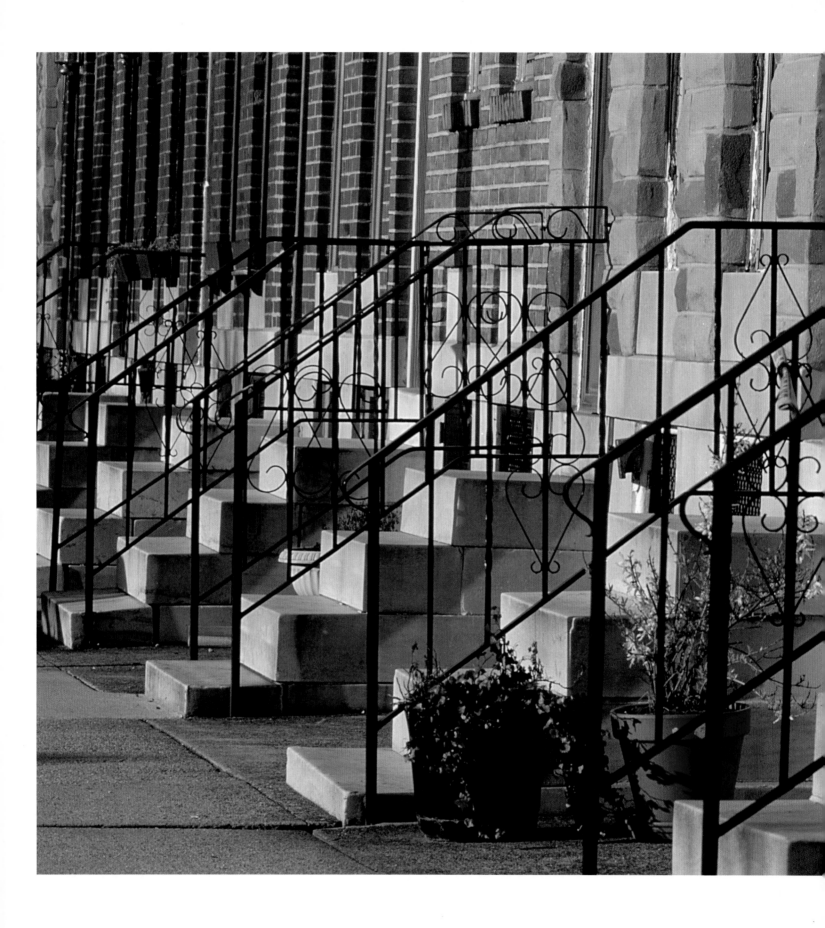

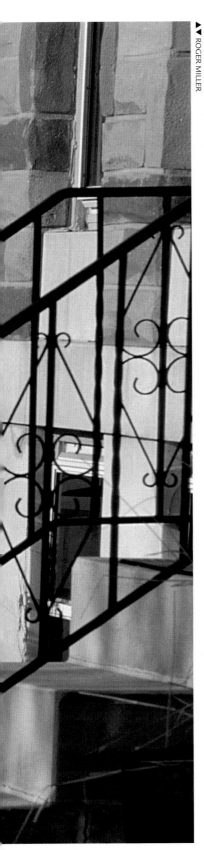

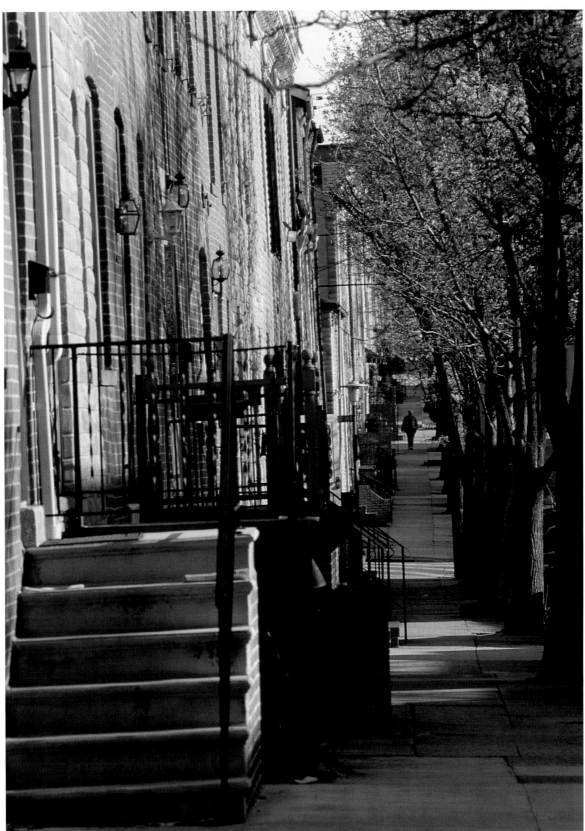

Baltimore's famous white marble steps came about because the material was both affordable and readily available. Folks at the time widely agreed that the marble accents lent a touch of elegance to the otherwise ordinary rowhouses.

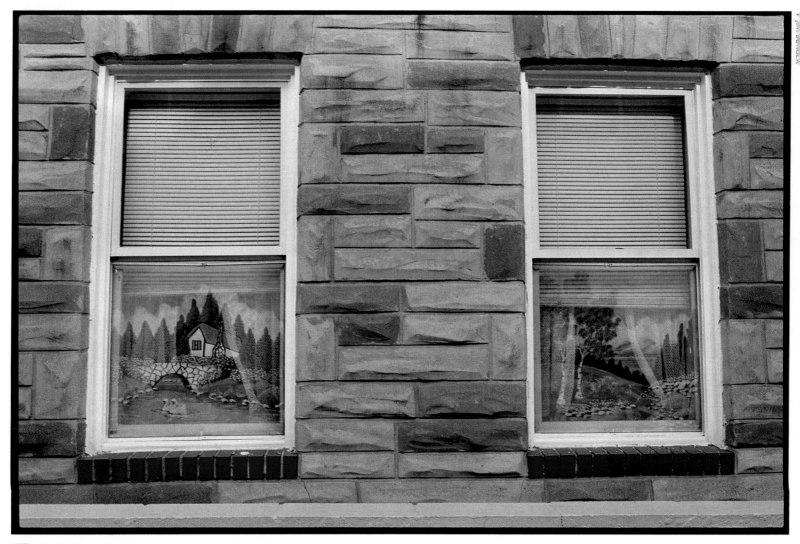

B EGINNING IN THE EARLY 1900S, screen painting became a major urban art form in Baltimore. Today, the practice is enjoying such a renaissance that its artists are displaying their work at local galleries, in addition to the traditional windows.

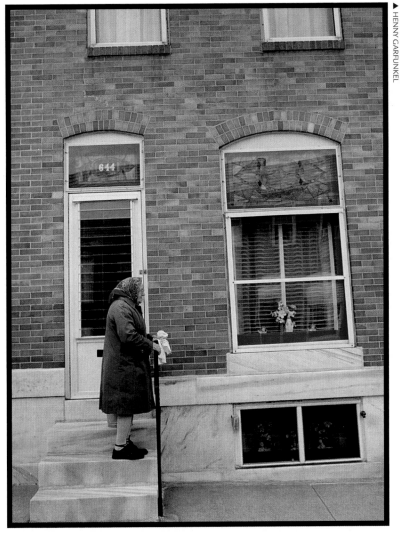

▶ HENNY GARFUNKEL

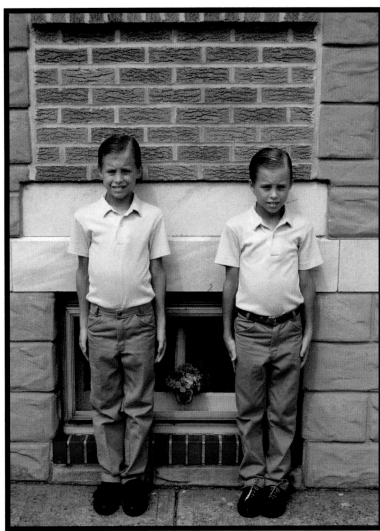

S TANDING OUTSIDE THEIR RESPECTIVE homes, a couple of boys and an elderly matriarch offer a glimpse into the real character of the city.

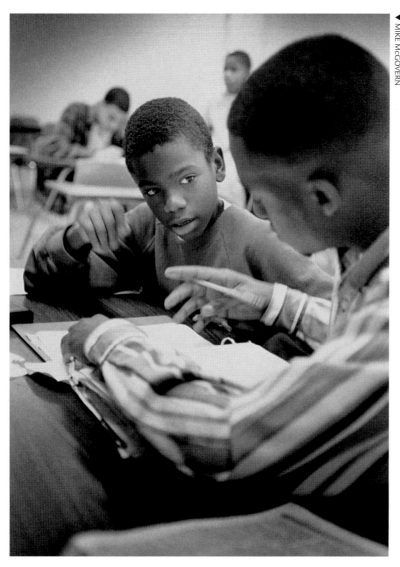

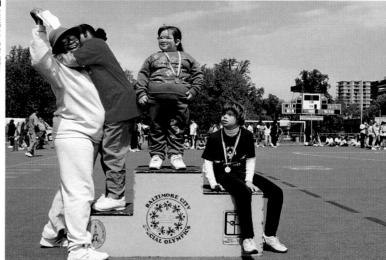

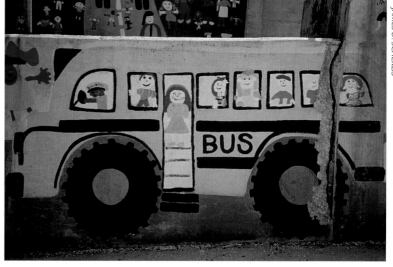

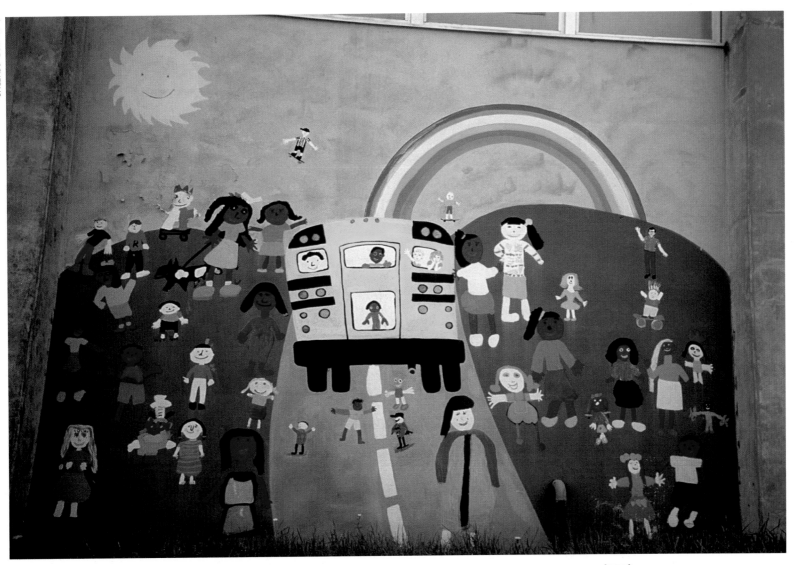

THE FUTURE OF BALTIMORE STARTS with its children, and city leaders have found a number of ways to nurture the talents and dreams of local youth. Examples of their creativity and determination abound.

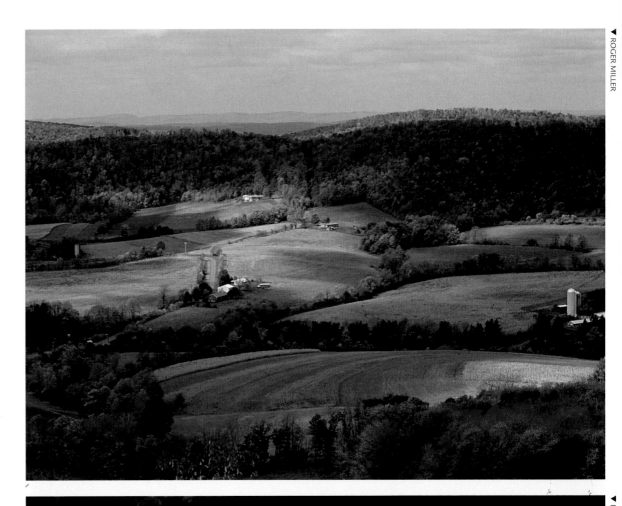

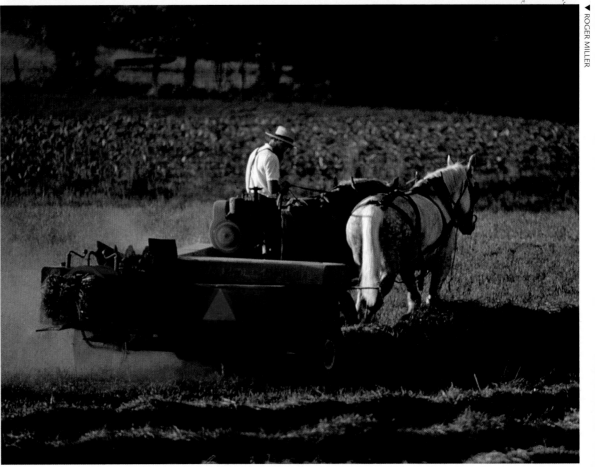

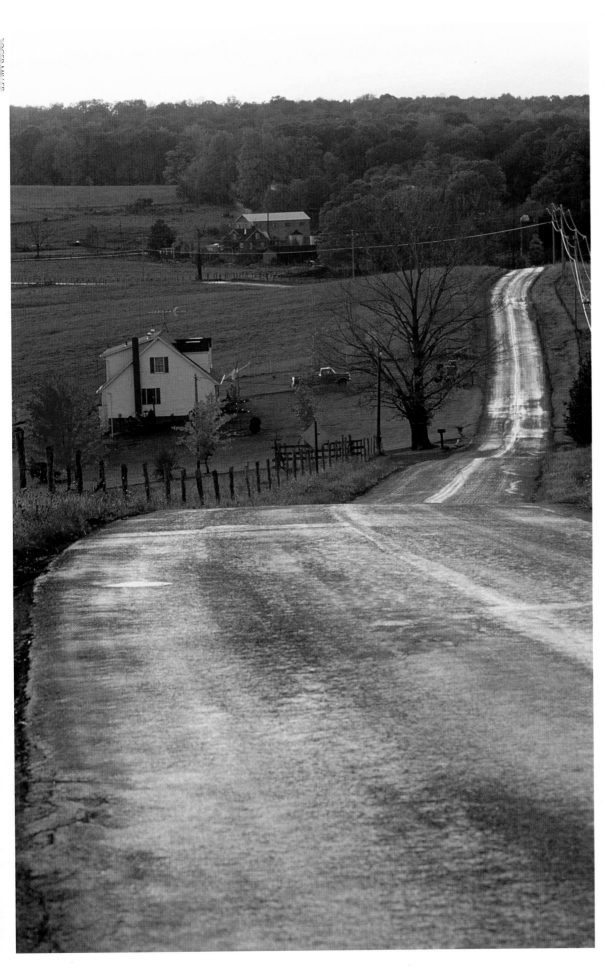

I N THE 18TH AND 19TH CENTURIES, farming drove the development of Baltimore's port. Today, although the city is no longer known primarily for agribusiness, rural scenes like these are still very much a part of life in the area.

NNOCENT FUN: A GROUP OF adventure-seeking boys dive courageously into the Patapsco River, circa 1930.

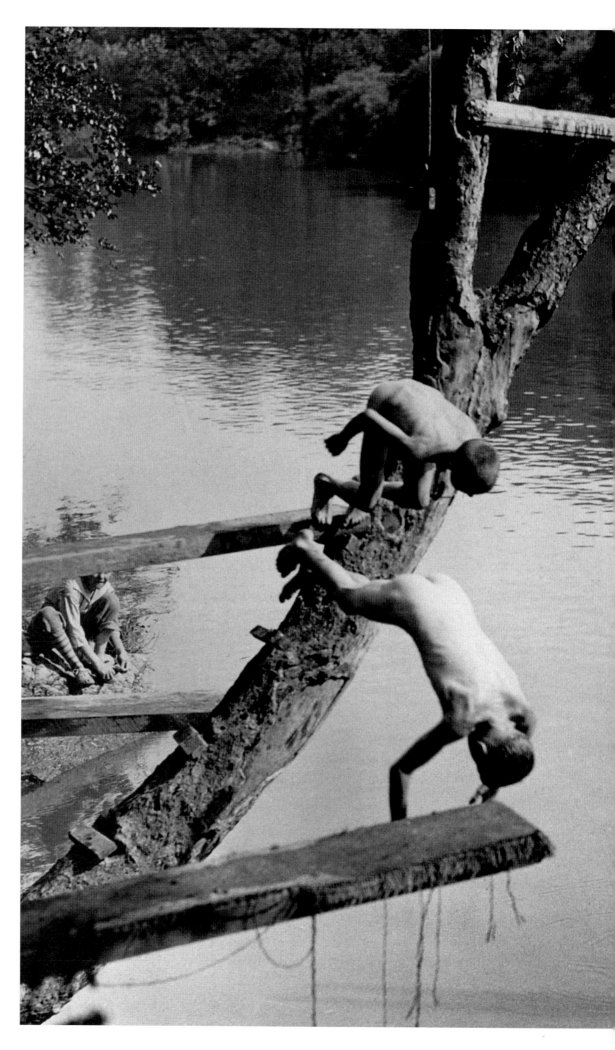

168

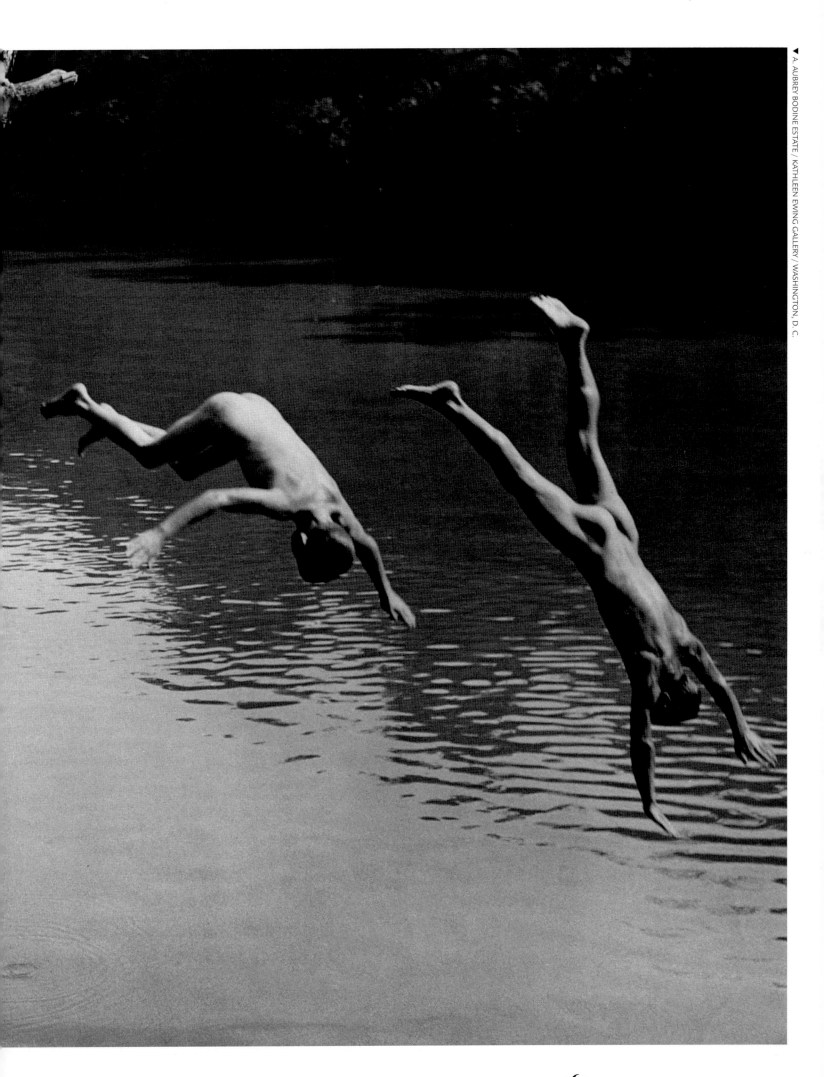

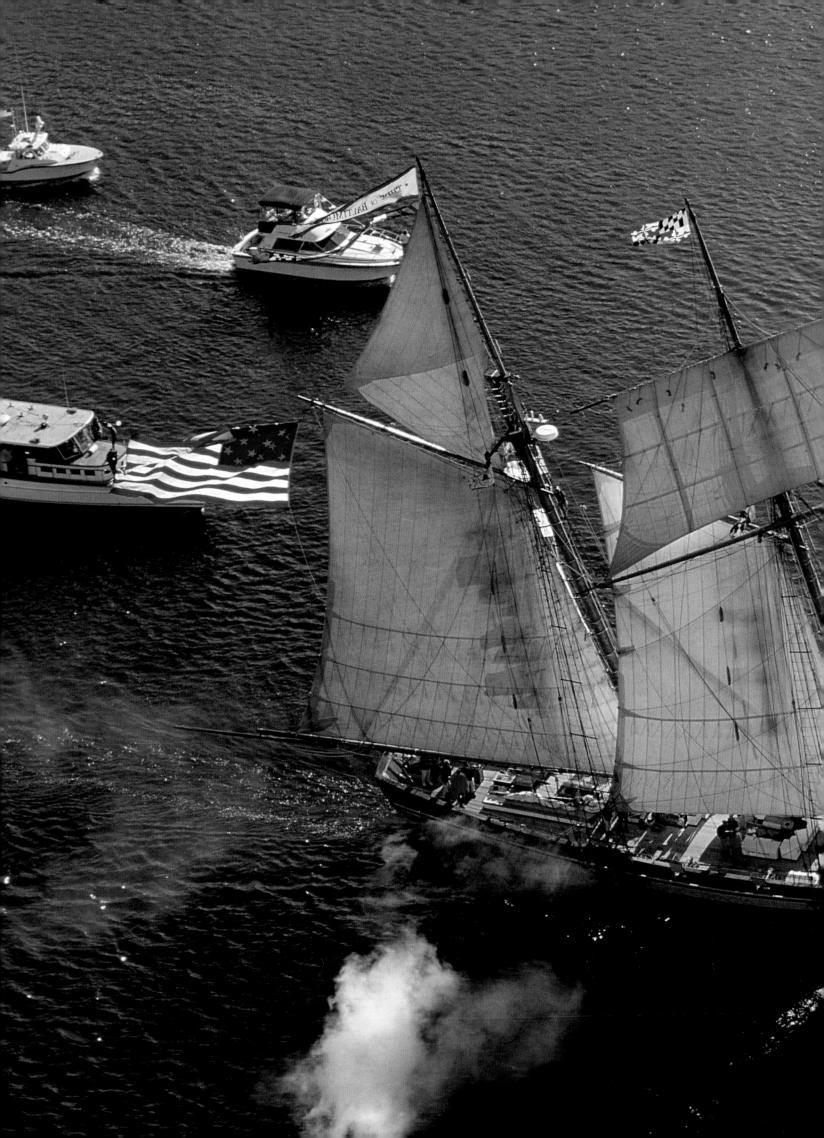

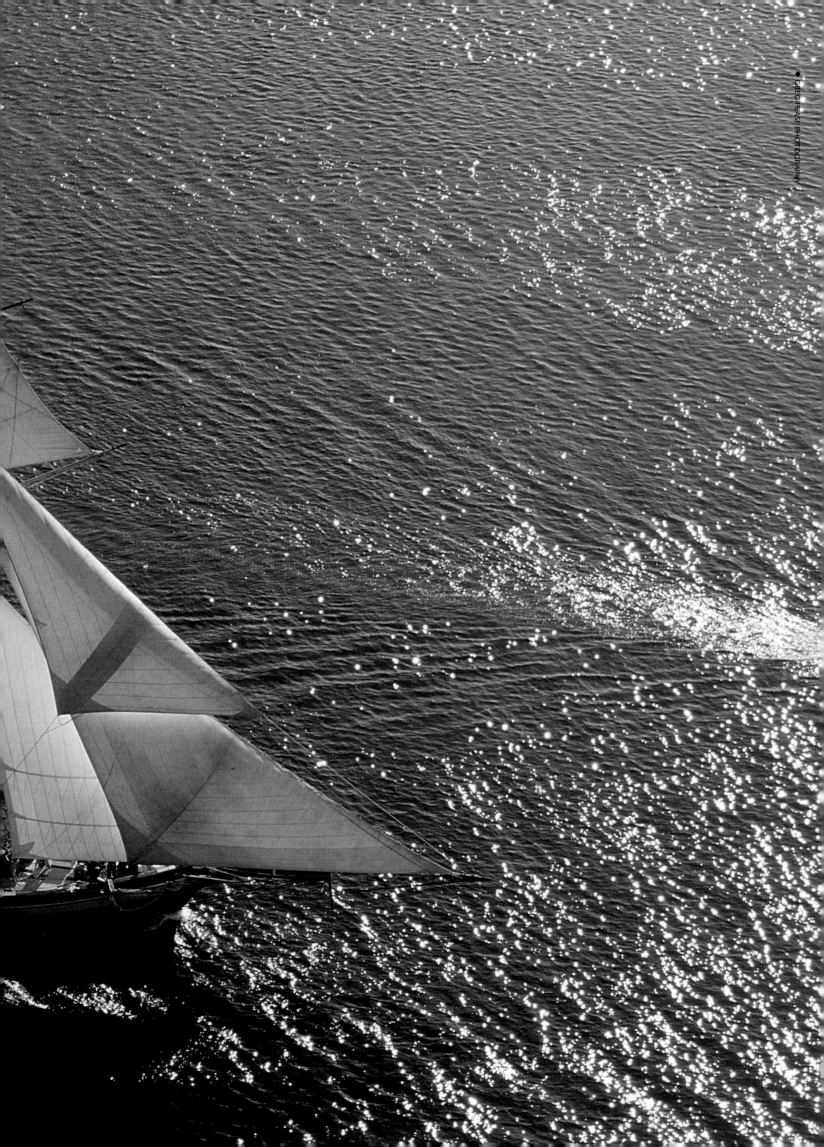

THE *Pride of Baltimore II*, A replica of an 1812-era clipper, serves as the city's goodwill ambassador (PAGES 170 AND 171). When it's not sailing the open seas, the ship is docked in downtown's Inner Harbor.

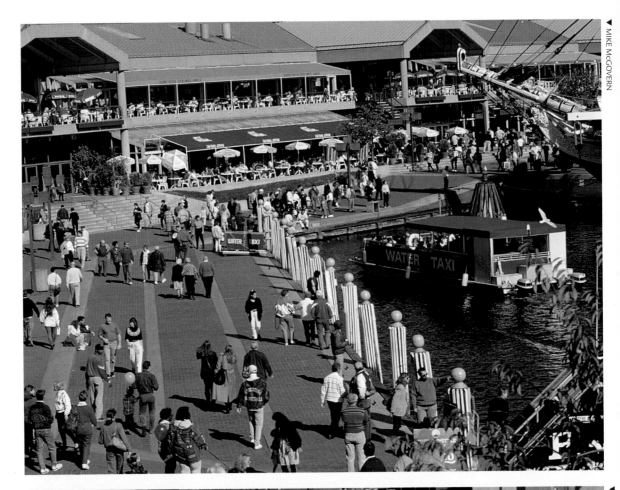

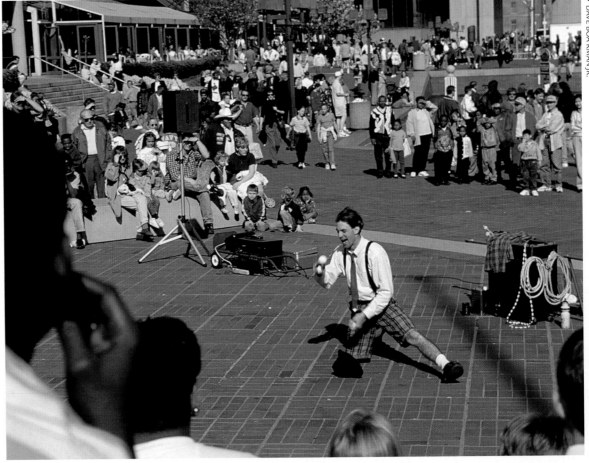

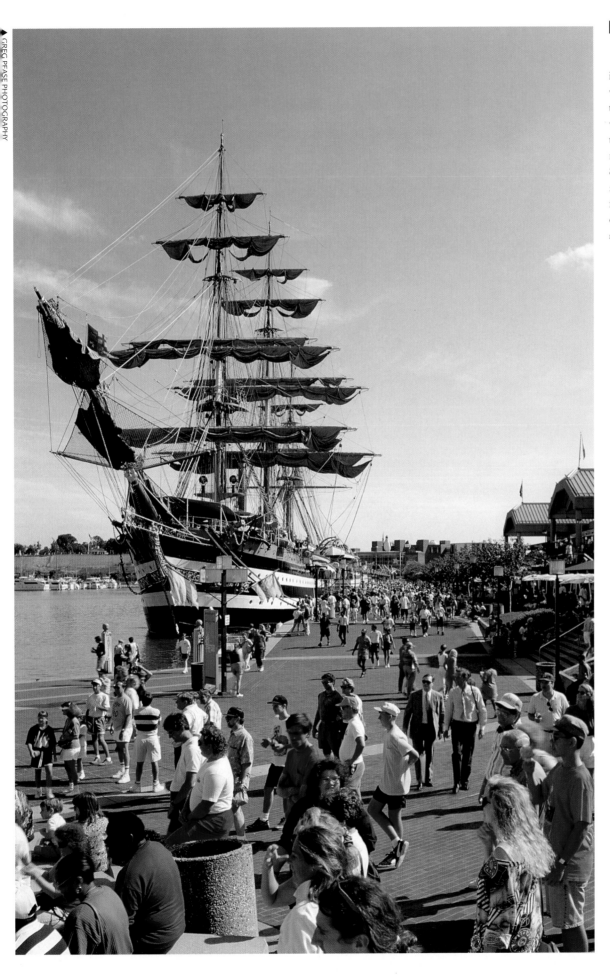

THE RENEWAL OF DOWNTOWN
Baltimore began in 1950, but
it wasn't until the 1980 opening of Harborplace—one of the first
waterside festival marketplaces in
the United States—that Charm City
was transformed into an international
tourist destination. The brainchild of
native Marylander James Rouse, the
85-acre complex houses more than
200 shops, restaurants, and eateries;
features several historic vessels on
display; and hosts more than 100
special events throughout the year.

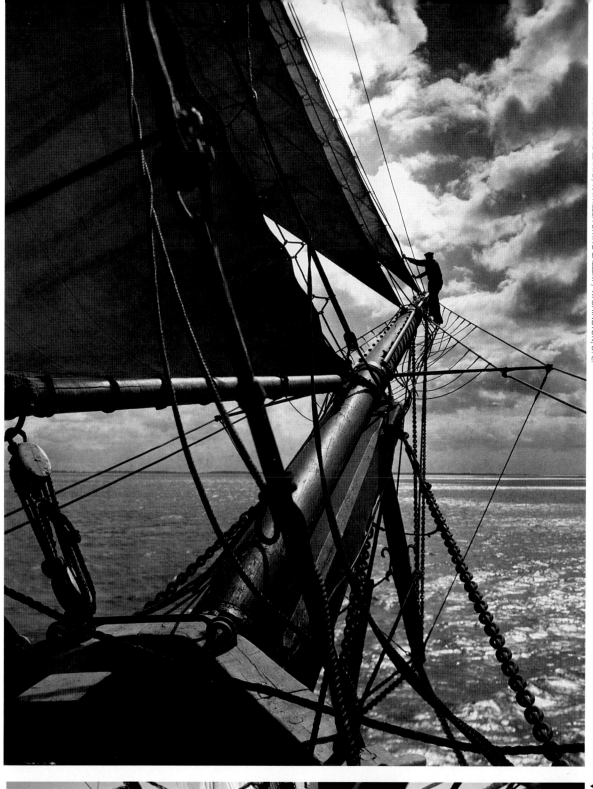

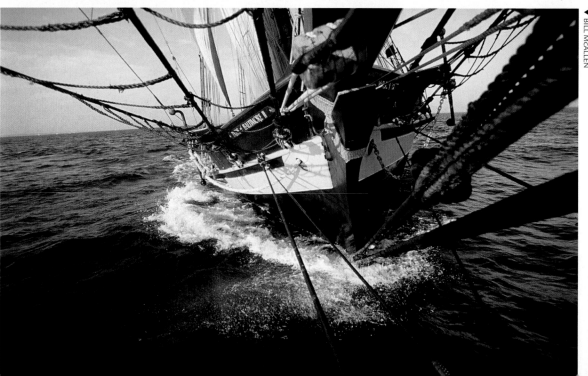

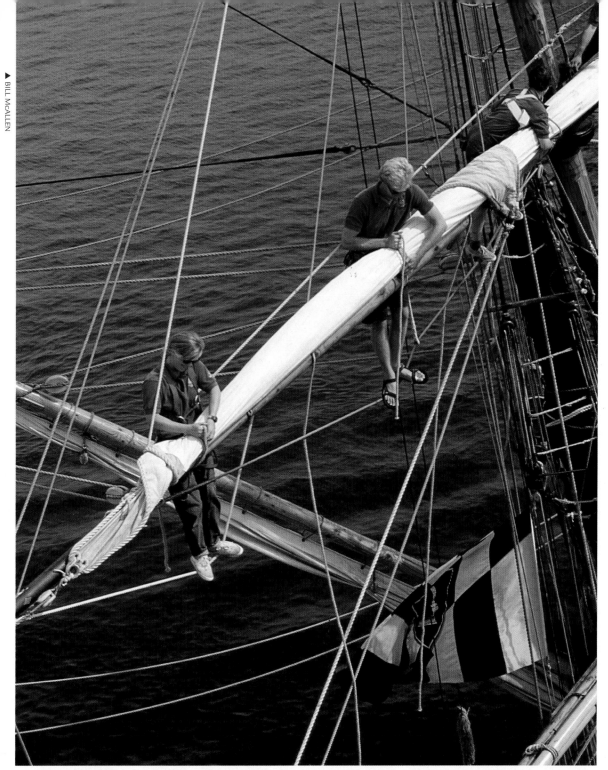

B OATS OF ALL SHAPES AND SIZES— and with all manner of ornamentation—ply the waters of the Chesapeake Bay.

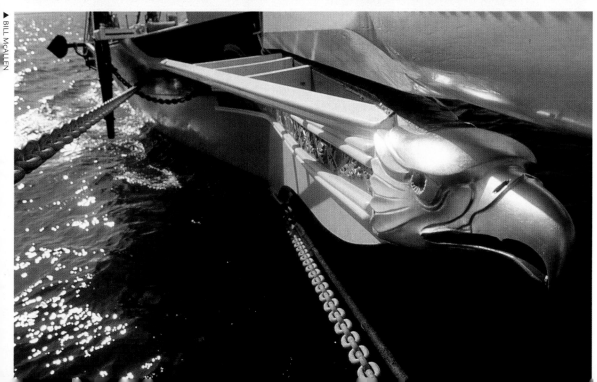

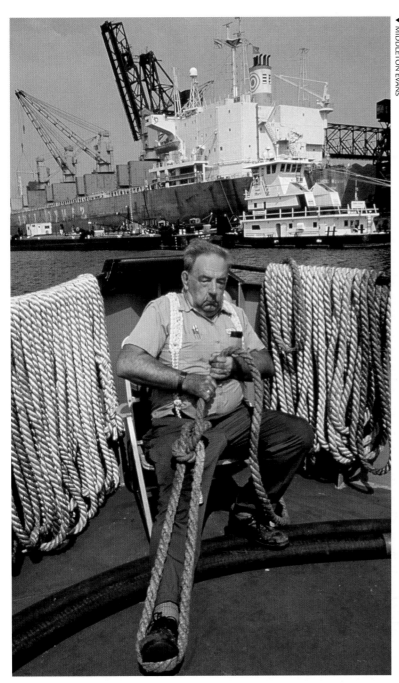

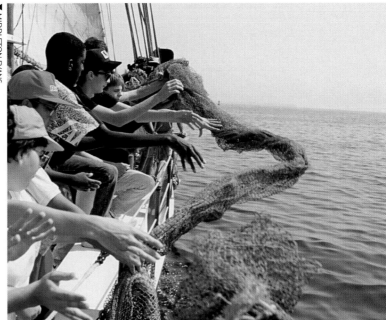

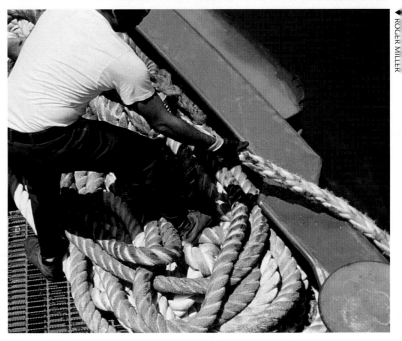

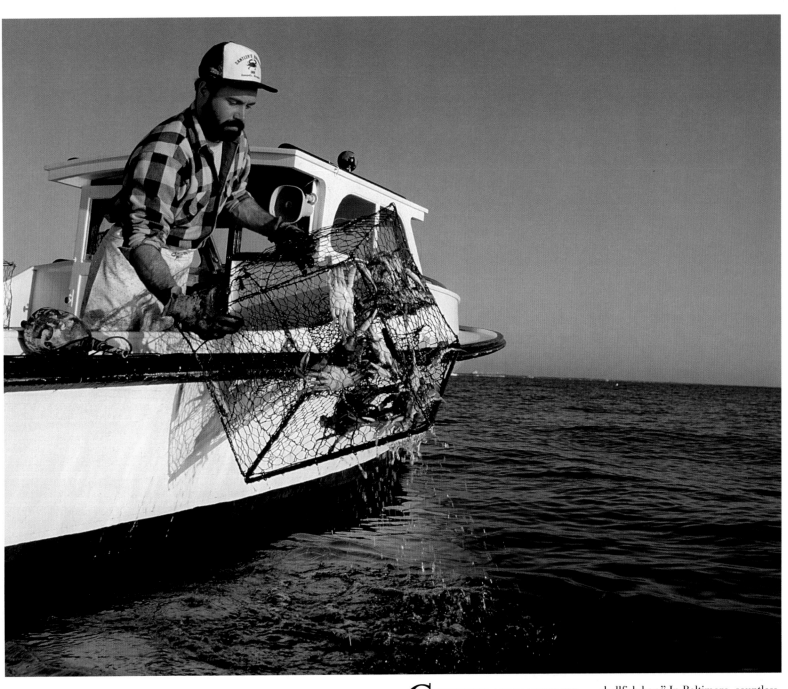

C HESAPEAKE, A NAME ORIGINATED by the Algonquians to describe the waters off the coast of Maryland and Virginia, means "great shellfish bay." In Baltimore, countless fishermen and tourists spend their days trying to net their share of the bay's plentiful creatures of the sea.

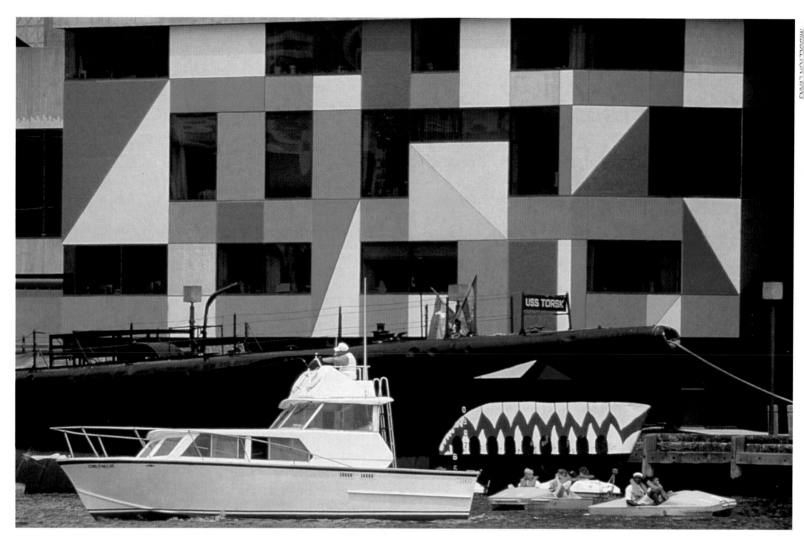

A TYPICAL INNER HARBOR regatta: Two paddleboats, a cabin cruiser, and the World War II-era submarine USS *Torsk*—now part of the Baltimore Maritime Museum—are framed against the National Aquarium.

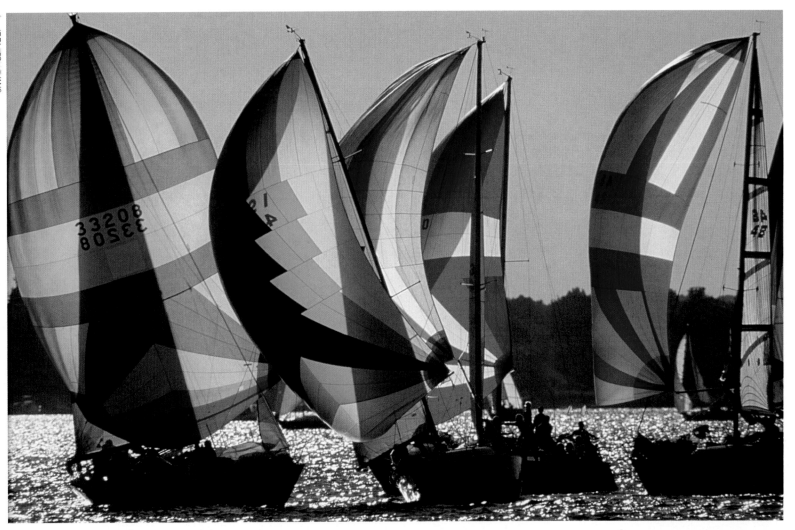

A genuine Chesapeake Bay regatta: A number of graceful boats try to capture the wind in their brightly colored sails.

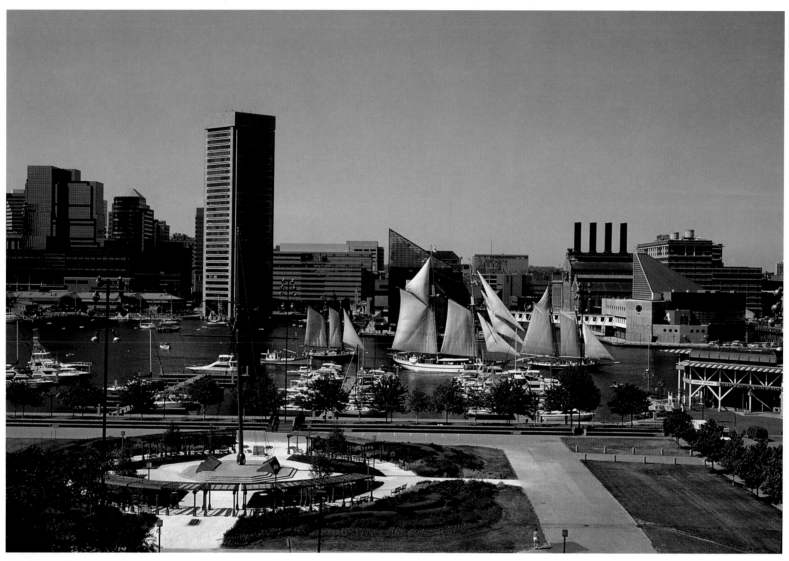

F ROM THIS MAJESTIC FEDERAL HILL
vantage point, it's easy to see
why Baltimore is sometimes
called the San Francisco of the East.

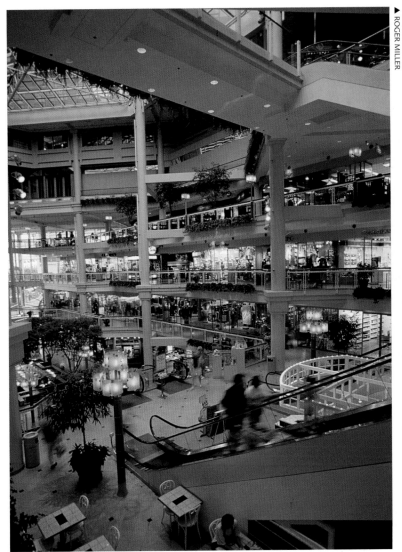

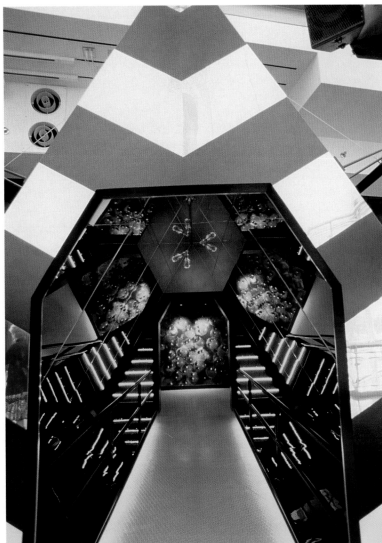

THE INNER HARBOR'S NUMEROUS attractions offer something for everyone, from the Gallery at Harborplace, a sleek urban mall that satisfies even the most avid shopper's cravings (LEFT), to the Columbus Center, a national facility for marine biotechnology research and education (RIGHT).

Each year, millions of tourists visit the Columbus Center, a nonprofit institute that strives to educate the public about science. The facility houses the University of Maryland Biotechnology Institute's Center of Marine Biotechnology, not to mention the Science and Technical Education Center, the food and water safety research units of the Food and Drug Administration, and the recently opened Hall of Exploration, which features hands-on, interactive exhibits.

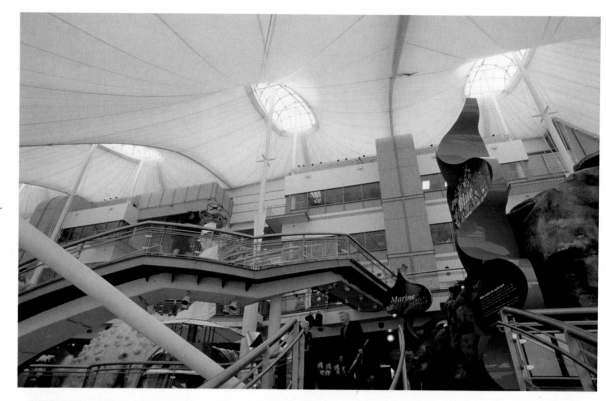

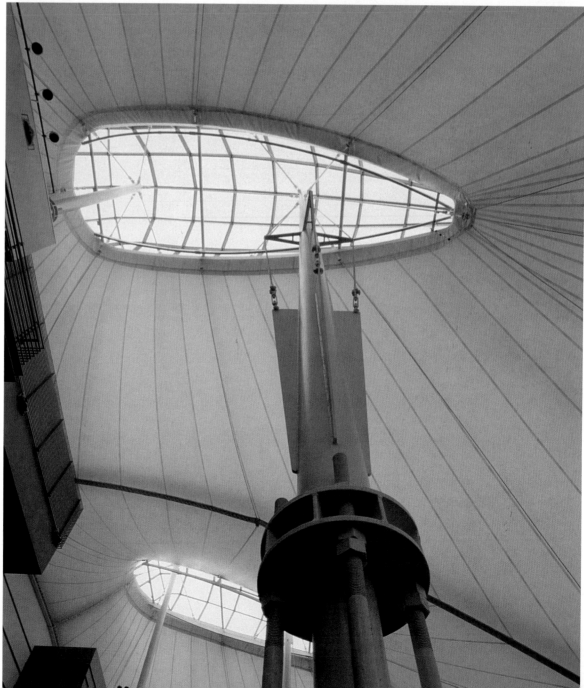

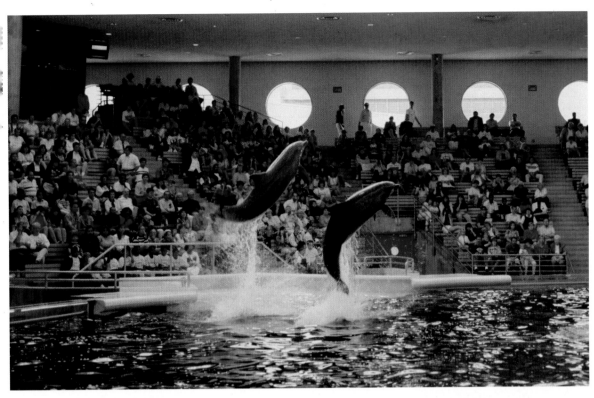

NOT SURPRISINGLY, BALTIMORE IS home to a number of attractions that showcase animals from the sea, including the National Aquarium (TOP) and The Baltimore Zoo (BOTTOM).

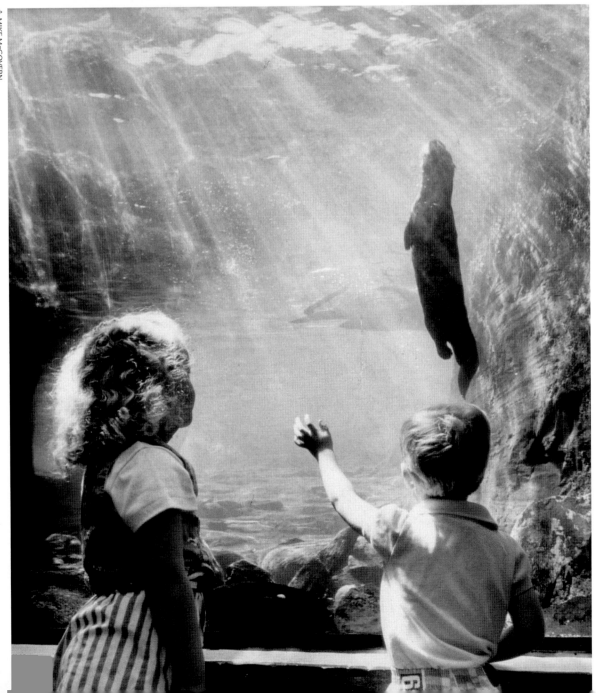

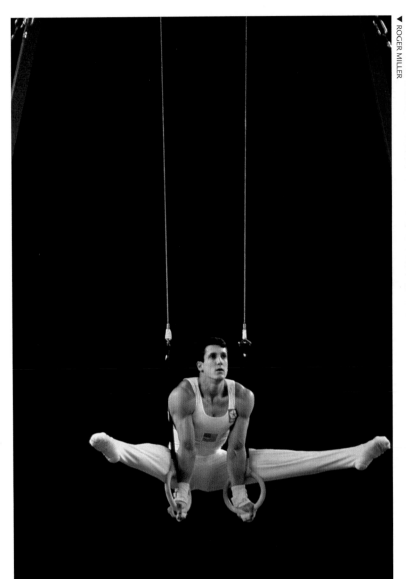

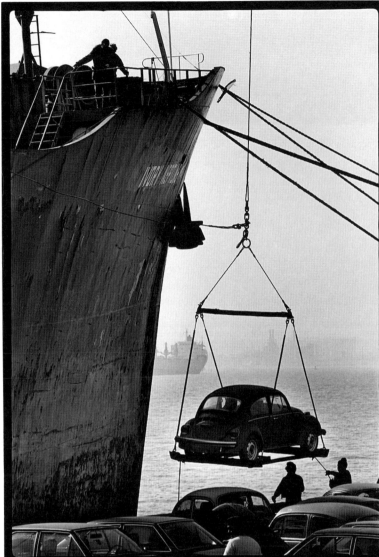

Hanging in the balance: John Roethlisberger and other American gymnasts thrilled local crowds during the 1992 Olympic trials; for decades, the Port of Baltimore has been a point of entry for the foreign auto industry's latest models.

COFF PEAFF PHOTOGRAPHY

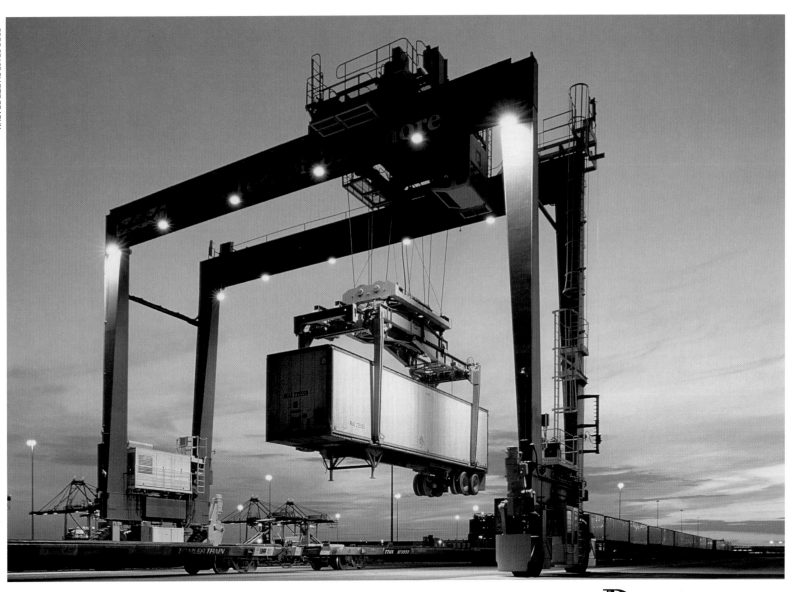

BALTIMORE'S PORT HAS ALWAYS been central to the city's commercial and industrial growth. In fact, when the township was created in 1729, the area located northwest of the Patapsco River had already been engaged in port activity for two decades.

ONE OF THE MOST SOPHISTICATED and technologically advanced facilities of its kind in the world, the National Aquarium in Baltimore features more than 10,000 marine and freshwater life-forms, from dart frogs to dolphins and everything in between. More than 22 million people have visited the aquarium since it opened in 1981, and its economic impact is pegged at $128.4 million annually.

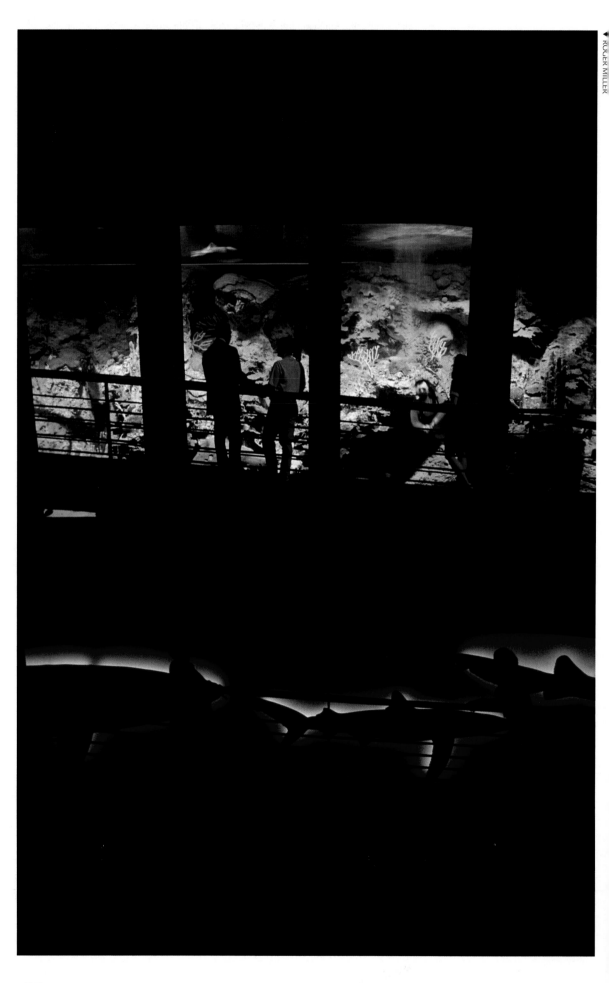

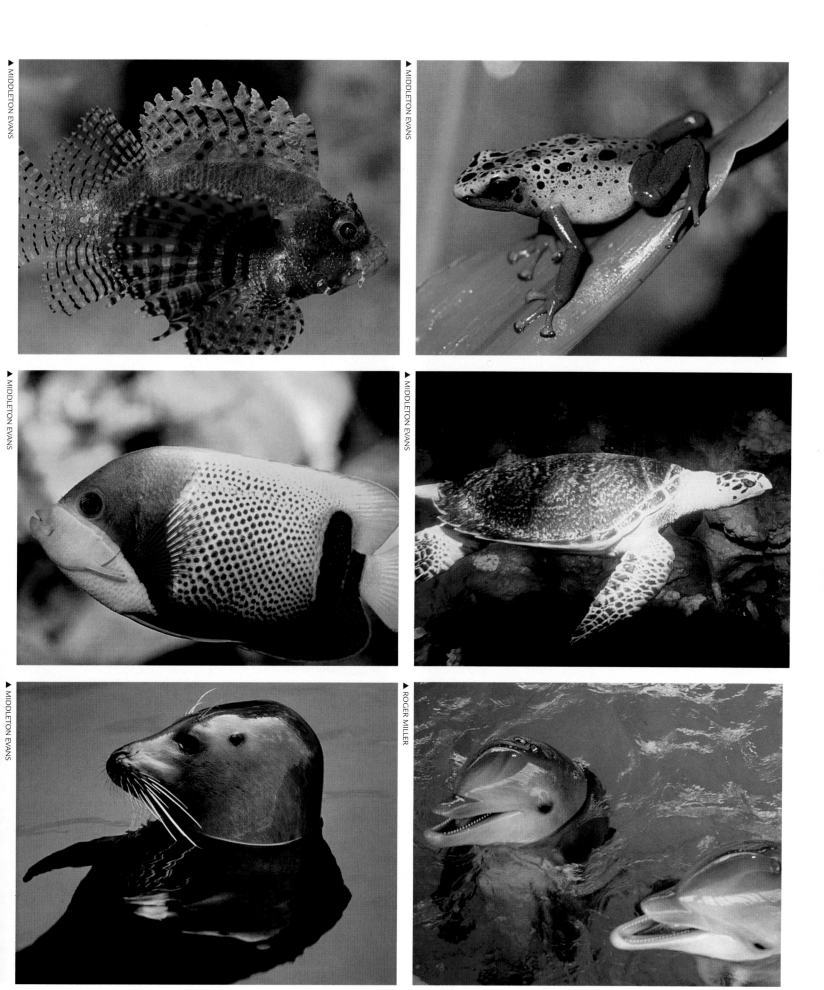

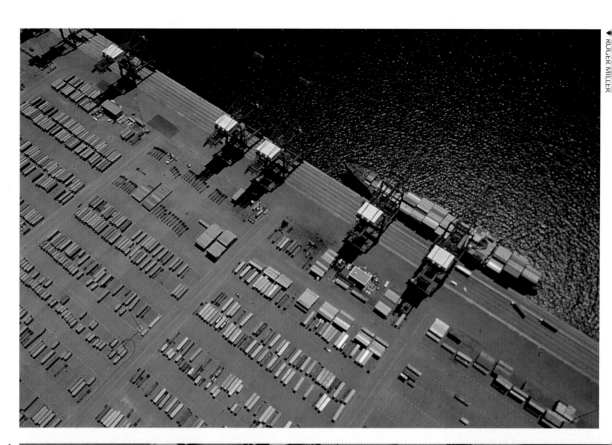

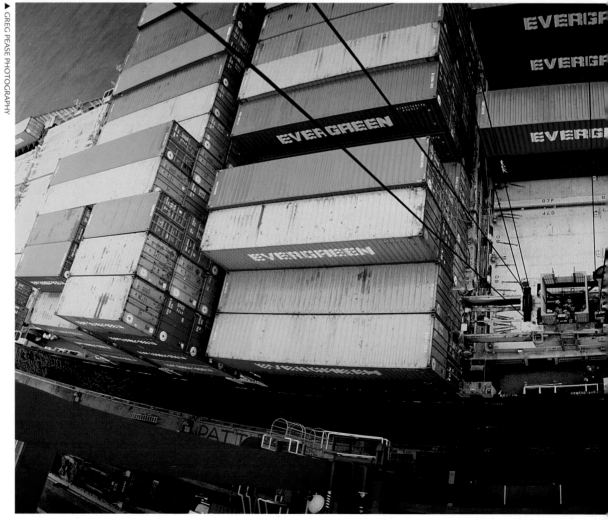

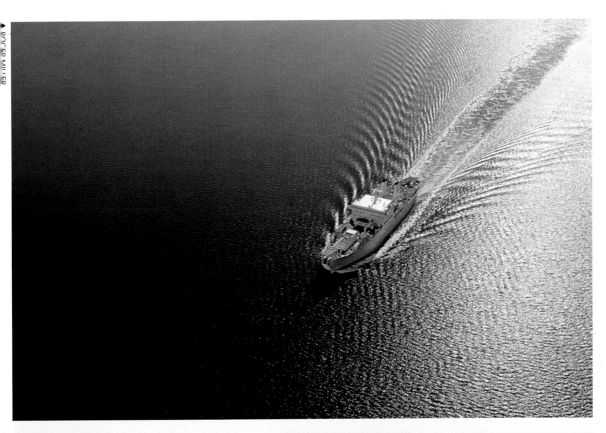

FOR NEARLY THREE CENTURIES, the Port of Baltimore has grown with the city. Today, more than 2,500 cargo ships annually import and export goods through the historic port, which boasts some 45 miles of improved waterfront; increased container capacity, thanks to the 1990 opening of the Seagirt Marine Terminal; and docking facilities that can handle up to 96 vessels at one time.

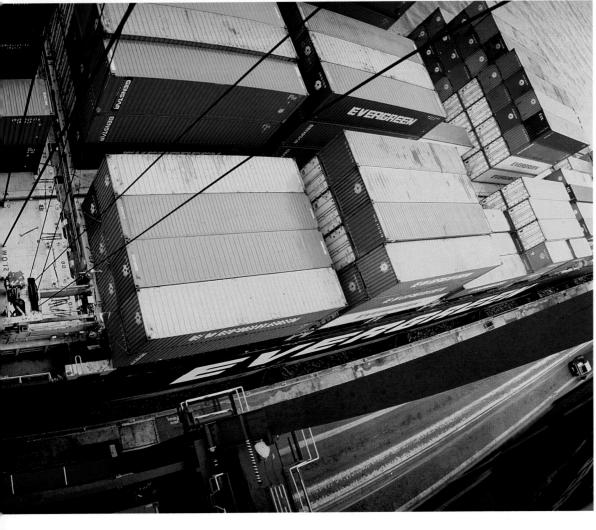

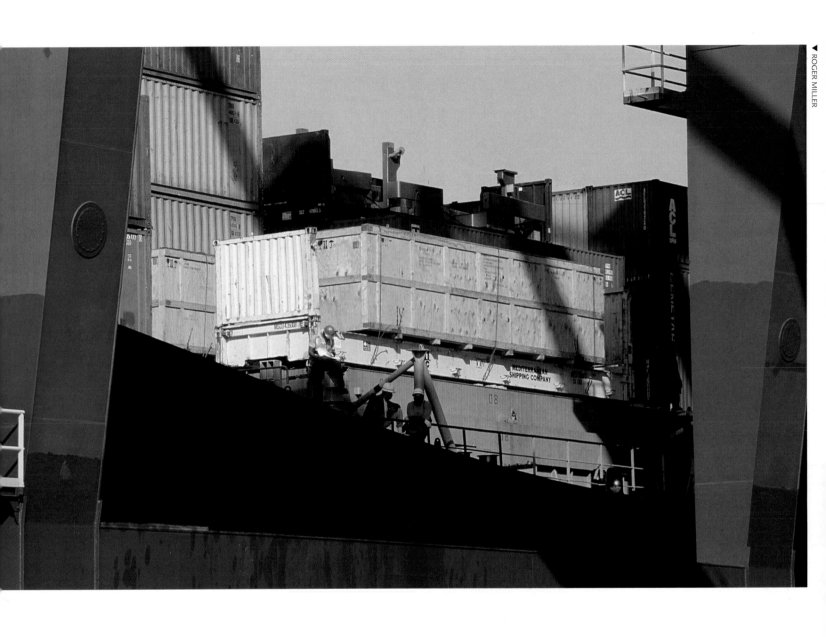

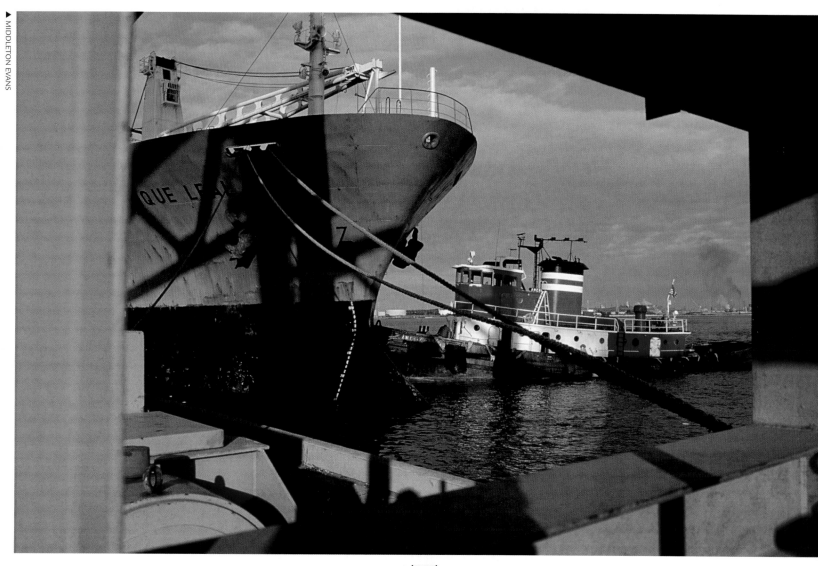

T HE GREAT COMPETITIVE ADVAN-
tage of the Port of Baltimore
is its geographic proximity to
the Midwest; it's located 200 miles
farther inland than any other Atlantic

harbor. Millions of dollars have been
invested in the seaport in recent years
to deepen the channel and modernize
facilities.

G IANT FREIGHTERS, CARGO SHIPS, tugboats, Coast Guard cutters, and countless other vessels find a temporary home at the Port of Baltimore.

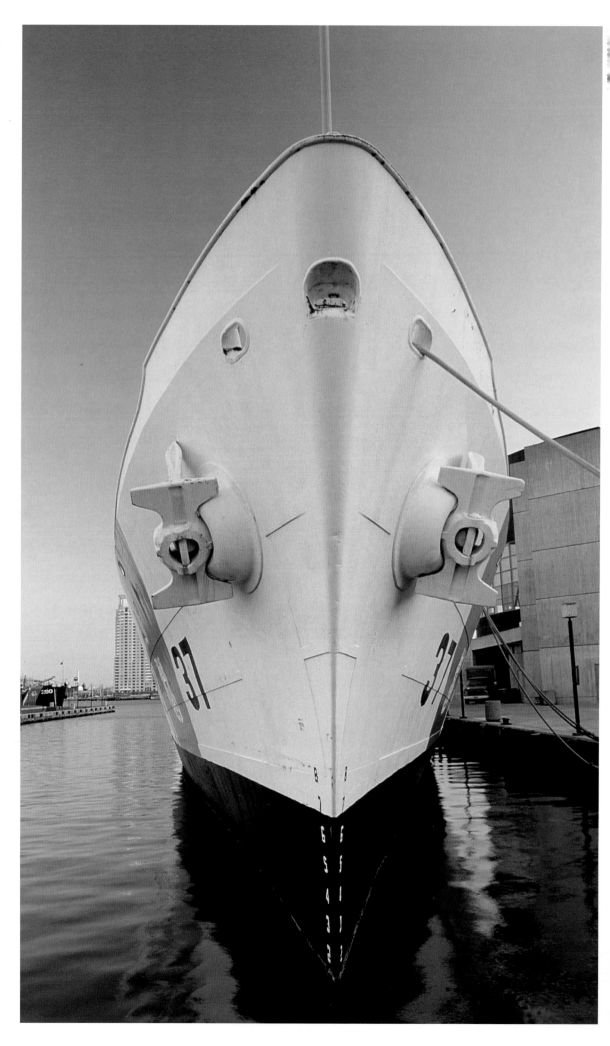

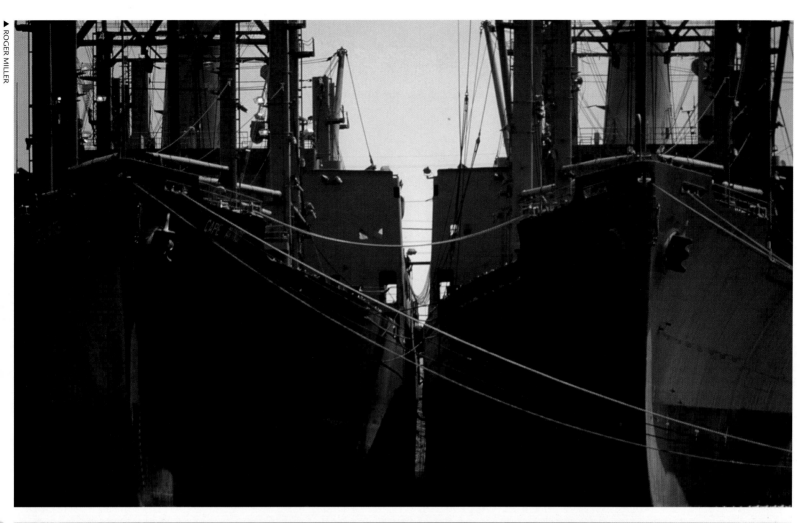

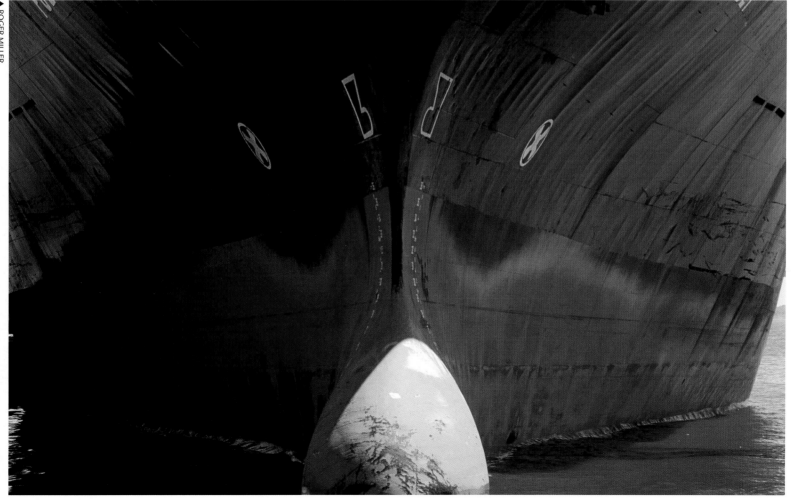

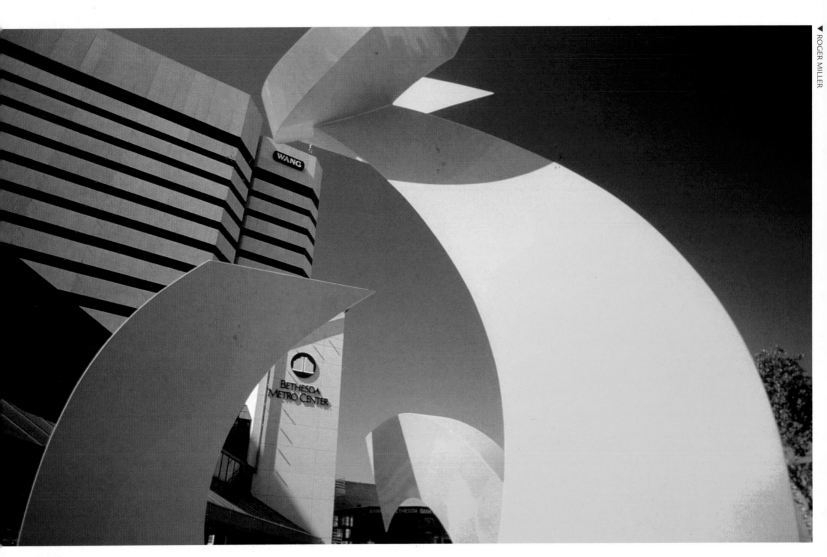

BETHESDA
METRO CENTER

THE BETHESDA METRO CENTER office complex is just one of the draws for businesses and tourists in nearby Bethesda, which also boasts countless ethnic restaurants and state-of-the-art health care facilities—all within a stone's throw of Washington, D.C.

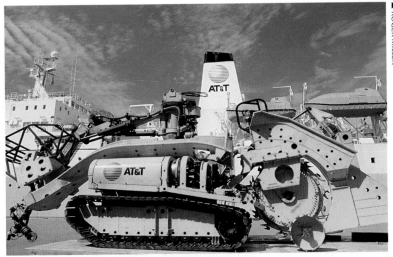

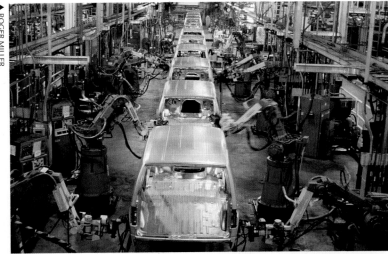

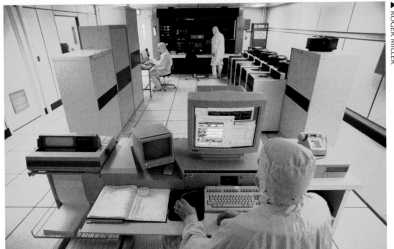

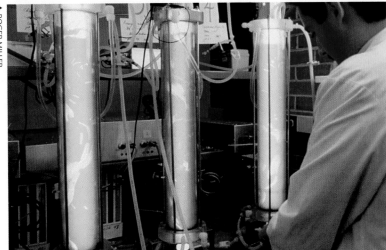

Many corporations in Balti-more are operating in the . . . yellow? Such familiar names as AT&T and General Motors join other giants of industry to create a well-rounded, healthy economy.

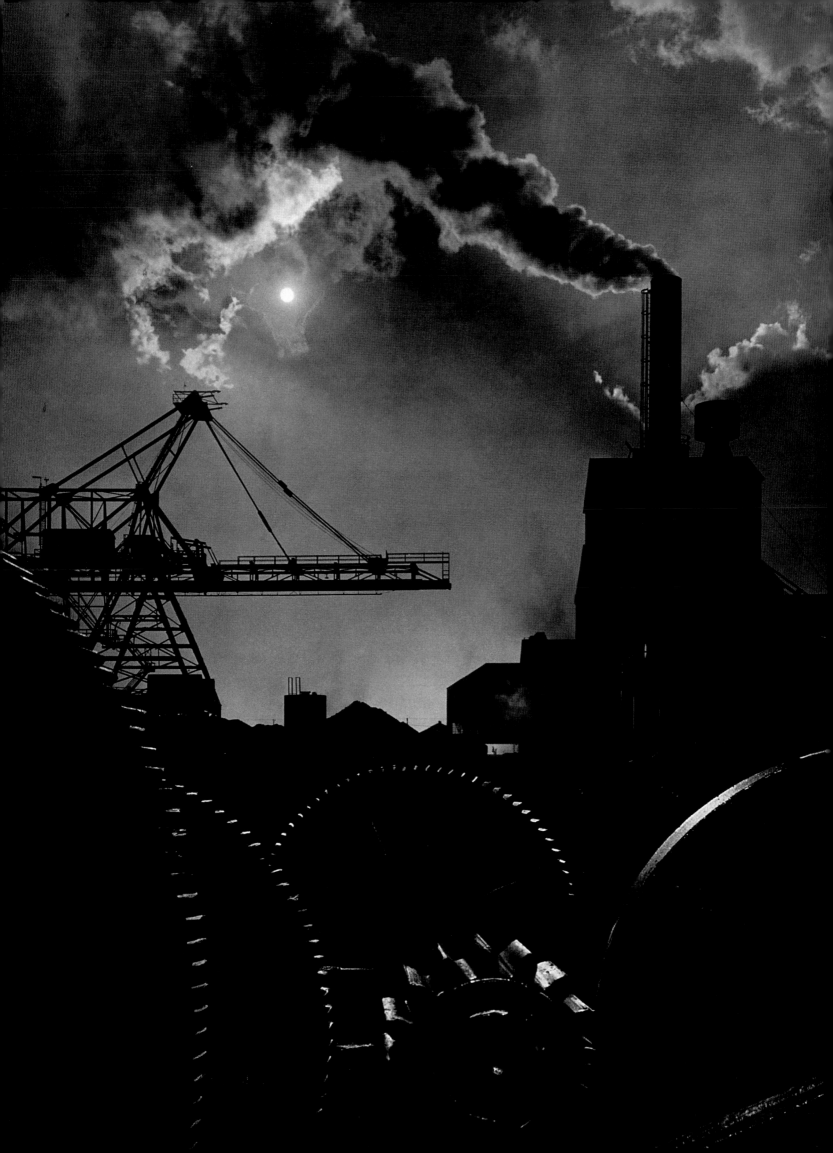

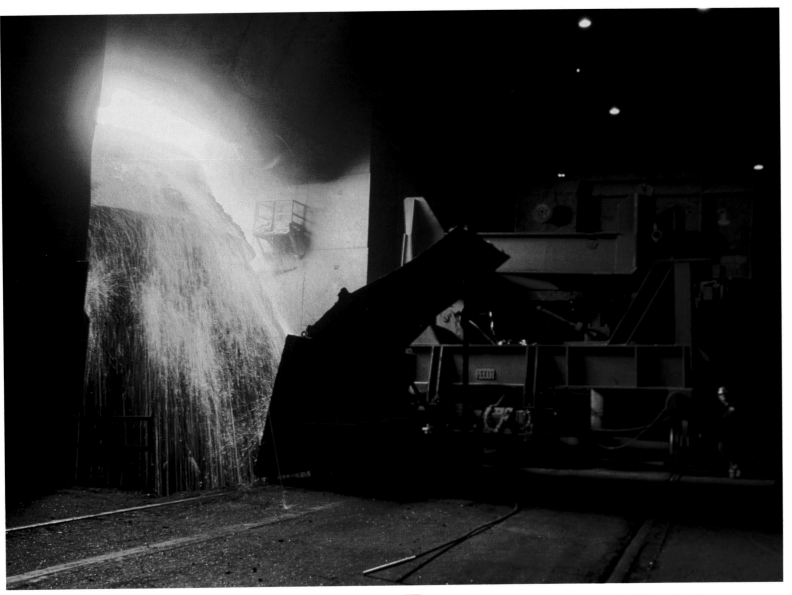

I N THE 1800S, BALTIMORE TOOK ITS place among the world's manufacturing centers as iron, steel, and textile companies cropped up in the area. Today, the city's industrial influence can still be felt worldwide.

Bethlehem Steel Corporation, which has had a local presence for decades, is currently the nation's second-largest steel manufacturer, producing hot rolled sheet, tin mill, and steel plate (ABOVE).

O N ANY GIVEN DAY, BALTIMORE'S laborers are hard at work, whether they're removing asbestos from a site, tackling a welding project at Ellicott International, surveying the scene at a Bethlehem Steel shipyard, or delivering iron ore to a local storage facility.

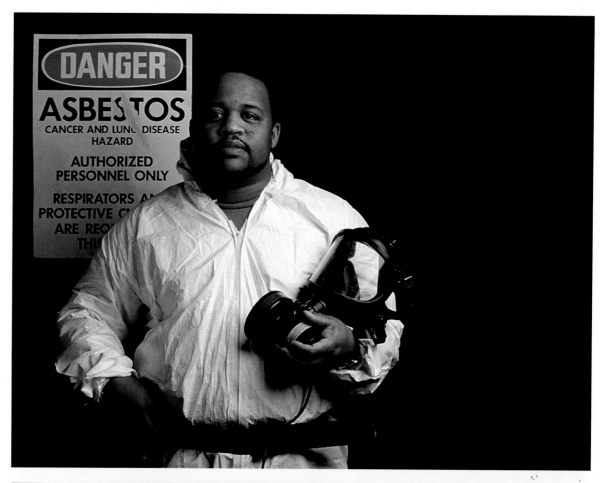

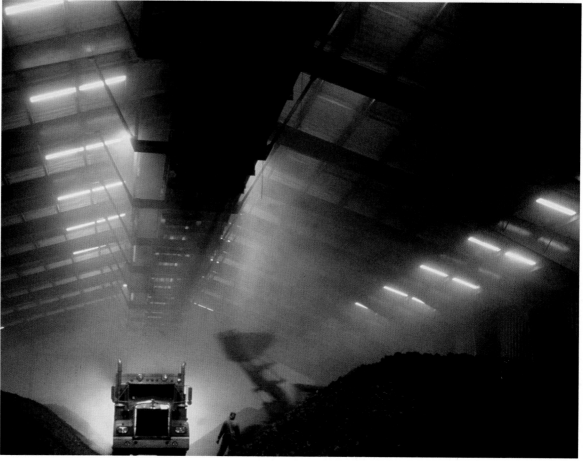

198

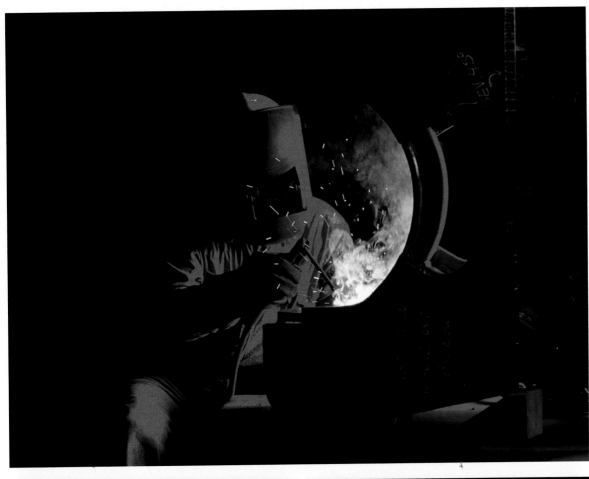

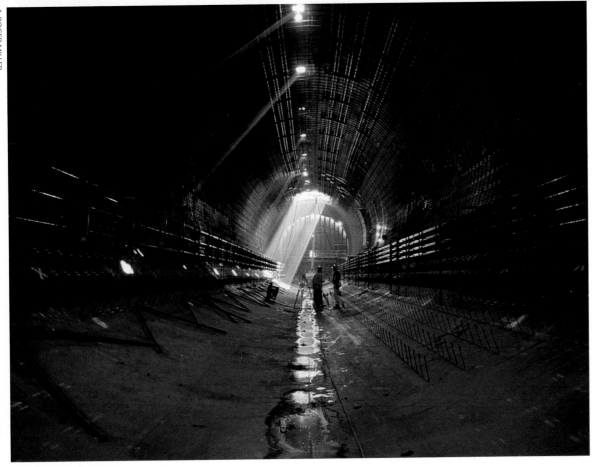

N EON OR NOT, BALTIMORE'S SIGNS point the way—in this case to a Domino Sugar plant and the *Energy* exhibit at the Maryland Science Center.

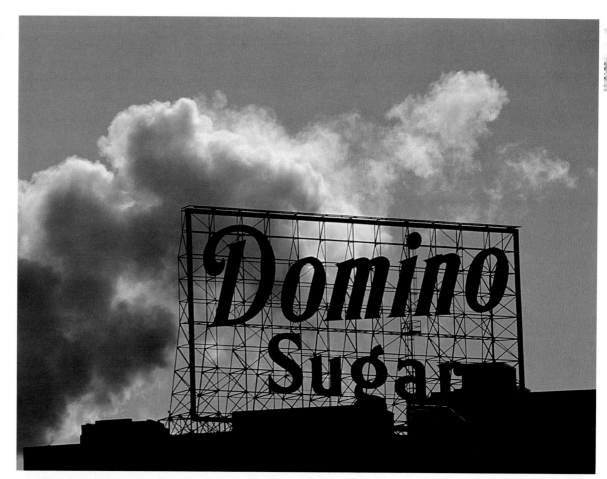

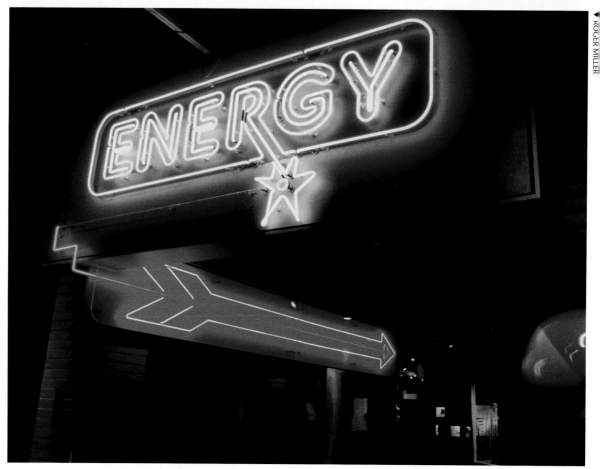

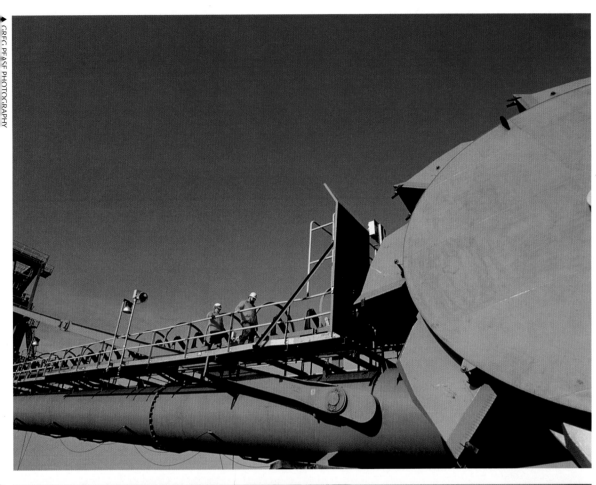

A HARD HAT IS OFTEN A NECESSARY accessory in the city's industrial sector. Employees of Conoco Coal Development get an overview of the company's operations at the Port of Baltimore (TOP), while a lone worker monitors the controls at the Calvert Cliffs nuclear plant in Calvert County (BOTTOM).

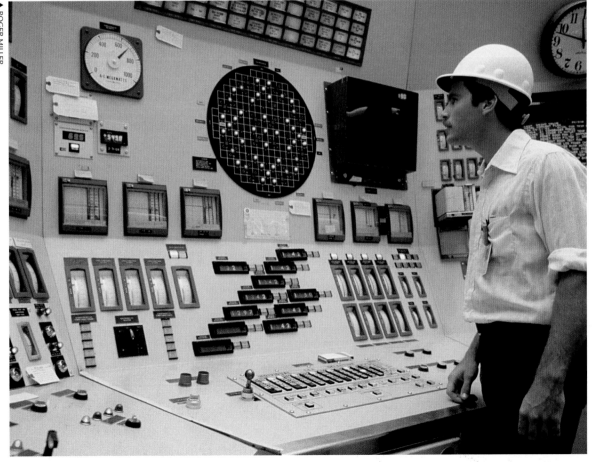

ENERGY HAS MYRIAD MEANINGS and manifestations in Baltimore, from a giant propeller standing ready for duty (RIGHT) to the high-flying swings at the Maryland State Fair (OPPOSITE TOP). For an energized moviegoing experience, the place to be is the IMAX Theater at the Maryland Science Center (OPPOSITE BOTTOM).

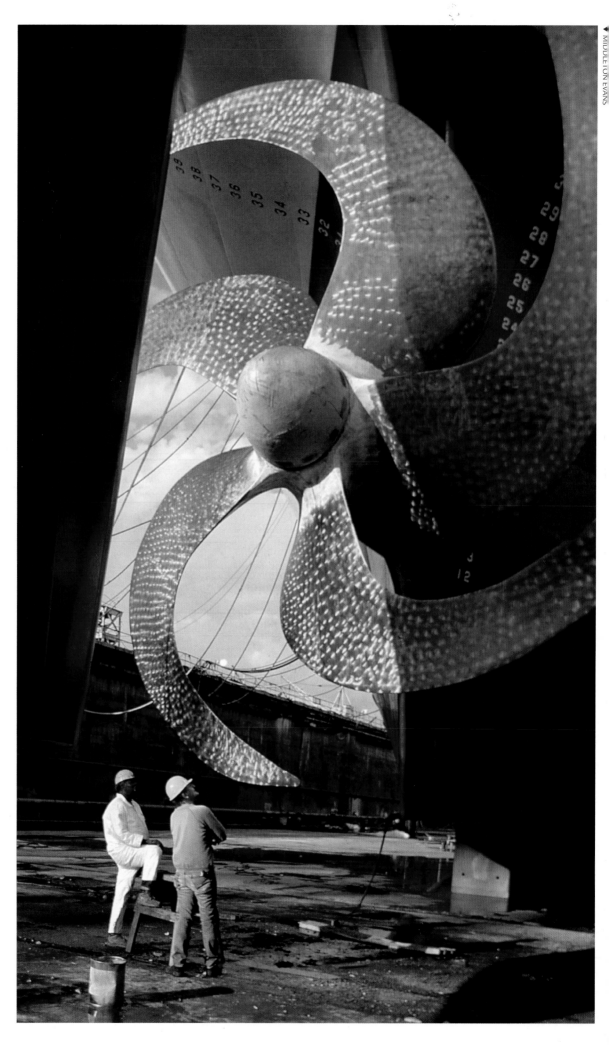

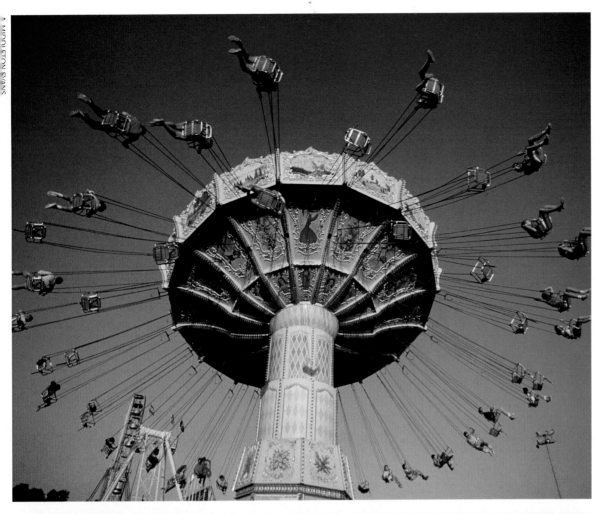

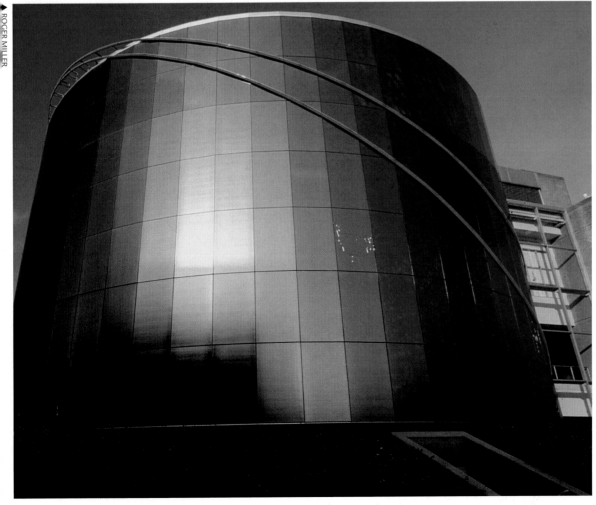

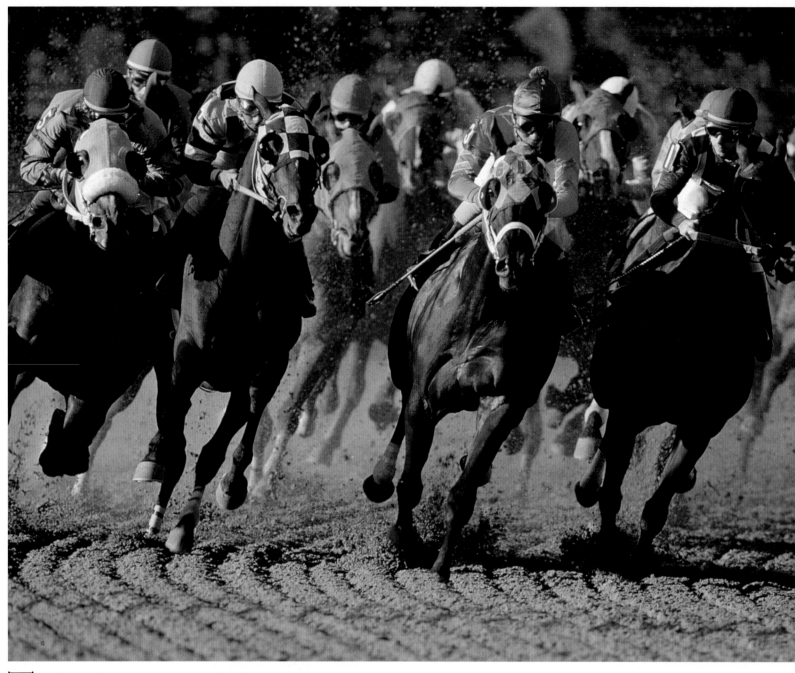

THE PIMLICO RACECOURSE IS home to the Preakness Stakes, the middle leg of the famous Triple Crown, which also includes the Kentucky Derby and the Belmont Stakes. Begun in 1873, the annual Thoroughbred horse race is the culmination of a nine-day festival that features hot-air balloons, live music, a parade, and countless parties.

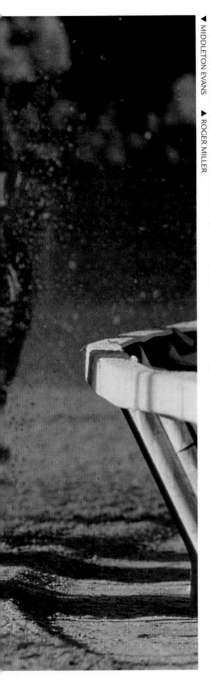

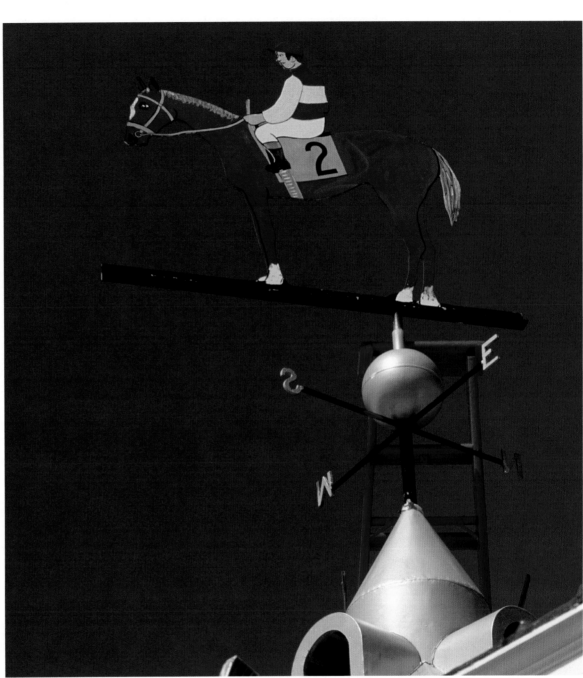

L OCAL KIDS KNOW THAT THERE'S NO
better way to beat the summer
heat than by frolicking in a
makeshift fountain.

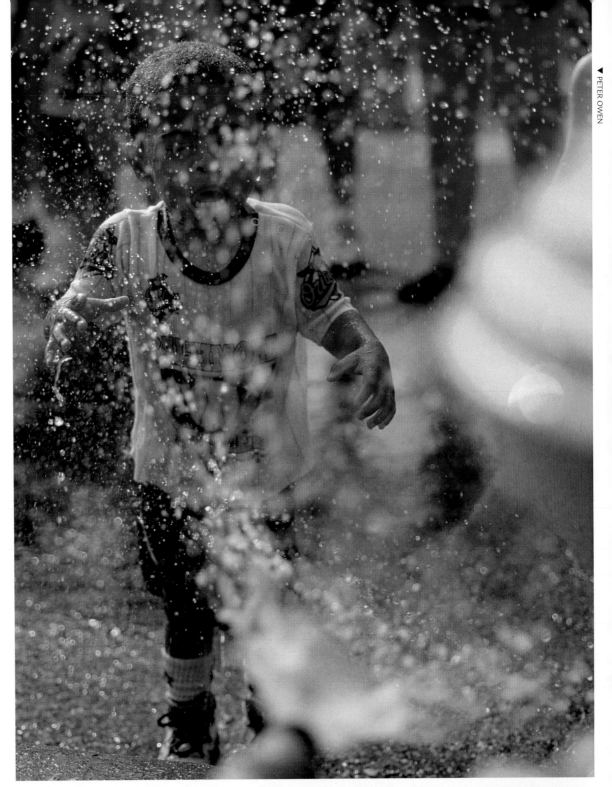

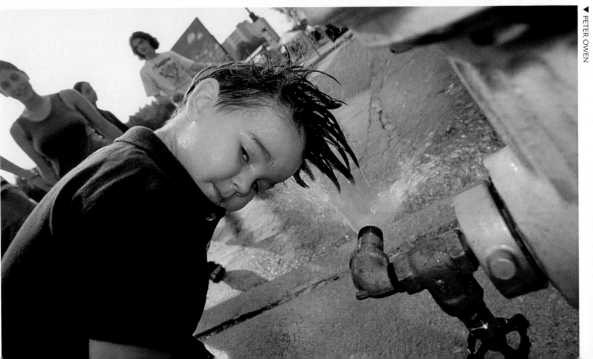

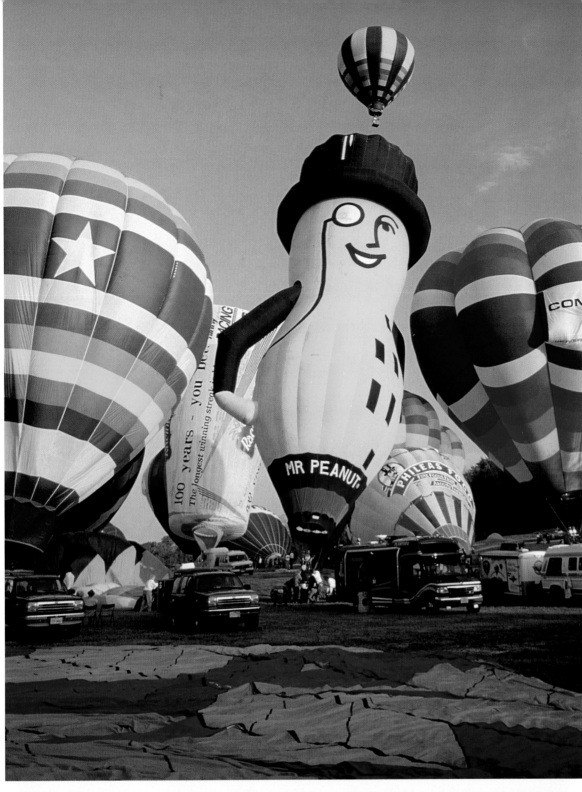

During the Preakness celebration leading up to Baltimore's own Triple Crown event, several hot-air balloon festivals draw a number of colorful craft and a few familiar faces.

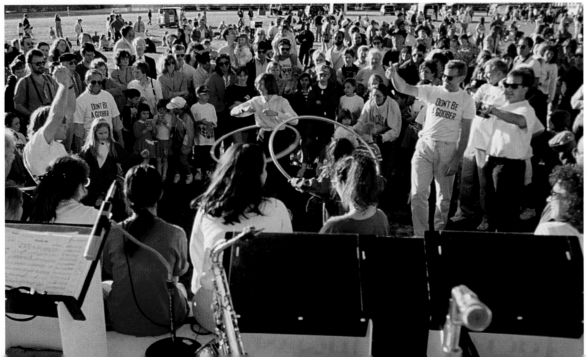

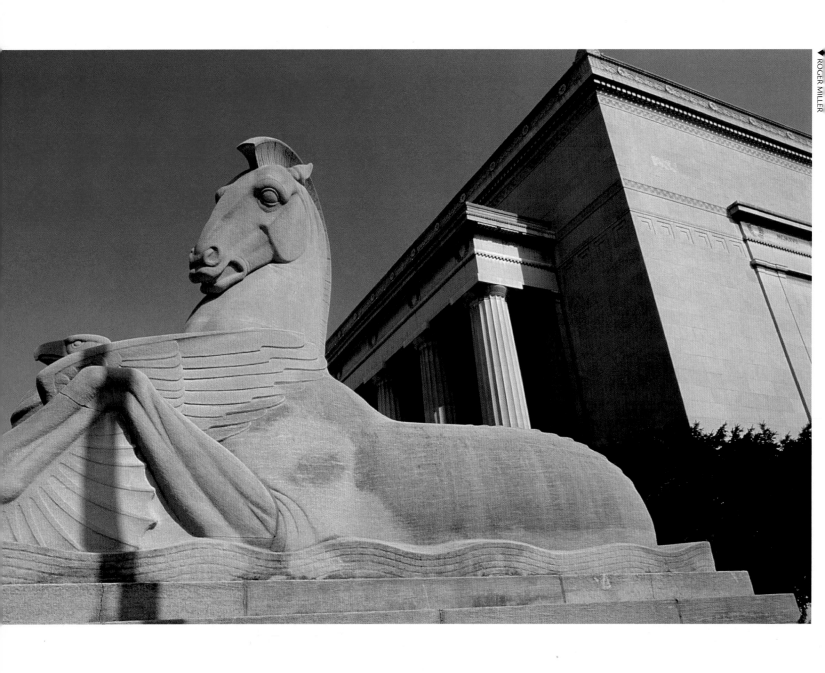

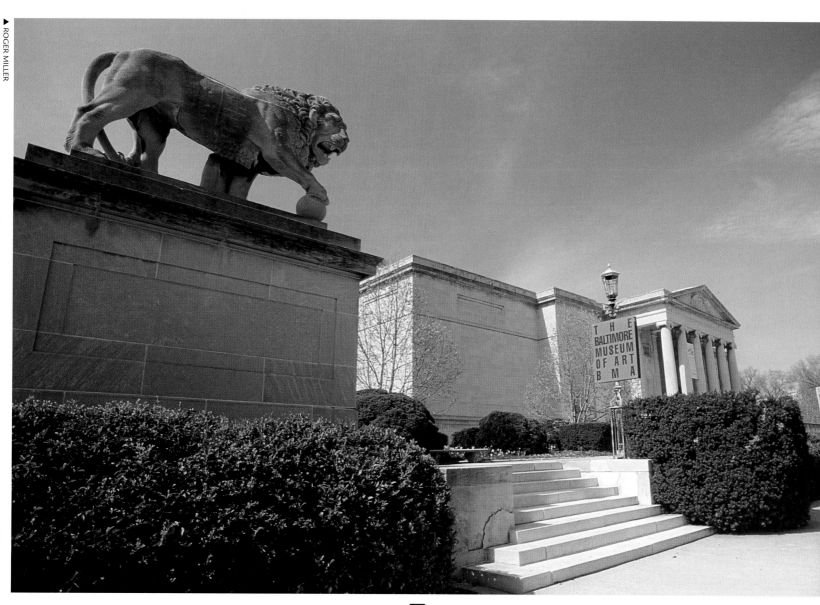

IMPRESSIVE SCULPTURES STAND GUARD over several of Baltimore's public spaces. Jeffrey Schiff's bronze horse, embedded in a granite and concrete base, greets visitors to War Memorial Plaza (OPPOSITE), and a regal lion, created in 1847 by Antoine-Louise Barye, is on the prowl outside the Baltimore Museum of Art (ABOVE).

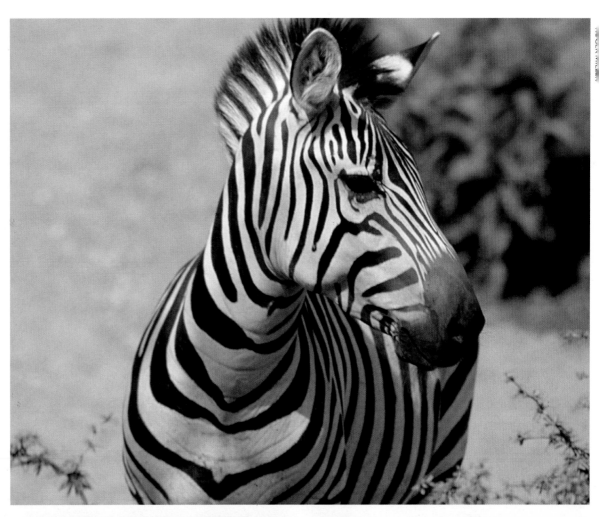

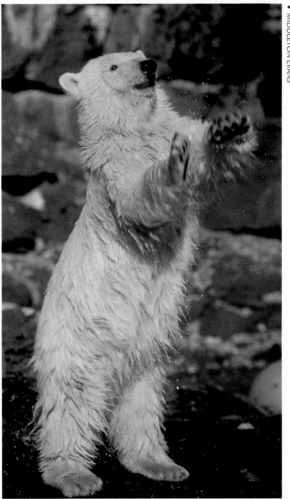

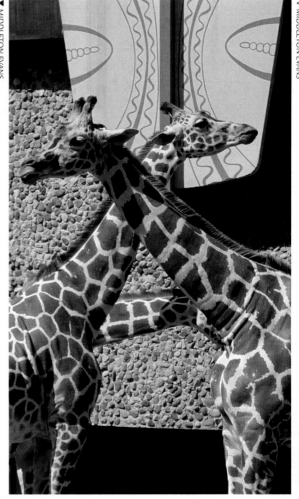

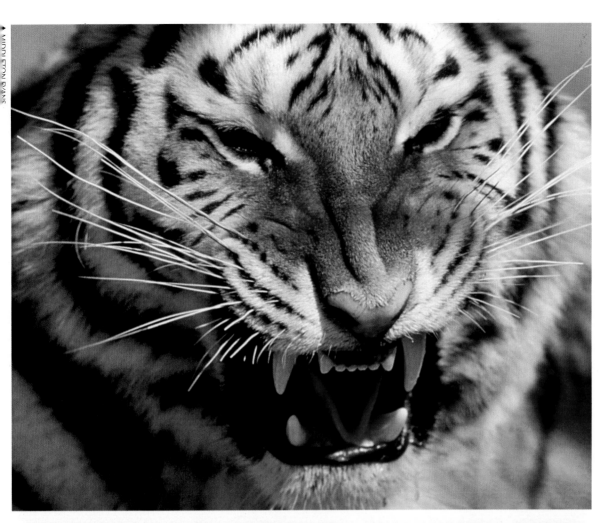

THE BALTIMORE ZOO, THE THIRD-oldest in the nation, is tucked away in historic Druid Hill Park. Chartered to the city in 1876, the zoo houses more than 2,000 mammals, birds, and reptiles.

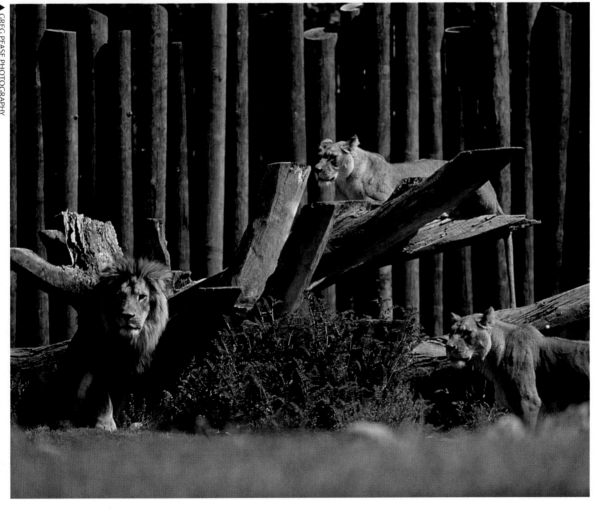

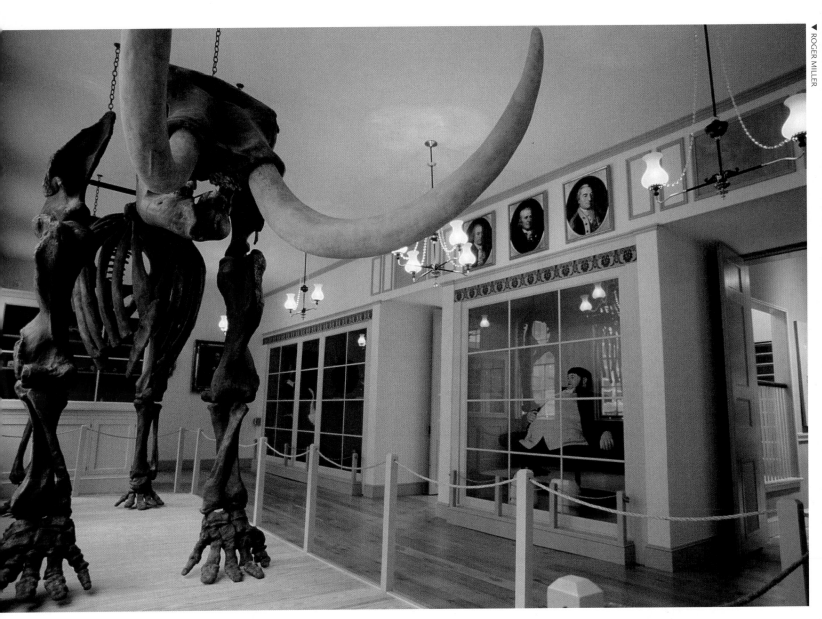

THE PEALE MUSEUM WAS THE FIRST
American venue to be designed
specifically as a place to exhibit
antiquities. Opened in 1814, it was
built by Baltimore painter Rembrandt
Peale to honor his father, Charles
Willson Peale.

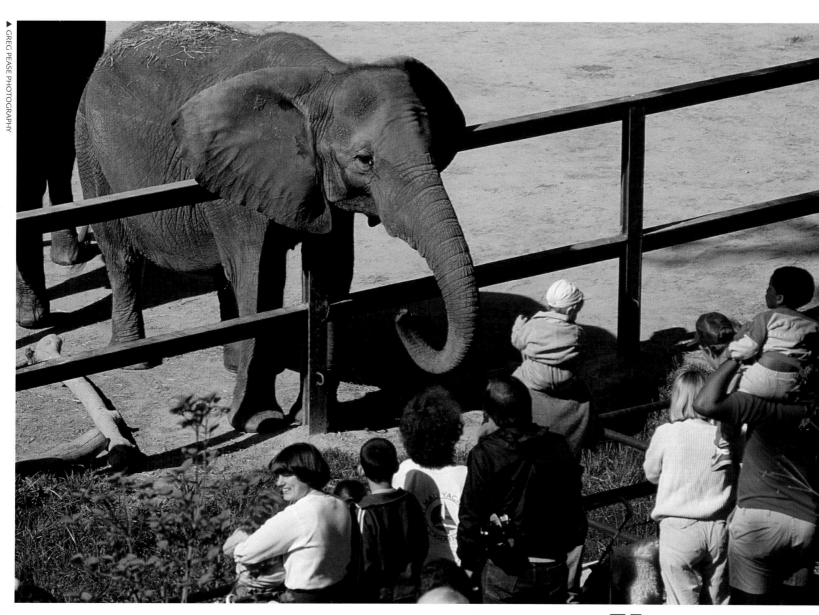

Y OU DON'T HAVE TO BE A KID TO enjoy the elephant exhibit at the Baltimore Zoo. Each year, more than half a million visitors of all ages marvel at the facility's exotic residents and naturalistic habitats.

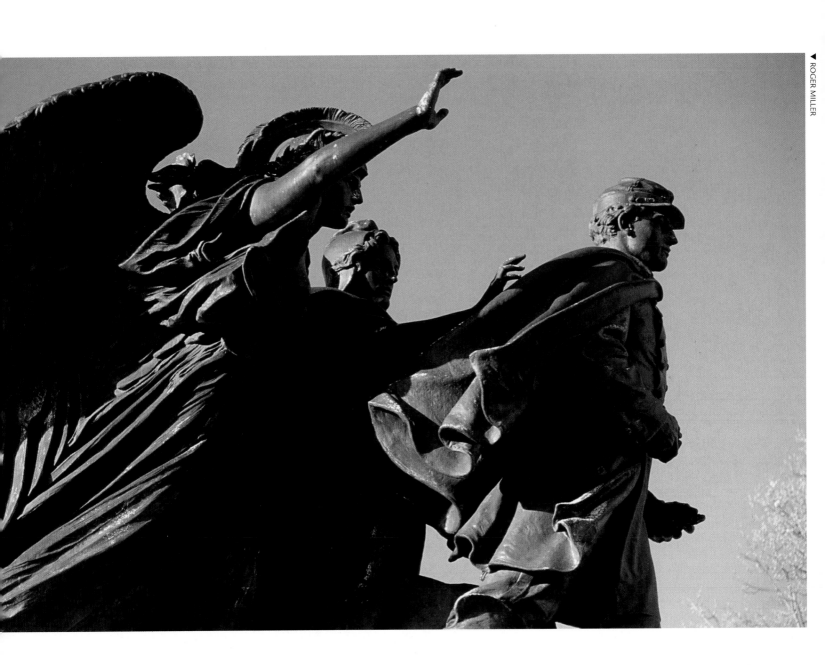

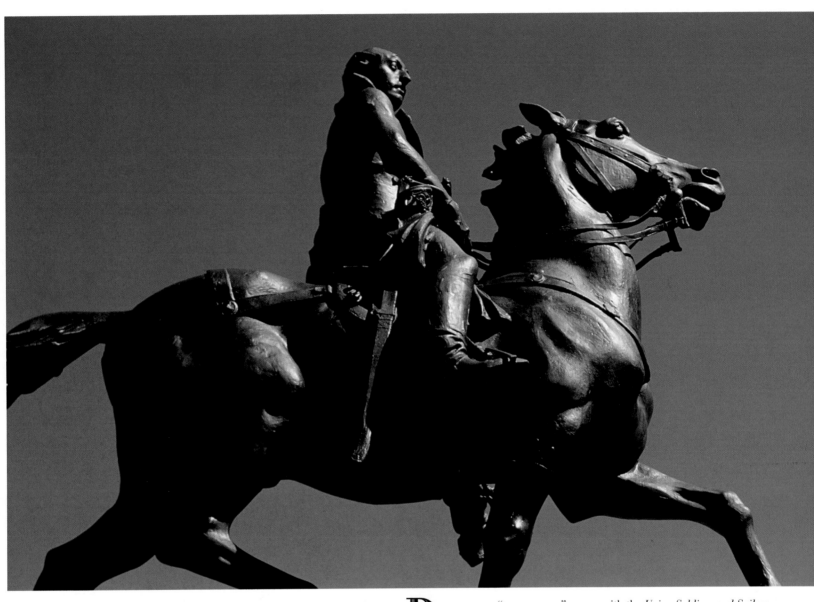

B ALTIMORE IS "MONUMENTAL" for countless reasons, and the proof is in the pudding: The city celebrates the past in grand style with the *Union Soldiers and Sailors* monument in Wyman Park (OPPOSITE) and the statue of Marquis de Lafayette in Mount Vernon Square (ABOVE).

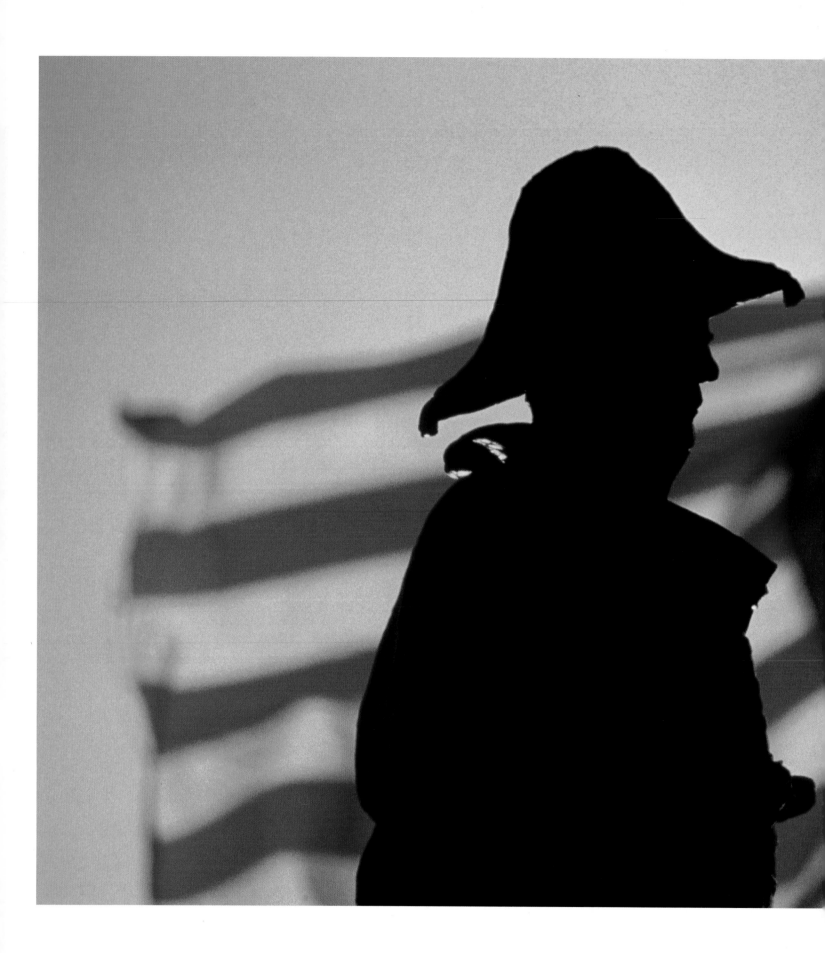

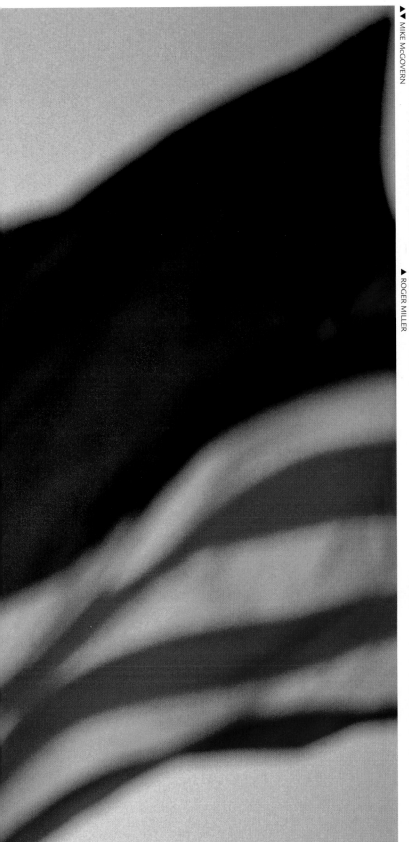

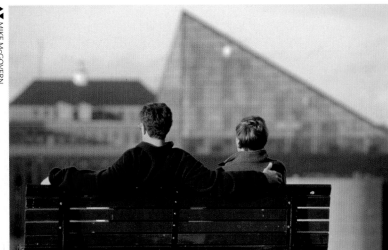

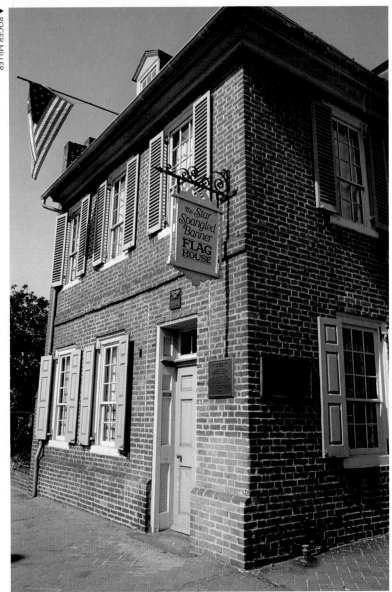

Just after midnight on September 13, 1814, British naval forces began their famous attack on Major General Samuel Smith and his stalwart American troops. Francis Scott Key, a lawyer from Frederick who witnessed the failed invasion at Fort McHenry, was so moved that he penned *The Star-Spangled Banner*. Today, Baltimore's Federal Hill, where a statue of Smith stands proudly (OPPOSITE), is still one of the best places to watch fireworks over the harbor (TOP), while the Star-Spangled Banner House, near Little Italy, is the only place to see the original 15-star, 15-stripe flag that survived the British attack (BOTTOM).

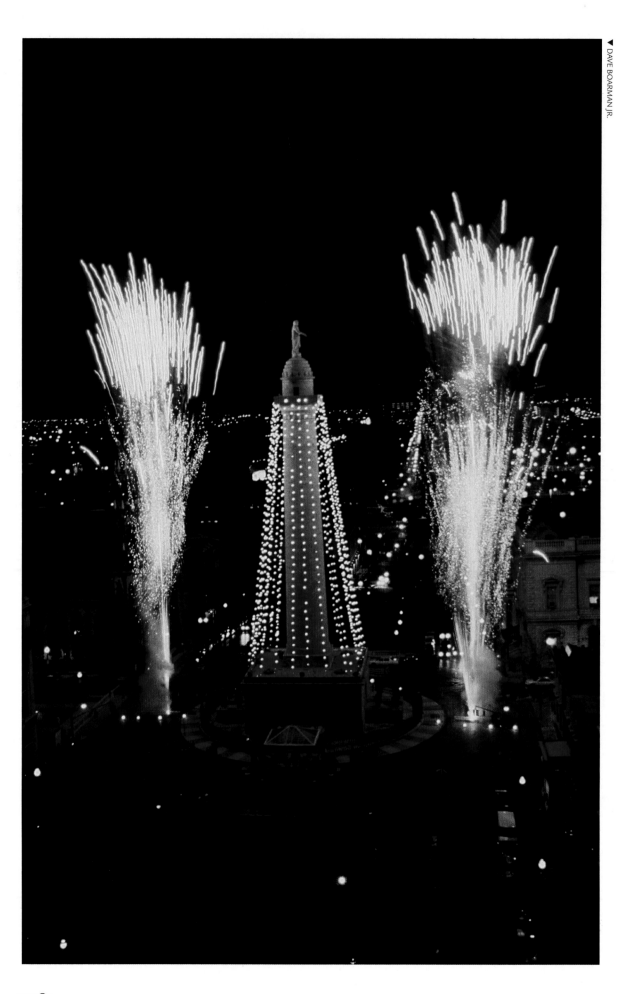

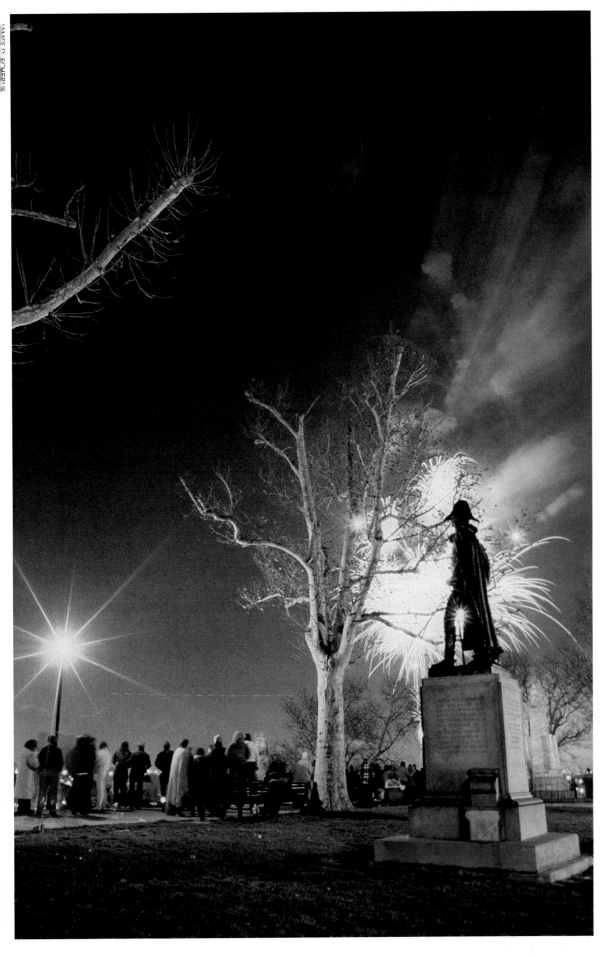

PATRIOTIC BALTIMORE CELEBRATES its prominent role in American history with spectacular fireworks displays near the Washington Monument in Mount Vernon Square (OPPOSITE) and in view of the statue honoring Major General Samuel Smith on Federal Hill (LEFT).

U SED AS A CIVIL WAR PRISON AND hospital, not to mention the famous fortress in the War of 1812, Fort McHenry today is a national monument topped by a replica of the flag that inspired the national anthem.

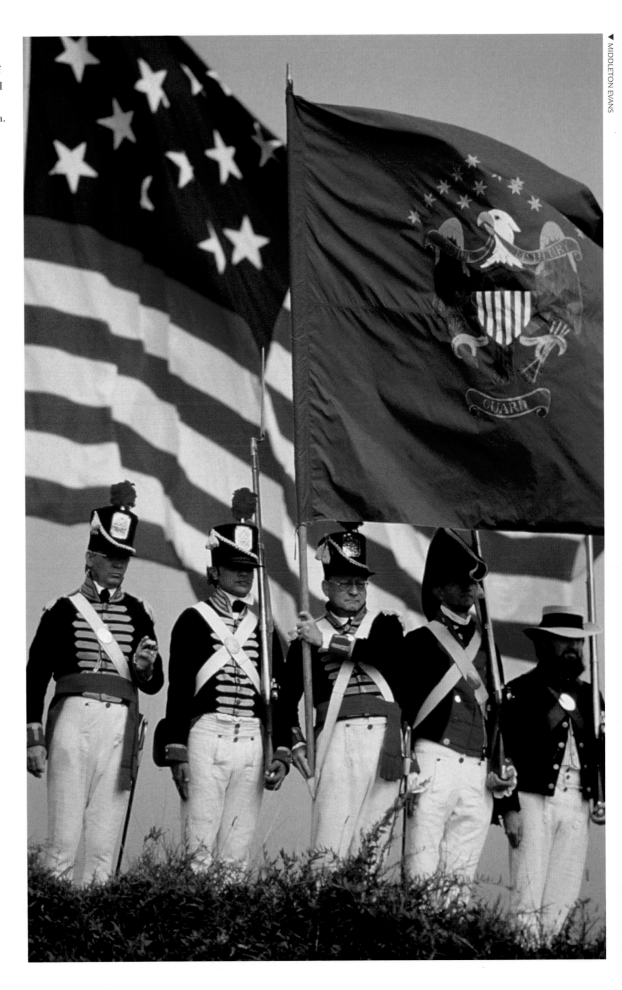

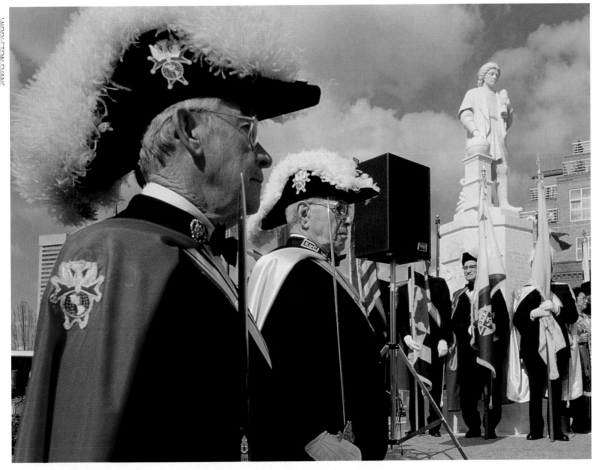

COMMEMORATIONS OF HISTORIC events are commonplace in Baltimore, from a Columbus Day celebration around the marble statue of Christopher Columbus at Eastern Avenue and President Street (TOP) to a reenactment of the Battle of North Point at Fort McHenry (BOTTOM).

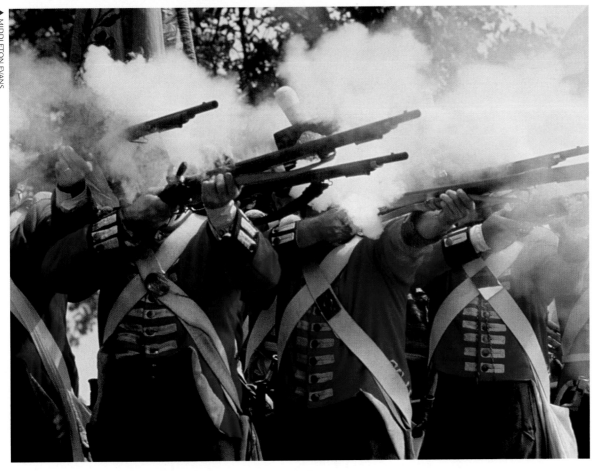

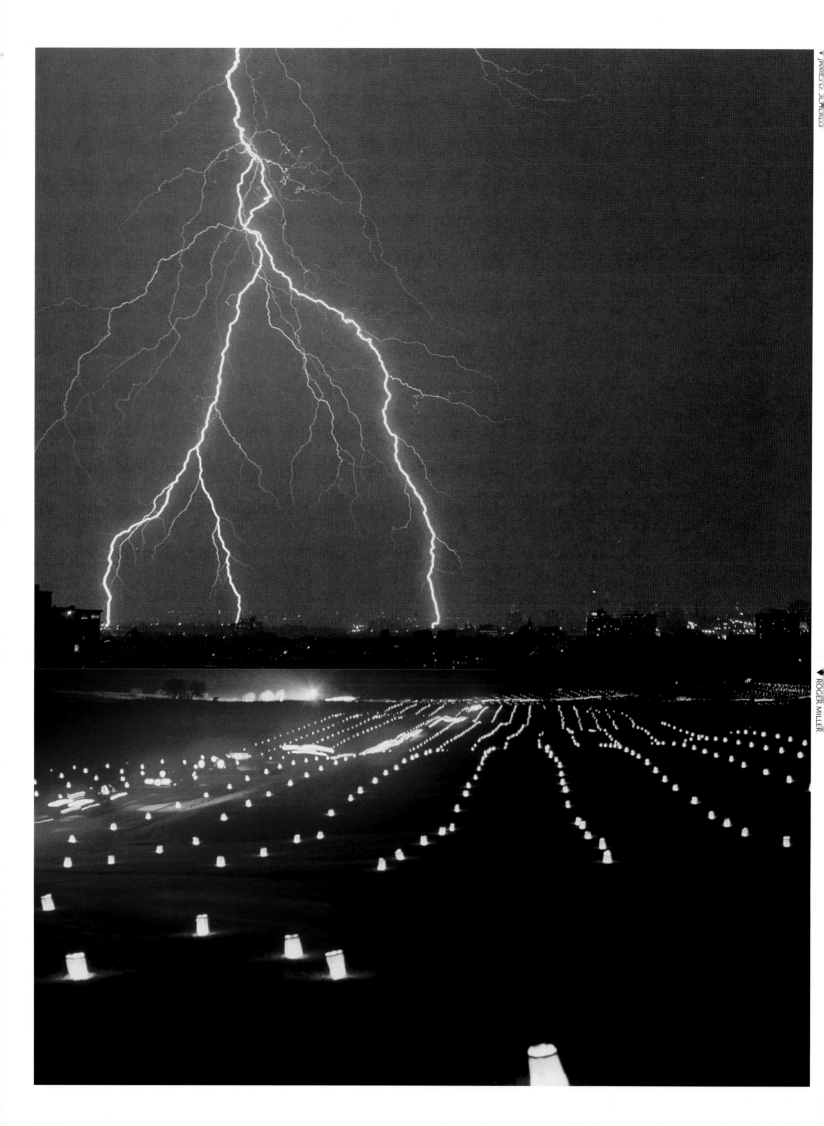

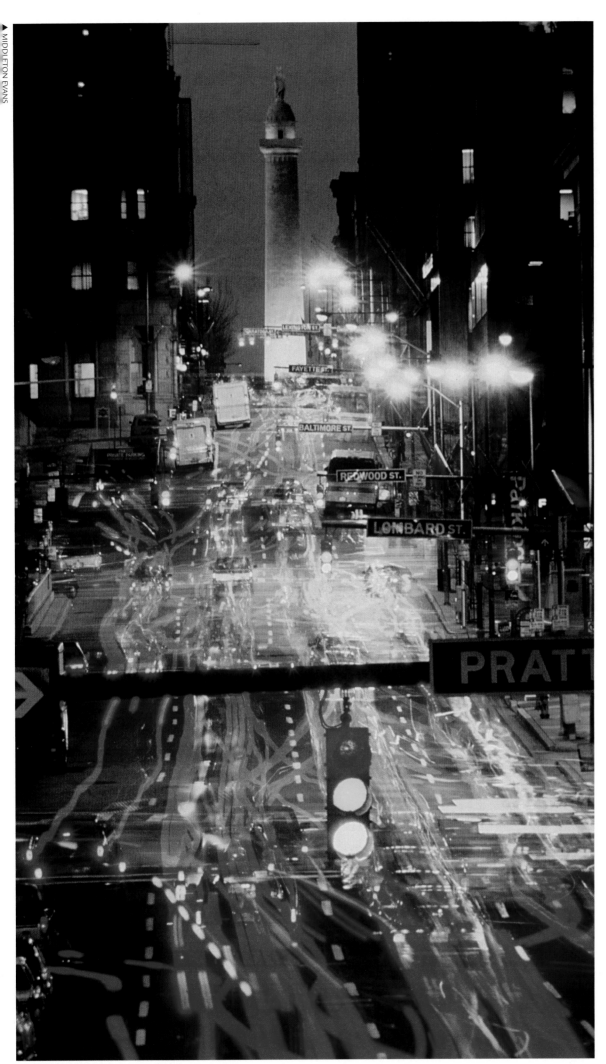

LIGHT HAS MANY SOURCES AND MANY meanings in Charm City. A dramatic bolt of lightning warns of stormy weather, thousands of headlights on Charles Street foreshadow an unusually long commute, and luminarias at the Antietam National Battlefield Site evoke a haunting nostalgia for the bloodiest conflict in the Civil War.

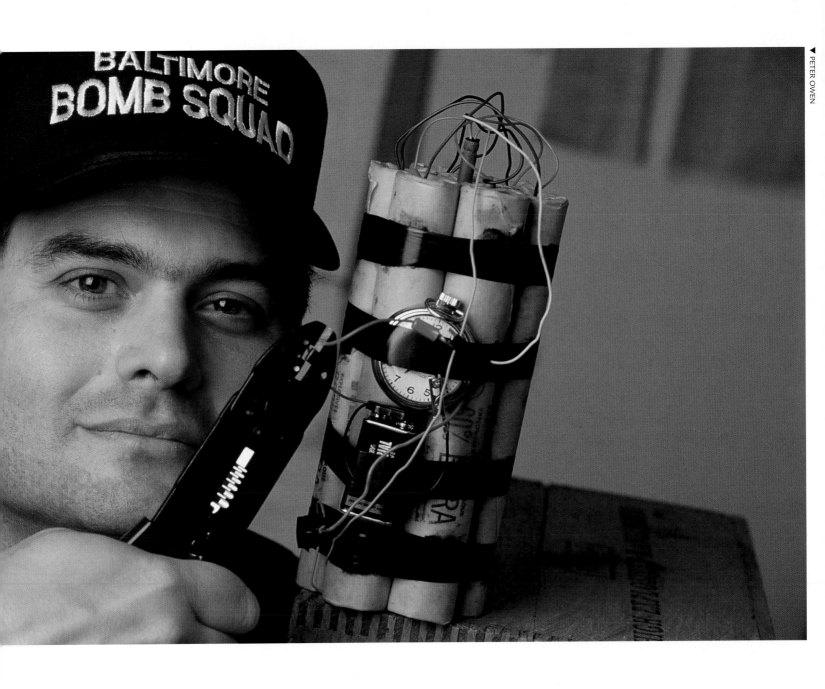

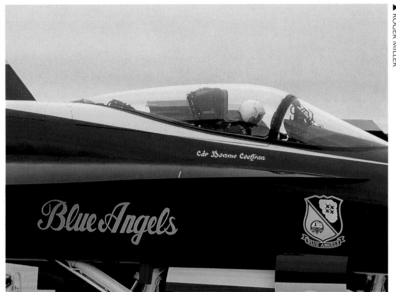

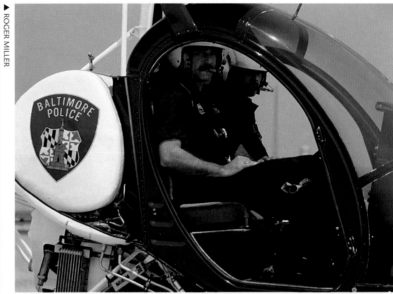

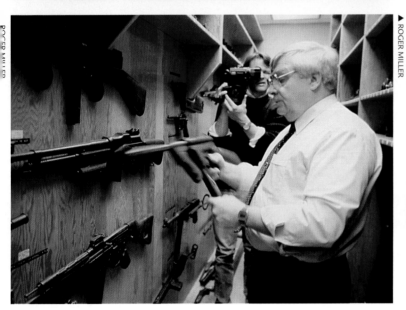

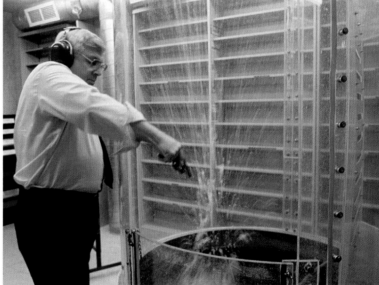

S INCE *Homicide: Life on the Street* first aired in 1991, Baltimoreans have gained new respect for the city's public servants, who risk it all to protect and serve. But the Baltimore Police aren't the only men in blue. The U.S. Navy's Blue Angels defy gravity and thrill audiences with their high-flying maneuvers (TOP LEFT).

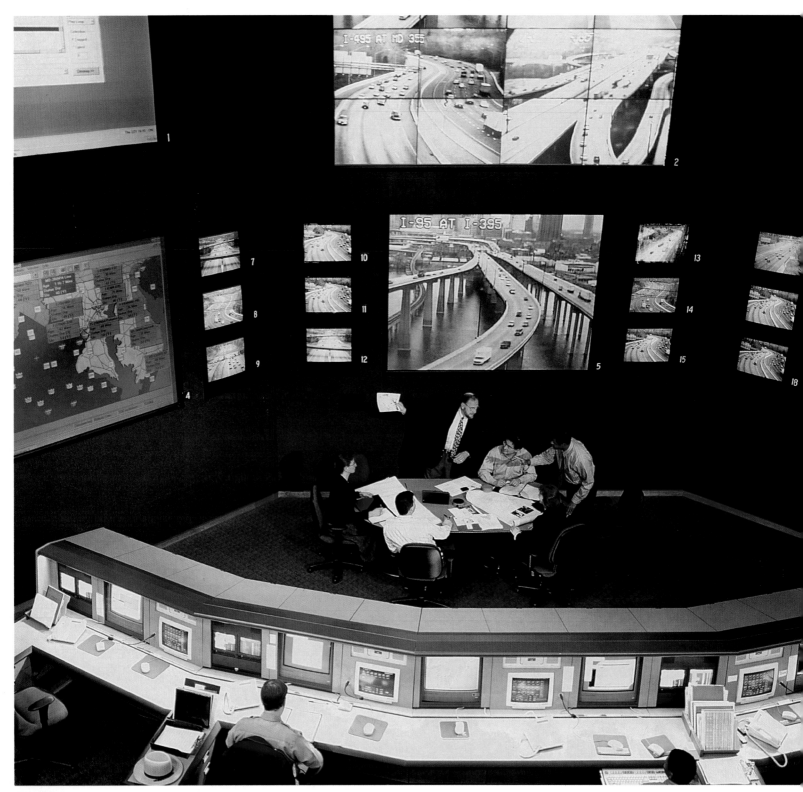

MARYLAND'S DEPARTMENT OF Transportation employs modern technology to monitor the state's highways (ABOVE), while the famed R. Adams Cowley Shock Trauma Center benefits from cutting-edge equipment that keeps up-to-the-minute tabs on medical emergencies (OPPOSITE BOTTOM). For the perfect blend of technology and style, Baltimoreans can look to Lynnette Young, chief of staff for Mayor Kurt Schmoke, as she test-drives a snappy BMW Z3 (OPPOSITE TOP).

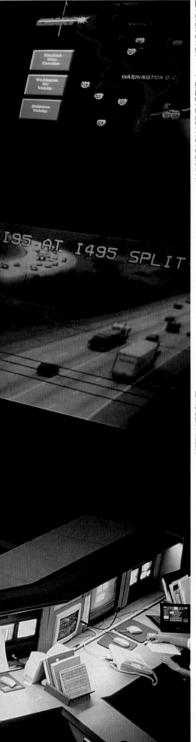

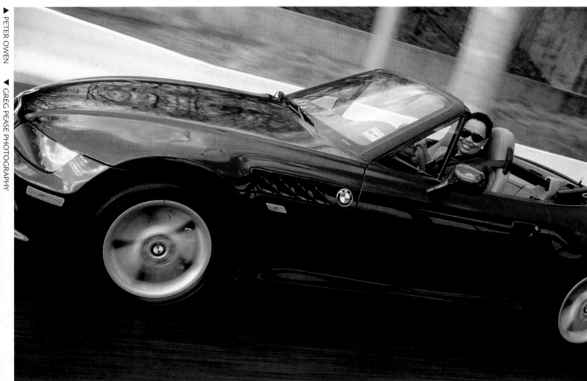

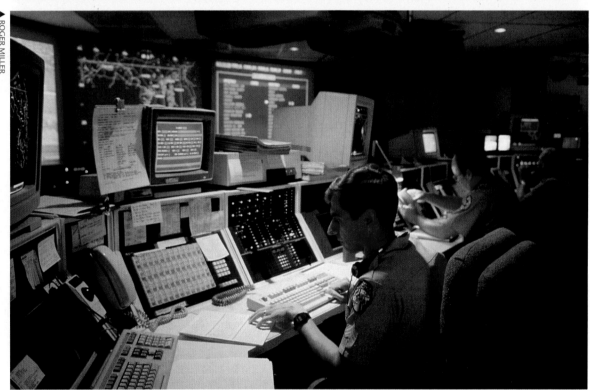

I N CHARM CITY, THERE'S NO SHORTAGE of ways to get around. Baltimore Washington International Airport, one of the fastest-growing airfields in the United States, saw some 13 million people pass through its terminals in 1996 on their way to one of 200 foreign and domestic destinations. For those who need to get from here to there within the city, the 15-mile Baltimore Metro system stretches from Owings Mills to the Charles Center (PAGES 228 AND 229).

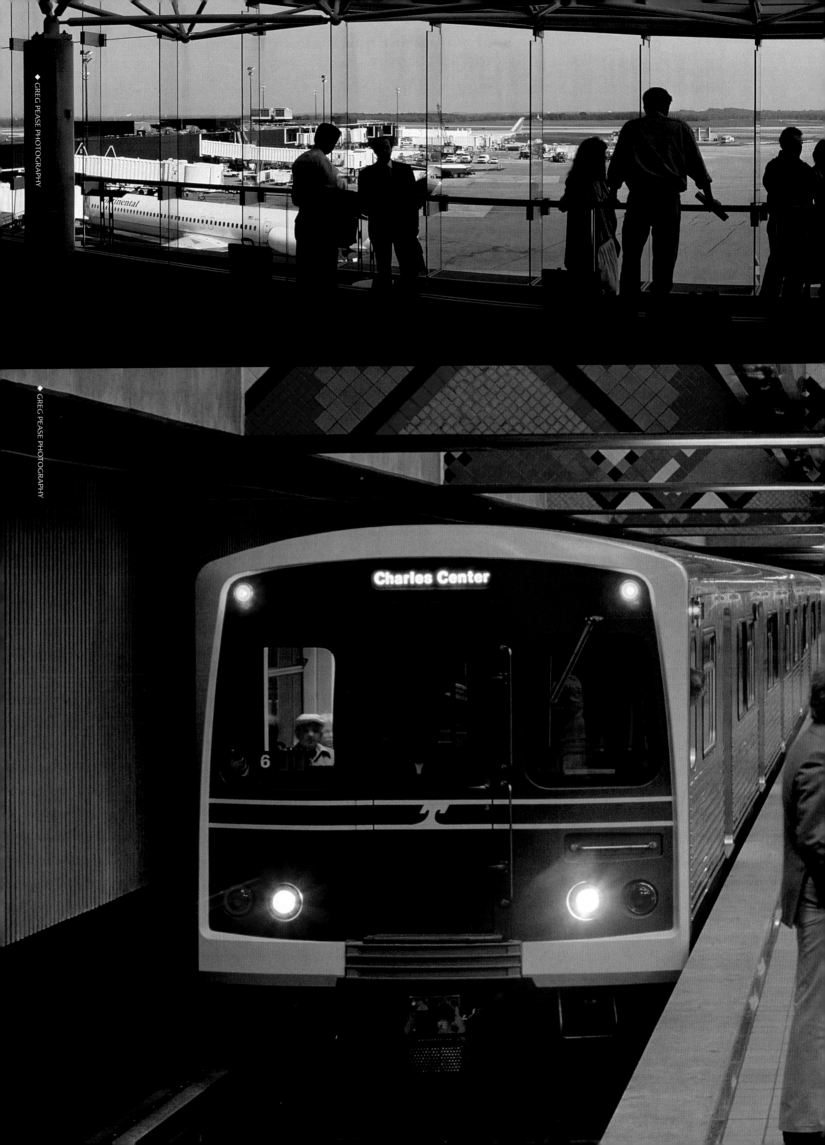

Charles Center

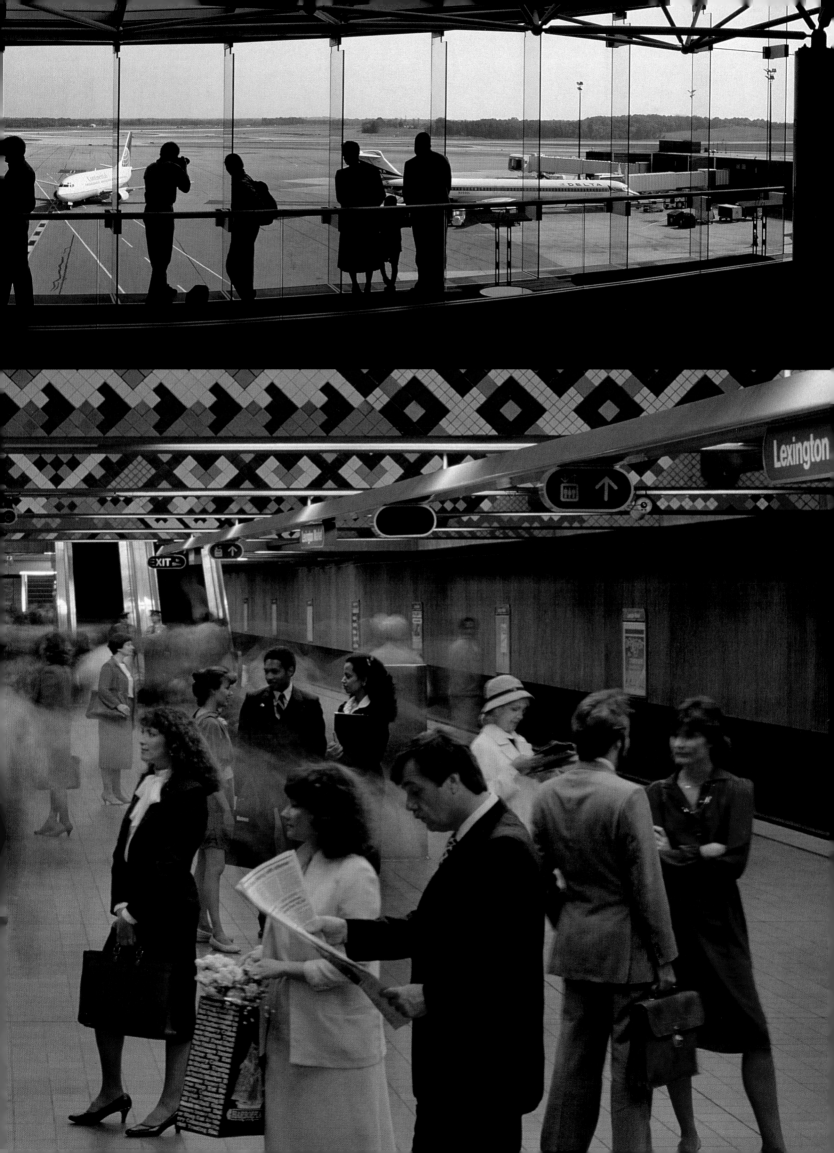

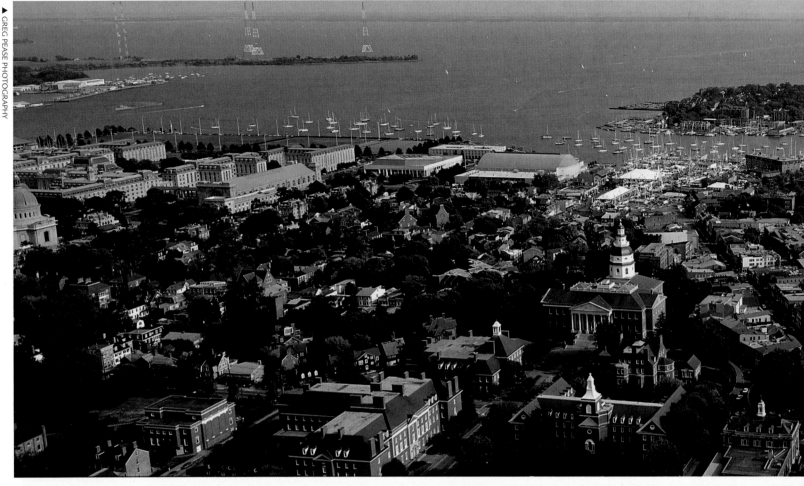

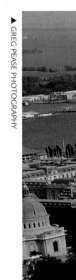

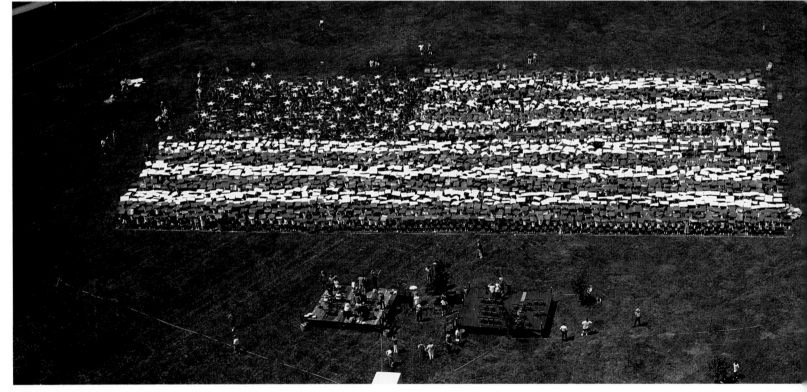

L ocated south of Baltimore, colonial Annapolis is not only the capital of Maryland, but also home to the United States Naval Academy and the site of several boat shows in the fall (top).

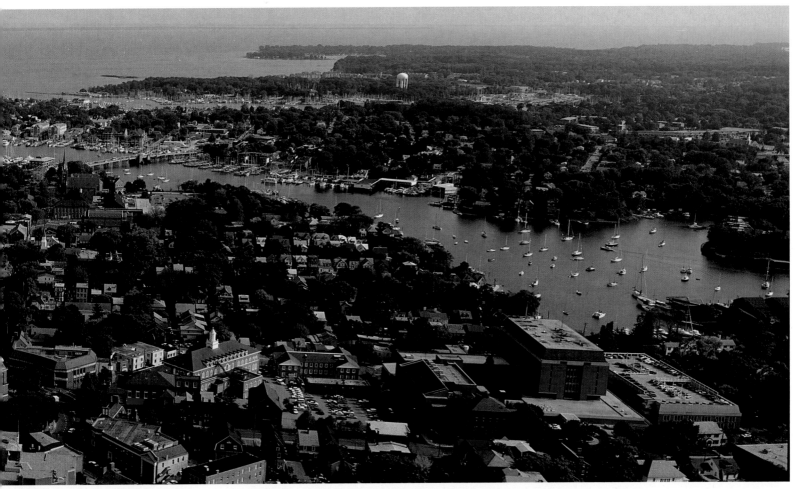

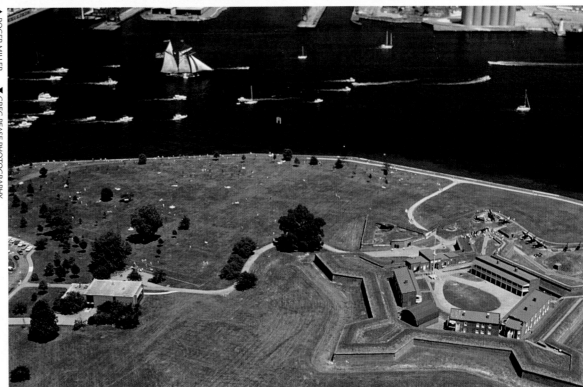

ROGER MILLER ▲

GREG PEASE PHOTOGRAPHY ▲

F IRST IN 1914, AND THEN IN EVERY
year since 1985, the pentagonal
Fort McHenry has created a
living American flag along the green
parkland that surrounds the historic
site (BOTTOM).

Life at the United States Naval Academy, the undergraduate college of the U.S. Navy, provides a unique combination of military training and academics. In return for four-year scholarships plus a monthly salary, students serve a minimum of five years in the navy or marine corps after graduation. Dubbed "four years by the Bay," this Annapolis institution has educated more than 60,000 men and women since its inception in 1845.

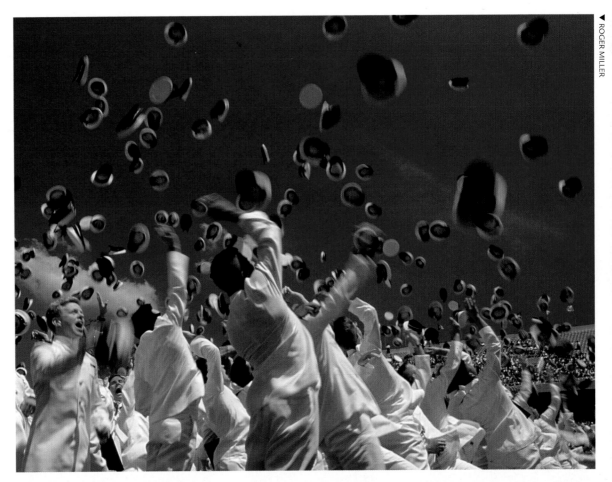

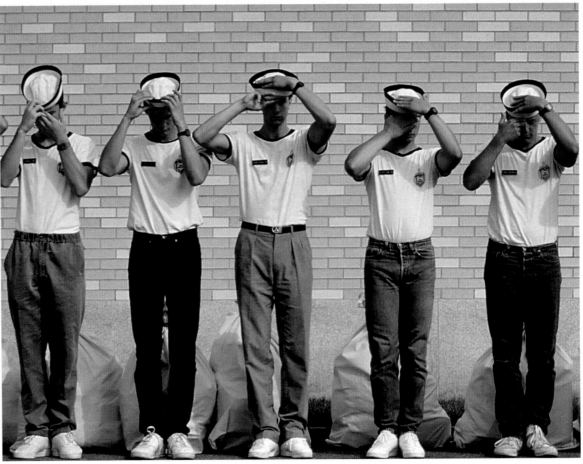

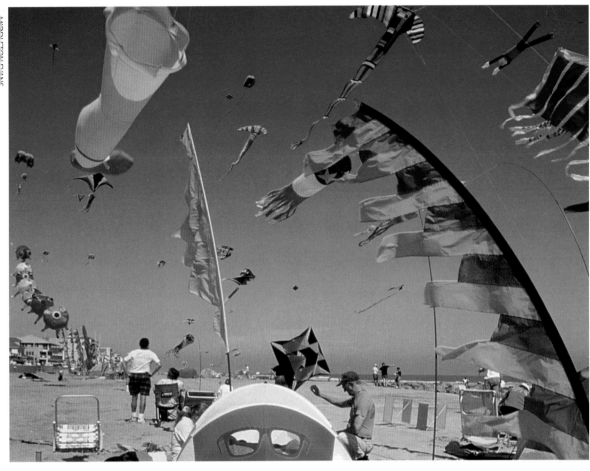

Ocean City, a seaside resort located only 120 miles from Baltimore, is a long way from the Naval Academy, at least in spirit. Equal parts scruffy, tacky, and electric—but always 100 percent fun—this beach community has its own ideas of what a lineup should be.

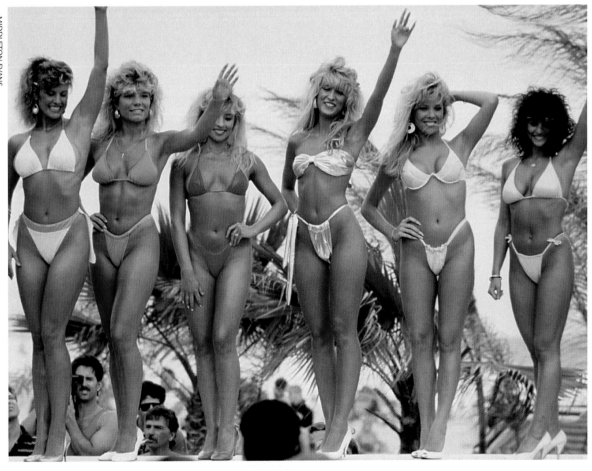

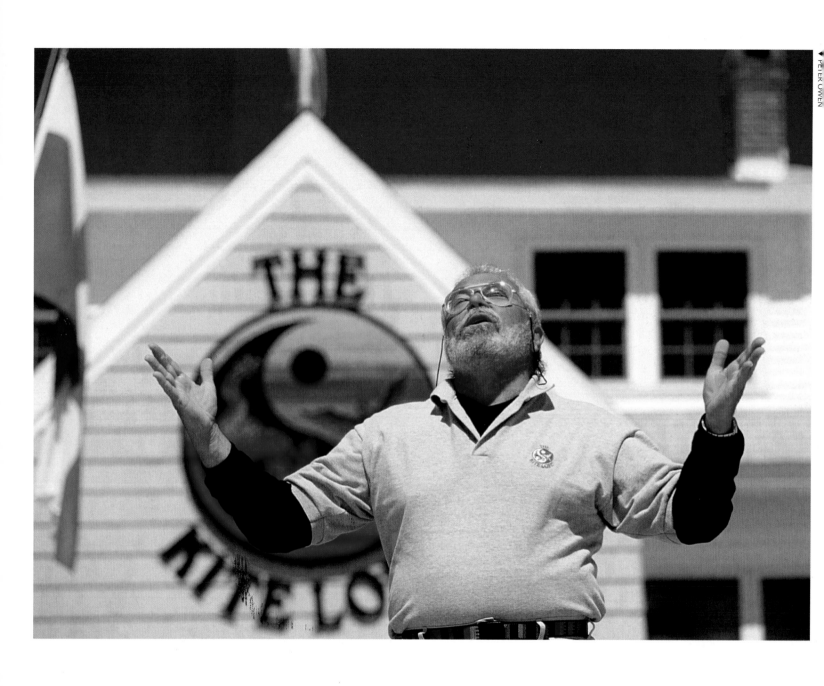

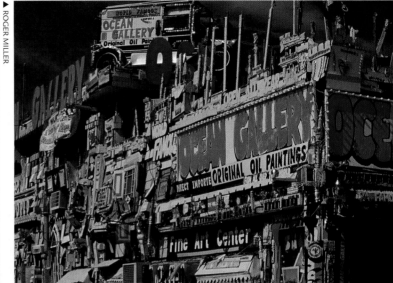

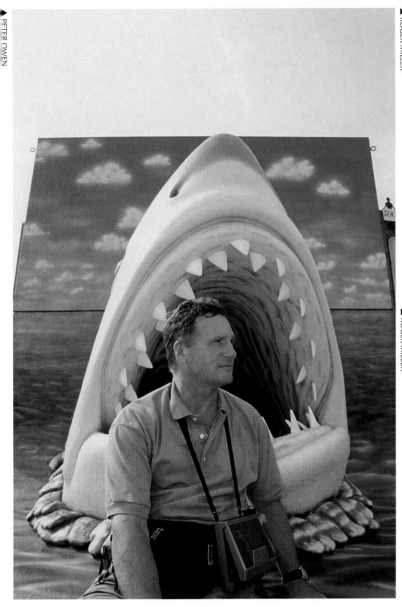

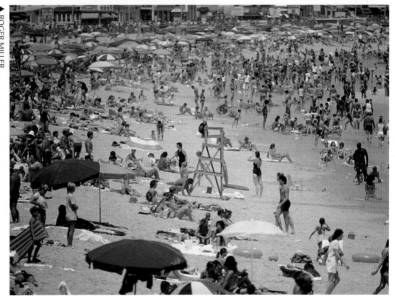

Baltimoreans can look forward to more than just the salt air in Ocean City. Local attractions range from the Kite Loft, the world's largest retailer of kites, to Ocean Gallery's eclectic selection of prints and paintings, but the town's heart is still its boardwalk and beach.

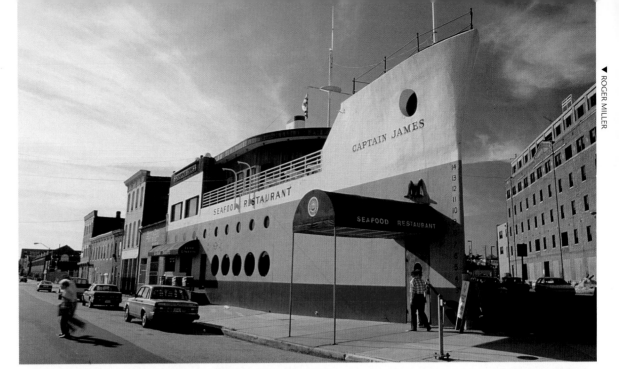

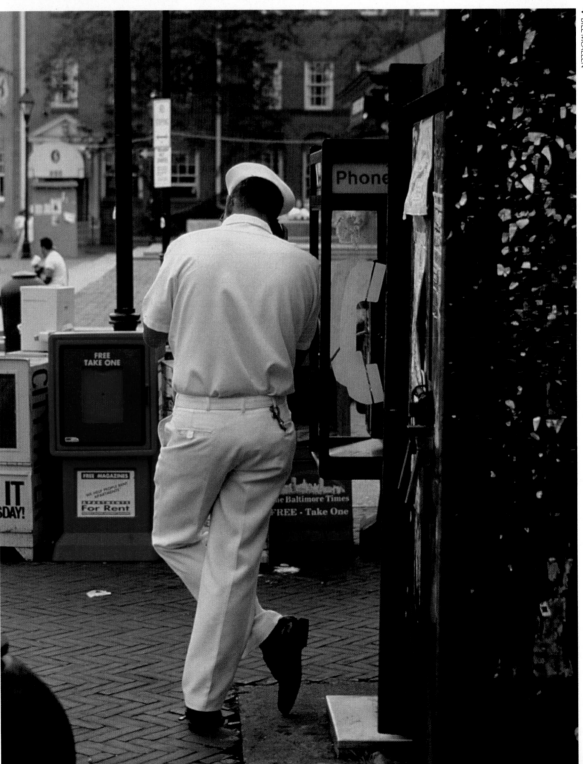

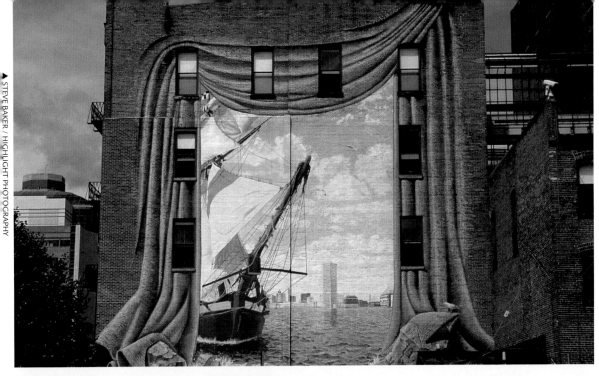

B ALTIMORE'S CONNECTION TO THE sea is reflected in scenes all over town, from the "ship-shape" Captain James seafood restaurant to a nautical-themed wall mural, and from a maritime window display in Fells Point to a uniformed sailor on shore leave.

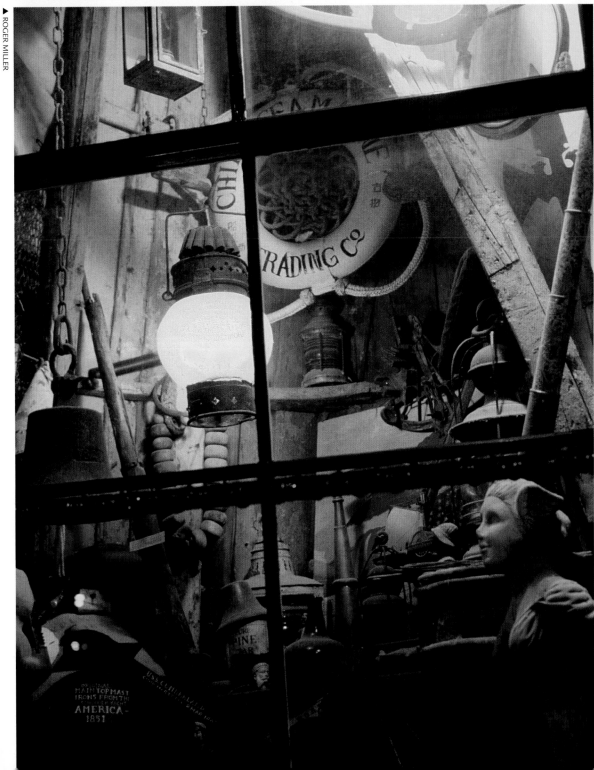

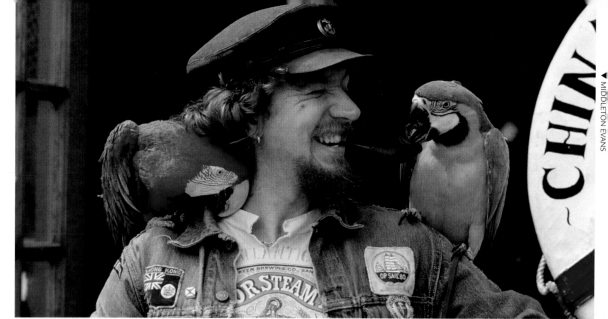

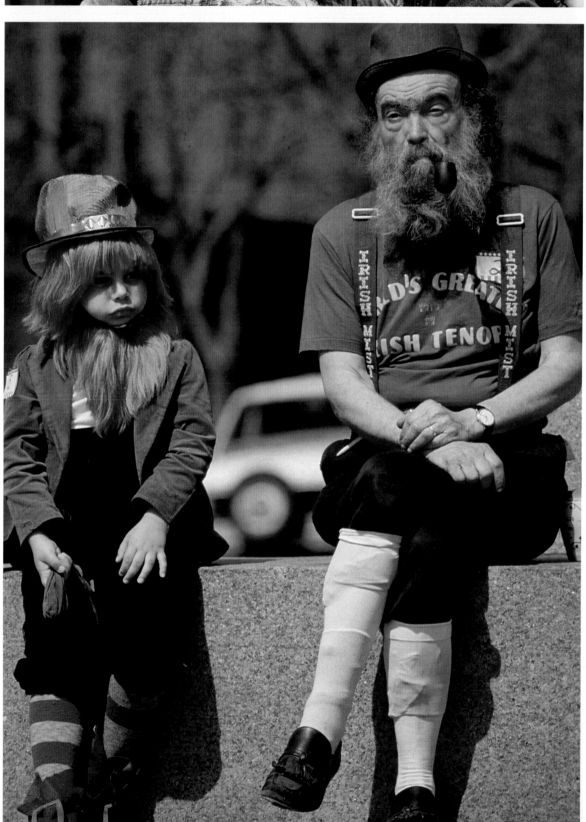

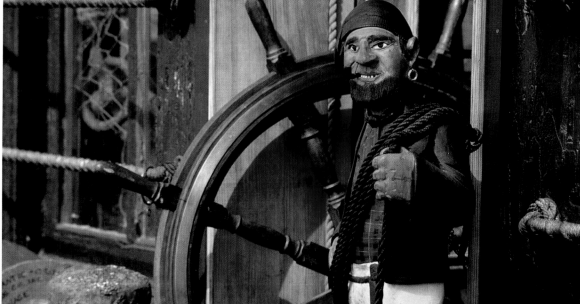

A NYTHING GOES IN FELLS POINT, where wooden sailors and real-life leprechauns are as commonplace as pipes and beards. Characters from all walks of life have converged on the historic neighborhood for centuries.

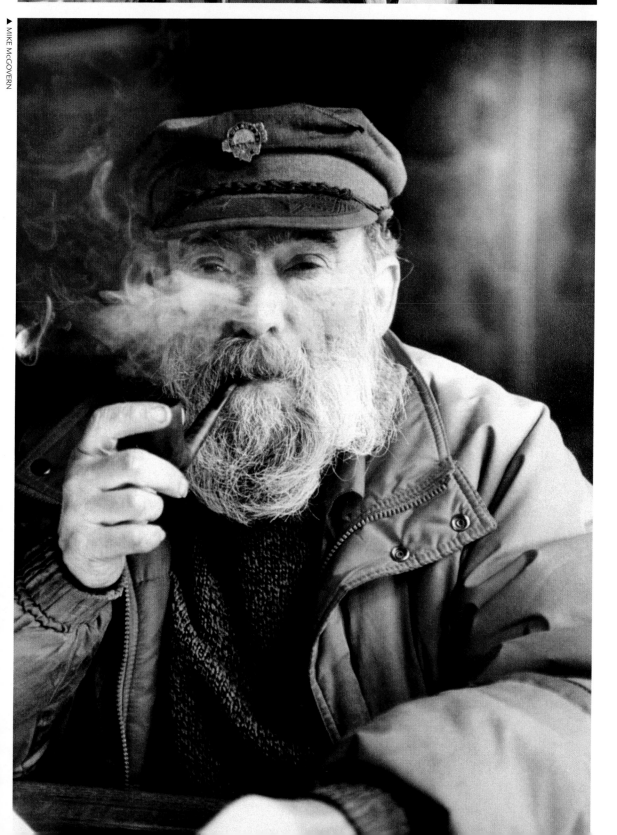

I N THE MID-1900S ON MARYLAND's
Eastern Shore, the Ward brothers
elevated the carving of decoys
to a fine art (TOP). Today, the Ward
Museum of Waterfowl Art in Salisbury
inspires present-day carvers like Joe
Leener (BOTTOM) to carry on the
tradition.

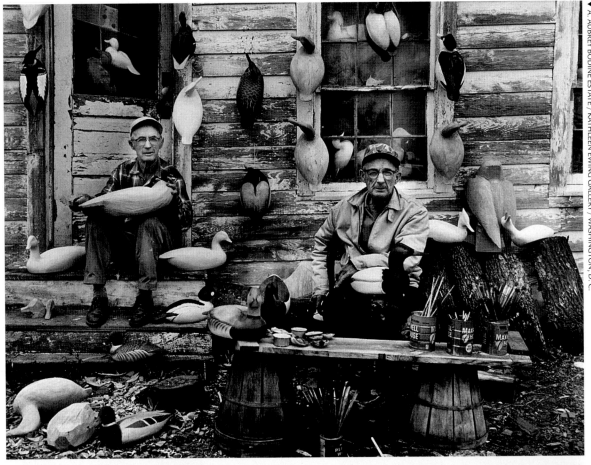

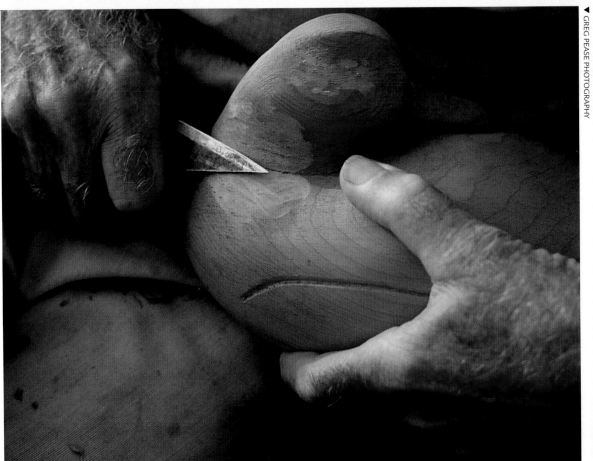

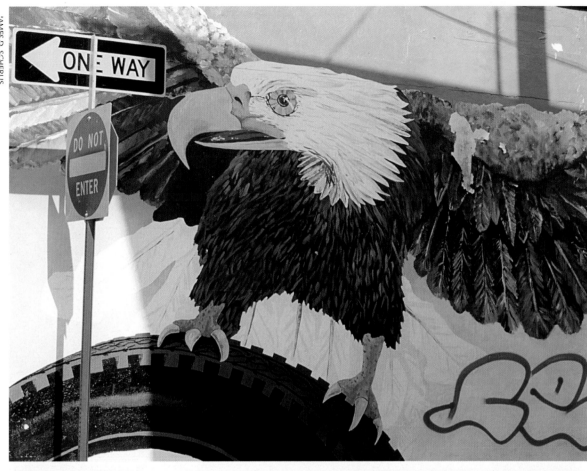

BALTIMOREANS HAVE A GREAT
admiration for their winged
friends, as evidenced by this
larger-than-life mural on the side of
a local building (TOP). Affectionately
dubbed the Canary Lady, native
resident Robin Wallace, founder of
Robin's Nest Aviaries, has made her
living creating bird sanctuaries for a
number of businesses—especially
nursing and retirement homes—in
Pennsylvania, New Jersey, Virginia,
and Maryland (BOTTOM).

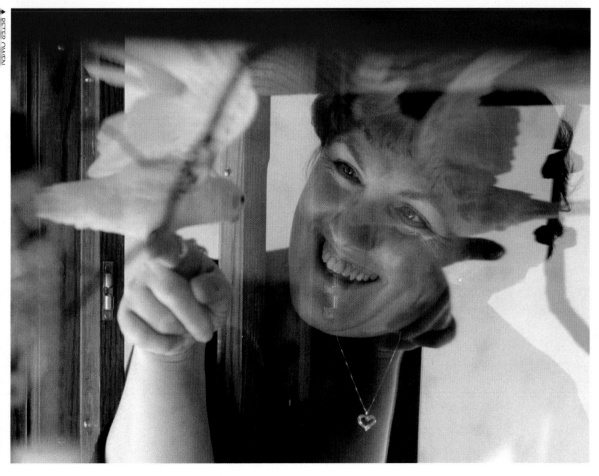

EDGAR ALLAN POE MAY HAVE SPENT much of his life in Richmond, but it was Baltimore that defined his beginnings and end. Known as the father of detective fiction, the poet is often celebrated through performances of his work and exhibits at the house he occupied from 1832 to 1835. Every January since 1949, a stranger has commemorated Poe's birthday by leaving a partial bottle of cognac and three roses at his grave site in Westminster Cemetery and Catacombs.

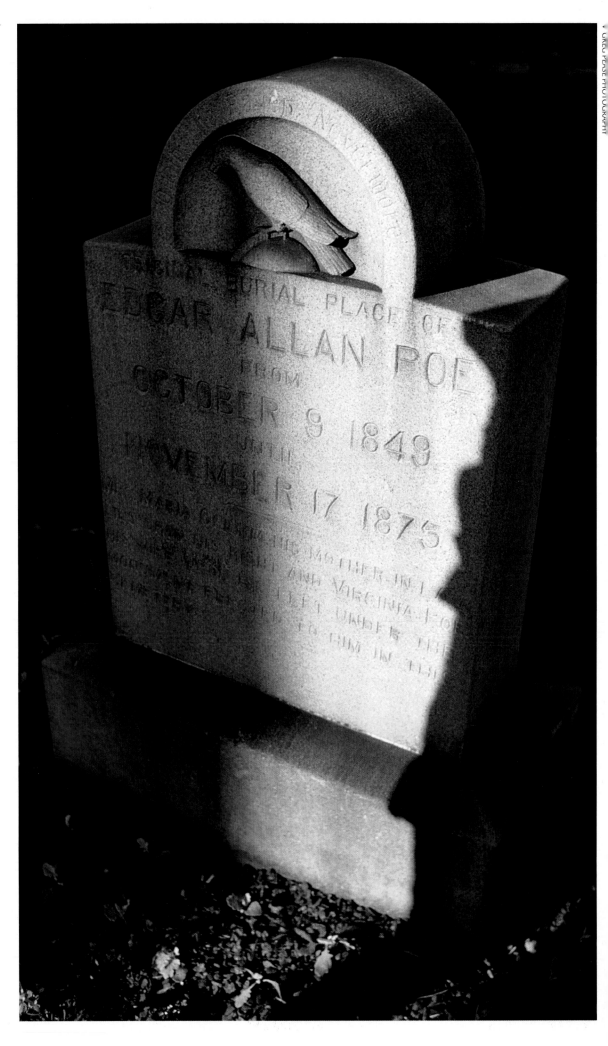

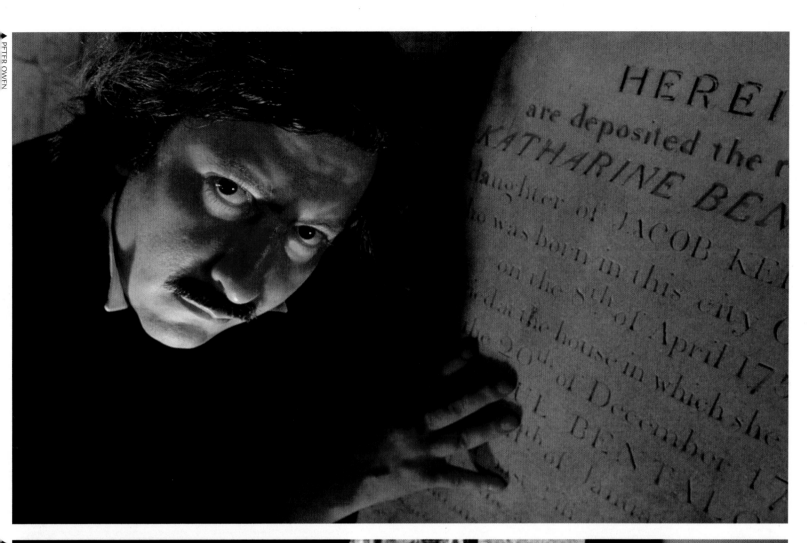

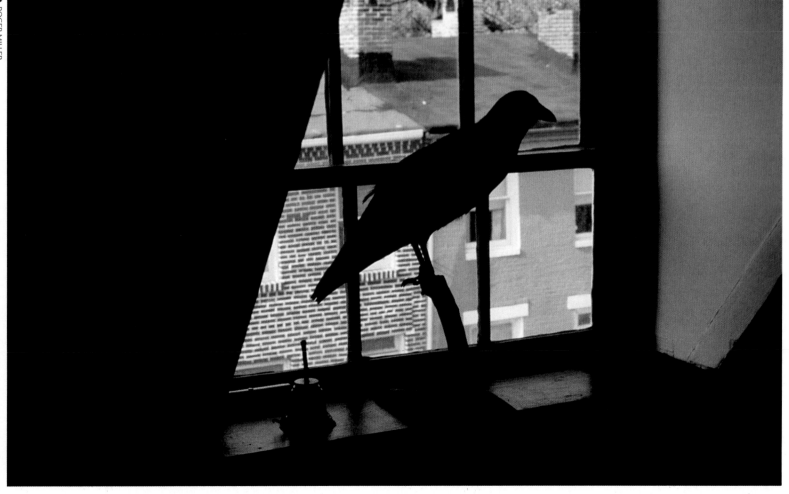

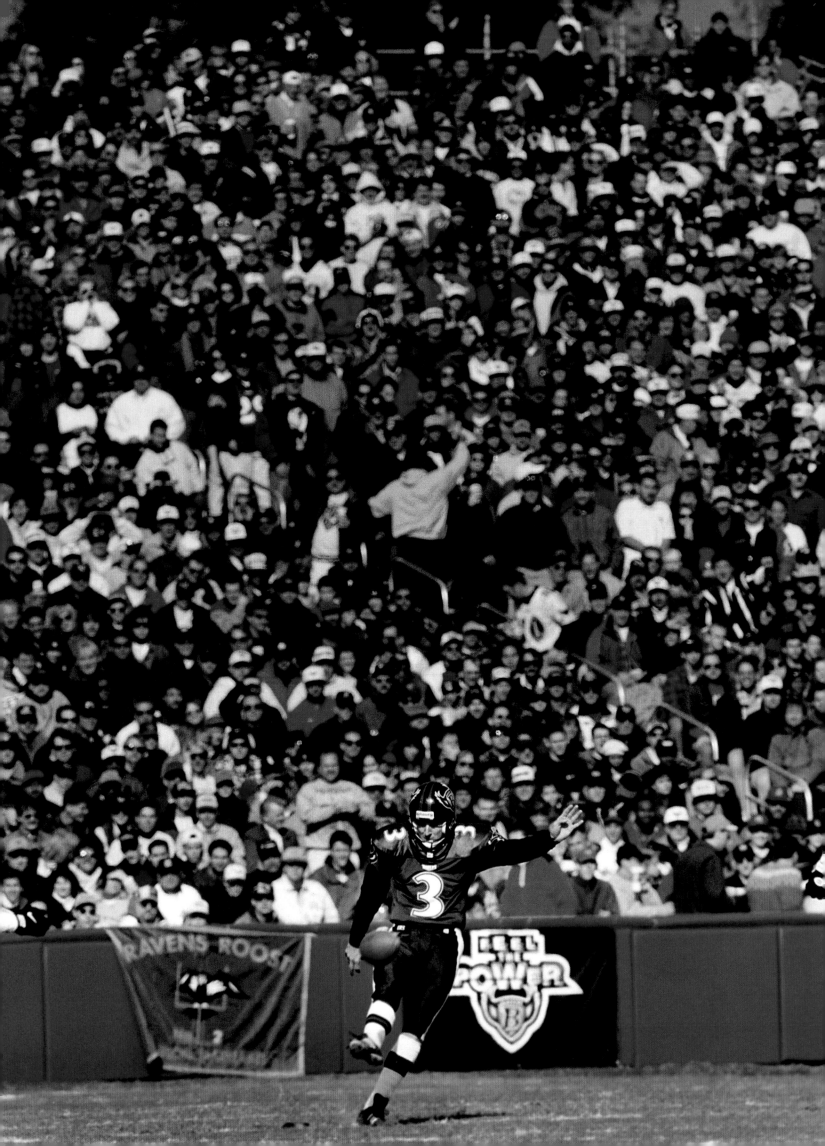

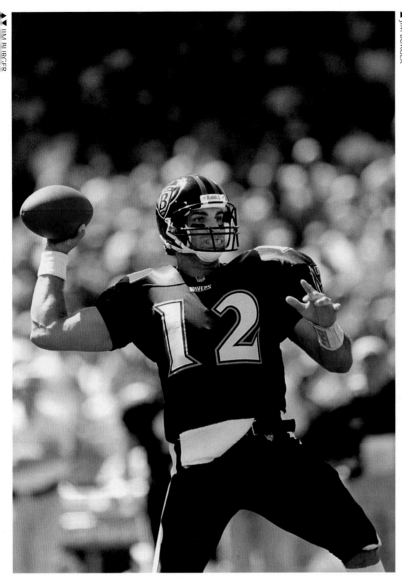

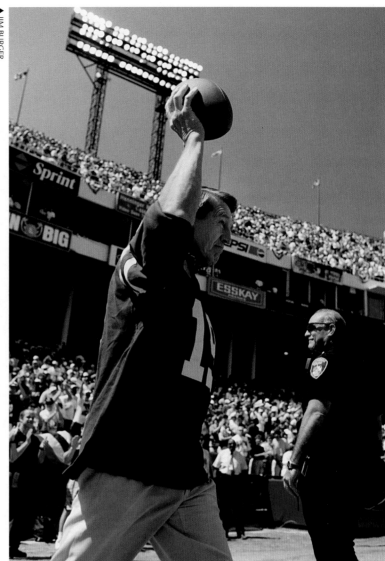

Named for Poe's masterpiece *The Raven*, Baltimore's NFL team started play in 1996, ending a 13-year drought caused by the Colts' defection to Indianapolis. In their inaugural game, famed Colt Johnny Unitas helped welcome the new team to town (RIGHT). That season, the Ravens had 10 sellouts in 10 games and sold more than 56,000 season tickets.

THE OPENING DAY PARADE COM-
memorating the start of the
Orioles season is an on-again,
off-again event that began when the
team moved to Baltimore from St.
Louis in 1954 (TOP). Regardless, fans
turn out by the thousands to Oriole
Park to cheer on their beloved team.

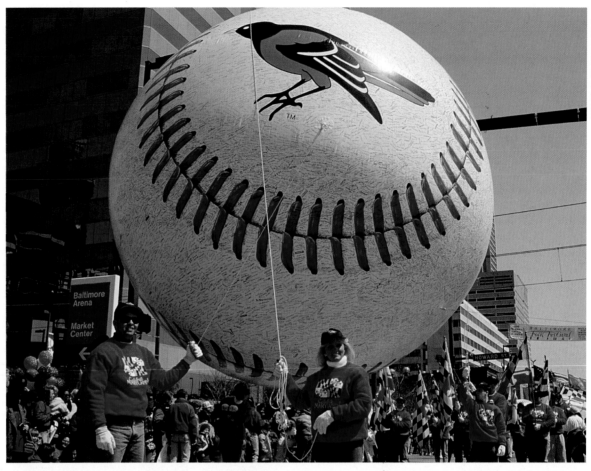

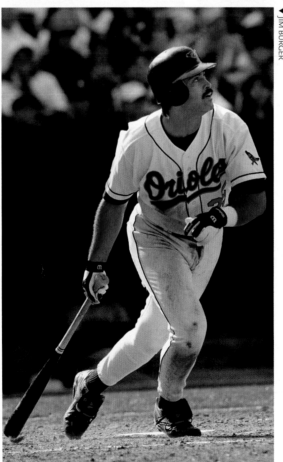

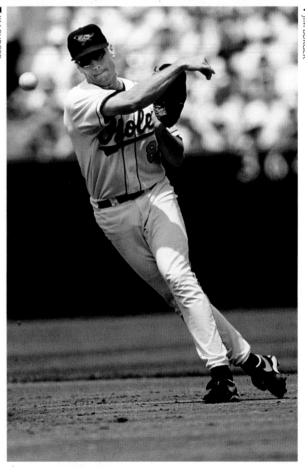

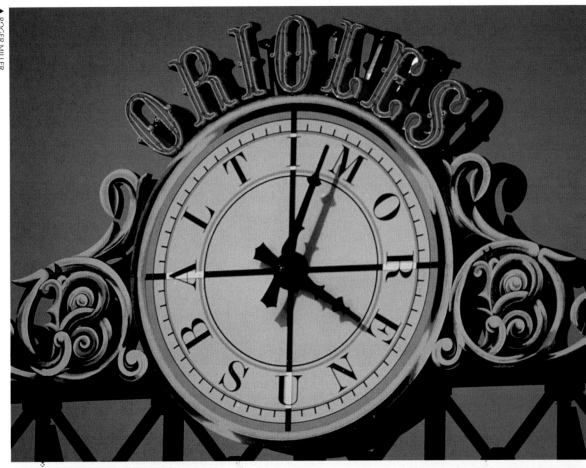

LOCATED AROUND THE STADIUM ARE a number of sights that inspire fans and help build team spirit. The old-fashioned clock that sits atop the scoreboard blends well with the ballpark's traditional design (TOP), while a rendering of Maryland's state bird and the team's namesake draws Orioles fanatics young and old (BOTTOM).

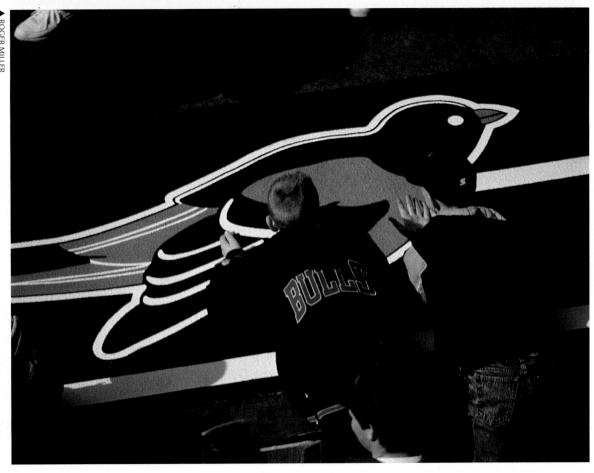

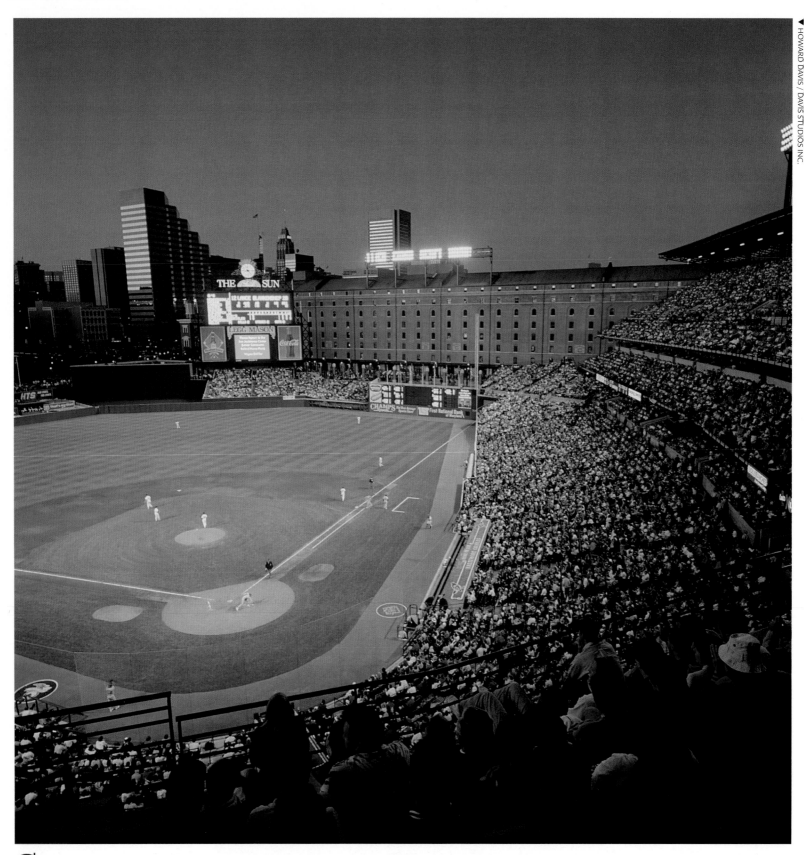

S ELLOUT CROWDS AT ORIOLE PARK have been the rule rather than the exception since it opened in 1992. Even when the stands are empty and the dugout's quiet, you can almost hear the fans cheering.

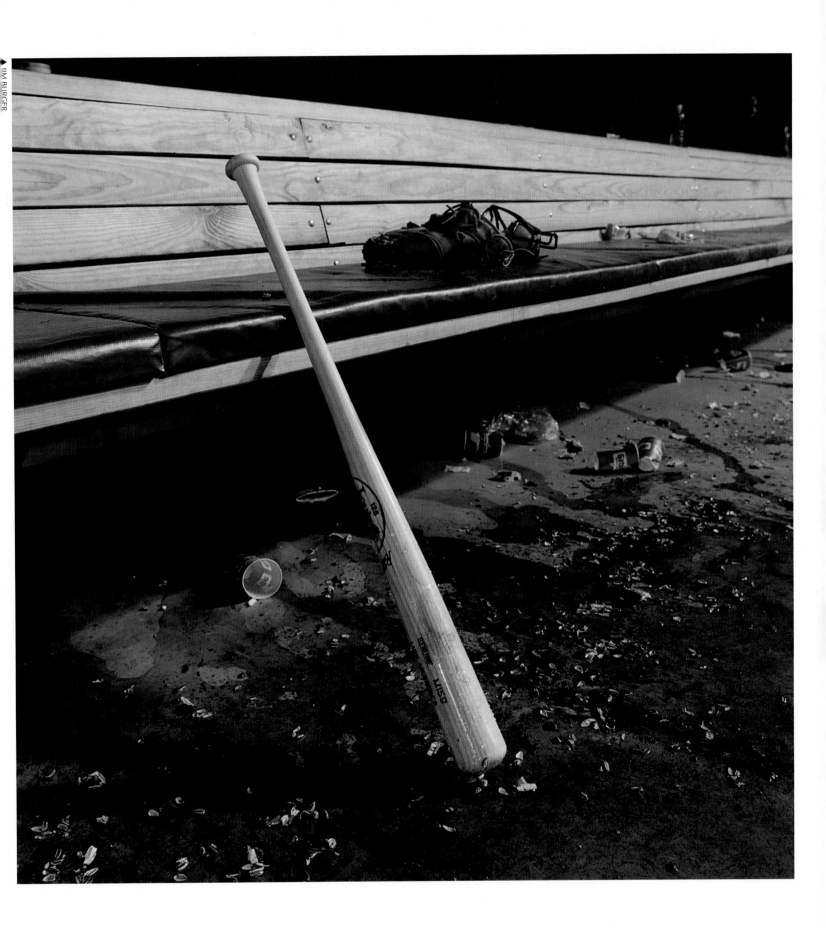

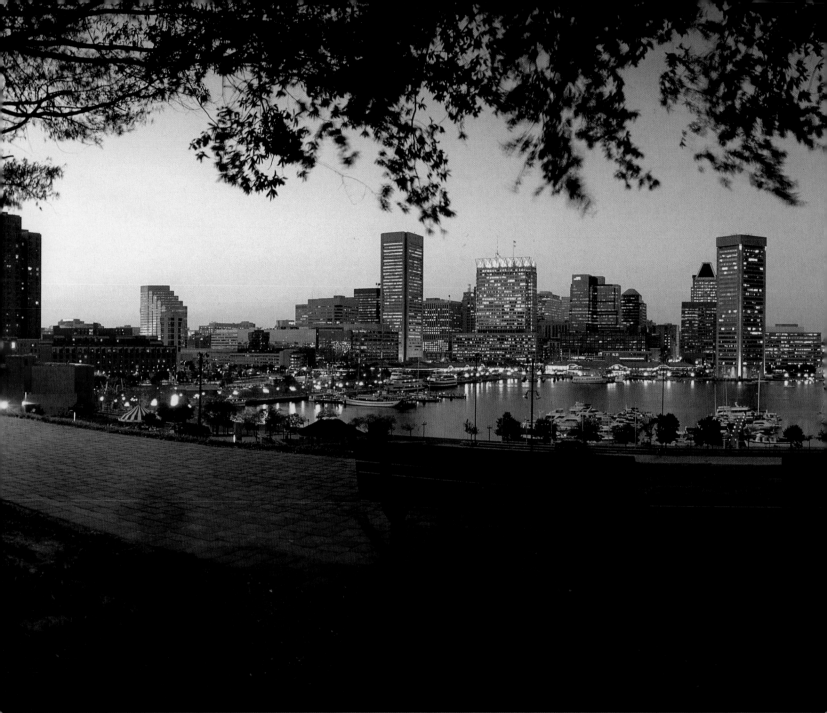

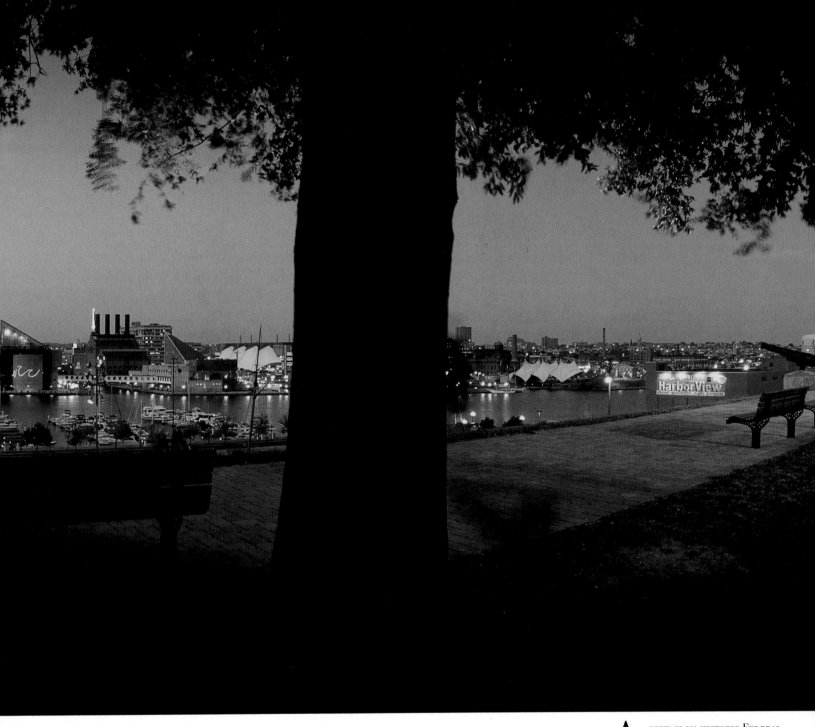

A VIEW FROM HISTORIC FEDERAL Hill reveals a city on the move. From the glow of the Inner Harbor to downtown's sleek office towers to the suburbs that stretch for miles, Baltimore proclaims its enduring charm time and again.

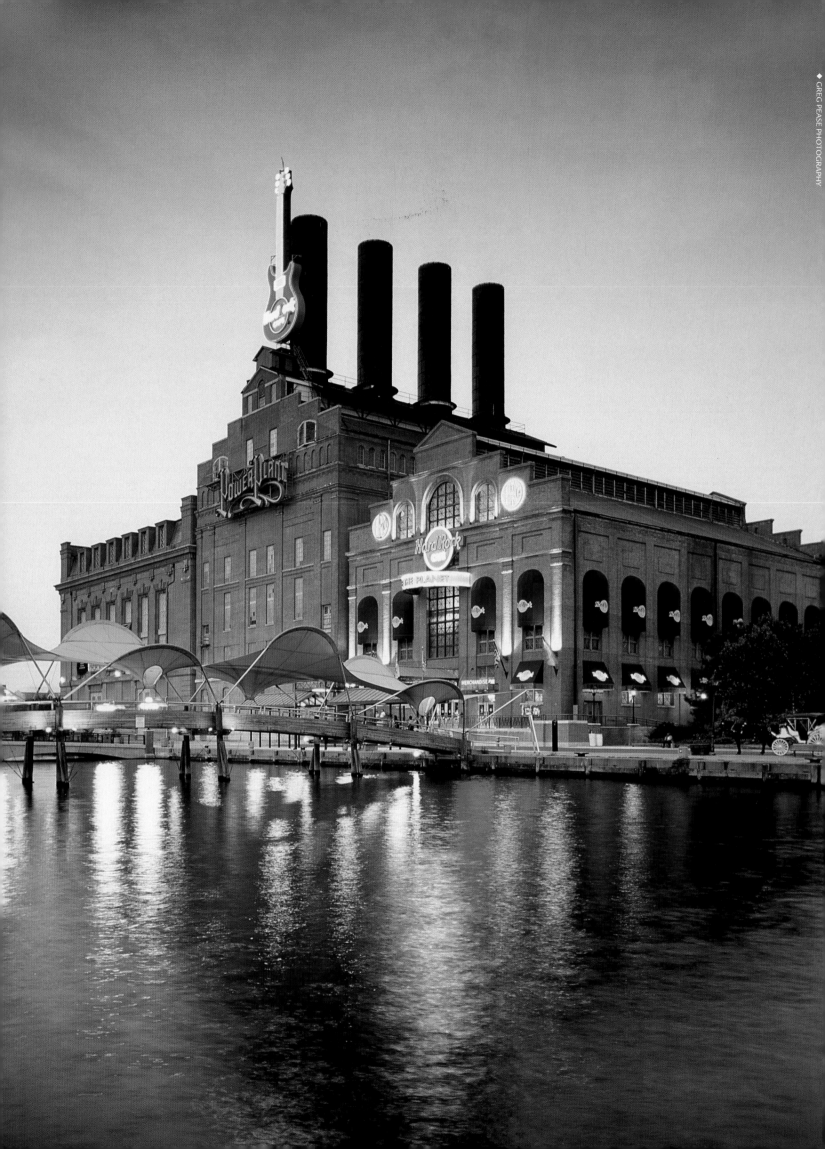

Baltimore

PROFILES IN EXCELLENCE

A LOOK AT THE CORPORATIONS, BUSINESSES, PROFESSIONAL GROUPS, AND COMMUNITY SERVICE ORGANIZATIONS THAT HAVE MADE THIS BOOK POSSIBLE. THEIR STORIES—OFFERING AN INFORMAL CHRONICLE OF THE LOCAL BUSINESS COMMUNITY—ARE ARRANGED ACCORDING TO THE DATE THEY WERE ESTABLISHED IN BALTIMORE.

THE AFRO-AMERICAN COMPANY OF BALTIMORE CITY, INC. ∾ ALBAN TRACTOR CO. INC. ∾ ANNIE E. CASEY FOUNDATION ∾ AVESTA SHEFFIELD EAST INC. ∾ BALTIMORE BUSINESS JOURNAL ∾ BALTIMORE LIFE INSURANCE CO. ∾ BALTIMORE MARRIOTT INNER HARBOR ∾ THE BALTIMORE MUSEUM OF ART ∾ BALTIMORE OPERA COMPANY ∾ BALTIMORE RAVENS ∾ BALTIMORE SPICE, INC. ∾ THE BALTIMORE SUN ∾ BALTIMORE SYMPHONY ORCHESTRA ∾ THE BALTIMORE ZOO ∾ BROADMEAD, INC. ∾ CELLULAR ONE ∾ CIENA CORPORATION ∾ COLLIERS PINKARD ∾ ECS TECHNOLOGIES, INC. ∾ EDENWALD/GENERAL GERMAN AGED PEOPLE'S HOME, INC. ∾ EISNER COMMUNICATIONS ∾ FILA U.S.A., INC. ∾ GREAT BLACKS IN WAX MUSEUM, INC. ∾ GUILFORD PHARMACEUTICALS INC. ∾ H&S BAKERY ∾ HARBOR COURT HOTEL ∾ HELIX HEALTH ∾ HS PROCESSING ∾ INPHOMATION COMMUNICATIONS, INC. ∾ INTEGRATED HEALTH SERVICES, INC. ∾ INTERNATIONAL YOUTH FOUNDATION ∾ JOHNS HOPKINS ∾ KAISER PERMANENTE ∾ LEGG MASON, INC. ∾ LEVER BROTHERS COMPANY ∾ LOYOLA COLLEGE IN MARYLAND ∾ MANAGEMENT RECRUITERS OF BALTIMORE/TIMONIUM ∾ MARYLAND HISTORICAL SOCIETY ∾ MARYLAND OFFICE RELOCATORS ∾ MARYLAND SCIENCE CENTER ∾ McENROE VOICE & DATA CORPORATION ∾ MY CLEANING SERVICE ∾ NATIONAL AQUARIUM IN BALTIMORE ∾ NATIONSBANK ∾ OMNI INNER HARBOR HOTEL ∾ P. FLANIGAN & SONS, INC. ∾ POLY-SEAL CORPORATION ∾ PORT OF BALTIMORE ∾ PRICE-MODERN, INC. ∾ PRO STAFF ∾ PROCTER & GAMBLE ∾ RE/MAX ADVANTAGE REALTY ∾ RIGGS, COUNSELMAN, MICHAELS & DOWNES, INC. ∾ ROLAND PARK PLACE ∾ THE ROUSE COMPANY ∾ SCHMIDT BAKING CO. INC. ∾ SHEPPARD PRATT HEALTH SYSTEM ∾ SNELLING STAFFING NETWORK ∾ SWEETHEART CUP CO. INC. ∾ SYLVAN LEARNING SYSTEMS, INC. ∾ SYSCOM, INC. ∾ SYSTEMS ALLIANCE INC. ∾ T. ROWE PRICE ASSOCIATES, INC. ∾ TAYLOR TECHNOLOGIES, INC. ∾ TOWN AND COUNTRY APARTMENTS ∾ TOWSON UNIVERSITY ∾ TREASURE CHEST ADVERTISING ∾ TRIGEN ENERGY BALTIMORE ∾ UP-TO-DATE LAUNDRY INC. ∾ VISITING NURSE ASSOCIATION OF MARYLAND ∾ THE WALTERS ART GALLERY ∾ WARD MACHINERY COMPANY ∾ WASHINGTON ALUMINUM COMPANY ∾ WBAL RADIO ∾ WBAL-TV 11 ∾ WJZ-TV ∾ WMAR-TV ∾ WOODBOURNE ∾

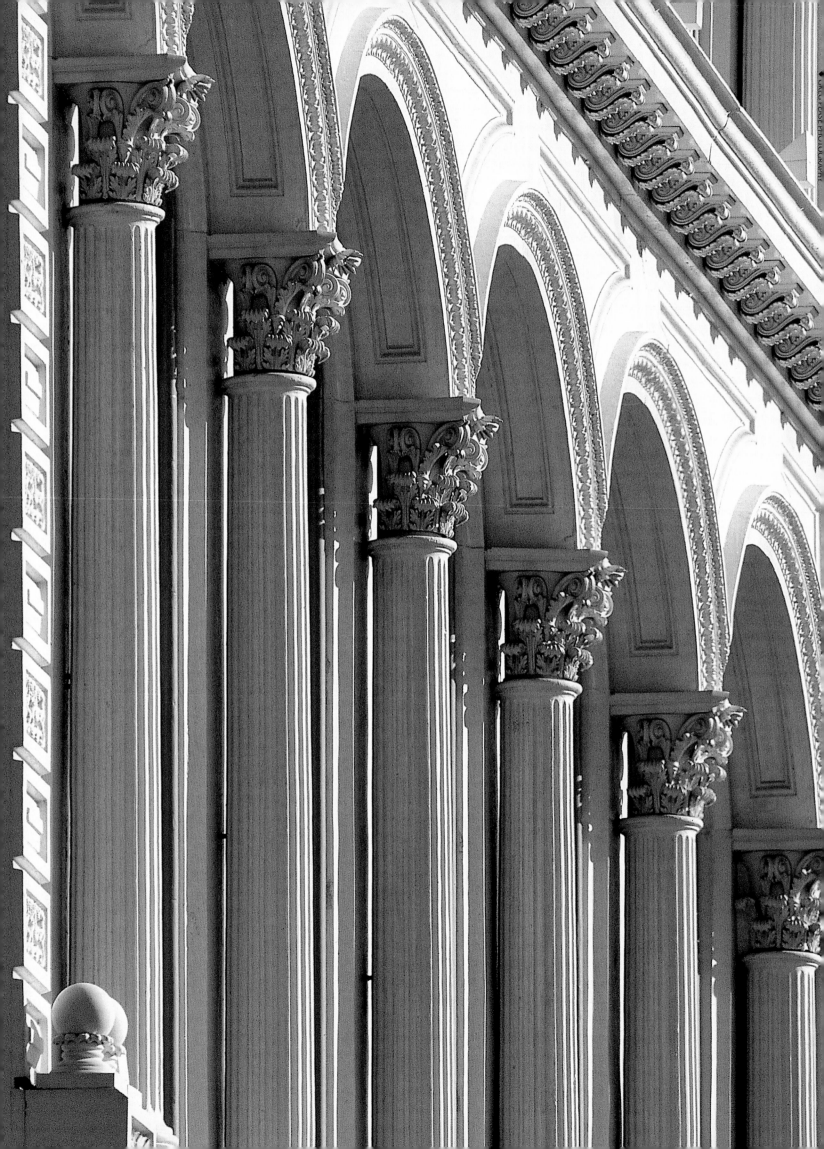

1706-1938

PROFILES IN EXCELLENCE

Port of Baltimore

Founded in 1706 on the banks of the Patapsco River, the Port of Baltimore has grown to become one of the busiest ports on the East Coast. Originally established to transport farmers' crops along the eastern seaboard, as well as cargoes to and from international destinations, today the port thrives on diversity. From automobiles to zinc, from Akron to Zhenjiang, the maritime center handles more than 30 million tons annually of all types of cargoes from around the world.

Modern Evolution

Nestled on the northwest branch of the Patapsco River, a tributary of the Chesapeake Bay, the Port of Baltimore consists of 45 miles of waterfront dotted with publicly and privately owned facilities, including Seagirt, Dundalk, North and South Locust Point, Fairfield Auto Terminal, and the Intermodal Container Transfer Facility.

It has long been said that one of the Port of Baltimore's greatest advantages is its strategic Mid-Atlantic location—and an inland setting that has made it the closest Atlantic port to major midwestern population and manufacturing centers. Its natural 14-state market area is comprised of Delaware, Illinois, Indiana, Iowa, Kentucky, Maryland, Michigan, Minnesota, Missouri, Ohio, Pennsylvania, Virginia, West Virginia, and Wisconsin, along with Washington, D.C.

In addition to its convenient geographical location, the Port of Baltimore has long maximized its enviable locale by combining on-site, state-of-the-art facilities with efficient connection to points north, south, and west. Proximity to major

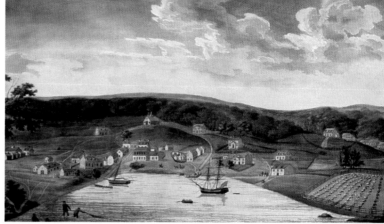

highway systems, such as Interstates 95 and 70, and a relationship dating back to 1827 with the nearby Baltimore & Ohio Railroad have been key elements in the growth of the Port of Baltimore over nearly three centuries.

As a result, it is recognized as one of the world's leading ports, routinely handling nearly 30 million short tons of foreign commerce representing more than $20.8 billion annually. Its cargoes have included aluminum oxide, coal, fertilizers, limestone, petroleum products, corn, fuel oils, soybeans, automobiles, farm equipment, iron, steel, and paper products.

But the Port of Baltimore did not achieve such growth overnight. Just as it was created 23 years before the founding of Baltimore itself, its modern evolution was also a step ahead of its time. In 1950, a group of local engineering experts, who recognized the potential economic impact of the port to the city, recommended a $129 million improvement plan. This plan, initiated six years later, resulted in the creation of the Maryland Port Authority (MPA) as a state agency.

The MPA developed the Dundalk Marine Terminal on a former harbor airfield; launched a $30 million reconstruction program on the Locust Point piers that created 15 modern berths to accommodate both rail and truck traffic; and purchased the Pennsylvania Railroad Pier I terminal in Canton. In another significant development, the MPA, whose name was changed in 1971 to the Maryland Port Administration, opened the World Trade Center. This unique, five-sided, I.M. Pei-

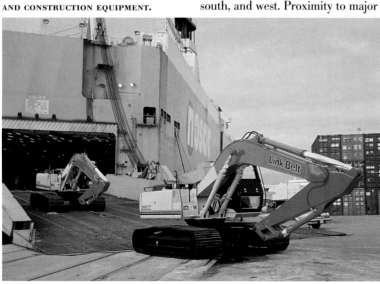

P.C. PIDLAOAN

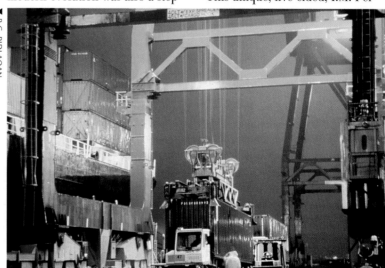

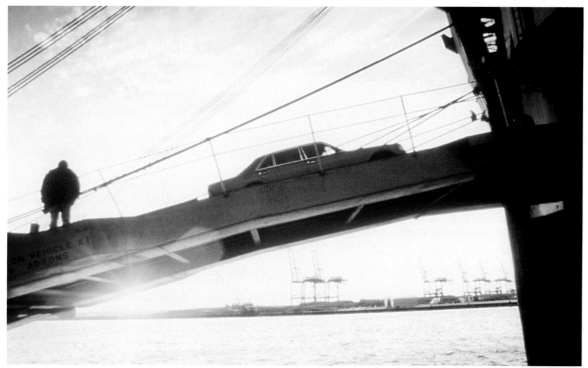

designed skyscraper, a landmark
on the city's skyline, marked the
renaissance of Baltimore's Inner
Harbor. Today, it houses an international mix of maritime agencies,
law firms, advertising agencies, customs brokers, freight forwarders,
the U.S. Export Assistance Center,
and the World Trade Center Institute,
among others.

The improvement program
begun nearly half a century ago
has continued. The Fairfield Auto
Terminal, opened in 1988 as a turn-
key project for Toyota Motor Sales,
USA, was an indispensable addition,
positioning the port as a major center
for East Coast auto distribution. And
the Seagirt Marine Terminal, completed in 1990, is regarded as one
of America's top container terminals, sparking technological advances
that have transformed port operations
from clipboard to keyboard.

The port now boasts computerized gate complexes, handheld
computers and scanners, and the
Electronic Data Interchange—all
of which have greatly increased its
efficiency, cost-effectiveness, and
focus on cutting-edge paperless
delivery systems.

Working with Labor

This focus on the development
of new facilities and introduction of state-of-the-art technology in the Port of Baltimore's
more modern history does not,
however, preclude the importance

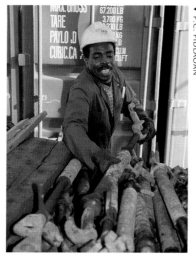

P.C. PIDLAOAN

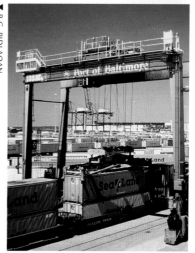

of its workforce. While justifiably
proud of its computerized cranes
and automated gate complexes, it
is the men and women who operate the high-tech equipment that
make it work.

Integral to the port's standard
of excellence, as well, are the state's
longshoremen. Baltimore's International Longshoremen's Association
(ILA) and the Steamship Trade
Association (STA) have formed a
progressive partnership that enhances
both the state's competitive position
and the skills of the port's workers.
In today's global market, service
dictates where the cargo flows. The
ability to handle any shipment—at
any time and in any weather—keeps
cargo moving and customers coming back. A commitment by labor
and management to that philosophy
has resulted in flexible scheduling,
ranging from unlimited midnight

starts—so vessels can work after most
other ports have closed up shop for
the night—to a flextime policy that
allows gate complexes to operate
continuously from 7 a.m. to 6 p.m.
for the receipt and release of cargo.

A tradition of excellence involves,
in addition to a commitment to serving maritime customers, an emphasis
on continuing education. Longshoremen work closely with other members of the port team, discussing
mutual concerns with the trucking
community, participating in joint
marketing calls, and playing an active
role in the influential Private Sector
Port Committee (PSPC).

As it nears its third century
of service, the Port of Baltimore,
under the direction of the Maryland Port Administration, continues to maintain its tradition of
staying a step ahead of the
times.

CLOCKWISE FROM TOP:
THE DUNDALK MARINE TERMINAL
HANDLES THOUSANDS OF AUTOMOBILES
AND CONTAINERS.

THE PORT'S INTERMODAL CONTAINER
TRANSFER FACILITY IS LOCATED
ADJACENT TO THE SEAGIRT MARINE
TERMINAL.

THE BALTIMORE INTERNATIONAL
LONGSHOREMEN'S ASSOCIATION AND
THE STEAMSHIP TRADE ASSOCIATION
HAVE FORMED A PROGRESSIVE PART-
NERSHIP WITH THE PORT TO ENSURE A
HIGH STANDARD OF FLEXIBLE SERVICE.

Woodbourne

FOR 200 YEARS, WOODBOURNE, A PRIVATE, NONPROFIT AGENCY, HAS HELPED at-risk children and adolescents grow into productive and self-sufficient adults by providing a comprehensive range of programs and services tailored to fit their needs. A group of Baltimore women established the organization in 1798, when they banded together to

provide food, shelter, and clothing for mothers and children, destitute and orphaned by the Revolutionary War. As this need declined, the group worked exclusively with orphaned children. The unique story of Woodbourne's survival began with this first instance of anticipating and meeting society's changing needs.

WOODBOURNE HAS A LONG AND PROUD HISTORY OF SERVING THE CHILDREN AND FAMILIES OF MARYLAND. ITS PROGRAMS TODAY ARE A REFLECTION OF THE AGENCY'S 200-YEAR COMMITMENT TO VULNERABLE CHILDREN AND ITS ONGOING EFFORTS TO MEET THE HIGHEST STANDARDS OF CARE.

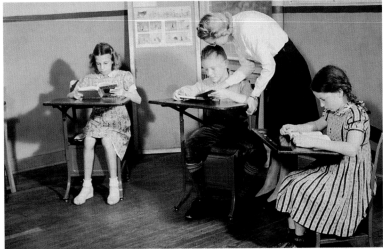

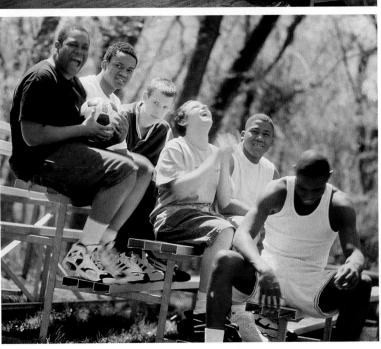

A Long History of Service

One of the five oldest child care institutions in the United States, Woodbourne has a long and proud history of serving the children and families of Maryland. For more than a century, Woodbourne remained an orphan-age. The last three decades, however, have been a time of dramatic transition and growth. By 1970, when it became a licensed residential treatment center, Woodbourne had focused its mission on the treatment of children with emotional disabilities. In the 1980s, the organization transformed its child-based approach to one that included the family in the treatment process. The 1990s brought even further change as Woodbourne realized that families need easy access to health, recreation, and social services in order to become productive and self-sufficient.

Woodbourne's programs today are a reflection of the agency's 200-year commitment to vulnerable children and its ongoing efforts to meet the highest standards of care. The agency is best known for the development of specialized education and clinical programs for Maryland's most emotionally challenged youngsters. Its wide array of residential and community-based programs form a comprehensive progression from the most to the least restrictive options for care. Programs for the most high-risk populations include residential treatment, therapeutic foster care, respite care, regular and special education, in-home services,

and outpatient clinical services. At the other end of the spectrum, school-based, community outreach programs build self-esteem, achieve academic progress, and teach problem solving among vulnerable children and families.

In the planning stages are programs to provide career education, long-term aftercare, and more education programs for adults and children in kindergarten through 12th grade. Woodbourne has been a benchmark for model programs across the country, and has made a commitment to documenting program and student outcomes.

Supportive Programs

In addition to direct human service programs, two related corporations support Woodbourne's goals: Advanced Resources Management Systems (ARMS) and the Woodbourne Foundation. The three entities are known as the Woodbourne Group. Established in 1992, ARMS, a for-profit corporation, specializes in training and placement of temporary, medical, counseling, and direct care staff to child care organizations, hospitals, and nursing homes. ARMS also offers psychological testing and evalu-

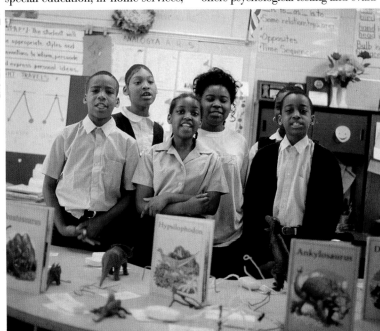

CHRIS HARTLOVE

ation to school systems. A third element provides staff development in organizational management through seminars offered to area businesses, public agencies, and nonprofit organizations. In its newest initiative, ARMS will train individuals formerly receiving welfare to enter and remain in the workforce.

The Woodbourne Foundation, founded in 1994, is a private, nonprofit organization established to support the Woodbourne Center through public relations management, program and resource development, fund-raising, and volunteer and intern management.

The Woodbourne Group has more than 600 employees representing a broad range of disciplines. These include physicians, registered and practical nurses, teachers, aides, child care counselors, social workers, therapists, and a full complement of administrative and support staff. A volunteer board of trustees governs the organization.

In 1998, Woodbourne celebrates its 200th anniversary. In addition to a series of yearlong special events, Woodbourne has launched a major fund-raising campaign: For Children, For Families, For Community. Funds raised in the campaign will support Woodbourne's innovative community-based program, the Woodbourne Community Partnership, and the construction of new residential facilities. The campaign is an important new step in Woodbourne's evolution in the development of comprehensive educational opportunities for children, adolescents, and families.

Making a Difference

The laughter of children fills Bert and Joyce Culton's home in Northwood. But for Bert, now retired, and Joyce, who works part-time, their household is far from typical. This is a house where biological offspring and foster children are treated the same. For a decade, the Cultons have acted as parents to a dozen kids in the Woodbourne Treatment Foster Care Program—one of Maryland's six original therapeutic foster care programs for emotionally and/or physically handicapped children. The program is working. Woodbourne's Treatment Foster Care

kids attend school regularly, make friends, and learn to trust adults. Several youngsters have gone on to college. Many others hold down jobs in the community. Some have been adopted, a number by the Treatment Foster Care families with whom they have been placed.

It is impossible to visit the Woodbourne Day School, a middle school for students with severe emotional disabilities, without feeling inspired, uplifted, and excited. Standards are high, and so is the school's success rate. In 1996, its 108 students had an overall attendance rate of 86 percent. Ninety percent of its students successfully met graduation requirements in academics, behavior, attendance, and clinical goals. The staff attendance rate is 95 percent. In giving the kids and their families the expectation, training, and hope for a positive future, Woodbourne has found a new way to give them life.

Moving Forward

The organization, too, has great expectations as it moves into its third century. As Woodbourne maintains its commitment to existing services, it reaches out to serve new needs as well. Primary among these is the Woodbourne Community Partnership, a coalition of public and private entities. The partnership provides a wide array of education, health, and career services to strengthen and enhance the quality of life in Baltimore. Through the partnership,

several schools in west Baltimore will become neighborhood hubs, where residents and educators are cooperating with Woodbourne to improve academic achievement and provide a host of learning opportunities for children in kindergarten through 12th grade.

In the future, Woodbourne will focus more of its resources at the community level to provide the full range of services needed to strengthen the quality of life for all children and families. This means achieving higher employment, higher graduation rates, better school performance, improved health, and lower crime rates and incidence of substance abuse. A hallmark of Woodbourne is its commitment to excellence—in its staff, its programs, and all that it does. This commitment, coupled with Woodbourne's historical creativity and ability to adapt to changing needs, will continue to produce positive results.

CLOCKWISE FROM TOP:
STUDENTS AT ROBERT COLEMAN ELEMENTARY SCHOOL ARE PART OF THE WOODBOURNE COMMUNITY PARTNERSHIP.

DR. JOHN HODGE-WILLIAMS SERVES AS PRESIDENT AND CEO OF THE WOODBOURNE GROUP.

THE HISTORIC TIVOLI ADMINISTRATION BUILDING IS LOCATED ON WOODBOURNE'S MAIN CAMPUS.

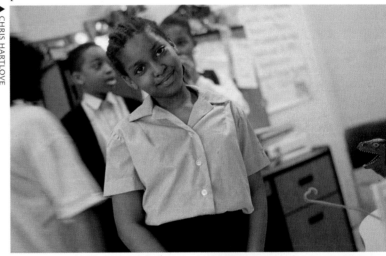

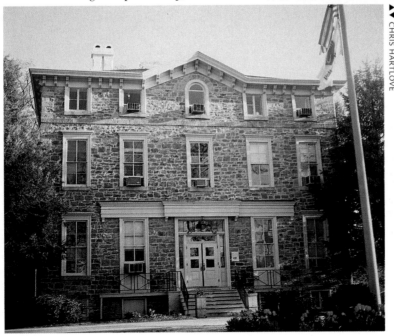

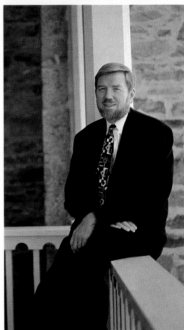

The Baltimore Sun

FOR MORE THAN 160 YEARS, *The Baltimore Sun* HAS BROUGHT THE WORLD to Maryland, earning a national reputation as "a newspaperman's newspaper." From its first issue on May 17, 1837, *The Sun* established its course: "We have resolved upon the experiment of publishing a penny paper, entitled *The Sun* . . . the publication of this paper will be continued

for one year at least, and the publishers hope to receive, as they will strive to deserve, a liberal support."

From its founding by Arunah S. Abell through its 1986 sale to the Times Mirror Company for the highest price ever paid for a newspaper at that time, *The Baltimore Sun* has consistently provided award-winning, in-depth, and independent-minded news coverage for readers throughout the state and beyond.

The Penny Paper

Baltimore in the late 1830s had already established a reputation as a mob town. "The Baltimore of that era was a smelly, unsanitary place of roust-abouts and roughnecks, a warren of 90,000 people where the municipal treasury was weighted with debt and the cobbled streets were littered with horse dung and the occasional dead dog," wrote *Sun* staff reporter Dan Fesperman in a recent 160th anniversary feature. "As for public

safety, stabbings were common-place. . . ."

The city's rough-and-ready days in 1837 provided the perfect setting for 30-year old Abell, a Rhode Island-born printer, who thought he could make a buck by starting a penny newspaper called *The Sun*—

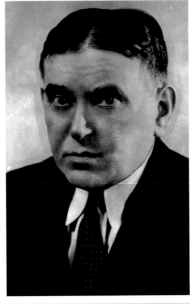

in a town where six other competing dailies were charging six cents a copy. Unlike his competitors, who strived to appeal to the wealthy, Abell designed his newspaper to attract the middle class.

In the early years, *The Sun* was a pioneer in transmitting news by overland horse express, railroad, and telegraph. It joined New York papers in a cooperative news-gathering effort that was the forerunner of the Associated Press. The newspaper dispatched its first correspondent overseas in 1887, and since then its foreign bureaus have come to rank among the most numerous and prestigious of American newspapers.

In 1910, *The Evening Sun* began as a late-day edition of the then 73-year-old *Sun*. It quickly established its own identity. In his 1987 history of the newspaper, Harold Williams, a 40-year *Sun* veteran, described *The Evening Sun*, in its glory days of the 1920s

H.L. MENCKEN, THE "SAGE OF BALTI-MORE," GOADED COLLEAGUES, SUPERI-ORS, AND READERS ALIKE DURING HIS 40 YEARS ON *The Evening Sun*'s EDITORIAL PAGE (TOP).

Today, *The Baltimore Sun* IS PRINTED AND ASSEMBLED AT A DEDICATED FACIL-ITY CALLED SUN PARK (BOTTOM).

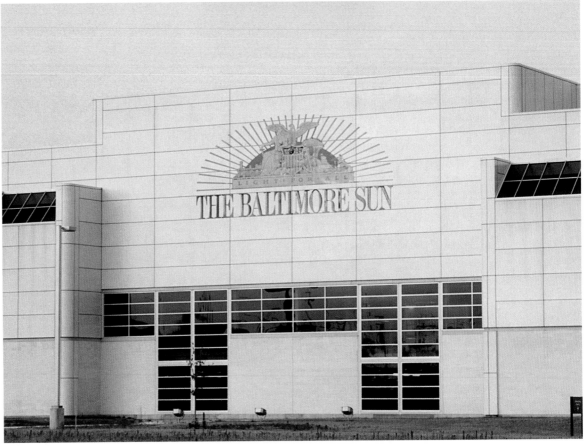

and 1930s: ". . . at once rambunctious, breezy, imaginative, visionary, mocking, whimsical, mischievous, saucy, and sometimes irreverent. It liked to think of itself as the rollicking son of the staid old lady, the morning *Sun*. . . ." *The Evening Sun* was published until 1995, when it was folded back into *The Sun*.

The Evening Sun's editorial page was the brainchild of H.L. Mencken, the irreverent, iconoclastic "sage of Baltimore" whose acerbic prose became a tradition. For more than 40 years, Mencken goaded his colleagues and superiors at least as much as he provoked his readers. *The Sun* was a magnet for other talented writers as well. Before beginning his career as a novelist, James M. Cain made a name for himself investigating labor conflicts in the West Virginia coalfields. In his first job as a journalist, a young Russell Baker moved up from covering police districts and YMCA shindigs to reporting from London on the coronation of Queen Elizabeth. At one time or another, *The Sun*'s staff has included Gerald W. Johnson, William Manchester, Jim McKay, Louis Rukeyser, and J. Anthony Lukas.

Throughout the years, *The Sun* has chronicled Baltimore's great and tragic events, from the glorious maritime era when signal flags were raised on Federal Hill and boatloads of immigrants arrived at a rate of 8,000 a year, to an established city rife with Civil War tension, to the Great Fire of 1904, and the civil rights riots of the 1960s.

A New Legacy

As much as *The Sun* today reveres its richly textured past, it believes in looking forward. Change has long been an important facet of the newspaper's design, reporting, and interpretation of the news, reflecting the changing nature of the world reported on each day.

Today, *The Sun*, which has been recognized with 13 Pulitzer Prizes, has more than 400 journalists and is Maryland's largest newsgathering operation. The newspaper operates five international bureaus and a state-of-the-art computerized printing press facility in South Baltimore. The company employs a total of 1,600 people, and enjoys a circulation of more than 310,000 for its daily editions and nearly a half-million for Sunday editions.

But the newspaper's real focus, as never before, is on local and state news. Zoned news editions and editorials cover Anne Arundel, Howard, Carroll, Baltimore, and Harford counties. The company's acquisition in 1997 of Patuxent Publishing, which produces weekly, community-based newspapers throughout the Baltimore metropolitan area, is another step in that direction. And still, reporters and editors of *The Sun* continue to probe, investigate, challenge, and entertain as they have in the past.

In the last 160 years, scores of daily newspapers have appeared on the streets of Baltimore. That *The Sun* alone among them remains standing imparts a sense of pride. The newspaper celebrates a history of Pulitzer Prize winners and foreign correspondents, police reporters and feature writers, editors and copy editors, printers and pressmen, and ad clerks and cartoonists. Today, *The Baltimore Sun* remains committed to a tradition of excellence, and looks forward to many years of doing what it does best—delivering the news.

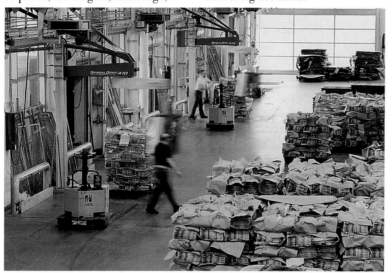

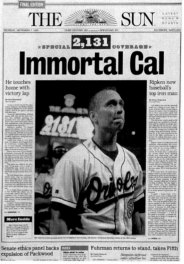

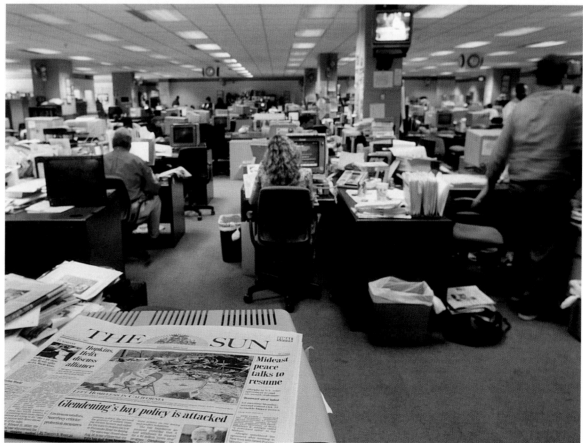

Maryland Historical Society

IN 1844, LEADERS OF BALTIMORE'S BUSINESS AND INTELLECTUAL COMMUNITY— concerned about preserving the state's history and providing its citizens educational and cultural resources—formed a historical society. Immediately, the new institution began collecting books, manuscripts, and objects of local interest, and soon initiated its noted publishing and exhibition activities.

More than 150 years later, the Maryland Historical Society (MHS) contains a profusion of treasures that illuminate the lives and events that have shaped the state and nation for nearly four centuries. With more than 6.2 million books and documents and 200,000 objects, the MHS has the most significant collection of Maryland cultural artifacts in the world. The richness, scope, and diversity of these collections are found in examples ranging from Charles Willson Peale's eyewitness painting *Washington and his Generals at Yorktown* to the archives and memorabilia of renowned jazz composer Eubie Blake. Its collection of American decorative arts is one of the largest and finest in the nation, and the institution is acclaimed for its fine art, folk arts, and maritime artifacts. It is the only museum of Maryland history in the state.

"Maryland's history is not just the story of white, Anglo-Saxon Protestants," says Dennis Fiori, executive director of the society. "It's also the history of Greeks, Italians, Poles, Germans, and African-Americans, among others. People of all heritages have built Maryland and we want to tell their stories. It's our mission to connect the past to the present and future." As a result, the museum features temporary exhibits, such as *Baltimore, Inc.: From Mobtown to Charm City*, in addition to permanent collections ranging from the *Gallery of Early Maryland Life, 1634-1800*, and *A House Divided: Maryland in the Civil War*, to the *Symington Sporting Arts Gallery and Library*.

The Maryland Historical Society enjoys strong support and currently has approximately 5,000 members. Its school tour program, much of which is funded through its Buses for Kids program, attracts more than 15,000 students annually. The Society's educational outreach programs embrace more than 30,000 individuals annually and include traveling trunks on 12 topics, ranging from a sailor's life to African-American artist Joshua Johnson. Fund-raising events, including the popular annual Maryland Antiques Show and the Maryland Hunt Cup Luncheon, attract wide support and much-needed capital.

Linking Past, Present, and Future

Today, the Maryland Historical Society has grown to more than three-quarters of a city block in the heart of the historic Mount Vernon/Howard Street neighborhoods. When the City of Baltimore recently donated the historically significant Art Deco Greyhound Bus Garage to the MHS, it renovated and reopened the building as the Heritage Gallery exhibition facility. The new gallery illustrates an important new goal for the Maryland Historical Society. "We are as dedicated to facilitating a renaissance of the Mount Vernon cultural district as we are to preserving historic artifacts," Fiori says. This goal is the guiding principle of the Maryland Historical Society, as it strives to link Maryland's past with its present and future.

MARYLAND HISTORICAL SOCIETY GALLERIES SHOWCASE ITS WIDE COLLECTION OF FINE AND DECORATIVE ARTS, THE MOST SIGNIFICANT COLLECTION OF MARYLAND CULTURAL ARTIFACTS IN THE WORLD.

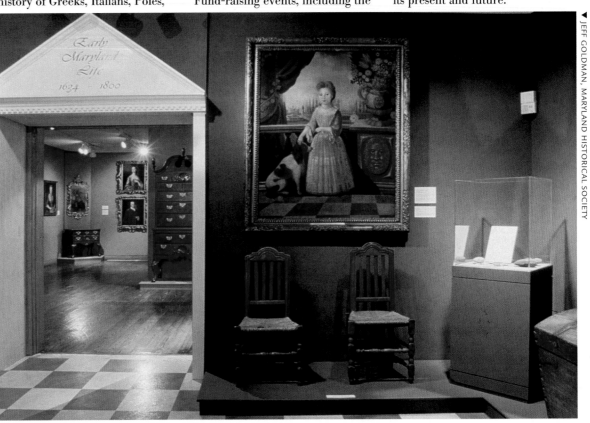

▼ JEFF GOLDMAN, MARYLAND HISTORICAL SOCIETY

Loyola College in Maryland

THE STORY OF LOYOLA COLLEGE IN MARYLAND IS LINKED TO A SERIES OF strategic plans that have profoundly altered the character of the college and helped to ensure its continued growth in size and strength while maintaining its Jesuit traditions. The result has been the emergence of Loyola College as a highly competitive regional and residential institution,

with a strong reputation for excellence in liberal arts education at the undergraduate level and professional programs at the graduate level.

As it approaches its sesquicentennial year in 2002, Loyola has unveiled its latest five-year strategic plan, focusing on learning, teaching, and scholarship. The college has also embarked upon a comprehensive capital building program, which will result in more than $70 million in new construction and renovation on its main Evergreen campus in North Baltimore by 2000.

Loyola College, established by members of the Society of Jesus in 1852, was the first Jesuit college in the United States to bear the name of St. Ignatius Loyola. The second-oldest chartered college in Baltimore, Loyola merged in 1971 with Mount St. Agnes College, an institution operated by the Sisters of Mercy, and has been fully coeducational in all programs ever since.

Now the largest private undergraduate college in Maryland, Loyola offers a curriculum that features a traditional academic program central to the Jesuit tradition, emphasizing the liberal arts and offering majors and minors in 31 academic fields. Its curriculum, which features a traditional academic program that is central to the Jesuit tradition, emphasizes the liberal arts and offers majors and minors in 31 academic fields. With

more than 200 full-time faculty and a student-teacher ratio of 14 to 1, the college currently attracts 6,000 undergraduate and graduate students, representing two-thirds of the United States and numerous foreign countries. More than 75 percent of undergraduate students are from other states. Some 25 percent study at least one semester abroad in Belgium, Thailand, or England.

Exercise of Reason, Practice of Faith

Several developments over the past 30 years have proved instrumental in defining present-day Loyola. The establishment of a separate school of business and management resulted in important alliances with Baltimore's business community. Recognizing the importance of expanding its core of advisers, the college—following Vatican II—invited laity from the business community to become

members of its board of trustees. This helped Loyola develop a greater strategic focus in terms of the governance of the institution and eventually led to its transformation from a local to a regional, residential institution.

As the college embraces its strategic blueprint for the 21st century, inseparable from its academic mission is the call for Loyola and its community to infuse the exercise of reason with the practice of faith. Such a combination will enable the college to cultivate leaders committed to serving in a rapidly changing world. A robust worship and retreat calendar is augmented by a strong community service program aimed at helping the underprivileged in Baltimore and other urban centers in the United States and Mexico. Two-thirds of all Loyola students participate in the volunteer program. This melding of study and service is what defines today's Loyola College in Maryland.

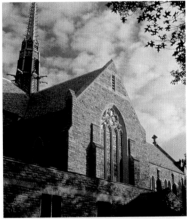

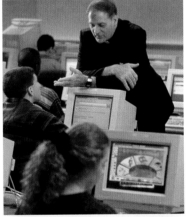

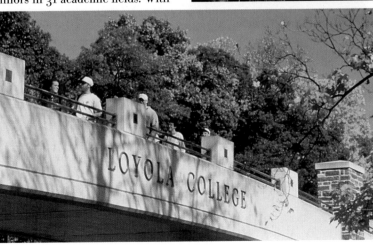

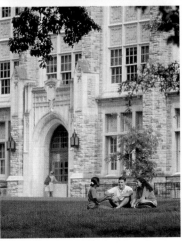

CLOCKWISE FROM TOP LEFT: THE ALUMNI MEMORIAL CHAPEL AT LOYOLA COLLEGE COMMEMORATES THOSE ALUMNI WHO GAVE THEIR LIVES TO THE COUNTRY IN WORLD WAR II. THE CHAPEL ANCHORS THE ACADEMIC QUADRANGLE AND HAS BEEN THE FOCAL POINT OF LOYOLA'S SPIRITUAL LIFE SINCE ITS 1952 CONSTRUCTION ON THE NORTH CHARLES STREET CAMPUS.

ALTHOUGH THE MEANS BY WHICH THEY ARE DELIVERED HAVE CHANGED TO MEET THE NEEDS OF SUCCEEDING GENERATIONS OF STUDENTS, THE LIBERAL ARTS STILL FORM THE FOUNDATION OF JESUIT EDUCATION AT LOYOLA COLLEGE, THE CITY'S LARGEST PRIVATE UNDERGRADUATE COLLEGE WITH NEARLY 3,200 STUDENTS.

GOTHIC STONE ARCHITECTURE AND A VERDANT ACADEMIC QUADRANGLE FORM THE BACKDROP OF THE EVERGREEN CAMPUS ON NORTH CHARLES STREET.

THE USF&G PEDESTRIAN BRIDGE SPANNING NORTH CHARLES STREET IS PERHAPS THE MOST VISIBLE SYMBOL OF LOYOLA COLLEGE FOR THOUSANDS OF VISITORS AND MOTORISTS EACH DAY. CONSTRUCTED IN 1989, IT CONNECTS THE RESIDENTIAL CAMPUS NEAR HISTORIC GUILFORD WITH THE ACADEMIC QUADRANGLE OF THE JESUIT INSTITUTION.

Sheppard Pratt Health System

CARING FOR PEOPLE IN MORE LOCATIONS THAN EVER BEFORE IN its history, Sheppard Pratt Health System responds to the rapidly changing behavioral health care market by offering a full continuum of mental health care for all members of the community. Today, Sheppard Pratt provides a vast array of programs and services that range from traditional inpatient care to innovative behavioral health plans and community-based treatment centers.

On its historic, tree-shaded, Victorian campus, Sheppard Pratt's psychiatric hospital consistently ranks among the nation's 10 best according to *U.S. News & World Report*, and patients from all backgrounds and income levels receive superior mental health treatment from this not-for-profit organization.

Building a Tradition of Quality Care

Sheppard Pratt was founded in 1853 by Moses Sheppard, a Quaker merchant in Baltimore, whose estate was transformed into an institution where studies were conducted in an effort to increase the cure rates among mental patients. "I wish everything done for the comfort of the patient," wrote Sheppard.

The first patient was admitted in 1891. Five years later, Enoch Pratt, another Baltimore philanthropist, left $1 million to extend the activities of the Sheppard Asylum, which was then renamed the Sheppard and Enoch Pratt Hospital.

From the beginning, Sheppard Pratt's commitment to serving patients with the highest quality of behavioral health care has resulted in a progressive, innovative institution. Because of the rapidly changing world of health care, at no other time has such an approach been more crucial. As a result, Sheppard Pratt has reinvented itself to fit modern times by expanding the communication lines among referring physicians, insurance companies, and managed care organizations. Through forward-thinking changes in treatment approaches and patient management, Sheppard Pratt has reduced the average length of inpatient stays from 38.8 days in 1991 to 14.6 days in 1995. In addition, the number of inpatient admissions has increased 41 percent during this period.

Strategic Initiatives

Key to the institution's strategic approach has been its successful efforts to develop more cost-effective alternative treatment programs. Sheppard Pratt has established a network of satellite facilities, which include day treatment programs and counseling centers in the city, as well as Anne Arundel, Baltimore, Frederick, Harford, and Howard counties. On its Towson campus, it has instituted a number of day treatment programs, which offer a cost-effective alternative to inpatient care for people who are making the transition from a hospital stay to the community, or for those who require an additional therapeutic structure and medical attention. In addition, Sheppard Pratt offers three community mental health centers in Baltimore and Harford counties, meeting the needs of a publicly funded population.

Initiating strategic partnerships with major area medical centers

SINCE ITS FOUNDING IN 1853 BY QUAKER MERCHANT MOSES SHEPPARD, SHEPPARD PRATT'S COMMITMENT TO SERVING PATIENTS WITH THE HIGHEST QUALITY OF BEHAVIORAL HEALTH CARE HAS RESULTED IN A PROGRESSIVE, INNOVATIVE INSTITUTION.

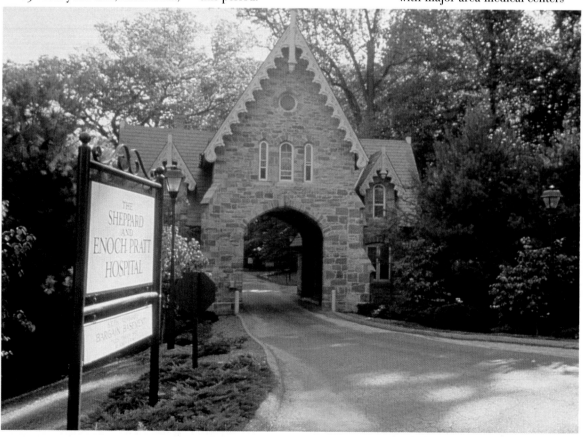

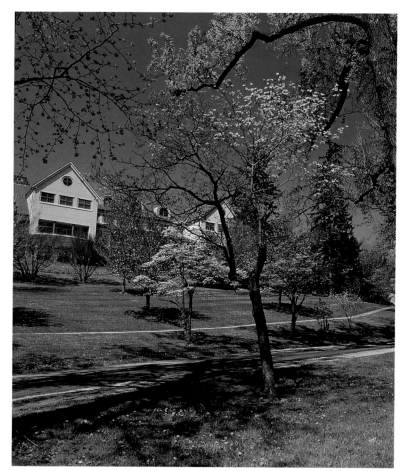

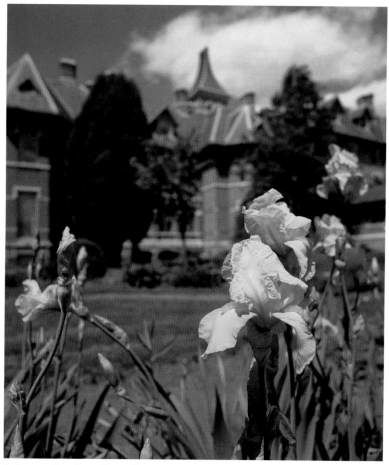

allows Sheppard Pratt to provide community-oriented mental health services in other ways. These alliances broaden Sheppard Pratt's reach, extend its base of services, and increase the number of people who have access to its treatment programs. Under an agreement with Upper Chesapeake Health System in Harford County, Sheppard Pratt manages Harford Memorial Hospital's 24-bed inpatient behavioral health unit, and provides emergency room psychiatric coverage for both Hartford Memorial and Fallston General Hospital.

The institution has a similar arrangement with St. Agnes Hospital, where it provides evaluation and treatment, crisis intervention for patients and staff, and in-service education for St. Agnes' health care providers, along with the management of psychiatric services. In Anne Arundel County, Sheppard Pratt manages a 17-bed inpatient behavioral health unit under contract with North Arundel Hospital.

Another expansion effort includes The Jefferson School, a $9.1 million, 40-bed residential treatment center and special education school for children and adoles-

cents. This K-12 facility, located in Frederick County, provides an additional resource for Maryland's youth.

Serving Business

According to the latest statistics, 18 to 20 percent of a company's workforce delivers only 75 percent of its potential. Much of the lost productivity is attributed to mental health problems, drug and alcohol abuse, stress, and other problems of daily living. As a result, Sheppard Pratt has also increased its efforts to meet the needs of local, regional, and national businesses by specializing in behavioral health care management on an at-risk or administrative-services-only basis. Through the Sheppard Pratt Health Plan, the institution provides employee assistance programs, managed care, and training and consulting services to more than 100 clients with approximately 200,000 enrollees in North America. This includes an at-risk contract to manage and provide mental health services to Kaiser Permanente's 40,000 members in the Baltimore area.

Companies such as Alex, Brown & Sons; Procter & Gamble; Miles

Laboratories, Inc.; Perot Systems; and the Federal Reserve Bank have contracted with Sheppard Pratt to increase profitability by providing comprehensive employee assistance and managed care programs.

Serving the Medical Community

From its earliest beginnings, Sheppard Pratt has been dedicated to education and research. In 1996, the institution entered a new era by creating a joint residency training program with the University of Maryland Medical Center. The four-year program offers medical school graduates an opportunity to master their skills in diverse settings, with clinical training facilities including the University of Maryland Medical Center, Sheppard Pratt, Walter P. Carter Center, and VA Medical Center.

Sheppard Pratt's ultimate goal is to help people improve their quality of life. The institution is committed to providing the highest-quality mental health and addictions services, aiding patients in managing their health care, and providing access to care for everyone.

TODAY, SHEPPARD PRATT PROVIDES A VAST ARRAY OF PROGRAMS AND SERVICES THAT RANGE FROM TRADITIONAL INPATIENT CARE TO INNOVATIVE BEHAVIORAL HEALTH PLANS AND COMMUNITY-BASED TREATMENT CENTERS (LEFT).

MOSES SHEPPARD'S VICTORIAN ESTATE WAS TRANSFORMED INTO AN INSTITUTION WHERE STUDIES WERE CONDUCTED IN AN EFFORT TO INCREASE CURE RATES AMONG MENTAL PATIENTS, IN COMPLIANCE WITH SHEPPARD'S DESIRE THAT "EVERYTHING [BE] DONE FOR THE COMFORT OF THE PATIENT" (RIGHT).

Towson University

THE LARGEST COMPREHENSIVE UNIVERSITY IN THE BALTIMORE AREA, Towson University offers undergraduate, graduate, and extended education programs in the arts and sciences, communications, business, health professions, education, fine arts, and computer information systems. Towson is Maryland's premier educator of teachers, as well as the home of the

Regional Economic Studies Institute (RESI), the largest university-based business and economic research center in the United States. Towson is also one of the largest producers of bachelor's and master's degree graduates in the health professions in both Maryland and the Mid-Atlantic area.

Its extensive curriculum, which includes 40 undergraduate and 25 graduate degree programs, attracts approximately 15,000 full- and part-time students. Towson recently added new degree programs, including the Master of Science in Information Technology Management and the Bachelor of Science in Special Education. It has created community-oriented partnerships with such diverse organizations as the Motor Vehicle Administration, Comcast Cable, St. Joseph Medical Center, and Sylvan Learning Systems.

Known since 1976 as Towson State University, the university adopted a new name in July 1997—one that reflected its status as a state-assisted, rather than state-supported, institution. This is an important distinction, one that allows Towson University to reintroduce itself, its new programs, and its initiatives. In 1996, *U.S. News & World Report* named Towson University a "best value" school, a designation that measures the

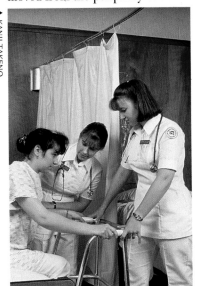

quality of students' educational experiences against tuition and fees.

Traditions of Growth

In 1866, Towson University opened its doors as the State Normal School. Located on a campus in downtown Baltimore, it was Maryland's only institution devoted exclusively to preparing teachers for public school careers. The inaugural class consisted of just 11 students.

The school moved to Towson in 1915. Subsequent changes throughout the early and mid-20th century included the introduction of a Bachelor of Science in Education degree and, later, an arts and sciences program. Its modern-day evolution began

in 1963, when the institution became known as Towson State College. The college was granted university status 13 years later in recognition of its development into a comprehensive university. Another milestone occurred in 1988, when Towson joined the new University System of Maryland, becoming part of the nation's 12th-largest public university system.

For more than 130 years, Towson University has embraced a strategy that emphasizes an ongoing focus on quality education in concert with expansion and change. At no other time in its history has the willingness to embrace new roles been more important.

"The vital university today has moved from the periphery of the

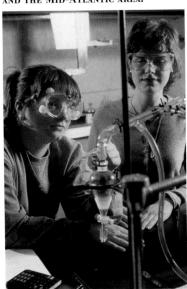

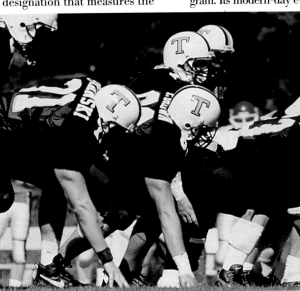

world and its day-to-day concerns to the center," says President Hoke L. Smith, who has guided the university for 18 years. "The university's primary purpose, the creation and transmission of knowledge in the interest of human development, has never been more essential to society. In the information age, knowledge is not merely power; it is the fuel that energizes the world. We understand that we can only fulfill our mission by involving the entire institution as a full partner in the Baltimore metropolitan community."

Partnerships with the Community

Community-based partnerships are a major emphasis of Towson University's new focus. In the past year alone, new partnerships were created with Comcast Cablevision of Maryland to provide the university with the state's fastest Internet access for residential students; the service, called Comcast@Towson University, is afforded to more than 3,000 students. Other partnerships, some of them involving the tristate region, are the Maryland Arts Festival, Towson's Professional Development Schools, and the Children's Dance Program.

In 1996, Towson University attracted the Regional Economic Studies Institute (RESI) to the campus. Affiliated with the College of Business and Economics, RESI, through contracts with organizations such as the state's Motor Vehicle Administration, offers students the opportunity to participate in problem-solving simulations on issues

ranging from customer relations to computer systems. In effect, RESI merges the classroom with real-world business.

In conjunction with Sylvan Learning Systems, Inc., Towson University has created a forum for students who need updating on mathematical concepts before they are ready for undergraduate level classes. And in other partnerships, Towson has expanded its relationship with the St. Joseph Medical Center in cardiac rehabilitation education and intervention.

The Quality Experience

An additional component of Towson's success has been its ability to embrace progressive programs while also honoring traditional aspects of quality education. As a result, many of its 1,000 full- and part-time faculty are recognized nationally and internationally for their scholarship. Their commitment to teaching and the university's dedication to small class sizes are also marks of what

Towson calls its student-centered university.

Each year, Towson's faculty authors many books and publishes hundreds of articles in academic journals. Its members also present hundreds of performances and creative exhibits, and hold offices in more than 200 professional organizations. Towson's faculty created the first occupational therapy program in the state, introduced "writing across the curriculum" into Maryland universities, and took a leading role in the development of women's studies.

To quote Henry Adams, an American historian admired by Smith: "A teacher affects eternity; he can never tell where his influence stops." Higher education ends with a degree, but a Towson education continues for life. Towson University enriches lives. As the 21st century unfolds, the influence of Towson University's teachers—as well as its progressive outlook on education—will be seen in the accomplishments of its graduates.

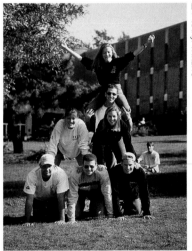

KANJI TAKENO

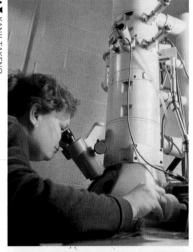

TOWSON IS A STUDENT-CENTERED UNI-VERSITY, WITH SMALL CLASSES IN A BROAD RANGE OF PROGRAMS. THE UNIVERSITY HAS ESTABLISHED ONGOING PARTNERSHIPS WITH THE MARYLAND ARTS FESTIVAL, TOWSON'S PROFESSIONAL DEVELOPMENT SCHOOLS, AND THE CHILDREN'S DANCE PROGRAM.

KANJI TAKENO

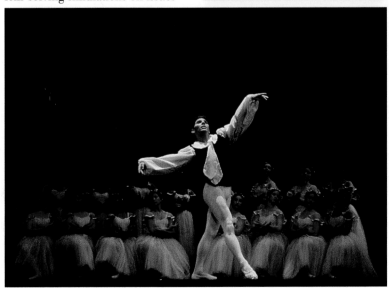

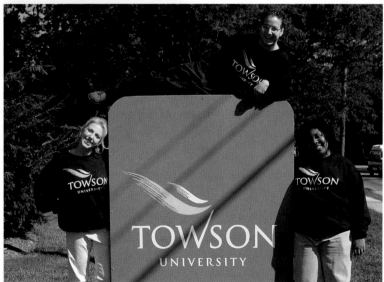

The Baltimore Zoo

JUST MINUTES FROM DOWNTOWN, AMID THE ROLLING, TREE-COVERED TERRAIN of Druid Hill Park, are Baltimore's wildest residents: elephants, zebras, penguins, tigers, crocodiles, and more. Over 2,000 animals make their home at The Baltimore Zoo, one of the nation's oldest zoos and a treasured part of the city's cultural heritage. ❧ Founded in 1876, The

Baltimore Zoo has a long and proud history of bringing people and animals together. For generations of Baltimoreans, the Zoo has provided an awesome and unforgettable introduction to the wonders of the animal kingdom—whether it be the lion's majestic roar, the quick-witted antics of chimpanzees at play, or the graceful beauty of giraffes towering above the treetops. Today's Baltimore Zoo, with its naturalistic habitats, innovative programming, and hands-on approach to learning, develops within visitors an even deeper appreciation for wildlife and the conservation efforts necessary to ensure survival within the animal kingdom.

"The appeal of the Zoo is timeless," explains Roger Birkel,

executive director. "I see it when a young child stands spellbound, absolutely mesmerized by the sheer massiveness of an elephant, or when an older couple hops hand in hand across the lily pads in our Children's Zoo. There's a magic here, an excitement that no one is immune to," Birkel continues. "The Zoo is irresistibly fun for kids, families, singles, seniors—virtually everyone in our community. But it's fun with a purpose. Our goal is to get people so enthralled with wildlife that they want to learn more and do more to help save species around the world."

At The Baltimore Zoo, the sights and sounds of the animal kingdom come to life when visitors venture deep into a tropical forest,

cross the grassy plains of an African savanna, or explore more familiar ground—from the rolling hills and caves of western Maryland to the shores of the Chesapeake Bay—in the nation's number one Children's Zoo. On-grounds programs, like the new and popular Keeper Encounters, enable visitors to learn more about animals and their caretakers. Special events and outreach efforts, including ZooMobile (the Zoo's traveling animal ambassadors and animal artifacts), attract new audiences and increase the Zoo's presence within the community.

Behind the scenes, Zoo staff are actively involved in conservation and research projects of local and international significance. In conjunction with the American Zoo and Aquarium Association, the Zoo participates in Species Survival Plans for 21 threatened and endangered species. The Zoo's birds-of-prey rehabilitation program enables injured eagles and other raptors to be released back into the wild. Already an international leader in assisted reproductive techniques for India's lion-tailed macaque, the Zoo is developing the first vaccine for avian malaria, a common and deadly threat to North America's captive penguins.

With the next century fast approaching, The Baltimore Zoo has renewed its commitment to wildlife and the community with a strategic plan to create a new zoo. Building upon the successes of nearly 125 years, The Baltimore Zoo faces a bright and thrilling future—the most spectacular chapter yet to be written in the history of this cherished institution. "The new Baltimore Zoo will be an incredible place where everyone can experience the amazing splendor of the animal kingdom," Birkel concludes, "a place where the diversity of all things wild is celebrated and preserved—not only for today's generation but for generations to come."

CLOCKWISE FROM TOP:
THE 2.5-ACRE AFRICAN PLAINS EXHIBIT PREMIERED AS THE BALTIMORE ZOO'S FIRST NATURALISTIC HABITAT IN THE AFRICA REGION. THE EXHIBIT FEATURES LIONS AND ANGOLAN AND RETICULATED GIRAFFES—NATURAL ENEMIES SEPARATED BY A 30-FOOT MOAT.

FOUND THROUGHOUT AFRICA AND ASIA, IN HABITATS RANGING FROM FORESTS TO SAVANNAS, SEMI-DESERTS TO MOUNTAINS, AFRICAN SPOTTED LEOPARDS ARE AMONG THE LARGEST CATS LIVING TODAY.

AS ONE OF THE ZOO'S MOST HIGHLY INTELLIGENT AND SOCIAL RESIDENTS, CHIMPANZEES ARE ACTIVE PARTICIPANTS IN BEHAVIORAL ENRICHMENT STUDIES, COMMUNICATING WITH KEEPERS AND EACH OTHER USING A VARIETY OF FACIAL EXPRESSIONS, POSTURES, TOUCHING AND GROOMING TECHNIQUES, AND SOUND.

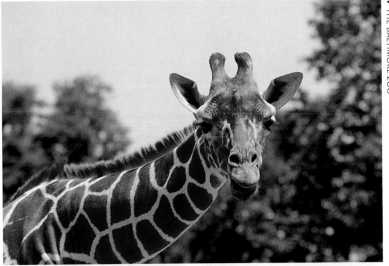

◄ THE BALTIMORE ZOO

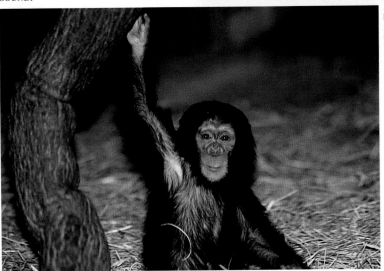

◄ ▶ THE BALTIMORE ZOO

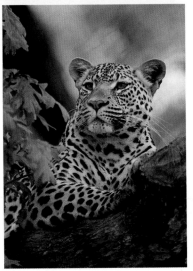

Edenwald/General German Aged People's Home, Inc.

AT EDENWALD, HOME IS MORE THAN A PLACE MERELY TO HANG YOUR HAT. Within this sleek, modern high-rise apartment building, located in the heart of Towson, home is much more: a full-service, continuing-care retirement community, as well as an entire neighborhood housed under one roof. It is a place where residents can take advantage of quality health care, a warm social atmosphere, and daily conveniences, all in an elegant setting.

"Edenwald's comfortable apartments and assisted living facilities provide a complete continuum of care in an atmosphere that emphasizes freedom and independence in a secure environment," says Sal J. Molite Jr., executive director.

A Legacy of Caring

When Edenwald opened in 1985, it had behind it a long legacy of caring for the elderly. In 1881, a group of Baltimoreans, concerned for the welfare of elderly Germans, created a home. Its focus, offering a caring community, is the backbone that sustains Edenwald today. Over the years, as demand grew, the General German Aged People's Home of Baltimore, Inc. relocated and expanded its facilities. During the 1980s, the organization reevaluated its mission and purpose, and decided to embark on a growth program that would embrace a more varied population. The result was the creation of Edenwald, designed to fulfill the need for a community that provided a full continuum of care, ranging from independent to assisted living to comprehensive nursing care.

Edenwald Today

Inside Edenwald's elegant lobby, cozy and quiet living room-style sitting areas coexist comfortably with the general hubbub of residents on the move. The contrast points out Edenwald's most delightful characteristic: this is a community where one can enjoy both moments of repose and days full of activity.

Amenities include workout facilities, a bank, woodworking shop, library, billiards room, and general store. There's a barber shop and beauty parlor, as well as an on-premises outpatient clinic,

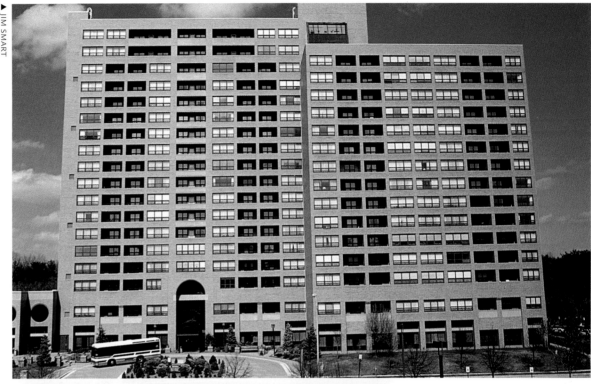

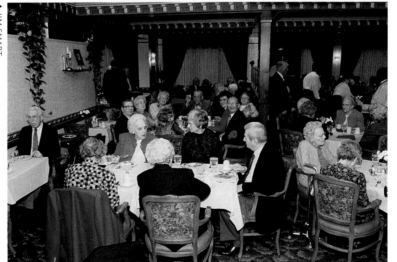

where residents can make appointments for ophthalmology, dentistry, podiatry, and physical and occupational therapy. For dining, residents who don't wish to cook in their own kitchens may eat at either the Garden Court Cafe, a cafeteria-style restaurant, or at Edenwald's luxuriously appointed resident center dining room.

In addition, Edenwald's Resident Association spurs new friendships, shared hobbies and interests, and traveling. Through this association, residents also have a voice in the operation of their community, serving on committees that range from health care to dining and from landscaping to trips.

For more than 100 years, the General German Aged People's Home, Inc., now Edenwald, has offered the finest in independent and assisted living as well as excellent health care. Under one roof, residents can fulfill all their needs and remain free to continue enjoying an excellent quality of life.

EDENWALD, A LUXURIOUSLY APPOINTED, 18-STORY HIGH-RISE WITH AN ADJOINING HEALTH CARE CENTER, IS CONVENIENTLY LOCATED IN THE HEART OF TOWSON (TOP).

EDENWALD RESIDENTS CAN TAKE ADVANTAGE OF QUALITY HEALTH CARE, A WARM SOCIAL ATMOSPHERE, AND DAILY CONVENIENCES, ALL IN AN ELEGANT SETTING (BOTTOM).

JIM SMART

JIM SMART

Johns Hopkins

Acentury and a quarter ago, Johns Hopkins, a son of Quaker tobacco farmers who raised himself from grocer's helper to millionaire financier, performed an act of generosity unprecedented in both size and impact. He provided in his will—with a bequest of $7 million, then the largest private donation of any kind in the United States—

for the founding of a university and hospital that transformed higher education in America and the practice of medicine worldwide. Hopkins' gift led to the creation in Baltimore of a new model for the pursuit of scholarship, teaching, and patient care together in a single place, a tremendously synergistic combination that seems obvious now, but had never been tried before.

Today, Johns Hopkins University and Johns Hopkins Medicine remain rooted in Baltimore; together, they are the city's and the state's largest private employer. But they are at work around the world—and, in fact, deep into space—making new discoveries, putting that knowledge to work for humanity, and preparing the next generation of scholars, scientists, caregivers, and other professionals.

Johns Hopkins University

When Johns Hopkins University opened in 1876, its first president, Daniel Coit Gilman, had something new in mind. This university, he determined, would not just impart the wisdom of the ages to its students. Its faculty and students would seek to make new discoveries, to create new knowledge. "What are we aiming at?" Gilman asked. "The encouragement of research . . . and the advancement of individual scholars who, by their excellence, will advance the sciences they pursue and the society where they dwell." Gilman's idea caught fire across America, leading to the creation of today's research university system.

Today, Johns Hopkins remains a world leader in teaching and scholarship. But it is also a vital contributor to the cultural and economic well-being of Baltimore, providing 8 percent of the jobs in its hometown. Hopkins faculty and researchers annually attract more federal research funding than any other American university, bring-

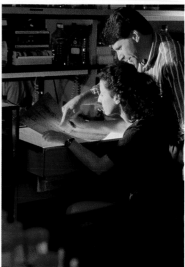

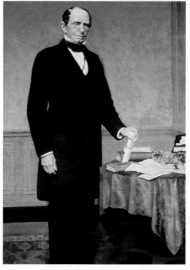

ing hundreds of millions of dollars into the Baltimore area. And the university's students and visitors add scores of millions of dollars more to the local economy.

The university's eight academic divisions enroll more than 16,000 students on three major Baltimore campuses; in Washington, D.C.; in additional classroom facilities throughout the Baltimore-Washington area; and in Italy and China. Approximately half of Hopkins' students study part-time, most enrolled in programs that bring the power of a Hopkins education to bear immediately on the needs of their employers in the technol-

ogy, financial, health, or public sectors.

The Zanvyl Krieger School of Arts and Sciences, the G.W.C. Whiting School of Engineering, and the School of Continuing Studies are based on the Homewood campus in northern Baltimore. The School of Medicine, School of Public Health, and School of Nursing share an east Baltimore campus with the Johns Hopkins Hospital. The Peabody Institute, one of the nation's leading professional schools of music, is located with other major cultural institutions in the city's Mount Vernon district. And the Paul H. Nitze School of

Advanced International Studies is in Washington, D.C.

Other affiliated institutions include the Applied Physics Laboratory, noted for contributions to national security, space exploration, and civilian research and development; the Johns Hopkins University Press, the oldest continuously operating university publisher in North America; and the Space Telescope Science Institute, a NASA facility located on the Homewood campus that serves as the science ground station for the Hubble Space Telescope. Also playing an integral role at the university are the Kennedy Krieger Institute, the Howard Hughes Medical Institute, the Carnegie Institution's Department of Embryology, the Dome Corporation, and the Lacrosse Foundation.

Johns Hopkins Medicine

Since its inception, Johns Hopkins has enjoyed a reputation for excellence. Its physicians and scientists are leaders and pioneers in their fields, responsible for many of this century's key discoveries and innovations in patient care.

Patients are the first to benefit from the new technologies and treatments developed by Hopkins physicians. Recent advances include the first successful treatment for sickle-cell anemia; new sight-saving procedures for disorders of the eye; nerve-sparing surgery for prostate cancer; new treatment for chronic fatigue syndrome; and new diagnostic, treatment, and prevention techniques for colon and other cancers.

For seven consecutive years, Johns Hopkins has been ranked the number one hospital in America by *U.S. News & World Report*. More of its physicians are listed in *Best Doctors in America* than any other medical center. Its medical school wins more federal research funds than any other institution. Among its staff of more than 15,000 are recipients of the Nobel Prize and virtually every other major award in science and medicine.

As a result of the recent creation of Johns Hopkins Medicine (JHM), operations and planning covering a full spectrum of activities in teaching, research, and patient care now fall under one umbrella. Participating organizations are the Johns Hopkins University School of Medicine and the Johns Hopkins Health System, which includes the Johns Hopkins Hospital, Johns Hopkins Bayview Medical Center, Johns Hopkins Geriatrics Center, and Johns Hopkins Medical Services Corporation. Also part of JHM are Johns Hopkins Bayview Physicians, Johns Hopkins Health Care, Johns Hopkins Home Care Group, and Employer Health Plans (EHP).

The organization is meeting the challenges of a new era, developing an integrated delivery system with a growing network of faculty and community practitioners, allied hospitals, new and more widely accessible facilities, and new models of care. At the forefront of sophisticated new quality control and outcomes measurement programs, Johns Hopkins now is providing cost-effective health services in the region and throughout the world.

STEPHEN SPARTANA

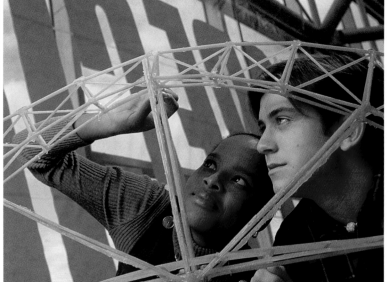

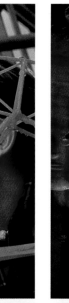

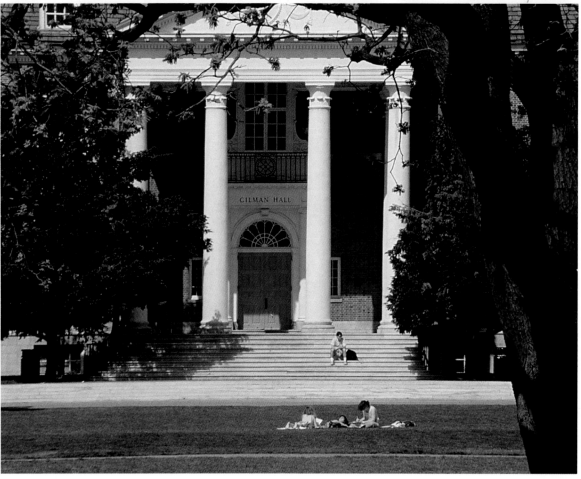

The Baltimore Life Insurance Company

I N 1882, BALTIMORE WAS ENJOYING ONE OF ITS GREATEST PERIODS OF GROWTH and prosperity. A hard-working man could earn $8 or $9 a week. It also was the year that five businessmen founded the Baltimore Mutual Aid Society of Baltimore City to "benefit members in case of disability from sickness or accident, bury the dead, and relieve widows and orphans." The company,

now called The Baltimore Life Insurance Company, still protects families throughout Baltimore and nationwide.

About Baltimore Life

Ever since, Baltimore Life has provided employment for people in the area. Baltimore Life is the oldest and largest mutual life insurance company in Maryland, and the 38th oldest in the United States. The company is currently licensed in 47 states and the District of Columbia.

Baltimore Life is a mutual company, owned by its policyowners and managed for their benefit. To provide financial stability to its policyowners, the company maintains high standards of conservative financial management. Profits are either returned to policyowners or reinvested in the company to increase the protection of their investment. As a measure of its financial strength, both Baltimore Life and Life of Maryland maintain excellent financial ratings from A.M. Best Company and Standard & Poor's. The financial strength of the company and its subsidiary is greater now than at any time in their history. Baltimore Life's surplus as a

percent of assets ranks well above industry averages.

Community Service

Community service continues as an important outreach. For many years, Baltimore Life has supported the United Way: Joseph E. Blair Jr., CLU, ChFC, has served as chairman of the board of the United Way of Central Maryland, and currently is chairman of the board of Baltimore Life and its subsidiary, Life of Maryland. In addition, numerous employees volunteer service to United Way agencies as well as

JOSEPH E. BLAIR JR., CHAIRMAN OF THE BOARD, AND L. JOHN PEARSON, PRESIDENT AND CEO OF BALTIMORE LIFE, MAINTAIN HIGH STANDARDS OF CONSERVATIVE FINANCIAL MANAGEMENT TO PROVIDE FINANCIAL STABILITY FOR POLICYOWNERS.

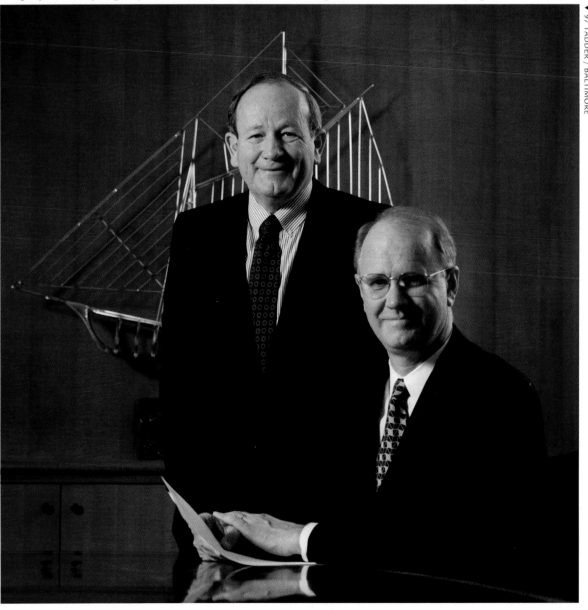

other community organizations, including churches, schools, and colleges.

Baltimore Life agents also carry out this tradition of community service: They offer child fingerprinting and photo identification services to area parents many times a year. This service can prove invaluable to parents searching for a lost child.

From Small Beginnings

When the company was founded in 1882, Baltimore was the sixth-largest city in the 38 United States. Five businessmen founded the Baltimore Mutual Aid Society of Baltimore City; Frank Strobridge was president. The new society boasted a scant $260.93 in assets.

Two years after its founding, the company passed a novel resolution that was to change the face of insurance in America: "Moved by Mr. Strobridge and seconded . . . that on and after the first day of July 1884, death claims be paid within 24 hours after satisfactory proofs are furnished." This action, unusual because most insurance companies took up to 60 days to settle a death claim, was named The Resolution of 1884. It has been in effect ever since.

In 1900, the company changed its name to The Baltimore Life Insurance Company of Baltimore City. Another milestone in the company's history was the stock market crash of 1929, when thousands of people turned to their life insurance companies for ready cash. The company helped its policyowners and showed its faith in the future by demolishing its four-story home office and erecting a 12-story tower in its place.

In the 1950s, Baltimore Life again demonstrated its faith in the city by building a new headquarters office on Howard Street, beginning an urban renewal project for its hometown. When the city built its light-rail line in 1992, the company moved to a new building in Owings Mills. The structure is the first commercial building to earn the National Association of Home Builders' Global Re-Leaf Award. Baltimore Life made a special effort to preserve the forested character of the site by carefully locating the

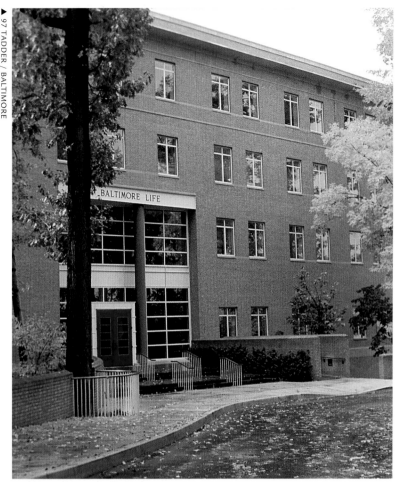

THE BALTIMORE LIFE HOME OFFICE MOVED TO A NEW BUILDING IN OWINGS MILLS IN 1992.

building and entrance drive among mature hardwood trees.

Expanding Markets

For its first century, Baltimore Life specialized in offering individual life insurance products through a home service system, serving families in the Mid-Atlantic states. In response to rising interest rates and changing competitive pressures, the company formed a subsidiary in 1981. Life of Maryland specializes in interest-sensitive products.

At the beginning of its second century, in 1982, Baltimore Life formed a new sales division to offer interest-sensitive products through general agents and brokers. Today, the Independent Sales Division targets special markets through independent marketing organizations throughout the United States.

Under the leadership of L. John Pearson, CLU, the company's 10th president and chief executive officer, marketing efforts have been expanded to substantially increase growth and services offered to policyowners. Pearson initiated several new strategies to position the company to move into the 21st century

from a position of strength. These strategies include establishing the Worksite Sales Division, to offer employer groups nationwide a unique package of services; beginning a new team approach to marketing in the company's Career Sales Division, which uses teams to increase productivity and provide better service to policyowners; reorganizing internal company operations to streamline service and reduce expenses; and investing in an expanded computer system to support substantial growth and excellent customer service.

These strategies will both support the substantial growth the company has experienced in recent years and position it for the future. In 1996, Baltimore Life achieved record sales and increased assets, surplus, and net income to the highest levels in the company's history.

Baltimore Life has proudly fulfilled its financial responsibility to the six generations of customers who have invested their trust in the company. With its tradition of growth, reliability, and service, Baltimore Life will continue to serve Baltimore and the nation for generations to come.

P. Flanigan & Sons, Inc.

SINCE 1885, P. FLANIGAN & SONS, INC. HAS PIONEERED INNOVATION AND technology in building Baltimore's foundations. The company, which constructs streets, highways, parking lots, terminals, and site developments, specializes in asphalt and concrete pavement, stone bases, excavation, storm drainage, and utilities. To follow its progression is to witness more

than a century of history, from Baltimore's Great Fire of 1904 to the city's expansion in the latter part of the 20th century.

Today, the family-owned and -operated P. Flanigan & Sons is a leader in new asphalt technology, continuing a tradition that draws on state-of-the-art processes, custom materials, sophisticated quality control, and laboratory design to produce durable roadways as ubiquitous as the Baltimore Beltway and the Jones Falls Expressway.

Coming to Baltimore

In 1880, Patrick Flanigan emigrated from Ireland. His principal assets were a collection of small tools and a burning desire to succeed in life. Also important were his friendships, fostered through active membership in the Hibernian Society of Baltimore, a group of young Irish workmen who had come to America in search of a better life.

When, five years later, Flanigan launched his contracting business, he could not have chosen a better time. The lack of public sewerage in Baltimore resulted in a competitive market for methods of piping household wastes to a location distant from local homesites.

Flanigan's ingenuity in the building of sewers established his company as the leader in the new industry.

The work also taught him skills in excavation and in repairing the cobblestoned streets of the period. In 1908, asphalt paving was introduced for street surfacing, and, soon thereafter, a plant was opened and running.

Modern Days

Nearly 90 years and 10 asphalt plants later, the P. Flanigan & Sons complex at Westport is still an important part of the business. Today, the company, headed by Pierce Flanigan

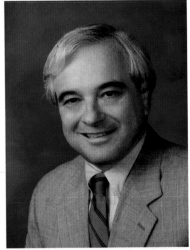

III, has branched out into myriad fields. For the *Baltimore Sun*'s printing plant, the company provided a full range of services, such as excavation, stone base preparation, concrete curb and slab pours, storm drainage and utilities installation, and asphalt paving.

Flanigan was the prime contractor on five parts of the Seagirt Marine Terminal, constructing the intermodal rail yard and much of the excavation, storm drainage, utilities, lighting, and paving for the rest of the facility. The company helped to transform the old Maryland Dry Dock Facility into the Toyota Terminal, a major auto distribution center. Flanigan handled the asphalt duties for the Baltimore Ravens' artificial turf practice field and built the warning track inside Oriole Park at Camden Yards.

The key to the company's enduring success has always been an ability to combine sophisticated project management with the aggressive pursuit of the leading edge in construction methods, machinery, and materials. With the fourth generation of Flanigans at the helm, P. Flanigan & Sons will continue to provide firm foundations for the Baltimore community well into the next century.

CLOCKWISE FROM TOP:
STILL A FAMILY-OWNED COMPANY, P. FLANIGAN & SONS IS TODAY HEADED BY PRESIDENT PIERCE FLANIGAN III.

FLANIGAN CONTRACTORS PLACE ASPHALT FOR A GROCERY STORE PARKING LOT.

A 1912 ROAD PROJECT SHOWS FOUNDER PATRICK FLANIGAN IN THE CENTER. WHEN HE EMIGRATED FROM IRELAND IN 1880, FLANIGAN'S PRINCIPAL ASSETS WERE A COLLECTION OF SMALL TOOLS AND A BURNING DESIRE TO SUCCEED IN LIFE.

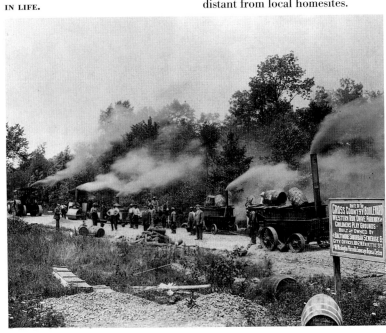

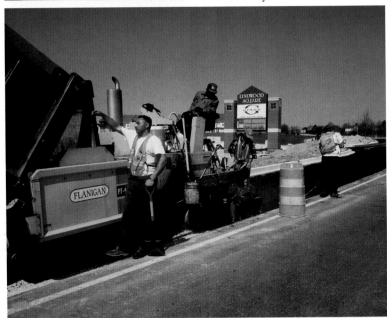

Riggs, Counselman, Michaels & Downes, Inc.

RIGGS, COUNSELMAN, MICHAELS & DOWNES, INC. (RCM&D) TRACES its Baltimore roots to 1885, when R.E. Warfield, a local insurance executive, was appointed resident manager for the Royal Insurance Company. In the ensuing 112 years, the company that today is RCM&D has continually evolved through growth and acquisition—establishing itself as a local leader offering full insurance protection to business, industry, and individuals. Over the years, even as the business world has changed exponentially, RCM&D has remained committed to two basic principles: loyalty and client service.

"Every client's needs are different to some degree," says Albert R. Counselman, CPCU, president and chief executive officer. "In today's fast-moving and sophisticated business world, an in-depth variety of specialists is often required to respond to those needs with the precise solution. That's why we believe in and practice the team approach."

Recognizing Changing Times

In 1923, the now-thriving insurance business was incorporated as The Henry M. Warfield-Roloson Company. Warfield served as the company's president while F. Albert Roloson, Counselman's grandfather, was one of its first officers. By 1946, the company was ready for growth and purchased the assets of Riggs, Rossman and Hunter, Inc., changing the firm's name to Riggs, Warfield, Roloson, Inc. (RWR). In 1969, RWR merged with Michaels, Fenwick & Downes and adopted the company's current name.

Today, Towson-based RCM&D offers a vast range of property/casualty coverages. Each member of its team of 165 employees specializes in areas of expertise and has an understanding of all the fundamentals of insurance coverage.

RCM&D's Commercial Insurance department handles questions relating to sales, marketing, risk prevention, loss control engineering, and claims. The same intensely focused effort applies to RCM&D's health care clients, who require services such as exposure to loss, negotiation and settlement of claims, leases and indemnity contracts, and establishment of risk management goals.

Other areas of specialty at RCM&D include financial institutions and special accounts, which are targeted to small and mid-sized businesses, and individual accounts for homeowners' coverage, as well as a myriad of ancillary areas, such as auto, watercraft, and recreational vehicles.

Reaching Out

As a founding member of Assurex International, a worldwide network of brokerage firms, RCM&D is becoming ever more innovative. Through this organization, the world's top brokerage firms work together to share information, insights, and educational programs, and, most important, to service clients with multistate locations as well as foreign operations.

The organization reaches out in other ways. RCM&D has long-standing relationships with major underwriters around the world. And in keeping with Counselman's belief that "only through growth can opportunities be provided for employees to move forward in an organization and enable the company to retain its valuable skills and experience," RCM&D is creating new lines of business.

Its New Business Development department is focusing on burgeoning industries in the fields of technology and the environment. Through new products like the firm's Self Insured Services Company (SISCO), formed in 1979, it is establishing itself as an indispensable resource for self-insured companies.

Facing the future aggressively and honoring its founding principles has been the key to RCM&D's enduring growth. For more than 100 years, clients seeking specialized care and services have found a home with RCM&D.

OFFICERS FOR RIGGS, COUNSELMAN, MICHAELS & DOWNES, INC. ARE (FROM LEFT) PRESIDENT AND CEO ALBERT R. COUNSELMAN, EXECUTIVE VICE PRESIDENT FRANCIS G. RIGGS, CHAIRMAN OF THE BOARD L. PATRICK DEERING, AND EXECUTIVE VICE PRESIDENT THOMAS P. HEALY.

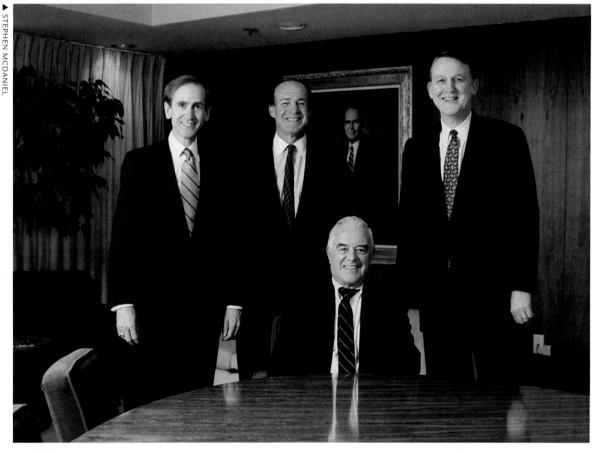

▶ STEPHEN MCDANIEL

Schmidt Baking Company

For Elizabeth Schmidt, a German immigrant who arrived in Baltimore in the 1860s, baking up loaves of bread for neighbors was a simple gesture of hospitality. The bread, which Elizabeth made according to her own precise standards for quality and taste, was so popular that she and her husband Peter opened a small bakery in their home. Elizabeth baked the bread, and Peter delivered it.

More than a century later, Schmidt Baking Company is still providing Baltimore with the homegrown taste of its founders' signature Schmidt Blue Ribbon Bread. From its modest beginnings, the company, now in its fourth generation of family ownership, has grown to become one of the 15 largest independent wholesale bakeries in the nation. Schmidt employs more than 1,100 people at three baking plants—in Baltimore and Fullerton, Maryland; and Martinsburg, West Virginia—and has expanded its product line to include such brands as Sunbeam, Old Tyme, Roman Meal, and Schmidt's potato breads and rolls. Locally, the company distributes its product to a vast range of retailers, restaurants, and institutional accounts.

In spite of its growth, Schmidt Baking Company remains very true to its founders' ideals. "We have always been committed to the fundamentals of quality, freshness, and service," says C. Peter Smith, president and chief executive officer, a fourth-generation descendant. "It's a matter of family pride. And although we've grown beyond the wildest

dreams of great-grandmother Schmidt, one thing hasn't changed. We still care about the quality of our product."

Modern Evolution

At a lunchtime meeting in the executive suite at Schmidt Baking Company, Smith and his management team dine on fresh-out-of-the-oven potato rolls and Blue Ribbon bread. Hold the mustard, hold the peanut butter and jelly. This is a "bread tasting." Much as a connoisseur savors wine, John Stewart, vice president of sales, tests a slice, checking for

a full-bodied aroma, judging for the perfect blend of salt and sugar, looking for a delicate sweetness. "People regard us as a local treat," he says, "and also a homegrown company that shares in Baltimore's history."

A company that is still very much a part of the fabric of the community in which it originated, Schmidt is proud to evoke a feeling of nostalgia in Baltimore by representing a treasured era. At the same time, Schmidt is a modern business. Integral to its success is the ability to pay homage to its traditional values while also applying innovative business techniques.

The company, which is the only wholesale pan-bread baker in Maryland, still uses Elizabeth Schmidt's recipe. Modern improvements have focused on establishing retailer delivery systems that ensure a loaf of bread baked at 4 a.m. is on the store shelf by late morning. Via state-of-the-art technology, Schmidt's products are always fresh, even as they are distributed throughout much of the Mid-Atlantic region, particularly Baltimore; Washington, D.C.; and Philadelphia.

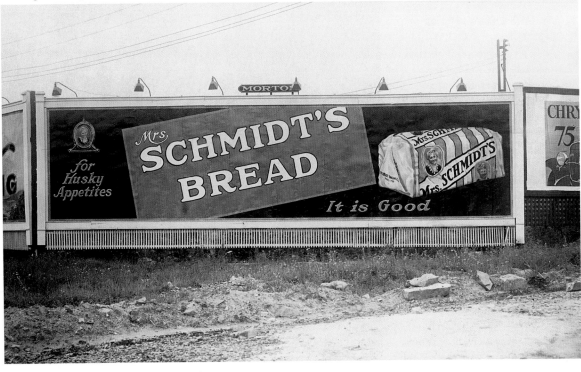

Upgraded technology is just one way to provide service. Another is by establishing personal relationships between company salespeople and retailers. In many cases, Schmidt's sales employees actually live—and shop for groceries—in the communities they serve. The intimate connection has meant a lot to the company's growth. At no time is Schmidt's local presence more keenly felt, for instance, than during the occasional snowstorm. "Nothing can generate a sale more potently than the threat of snow," Smith says, laughing.

The Blizzard of 1996 was indeed a challenge—one that Schmidt met by calling in extra bakers, switching roll line people to bread lines to increase capacity, and making extra delivery runs before and during the series of snowstorms. In just a five-day period, the company sold more than 1 million loaves of bread. "During that time, everyone in Baltimore ate two loaves of Blue Ribbon," Smith figures, sporting an "I Survived the Blizzard of '96" T-shirt, a gift from a grateful grocery chain that never ran out of bread.

Another component of Schmidt's enduring success is its willingness to reinvest in the business. A few years ago, the company opened its third baking facility—a state-of-the-art bakery in Fullerton, with half-a-block-long ovens. This expansion enabled Schmidt to increase production while also maintaining the traditional levels of quality.

When Elizabeth and Peter Schmidt founded their company in 1886, they were one of a number of family-run bakeries in Baltimore. Very few of those exist today. "Companies faded because of a lack of family commitment, or they sold their brands," Smith says. "We have taken a different approach, one that I believe is integral to our staying power. We have always believed that this is a business we want to pass on to following generations, a company that regards as our primary measuring stick our commitment to our employees and our customers."

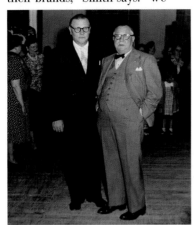

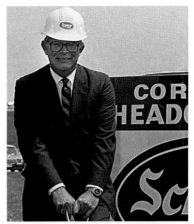

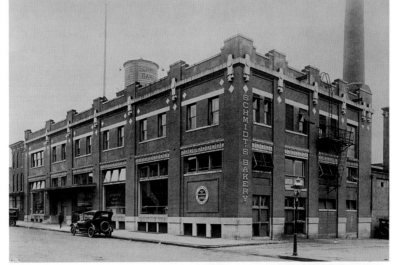

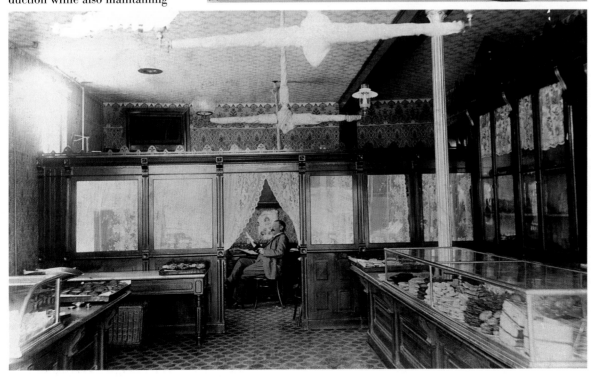

Afro-American Newspaper Company of Baltimore, Inc.

THE NEWSPAPERS PUBLISHED BY THE AFRO-AMERICAN NEWSPAPER Company of Baltimore, Inc. have long been among the nation's leading voices for racial equality and economic advancement for African-Americans. The country's oldest continuously published African-American newspaper chain, the company was founded in Baltimore in 1892.

Over the years, the Afro-American Newspaper Company has produced as many as 13 editions, serving readers from New Jersey to South Carolina, and has featured the bylines of great African-Americans who have gone on to become national figures in the struggle for civil rights. Today, with a combined readership of 135,000, the company publishes editions in Baltimore and Washington, D.C., as well as a Wednesday weekly.

Answering the Call

When President Abraham Lincoln issued a call for "colored troops" in the Civil War, John Henry Murphy, only 16 years old, enlisted in Company G of the 30th Regiment Infantry, U.S. Colored Troops, Maryland Volunteers. Quickly, he rose to the rank of first sergeant.

Twenty years after the end of the Civil War, the ex-military man and former slave purchased a one-page weekly called the *Afro-American* at public auction for $200. Murphy transformed that publication into a 12-page journal with a readership of 14,000. By 1922, the *Afro-American*'s circulation was the highest of any African-American publication in the nation.

Murphy's son, Carl, then took the helm. Under his tenure, the paper became the preeminent mirror of African-American life. For 45 years, Carl Murphy used the editorial pages to attack Jim Crow practices in Maryland and to challenge African-Americans to organize in the struggle for equality.

Casting a Wider Net

Ever a family business, the Afro-American Newspaper Company was headed in the 1970s by Carl Murphy's daughter, Frances, before the baton was passed to Carl's nephew, John Murphy III. And just as their great-grandfather was a pioneering newspaperman more than 100 years ago, current publisher John J. Oliver, and Frances Murphy Draper, president, are taking the family dynasty into new territory: the Internet. The company's Web site, AFRO-Americ@ (www.afroam.org), offers current news from the company's two newspapers, as well as from a growing consortium of other African-American newspapers around the nation.

The on-line National News Edition helps to keep people abreast of current events that impact the African-American community, featuring regional news, commentaries, entertainment, sports stories, lifestyle topics, the highly regarded Job Vault, and the Christian Singles Network.

The Black History Museum is one of the most popular areas of the site. Articles and exhibits on such topics as the Tuskegee airmen, the Scottsboro boys, baseball hero Jackie Robinson, and the Million Man March help to educate and raise awareness of the historical contributions of African-Americans, making use of the abundant reference material in the *Afro-American* archives.

For more than 100 years, the voice of Afro-American Newspaper Company publications has spoken clearly to and for African-Americans. And true to its pioneering tradition, it will continue to be on the front lines for its readership nationwide.

FOR 45 YEARS, CARL MURPHY USED THE EDITORIAL PAGES OF THE AFRO-AMERICAN NEWSPAPER TO ATTACK JIM CROW PRACTICES IN MARYLAND AND TO CHALLENGE AFRICAN-AMERICANS TO ORGANIZE IN THE STRUGGLE FOR EQUALITY (LEFT).

TODAY, THE NEWSPAPER IS UNDER THE LEADERSHIP OF PUBLISHER JOHN J. OLIVER JR. (MIDDLE) AND PRESIDENT FRANCES MURPHY DRAPER (RIGHT).

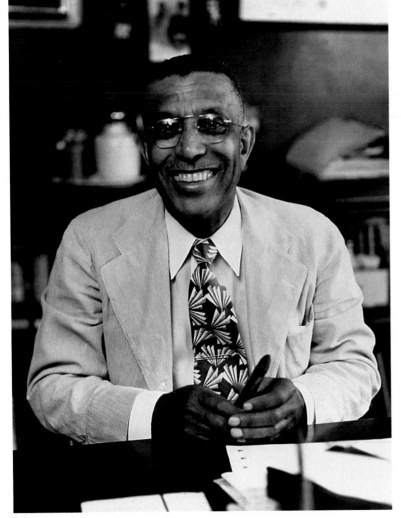

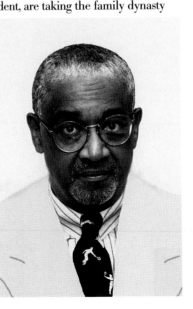

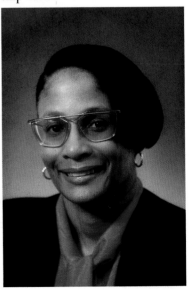

Baltimore Symphony Orchestra

THE BALTIMORE SYMPHONY ORCHESTRA IS INTERNATIONALLY RECOGNIZED as having achieved a preeminent place among the world's most important orchestral ensembles. Renowned for its imaginative interpretations of masterworks and uncompromising artistic innovation, the Baltimore Symphony Orchestra (BSO) has been hailed as a prototype

for classical music in the 21st century.

The BSO has also earned unqualified acclaim on the local, national, and international levels for its imaginative musical formats. Through the Concert and Conversation, Casual, and Discovery concerts, audiences gain a unique perspective through lively interaction with conductor, musicians, and guest artists.

Committed to influencing the future of orchestral performance, the BSO, through numerous commissions of original symphonic works, has earned a reputation as a haven for the newest generation of American composers. Additionally, world-renowned artists such as Yo-Yo Ma, Isaac Stern, James Galway, Emanuel Ax, and Andre Watts regularly perform with the Baltimore Symphony Orchestra. International stars such as violinist and conductor Pinchas Zukerman and legendary composer Marvin Hamlisch have joined the artistic leadership of the BSO as Summer MusicFest artisitic director and principal Pops conductor respectively.

A Long, Rich History

Organized in 1916, the Baltimore Symphony Orchestra is the only major American orchestra originally established as a branch of the municipal government. Reorganized as a private institution in 1942, it retains close relationships with the governments and communities of the city and surrounding counties, as well as with the state of Maryland.

The BSO's modern history dates from 1965, when Baltimore arts patron Joseph Meyerhoff became president of the symphony orchestra, a position he held for 18 years. Meyerhoff appointed Romanian-born conductor Sergiu Comissiona as music director; together, the visionary philanthropist and the charismatic conductor ensured the creation of an artistic institution

that has become an integral part of the arts community.

With the appointment of David Zinman as music director in 1985, the BSO's reputation for musical excellence and high artistic achievement spread far beyond the shores of the Chesapeake to a new and devoted international audience. With the first visit to east Asia in 1994, Zinman and the Baltimore Symphony Orchestra became the hit of Tokyo's star-filled concert season. The newspaper *Yomiuri Shimbun* proclaimed the BSO's presentation as "the performance which can be considered the best of all the overseas orchestras that have visited Japan this year," in a field that included the Berlin, Vienna, and New York philharmonics. An invitation to return to Japan was promptly extended, resulting in a second tour during the fall of 1997.

Music for the Masses

The BSO has also achieved critical success for its growing collection of recordings, with a discography of more than 20 highly acclaimed CDs on such major labels as Argo/London, Telarc, and Sony Classical. The orchestra and Zinman won their first Grammy Award in 1987 for a Sony Classical recording of cello concertos by Samuel Barber and Benjamin Britten with soloist Yo-Yo Ma. The BSO's stature as one of America's most admired orchestras was further enhanced in 1994 when *The New York Album*, recorded under the direction of Zinman and again featuring Yo-Yo Ma, won two Grammy awards.

Millions of listeners nationwide tune in to hear the BSO's *Casual Concert* radio broadcasts, an innovative 13-week series produced by WJHU-FM and aired on more than 150 Public Radio International and commercial classical stations. Combining warmth, wit, and informality

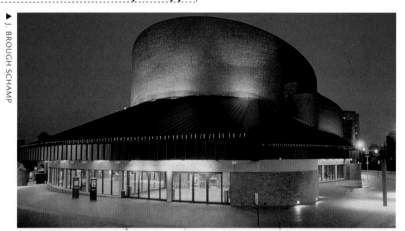

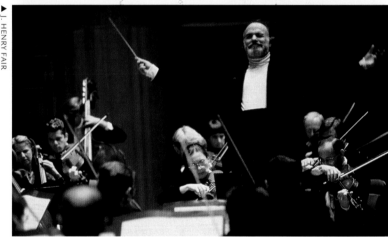

with outstanding orchestral performances, Zinman and the BSO have earned unqualified praise for their fresh and stimulating approach to classical music broadcasts.

The Baltimore Symphony Orchestra gives back to the community not only through its concerts, recordings, and nationally acclaimed radio programs, but also through its community outreach efforts and the Arts Excel initiative. This model school partnership program uses music and the arts to teach curriculum subjects to city and county students from preschool to high school age.

"We are delighted and proud that our orchestra has triumphed on the world stage," says BSO President John Gidwitz. "However, the primary mission of the Baltimore Symphony Orchestra is, as it has always been, serving the artistic, civic, and educational life of the Maryland community."

PLAYING IN THE JOSEPH MEYERHOFF SYMPHONY HALL, THE BALTIMORE SYMPHONY ORCHESTRA IS RENOWNED FOR ITS IMAGINATIVE INTERPRETATIONS OF MASTERWORKS AND ITS UNCOMPROMISING ARTISTIC INNOVATION. THE BSO HAS BEEN HAILED AS A PROTOTYPE FOR CLASSICAL MUSIC IN THE 21ST CENTURY (TOP).

WITH THE APPOINTMENT OF DAVID ZINMAN AS MUSIC DIRECTOR IN 1985, THE BSO'S REPUTATION FOR MUSICAL EXCELLENCE AND HIGH ARTISTIC ACHIEVEMENT SPREAD FAR BEYOND THE SHORES OF THE CHESAPEAKE TO A NEW AND DEVOTED INTERNATIONAL AUDIENCE (BOTTOM).

VNA of Maryland

THE VISITING NURSE ASSOCIATION (VNA) OF MARYLAND IS THE STATE'S oldest and largest home health care organization. Established in 1895, its mission was to provide home health care to the neediest residents of Baltimore. The VNA is a vital and thriving part of the fabric of this city, having provided care to the multitudes affected during past epidemics:

TB, polio, typhoid and the flu, and now the HIV/AIDS epidemic. The VNA has a history of involvement in caring for children and the elderly in their homes, as well as in expansive outreach programs to the underserved in Baltimore. Today's Visiting Nurse Association serves all residents of Maryland and is not only Medicare/Medicaid Assistance certified as a home health care agency and hospice, but also has been accredited with commendation by the Joint Commission on Accreditation for Healthcare Organizations (JCAHO).

The VNA continues to maintain its century-old mission of ensuring the availability of quality health care. As VNA President and Chief Executive Officer Jim Elmslie states, "Our mission is to improve the clinical outcomes for all patients by assisting them in maintaining or regaining optimal health and independence." During 1996, the VNA provided home care to more than 6,000 individuals. "The VNA was formed in response to community health needs and, generation after generation, we remain committed to serving all," says Elmslie. "We believe strongly that people recover better at home where they can be close to family and friends."

Comprehensive Home Care

Home health care has expanded rapidly over the past several years. The VNA provides an array of comprehensive services throughout the state of Maryland that includes registered nursing, home health aides, physical/occupational/speech therapies, social work, respiratory therapy, durable medical equipment, and medical supplies. In response to the ever changing health care environment, the VNA has specialized care programs including hospice, infusion therapy, behavioral health management, HIV/AIDS care team, transplant, oncology and chemotherapy services, high-risk pregnancy, pediatrics, and prenatal care. All services are available 24 hours a day, 365 days a year.

In 1988, the VNA Hospice of Maryland was established. "Hospice is a philosophy of care that helps patients and families make choices about care in life's final stages," says Elmslie. "Our goal is to help the patient and his or her family live as comfortably as possible, and find meaning and a sense of peace." The VNA's approach is to look at the whole person—the physical, psychological, spiritual, and social needs—and place importance on comfort, peace of mind, and quality of life. Patients are cared for by a team of medical professionals, volunteers, and spiritual care providers in their own homes. A program for residents of long-term care facilities has been established to address these unique needs. Personalized Bereavement Services help family survivors cope with their unique loss.

VNA's Home Support Services program assists individuals in maintaining their independence by providing personal care services in the home. Services include companions, assistance with shopping, and personal hygiene/grooming. Specialized programs have been developed that assist those dealing with the effects of Alzheimer's,

THE VISITING NURSE ASSOCIATION OF MARYLAND HAS BEEN PROVIDING HOME HEALTH CARE TO THE NEEDIEST RESIDENTS OF BALTIMORE SINCE 1895.

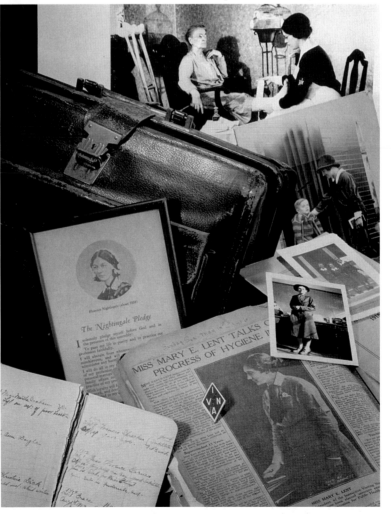

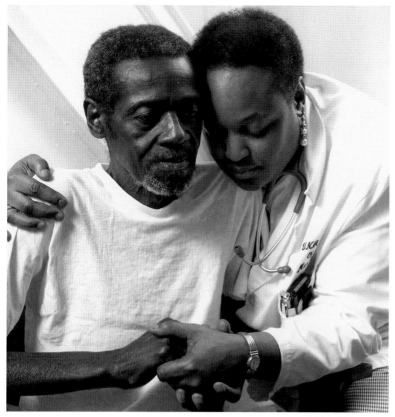

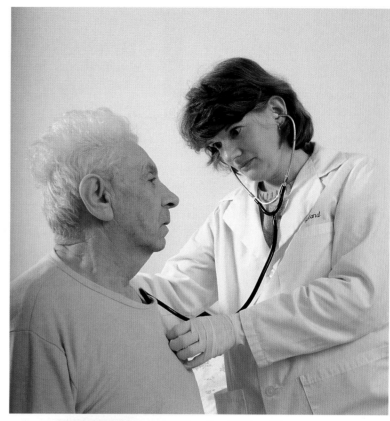

chronic diseases, or the ongoing effects of aging.

Vision 2000

As the 21st century approaches, making quality health care affordable requires a partnership with business, as well as with patients. Elmslie has been influential in moving the VNA forward through strategic alliances with other health care systems in the state of Maryland. "Our approach is to utilize state-of-the-art information systems to monitor care and measure outcomes. We will focus on the quality management of diseases and its impact upon the individual and caregiver.

"We recognize our responsibility to the changing needs of our community. We will continue to deliver the most effective, efficient home health and hospice services to our patients," says Elmslie. The VNA of Maryland is as committed to the future of health care as it has been in the past. "We take pride in our long, rich history of providing high-quality home health and hospice care to our neighbors and patients," he adds, "and will strive to continue to be faithful to our mission of service to the community."

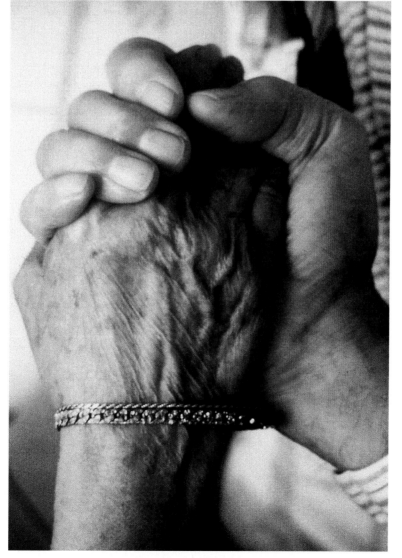

THE VNA OF MARYLAND ASSISTS INDIVIDUALS IN MAINTAINING THEIR INDEPENDENCE BY PROVIDING HEALTH CARE SERVICES IN THE HOME (TOP).

THE VNA OF MARYLAND IS COMMITTED TO THE FUTURE OF HEALTH CARE, AND WILL STRIVE TO CONTINUE TO BE FAITHFUL TO ITS MISSION OF SERVICE TO THE COMMUNITY (BOTTOM).

Legg Mason, Inc.

LEGG MASON, INC. IS A DIVERSIFIED, PUBLICLY OWNED FINANCIAL services firm with a strong presence in securities brokerage, asset management, investment banking, and related financial services. ∾ The firm traces its roots back to 1899, when a predecessor firm to Legg & Co. was founded in Baltimore. ∾ Newport News-based Mason & Co.

was founded in 1962 by Legg Mason's current chairman and CEO, Raymond A. "Chip" Mason. In 1970, the two firms merged and the newly created company was named Legg Mason. Mason & Co.'s first employee, James W. Brinkley, now serves as president of Legg Mason Wood Walker, Inc., Legg Mason's principal securities brokerage subsidiary that serves both corporate and individual investors.

Growth and Acquisitions Fuel Success

In 1982, Legg Mason entered the investment advisory business, introducing its first mutual fund, Legg Mason Value Trust. In the same year, two new subsidiaries were established to provide separate account management for small institutions and wealthy individuals, as well as advisory services for mutual funds. Since that time, assets under management have grown to more than $50 billion, including $12 billion in 41 proprietary mutual funds.

Since its initial public offering in 1983, Legg Mason's revenues have increased from $50 million to more than $700 million annually. Its total equity has increased from under $30 million to more than $450 million. Legg Mason Wood Walker has also grown dramatically in recent years, expanding its branch network to approximately 1,000 Financial Advisors in more than 100 offices along the east coast from Maine to Florida, and across the South to Texas, as well as internationally in London, Paris, and Geneva.

Securities Brokerage

Since Legg Mason's inception, securities brokerage has represented the largest segment of its business. As the firm's principal brokerage subsidiary, Legg Mason Wood Walker serves more than 450,000 investors and adheres to a client-conscientious mission. "Our primary objective is to help our clients acquire and maintain financial independence," says Brinkley.

To this end, the Equity Research Department has dedicated significant resources to assembling a senior research team of experienced analysts in attractive industry sectors. Utilizing extensive industry experience and fundamental company analysis, Legg Mason analysts identify timely and attractive investment opportunities in the equity markets.

Investment Advisory Services

Managing domestic and international equity and fixed-income assets for institutions and individuals is key to Legg Mason's business strategy, accounting for approximately 30 percent of total revenues. In fact, Legg Mason derives a higher percentage of its total revenues from asset management activities than any other publicly owned securities firm.

Legg Mason manages 41 proprietary stock, bond, and money market funds, including the Legg Mason Family of Funds, the firm's domestic funds family, and the LM Global Offshore Funds, an offshore funds family available to non-U.S. investors. The firm also offers investment advisory services through nine subsidiaries: Bartlett & Co. (Cincinnati); Batterymarch Financial Management, Inc. (Boston); The Fairfield Group, Inc. (Horsham, Pennsylvania); Gray, Seifert & Co., Inc. (New York); Legg Mason Capital Management, Inc. (Baltimore); Legg Mason Real Estate Services (Philadelphia); Legg Mason Fund Advisers, Inc. (Baltimore); Western Asset Global Management Limited (London); and Western Asset Management Company (Los Angeles). Legg Mason also established a *de novo* trust company in 1993.

Investment Banking Services

Legg Mason Wood Walker offers a broad range of investment banking services to corporations, state and local governments, and public agencies. Legg Mason's corporate finance division offers multidisciplinary resources

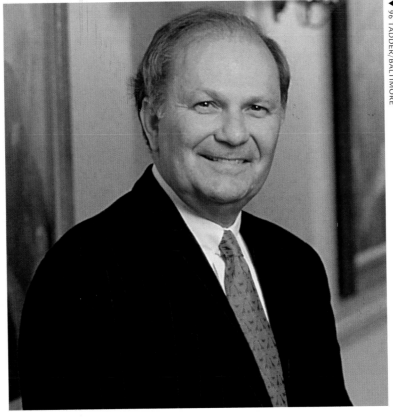

RAYMOND A. "CHIP" MASON IS LEGG MASON'S CHAIRMAN AND CEO.

◄ 96 TADDER/BALTIMORE

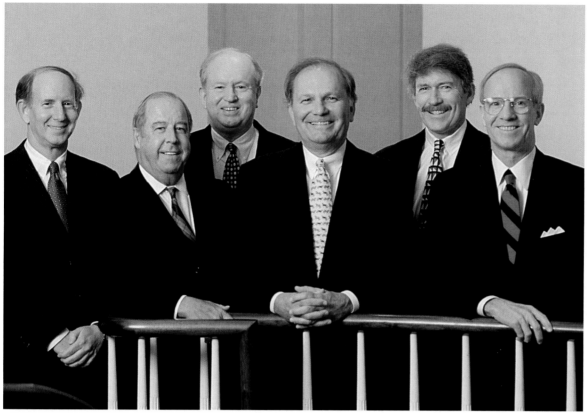

in research, trading, and sales that enable its investment bankers to recommend and execute a broad range of integrated, innovative solutions to the challenges of today's complex and rapidly evolving capital markets. These include mergers, acquisitions and divestitures, public offerings, and private placements.

Using the firm's own capital and extensive distribution net-

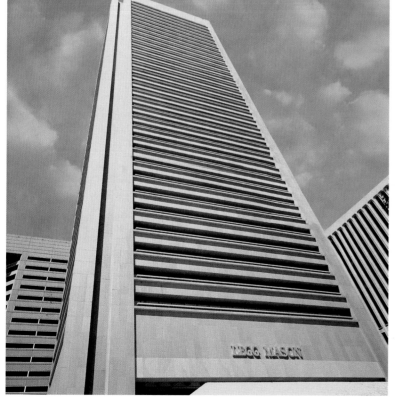

work, Legg Mason Wood Walker and its affiliate Howard, Weil, Labouisse, Friedrichs Inc. (New Orleans) make secondary markets in many of the securities they underwrite, as well as in more than 400 Nasdaq stocks. The breadth of Legg Mason's expertise serves a traditional middle-market client base, as well as larger companies in the following core areas: real

estate, health care, capital goods, education, financial institutions, retail and consumer, utilities, business services, and technology and communications.

Meeting Financial Needs on the Web

Introduced in 1996, Legg Mason's World Wide Web site—www.leggmason.com—provides general information about the fundamentals of financial planning and investing in stocks, bonds, and mutual funds; current market commentaries and recommendations regarding the economy and stock and bond markets; and detailed information regarding the wide variety of products and services available to individual investors through Legg Mason.

The firm's site is also interactive, permitting users to ask Legg Mason experts a range of specific investment questions. In addition, it offers a multipurpose financial planning calculator that can help investors calculate their retirement, college, estate, and other financial planning needs.

It's all part of Legg Mason's commitment to build and maintain a highly successful investment firm that places its clients' interests first and rewards its shareholders and employees.

Price-Modern, Inc.

IN 1904, BALTIMORE WAS A RAPIDLY GROWING COMMERCIAL CENTER. IT WAS A natural seaport, attracting merchant traders from around the world. It was a market hub, where seafood and produce were packed for shipment west. It was home to growing numbers of financiers, manufacturers, merchandisers, and tradesmen of every sort. ∾ In that year, when Charles Street was the city's

main thoroughfare and Mount Vernon Square was lined with the granite mansions of Baltimore's elite, Price-Modern, Inc. first opened its doors. Originally a printer and stationer, the firm quickly became known for its fine workmanship, distinctive products, and courteous, capable staff.

A Foundation for Success

This original reputation has served as Price-Modern's foundation for success. It spurred its evolution into a full-service commercial interiors firm, with business supplies and beverage service operations, and directed its market expansion throughout the Mid-Atlantic region. It is the basis

of the firm's long-standing relation-ships with the region's premier insti-tutions—Waverly Press, Johns Hopkins University and Johns Hopkins Hospital, Alexander & Alexander, Blue Cross/Blue Shield, Maryland Insurance Group, MCI, Northrop Grumman, Sylvan Learning Centers, and Riggs Bank, to name a few. And maintaining this reputation is the primary mission of Price-Modern's 200 employees working from the firm's four locations in Baltimore; Washington, D.C.; and Richmond and Norfolk, Virginia.

Furnishings That Work

Productivity is the bottom line in the current corpo-rate environment. Space design and furnishings play an important role in enhancing em-ployee effectiveness and output. As Price-Modern President Milford H. Marchant puts it, "To gain produc-tivity today requires efficient design, flexible and functional furnishing systems, and an intense level of before and after service."

Functional. Versatile. Sturdy. Affordable. These are the criteria today's office furnishings must meet. Price-Modern fulfills these criteria

by representing more than 100 manufacturers of distinctive, high-quality products and matching these products to a business' objectives and budget parameters.

Planning and Design Services

Price-Modern has the capa-bilities to manage interior design and furnishing projects from beginning to end.

Long before product selections are made, the firm's planning and design specialists analyze a business' space requirements, evaluate the feasibility of alternative solutions, and develop preliminary designs. Price-Modern was the first furniture dealer in Baltimore to invest in a computer aided design (CAD) unit. Today, CAD is considered standard technology in every facet of the office furniture business. The installation drawings and specifications it gen-erates match office furnishings to floor plans with electronic precision.

Price-Modern consultants make recommendations and guide businesses through the furnishings selection process. When it comes to choosing furniture, there are many options to consider: purchas-ing from manufacturers' standard

CAREFUL PROJECT MANAGEMENT GUAR-ANTEES AN ON-TIME, ON-BUDGET IMPLEMENTATION PROCESS (RIGHT).

PRESIDENT MILFORD H. MARCHANT (ON LEFT) AND SENIOR VICE PRESI-DENT ROBERT S. CARPENTER

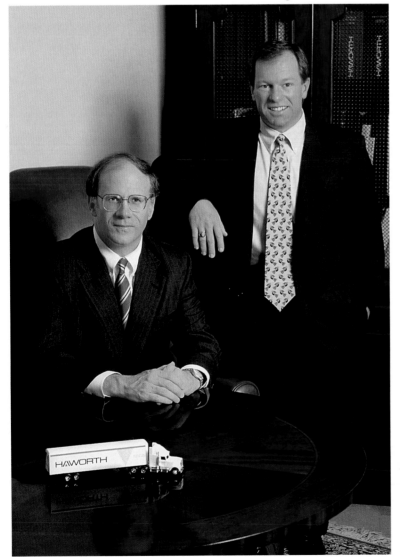

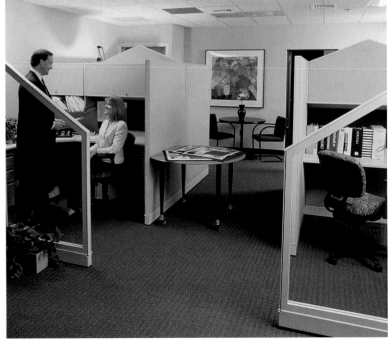

lines; investing in custom-designed pieces; leasing furniture; and refurbishing, refinishing, and reupholstering existing furniture.

No matter what options a business selects, Price-Modern has services to match. From order placement to delivery and installation, every project detail is expertly managed. Timing and other logistical considerations are addressed. If needed, warehousing is provided. Furniture trade-ins or liquidations can be arranged. And new furnishings are installed by factory-certified professionals who are trained in optimal furniture-handling techniques.

Price-Modern's services don't end when the installers' work is finished. The firm provides ongoing maintenance and repair services to back up its 100 percent customer-satisfaction guarantee.

From Paper Clips to Conference Tables to Coffee

Price-Modern meets the office supply needs of commercial customers throughout the region. The firm's catalog of office supplies features 24,000 items. A sophisticated order management system links the firm with suppliers and customers. Bringing it all together is the firm's courteous, knowledgeable staff. Thanks to their hard work and efficiency, most of the 1,000 daily orders Price-Modern receives reach customers within 24 hours.

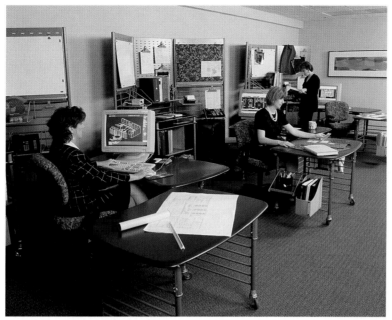

Price-Modern provides a full line of beverage products and services. The beverage menu includes gourmet coffees and teas, hot chocolate, instant soup, juices, cold beverages, and more. Sugar, sweetener, creamer, stirrers, cups, and other products are provided as well. Deliveries are made by Price-Modern's courteous, uniformed staff, who also check inventory levels to ensure that items are not overstocked or running short in between deliveries.

Strategic Growth

Price-Modern has engaged in a number of mergers, acquisitions, and alliances over the last three decades. In each case, the catalyst has been management's philosophy that strategic growth enhances the firm's stability and increases its buying clout on behalf of customers.

In the 1970s, Price-Modern merged with two regional office products firms, Modern Stationery Company and H.L. Marchant Company. In 1981, the firm formed a strategic partnership with Haworth, an organization regarded as the industry's most innovative manufacturer of high-quality office furnishings. The year 1986 saw the firm's expansion throughout the Mid-Atlantic region, with new offices in Washington, D.C., and Richmond and Norfolk, Virginia. Most recently, Price-Modern merged in 1996 with U.S. Office Products, a $3.3 billion corporation based in Washington, D.C.

Commenting on the firm's growth, Marchant again refers to the values instilled by Price-Modern's original founders. "Through these years of acquisition and expansion," Marchant states, "we've also enjoyed organic growth. This results from an ongoing tradition of quality customer service, an innovative product, competitive pricing, and a staff of dedicated professionals who take their responsibilities personally."

Much has changed since Price-Modern first opened its doors, but these core values remain the same. They have been the firm's guiding principles for nine decades, and they will provide direction and focus as Price-Modern moves into the next century and beyond.

WITH PRODUCTIVITY AND TECHNOLOGY IN MIND, AN EFFICIENT DESIGN BRINGS FURNISHINGS AND FUNCTIONS TOGETHER.

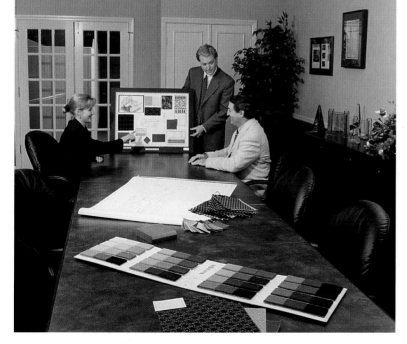

PRICE-MODERN CONSULTANTS ASSIST BUSINESSES THROUGH THE PROGRAMMING AND FURNITURE SELECTION PROCESS.

The Baltimore Museum of Art

ONE OF THE REGION'S GREATEST CULTURAL TREASURES, THE BALTIMORE Museum of Art (BMA) is Maryland's largest art museum. Contributing to the exceptional quality of life in Baltimore, the BMA welcomes more than 350,000 visitors annually, and offers a world-class permanent collection, ever changing exhibitions, exciting performances and special events, and a spectacular array of educational programs for children and adults alike.

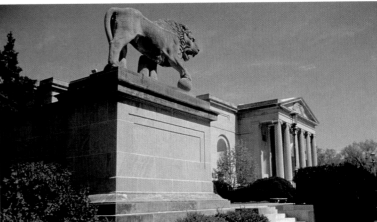

A Collection of Collections

Boasting a collection of more than 100,000 objects ranging from ancient mosaics to contemporary art, the BMA is acclaimed for the extraordinary private collections that have been donated to the museum over the years. The keystone of the BMA's permanent collection is the Cone Collection, celebrated as one of the most outstanding holdings of modern art in the world. Attracting visitors from around the globe, the Cone Collection features incomparable works by Matisse, Picasso, Cézanne, Gauguin, van Gogh, Renoir, and other masters of the late 19th and early 20th centuries. The Cone Wing's central Matisse Gallery, with dozens of works by the famed artist aligned in symphony, is a must-see destination in Baltimore. Altogether, the collection includes some 3,000 pieces acquired by Baltimore sisters Dr. Claribel and Miss Etta Cone between 1898 and 1949.

The BMA's distinguished collection of American and European decorative arts finds a fitting home in the museum's original 1929 building, grandly designed by the great neoclassical architect John Russell Pope. Spanning three floors, the BMA's newly renovated Pope Building showcases elegant exhibits of American paintings and sculpture of the 18th and 19th centuries, American and European decorative arts, textiles and American folk art, period rooms from six Maryland historic houses, and 12 miniature rooms. A stroll through these galleries offers a wonderful encounter with style, ornament, and craftsmanship.

The Baltimore Museum of Art houses one of the most notable collections of prints, drawings, and photographs in the country, with works spanning from the 16th to the 20th centuries. Prints and drawings by such distinguished artists as Rembrandt, Matisse, Picasso, Cézanne, Vuillard, Bonnard, Toulouse-Lautrec, Degas, Manet, Whistler, Cassatt, and Seurat are represented. The BMA also holds an exceptional range of photographs and numerous rare, vintage prints by many of the major photographers of the 20th century.

Exquisite African masks and brilliant Native American headdresses are among the objects found in the BMA's vast collection of the Arts of Africa, the Americas, and Oceania. This exceptional gallery displays the diverse cultures outside the Euro-Asian continent including African, pre-Columbian, Native American, and Oceanian.

Modern and Contemporary Art

The BMA has been dedicated to gathering the art of the 20th century since its founding. Exemplifying the museum's dedication to 20th-century art is the West Wing for Contemporary Art, which opened with much fanfare in October 1994. This striking aluminum and concrete structure houses 16 galleries for the display of the BMA's expanding and diverse permanent collection of post-1945 art. The West Wing's grand central gallery is a favorite of BMA's visitors; it is given entirely to the works of Andy Warhol, making the BMA home to the world's second-largest collection of paintings by the artist on regular public display. Other highlights include famous works by

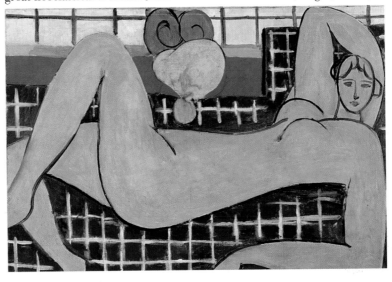

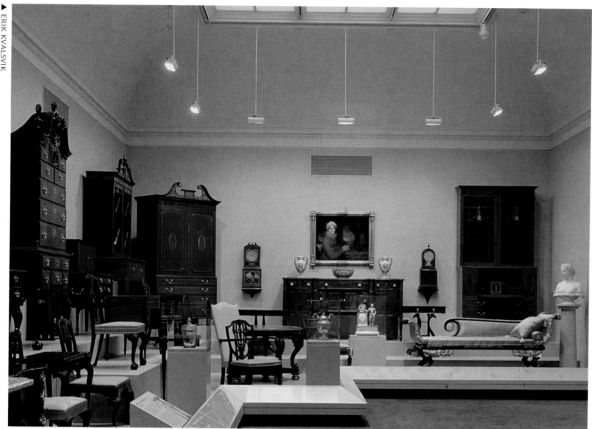

THE BMA'S DISTINGUISHED COLLECTION OF AMERICAN AND EUROPEAN DECORATIVE ARTS FINDS A FITTING HOME IN THE MUSEUM'S ORIGINAL 1929 BUILDING, GRANDLY DESIGNED BY THE GREAT NEOCLASSICAL ARCHITECT JOHN RUSSELL POPE.

Willem de Kooning, Grace Hartigan, Jasper Johns, Ellsworth Kelly, Roy Lichtenstein, Barbara Kruger, and Frank Stella, among others.

Those looking for a quiet haven can stroll through the BMA's outdoor sculpture gardens, among the nation's largest in an urban setting. The Ryda and Robert H. Levi Sculpture Garden and the Janet and Alan Wurtzburger Sculpture Garden feature modern and contemporary sculpture amid some 90,000 square feet of elegant landscaping. The two gardens include 20th-century works by artists from Auguste Rodin to Ellsworth Kelly, from Alexander Calder to Henry Moore.

Art in Action

All year long, the BMA offers Family Art Adventures, an array of programs for children and families. From Drop-In Workshops to Family Days, from Art-Ful Grandparenting to Family Gallery Games, the BMA uses its collections to introduce thousands to the world of art every year. The BMA's Department of Education and Community also offers a series of adult programs ranging from minicourses to Single Sundays.

The BMA hosts an abundance of performances and special events every year. Highlights include Black History Month, Summer Jazz Series, African Spirit Series, and the Baltimore Museum Antiques Show. The museum's popular FREESTYLE program features a festive, free-for-all evening on the first Thursday of each month that attracts thousands of visitors for a night of art, film, dance, gallery talks, children's workshops, and much more.

Since its founding in 1914, The Baltimore Museum of Art—with its remarkable collections, special exhibitions, and inviting programs—has served as a vital, enriching member of the community; it is a role that the BMA will fulfill for many years to come.

CONTRIBUTING TO THE EXCEPTIONAL QUALITY OF LIFE IN BALTIMORE, THE BMA WELCOMES MORE THAN 350,000 VISITORS ANNUALLY, AND OFFERS EVER CHANGING EXHIBITIONS AND A WORLD-CLASS PERMANENT COLLECTION (RIGHT).

BOASTING A COLLECTION OF MORE THAN 100,000 OBJECTS RANGING FROM ANCIENT MOSAICS TO CONTEMPORARY ART, THE BMA IS ACCLAIMED FOR THE EXTRAORDINARY PRIVATE COLLECTIONS THAT HAVE BEEN DONATED TO THE MUSEUM OVER THE YEARS (LEFT).

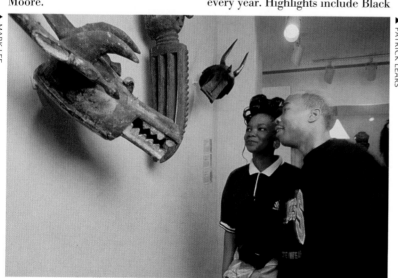

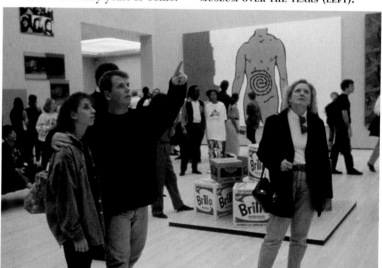

Procter & Gamble

IN 1914, A HAMPDEN PHARMACIST INVENTED A MEDICATED SKIN CREAM TO REMEDY sunburn pain. Dr. George A. Bunting's miracle cream acquired its name after a customer praised its many uses, exclaiming, "Your sun cream really knocked my eczema!" Today, Noxzema, Bunting's unique creation, has become one of the cosmetics industry's most enduring classics. ∾ With the multiuse skin

cream as its core product, the Bunting family operated Noxzema Chemical Company—renamed Noxell Corporation in 1966 when headquarters were moved to Hunt Valley, Maryland. Throughout the years, the company established itself as one of the nation's leading manufacturers of skin care products.

The Cover Girl Story

The introduction of Noxell's Cover Girl line of cosmetics, which blended Noxzema's medicated creams with makeup, revolutionized the company almost as much as Bunting's initial invention. The first Cover Girl product, a foundation that was manufactured in cream, powder, and liquid forms, was unveiled in 1961. Throughout that decade, other products appeared, including lip colors, mascaras, eyeliners, and nail polishes. Positioned as a glamour product rather than a medicinal one, Cover Girl was an immediate success. And indeed, famous beauties, such as Cybill Shepherd, Cheryl Tiegs, and Jennifer O'Neill, were among its beguiling spokesmodels. Cover Girl wasn't the only Noxell product to get celebrity treatment. Before Farrah Fawcett became one of ABC-TV's *Charlie's Angels*, she could be seen during NFL commercial breaks promoting Noxzema Instant Shave's "Great Balls O' Comfort."

A New Future

For six decades, Noxell Corporation had remained a private, family-owned business. Bunting's son Lloyd stepped in as president when his father retired, inheriting what essentially was a two-product company. Lloyd's son George, a member of the third generation of Buntings, took over the business in 1974.

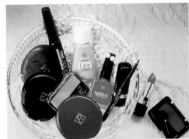

In 1989, Noxell Corporation took a new leap, merging with Procter & Gamble, one of the world's leading manufacturers in the development and marketing of consumer products. The move was positive for both companies. It enabled Procter & Gamble to immediately enter the cosmetics industry, and Noxell gained access to vast distribution channels and capital for expansion.

The partnership was such a success that, in 1991, Procter & Gamble acquired Max Factor, a major cosmetics seller in the drugstore marketplace. Max Factor, like Noxell, had a glamorous pedigree; its namesake had transformed his father's Hollywood-based movie-star makeup company into a global, mass-market enterprise. The combined businesses became known as Procter & Gamble Cosmetics.

Today, Procter & Gamble Cosmetics is one of the world's leading beauty products companies. Cover Girl is the best-selling mass cosmetics brand in the United States, employing such international supermodels as Niki Taylor and Tyra Banks, while Max Factor is sold in more than 50 countries around the world.

CLOCKWISE FROM TOP RIGHT: THE FIRST COVER GIRL PRODUCT WAS A FOUNDATION THAT WAS MANUFACTURED IN CREAM, POWDER, AND LIQUID FORMS. TODAY, THE COVER GIRL LINE OF COSMETICS INCLUDES LIP COLORS, MASCARAS, EYELINERS, AND NAIL POLISHES.

MAX FACTOR IS SOLD IN MORE THAN 50 COUNTRIES AROUND THE WORLD.

COVER GIRL IS THE BEST-SELLING MASS COSMETICS BRAND IN THE UNITED STATES, EMPLOYING SUCH INTERNATIONAL SUPERMODELS AS NIKI TAYLOR.

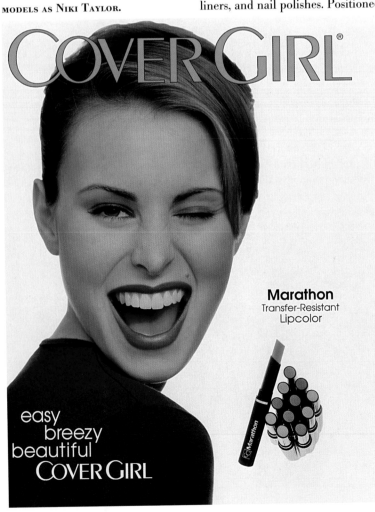

COVER GIRL®

Marathon
Transfer-Resistant
Lipcolor

easy
breezy
beautiful
COVER GIRL

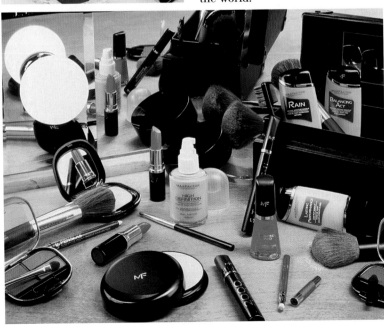

Lever Brothers Company

FOR MORE THAN 100 YEARS, THE LEVER BROTHERS COMPANY, WHICH marketed America's first brand of soap, has maintained a tradition of providing consumers with quality products at a sensible price. Today, Lever offers a wide range of family and home care products for the bath, laundry, and kitchen. ∾ Lever Brothers was originally established

in England by brothers William and James Lever. The U.S. arm of the company dates back to 1895, when William Lever traveled to New York to establish an American sales office. At that time, the company was known for Sunlight, a pure laundry soap. Soon after, it introduced Lifebuoy, the first deodorant soap. Today, Lever Brothers, a worldwide leader in the consumer products industry, manufactures brands such as Wisk®, all®, and Surf® laundry detergents; Snuggle® fabric softeners; and Dove®, Caress®, and Lever 2000® bars and shower gels.

A Baltimore Beginning

The opening of the Lever Brothers plant in Baltimore in 1938 marked a new era in the company's history. The plant, located on a onetime dairy farm, was first operated in 1926 by the Gold Dust Corporation. Since its acquisition by Lever Brothers, the original five-story building has been modernized and expanded into a large manufacturing complex, including a 460,000-square-foot distribution center.

From the beginning, the Baltimore plant has been a trendsetter in work practices and employee recognition. In 1939, the first "office girls club," called the Colony Club, was established. The Quarter Century Club, marking employees with 25 years of service to Lever, began in 1940 and is still in operation today. Baltimore employees also enjoyed then-progressive benefits, such as pension plans.

Lux Flakes and Lifebuoy were the first Lever brands produced at the Baltimore plant. The manufacturing center scored a number of firsts in new product development, including the 1950 production of Dove, a non-soap, moisturizing beauty bar, and Wisk, an all-purpose, heavy-duty laundry detergent. Currently, the Baltimore facility, which employs 525, manufactures the liquid laundry detergent for

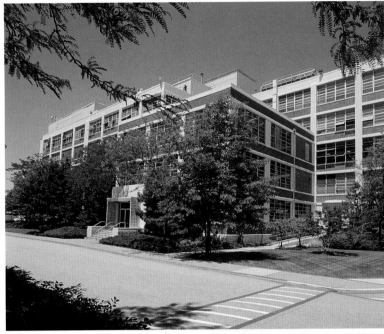

BOB STOCKFIELD

popular household brands Wisk, all, and Surf, as well as Dove and Caress beauty bars.

Commitment to Community

Lever's commitment to its Baltimore manufacturing center also extends to the local community—so much so that the company was honored in 1996 with the Mayor's Business Recognition Award for outstanding service.

Recognizing the importance of environmental initiatives, Lever Brothers was the first corporate sponsor of Tree-Mendous Maryland, a statewide conservation program. It also has underwritten programs like Project C-Wrap, a wetlands conservation and environmental education project benefiting Baltimore-area schools. Lever employees also have joined community volunteers for worthwhile projects with the National Park Foundation at Fort McHenry to promote recycling, and with the Mayor's Office for a cleanup project at Gwynn's Falls Park.

In addition, Lever supports, through charitable donations, such organizations as the Johns Hopkins Children's Center, Our Daily Bread, Dundalk Family

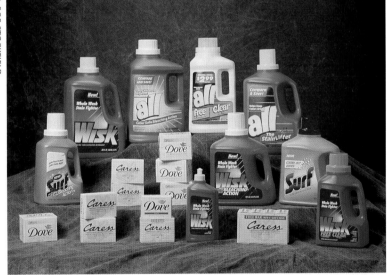

BOB STOCKFIELD

Crisis Center, and My Sister's Place. Likewise, the company has been active in community initiatives such as the Southeast Middle School Partnership, Hannah More School, food and clothing collections, and Red Cross blood drives.

From Lever Brothers Company's historic beginnings to its innovative products, its progressive systems development, and its environmental and community initiatives, the Baltimore manufacturing plant is poised to meet the 21st century with an eye on the future, while honoring its rich heritage.

PRODUCTS MANUFACTURED AT THE LEVER BROTHERS COMPANY FACTORY IN BALTIMORE INLCUDE, WISK®, ALL®, AND SURF® LAUNDRY DETERGENTS, AND DOVE® AND CARESS® BEAUTY BARS.

Sweetheart Cup Company Inc.

SWEETHEART CUP COMPANY INC., ONE OF BALTIMORE COUNTY'S LARGEST employers, has a proud tradition that dates back more than 75 years. Sweetheart, America's largest maker of disposable food service products, manufactures paper and plastic cups, plates, forks, and other utensils from its 11 factories in the United States and Canada, including its sprawling, 1.1 million-square-foot plant in Owings Mills.

The Man with a Vision

In the beginning, circa 1911, the Shapiro brothers of Boston opened a small grocery store in Chelsea, Massachusetts. Nearby, they established a tiny bakery to produce ice-cream cones. In 1920, the cone bakery was relocated to Baltimore. The city's appeal? A warmer climate and a diverse, growing population. According to company legend, Joseph Shapiro boarded a southbound train from Boston looking for a more prosperous locale, hopping off at Baltimore, the first stop below the Mason-Dixon Line.

Joseph Shapiro was an unusual man. A turn-of-the-century Russian immigrant, he created a benevolent, innovative, and profitable corporate giant that was first named Maryland Baking Co. Employees were treated like family, an atmosphere that encouraged many to stay for decades. The company, which soon expanded its product line to include straws, cups, and other picnic products, was paternalistic; layoffs and firings were discouraged. Executives led seasonal celebrations, handing out candy canes at Christmas and popsicles in the summer.

"Uncle Joe," a self-made man with only a basic education, established Shapiro Scholarships, which provided educational grants to children of poor families. While he stayed in Baltimore, his newly adopted home, the rest of the Shapiro family branched out across the United States, establishing bakeries in major cities.

During the depression, the Shapiros saw the ice-cream-soda-sipping straw as a natural addition to their product line of cones. Two wrapped straws were perfect for a boy and girl to share one soda; hence, the name Sweetheart—and its unforgettable logo—was born.

The Disposable Revolution

In 1947, Uncle Joe, a master of innovation, was poised to join the "disposable revolution," adding paper cups to his roster of products. He believed that paper cups would fit with the other Sweetheart products: they were inexpensive, nonreusable, and open to imaginative marketing. Uncle Joe convened family members for a vote. Accord-

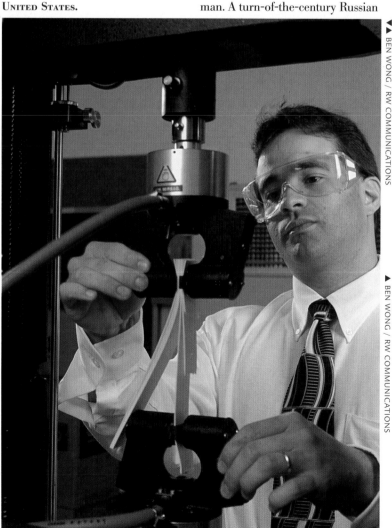

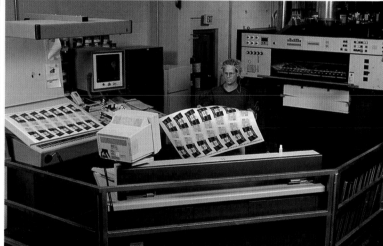

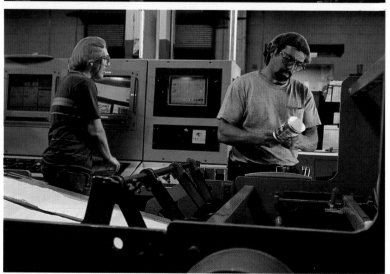

BEN WONG / RW COMMUNICATIONS

BEN WONG / RW COMMUNICATIONS

ing to company lore, he lost: 14 to one. It is said that he responded, "Good. We've got a majority of one." And, indeed, Sweetheart Cup entered the disposable marketplace at its very beginning. The result was the creation of products that became part of American life—the first yellow banana split dish, the revolutionary McDonald's foam "clamshell" (used until recently to keep hamburgers warm), and glossy plastic containers for yogurt.

Even as the company expanded, Uncle Joe continued to create a warm, family atmosphere. Under his tutelage, employees carved out a premium reputation for quality products and nutty promotions. There was the infamous Redcoat Revolution, in which teams of salesmen mimicked Paul Revere's fabled ride through the villages of New England; clad in red coats, these folks were actually on a mission to sell Sweetheart products. Another sales promotion was the Win a Rolls-Royce for a Day or a Week contest. The company purchased a Rolls-Royce and hired a French chauffeur from Brooklyn. The popular promotion finally folded after one Connecticut jobber, who'd won the car for the weekend, piled his family and luggage into the auto and ordered the driver to head for Montreal. "I think back to the days when I referred to Sweetheart as 'Disneyland East,' " remembers Richard D. Folkoff, a 32-year employee. "There was a forward-looking atmosphere of excitement, enthusiasm, and style—an atmosphere that was viewed first with tolerant amusement by the older, more established areas of the company. But as the years passed, amusement turned to admiration and tolerance turned to respect."

New Ownership

Throughout three decades, from the 1950s through the 1970s, Sweetheart Cup Company continued to create innovative disposable products. It introduced the now famous casual cup and holder, injection-molded "crystal" cups, and Silent Service dinnerware. By the time Shapiro died in 1968, the company was firmly established—32 Shapiro-owned operations had been combined in 1961 for a public offering of Maryland Cup stock. By

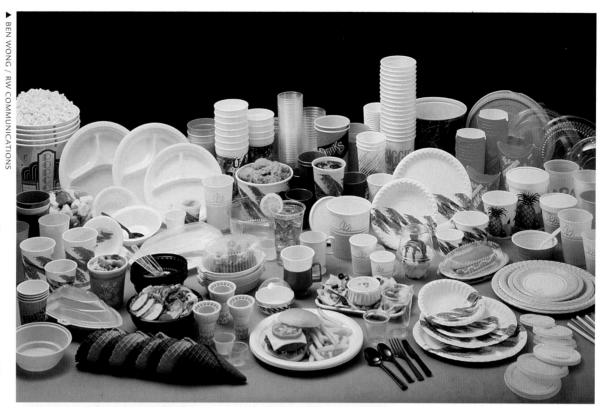

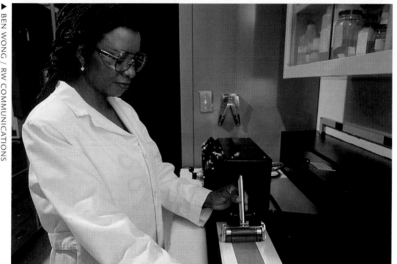

the 1980s, members of Sweetheart's senior executive staff were nearing retirement, and issues of succession were delicate among the close relatives who held the majority of the stock.

In 1983, the company was sold to Fort Howard Corporation. The years that followed brought with them management reorganization, plant consolidation, and a streamlining of operations. Fort Howard merged Sweetheart with Lily-Tulip, Inc., then spun off the company to investment banking giant Morgan Stanley. Sweetheart was acquired from Morgan Stanley in 1993 by American Industrial Partners Capital Fund, L.P. (AIP), which returned the company to independent status, returned its headquarters to Baltimore,

and reinstituted the company's commitment to quality, innovation, and customer service that had originally propelled Sweetheart to its leadership position.

Since then, Sweetheart Cup has enhanced its position in the industry. The Owings Mills facility once more is the heart of the company. With 2,200 employees, producing paper, plastic, and bakery items in Baltimore County, it is Sweetheart's largest manufacturing and warehousing complex, and serves as the administrative headquarters for 18 production and storage facilities throughout the United States.

Since its first set of straws, Sweetheart Cup Company has maintained its commitment to quality products and its Baltimore home.

SWEETHEART IS AMERICA'S LARGEST MAKER OF DISPOSABLE FOOD SERVICE PRODUCTS, MANUFACTURING PAPER AND PLASTIC CUPS, PLATES, FORKS, AND OTHER UTENSILS (TOP).

FROM THE COMPANY'S R&D LABS, SWEETHEART CONDUCTS A VARIETY OF TESTS AIMED AT ENSURING PRODUCT QUALITY (BOTTOM).

BEN WONG / RW COMMUNICATIONS

BEN WONG / RW COMMUNICATIONS

Colliers Pinkard

FOR 75 YEARS, COLLIERS PINKARD HAS PROVIDED REAL ESTATE SERVICES to maximize opportunities for its clients, whether focusing on local investments or multinational strategies. The firm has remained committed to forming partnerships with its clients and achieving unparalleled results on their behalf. ∾ The Colliers Pinkard of today is a diversified real estate company offering a full range of services to property owners, users of real estate, and all others connected with the commercial real estate industry. Services include asset management, leasing, building operations, construction, consulting, project marketing, appraisal, development, and investment sales, and are provided in the Baltimore region or wherever client needs dictate.

A Family History

In 1922, Walter Clyde Pinkard opened a small real estate office in Baltimore at 12 East Lexington Street, concentrating on rural and residential real estate. In those days, Baltimore did not include extensive suburbs, and much of the land bordering the city consisted of rural estates—the company's first specialty. In the 1930s, the firm took on property management when lenders foreclosed on struggling hotels and apartments.

Pinkard is remembered for helping to form the Governmental Efficiency and Economic Commission and for his services as president of the Real Estate Board of Baltimore (now the Greater Baltimore Board of Realtors) in 1940 and 1941. Through his association with the latter, he was instrumental in originating the first multiple listing service in the area.

Walter D. Pinkard joined his father at W.C. Pinkard & Co., Inc. in 1945, after graduating from Princeton and serving in the army during World War II. The younger Pinkard was instrumental in moving the firm to focus on commercial and industrial real estate. He soon became active in the Baltimore business community, serving the Junior Association of Commerce, Mortgage Bankers Association, and Citizens' Planning and Housing Association.

In 1959, Philip C. Iglehart became associated with the company, and played a major role in its evolution into one of the region's leading commercial and industrial real estate companies. Iglehart was elected president of the company in 1978, becoming the first nonfamily stockholder in the firm's history. This trend of expanded ownership has continued since, and today finds the firm owned by a large group of its key professionals.

In 1974, after graduating from Yale and Harvard Business School, Walter D. Pinkard Jr. became the third generation of Pinkards to become associated with the well-known firm. The company's president since 1982, he has been central to the firm's present-day positioning as a primary force in the real estate marketplace. Appraisal, consulting, investment, and corporate services units have been added since Pinkard took the helm, while the property management division has grown considerably. He has also continued the family tradition of civic leadership, serving on numerous boards, including the Greater Baltimore Committee, Johns Hopkins University, and the Baltimore Community Foundation, which he currently chairs.

In 1984, Pinkard took the firm to a new level, joining the prestigious Colliers International group, prompting the company's name change to Colliers Pinkard. As a corporation built on the collective expertise of local experts, Colliers International is uniquely able to operate across cultures, languages, customs, and business practices. The international company harnesses the resources, skills, experience, and capabilities of more than 5,000 professionals in more than 200 markets worldwide. This collective knowledge, ability, and experience can be brought to bear in any client relationship and on any assignment.

Today, Colliers Pinkard is a team of some 60 professionals and 20 support staff in the company's three offices in downtown Baltimore, Columbia, and Towson, as well as

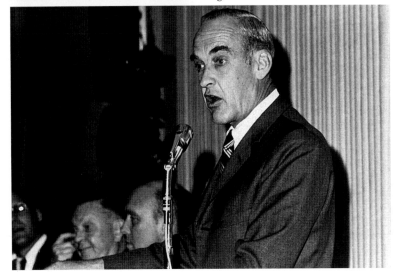

WALTER CLYDE PINKARD OPENED A SMALL REAL ESTATE OFFICE IN 1922 THAT BECAME TODAY'S COLLIERS PINKARD.

WALTER D. PINKARD JOINED THE COMPANY IN 1945 AFTER SERVING IN THE ARMY AND GRADUATING FROM PRINCETON.

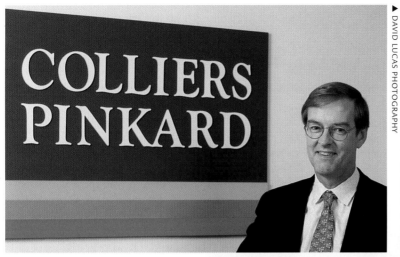

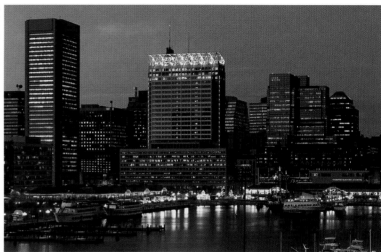

DAVID LUCAS PHOTOGRAPHY

being an equity owner of Colliers' offices in Eastern Europe.

Advisory Relationship Strategy

Operating more along the lines of an accounting firm or law firm, Colliers Pinkard has concentrated on developing advisory relationship business with owners, users, and corporations. The firm views its approach as distinctly different from the transaction-driven brokerage business of many real estate companies. To better provide this advisory relationship, Colliers Pinkard has dramatically expanded and diversified the services it offers and continues to change in response to the needs of its clients.

Calling upon its diversity, from consulting to sales, valuation to management, Colliers Pinkard professionals bring a unique perspective to problem solving. Corporations such as T. Rowe Price, BT Alex. Brown, Legg Mason, Black & Decker, IBM, Procter & Gamble, and Rite Aid have benefited from the strong foundation and presence of Colliers Pinkard in the community.

A Crucial Role in the Community

Employees of Colliers Pinkard are strong proponents of investing in the community. Throughout its 75-year history, the firm has encouraged its employees to donate time, money, and intellectual capital to charities and organizations that improve the quality of life for people in Baltimore and, indeed, around the world.

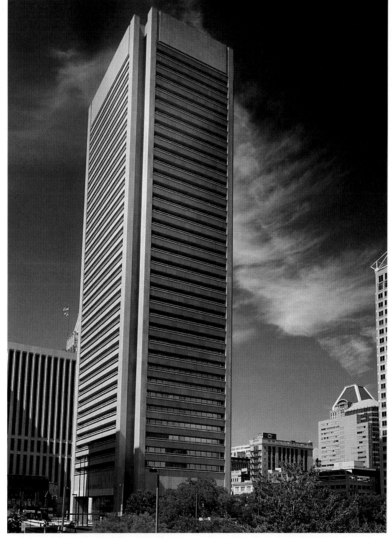

The American Heart Association, Salvation Army, United Way of Central Maryland, Make-A-Wish Foundation, and Goodwill Industries have seen the beneficence of Colliers Pinkard. Baltimore Institutions such as the Johns Hopkins Institutions, Baltimore Zoo, Baltimore Symphony Orchestra, Maryland Science Center, and Walters Art Gallery have also benefited

from the generosity of the company and its employees.

Today, Colliers Pinkard and its employees are involved in a partnership with City Springs Elementary School. Their donation of time, money, expertise, and materials has helped to create a more vibrant and hopeful atmosphere at this important inner-city school.

CLOCKWISE FROM TOP LEFT: WALTER D. PINKARD JR. IS THE THIRD GENERATION OF THE PINKARD FAMILY TO BE ASSOCIATED WITH THE FIRM.

THE BALTIMORE SKYLINE

COLLIERS PINKARD'S HEADQUARTERS OFFICE IS LOCATED AT 100 LIGHT STREET.

Baltimore Opera Company

BALTIMORE LOVES OPERA. WHETHER IT IS *The Beggar's Opera*, WHICH was the city's first operatic performance on record in 1752, or more recent productions of works by Beethoven or Verdi, Baltimoreans have embraced the art form. "Opera is beautiful," says Michael Harrison, general director of the Baltimore Opera Company. "Its appeal is in the

blending of art forms—drama from the theater, music from the symphony, spectacular singing from musical theater, and magnificent sets and costumes thrown in for good measure. Opera is a treat that satisfies all the senses, one that is every bit as entertaining as a Broadway show. Opera is a spectacle."

Baltimore's love for opera has evolved throughout a long heritage. During the 19th century, traveling opera companies regularly per-

formed in the city, supplying Baltimore's first performances of works such as *Faust*, *La Sonnambula*, *Norma*, and *La Favorita*. World-renowned divas such as Clara Kellogg, Marcella Sembrich, and Jenny Lind were among the performers.

"Imported" opera was a Baltimore staple for many years until 1924, when Eugene Martinet founded the Martinet School of Opera, which played at the Maryland Casualty Audi-

torium in what is now the Rotunda. Dedicated to spotlighting local talent, the school blossomed into the Baltimore Civic Opera Company.

It was out of this hardworking organization that the present-day Baltimore Opera Company was formed. Incorporated in 1950, its first performance was *Aïda*, and its first artistic director was Baltimore's own great diva, Rosa Ponselle. The company's original goals of developing talented artists and educating the public in the appreciation of opera and fine music provide a solid foundation for the continued growth of the company today.

Baltimore's Modern Opera

The Baltimore Opera Company quickly established a reputation for developing high-quality productions featuring many of the world's top performers. In the 1960s, the company's repertoire, which had been primarily the operatic warhorses, diversified with such productions as *Der Rosenkavalier*, featuring noted conductor Kurt Adler. Major opera stars appeared, including Sherrill Milnes in *Rigoletto*, Anna Moffo in *Lucia di Lammermoor*, Birgit Nilsson and Teresa Stratas in *Turandot*, and Beverly Sills, Placido Domingo, and Norman Treigle in *Tales of Hoffmann*.

The year 1963 marked the first Baltimore Opera Vocal Competition. Second only in size to the Metropolitan Opera's Audition of the Air, Baltimore's competition has given many talented young singers recognition and financial help to support their careers. Many winners have found major operatic careers, among them Paul Plishka, Maria Ewing, Shelia Nadler, Florence Quivar, Carmen Balthrop, and Baltimore native James Morris, who got his start in the Baltimore Opera Chorus and is considered one of the world's premier basses.

In the 1980s, the company, like many arts organizations of that time, found its future endangered

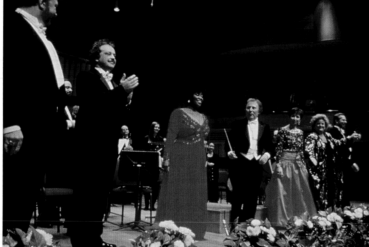

A GALA BENEFIT FOR THE EDUCATION AND OUTREACH PROGRAM STARRED CHRIS MERRITT, STEFAN PIATNYCHKO, FLORENCE QUIVAR, MAESTRO ANTON GUADAGNO, SUSAN POWELL, DEBORAH VOIGT, AND JAMES MORRIS (TOP).

THE BALTIMORE OPERA COMPANY'S ORIGINAL PRODUCTION OF *Samson et Dalila* WAS DESIGNED BY ROBERTO OSWALD AND ANIBAL LAPIZ (BOTTOM).

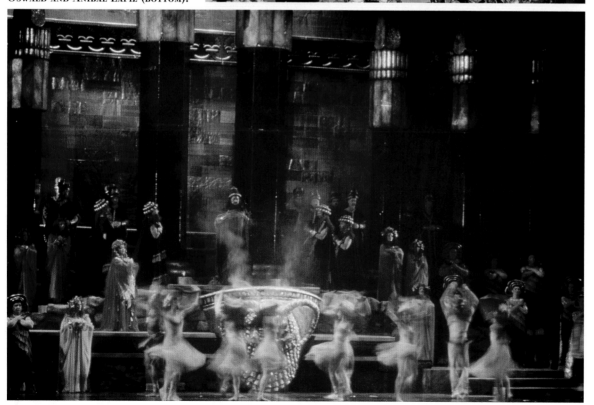

by a financial crisis. Harrison was hired as the company's new general director, and the Baltimore Opera Company set out to charter a new course, rejuvenating itself by repositioning the business and by enhancing awareness of the art form.

The goal of the revamped company was threefold: to attract new audiences with blockbuster productions, to continue tantalizing patrons—veterans and newcomers alike—with innovative interpretations of classics, and to produce important and wonderful works that hadn't yet achieved mass popularity.

Under Harrison's tutelage, the Baltimore Opera Company regained—and has maintained—its financial footing. In the last five years, audience levels have increased by 70 percent. The Baltimore Opera Company is recognized as a premier organization by artists and businesses alike.

One important factor in opera's resurgence of popularity is the widespread use of surtitles. "At the Baltimore Opera, we project translations above the stage so people are able to follow the action and drama while experiencing the opera in its language of composition," Harrison explains. "We've found that reassuring the public that they will understand the plot dramatically increases the likelihood that they will attend the opera."

Opera for the Community

In stabilizing its base, the company has recognized that strenuous efforts should be directed toward the community that supports it. Its comprehensive touring program, which consists of a half-dozen different programs that reach an audience of 70,000 public school students annually in the city and county of Baltimore, features everything from Puppets & *Pagliacci*, geared to pre-elementary-level children, to Create & Produce, an operative venture in which high school students create their own productions.

Baltimore Opera has not limited its influence to the Mid-Atlantic region. The company has also entered into partnerships with major U.S. and European opera companies to collaborate in the development of

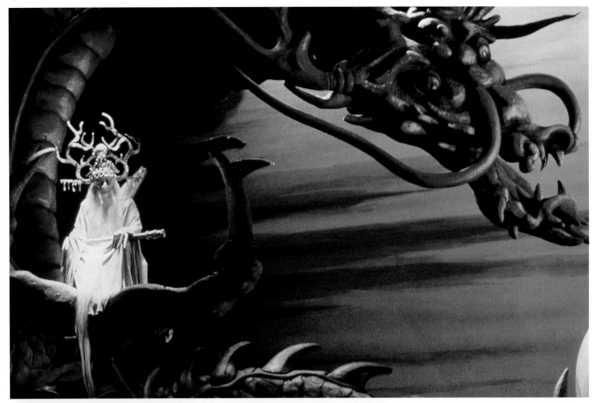

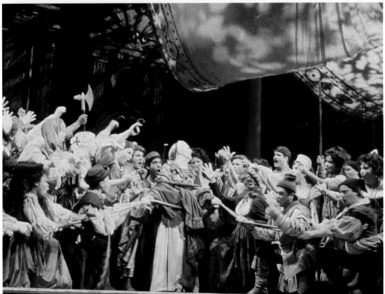

THE COMPANY WOWED AUDIENCES WITH ITS 1992 PRODUCTION OF *Turandot* (TOP).

THE 1996 PRODUCTION OF AMILCARE PONCHIELLI'S *La Gioconda* STARRED GHENA DIMITROVA (BOTTOM).

new grand operatic productions, which will be presented to Baltimore audiences in coming seasons.

Designers and directors from theater and film, as well as noted choreographers, are engaged for future operas. Additionally, the company's administrative office relocated to the Lyric Opera House—further evidence of the growth and stability of the organization.

An Amazing Resurgence

Onstage and off, the Baltimore Opera Company is committed to conveying the excitement of this dramatic form to new audiences and seasoned opera fans.

"The success of this company is due to the concerted efforts of dedicated individuals who believe that a thriving art and cultural scene is crucial to the life of a community," says Harrison. "Without the support of a viable board of trustees, business partners, government agencies, supporting foundations, staff, and volunteers, the company could not have achieved the level of artistic and financial success it enjoys today."

From the early performance of *The Beggar's Opera* to Rosa Ponselle's *Aïda* to current productions, the Baltimore Opera Company is making sure opera remains a thriving art form.

WBAL Radio

WBAL Radio is Baltimore's dominant and most powerful radio station. Since 1925, generations of Marylanders have turned to WBAL Radio for news, weather, thought-provoking discussions, and sports. As Maryland's only 50,000-watt AM station, WBAL's signal travels substantially farther than any other

station in the state and beyond.

WBAL Radio is recognized as one of the most successful stations in America and has dominated the Baltimore market for decades. The station's news/talk format is a source of both information and entertainment. WBAL, according to the Arbitron ratings service, is consistently the radio station most listened to in Maryland. WBAL Radio's target audience is adult listeners aged 25 and older.

Where Baltimore Turns for News, Talk, and Sports

WBAL Radio employs the largest news staff of any radio station in the state, providing in-depth reports on local and regional issues. When something important happens, people know they can hear about it on WBAL Radio. In addition, the station's talk programming provides lively discussions and frank opinions

about what is happening down the block and around the world.

WBAL Radio is a unique news/talk/sports station. It provides a rich source of information and entertainment. The talk shows on WBAL Radio are like town meetings. From the deficit to Darwinism, from politics to pornography, hosts Allan Prell, Ron Smith, and

Rush Limbaugh talk about it. WBAL Radio covers the topics people care about and has the guests people want to hear.

WBAL Radio positions and markets itself as the station "Where the news comes first." The station has Baltimore's largest radio news staff, comprised of 10 anchors and reporters, three meteorologists, a

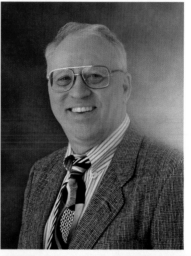

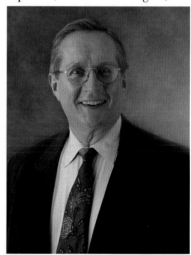

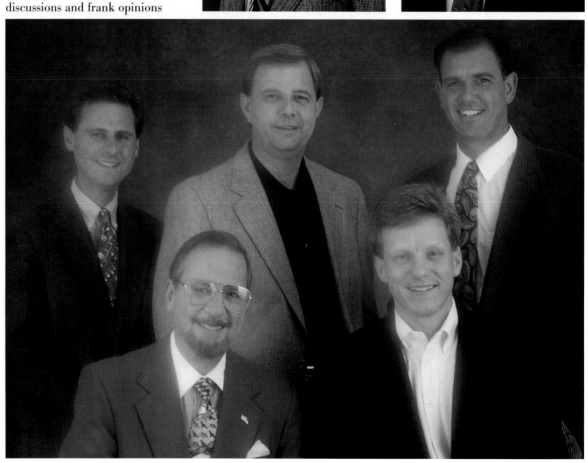

CLOCKWISE FROM TOP LEFT: WBAL RADIO'S ALLAN PRELL IS ON THE AIR WEEKDAY MORNINGS FROM 9 A.M. UNTIL NOON.

RON SMITH TAKES TO THE AIRWAVES WEEKDAY AFTERNOONS FROM 3 P.M. UNTIL 6 P.M.

DAVE DURIAN AND THE WBAL MORNING TEAM ENTERTAIN AUDIENCES WEEKDAYS FROM 5 A.M. TO 9 A.M.: (FRONT ROW, FROM LEFT) ALAN WALDEN, MORNING NEWS ANCHOR; TOM TASSELMYER, CHIEF METEOROLOGIST; (BACK ROW, FROM LEFT) DAVE SANDLER, TRAFFIC REPORTER; DAVE DURIAN, MORNING SHOW HOST; AND MARK VIVIANO, SPORTS REPORTER.

traffic reporter, a large sports staff, and specialists in business and political reporting.

There is a lot more to sports than just knowing the score. That's why WBAL Radio is Baltimore's sports voice. Weekday evenings and on weekends the station conducts sports talk shows with a great menu of hosts. In addition, WBAL Radio covers all sports, from prep to pro. As the voice of the Baltimore Orioles, WBAL Radio provides exciting play-by-play coverage of every game, including informative and entertaining pre- and postgame shows. WBAL Radio also provides play-by-play coverage of collegiate sports, including University of Maryland football and basketball. In addition, the station airs coverage of the World Series, the Super Bowl, the NCAA Basketball Tournament, and the Preakness.

Involved in Baltimore

WBAL Radio's ratings superiority is not just the result of the station's programming. WBAL Radio is a Baltimore institution. The station believes that it is good business to be a good citizen, and is committed to the community. WBAL

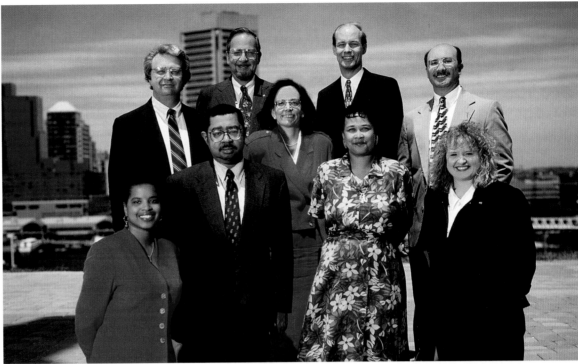

Radio's community involvement has been honored with numerous awards, including the National Association of Broadcasters' prestigious Crystal Award for excellence in local achievement. The station also has been the recipient of awards from the Greater Baltimore Committee and has received the Mayor's Business Recognition Award.

The WBAL Radio Kids Campaign is an ongoing partnership between the station and its listeners to provide needy children with coats, books, eyeglasses, medical help, and even some fun. Several million dollars have been distributed in recent years. In addition to raising funds, WBAL Radio has been instrumental in collecting items for the needs of people.

THE AWARD-WINNING WBAL RADIO NEWS DEPARTMENT INCLUDES (FRONT ROW, FROM LEFT) LINDA FOY, LEONARD ROBERTS, SUE KOPEN, ROSEARL JULIAN, ANNE KRAMER, (BACK ROW, FROM LEFT) JACK SHAUM, ALAN WALDEN, MARK MILLER, AND JOHN PATTI.

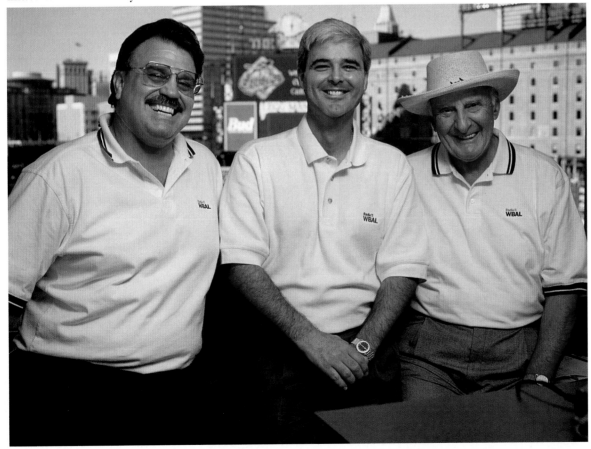

THE WBAL RADIO ORIOLES PLAY-BY-PLAY BROADCAST TEAM: FRED MANFRA, JIM HUNTER, AND HALL-OF-FAMER CHUCK THOMPSON

Alban Tractor Company Inc.

ALBAN TRACTOR COMPANY INC., A FOURTH-GENERATION FAMILY FIRM THAT celebrated its 70th anniversary in 1997, is one of America's oldest and largest distributors of Caterpillar construction equipment. Additionally, the Baltimore-based company has been rebuilding the products it sells—from bulldozers to excavators to trucks—for some 40 years.

Under the leadership of James "Jamie" Alban IV, Alban Tractor Company today employs more than 460 people—a third of whom have worked at the company for more than two decades. As he guides the company through a period of aggressive growth, Alban—like his father, grandfather, and great-grandfather before him—remains committed to honoring time-tested traditions. "We're a 1990s company with an old-fashioned family sense," he says.

The Early Years

In 1917, James C. Alban was an automotive toolmaker with an entrepreneurial spirit. During a time when commercial equipment focused mainly on farming, the Pennsylvania native recognized that along with the invention of the car came a need for good roads and the equipment it would take to build them. He left his job at a local Cadillac dealership and went to work for a tractor wholesaler.

Alban joined forces with Zachariah Johnson in 1922 to form Alban & Johnson. Three years later, as the Caterpillar Corporation emerged as an industry giant, Alban & Johnson became a dealer for a New York-based Caterpillar distributor. Johnson retired in 1927, and Alban formed his own company.

In its first year, Alban's only employee was his wife, Clara. Operations netted just $20,000. But despite the Great Depression, the business began a long history of steady growth, eventually being named direct Caterpillar distributor for Maryland, Delaware, the District of Columbia, and Virginia's eastern shore.

The World War II era marked an explosion of construction projects related to the military and spin-off projects following the war's end. Soldiers, who had learned to use industrial equipment during the war, returned home and opened their own construction companies. And, perhaps more important, the era marked the creation of the interstate highway system.

Alban Tractor's own growth spurt began in 1940, when it opened a sales and service facility in Salisbury. In 1945, the company took on responsibility for sales and service in northern Virginia, opening a branch in Arlington. A few years later, Alban Tractor dedicated itself exclusively to Caterpillar.

The postwar era also included the creation of Alban's Undercarriage Repair Division. While most companies were replacing undercarriages, Alban became one of the first distributors to economically and efficiently rebuild the undercarriages of Caterpillar's track-type tractors.

Other milestones included the construction of a new facility on Pulaski Highway in 1948; westward expansion into Frederick in 1955; and adoption of a profit-sharing plan for employees in 1957. Throughout the next three decades, Alban Tractor continued to open new facilities throughout Maryland and Virginia. Alban Engine Power Systems, a sales and service facility for marine and industrial truck engines, was created in the 1970s.

Today, the company is one of the East Coast's largest distributors of Caterpillar construction equipment, as well as a leader in the field of industrial reconstruction and repair. In 1997, Alban created its state-of-the-art Remanufacturing Center, which has enabled Alban to offer new services to new customers, including hydraulic repair for SCM Chemicals and Bethlehem

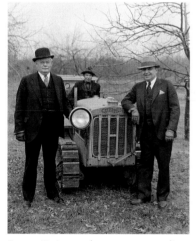

JAMES C. ALBAN (ABOVE, AT RIGHT) FOUNDED ALBAN TRACTOR IN 1922.

FOUR GENERATIONS OF ALBANS HAVE LED THE FAMILY BUSINESS. THREE OF THOSE GENERATIONS INCLUDE FROM LEFT: JAMES "JAMIE" ALBAN IV, JAMES C. "BUCK" ALBAN JR., AND JAMES C. ALBAN III (RIGHT).

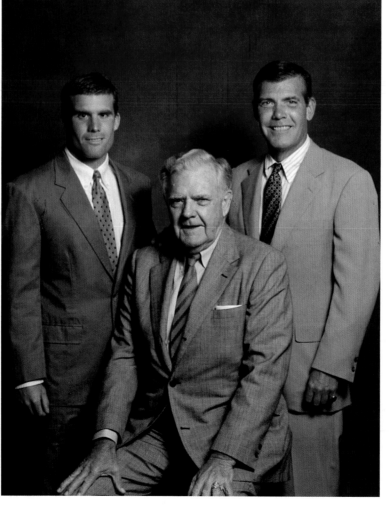

Steel's shipyard, component rebuilding for General Motors factory equipment, and cylinder rebuilding for Dundalk Marine Terminal.

Honoring Community and Family Roots

Ever since James and Clara Alban founded Alban Tractor Company, the family has continued its rich tradition of leadership. James and Clara's son, James C. "Buck" Alban Jr., joined the family firm in 1938. James C. Alban III joined the company in 1961 and became president in 1983. His son, Jamie Alban, came to work for Alban Tractor Company in 1992. Upon his father's retirement in 1997, Jamie Alban assumed the post of company president.

Through four generations of Alban leadership, the company has maintained close ties to both its employees and its hometown. "As a family, we are very visible and very involved," Jamie Alban says. At the same time, company employees are treated as family. Benefits are generous; for more than 40 years, Alban Tractor Company has maintained a pension and profit-sharing plan for employees, and it added a 401(k) provision a few years ago. End-of-year bonuses are common for all employees, including those who work for an hourly wage.

A wide range of programs—from athletics to safety seminars to valued service awards—keeps the family way of doing business alive. The approach pays off: In addition to the Albans, the staff itself is made up of quite a few second-generation families.

Alban Tractor is also committed to community causes, supporting the United Way Campaign for Central Maryland for many years. Individual family members concentrate their community efforts in the health and education arena, with family involvement in the Kennedy-Krieger Institute, Make-A-Wish Foundation, Boys' Latin School, Franklin Square Hospital, Maryland Historical Society, and Associated Catholic Charities. Alban Tractor Company also donates generously to the Baltimore Community Foundation, which specializes in funding for education and health care.

Since its beginnings in 1927, Alban Tractor has served the Baltimore area and much of the East Coast by distributing, servicing, and rebuilding the construction equipment that has kept a country on the move.

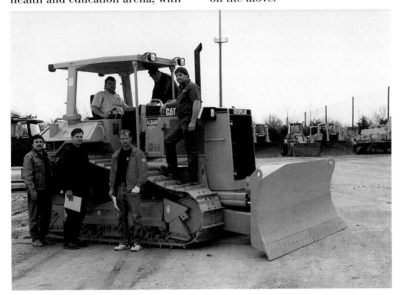

ALBAN TRACTOR COMPANY, A FOURTH-GENERATION FAMILY FIRM THAT CELEBRATED ITS 70TH ANNIVERSARY IN 1997, IS ONE OF AMERICA'S OLDEST AND LARGEST DISTRIBUTORS OF CATERPILLAR CONSTRUCTION EQUIPMENT.

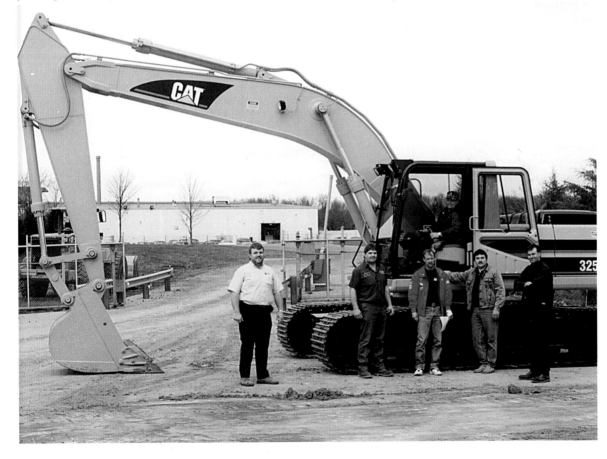

Taylor Technologies, Inc.

IN 1930, WHEN DR. WILLIAM A. TAYLOR SET UP A SMALL LAB TO MAKE WATER test kits in downtown Baltimore, he likely did not anticipate that W.A. Taylor & Company would eventually become one of the area's fastest-growing technology firms. Renamed Taylor Technologies 50 years after its founding, the company still manufactures products for water analysis, but now its

reagents and testing apparatus are employed by water analysts world-wide in an amazing variety of applications.

At the time of its inception, Taylor targeted industrial customers, helping boiler operators extend the life of their equipment and improve its efficiency by providing simple color-matching and drop tests to determine pH, alkalinity, and other aspects of boiler water treatment. Over time, the business has grown to keep pace with changes in society that have brought about an ever-increasing need to monitor water quality—at home, in the workplace, and in the natural environment.

While the company continues to manufacture test kits for boilers and cooling systems, its product line also includes kits for numerous other uses: swimming pool and spa maintenance; paper manufacturing, surface finishing, and many other water-dependent industrial operations; municipal water and wastewater treatment; stormwater monitoring and related water pollution control activities; residential and commercial water conditioning; food and beverage production; aquaculture; even as teaching aids for high school ecology classes. Nearly 600 different test kits are currently offered.

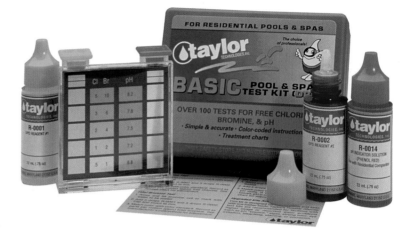

CLOCKWISE FROM TOP: TAYLOR TECHNOLOGIES' POOL/SPA TEST KIT LINE HAS SEEN THE MOST GROWTH IN RECENT YEARS.

MANY FORMULAS FOR THE COMPANY'S LIQUID COLOR STANDARDS, WHICH ARE GUARANTEED NEVER TO FADE, WERE DEVELOPED IN THIS TOWSON LAB.

TAYLOR NOW MAKES ITS OWN PLASTIC KIT COMPONENTS TO BETTER CONTROL QUALITY AND AVAILABILITY.

Continuing a Tradition of Great Customer Service

What hasn't changed over the years is the emphasis placed on customer service. "We don't compete on price," says Paul F. Wooden Jr., president and CEO. "Never have, never will. We make a good product, we make it easy to buy, and we provide technical support to our users." Clearly, the marketplace has responded. In 1995, Taylor was named to the Baltimore Fast 40, the first-ever ranking of the top technology firms in the region, based on its growth rate of 67 percent over the previous five years.

The evolution of Taylor Technologies into the modern era of water testing can be traced back to 1980, when Wooden, a CPA-turned-entrepreneur, purchased the firm. It was then called Taylor Chemicals, and business was conducted out of the basement and ground floor of a modest residence in suburban Towson by Dr. Taylor's successor, John Lambrecht. Wooden's first move was to rename the company to reflect its broader mission, his next, to leave the outmoded facility at York Road and Stevenson Lane. Ever since, Wooden, who received the 1995 Maryland Entrepreneur of the Year® award for manufacturing, has continued to transform the company into a world-class supplier of tools for water-quality monitoring.

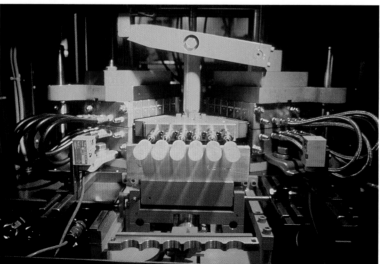

◀ ROGER MILLER

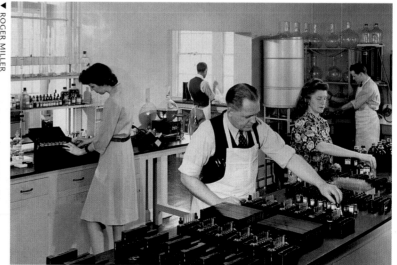

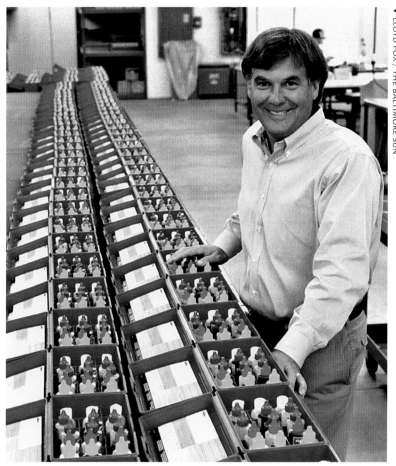

1995 Entrepreneur Of The Year®

PAUL F. WOODEN, JR.

TAYLOR TECHNOLOGIES, INC.

ERNST & YOUNG LLP   Inc.   Merrill Lynch

"For over 65 years, people involved in all facets of water testing have come to depend on the excellence built into every Taylor product," Wooden says. "Taylor Technologies' reputation is based on thorough research and development, high-quality materials, and dedicated customer service. While our brand recognition is very gratifying, particularly in the commercial pool and boiler/cooling system markets, our focus is on constantly upgrading the value we provide to our customers."

Under Wooden's leadership, Taylor Technologies now occupies a modern, 60,000-square-foot plant in the Loveton Center industrial park; boasts state-of-the-art management information systems, computerized workstations, and a sophisticated call center for sales and customer service; and employs a skilled workforce to design its products and operate complex machinery for molding plastic components, filling and labeling reagent bottles, and shipping the kits around the globe. (To maintain quality control, chemical make-up and kit assembly are still largely manual operations.) According

to Cliff Mauler, vice president of production, the firm is presently undertaking an ambitious series of improvements in its receiving areas and warehouses.

Environmental Awareness

Wooden credits Taylor's steady growth to heightened public awareness of the importance of water quality generally and its managers' clear vision for the company specifically. "Since the National Environmental Policy Act of 1969, better stewardship of our water resources has been a national priority," says Wooden. "Recognition of the risk of waterborne diseases has also increased. Taylor has prospered by resisting the temptation to expand outside of our area of expertise. We have chosen to be uniquely dedicated to water testing."

Within that sphere, however, Taylor has been highly visible. Part of the company's success stems from its creation in the mid-1970s of an alternative to the awkward tablet form of DPD, a chemical used to measure the effectiveness of chlorine as a sanitizer in water. Company scientists invented a liquid

version, which has since become a testing standard. Taylor's DPD test kits are particularly popular with the public health officials who monitor commercial pools and spas because they are portable, easy to use, and—most importantly—highly accurate.

In fact, sales to the commercial and residential pool/spa markets now account for half of Taylor's business, and the potential for continued growth here is strong as the firm targets international customers. In 1997, Taylor began a push to expand its pool/spa kit sales in French-speaking Canada, Mexico, and western Europe with the introduction of kits in French, Spanish, and German.

"A test kit is just chemicals and plastic," Wooden maintains, "unless the results can be trusted." Closely adhering to this philosophy has been smart business for nearly 70 years; historically, upwards of three-quarters of the company's revenue comes from repeat customers. Taylor Technologies will enter the new century armed to compete globally with three proven weapons in its arsenal: a laserlike business focus, a consistently dependable product, and excellent customer service.

TAYLOR TECHNOLOGIES PRESIDENT AND CEO PAUL F. WOODEN JR. RECEIVED THE MARYLAND ENTREPRENEUR OF THE YEAR® AWARD FOR MANUFACTURING IN 1995.

Poly-Seal Corporation

TRACING ITS HISTORY TO 1934, POLY-SEAL CORPORATION IS ONE OF THE nation's leading manufacturers of injection- and compression-molded closures for consumer products such as toiletries and cosmetics, drugs and pharmaceuticals, foods and beverages, household chemicals, and automotive products. "Our mission is to create innovative packaging that enables our customers to differentiate and add value to their products," says Karl Mauck, market manager. "We do this through market-driven manufacturing principles that combine factors such as consumer preferences, optimal designs, and years of production expertise."

First organized in Baltimore as Standard Cap and Molding Co., Poly-Seal was originally a compression molder of closures for the liquor industry. Reorganized in 1969, the company has grown in size and scope—through acquisitions and product development—to become a premier manufacturer.

Molding Plastics

A train pulls along-side the tracks that run behind Poly-Seal's giant manufacturing plant. Pellets of plastic, resembling extremely coarse grades of salt and pepper, are funneled into different silos. The actual materials—polypropylene, polystyrene, and polyethylene—eventually will be transferred into the facility. In a variety of molds and machines, they then will be transformed into closures and related components, many of which are seen on today's store shelves.

At Poly-Seal, there are two primary processes for molding plastics: injection and compression. While injection molding is more commonplace in the industry, compression processing can yield a component with a richer, more distinctive finish and a superior function, used for a variety of products from cosmetics to chemicals. Both processes offer the company's trademark quality and innovation. Some of the products using Poly-Seal packaging components include hand soap, olive oil, soy sauce, mouthwash, bleach, and cosmetics. Closures range in size from eight millimeters for a vial or tube to 120 millimeters for foodstuffs.

A Baltimore Tradition

Since its founding, Poly-Seal has established itself as an important Baltimore employer. Its first plant was located in East Baltimore. By 1981, the company had constructed a new manufacturing facility in the Dundalk area of the city. After several expansions, the facility now encompasses more than 220,000 square feet and operates on a seven-day, 24-hour schedule. Modern presses with state-of-the-art production monitoring systems, ranging in size from 75 to 500 tons, produce packaging components designed to meet the needs of the customer. Using the latest scheduling and warehouse management processes, Poly-Seal follows through with timely delivery for a customer base that extends throughout North America and abroad.

The success of this privately owned firm, Mauck says, is based on a commitment that extends not only to quality production, but also to superior customer service and product innovation. "We don't sell on purely a price basis," he adds. "Where Poly-Seal has carved its niche is in products that help our customers realize the maximum return on their packaging investment."

Poly-Seal's growth in the industry has been aided by strategic acquisitions. In 1990, the firm acquired Mold-Craft Plastics. Two years later, Poly-Seal purchased the injection molding closure division of American National Can and moved the Midwest-based operation to Baltimore. This increased Poly-Seal's employee base by more than 20 percent and gave the company an even larger share of the closure market.

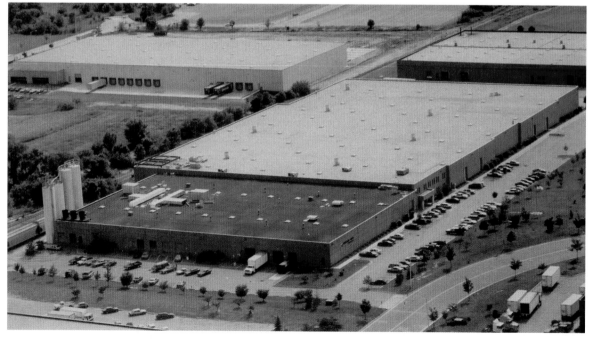

POLY-SEAL'S MAIN MANUFACTURING FACILITY IS MORE THAN 220,000 SQUARE FEET AND OPERATES ON A SEVEN-DAY, 24-HOUR SCHEDULE.

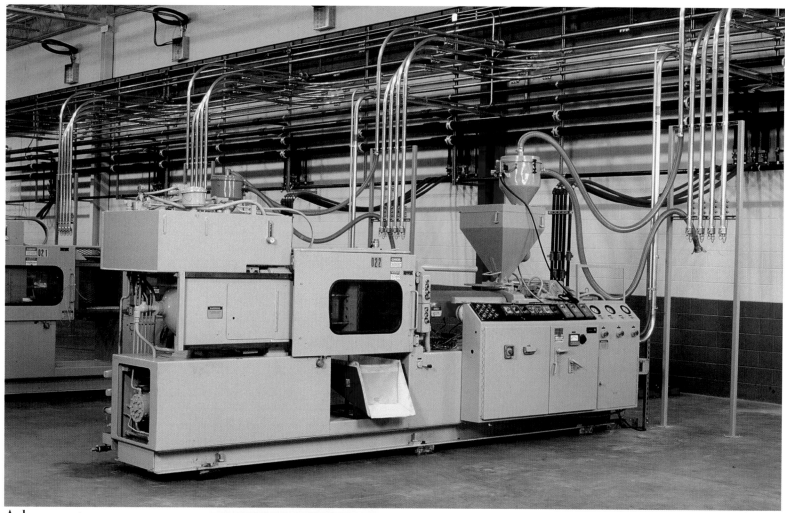

Achievements

Poly-Seal counts among its achievements the creation of an extensive line of stock closures that vary widely in size. The company's patented design and manufacturing of Poly-Seal® lined closures, as well as Puncture and Tear induction seal closures, have attracted important clients from the pharmaceutical marketplace. Poly-Seal has been recognized for launching Poly-Tab lining technology for tamper-evident sealing, and for new product designs such as its Em-Press™ and Accu-flo™ Dispensing systems.

The company is equally proud of its commitment to employees and to the community. In the past five years, employees, in conjunction with the corporation, have contributed $100,000 to the Johns Hopkins Children's Center—an organization chosen because of its policy of serving the Baltimore community. As important business partners, Poly-Seal's suppliers have gotten involved in such efforts, as well, remitting a portion of dollar purchases to the charity.

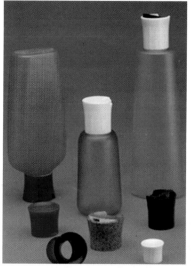

The company also notes its commitment to the community in other ways. "We are always proud that in an era in which manufacturing jobs are decreasing, Poly-Seal remains committed to growing and thriving as a viable force in the Baltimore economy," Mauck concludes.

One of the keys to the company's success over the years has been its distribution system. Poly-Seal's distributors help bring additional expertise and service to the packaging marketplace. To help

service and strengthen this important segment of its business, the company implemented an innovative inventory program guaranteeing next-day delivery of up to 35 different items. Technical seminars and regular product information mailings have supported the sales effort further. Poly-Seal is extremely proud that the National Association of Container Distributors, at its 22nd annual convention in April 1997, presented the company with its prestigious Supplier of the Year Award.

Future

In 1994, William R. Herdrich assumed the presidency of Poly-Seal. During his tenure, the company has placed renewed emphasis on new product development and manufacturing responsiveness. Poly-Seal also has worked to respond to the demanding marketplace by emphasizing market research, design, and technical expertise. As in its formative years, the Poly-Seal focus remains: "Innovation by design; quality in product and distribution."

POLY-SEAL USES STATE-OF-THE-ART MATERIAL HANDLING AND MOLDING MACHINES TO CREATE CLOSURE AND RELATED PACKAGING USED FOR A VARIETY OF CONSUMER PRODUCTS (TOP).

AS WITH OTHER POLY-SEAL PRODUCTS, THE EM-PRESS™ DISPENSING CLOSURE AND RELATED COMPONENTS BRING A DISTINCTIVE LOOK TO CONSUMER PACKAGING (BOTTOM).

Walters Art Gallery

Traveling back in time to ancient Egypt, Greece, and Rome. Viewing the arms and armor of medieval warriors. Watching the Middle Ages spring to life on the pages of illuminated manuscripts. Reliving the Renaissance and the French Revolution. Enjoying Paris in the afternoon and Venice at sunset. These and other spectacular experiences are just a sampling of the worlds to explore at the Walters Art Gallery.

For more than 60 years, the internationally acclaimed Walters Art Gallery has offered art lovers a unique museum-going experience that encompasses a breathtaking range of styles and eras. The Walters has achieved national prominence for its collections of old masters, Asian art, Renaissance and post-Renaissance sculpture, tapestries and decorative arts, 19th-century French painting, and illuminated manuscripts and rare books.

Father and Son Team

Born in 1819, William Walters was one of America's great 19th-century tycoons. The shrewd businessman made his fortune in shipping, liquor sales, and the development of railroads. His rough diamond demeanor belied the genteel aspirations of a man who spent the first $5 he ever earned on a Swiss artist's rendering of *Napoleon Crossing the Alps*.

Walters credits his mother, and later his wife, with fostering his love of art. In the 1850s, he began to fill his fashionable residence on Baltimore's Mount Vernon Place with American genre paintings of the schools of New York, and with the works of local painters and sculptors who portrayed such subjects as the Chesapeake Bay and the West.

When the Civil War broke out, Walters, like many Baltimoreans of the time, was conflicted. Even though Maryland was considered a northern state, much of Walters' commercial enterprise lay in America's South. After witnessing the arrest of such prominent local citizens as the mayor and the chief of police for their Confederate leanings, Walters moved his family to France for the duration of the war.

There, Walters learned about art collecting from George Lucas, another Baltimore expatriate, and was soon purchasing works from the leading artists of the time, such as Jean-Baptiste-Camille Corot, Honoré Daumier, and Jean-Léon Gérôme. He also became the chief patron of A.L. Barye, a French master of bronzes, and began contracting pieces that now fill Baltimore's public squares.

Return to Baltimore

When the family returned to Baltimore in 1866, Walters began developing an interest in Oriental porcelains, and by 1886, when he obtained the renowned Ching dynasty *Peachbloom Vase*, he was recognized as the leading American collector of Asian ceramics. He was also a leading supporter of introducing art to the people. During the spring of 1877, Walters opened his gallery three days a week, charging 50 cents admission. All proceeds were donated to the poor.

After Walters died in 1894, his son Henry began to build on his father's collection. Initially expanding on the 19th-century collection by acquiring significant works by Ingres, Delacroix, and Géricault, Henry Walters also turned his attention to the 17th-century old masters and then added substantially to the collection when he purchased the contents of the Roman Massarenti collection in 1902. Including more than 800 paintings, 500 antiquities, and various decorative art objects, this major purchase inspired Walters to complete construction of a new exhibition gallery, based on a Genovese palazzo, behind the family's Baltimore home. It was completed in 1909.

For more than 60 years, the internationally acclaimed Walters Art Gallery has offered art lovers a unique museum-going experience that encompasses a breathtaking range of styles and eras, including such treasures as this Tiffany iris corsage ornament (left).

The Green Gallery features Italian Renaissance and mannerist paintings (right).

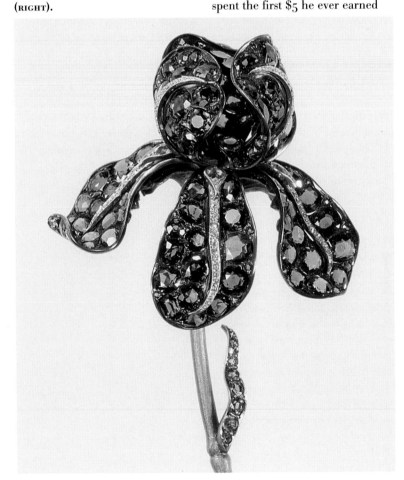

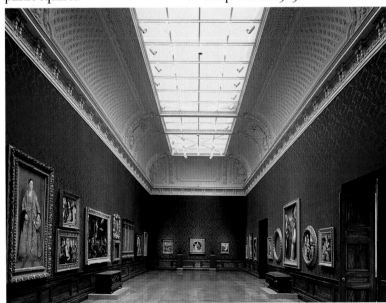

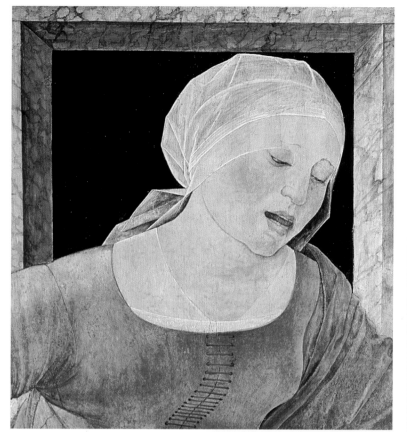

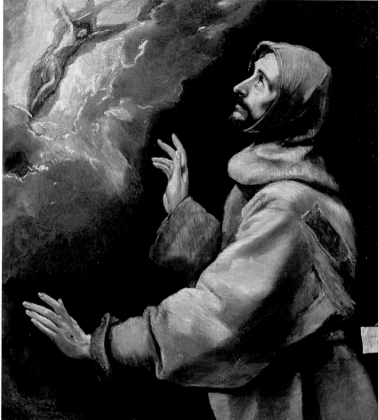

The arts community was shocked when, upon Henry Walter's death in 1931, his 22,000-piece collection was bequeathed to the people of Baltimore. In 1974, a new wing was added to the gallery to display ancient and medieval art and 19th-century paintings.

Further expansion occurred in 1991, when the $7 million Museum of Asian Art opened in the Hackerman House. Located on the corner of Charles Street and West Mount Vernon Place, it features a collection of sculpture, lacquerware, porcelain, and paintings totaling more than 7,000 pieces.

Modern-Day Museum

Today, the legacy of William and Henry Walters has evolved into a modern museum poised for the rewards and challenges of the 21st century. In addition to showcasing the family's collections, it generates crowd-pleasing excitement via highly acclaimed temporary exhibitions, such as *Russian Enamels*; *The First Emperor: Treasures from Ancient China*; and 1998's *Monet: Paintings of Giverny from the Musée Marmottan*.

Like the Walters family, which took pleasure in art of all forms and shared that joy with the citizens of

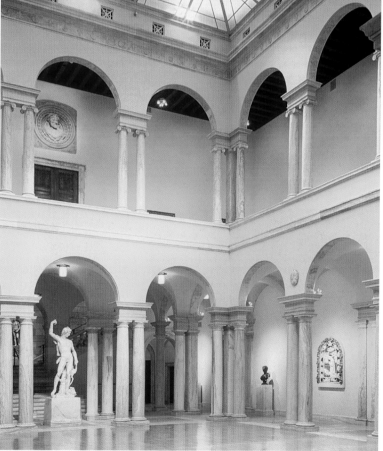

The Walters Art Gallery permanent collection includes *A Mourning Woman* by Ercole de' Roberti (top left) and *St. Francis Receiving the Stigmata* by Domenikos Theotokopoulos, known as El Greco (top right).

Modeled after Italian Renaissance and Baroque palace designs, Walters Art Gallery's central court is a replica of Genoa's Palazzo Balbi, designed in the 1630s by Bartolomeo Bianco.

Baltimore, the museum also is renowned for its dynamic programs for young children, adult learning series, and classical music concerts.

"We have always believed that our role as a museum is to communicate the joy and passion

of living and loving art," says Gary Vikan, director of the Walters Art Gallery. "Today, as in earlier eras of history, art comes in many different shapes, forms, and sizes. We delight in sharing them with our museum-goers."

T. Rowe Price Associates, Inc.

WHEN THOMAS ROWE PRICE JR. MADE THE DECISION 60 YEARS AGO to start his own investment counsel firm, he did so with considerable trepidation. America was still recovering from the Great Depression, and Price's vision for his new enterprise was based on an investment philosophy that was generally unknown and untested.

"I may be a darn fool for taking this unnecessary risk," he wrote in his diary in 1937, "but I am going to have the satisfaction of knowing that I tried to build my own business. If I later fail, I will have no regrets."

Price was willing to undertake such a challenge because he was convinced that his real calling was to provide a new, almost unheard-of service: investment counseling. He would provide this service for a fee—rather than relying on commission income—which would allow him to recommend stocks on the basis of his judgment.

Growth and Prosperity

Price would later become an investment legend with his growth-stock theory of investing. In essence, he believed that corporations, like people, have life cycles of growth, maturity, and decline. Price defined a growth company as one still in the early stages of exploiting new technology or products, or of exploring new uses for old products. Price believed that investors who could identify growth stocks could hold and profit from the shares for many years. Over time, the company's superior earnings growth would be reflected in both market value and growth of dividend income.

Price's growth-stock theory of investing has withstood the test of time. His original goals of building a company with 25 employees and $60 million in assets under management were surpassed years ago. Today, T. Rowe Price and its affiliates are the industry's third-largest manager of no-load mutual funds, the third-largest full-service mutual fund manager of 401(k) retirement plans, and the largest manager of no-load international funds. Among the firm's clients are pension, profit sharing and other employee benefit plans; endowments; and foundations.

Broad Services

Through its more than 70 equity, bond, and money market funds, as well as its private account management services, T. Rowe Price provides a broad selection of investment services. Keys to the firm's success have been consistently strong performance, sensitivity to investment risk, low costs, and high-quality services to shareholders.

T. Rowe Price's joint venture with the Fleming Group currently manages more than $33 billion, including $19.2 billion in no-load

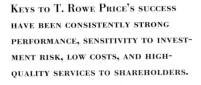

KEYS TO T. ROWE PRICE'S SUCCESS HAVE BEEN CONSISTENTLY STRONG PERFORMANCE, SENSITIVITY TO INVESTMENT RISK, LOW COSTS, AND HIGH-QUALITY SERVICES TO SHAREHOLDERS.

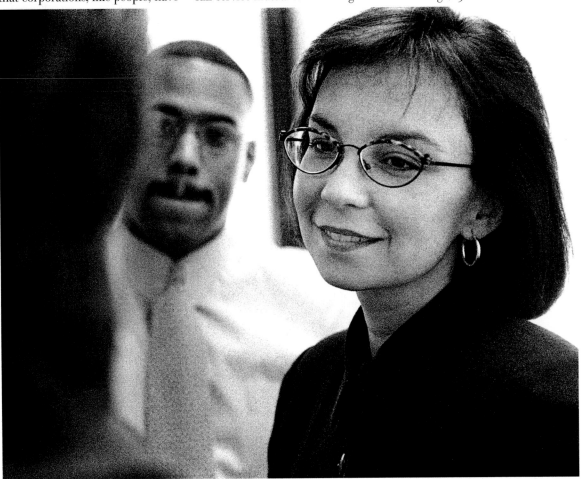

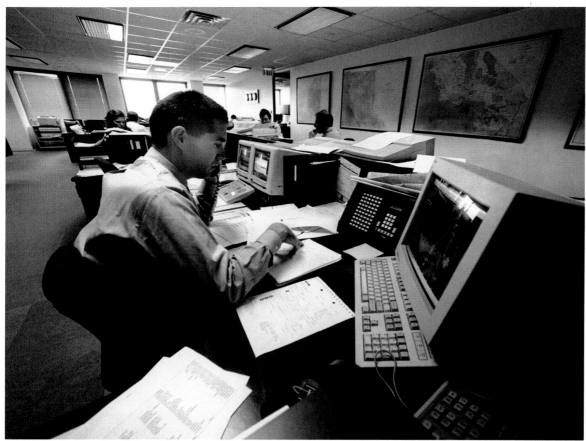

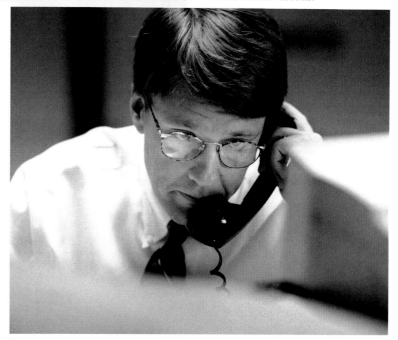

international funds, making Rowe Price-Fleming International one of the largest managers of international funds nationwide. Rowe Price-Fleming has access to more than 100 analysts worldwide, carrying the firm's tradition of rigorous, independent, on-site research.

As a leading provider of investment and administrative services for defined contribution plans, T. Rowe Price provides investment management, state-of-the-art record keeping, and participant communication services to more than 1,500 corporate and public retirement plans nationwide. The firm pays particular attention to the individual institution's needs. This tailor-made approach might include customized investment alternatives and communications, special reporting, or flexible processing.

The firm also operates a discount brokerage service that lets investors buy and sell individual stocks, bonds, precious metals, and other securities.

As of September 1997, the firm that was incorporated in 1947 as successor to the investment counseling business Price formed a decade earlier managed $125 billion in total assets for more

than 6 million individual and institutional investor accounts, and had $82 billion in mutual fund assets under management. The company employs more than 2,900 people, with offices in Baltimore; Owings Mills, Maryland; Chicago; Los Angeles; Richmond, Virginia; San Francisco; Tampa; and Washington, D.C.

The overriding strength of T. Rowe Price remains its people. The 45 portfolio managers, who have an average of 10 or more years' tenure at the firm, work closely with more than 40 equity and credit analysts to uncover investment opportunities. T. Rowe Price strives to achieve superior investment performance for its investors, but is always mindful of the risks incurred versus the potential reward. In addition, more than 400 highly trained service representatives are available, seven days a week, through the firm's toll-free number to answer investors' questions.

T. Rowe Price has evolved dramatically in the more than half a century since Price founded the company. Its growth has reflected changes in the country and in the financial arena. Nevertheless, T.

Rowe Price continues to be guided by the principles that formed the cornerstone of its tradition. Chief among these is the commitment to provide high-quality investment services that meet the needs and goals of its investors. "Profitable operations are essential," Price advised his clients many years ago, "but profits must follow a job well done and result from the goodwill of the investment public."

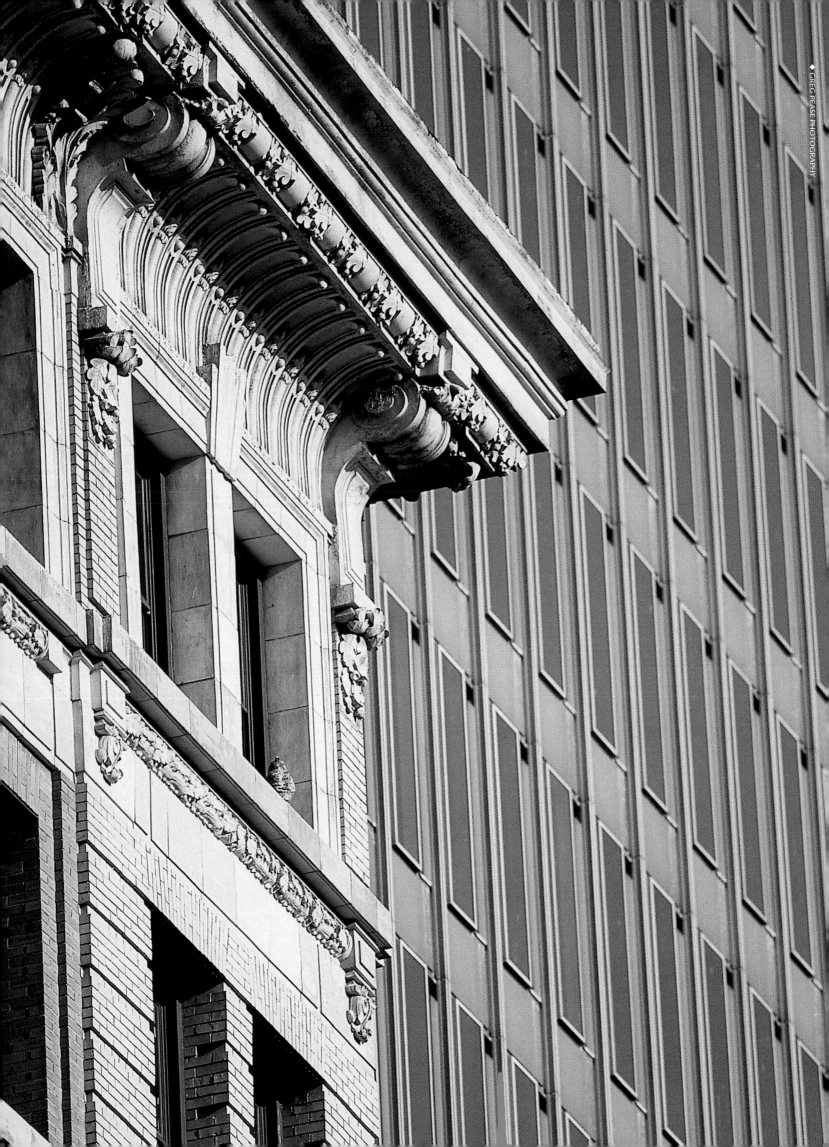

1939-1979

PROFILES IN EXCELLENCE

Eisner Communications

WITH TODAY'S FIERCELY COMPETITIVE AND RAPIDLY CHANGING BUSINESS environments, marketing isn't just about making ads anymore. It's about reaching the consumer on a multitude of levels. It's about building brands. It's about having all of the right resources under one roof. And it's why Eisner is on the cutting edge.

Eisner's Special Culture

Eisner Communications has enjoyed steady and rather dramatic growth of approximately 15 percent a year for the last five years. Of course, that kind of success is always due to a variety of factors. Part of the agency's growth, however, is certainly owed to the high premium it places on supporting an environment conducive to creating inspired, effective work.

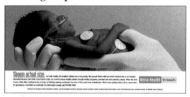

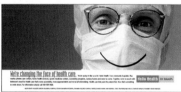

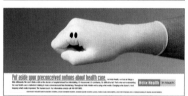

After all, the only real commodity an ad agency has to sell is talent. That's why Eisner has had a concerted and deliberate effort in place for some time to attract and keep some of the most creative, intelligent, and skilled advertising professionals in the country. In order to achieve that goal, Eisner recognized the need to build an impressive and diverse roster of blue-chip clients who demand the highest level of creativity, energy, and expertise. And Eisner has been quite successful in doing so.

Eisner Communications is the agency that brought the Black & Decker account back to Baltimore after the business left the market 15 years ago in search of bigger talent. Eisner is the agency that launched the Go RVing Coalition's national marketing effort to sell recreational vehicles. It is the agency that moved the *Scientific American* magazine account away from Madison Avenue.

Eisner is also the only agency the Detroit-based shopping center giant, The Taubman Company, has entrusted with the greatest share of its properties across the country. And just recently, Eisner won the coveted Maryland State Lottery and Baltimore-Washington International Airport accounts.

Eisner's Partnership with the Consumer

Eisner's growth is inextricably tied to its clients' successes. The agency takes the responsibility and trust that comes with a client/agency relationship very seriously. It considers results as a collective bottom line. Eisner realizes that in order to deliver results, consumer behavior must be influenced. The agency's first and most important task, therefore, is to always listen carefully to the consumer—a marketer's most important audience and source of guidance.

After all, the most creative idea in the world is useless unless it is strategically sound. That's why

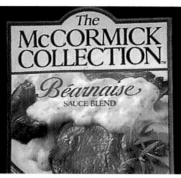

Eisner's full-time account-planning team, including professional focus group moderators, are in the field on a weekly, even daily basis conducting quantitative and qualitative, traditional and nontraditional research to better understand the mind-set of its clients' target audiences.

Eisner is helped in this process by its location in the heart of Baltimore. The city—with its blue-collar roots, its emerging service industry, and its rich and widely diverse ethnic heritage—was named by *American Demographics* magazine as the most representative of the U.S. population.

Eisner's Competitive Spirit

By design, Eisner does not specialize in accounts from one particular industry category. In fact, the agency has worked hard to always maintain a highly diverse client list so that it can

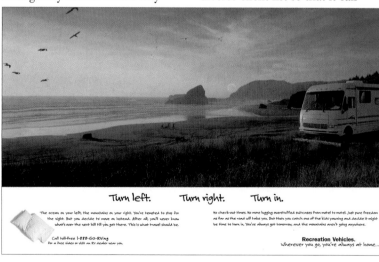

Turn left.   Turn right.   Turn in.

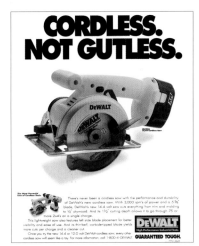

year, Eisner brought an unknown new health system, Helix Health, to a level of awareness on the scale of Johns Hopkins, the 150-year-old giant.

Eisner has helped clients in many different categories achieve success against formidable odds. If the company has a specialization, it is this.

Eisner's Client Relationships

Eisner Communications exists to serve today's forward-thinking managers, who live and thrive in competitive, complex business environments. Their success, and the agency's, depends on their collective ability to be resourceful, imaginative, innovative, and nimble problem solvers. Eisner people regard themselves as mar-

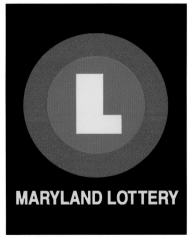

MARYLAND LOTTERY

keting partners to their clients, bringing to every client challenge the full weight of the company's entirely integrated communications services, state-of-the-art business resources, and passionate dedication to winning. It's all a part of the art of brand building.

bring a broader and more realistic perspective to each client challenge. If there is one kind of account Eisner does specialize in, however, it is working for clients who face fiercely competitive challenges. It is this kind of situation that allows the agency to be the most resourceful and, according to account executives and the creative staff, motivates them to be smarter than the next guy.

It was just this kind of circumstance that propelled Eisner to develop a highly successful shopper loyalty program for its Taubman shopping centers. Eisner also led the pharmaceutical industry's fight against the federal government's attempt to install price controls, which would have crippled critical research and development efforts. The agency developed strategies that enabled Black & Decker's DeWalt tools to overwhelm dominant Makita and become the market share leader. And in just one short

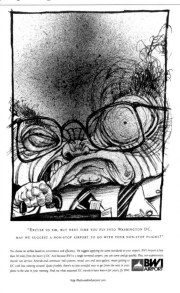

"EXCUSE US SIR, BUT NEXT TIME YOU FLY INTO WASHINGTON DC, MAY WE SUGGEST A NON-STOP AIRPORT TO GO WITH YOUR NON-STOP FLIGHT?"

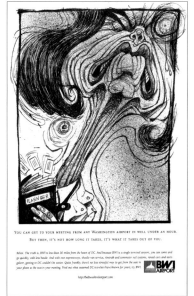

YOU CAN GET TO YOUR MEETING FROM ANY WASHINGTON AIRPORT IN WELL UNDER AN HOUR. BUT THEN, IT'S NOT HOW LONG IT TAKES, IT'S WHAT IT TAKES OUT OF YOU.

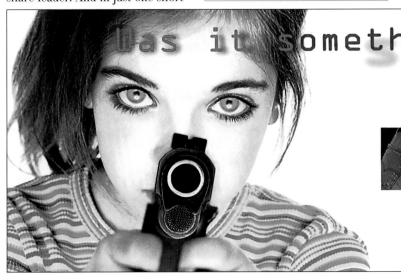

Baltimore Spice, Inc.

AN INNOVATIVE COMPANY ON THE LEADING EDGE OF SPICE TECHNOLOGY, Baltimore Spice, Inc. has long been one of the nation's leading purveyors of herbs, spices, seasonings, and mustards to Fortune 500 food processors. It has been noted that one cannot walk down a grocery aisle in the United States without passing a food item containing Baltimore Spice products. A presence in Baltimore for more than a half-century, its modern spice technology and seasoning innovations are backed by its founder's old-fashioned values.

Tasteful Beginnings

Gustav Brunn came to Baltimore from Germany with just a few possessions, including a small spice grinder. With such basic equipment, he founded the Baltimore Spice Company in 1939, occupying a small office upstairs from a city wholesale fish market, on land now occupied by Oriole Park at Camden Yards.

From the early days, Brunn sold spices to wholesalers. His products—particularly his black and red peppers, mustard, and celery seed—were much in demand by seafood steamers coming to the fish market. The entrepreneur began experimenting with various proportions of these and other spices, and eventually created his signature spice, which he named Old Bay after a steamship line that ran from Norfolk to Baltimore. Old Bay has since become a national classic and is lauded as a seasoning for steamed crabs.

As a result of the success of Old Bay, as well as the popularity of Brunn's other products, the entrepreneur quadrupled the size of his plant in just 10 years. By 1960, the company was expanding again, this time into its own facility on Reisterstown Road in the western suburbs of Baltimore. A new warehousing facility was constructed in Grand Forks, a geographically strategic location because of its proximity to America's mustard harvest land.

Baltimore Spice remained a family-owned business until 1985, when it was acquired by SCM Corporation. But it wasn't until 1990, when the company was sold to the Fuchs Group, that Baltimore Spice found its modern-day home.

Spicy Innovations

The Fuchs Group was founded by German businessman Dieter Fuchs in 1952 to service Europe's industrial spice and seasoning markets. In addition to the retail-oriented Old Bay seasoning, which was sold in 1990 to McCormick & Company, Baltimore Spice Company had also become focused on industrial spice and seasoning production. Fuchs had found the perfect American partner.

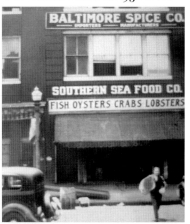

The acquisition by the Fuchs Group—known throughout the world for its emphasis on innovative technology, state-of-the-art research and development, and quality control—resulted in enormous capital improvements for Baltimore Spice. The company recently introduced its patented Encapsulated Spices, which are created by a process that protects the flavor and aroma of commonly used products such as black pepper, cinnamon, and garlic. And in 1997, the company launched its new food service division, which provides its high-quality spices and seasonings to the away-from-home eating industry, including restaurants, hospitals, hotels, schools, and caterers.

At Baltimore Spice, the merger of technology and tradition has transformed the company into a leader in the industrial spice marketplace.

CLOCKWISE FROM TOP:
WITH SUCH BASIC EQUIPMENT AS A SPICE GRINDER, GUSTAV BRUNN FOUNDED THE BALTIMORE SPICE COMPANY IN 1939, OCCUPYING A SMALL OFFICE UPSTAIRS FROM A CITY WHOLESALE FISH MARKET, ON LAND NOW OCCUPIED BY ORIOLE PARK AT CAMDEN YARDS.

BALTIMORE SPICE INTRODUCED ITS NEW FOOD SERVICE PACKAGING LINE IN 1997.

SEASONINGS ARE BLENDED IN 10,000-POUND BATCHES AT THE COMPANY'S OWINGS MILLS FACILITY.

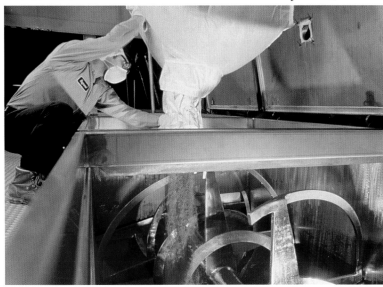

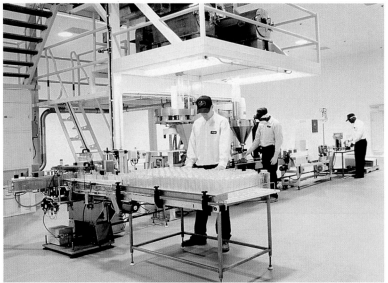

H&S Bakery

THE STORY OF H&S BAKERY READS LIKE A CLASSIC AMERICAN SUCCESS story. It is a tale of the Paterakis and Tsakalos families, who came from Greece to make a new and better life. ❧ Isadore "Steve" Paterakis came to America in 1921 with his wife, Kyriaki, and daughters, Despina and Liberty. Their son John was born in 1929. Also emigrating from Greece were Roanthi and Nikolas Tsakalos, whose son, Harry, married Liberty Paterakis. After this union merged the two families, Harry and Steve, for whom H&S is named, opened their new bakery for business in 1943. They started by making Italian bread by hand and baking it in an old brick flat-hearth oven.

Embracing the Food Service Industry

H&S Bakery was incorporated in 1962, setting its sights on the rapidly growing food service industry in which it plays a dominant role today. In 1965, the Athens Automatic Rolls division opened as the company's first fully automated roll plant, which eventually grew into the multistate Northeast Foods, a division that specializes in food service.

The family continued to grow, too. When John Paterakis was 23, he inherited his father's interest in the bakery. In 1950, he wed Antoinette Apostolou, and a new generation of six children came along. This third generation is also actively involved in the business.

Still family-owned and -operated to this day, H&S Bakery has nine divisions operating in seven states, with distribution in 23 states and still growing. The company is made up of more than 2,000 employees systemwide, in addition to a fleet of 110 delivery vans and more than 200 tractor trailers. It has carved a niche for itself in the specialty bread category, and many of its products are still hearth baked for traditional European flavor and crust. H&S Bakery continued its growth in the food service industry with the production of rolls, bagels, and English muffins.

The company's divisions bake a variety of products for restaurants and supermarkets, including customized private label programs for European specialty bread products. H&S also operates its own outlet store just across the street from the bakery premises. One can smell such appetizing aromas as cinnamon and rye bread wafting throughout the Fells Point neighborhood, as row after row of baked goods come off the production line.

Bettering Baltimore

Neither H&S Bakery, with all its extensive divisions and holdings, nor its family members have strayed from their Baltimore roots. The family continues to contribute to Baltimore's waterfront growth through economic development projects including Inner Harbor East. They are also the advocates of a wide variety of community activities.

Lured to America by a dream for a better life, the family continues to give back to the people that helped make it possible for them to realize their dream. H&S Bakery continues to flourish because its people share the same core values of hard work, dedication to community, and pride of achievement.

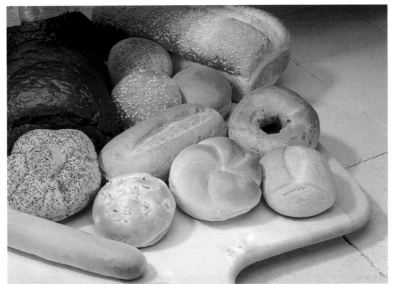

THIS ARRAY—WHICH INCLUDES CRUSTY ITALIAN BREAD, ONION ROLLS, BAGELS, KAISER ROLLS, AND SOUR DOUGH ROLLS—SHOWS WHY H&S IS KNOWN AS "THE VARIETY BAKER." H&S BAKERY'S WEBSITE CAN BE FOUND AT WWW.HSBAKERY.COM (TOP).

BREAD OFTEN CREATES THE FIRST IMPRESSION OF A RESTAURANT'S FARE WITH ITS PATRONS. H&S BAKES ITS BREADS AND ROLLS DAILY AND PROVIDES COMMITMENT SEVEN DAYS A WEEK TO ENSURE FRESHNESS AND QUALITY FOR ITS CLIENTS AND THEIR CUSTOMERS (BOTTOM).

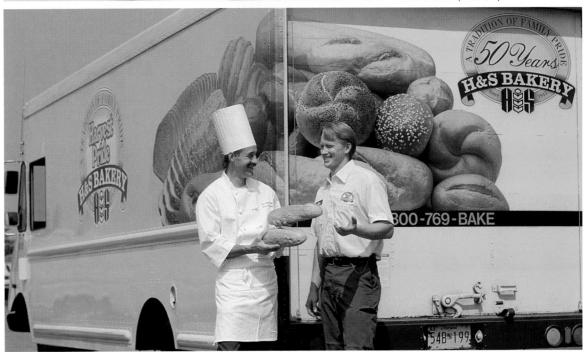

The Rouse Company

ONE OF AMERICA'S LARGEST PUBLICLY HELD REAL ESTATE DEVELOPMENT and management companies, The Rouse Company operates more than 250 properties encompassing office, retail, research and development, industrial and hotel space. The company has received international recognition for its creation of Columbia, an innovative,

planned community where 14,000 acres of rural land have been transformed into a city of approximately 83,500 residents, with 2,500 businesses, more than 59,000 jobs, and 3.5 million square feet of commercial space. Understandably proud of its creation, The Rouse Company is headquartered in Columbia.

Since its founding, The Rouse Company leadership has operated on the premise that a successful business requires a delicate balance of diverse needs and objectives. As a result, the company has incorporated three goals into its business philosophy: to improve the quality of life in communities in which it

operates, to provide its employees with opportunities for fulfillment, and to produce rewarding financial results for investors and partners.

From the Beginning

In 1939, James W. Rouse and Hunter Moss founded the Moss-Rouse Company in Baltimore to originate Federal Housing Administration loans for single-family housing. Following World War II, when returning veterans created an increased housing demand, the company benefited from the government-financed residential real estate boom.

In 1954, Moss withdrew from the firm, which then became James

W. Rouse & Company, Inc. The organization soon expanded its capabilities to arranging financing for commercial real estate projects, such as strip shopping centers. Rouse then became interested in the concept of a high-quality, well-designed retail facility, and, in 1958, opened Harundale Mall.

During the 1960s, the firm, which was renamed The Rouse Company, dramatically broadened its scope. The first new venture focused on community development activities, resulting in the creation of The Village of Cross Keys in Baltimore. In 1963, the company purchased rural land in Columbia and began creating the planned community.

Having successfully developed major suburban malls across the United States, including White Marsh and Owings Mills, both in Baltimore County, in the late 1970s and through the 1980s, The Rouse Company embarked on the development of a series of downtown retail and mixed-use urban marketplaces. Some of its highly acclaimed projects include Harborplace and the Gallery in Baltimore; Faneuil Hall Marketplace in Boston; South Street Seaport in New York City; the Gallery at Market East in Philadelphia; Westlake in Seattle; the Grand Avenue in Milwaukee; Bayside Marketplace in Miami; Pioneer Place in Portland, Oregon; and St. Louis Union Station in St. Louis.

In addition to its urban shopping places, The Rouse Company has become a recognized leader in regional retail-center development and management. Its innovative specialty retailing, open storefronts, interior landscaping, cooperative advertising and merchandising programs, and food courts have earned acclaim.

The Vision of Columbia

Since its inception, Columbia has been seen in terms of human values, not just as an economics and engineering project.

BALTIMORE'S HARBORPLACE AND THE GALLERY, TWO OF THE ROUSE COMPANY'S PREMIER URBAN MARKETPLACES, ATTRACT MILLIONS OF VISITORS EACH YEAR.

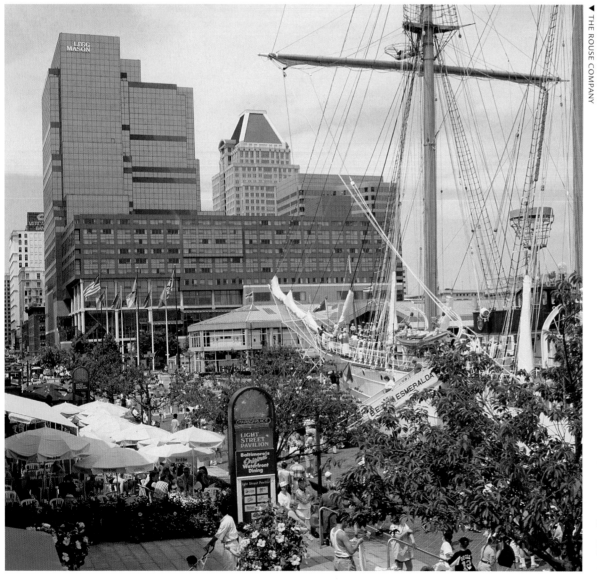

THE ROUSE COMPANY

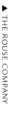
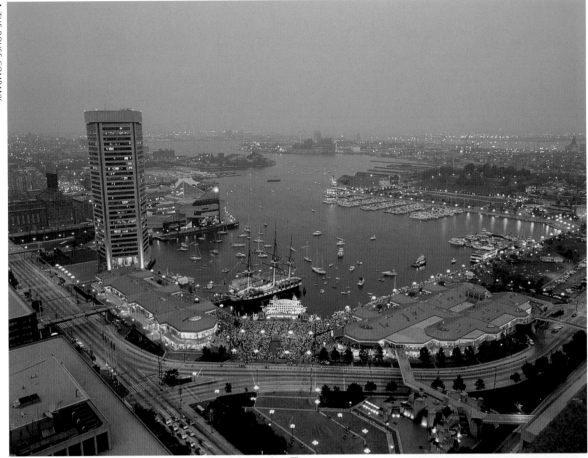

Begun in the early 1960s, this "new town" was designed to eliminate uncontrolled sprawl and the inconveniences of typical subdivision design. Even more, Columbia was built on the premise that a community could foster a true coming together of its residents as a place for all people, embracing different races, religions, and income groups.

To achieve these goals, the city's master plan called for a series of self-contained villages, around which day-to-day life would revolve. Today, nine such villages each contain several neighborhoods, schools, a shopping center, community and recreational facilities, and houses—ranging in style from single-family homes and town houses to apartments and condominiums.

Complementing the community development in Columbia are more than 5,000 acres of parks, playgrounds, and natural open space. In addition, each village community is designed for easy access to schools, recreational facilities, and neighborhood centers with child care. The city's extensive pathways give ready access to village centers and connect homes to tot lots and open spaces.

Building the Future

The 1990s have been a time of continued growth for The Rouse Company. Occupancy levels at the firm's retail and office properties are more than 90 percent—well above industry averages. The company's development efforts have centered primarily on the Sun Belt, with the construction of Oviedo Marketplace in Orlando, as well as on expansions of existing centers from Atlanta to Portland, Oregon, to Columbia.

In 1996, The Rouse Company acquired The Howard Hughes Corporation of Las Vegas. This acquisition enhanced The Rouse Company's geographic diversification and complemented its existing business lines through the addition of four large-scale, master-planned business parks; a 75 percent interest in Fashion Show Mall; a regional shopping center anchored by five department stores; Summerlin, a 22,500-acre, master-planned community, which is home to nearly 24,000 residents; and numerous other land parcels and commercial properties in Nevada and California.

The company also continues to enhance and expand closer to home. In Columbia, it is develop-

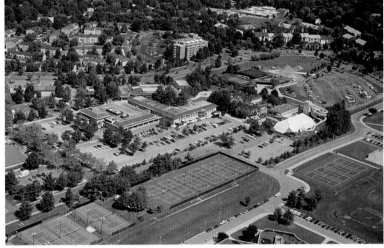

ing Columbia Crossing, a 400,000-square-foot power center; Columbia Gateway, a 600-acre corporate park; four new residential neighborhoods; and an expansion of the mall in Columbia that will include new small shops as well as Nordstrom and Lord & Taylor department stores. Lord & Taylor stores will be added to White Marsh and Owings Mills, which will also get a new Sears department store.

As The Rouse Company looks toward the next century, it continues to grow through innovative efforts and a commitment to enhancing quality of life in all communities it serves.

AN AERIAL VIEW OF HARBOR PLACE REVEALS THE DEVELOPMENT THAT WAS THE CATALYST FOR THE REVITALIZATION OF BALTIMORE'S DOWNTOWN AREA (TOP).

THE VILLAGE OF WILDE LAKE WAS THE FIRST OF NINE SELF-CONTAINED VILLAGES IN THE COMPANY'S NEW COMMUNITY OF COLUMBIA (BOTTOM).

Up-To-Date Laundry Inc.

IT's 5:15 A.M. WHILE FREDERICK AVENUE IN WEST BALTIMORE IS STILL sleeping, employees begin to trickle into Up-To-Date Laundry. By 5:30 a.m., the boilers have been started, the tunnel—a 40-foot, 16-chamber washer—is gearing for a 55,000-pound day. The dryers are heating up for 400-pound loads and ironers are racing to feed more than 800

sheets an hour. By 6 a.m., 75 of 180 employees have started processing everything from doctors' scrubs to hotel bed sheets, which will by day's end be 55,000 pounds of sweet-smelling, neatly packed linen.

Up-To-Date, which in 1996 cleaned more than 14 million pounds of laundry, is one of the largest independent commercial laundries in the region, serving major institutions in Maryland; Washington, D.C.; and Virginia. Up-To-Date specializes in challenging-to-clean industries. Its biggest customers are hospitals, including University of Maryland Medical Systems, Georgetown University Hospital, George Washington University Hospital, Anne Arundel Medical System, and Columbia Arlington; hotels such as Sheraton Inner Harbor Hotel and the Hyatt Regency Inner Harbor; and the area's maritime industries.

A Family Business

Nancy Stair, CEO of Up-To-Date, credits the company's success to being a family-operated business. As a matter of fact, she is known throughout the plant as Mom. The firm was acquired in 1946 when her father, William Stair Sr., a successful salesman for Wyandotte Chemical Corporation—which specialized in commercial laundry clients—was offered an opportunity to purchase Up-To-Date. He borrowed $3,000 from his mother and launched what has since become a family dynasty.

In the early days, Up-To-Date was servicing the ships from New York docked in the harbor, as well as residential laundry and dry

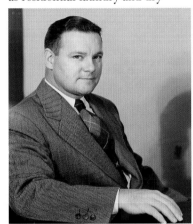

cleaning. State-of-the-art equipment was purchased in the 1960s and the service was extended to hospital linen.

William Stair, a Baltimore-area civic leader, actively worked until 1993. He died in 1994 at the age of 84. Stair bequeathed Up-To-Date to his daughter. An entrepreneur in her own right, Nancy Stair co-owned and operated a metal fabrication business in West Virginia for nearly two decades. Despite the differences between metal and laundry, it was the experience that prepared her for operating the family firm. In West Virginia, she handled the full range of company responsibilities, including bookkeeping, office and employee management, and accounting and legal issues.

Good for Baltimore

Since taking the helm, Nancy Stair has continued to expand Up-To-Date's client base, creating additional jobs for Baltimore residents. In the July 1996 issue of the *Baltimore Business Journal*, she was listed in the top 25 women's businesses in Baltimore. Stair has also introduced the family's third generation to the business. As company president, her son Bradley Minetree oversees the marketing and operations. A second son, David Minetree, serves as vice president and oversees the traffic and transportation of the product.

Due to a increase in customers, Up-To-Date Laundry will relocate in 1998 to a new facility three times the size of its current site. The company has purchased a second tunnel and has plans to acquire additional equipment that will bolster its capabilities to 80,000 pounds of laundry per day.

"Up-To-Date shall always be a family business," Nancy Stair says. "This is an industry where personal relationships mean everything—to us and to our clients."

UP-TO-DATE LAUNDRY WAS ACQUIRED IN 1946 BY WILLIAM STAIR SR., NANCY STAIR'S FATHER, A SUCCESSFUL SALESMAN FOR WYANDOTTE CHEMICAL CORPORATION (TOP).

NANCY STAIR, CEO OF UP-TO-DATE LAUNDRY INC., CREDITS THE COMPANY'S SUCCESS TO BEING A FAMILY-OPERATED BUSINESS (BOTTOM).

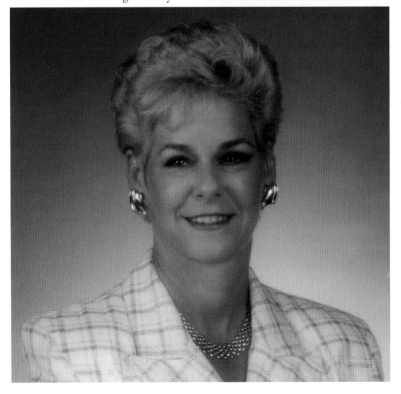

My Cleaning Service, Inc.

MY CLEANING SERVICE, INC., A SECOND-GENERATION COMMERCIAL janitorial company, is one of the largest women's business enterprises in Baltimore. Lisa R. Bands, owner and president since 1993, continues the same basic company philosophy of personal service and controlled, steady growth initiated by her parents, Gerald "Gerry" and Margaret Rogers, the company's founders.

Gerry and Margaret Rogers began with the hopes of bringing high-quality janitorial service to Baltimore. Gerry realized the need for a partnership with property managers and building owners to provide complete customer satisfaction. Customer relations were developed through daytime inspections, listening to tenant needs, and providing quick response to requests.

The American dream came true for Gerry Rogers in July 1970, when he started My Cleaning Service, Inc. with the help of Margaret. It began in the basement of their northeast row house with borrowed equipment. It has grown to become one of the premier cleaning services in the metropolitan Baltimore area, employing more than 400 people.

Commitment to Quality

Today, Lisa and her husband, Daniel A. Bands—who serves as vice president and is active in managing the business administration—service accounts that range from an old, historical building such as St. Mary's Seminary, to ultramodern downtown high-rises. Customers include Colliers Pinkard, Rouse Company, Fidelity & Deposit, and the Maritime Institute located near Baltimore/Washington International Airport.

"We believe that total quality is achieved through respect, continuous education, and training of all employees," Lisa Bands says. "Our management team is committed to setting the standard for leadership within the building service industry."

Promotions are made from within whenever possible; current managers started at entry level. Ongoing training facilitates their advancements.

My Cleaning Service, Inc. is committed to making a long-term impact on the image and professionalism of its customers' buildings. Management partners with customers and employees, matching building needs with the right personalities and skills to ensure total customer satisfaction.

My Cleaning Service, Inc. implements high-quality systems and excellent customer service through company goals and award programs.

Special Services

The Specialty Cleaning Division was formed as a support group in 1981. Now managed by Terry B. Froehlich, it has evolved to offer diversified services for a varied list of customers, including construction companies, schools, government, and commercial buildings located in Maryland; Washington, D.C.; and northern Virginia.

Supervised specialty crews are equipped for any size job. They are uniformed personnel who are thoroughly trained in all phases of building service needs, bonded, and insured. Employees are screened for criminal backgrounds as a condition for employment companywide.

Work crews provide an array of services 24 hours a day, including construction cleanup, carpet and upholstery cleaning, emergency cleanup, professional floor care, industrial cleanup, marble restoration, acoustical tile cleaning, and low-rise window cleaning.

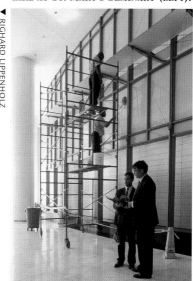

THE SPECIALTY CLEANING CREW GIVES PERSONALIZED ATTENTION TO DETAILS AND DIRECT CUSTOMER COMMUNICATION FOR EACH PROJECT (RIGHT).

EVELYN MOODY, SUPERVISOR AND ONE OF THE FIRST EMPLOYEES OF MY CLEANING SERVICE, INC., PROVIDES LOVING CARE AT ST. MARY'S SEMINARY (LEFT).

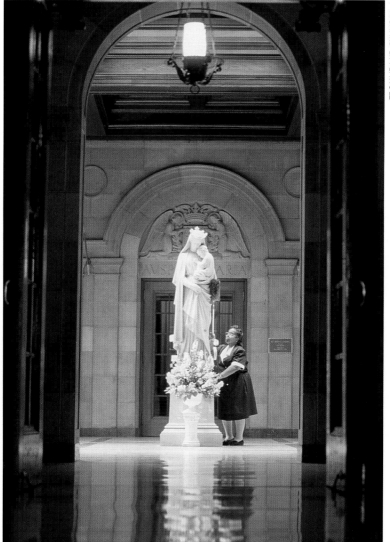

RICHARD LIPPENHOLZ

Washington Aluminum Company

WASHINGTON ALUMINUM COMPANY (WACO) WAS FOUNDED IN 1947 to design and manufacture aluminum gangways and ladders for the U.S. Navy. In the ensuing half-century, the company has developed expertise and broad capabilities for high-quality custom fabrication, and today WACO designs, fabricates, and installs engineered components and products for industrial, commercial, and government applications. The company, which operates from a 65,000-square-foot facility in Baltimore, has established itself as a market leader in innovation, industrial flexibility, and reliability for engineering and fabrication solutions.

A Successful Transition

Until the 1980s, Washington Aluminum specialized primarily in defense industry contracts, which comprised two-thirds of its business. But that decade marked a time of defense industry spending cutbacks; WACO's management team turned the downshift into an opportunity for change.

Through a cohesive program that combined acquisitions with an expansion of product lines, Washington Aluminum targeted industrial and municipal markets. Today, these markets make up more than 75 percent of WACO's annual revenue. At the same time, the company continues to produce its traditional maritime/government line, which represents a still-healthy quarter share.

"Business has actually grown," says Kenneth A. Walker, president of Washington Aluminum. "We've been fortunate, but also quite flexible and adaptable. We've filled in the holes."

Washington Aluminum now offers seven different product lines. Its marine products category serves naval and commercial ship applications, with specific expertise in aluminum and fiberglass access systems. These include gangways, accommodation ladders, and vertical ladders for clients such as the U.S. Navy. The company's environmental products, which serve large and complex treatment plants and small pump stations, are installed in water and wastewater systems. These products include slide gates for water shutoff and weir gates for balancing flows.

A variety of custom structural components make up the industrial products line. These include extension booms for fire trucks, specialty containers, and enclosures, as well as custom fabrications for defense contractors. Complementing these items are Washington Aluminum's fan products. These consist of high-performance propeller fan blades used for radiator cooling and ventilation in off-road vehicles, locomotives, diesel generator sets, and heat exchangers.

More recent introductions include WACO's development of Duralite shoring products to serve

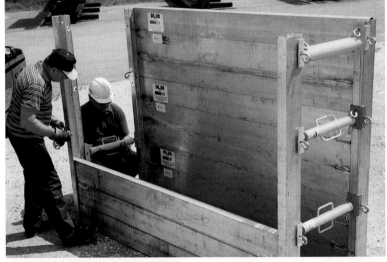

CLOCKWISE FROM TOP:
WASHINGTON ALUMINUM COMPLETES THE NO-TOOL ASSEMBLY OF DURALITE SAFETY TRENCH SHORING THAT WILL BE USED TO PROTECT WORKERS IN A PIPELINE EXCAVATION.

EMPLOYEES OVERSEE THE SEMIAUTOMATIC WELDING OF LARGE, ALUMINUM STRUCTURES TYPICALLY FOUND AT THE WACO FACILITY.

THE COMPANY EXPERTLY MACHINES A LARGE, STAINLESS STEEL COMPONENT FOR AN INDUSTRIAL CLIENT.

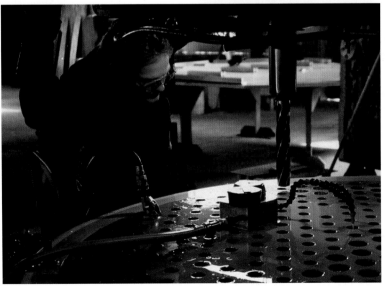

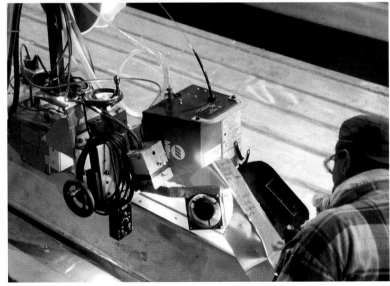

the construction industry, with trench shielding applications. The shoring line features a proprietary design that incorporates the strength and lightweight advantages of aluminum to protect workers' lives and increase productivity in pipeline installation and maintenance.

In the early 1990s, Washington Aluminum acquired TriFab, Inc., a Waynesboro, Pennsylvania-based company that specializes in steel fabrication. As a result, WACO was able to further expand its product lines to include steel components for major equipment producers; industrial products, such as air pollution systems and maintenance fabrication; and Dixie Air Systems, which handles material collection and movement in the wood products and finished paper industries.

Looking Forward

WACO's client list reflects the company's national and international diversity, and includes Bethlehem Steel; Exxon; Litton; Lockheed Martin; NASA; the U.S. Army, Coast Guard, and Navy; Northrop Grumman; Newport News Shipbuilding; and Bath Iron Works.

"While our markets are diverse, the common thread is the large, structural nature of all of our products, which utilize castings, extrusions, and heavy-gauge sheet and plate as primary raw materials," Walker explains.

In addition, WACO has carved out an identity in the marketplace for its adeptness at providing engineering and fabrication solutions for uncommon projects. The company's custom fabrication capabilities enable it to manufacture just about anything, regardless of product size or configuration.

One key element in WACO's success—whether in custom fabrication or in its trademark maritime applications—is the company's solid workforce. With 45 employees at its Baltimore facility and another 45 at TriFab, WACO operates management programs that emphasize the involvement of all staff and look ahead to innovative, new manufacturing practices.

"A lot of the credit for our success goes to our employees,"

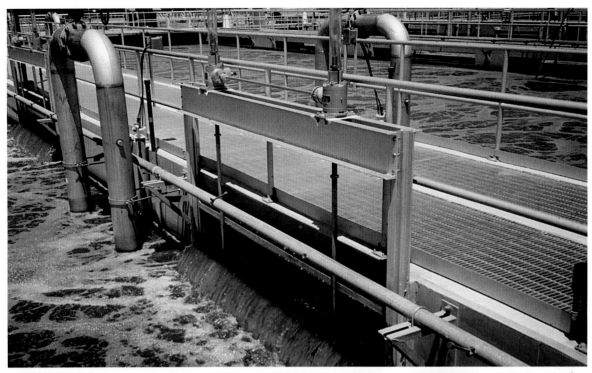

says Walker, noting that quite a few of WACO's employees have up to 35 years of tenure—an anomaly in today's business environment.

Longevity is important to WACO because the equipment, far from relying solely on the high-tech, computer-driven modules of many fabricators, is skill-based. This requires superior, trained employees. To achieve this base, WACO has introduced an innovative Work Team program, through which all employees—from production workers to office staff—join together to operate their team for each line of business. These groups meet monthly to discuss existing orders, customer needs, problems, goals for improved manufacturing processes, and ideas for new products.

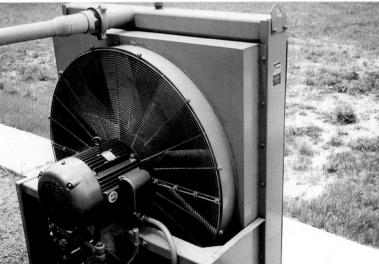

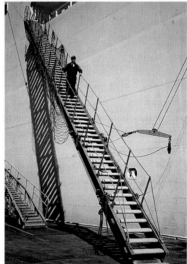

"This way," notes Walker, "all employees are responsible for building a product from start to finish. There is a sense of ownership and responsibility. The final product—whether it be a Duralite trench shield system, a fire truck extension boom, a slide gate for a water treatment plant, or an accommodation ladder for a navy frigate—very much belongs to them."

WACO's management practices, its commitment to innovative product development, and its eye for strategic acquisitions are just a few of the reasons why the company celebrated its 50th anniversary in 1997. These basic principles have guided Washington Aluminum's past successes, as they continue today to guide the company into the future.

CLOCKWISE FROM TOP:
A WACO WEIR GATE CONTROLS FLOW THROUGH A NEW JERSEY WASTEWATER TREATMENT PLANT.

ONE OF THE COMPANY'S ACCOMMODATION LADDERS PROVIDES ACCESS TO THE HOSPITAL SHIP USNHS *Comfort*.

WACO AIRFOIL ALUMINUM FANS PROVIDE HIGH-EFFICIENCY COOLING FOR A RADIATOR PACKAGE.

WMAR-TV

OCTOBER 27, 1947, IS A VERY IMPORTANT DAY IN THE HISTORY of Maryland. It is the day a television station first began broadcasting within the state. That station was WMAR-TV. The date also marks the beginning of a long, unrivaled history of firsts for WMAR. WMAR's premiere broadcast aired horse races from

"Old Hill Top"—Pimlico Race Course.

In 1997, WMAR-TV, Baltimore's ABC affiliate, celebrated its 50th anniversary. From its beginnings in an era of rebuilding after World War II, WMAR-TV has depended on the lenses of its cameras and the eyes and ears of its dedicated staff to become a part of Baltimore life—through momentous events in history, as well as through day-to-day news and events.

Early Days

Despite the acclaim received as the first television station to go on the air in Baltimore, the early days of the medium were a challenge. Television sets were not yet in every home. Instead, viewers were required to patronize the few area bars and restaurants that could invest in the sets. It wasn't until 1947,

when the World Series was telecast for the first time, that the general public embraced the concept of television.

Throughout the years, WMAR-TV has accomplished many technological firsts in the television market. It was the original station to televise direct pickups of major sporting events, from football to horse racing to regattas, and the pioneer in providing Maryland viewers with regularly scheduled religious, educational, children's, and talk-format public service programming. In fact, *National Review*, the country's first national talk show, premiered on WMAR-TV.

Additionally, WMAR-TV participated with CBS in broadcasting the first color television pictures in North America. WMAR-TV had the first color film processor

for television news and production and was the pioneer user of the zoom camera lens for film and tape cameras.

A commitment to cutting-edge technology was important to WMAR-TV, both then and now, but the company is equally known for the talented professionals—both behind and in front of the camera—who, early on, elevated the station's reputation. Jim McManus, better known as ABC Sports' beloved anchorman Jim McKay, started his career at WMAR-TV as a cub reporter for the city desk. Janet Covington, who in 1948 was the station's first woman director, went on to mastermind *National Review*, one of America's most dynamic daily variety shows.

Among the medical firsts was a broadcast from Johns Hopkins

CLOCKWISE FROM TOP RIGHT: NEWS CHANNEL 2 AT 6 P.M. ANCHOR TEAM (FROM LEFT): SPORTS DIRECTOR SCOTT GARCEAU, KEITH CATE, SANDRA PINCKNEY, AND METEOROLOGIST NORM LEWIS

NEWS CHANNEL 2 *First at Five* ANCHOR TEAM (FROM LEFT): SPORTS DIRECTOR SCOTT GARCEAU, MARY BETH MARSDEN, STAN STOVALL, AND METEOROLOGIST VERONICA JOHNSON

WMAR-TV ONCE OPERATED FROM FACILITIES ON REDWOOD STREET IN DOWNTOWN BALTIMORE.

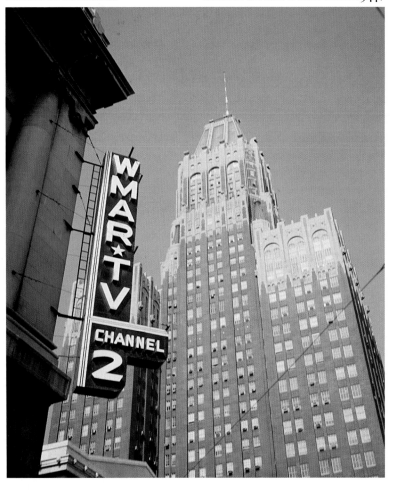

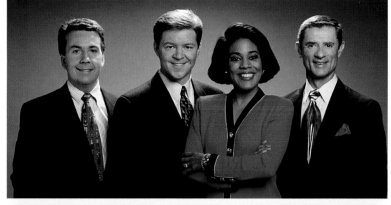

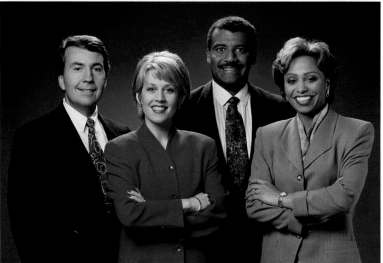

Hospital on the first blue baby operation. Hit shows throughout the decades that have been immortalized by Baltimoreans include *Romper Room* and *Professor Kool's Fun School*, which made stars out of characters "Miss Nancy" and, later, her daughter "Miss Sally," as well as Stu Kerr.

The Modern Era

For WMAR-TV, television's modern era has led to a major emphasis on news broadcasting. With newscasts that begin at 5:30 a.m. and wrap up at 11:30 p.m., WMAR-TV's around-the-clock commitment has given the station a leadership role as a news organization. WMAR-TV's signature programs provide a seamless blend of hard-hitting reports and news-you-can-use that has earned it recognition on the local, regional, and national levels.

As a result, in 1996, WMAR-TV was awarded 10 Emmys by the Capital Region Awards Committee and the Board of Governors of the Washington, D.C., chapter of the National Academy of Television Arts and Sciences. It has received awards as well from the Maryland Society of Professional Journalists; PROMAX International, the world's foremost association of electronic media promotion and marketing professionals; and the National Association of Black Journalists, to name a few.

Community Leadership

WMAR-TV's commitment to the community is what sets it apart from its competitors. Since its inception, WMAR-TV has been committed to addressing social and health issues that affect the community—both on and off camera. For more than 30 years, WMAR-TV has donated 21 hours of airtime to the Jerry Lewis Labor Day Telethon, an annual national tradition that benefits the Muscular Dystrophy Association. In addition, WMAR has also helped to raise nearly $20 million for the Johns Hopkins Children's Center, a comprehensive pediatric institution recognized internationally as a leader in pediatric research, treatment, and education.

One of WMAR-TV's biggest community outreach initiatives is Talking 2 Us. Each month, station managers and employees visit local community associations to hear what viewers have to say about the problems within their community. This open forum is designed to keep the station in touch with the communities it serves.

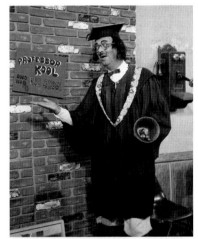

For more than a decade, WMAR-TV has helped raise funds for the Maryland Food Committee, the Baltimore School for the Arts, the Fuel Fund of Central Maryland, and Afram Expo, a forum for recognition of the accomplishments of area African-Americans. Other important programs supported by WMAR-TV include Contact 2, the station's free-to-the-community consumer information and referral service spearheaded by the National Council of Jewish Women.

WMAR broadcasts more than 20 hours of local news per week, as well two public affairs programs and *Rodricks for Breakfast*, a live program featuring *Baltimore Sun* columnist Dan Rodricks. Throughout the year, the station also features a variety of local specials, including live, day-long coverage of the Preakness and WMAR-TV's annual drama competition in honor of Black History Month.

WMAR-TV is owned by the E.W. Scripps Company. The vice president and general manager is Steven J. Gigliotti.

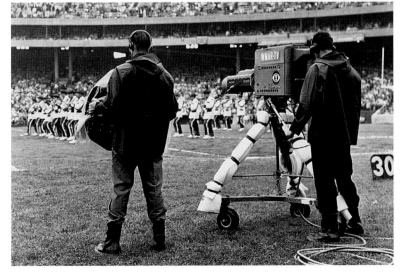

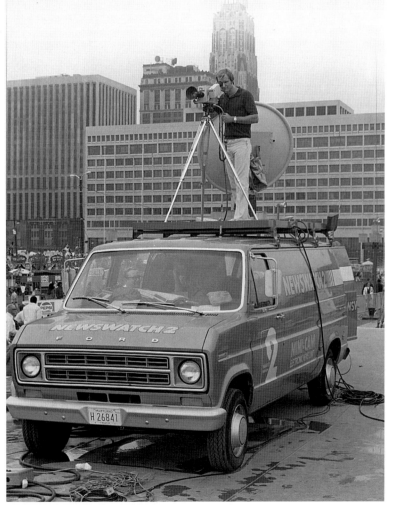

WBAL-TV 11

FROM ITS ORIGINAL HEADQUARTERS ON NORTH CHARLES STREET IN downtown Baltimore to today's Television Hill location, WBAL-TV 11 has become the most watched local television station in the Baltimore market. Hearst–Argyle Television, Inc., reaching viewers in the 23rd-largest market in the United States, currently owns WBAL-TV 11,

which began broadcasting on March 11, 1948.

In August 1981, Channel 11 became affiliated with the CBS network, ending a 22-year relationship with NBC. In 1995, the station rejoined the NBC network where it will mark its 50th year on-air in 1998, continuing to take an active role in community involvement while providing its viewers with quality news and entertainment programming.

Viewing History

The early days of Channel 11 meant few shows and frequent test patterns scattered throughout the day. During the late 1940s, WBAL-TV offered programs like *Musical Almanac*, *Look and Cook*, *Know Baltimore*, and western films such as *Billy the Kid*, as well as news and sports programming.

Local television buffs will remember other well-known shows of Channel 11's past like Baltimore's first live morning variety show,

Romper Room, an internationally syndicated program that originated on WBAL-TV in the 1950s.

Channel 11's news documentaries made their impact on the community in the early 1960s. *Dark Corner*, hosted by Rolf Hertsgaard and Larry Levin, was a series of prime-time specials focusing on timely issues and concerns of the Baltimore viewing audience. This critically acclaimed program won numerous honors, including national Emmy awards for excellence.

Throughout the mid-1960s and early 1970s, WBAL-TV introduced a variety of children's and entertainment programs including *Rhea and Sunshine*; *Pete the Pirate*, a program that boasted a lifelike replica of a ship as its set; and *P.W. Doodle*, appealing to children during the afternoon viewing hours. *Duckpin and Dollars*, a weekday bowl-for-cash show, was then Baltimore's most popular locally produced program. A spin-off, *Pinbusters*, was a youth championship bowling show.

And teens rocked and rolled to the latest sounds on *The Kirby Scott Show*.

A Station of Firsts

Throughout its 50 years of television, Channel 11 has made significant advances in the fields of equal employment opportunity and technology. Channel 11 employed Baltimore's first black anchorman and first black news director. Using homemade gear built by the station's engineers, Baltimore viewed the debut of color television on WBAL-TV. Channel 11 was the first station in Maryland to acquire a videotape cartridge machine, becoming the eighth station in the world to own this advanced piece of equipment.

WBAL-TV entered a new era in space technology with the acquisition of NEWSTAR 11, Baltimore television's first mobile satellite news-gathering system. In Baltimore and from around the country, wherever news is happening, WBAL-TV 11

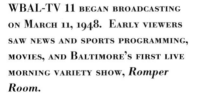

WBAL-TV 11 BEGAN BROADCASTING ON MARCH 11, 1948. EARLY VIEWERS SAW NEWS AND SPORTS PROGRAMMING, MOVIES, AND BALTIMORE'S FIRST LIVE MORNING VARIETY SHOW, *Romper Room.*

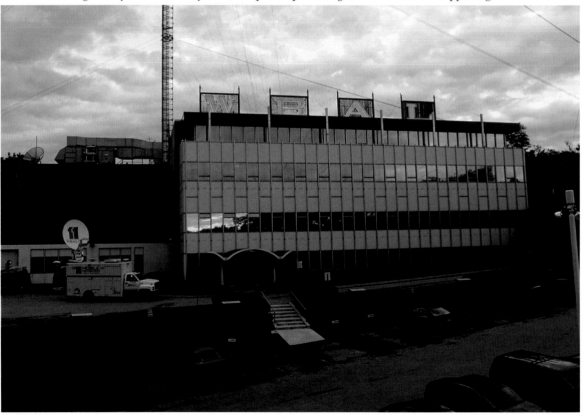

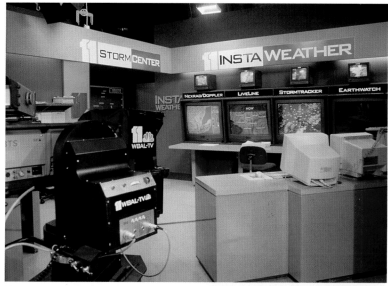

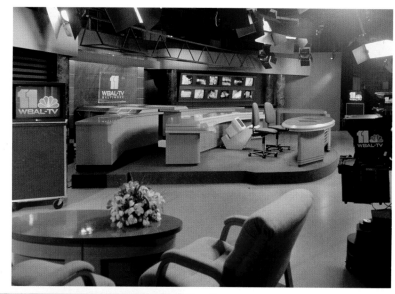

News and NEWSTAR 11 can quickly bring home complete, live news coverage.

This commitment to quality news has garnered the station several prestigious honors. WBAL-TV News earned the Edward R. Murrow Award for outstanding overall news coverage and presentation. The George Polk Award and the American Bar Association Gavel Award were presented to WBAL-TV News for excellence in reporting and journalism. Both the Associated Press and United Press International have named WBAL-TV as the outstanding television news operation in Baltimore.

Changing the Face of Baltimore Television

With exciting new programming acquisitions, a revitalized news effort, and an enhanced concern and involvement with the community, WBAL-TV has repositioned itself for growth and success in the 21st century. As of February 1997, WBAL-TV finished as Baltimore's number one television station for the 10th sweeps period in a row. This victory is certainly due in part to the station's celebrated 11 p.m. newscast. With a solid anchor team, compelling special assignments, and hard-hitting franchises, the product has never looked stronger. Behind the headlines, the investigative team uncovers the real story that no one else is reporting; and Chief Meteorologist Tom Tasselmyer leads the WBAL Forecast Center team in tracking severe weather.

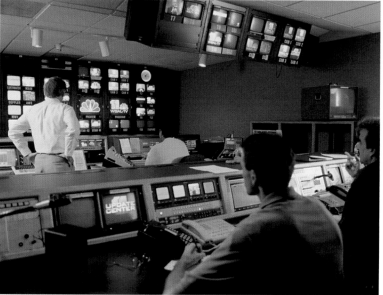

WBAL-TV airs Baltimore's only locally produced public affairs show, *The Bottom Line*, with a live audience. Hosted by Kweisi Mfume, president and CEO of the NAACP, the show tackles the issues facing families today, from education to abortion and from domestic violence to police brutality. The weekly hour-long show airs each Saturday at noon, following the award-winning weekend morning news.

Another exciting development at the station is The More You Know, a comprehensive community affairs campaign recognized by government and business leaders, medical professionals, parents, and teachers. NBC has produced more than 200 award-winning public service announcements featuring some of the network's biggest stars, such as Brooke Shields from *Suddenly Susan*, Eriq La Salle and Anthony Edwards from *ER*, Jennifer

Aniston and David Schwimmer from *Friends*, David Hyde Pierce from *Frasier*, and many more. The campaign is aimed at issues affecting health, children, and the future.

Broadcasting Dedication to Viewers

Through the years, WBAL-TV has also continued its commitment to the community it serves by providing major support to local charitable organizations, including the Maryland Food Bank, Greater Baltimore Committee, United Way of Central Maryland, and Baltimore Symphony Orchestra.

Spanning five decades of broadcasting, the cornerstones of WBAL-TV 11's mission have remained the same: to provide quality entertainment and informational programming, superior news reports, and a dedication to the community it serves.

CLOCKWISE FROM TOP LEFT: THE STATION'S INSTA-WEATHER CENTER PROVIDES UP-TO-THE-MINUTE METEOROLOGICAL UPDATES.

FROM ITS MODERN-DAY STUDIO IN BALTIMORE, WBAL-TV CELEBRATES 50 YEARS OF BROADCASTING IN 1998.

IN-HOUSE PROGRAMMING IS DIRECTED FROM THE WBAL-TV DIRECTOR BOOTH.

WJZ-TV

WHEN PEOPLE THINK ABOUT WJZ-TV, CERTAIN PHRASES COME TO mind: "Baltimore's favorite news team." "People who feel like family." "The station that's most like home." ℘ The address called home by many area television viewers is WJZ-TV, known for decades as the most-watched local news station in Maryland.

That sense of family began with a "WAAM"—as in WAAM-TV—the forerunner of WJZ-TV, founded by brothers Ben and Herman Cohen in 1948. WAAM's first broadcast on November 2 told an astonished public what the newspapers couldn't: Truman, not Dewey, had won the presidential race. That news scoop would come to define WJZ-TV's *Eyewitness News* and would prompt viewers to tune to WJZ-TV first when they want breaking news.

Initially, WAAM was a dual affiliate of ABC and the now defunct Dumont Network. In 1957, it became solely affiliated with ABC when Westinghouse Electric Corporation acquired the station, renamed it WJZ, and transformed it into an ABC affiliate powerhouse. That relationship lasted until January 1995, when WJZ-TV switched to an affiliation with CBS, a move that preceded the November 1995 purchase of CBS, Inc. by parent company Westinghouse.

Thorough News Coverage

WJZ-TV offers its viewers the day's first dose of news with the wake-up call of *Rise and Shine* weekdays at 5:30 a.m., followed by *Morning Edition* at 6 a.m., and then *This Morning Edition* at 7 a.m. *This Morning Edition* expanded by an hour in August 1996 to provide fans with even more of Don Scott and Marty Bass, the top-ranked local morning news team in Baltimore. WJZ provides the city's only local news program produced at 7 a.m. The station's *Eyewitness News at Noon* serves up anchor team Don Scott, Marty Bass, and Kellye Lynn.

Viewers already home by the 5 p.m. rush hour catch up on the day's news from the Emmy-award-winning *Eyewitness News at Five*, anchored by Sally Thorner and Richard Sher, along with weatherman Bob Turk, sportscaster John Buren, and "Health Watch" reporter Kellye Lynn.

At 6 p.m., Baltimore's veteran, Emmy-award-winning anchorwoman Denise Koch anchors the area's only hour-long 6 p.m. local newscast, along with Vic Carter, who became part of the *Eyewitness News* family in December 1995. The team of Koch, Carter, Turk, and Buren continues to drive audiences home to WJZ-TV for the late-night newscast at 11 p.m.

Eyewitness News is also hard at work on weekends, with the Saturday and Sunday morning anchor teams of Katie Leahan and Tim Williams, as well as evening news with anchors Pat Warren and Kal Jackson, Dr. Bob Sopka's weather, and Chris Ely's sports.

The Names in the News

Many careers have been launched at WJZ-TV. Oprah Winfrey made her talk-show debut at WJZ, sharing the mike with Richard Sher on the popular *People Are Talking* program. While Winfrey went on to international fame, many others made WJZ-TV their home.

Two standouts formed the anchor team once ranked by *Electronic Media* among the top three in the country: Jerry Turner and Al Sanders. Turner joined the station in the 1960s and was named one of the nation's top 10 local news anchors before dying of cancer in 1987. After Turner's death, Sanders assumed the unofficial title of Dean of Television in Baltimore and shared the news desk for a time with Koch. Sadly, Sanders was diagnosed with lung cancer in 1995, dying at the age of 54.

The First among Many

WJZ has built a reputation as a station that does things first. This started the day it opened as WAAM, housed in the area's first studio designed strictly for the then new medium of television.

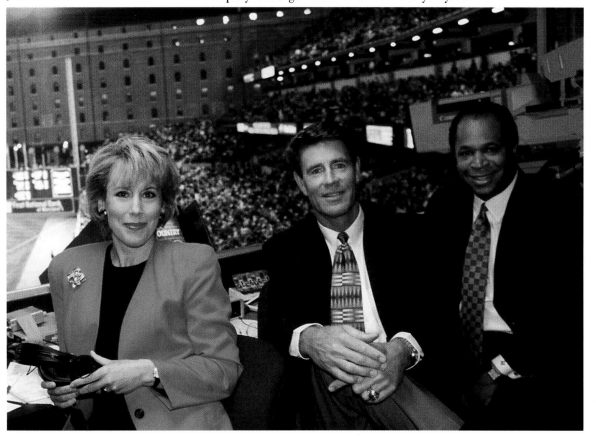

WJZ's Emmy-award-winning anchorwoman Denise Koch (left) anchors the area's only hour-long 6 p.m. local newscast, along with Vic Carter (far right). The two are joined here by baseball great Jim Palmer.

WAAM was the first station in the market to air a locally produced minority public affairs show, *The Fourth Man*. In 1965, the station became the first in the market to reflect diversity in its reporting staff with the hiring of Wiley Daniels.

WJZ, in 1976, was the first Baltimore station to expand its evening newscast to one hour, and the first to introduce a local morning news show back in 1982. Today, both of these news programs remain tops in their time periods.

Additionally, WJZ aired the first locally produced national weekday program in the coveted local access position next to the start of the 8 p.m. prime-time hour. Called *Evening Magazine*, the program ran from 1977 to 1990.

In the 1990s, WJZ became the first and only station in the market to provide real-time closed captioning of its newscasts, and the first and only Baltimore TV station to provide two hours of early evening local news when it launched *Eyewitness News at Five*, in January 1994, as the lead-in to its established 6 p.m. newscast.

In April 1997, WJZ became the only Maryland station offering live Doppler radar, known as First Warning Weather. Thousands of allergy sufferers received a break

the previous year when WJZ-TV became the first station to include an allergy watch in its weather reports.

A Community Success

First in news and technical innovations, the station is also a top performer in the programming arena. It is the flagship broadcast station for the Baltimore Orioles and has the area's number one locally produced program for children, *It's Academic*. News and programming topics can be tracked via the Internet at www.wjz.com on the World Wide Web.

The station is also one of the first to respond to the needs of the community, with such outreach programs as *Shaping Tomorrow*, a multipronged campaign designed to ensure a better tomorrow; and *Ask the Pharmacist*. WJZ is an active supporter of such community events as Artscape, a celebration of the arts drawing more than 1 million people each year; the Susan G. Komen Foundation's Race for the Cure; and AIDSWALK, among many others.

Over the years, the station has become part of Maryland's rich social fabric. It is the broadcast neighbor next door, the helping hand to those in need, the friendly voices and faces who bring viewers news in the unmistakable WJZ, real-people style.

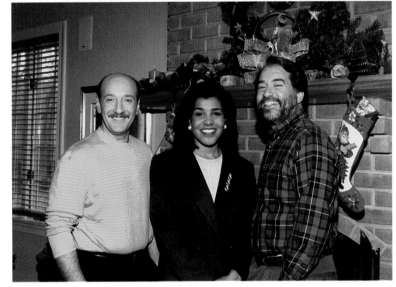

WJZ PROVIDES THE CITY'S TOP-RATED MIDDAY NEWS PROGRAM. THE STATION'S *Eyewitness News at Noon* SERVES UP ANCHOR TEAM (FROM LEFT) MARTY BASS, KELLYE LYNN, AND DON SCOTT.

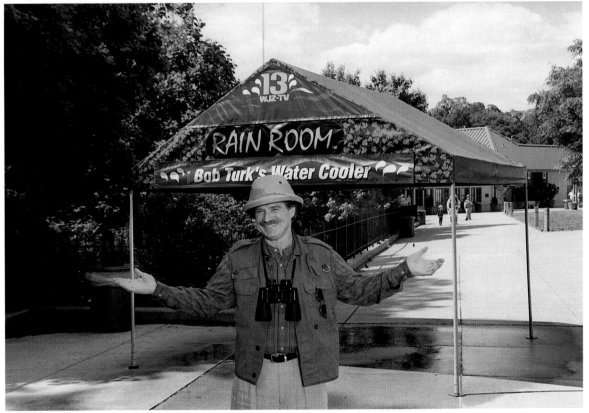

WEATHERMAN BOB TURK KEEPS BALTIMORE RESIDENTS CURRENT ON CHANGING WEATHER CONDITIONS WITH FIRST WARNING LIVE DOPPLER WEATHER.

Ward Machinery Company

N 1962, ENGINEER BILL WARD SR. HAD AN IDEA THAT HE COULD BUILD the proverbial better mousetrap. And he did. In his basement workshop, Ward invented the modern rotary die cutter. It was an innovation that went on to revolutionize an industry. ❧ Today, the Ward Machinery Company, based in Hunt Valley and helmed by CEO Bill Ward Jr., is a world leader in

the creation of machinery for the printing, folding, and cutting of corrugated board. And in the past 35 years, Ward Machinery has carved for itself an international reputation for innovation, precision manufacturing, and unsurpassed reliability. Every day, in all parts of the world, machines made by Ward are manufacturing product packaging, corrugated shipping containers, point-of-purchase displays, and more.

Ward Machinery is an integral part of a multibillion-dollar global industry. The company currently employs more than 600 people, with plants in Baltimore, Ireland, and Spain, as well as a worldwide sales and customer-support organization. Everything produced by Ward Machinery reflects its trademark qualities of technological leadership and manufacturing excellence. In addition to new product introductions, the com-

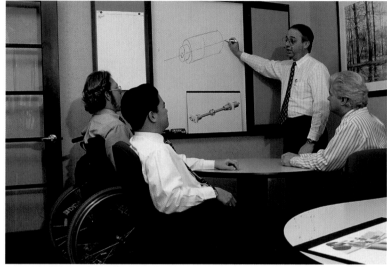

pany continually updates existing technology and processes.

State-of-the-Art Mechanics

Bill Ward Sr.'s idea was to create a more efficient and more capable machine for making die-cut boxes. This style of box is characterized by a series of

different flaps of varying sizes that can fold into a variety of shapes and add flexibility to design. Ward's creation of the modern rotary die cutter established a standard of efficiency that has transformed this Maryland-based company into a worldwide leader in the packaging industry. In the process, he founded a company that has always emphasized superior design from an engineering perspective; performance, precision, and reliability from a manufacturing standpoint; and customer-driven service to its clientele. Ward Machinery primarily markets to two groups: major paper companies like International Paper and Georgia Pacific, and small, independent box manufacturers who cater to the booming point-of-sale marketplace.

Ward Machinery's commitment to innovation has helped it maintain its leadership position as well. Ten years ago, the company integrated a high-quality, state-of-the-art printing process into its rotary die cutter. Now, the equipment can fold and cut corrugated board, and print up to seven colors simultaneously. The efficiencies designed by Ward Machinery are aimed at helping its customers operate in the most cost-efficient and cost-effective manner possible. The com-

WARD MACHINERY'S COMMITMENT TO INNOVATION HAS HELPED THE COMPANY MAINTAIN ITS LEADERSHIP POSITION IN A MULTIBILLION-DOLLAR GLOBAL INDUSTRY. EVERY DAY, IN ALL PARTS OF THE WORLD, MACHINES MADE BY WARD ARE MANUFACTURING PRODUCT PACKAGING, CORRUGATED SHIPPING CONTAINERS, POINT-OF-PURCHASE DISPLAYS, AND MORE.

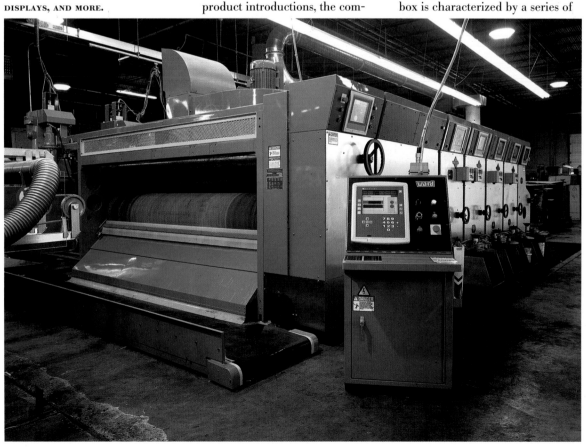

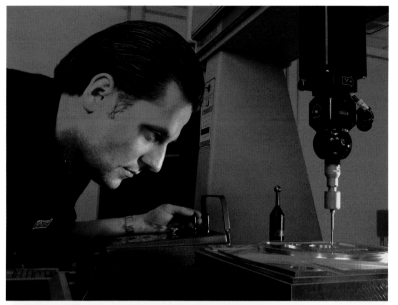

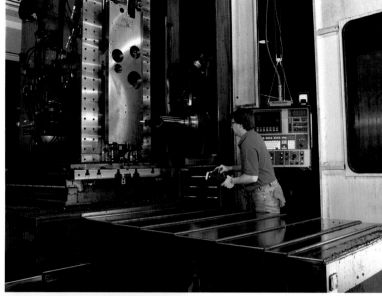

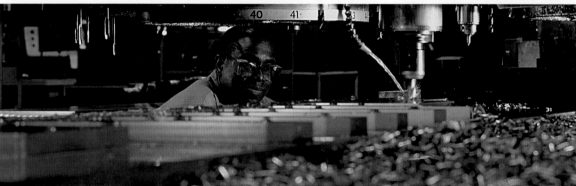

pany's innovations have consistently improved the way in which its clients operate, and clients credit Ward's machines with helping make them more profitable. Its equipment shortens production time and helps reduce the consumption of raw materials.

One important element of the company's customer-driven philosophy is to work with clients as a team. As a result, close communication with customers, which results in a better understanding of their manufacturing needs, has enabled Ward Machinery to be first in the market with many performance-enhancing innovations. "Our success comes directly out of the ability of our engineering and design teams to deliver the technologies and products that enhance our customers' competitiveness," says Bill Ward Jr. "Reliability and performance are built into all Ward products, from concept and design, through manufacture and customer service and support."

One key factor in this effort is the company's Information Services

department, which maintains Ward's extensive network of computers. From desktop systems to multiseat, minicomputer-driven CAD workstations, Ward uses the most advanced computer technology available. The company intranet, which connects its U.S. and overseas business, enables Ward to efficiently manage its far-reaching operations.

Impeccable Standards

In 1995, Ward Machinery received the International Organization for Standardization's coveted ISO 9001 certification. One of the first in its industry to win the classification, it further reinforces the company's effort to guarantee consistency in all of its machine products. Each piece of equipment that leaves Ward's manufacturing plants undergoes a quality audit at every stage of the manufacturing process. At each step, from the receipt of suppliers' materials to the checkout after final assembly, quality is meticulously monitored. To ensure compliance with the most exacting tolerances in the industry,

98 percent of the parts the company manufactures are produced on computer-driven machines.

Just as important as the technology, however, are company employees. "High-quality people produce high-quality products," says Bill Ward Jr. "It is our ongoing policy to recruit those who display leadership qualities in all areas, and to encourage and reward individual initiative, including promoting from within whenever possible."

In addition, the same entrepreneurial spirit and commitment to achievement that produced the founder's first successes remain a priority. "Because our continued success depends on our ability to seize an opportunity and respond quickly," says Bill Ward Jr., "we empower employees at all levels in the company to share ideas for improvement." As a result, Ward Machinery's consistently low employee turnover has contributed to the company's strategic, careful growth—a balance of innovation and conservation that would make its founder proud.

McEnroe Voice & Data Corporation

McENROE VOICE & DATA CORPORATION, HEADQUARTERED IN HUNT Valley, is celebrating its 25th year in business. McEnroe Voice & Data supports a variety of voice and data networks that include dictation systems, telecommunication and voice mail systems, voice logging, and specialized wide area networks for the health care industry.

The company provides voice and data transportation for the information superhighway.

The Voice in the Past

In 1972, Peter C. McEnroe founded McEnroe Business Systems Inc., the sole distributor for Lanier Dictation Systems in Maryland and Virginia.

Lanier captured the word processing marketplace in 1976, and this success was mirrored locally by McEnroe Business Systems. The company's growth continued through the end of that decade with success in the dictation and word processing divisions and eventual expansion into personal computer and network environments.

With telephone divestiture in 1983, the company capitalized on this market, providing state-of-the-art, reliable, and cost-effective telecommunications solutions. McEnroe Voice & Data now provides digital telecommunication products, integrating E-mail, voice mail, and the client's database.

In February 1996, McEnroe Business Systems changed its name to McEnroe Voice & Data Corpo-

ration to reflect the scope of its products and services, as well as the corporate mission of providing voice and data solutions to commercial customers.

Quality Products, Quality Service

Kathleen Del Monte succeeded her father, Peter McEnroe, as president of the company in 1987. Del Monte's leadership, combined with the strong support of the company's vice president, John Del Monte, led the company into the 1990s. "Our philosophy is to recommend the best combination of features and technology in a system to fit our customers' needs," says Kathleen Del Monte. McEnroe Voice & Data offers a strong blend of industry knowledge, technological expertise, and many years of experience in its senior management team. "We cannot rely on innovative technologies alone," says Del Monte. "We still believe in old-fashioned customer service."

McEnroe Voice & Data also provides specialized voice and data systems for the health care marketplace. This division has been a key

success for the company, with major installations in 95 percent of the hospitals in its markets. The company has formed numerous strategic partnerships with the largest health care providers in the region.

McEnroe Voice & Data's goal is to offer customers the highest-quality products, which include Lanier dictation, Toshiba and Lucent telephones, Active Voice call processing systems, Dynamic Instrument voice loggers, Sharp facsimile, and Novell network systems. The ability to sell, service, and support these state-of-the-art technologies translates into added value for the company's customers.

McEnroe Voice & Data is annually recognized as one of Baltimore's largest woman-owned businesses. The company has experienced a steady growth in revenues and profits during its 25 years in business and currently services more than 8,000 customers in Maryland, northern Virginia, and Washington, D.C. Committed to providing reliable and practical solutions to its customers, backed by the finest service and support available, McEnroe Voice & Data is proud to be Baltimore's business partner.

THE SENIOR MANAGEMENT TEAM OF MCENROE VOICE & DATA INCLUDES PHIL LAUCK, BOB REAVIS, PRESIDENT/ OWNER KATHLEEN DEL MONTE, VICE PRESIDENT/OWNER JOHN DEL MONTE, LORI WHALEY, PATRICK ZORZI, AND NICK VISSER (LEFT).

MARK KENDRICK, FACILITY AND PROJECT MANAGER FOR ADVANCED RADIOLOGY, AND PHIL LAUCK, DIVISION MANAGER AT MCENROE VOICE & DATA, DISPLAY THE LARGEST PRIVATE VOICE PROCESSING NETWORK IN THE STATE OF MARYLAND, SERVICING PHYSICIANS AT MORE THAN 35 REMOTE LOCATIONS (RIGHT).

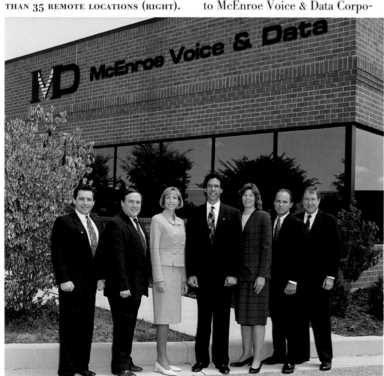

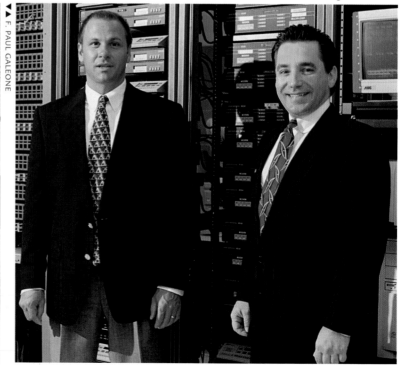

F. PAUL GALEONE

Maryland Science Center

I N THE LATE 1700S, AN AFFABLE GROUP OF CITIZENS, BROUGHT TOGETHER BY their shared interest in nature and the stars, founded the Maryland Academy of Sciences, the state's oldest scientific institution. The academy, inspired by founding member and impresario Charles Wilson Peale, opened the Museum of Natural History on April 6, 1797, at 45 South Charles Street.

A Dream Realized

The longtime dream of the Maryland Academy of Sciences was realized 129 years later with the opening of the Maryland Science Center at Baltimore's Inner Harbor on June 13, 1976. Today, three floors of interactive exhibits, the renowned Davis Planetarium, and the IMAX Theater—along with extensive educational programs—touch more than half a million Marylanders and out-of-state visitors each year.

The Maryland Science Center remains strongly committed to its mission of improving the public's understanding of science. Outreach programs attract more than 250,000 schoolchildren and teachers annually. The Davis Planetarium produces quality original productions and distributes them to planetariums worldwide. Exhibits such as *Chesapeake Bay, Beyond Numbers,* and the *National Visitors Center for the Hubble Space Telescope*, plus compelling visiting exhibitions, delight visitors of all ages. The IMAX Theater, with its five-story-high screen and 38-speaker sound system, offers a spectacular visual experience.

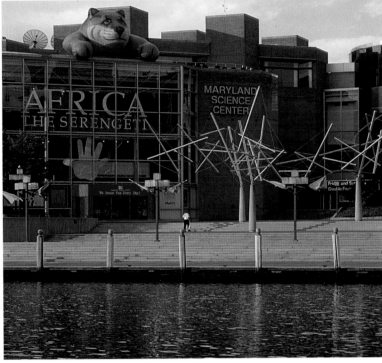

The Maryland Science Center continues to cultivate interest in, and understanding of science for all of the state's residents and out-of-town visitors. An important regional resource and national model for informal science education, the Maryland Science Center honors outstanding achievements in the fields of science and engineering, and seeks to inspire young and old alike by encouraging careers in science and science-related fields, especially in those areas of particular importance to the state's economic well-being.

The dream of the Maryland Academy of Sciences continues to shine brightly, touching the lives of children and adults, and helping them not only to be intrigued by science, but also to discover firsthand its awe-inspiring wonder.

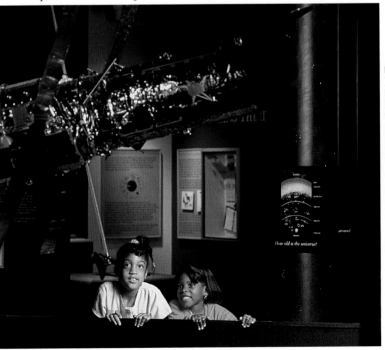

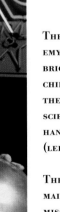

▲▼ PETER C. HOWARD

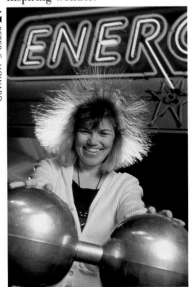

Broadmead, Inc.

TRUE TO THEIR QUAKER VALUES, BALTIMORE'S STONY RUN FRIENDS MEETING and the wider Religious Society of Friends founded Broadmead, a continuing care retirement community in Baltimore. Broadmead, Inc., which was incorporated as the Friends Lifetime Care Center of Baltimore, Inc. in 1976 and opened as a private, not-for-profit community in 1979.

Living at Broadmead is an opportunity limited only by the individual's interests, energy, and physical capacities.

Although the corporation must have a majority of trustees who are members of the Society of Friends, the Broadmead community is open to men and women aged 65 and older, regardless of race, color, creed, or national origin.

Concept of Community

A continuing care retirement community is distinguished from all other types of housing options for older persons by the offer of a continuum of care, a long-term contract that provides a residence, services, and nursing care. What makes Broadmead unique from other continuing care organizations is its concept of community.

From the beginning, Broadmead has served as a community that offers warmth and camaraderie as well as an intellectually stimulating atmosphere. It was designed for people who want to maintain maximum independence and yet be assured of health and personal support systems. With a setting in which costs are spread among all residents to minimize risk for each individual, and where input on issues is encouraged, Broadmead is a place where people recognize the needs of the community, as well as their own preferences.

An assurance of quality service is also a central theme within the context of community at Broadmead. Its commitment in this area has led to consistent accreditation by the Continuing Care Accreditation Commission since 1983.

Above all, Broadmead's community concept is manifested in its people. The partnership of a dedicated board of trustees, a committed Residents' Association, and a talented staff leadership group has guided and charted the community on a steady course, helping Broadmead grow through the many challenges that face a creative and vibrant continuing care retirement community.

Prime Amenities and Location

Broadmead is located in Hunt Valley on an historic, 84-acre estate that was once owned by Lord Baltimore. This area has long been known as Maryland's "horse country," with its riding stables, breeding farms, and steeplechases.

Broadmead's own property offers walking paths and a resident-designed nature trail. Nearby, restaurants and shops, ranging from elegant boutiques to major malls, abound. Within two miles is Oregon Ridge State Park, which, with a

EACH GARDEN-STYLE UNIT INCLUDES A PRIVATE PATIO AND A PLANTING AREA AROUND THE PATIO.

BROADMEAD'S COMMUNITY BUILDING FEATURES A BEAUTIFUL ROSE GARDEN CARED FOR BY ITS RESIDENTS.

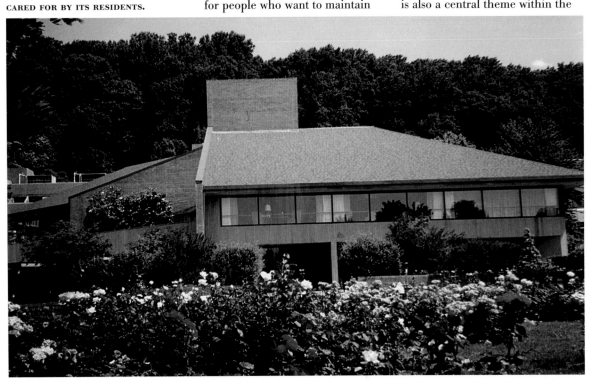

nature center, dinner theater, and summer concerts, satisfies a multiplicity of interests. Located just 10 miles north of Baltimore, Broadmead also offers easy access to all the city has to offer, including such attractions as the Inner Harbor, Oriole Park at Camden Yards, the Baltimore Symphony Orchestra, and numerous museums and theaters.

Broadmead is a community full of benefits, offering choices in accommodations, activities, and social functions, among others. The community as a whole offers a variety of entertaining and educational programs in the Broadmead Center, with its lounge, auditorium, and many meeting rooms. There are libraries, indoor and outdoor recreational areas, and craft areas used for ceramics, art, sewing, woodworking, photography, and various other interests.

Residents can select from five different garden-style and mid-rise units, ranging from studios to two-bedroom, two-bath homes. All units are equipped with resident safety features, resident-controlled heating and air-conditioning, walk-in closets, storage space, master television antennas, draperies, and wall-to-wall carpet. Each garden-style unit also includes a private patio and a planting area around the patio. Vegetable and flower plots are available on campus to all residents.

Also included in each resident's monthly fees are three meals a day, weekly housekeeping, routine maintenance services, scheduled trans-

portation for shopping, access to an indoor swimming pool with a Jacuzzi, full medical care, and processing of all medical claims.

Meals are served in three different dining rooms. For breakfast, residents eat at the informal Coffee Shop or in the Health Care Dining Room, both of which are also open for lunch and dinner. The elegant main dining room hosts lunch and dinner meals every day.

Broadmead's medical services are top-notch, and most of these services are included in the lifetime care contract at no additional cost. Included are the services of the full-service clinic, off-campus referrals, physical therapy, prescriptions, and much more. Physicians in the clinic are on call 24 hours a day, seven days a week. Also available to residents on campus are the services of a dentist, an

ophthalmologist, an audiologist, and a podiatrist.

When totally independent living becomes difficult, a resident can transfer to an intermediate care unit. Residents desiring restorative nursing care for posthospital recovery, temporary care for illnesses and injuries, or permanent care receive it on the comprehensive care floors. Unlimited use of both levels of care is included in the lifetime care contract at no additional cost.

Also available on-site are such professional services as a beauty shop, a travel agent, and a bank, as well as the Country Store.

Broadmead's continuum of care, coupled with its concept of community, makes it uniquely equipped to provide its residents with all facets of care and well-being.

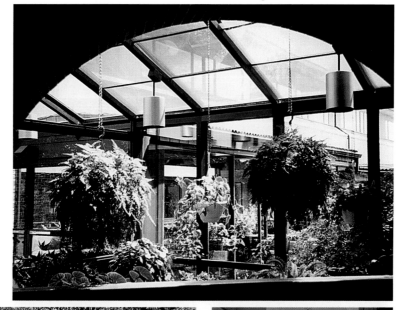

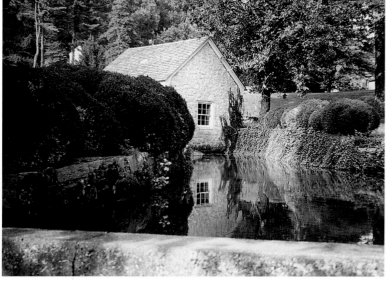

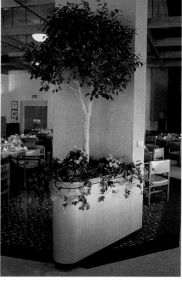

CLOCKWISE FROM TOP: BROADMEAD'S ATRIUM OF FERNS IS TENDED BY ITS RESIDENTS.

MEALS WHICH ARE INCLUDED IN MONTHLY RESIDENT FEES, ARE SERVED IN THREE DIFFERENT DINING ROOMS. THE MAIN DINING ROOM HOSTS LUNCH AND DINNER EVERY DAY.

A SPRINGHOUSE AND WARMING POOL GRACE THE BROADMEAD CAMPUS.

Management Recruiters of Baltimore/Timonium

SINCE 1976, MANAGEMENT RECRUITERS OF BALTIMORE/TIMONIUM HAS BEEN committed to establishing a partnership with its clients. It has been the premier provider of innovative and intelligent staffing solutions throughout the United States and worldwide. "Today, unprecedented changes are transforming every aspect of how people work and how companies hire," says Kenneth R. Davis, president and CEO.

The Baltimore/Timonium team is part of the Management Recruiters (MRI) network, the world's largest executive search firm, with more than 750 offices across the United States and in 32 countries. Not only is MRI of Baltimore/Timonium in the top 3 percent of all MRI offices nationally, but it is one of only 26 offices to be inducted into the President's Platinum Club. "We are Baltimore's largest executive search firm, and we are one of the most successful offices in the history of MRI," says Davis.

In any organization, strong leadership is the key to success. Davis and Linda Burton, vice president and general manager, have built MRI of Baltimore/Timonium into a company composed of more than 30 professionals whose foundation is based on a client-focused approach, needs analysis, and consultative selling. "We are professionals who are experts at identifying, qualifying, and attracting top-notch talent for our client companies," says Burton.

Davis and Burton lead Baltimore's nationally recognized, award-winning team with unprecedented tenure, knowledge, leadership, and professionalism. Their broad experience, expertise, and sound business solutions help clients adjust to the ever changing workforce climate.

Says Davis, "We staff vertically from top to bottom, from high-level executives or mid-level managers to office support. That breadth of service ensures that we don't merely supply companies with employees.

Instead, we enhance our services by identifying the clients' specific needs and, through continuous communication and follow-up, ensure a proper candidate/client match. These are the keys to our successful relationships."

Permanent Staffing

No one has more experience in finding and placing the best people for available positions," Davis says. "The client's account team manages the recruiting process through four specialized and comprehensive MRI divisions." Management Recruiters searches for individuals to fill professional and middle- to upper-management positions in the manufacturing and engineering industries. Sales Consultants concentrates on hiring for

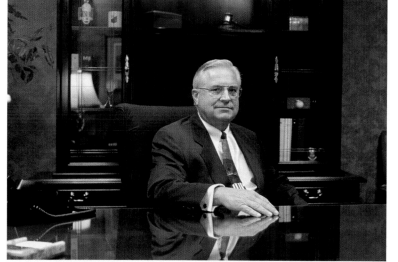

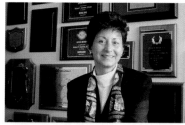

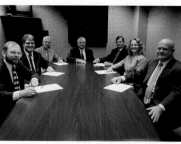

CLOCKWISE FROM TOP LEFT: KENNETH R. DAVIS, PRESIDENT AND CEO OF MANAGEMENT RECRUITERS, INC. OF BALTIMORE/TIMONIUM

SUSAN T. CREMEN, CERTIFIED SENIOR ACCOUNT MANAGER.

EACH CLIENT IS ASSIGNED AN ACCOUNT TEAM, WHICH MANAGES THE RECRUITING PROCESS THROUGH FOUR SPECIALIZED AND COMPREHENSIVE MRI DIVISIONS.

KENNETH R. DAVIS AND LINDA BURTON, MRI VICE PRESIDENT AND GENERAL MANAGER.

THE BALTIMORE/TIMONIUM TEAM IS PART OF THE MRI NETWORK, THE WORLD'S LARGEST EXECUTIVE SEARCH FIRM, WITH MORE THAN 750 OFFICES ACROSS THE UNITED STATES AND IN 32 COUNTRIES.

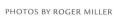

PHOTOS BY ROGER MILLER

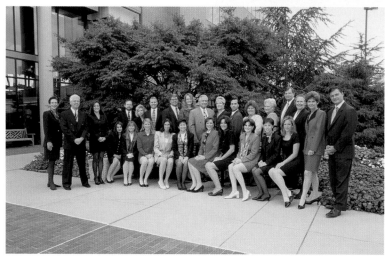

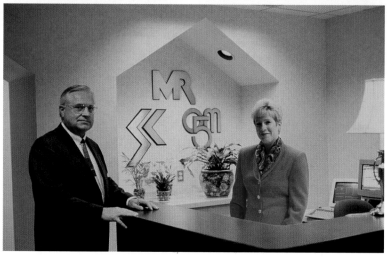

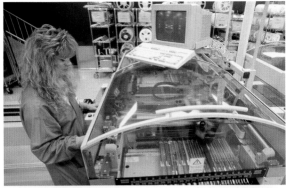

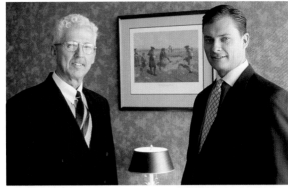

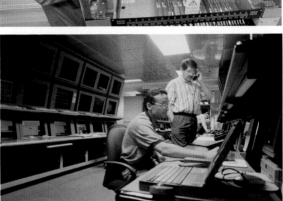

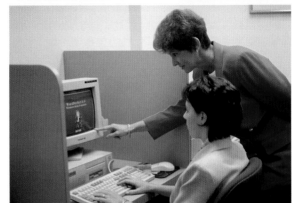

sales, sales management, and marketing professionals. CompuSearch provides information systems personnel, and Office Mates 5/DayStar focuses on finding permanent and interim administrative and office support personnel.

Flexible Staffing

Firms of the 1990s and into the millenium need alternatives to permanent placement. MRI's flexible staffing divisions have the systems, candidate networks, and national scope to meet any short-term staffing need, allowing the client to save recruiting, screening, and benefit costs. InterExec provides high-quality interim professional, technical, and managerial talent on an as-needed basis as an alternative to full-time

employees or traditional management consultants. Sales Staffers International trains, manages, and handles all payroll functions for temporary sales professionals to meet demands due to new product roll-outs, sudden growth opportunities, or test markets. DayStar sources the best and the brightest temporary/interim administrative and office support staff. Because of the success of these systems, MRI has thousands of topflight performers on the job every day.

Right-Fit Services

MRI commands state-of-the-art tools that help clients make the right decisions about their company's most important asset—its people. ConferView, MRI's interactive

Televideo Network enables a company to interview long-distance candidates without ever leaving town. SelecSys, MRI's reliable and action-oriented personality assessment tool, helps to evaluate the potential fit of prospective employees. Global Human Resources (GHR) puts the staffing expertise of MRI and its international alliance partners to work in order to provide a client with skilled candidates and professionals. Relocation Services provides cost-of-living analyses, home-finding assistance, mortgage services, and significant savings on moving and travel costs.

Whatever a company's personnel needs, Management recruiters of Baltimore/Timonium can fill them quickly and efficiently for a partnership that lasts.

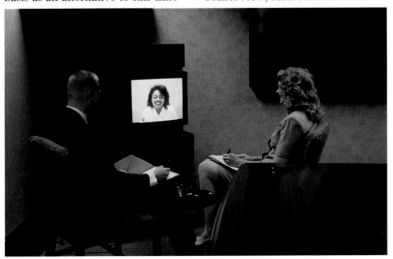

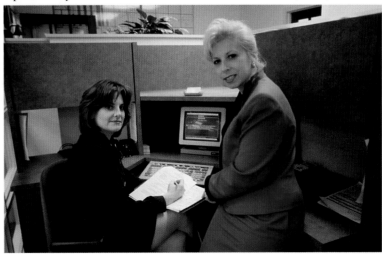

ECS Technologies, Inc.

ECS Technologies, Inc., established in 1979, is a solutions-driven systems integration firm that offers expertise in five competency areas: open systems integration, client/server computing, telecommunications, local and wide area networking, and scientific and engineering computing solutions. Founded by Eillen Dorsey, president, and Walter H. Hill Jr., vice president, who parlayed their experience in the engineering and technology consultancy fields into one of Baltimore's most successful computer firms, ECS' reputation extends nationwide.

Based in Baltimore, ECS, which counts among its clients such blue-chip firms as T. Rowe Price, Visa International, and the Naval Research Labs Effective Navy Electronic Warfare, is on the leading edge of technology—not only in Baltimore, but throughout the United States. In a nod to Dorsey's leadership, it is also, according to the *Baltimore Business Journal*, the number one computer reseller company owned by a woman. ECS, with a staff of more than 50 high-level technology professionals, enjoyed its most successful year ever in 1996, earning more than $43 million.

An Evolving Company

Today's success is quite a change from yesterday's challenge. When Dorsey and Hill founded ECS, which stands for electronic component sales, they envisioned a successful business in the sales of high-reliability aircraft components for the military—parts used in building missiles and aircraft. The company, based on the experience and technical sophistication of its two partners, thrived—until the U.S. government drastically reduced its defense budget. At that time, ECS could have been content to scale back its business. Instead, Dorsey and Hill took advantage of bad news to create new lines of business. "It was a tremendous opportunity to diversify," says Dorsey.

Intrigued by the constantly changing environment of the computer industry, the company transformed existing relationships with multinational technology manufacturers such as Digital, Sun Microsystems, Novell, and IBM into a highly specialized service-oriented firm. ECS also sought to provide corporate clients with expert advice on, and development of, new technologies. Today, ECS offers a one-stop solution for technology needs that range from highly classified to a simple networking of PCs.

Since its inception, ECS' team of committed professionals has demonstrated competency in emerging technologies and, armed with industry-specific knowledge, has delivered value-added solutions to its customers. "Our success can be attributed to our staff's technical competence," Dorsey says. "But we're also proud of our attention to detail, our integrity, and the firm's overall reputation of providing clients with the highest possible level of service."

As a small business, ECS recognized early on that it needed to

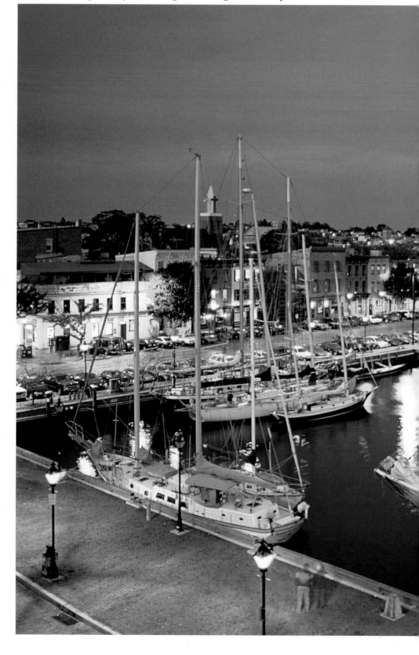

establish strategic business relationships with other system integration firms, manufacturers, and technology professionals. These partnerships have expanded the firm's technical depth and knowledge base, which has allowed ECS to address technology issues of the most complex type.

"Our clients are engaged in competition in the global marketplace," Dorsey says. "Survival in this arena requires efficient use of information and management technologies. Access to information is extremely important in keeping pace with the marketplace on a daily basis." The company also believes strongly that future business success is attained by those firms that integrate new technologies into their business operations. The integration of leading-edge technology improves the linkage between clients' needs and information technology solutions.

Multirange Service Provider

ECS has handled a wide variety of projects for a wide range of clients. For Visa International, ECS was awarded a new software conversion contract that requires its programmers to transform a legacy database application to one that is more up-to-date. The Carroll County Public Library asked ECS to correct issues with its frame relay network. Glass Jacobson & Associates, a medical practice, was in need of ongoing support for database applications.

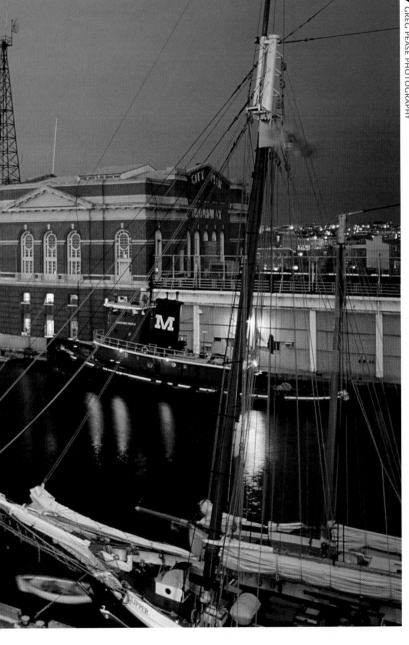

For the Rouse Company, ECS supplied a Sun Microsystems server and firewall technology. And Freddie Mac, a Virginia-based, federally chartered mortgage investment company, contracted with ECS for software consulting services.

In particular, ECS emphasizes four areas of technical expertise. Its professional and technical services division offers services such as certified engineers and administrators for both Novell NetWare and Windows.

There are Internet and intranet consultants, Visual BASIC programmers and system designers, and JD Edwards software implementation experts, to name a few.

ECS' advanced technology area provides expertise on DOS/Windows-based systems, coordination of local area network design and implementation, client/server network development, office automation, and desktop computer solutions. In telecommunications, dedicated staffers design and implement voice and data communication networks, work-group and enterprise messaging systems, and multiplatform network engineering and integration. Other services in this area include strategic product acquisition, analysis of system requirements, and system planning and design.

ECS' scientific and engineering solutions division, unique in the industry, offers a wide range of services. Among these include high-performance computing, image processing, database management, 3D visualization, virtual reality hardware and software solutions, and graphics and object-oriented programming.

For the folks at ECS, the most difficult challenge is not in coming up with simple solutions to highly complex needs. "In an industry that changes every day, a company that works on the leading edge of technology must keep constantly abreast with new developments," says Dorsey. "We relish the challenge." With its experience, expertise, and commitment to succeed, ECS will be meeting that challenge for many years to come.

Omni Inner Harbor Hotel

THE 707-ROOM OMNI INNER HARBOR HOTEL IS THE LARGEST HOTEL IN THE state of Maryland. With 30,000 square feet of meeting and convention space, the hotel attracts an impressive number of both large and small groups for all types of meetings. Connected by skywalks to the Inner Harbor and the Convention Center, the Omni is in the center of the city's business, financial, and entertainment districts.

Owned by Tavis Real Estate Group, Joint Venture, the Omni Inner Harbor is managed by Gencom American Hospitality under license by Omni Hotels Franchising Corporation. In 1979, The Gencom Group began acquiring and managing hotel properties for its own portfolio and has since emerged as one of the fastest-growing independent hotel companies in the industry. Gencom has built a sterling reputation, owning and operating a diverse portfolio of properties at profit levels well above industry averages. The Omni Inner Harbor Hotel has been among the company's top five, fastest growing properties in the past few years.

Just having undergone a $5 million renovation, all of the hotel's guest rooms have been upgraded. The Omni Inner Harbor Hotel has 187 king rooms, 133 queens, 365 two double-bed rooms, 11 classic living rooms (which connect one or two bedrooms), and 11 suites. There are 25 meeting rooms, an International Ballroom, and a smaller Liberty Ballroom to accommodate meetings and parties.

The hotel's renovated main lobby is majestic, with marble floors and walls with brass accents, round stone pillars, and domed chandeliers that highlight the new, vaulted lobby ceilings. The hotel's porte cochere includes elegant backlit signs to welcome hotel guests, extended overhead protection from bad weather conditions, and natural overhead skylights. The marble and brass of the hotel's facade are maintained throughout the first floor.

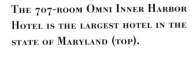

THE 707-ROOM OMNI INNER HARBOR HOTEL IS THE LARGEST HOTEL IN THE STATE OF MARYLAND (TOP).

WITH 30,000 SQUARE FEET OF MEETING AND CONVENTION SPACE, THE HOTEL ATTRACTS AN IMPRESSIVE NUMBER OF BOTH LARGE AND SMALL GROUPS FOR ALL TYPES OF MEETINGS (BOTTOM).

A Commitment to Service

But as hotel General Manager Peter Bheda cautions, "Nowadays, it's not the brass, the glass, and the marble that set the tone. It's the service and the understanding of what convention goers and visitors really need. This is where the Omni Inner Harbor Hotel really shines."

The Omni's room service provides all-day dining, snacks, and intimate, catered parties. A business center offers secretarial services dedicated to guests' needs, and a

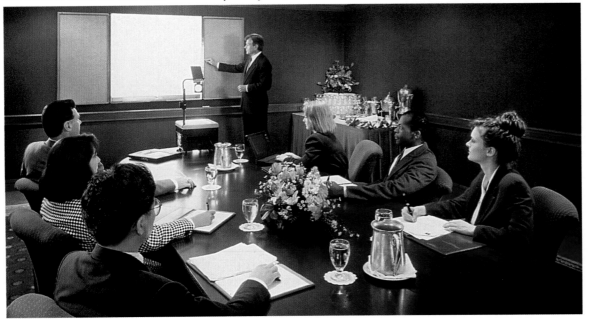

concierge is available from 7 a.m. to 11 p.m. to answer questions and make arrangements for local attractions, theaters, and restaurants.

The Omni Inner Harbor Hotel is home to two fine restaurants and a bar. The Baltimore Grille is its signature restaurant, featuring certified Black Angus beef, pasta, lamb, and seafood. Open for dinner only, the Baltimore Grille is a longtime winner of *The Wine Spectator*'s award of excellence for its outstanding wine list. Jackie's Cafe is casual dining at its best, with giant burgers, soups, salads, and a breakfast buffet. The Corner Sports Bar is a veritable library of liquors, featuring more than 200 premium labels and 55 beers. A light-fare menu is available nightly.

A gift shop is located in the main lobby, offering a variety of gifts, personal items, newspapers, magazines, and more. For added convenience to hotel guests, the Omni has installed an automated teller machine and a computerized printout system, which lists shopping and dining opportunities available in the Inner Harbor area.

An outdoor swimming pool is open daily from Memorial Day to Labor Day; an exercise facility offers Lifecycles, treadmills, and rowers; and jogging maps and neighborhood sports club memberships are available at the concierge desk.

The Omni prides itself on its ability to provide a one-stop business meeting service—from sleeping accommodations to audiovisual equipment, meeting room, food service, and every other necessary

detail. Directly across from the Baltimore Arena and Morris Mechanic Theater, as well as just a few blocks from Oriole Park at Camden Yards, the Omni Inner Harbor Hotel is ideal for business travelers as well as tourists.

A Hotel with a Future

In 1997, the Omni Inner Harbor Hotel received the coveted community service award from the Maryland Hotel and Motel Association. The award is partly in recognition of an innovative new program the hotel has instituted. FUTURE is an aggressive collaboration between the Omni, Goodwill Industries, and the Baltimore City Department of Social Services. The program seeks to provide employment opportunities to former welfare recipients in order to allow fair treatment and opportunity in the workplace. FUTURE identifies and actively

recruits prospective employees in the hotel/hospitality industry, who are then trained by a well-established organization and placed in jobs with career ladders.

Currently, a total of 14 of these individuals are full-time employees at the Omni, and include nine general room attendants, two maintenance workers, and three employees in the banquet housekeeping department. The program's achievements have received glowing endorsements from Mayor Kurt Schmoke. "We hope its success results in other hotels adopting similar programs to reduce unemployment in Maryland," notes Bheda.

While helping others to achieve success in their careers, the Omni Inner Harbor Hotel is assured of its own continuing success through its attention to detail, ambience, service, and the needs of its guests and visitors.

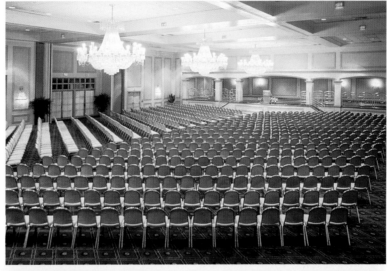

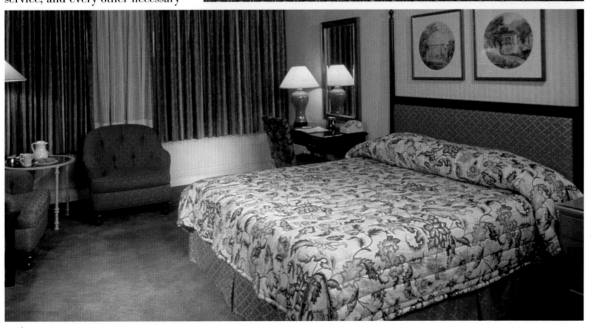

THE INTERNATIONAL BALLROOM EASILY ACCOMMODATES MEETINGS AND PARTIES.

JUST HAVING UNDERGONE A $5 MILLION RENOVATION, ALL OF THE HOTEL'S GUEST ROOMS HAVE BEEN UPGRADED. THE OMNI INNER HARBOR HOTEL HAS 187 KING ROOMS, 133 QUEENS, 365 TWO DOUBLE-BED ROOMS, 11 CLASSIC LIVING ROOMS (WHICH CONNECT ONE OR TWO BEDROOMS), AND 11 SUITES.

Town and Country Apartments

THE TOWN AND COUNTRY TRUST IS A LEADING OWNER-MANAGER OF multifamily residential communities throughout the Mid-Atlantic region. The Baltimore-based company values quality service, community stability, and long-term relationships throughout its communities in Maryland, Virginia, Pennsylvania, and Delaware. ∾ Town and Country was founded in 1979 when Alfred Lerner, a national real estate investor, and others purchased a group of residential communities from Monumental Properties, a local real estate development company. The purchase of this apartment division involved the acquisition of more than 10,000 units in 26 rental communities in Maryland and Pennsylvania. Aside from changing its name to Town and Country, Lerner relied on the existing management team to continue Monumental Properties' already successful operation.

Town and Country has grown from 10,000 units in two states to

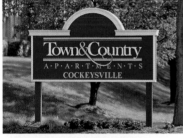

almost 14,000 in four states since becoming a Real Estate Investment Trust (REIT) in 1993.

Town and Country's success has much to do with the stability of its management team. Senior officers have been with Town and Country an average of 23 years. As a result, many of the 400+ staff, from its chief operating officer to its service staff, have been with the company since its inception. Longevity is remarkable at every level of the organization, thus creating a tight-knit, disciplined team dedicated to providing superior resident services, as well as efficient operations.

Service as the Ultimate Maxim

Michael H. Rosen, Town and Country's executive vice president and chief operating officer, sums up the company's service policy succinctly:

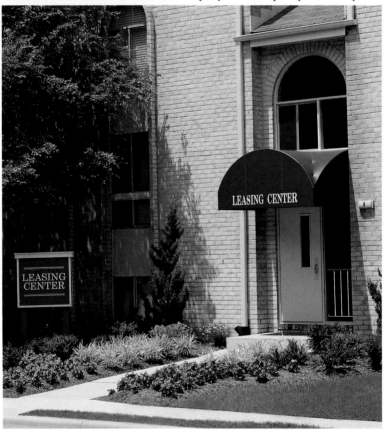

"Whatever it takes: WIT. It's our company philosophy—one that relies entirely on a team concept. Creating a family feeling is a big part of what has made us a success. It is a sense of pride and of commitment." All employees wear the WIT symbol. Every quarter, employees who have gone above and beyond the norm in service to the company are nominated for a special recognition.

One such employee's story has become a legend. During the blizzard of 1996, when the governor of Pennsylvania closed down all state roads, most citizens stayed in their homes and took a day off from work, but one devoted Town and Country employee, a member of the service team at the Colonial Park Harrisburg community, was mindful of his responsibility to clear roads and sidewalks in the community. He walked the seven miles to work that day. His story is one of many examples of employees who have provided extraordinary service, and, for residents at Town & Country communities, such dedication translates to high-quality living environments.

This strong commitment to serve the residents of its communities is precisely what distinguishes Town and Country properties from others. "This reputation for well-run communities with expert, caring managers is a crucial factor in our low resident turnover, high-quality residents, terrific occupancy rates, and steadily increasing rentals," Rosen says.

Service is the most important element for success in owning and managing apartment communities. "We also remain committed to maintenance and upgrade practices that encourage resident satisfaction," he says. Individual properties are superbly maintained and continually improved. In the past few years, more than $6 million has

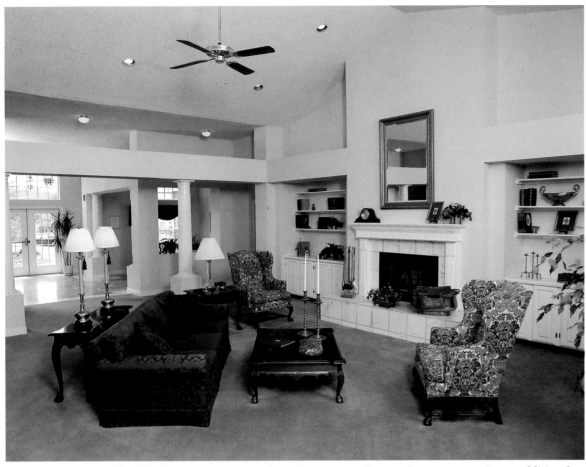

been spent on remodeling kitchens and bathrooms, as well as adding washers, dryers, dishwashers, monitored alarm systems, and other amenities to numerous communities—a process that directly results in rental increases. Enhancing common areas is important, too. Town & Country has added clubhouses, swimming pools, fitness centers, and day care centers to many properties. These improvements have added value to Town and Country properties, enhanced their competitiveness, generated impressive rental increases, and improved residents' lifestyles.

With more than 50 floor plans, the communities offer residents a variety of amenities, such as ceiling fans, fireplaces, dens, lofts, or sunrooms. All communities are centrally located and are close to shopping malls, schools, and public transportation.

Facing the Future

In the past 10 years, middle-income demand for apartment living has been rising. The emphasis for communities has been on safety and location—two factors that are consistently important. But, there is a growing market of apartment dwellers who have chosen this lifestyle over that of a home owner, not because of a lack of affordability, but because they appreciate the service, amenities, and convenience.

Town and Country's conversion in 1993 to a REIT has enabled the company to invest additional capital in its properties. "The Trust's key strengths continue to be our properties, our management team, and the markets in which we operate," Rosen says. He also adds, "The fundamentals to our long-term success are keeping our residents happy, occupancy high, turnover low, and rental income increasing."

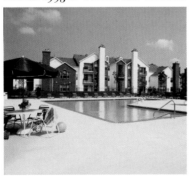

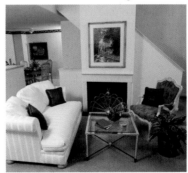

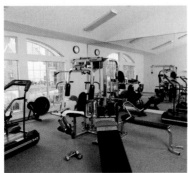

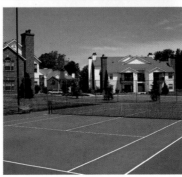

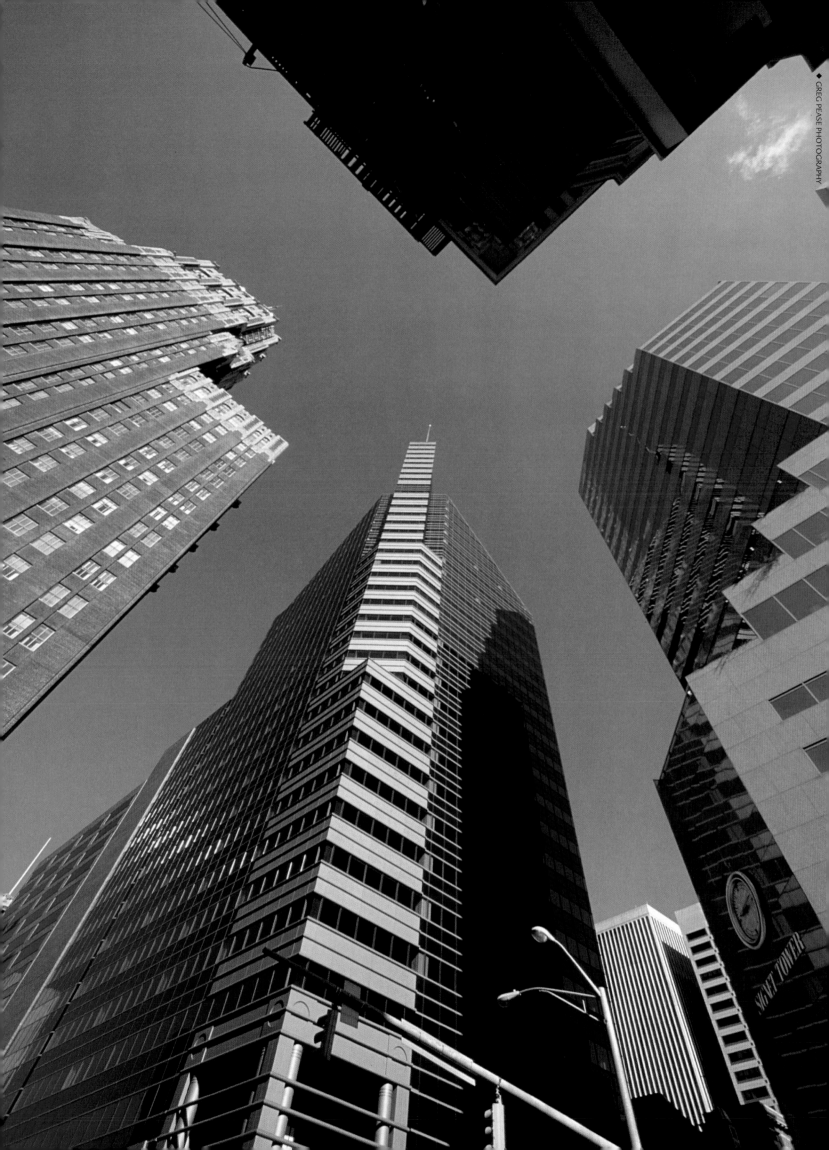

1980-1997

PROFILES IN EXCELLENCE

1981	NATIONAL AQUARIUM IN BALTIMORE
1982	SYSCOM, INC.
1983	BALTIMORE BUSINESS JOURNAL
1983	CELLULAR ONE
1983	GREAT BLACKS IN WAX MUSEUM, INC.
1984	FILA U.S.A., INC.
1984	MARYLAND OFFICE RELOCATORS
1984	ROLAND PARK PLACE
1985	BALTIMORE MARRIOTT INNER HARBOR
1985	KAISER PERMANENTE
1985	TRIGEN ENERGY BALTIMORE
1986	HARBOR COURT HOTEL
1986	INTEGRATED HEALTH SERVICES, INC.
1986	SNELLING STAFFING NETWORK
1987	HELIX HEALTH
1988	HS PROCESSING
1988	RE/MAX ADVANTAGE REALTY
1989	PRO STAFF
1990	INTERNATIONAL YOUTH FOUNDATION
1991	INPHOMATION COMMUNICATIONS, INC.
1992	CIENA CORPORATION
1992	NATIONSBANK
1993	GUILFORD PHARMACEUTICALS INC.
1993	SYSTEMS ALLIANCE INC.
1994	ANNIE E. CASEY FOUNDATION
1995	AVESTA SHEFFIELD EAST INC.
1995	TREASURE CHEST ADVERTISING
1996	BALTIMORE RAVENS
1996	SYLVAN LEARNING SYSTEMS, INC.

National Aquarium in Baltimore

A WORLD-CLASS AQUATIC MUSEUM DEDICATED TO EDUCATION AND CONSERVAtion, the National Aquarium in Baltimore uses sophisticated, themed exhibits; state-of-the-art technology; and exciting architecture to re-create underwater environments for the entertainment and education of its 1.5 million visitors each year. Located on a tributary of the Chesapeake Bay, the nation's largest estuary, the aquarium is a delight for children and adults of all ages. After all, where else can curious souls get nose-to-nose with the animal kingdom and live—and love—to tell about it?

Creating a Water World

As water is an integral part of the history and culture of Maryland, it is only natural that plans for the renewal of Baltimore's historic Inner Harbor area included the construction of the 115,000-square-foot aquarium. Ground was broken in 1978 for the aquarium on Pier 3 in the Inner Harbor. Designed by Cambridge Seven Associates of Massachusetts, the aquarium opened its doors on August 8, 1981, with considerable public attention in both local and national media. Within 10 months of opening, more than 1 million people had visited the aquarium, and it continues today as Maryland's top tourist draw.

In 1979, Congress granted the aquarium national status because it fell within the parameters of 1962 congressional legislation mandating that a world-class aquarium be built within 50 miles of the nation's capital. Despite its designation as the National Aquarium in Baltimore, it is not federally funded; the name reflects the aquarium's commitment to the highest standards of exhibitry and education.

Outstanding Exhibits

With a diverse collection of more than 10,000 animals representing more than 600 species of invertebrates, fish, birds, amphibians, reptiles, and marine mammals, the aquarium re-creates natural habitats from around the world. More than 2 million gallons of fresh and salt water are used in displays on seven levels of exhibition space in two buildings.

Free to the public, the 70,000-gallon outdoor rock *Seal Pool* provides a home for harbor and gray seals. Mammalogists train and feed seals daily.

Dozens of stingrays, a hawksbill sea turtle, and many small sharks can be seen from the surface or through underwater viewing windows of the 260,000-gallon *Wings in the Water*, which is one of the largest ray collections in the country. Divers feed rays underwater, and offer narrations above water daily.

Four exhibits titled *Maryland: Mountains to the Sea* depict local Maryland habitats. The water cycle is followed from an Allegheny pond, through a tidal marsh and coastal beach, and out to the continental shelf. Bullfrogs, diamondback terrapins, and sea robins show the diversity of Maryland's aquatic life.

The aquarium's multiexhibit *Surviving through Adaptations* gallery demonstrates how different adaptations allow a diverse group of animals to survive in the wild. A giant Pacific octopus devours a crab, green moray eels lurk in caves, seahorses slurp, jawfish burrow, and an electric eel audibly generates electricity.

In the *North Atlantic to Pacific* gallery, visitors explore Atlantic sea cliffs—home to playful puffins and the only black guillemots on display in the country, as well as an undersea kelp forest and a brilliant Pacific coral reef. In the *Children's Cove*, visitors of all ages can touch intertidal animals.

Tropical birds fly, poison dart frogs hop, piranhas swim, sloths hang, and tamarins scamper in the *South American Rain Forest* exhibit. The animals live among thousands of rain forest plants in this jungle habitat under a towering glass pyramid. The exhibit is introduced by a fiber-optic display that reminds visitors of the fragility of rain forests.

In the *Atlantic Coral Reef* exhibit, hundreds of colorful tropical fish swim and school on the most authentic reef ever fabricated.

THE NATIONAL AQUARIUM IN BALTIMORE IS LOCATED ON A TRIBUTARY OF THE CHESAPEAKE BAY.

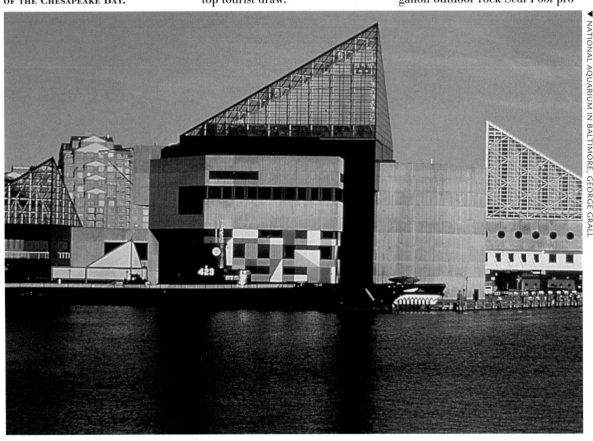

NATIONAL AQUARIUM IN BALTIMORE, GEORGE GRALL

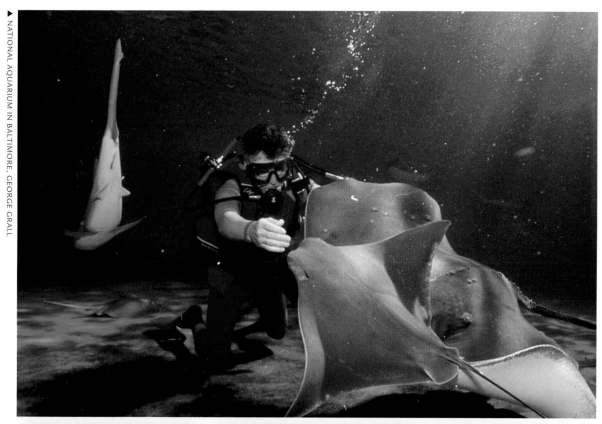
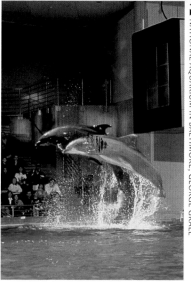

CLOCKWISE FROM TOP:
DIVERS FEED RAYS IN *Wings in the Water*, ONE OF THE LARGEST RAY COLLECTIONS IN THE COUNTRY.

VISITORS TO THE RING-SHAPED *Open Ocean* EXHIBIT GET UP CLOSE AND PERSONAL WITH SOME OF THE MOST FEARED CREATURES IN THE OCEAN.

BOTTLENOSE DOLPHINS DEMONSTRATE THEIR GRACE AND AGILITY IN DAILY SHOWS IN THE 1,300-SEAT AMPHITHE-ATER OF THE MARINE MAMMAL PAVILION.

As visitors descend, they are surrounded by a 335,000-gallon tank complete with grunts, triggerfish, surgeonfish, porcupine fish, hogfish, and dozens of other species. Divers feed the reef's fish several times each day.

Large sharks and small-toothed sawfish slowly encircle visitors inside the 225,000-gallon, ring-shaped *Open Ocean* exhibit. In perfect safety, visitors can get up close and personal with some of the most feared creatures in the ocean.

Bottlenose dolphins demonstrate their grace and agility in daily shows performed in the 1,300-seat amphitheater of the Marine Mammal Pavilion. In *Exploration Station*, a collection of high-tech displays, visitors can probe into the life and lore of marine mammals through interactive exhibits, videos, graphics, and innovative technology unrivaled elsewhere on the East Coast.

Window to the Majesty of the Ocean World

Today, the National Aquarium in Baltimore remains one of the most sophisticated and technologically advanced aquariums in existence. Its architecture, exhibits, programs, and management structure are considered definitive role models worldwide. Every week, the aquarium receives calls and visits from groups from around the world who come to see and learn from the accomplishments of its staff.

With the aquarium's mission, every effort is made to keep the exhibits dynamic, naturalistic, and educational. The aquarium's research activities continue to increase, particularly in captive breeding programs. Conservation education is emphasized in curricula, programs, exhibit graphics, and presentations, all with the goal of supporting the aquarium's mission of seeking to "stimulate interest in, develop knowledge about, and inspire stewardship of aquatic environments."

SYSCOM, INC.

BALTIMORE-BASED **SYSCOM, INC.** IS A DIVERSIFIED INFORMATION technology company, supplying progressive solutions to international corporations. SYSCOM's mission has been to excel in specific niche software services and product markets. It has evolved into a growing company of divisions directed to develop these market niches. A focused, profit-oriented, yet fluid organization allows SYSCOM to have greater overall breadth and strength while retaining management efficiencies. The customer-oriented, quality-driven philosophy of its employees, in conjunction with the efficacy of its business model, have made SYSCOM the growing company it is today.

History of SYSCOM

SYSCOM was founded in 1982 by Ted Bayer, a native of Baltimore, who recognized the business potential associated with providing key information technology (IT) expertise in support of large-scale, complex IT projects. Early on, the company distinguished itself with its support of customers within the local defense and steel industries. Early projects included the design of large-scale databases and the custom development of unique system utilities for supporting large, around-the-clock database systems. SYSCOM designed the first successful automated hierarchical to relational data propagation bridge for IBM's database management systems. Later efforts expanded into design review, technical project monitoring, and custom application development.

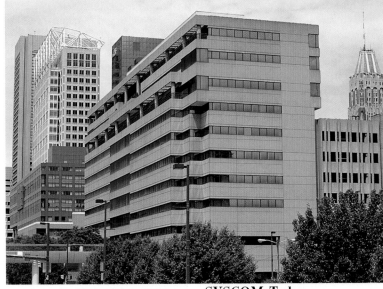

The recession of the early 1990s had a significant impact in the Baltimore area, particularly to the contractual services industry. The company's emergence from this period came with a resolve to expand its customer base nationally, improve diversification, and develop product offerings. Since 1991, SYSCOM has grown in leaps and bounds through internal growth and acquisition. Revenues have increased at an annual average compounded rate of more than 80 percent, to $14 million in 1997.

SYSCOM Today

SYSCOM currently provides specialized, comprehensive information technology services and products for large organizations, both public and private, from Tokyo to London. Current major areas of business include state systems support services, systems integration of work-flow and document management systems, complete project life-cycle software support services, and training and qualification management software.

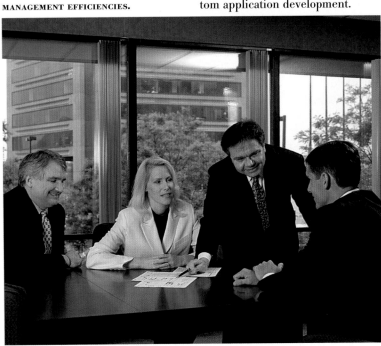

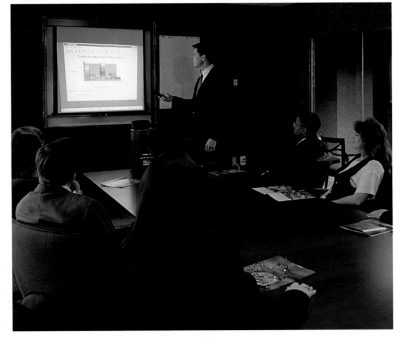

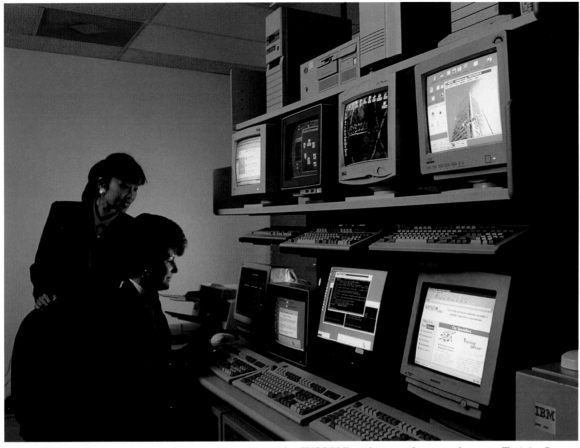

SYSCOM continues to provide the primary technical application support to the State of Maryland's Department of Human Resources in its implementation of one of the most complex, comprehensive, and the only fully integrated welfare, child support, and social services systems in the nation.

In addition, the company has achieved outstanding success in integrating work-flow and document management solutions within large public sector and Fortune 100 com-panies nationwide. SYSCOM's soft-ware products and tools for work-flow integration, such as AIS+ and FluxWorks, along with state-of-the-art expertise, place the com-pany at the industry's leading edge in large-scale work-flow systems integration.

Since its inception in 1992, SYSCOM's TrainingServer™ has consistently been the most advanced training administration software offering available. Citibank, MCI, the U.S. Strategic Air Command, and many others use TrainingServer in support of enterprisewide train-ing. Through its companion prod-ucts, TrainingServer continues to be the industry leader in the use of telephony with Training-Teleserver and Internet technologies with TrainingServer@Online, as well as providing the latest in business functionality for administering corporate training.

SYSCOM's Future

Even faster growth is on the horizon for SYSCOM. Expan-sion beyond Baltimore to sup-port its nationwide customer base is expected. Regardless of its growth, SYSCOM, INC. will remain headquar-tered at its scenic downtown Inner Harbor location in Charm City.

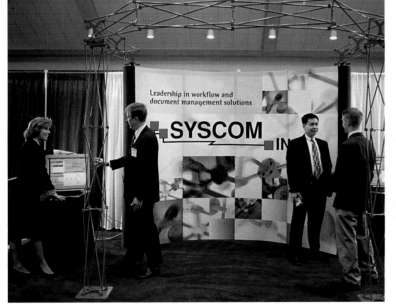

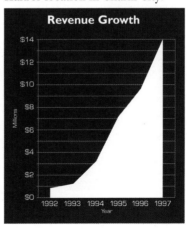

Revenue Growth

Baltimore Business Journal

SINCE 1983, THE *Baltimore Business Journal* HAS PROVIDED A WEEKLY marketplace of opportunities for businesspeople who want to stay competitive and grow their business. As the leading business publication in Baltimore, it provides comprehensive coverage of such industries as health care, banking, manufacturing, hospitality, real estate, marketing, high technology, and investing.

In addition to covering breaking business news stories, the *Baltimore Business Journal* (BBJ) provides a comprehensive *Record* section, with detailed lists of business transactions in the city and five-county metropolitan area, such as bankruptcy filings and liens; building permits, contracts, and bids; and personnel changes, awards, and announcements.

The BBJ's weekly Top 25 list, which ranks Baltimore's largest companies in dozens of industries, is among the publication's most popular features. The *Growth Strategies* section, geared to small-business owners, profiles entrepreneurs who have faced major challenges.

Each issue also features the *Special Report*, an in-depth look at one industry, such as commercial real estate, hospitality, or technology.

Targeting Its Readers

According to a recent survey, 76,000 of Baltimore's most influential executives read the *Baltimore Business Journal* every week. Local business journals are the proven source of local business information, with 55 percent of readers preferring the weeklies over daily newspapers for industry coverage.

The *Baltimore Business Journal* is a wholly owned subsidiary of American City Business Journals (ACBJ), based in Charlotte, North Carolina. ACBJ owns 35 weekly business publications and is the nation's leading publisher in the field.

Cutting-Edge Business Publishing

As part of its commitment to providing useful business information, the *Baltimore Business Journal* publishes a number of special publications. Among these are *The Book of Lists*, a compilation of the journal's weekly feature, and the *Health Care Resources Guide*, which is a compendium of health care facilities and companies ranging from nursing to HMOs. Others include *How-to Book, The Book of Money, Small Business Handbook, Book of Market Facts,* and *Maryland Meetings & Conventions*. Special features include *Women in Business,* and *40 Under 40*—a look at the area's next generation of leaders. The BBJ is also targeting the Internet via a Web site (http://www.amcity.com/baltimore), which provides readers with a comprehensive source of business news.

"Our role goes beyond reporting news and disseminating information," says James Breiner, publisher. "By publishing information useful to the business community, we're also stimulating economic growth."

CLOCKWISE FROM TOP LEFT: SEVERAL *Business Journal* STAFF MEMBERS HAVE BEEN RECOGNIZED FOR OUTSTANDING PERFORMANCE. THEY ARE PROUD TO PROVIDE A WEEKLY MARKETPLACE OF OPPORTUNITIES FOR BUSINESSPEOPLE WHO WANT TO STAY COMPETITIVE AND GROW THEIR BUSINESS.

THE *Business Journal* IS ESSENTIAL READING FOR BUSINESSPEOPLE.

AS PART OF ITS COMMITMENT TO PROVIDING USEFUL BUSINESS INFORMATION, THE *Baltimore Business Journal* PUBLISHES A NUMBER OF SPECIAL PUBLICATIONS.

PRODUCTION DIRECTOR JUDI ZAMZOW AND EDITOR MARGIE FREANEY WORK ON PAGE DESIGN.

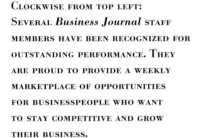

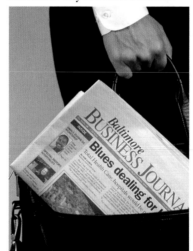

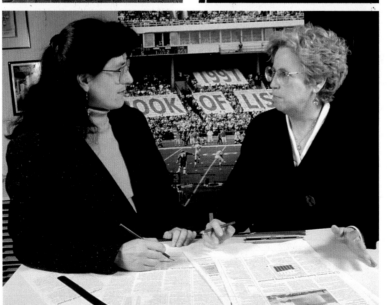

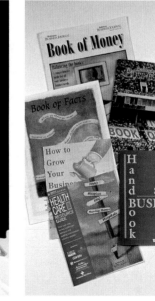

The Great Blacks In Wax Museum, Inc.

A TRIP TO FRANCE, WHERE DRS. ELMER AND JOANNE MARTIN REDISCOVered the importance of celebrating the history of a culture, was the genesis of The Great Blacks In Wax Museum, Inc. Today, The Great Blacks In Wax Museum is among America's most dynamic cultural and educational institutions. Its life-size, lifelike wax figures highlight

historic and contemporary personalities of African ancestry—starting with a replica of a 19th-century slave ship, which memorably captures the horror of captivity for passengers as they began life as American slaves.

But the museum also celebrates many accomplishments through the centuries. Wax figures are clad in appropriate historic attire and are part of displays that depict the struggles, achievements, and contributions of African peoples worldwide. Highlights focus on ancient Africa, the middle passage, the antebellum and postbellum periods, Reconstruction, the Harlem renaissance, the civil rights era, and the present.

Figures include such heroes and heroines as the writer Richard Wright, the athlete Jesse Owens, and African freedom fighters Stephen Biko, Winnie Mandela, and Nelson Mandela. Also represented are Islamic leaders, military leaders, and human rights activists. Other exhibits feature outstanding Marylanders, including Eubie Blake, as well as superlative educators, labor movement leaders, and modern civil rights era heroes.

"The personalities are those whose lives exemplify the African-American traditions of helping, up-lifting, and protesting," Dr. Elmer Martin says. "They are those of humble beginnings who have risen against tremendous odds, and those who have pioneered in particular fields of endeavor. Above all, they are those whose talents and genius reflect the gifts and skills of the African-American masses."

Building a Museum

The Martins initially opened the museum in a storefront in 1983. The tremendous response exceeded their wildest expectations. Fourteen years later, The Great Blacks In Wax Museum is housed in an expanded gallery on East North Avenue in Baltimore and attracts an average of 150,000 guests annually.

Why the appeal? "Our visit to France reminded us that in building monuments to your history, you can instill pride in people," says Dr. Joanne Martin, a former English professor at Coppin State College. "To know that your ancestry has a place in history offers a feeling of great comfort and confidence. And we both believed that, as a people, African-Americans had failed to build institutions to their history."

No longer. The Great Blacks In Wax Museum has been success-ful in achieving several objectives, not the least of which is the stimulation of interest in African-American history for all people, regardless of race. Using great leaders as role models to motivate youth to achieve, the museum is working to improve race relations by dispelling myths of racial inferiority and superiority.

Success is also measured by expansion. Currently, the museum is embarking on its second fundraising campaign (the first enabled it to move from its original space to a restored Victorian firehouse). The new funds will allow it to acquire an entire city block and add restaurants, banquet facilities, expanded galleries, and interactive exhibits.

The Martins have achieved their dream of celebrating the history of African-American culture—past, present, and future. And Baltimore is blessed with the fruits of their labor.

THE GREAT BLACKS IN WAX MUSEUM ACKNOWLEDGES THOSE WHO CONTRIBUTED TO SCIENTIFIC DEVELOPMENT, INCLUDING DR. CHARLES DREW, PIONEER IN BLOOD PRESERVATION; DR. GEORGE WASHINGTON CARVER, AGRICULTURAL CHEMIST AND DEVELOPER OF MORE THAN 300 PRODUCTS FROM THE PEANUT; AND DR. LEWIS LATIMER, PIONEER IN THE DEVELOPMENT OF THE ELECTRIC LIGHTBULB (LEFT).

THE MUSEUM'S LIFE-SIZE, LIFELIKE WAX FIGURES HIGHLIGHT HISTORIC AND CONTEMPORARY PERSONALITIES OF AFRICAN ANCESTRY, SUCH AS IDA B. WELLS, ANTILYNCHING CRUSADER, AND ROSA PARKS, CIVIL RIGHTS CHAMPION (RIGHT).

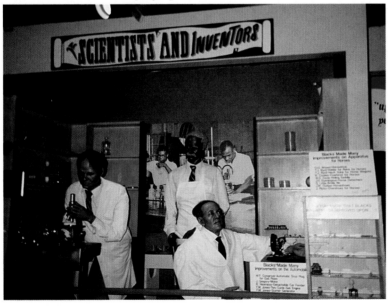

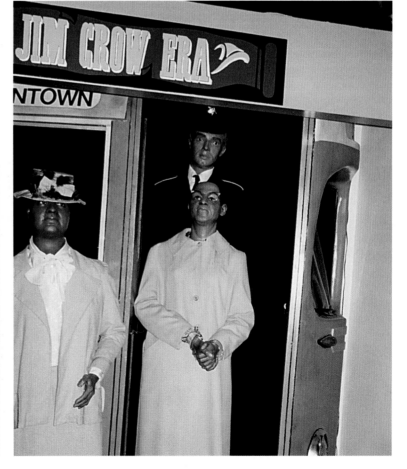

Cellular One

ON DECEMBER 16, 1983, A CELLULAR OPERATION IN THE BALTIMORE/ Washington, D.C., region known as Cellular One became the nation's first commercial wireless cellular phone company. Recognized as one of the most successful pioneers in the industry, Cellular One has since increased its employees from eight to more than 600 (with 50 percent of

that growth occurring since 1992) and has created a distribution network totaling more than 500 locations. These include company-owned stores, independent dealers, and well-known retailers such as Best Buy, The Edge, Ritz Camera, RadioShack, Wal-Mart, and Kmart.

The Company Evolves

Cellular One played a major role in the birth of the mobile communications industry. In 1987, Southwestern Bell Corporation (now known as SBC Communications, Inc.) acquired the Baltimore/Washington property from Metromedia. In addition, SBC acquired Cellular One's sister properties in Boston, New York, and Chicago, and the rights to the Cellular One service mark.

Cellular One, together with its Southwestern Bell affiliates, is the nation's second-largest wireless company, with an industry-leading 10.1 percent market penetration rate.

Cellular One is the brand under which SBC, one of the world's leading diversified telecommunications companies, markets its service outside its traditional service area. SBC's businesses include Southwestern Bell Telephone, Pacific Bell, and Nevada Bell; wireless services and equipment in the United States; wireless interests in Europe, Latin America, South Africa, and Asia; business and consumer telecommunications equipment; messaging; cable TV in domestic and international markets; and directory advertising and publishing.

The Cellular One Network

Cellular One Baltimore/Washington manages its extensive network from its operations center in Hanover, Maryland. Designed as the nerve center for the entire region, this 40,000-square-foot facility includes more than 90 employees working in the areas of

engineering, maintenance, switching, construction, and real estate. The Network Operations group builds cell sites on an ongoing basis to meet customers' needs by expanding the network and increasing the capacity of existing channels. In addition, this group analyzes new technologies for implementation in the market, such as installing a series of state-of-the-art minicells within downtown Washington.

Special Features

Cellular One has long been committed to enhancing its technology. Among its noteworthy accomplishments was the 1994 introduction of digital technology, which provides numerous customer benefits, including improved quality, greater privacy, increased call handling capability, and reduced exposure to fraud.

The company also launched FreedomLink, an in-building wireless system that serves as an extension

CELLULAR ONE CURRENTLY OFFERS ITS PRODUCTS AND SERVICES THROUGH A DISTRIBUTION NETWORK TOTALING MORE THAN 500 LOCATIONS, INCLUDING COMPANY-OWNED STORES.

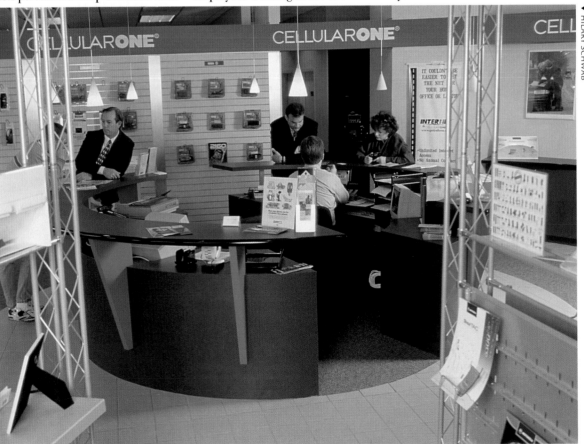

HILARY SCHWAB

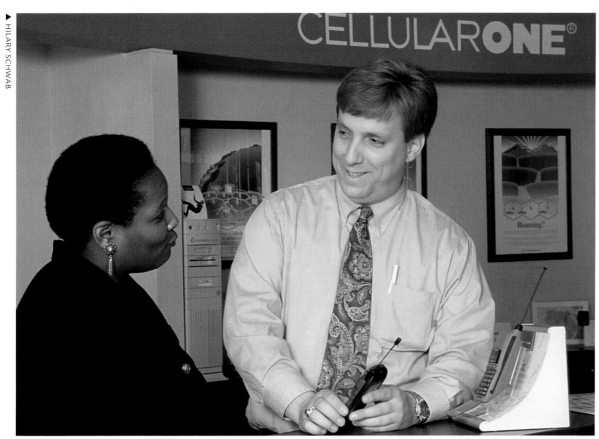

of an individual's office telephone console. FreedomLink, already used by employees at the headquarters of a major premier hotel chain based in the area, enables staff to travel freely throughout the office complex while placing and receiving calls.

In May 1995, as part of its commitment to education, Cellular One introduced a version of Freedom-Link for an elementary school in Washington. Called ClassLink, the system, which operates as an extension of the school's wireline telephone, enables teachers and other school employees to travel freely throughout their campus while placing and receiving calls. As a result of its success, the program has been expanded to schools in Maryland.

While Cellular One is aggressively improving wireless technology, it is also focusing on other products and services to be able to meet customers' communication needs. Within the past two years, Cellular One has added products like paging and long-distance services for home, office, and cellular phones. The company has broadened its cellular service options to include low-cost rate plans, like SafetyLink, that are geared toward the safety and security user, as well as enhancing its Value Plans for moderate,

occasional, and heavy users. In addition, Cellular One has added optional features like voice mail service, nationwide roadside assistance, and wireless data services that allow customers to be on the go and stay in touch.

Since Cellular One was founded 14 years ago, cellular phone service has grown enormously. More than

34 million Americans subscribe to the service, with approximately 31,000 more being added each day. This continual growth represents the changing attitudes of consumers throughout the world. Wireless communication, whether for business or personal use, enables people to stay in contact with those who are most important.

ESTABLISHED IN 1983, CELLULAR ONE EMPLOYS MORE THAN 600 PEOPLE WHO ARE COMMITTED TO MEETING THE NATION'S GROWING DEMAND FOR WIRELESS COMMUNICATIONS.

Fila U.S.A., Inc.

IT'S BEEN SAID THAT "WITHOUT VISION, THE PEOPLE PERISH." AT FILA U.S.A., Inc., the world's fourth-largest athletic footwear and apparel company, that philosophy rings true throughout the organization. With its U.S. headquarters and distribution center in Maryland, and offices in New York, Oregon, Massachusetts, and California, Fila's motto is Life Is Our Inspiration.

The company's designs merge fashion and function, attitude and technology—all the while reflecting people, places, and perspectives that are infused with energy, vitality, and creativity.

"We are in one of the most intensely challenging and competitive industries in business today," says Dr. Enrico Frachey, Fila president and CEO. "We have the products, the technologies, the promotions, the motivation, and the momentum to achieve continued success in the new millennium."

International Beginnings

In 1923, in the town of Biella at the base of the Italian Alps, the Fila brothers founded their company as a knitter of fine textiles and a maker of underwear. Over the years, the company's global appeal strengthened as Fila's creators moved toward the athletic apparel marketplace. There, they outfitted some of the world's best athletes competing in a wide range of sports, including basketball, tennis, soccer, running, golf, and beach volleyball.

In 1973, the Fila brand of athletic sportswear was launched, and became an international leader through superior design and quality manufacturing. In 1984, the company made its foray into the U.S. market under a Baltimore-based licensing agreement that lasted until the early 1990s. By 1991, Fila had decided to make a strategic move to gain direct control of the U.S. footwear line. The company bought back its license; consolidated apparel distributor Fila Sports Inc. and its production arm, Fila Footwear U.S.A., into Fila U.S.A., Inc.; and centralized its management facilities in the Baltimore area. Baltimore's proximity to the megacities of Washington and New York, its world-class sports organizations, a supportive state government, and an active port made the city a perfect choice for Fila.

Since 1991, footwear sales have exploded, and the company has propelled itself into the forefront as one of the few sportswear companies to successfully diversify into athletic footwear. Under Frachey's leadership, Fila has established itself as a major resource in the athletic apparel industry.

And while Fila may indeed be emphasizing new footwear lines, the company remains committed to its traditional strength in sports activewear. A renewed emphasis on windwear, outerwear, fleece, and warm-ups will result in fashion-forward fabrics, details, logo treatments, and silhouettes. For after-workout dress, Fila offers the Fila Sport line of casual dress for men, inspired by those who lead an active lifestyle.

FILA SUPPORTS ITALIAN SKI TEAM MEMBER ALBERTO TOMBA.

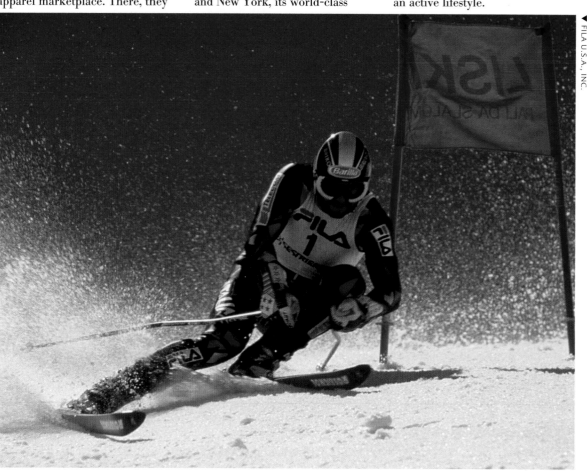

▼ FILA U.S.A., INC.

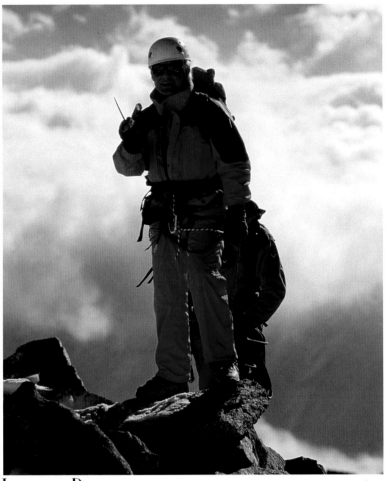

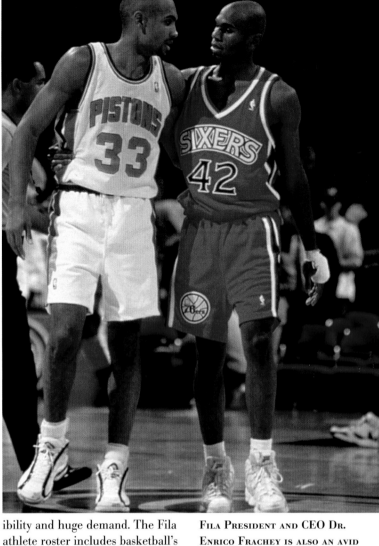

Innovative Designs and Products

In the past few years, Fila has achieved the top growth rate among market leaders. Much of this is due to the company's commitment to innovation, technological investment, and fresh designs. "Our creativity extends to every aspect of our business, from new product development to performance enhancement," says Frachey.

Fila footwear is legendary in the industry for its aggressive design and gotta-have-it style. Fila is also an innovative manufacturer, committed to developing new, better products. The patented 2A technology, the first controlled cushioning system, combines air and a high-tech compound in a unique pod that provides optimal levels of shock absorption, responsiveness, flexibility, and stability. Another technology in which Fila excels is the use of Carbon/Kevlar® fibers. Using a unique weaving process, these fibers form a matrix that greatly enhances shock absorption, stability, energy return, and flexibility.

The company is making great strides in other areas, as well. In 1997, Fila launched its debut collection of performance soccer footwear and apparel. Its new line of golf shoes offers classic styling and such technological components as breathable Pebatex™ inner membranes and 6-millimeter Cer-Mec™ extra-durability spikes.

The company's foray into the in-line skating category occurred in 1997. Tagged The Shoe That Rolls™, Fila in-line skates incorporate state-of-the-art performance technology, backed by extensive research and field testing. The team of experts who developed the Fila product line succeeded in redefining all aspects of in-line skates, from boot to wheel systems. The Shoe That Rolls will be on retailers' shelves in early 1998.

High-Performance Campaigns

Fila footwear and apparel are designed with the high-performance athlete in mind, and a number of the world's top athletes extol the virtues of Fila products. Endorsement agreements with athletes and others have ensured credibility in the athletic arena, while generating high visibility and huge demand. The Fila athlete roster includes basketball's Grant Hill, Chris Webber, Jerry Stackhouse, and Nikki McCray (Most Valuable Player in the ABL); tennis' Mark Philippoussis; baseball's Derek Jeter and Eddie Murray; football's Jim Harbaugh; golf's Lee Janzen; skiing's Alberto Tomba; long jump world record holder Mike Powell; two-time New York City Marathon champion German Silva and Boston Marathon champion Moses Tanui; speed skating's Olympic gold medalist Bonnie Blair; beach volleyball's Olympic gold medalist Kent Steffes; and soccer's Claudio Reyna, Juergen Sommer, and Carla Overbeck. In addition, Fila sponsors many world-class athletic events, including the Fila Summer Pro Basketball League and the Fila SkyMarathon Series.

As the company enters the 21st century, the free-spirited innovators at Fila plan to reach out to achieve a bold goal: to change the game in more markets, with more impact, than ever before.

FILA PRESIDENT AND CEO DR. ENRICO FRACHEY IS ALSO AN AVID MOUNTAIN CLIMBER (LEFT).

FILA SPONSORS ATHLETES SUCH AS DETROIT PISTONS STAR GRANT HILL AND PHILADELPHIA 76ERS PLAYER JERRY STACKHOUSE (RIGHT).

Maryland Office Relocators

ON A BALMY SPRING MORNING—THE PERFECT DAY FOR A MOVE—14 trucks emblazoned with the distinctive Maryland Office Relocators (MOR) logo are fanned out around the Baltimore and Washington, D.C., region. On the move today are companies, organizations, and institutions such as Catholic University, Smith Somerville & Case,

RTKL, and Northrop Grumman. MOR employees are also in planning stages on massive moves for the IRS, HCFA, and FBI. It's just an ordinary day at Maryland Office Relocators.

The company, one of the region's leading specialists in corporate relocation, was founded in 1984. Seven years later, Maryland Office Relocators was acquired by Henry Homes III and Michael S. Hoffberger, two Baltimore entrepreneurs who saw the potential for enhancing services and for growth and expansion. Since then, sales have doubled, and the company's list of clients ranges from NationsBank to Alex. Brown, from the National Institutes of Health to Baltimore Gas and Electric, and from CSX to Sylvan Learning Centers.

"What distinguishes Maryland Office Relocators is our commitment to servicing our customers in the most efficient and cost-effective way possible," says Homes, the company's president. "The type of moving we do is time critical. If a business is in the process of being moved, it is not generating revenue. The secret is to get the business relocated in off-hours—and as quickly as possible."

Growing the Company

Primarily known for its corporate office relocation capabilities, Maryland Office Relocators employs 50 full-time and 300 hourly workers, who are responsible for moving a diverse group of business clients, from a 1,000-square-foot doctor's office to a relocation of the Internal Revenue Service's 4,000 employees—a project so vast that it is spread out over a six-month period. The company also handles moves for delicate cargo, such as the Phase One computer from the Hubble Space Telescope program and medical lab work for hospitals.

To achieve success in an industry of such heavy responsibility, Maryland Office Relocators takes a unique approach with its staff, offering special training to maintain a skilled workforce. Quality control managers consistently review jobs in progress to ensure a high standard of performance. Periodic training sessions are mandatory for

BALTIMORE-BASED MARYLAND OFFICE RELOCATORS IS KNOWN PRIMARILY FOR ITS CORPORATE OFFICE RELOCATION CAPABILITIES, SERVICING A DIVERSE GROUP OF BUSINESS CLIENTS.

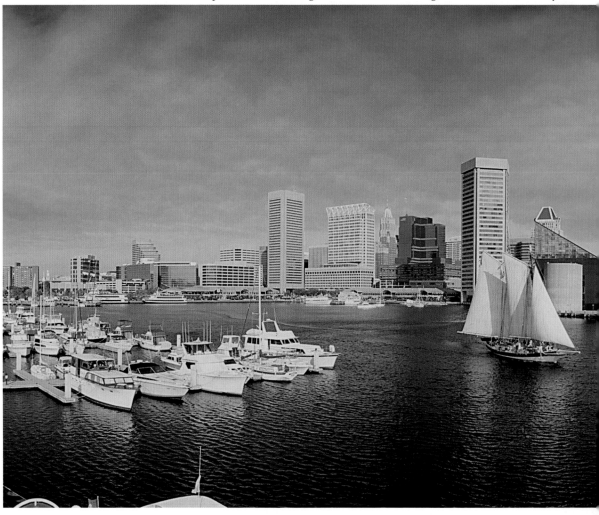

all employees. And part-time crews, consisting primarily of off-duty military personnel from Fort Meade (most of whom work for the National Security Agency), are of an especially high caliber.

Maryland Office Relocators also has carved a niche for itself in the factory/light industry/warehouse moving field. In addition, it offers extensive services in the areas of warehousing, storage, and inventory control. With more than 30,000 square feet of palletized storage facilities, the company provides long- and short-term storage, new furniture consolidation, and computerized inventory management and control. This enables management to easily access up-to-date information on receiving, back orders, and availability of goods. Capacities also include consolidation of new furnishings for subsequent delivery and installation.

Bearing in mind that an office move is no less traumatic for workers than a home move is for families, MOR's service program extends its capabilities beyond loading, unloading, setup, and teardown. Prior to each customer's move, the client is issued a number of helpful suggestions for ensuring a smooth transition. In particular, Maryland Office Relocators emphasizes its Purge Campaign—Chuck It, Don't Truck It—which offers tips on in-house file cleaning. The company also offers packing, storage, record retention, modular furniture installation and reconfiguration, and used furniture disposal.

Cycle of Customers

At Maryland Office Relocators, customers are drawn equally from Washington, D.C., and Baltimore. In particular, with the two cities growing together and forming the Baltimore-Washington business and industrial corridor, the region is rife with newly created corporate headquarters and warehouses.

The relocation of companies to the Baltimore-Washington area in general has ensured MOR of continuous growth over the past half decade. But the company's healthy customer base is also attributed to what Homes classifies as the "three to five cycle." Businesses in the Mid-Atlantic region typically sign leases of three to five years. If business is dynamic, they will expand. If it's slow, they'll contract. All require moves to some degree.

Homes and Hoffberger, whose own no-nonsense approaches mean they answer their own phones, pride themselves on a simple approach to corporate relocation. "We're straight with our customers," Homes says bluntly. "Our employees do good work and are responsible and accountable. You are not going to lose your eyesight reading our contracts. What we offer is good service."

And yet, the extra services, well-trained staff, and efficient processes have all contributed much to the company's growth over the past six years. Most of all, its success can be traced back to relationships. "Our best salesman is a satisfied customer," Homes says.

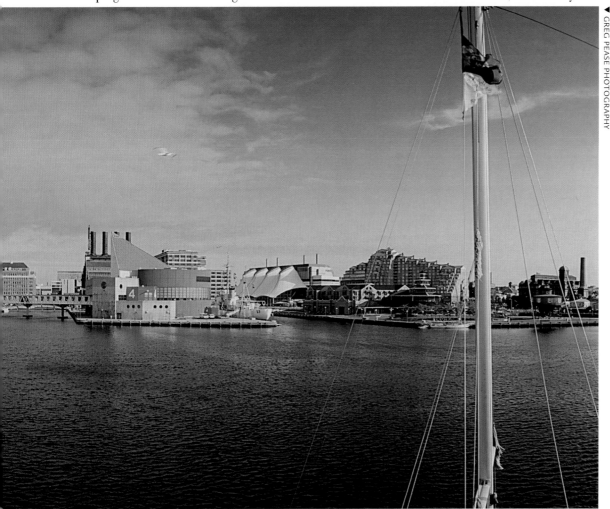

▲ GREG PEASE PHOTOGRAPHY

Roland Park Place

T HOSE FAMILIAR WITH THIS UNIQUE CONTINUING CARE RETIREMENT community affectionately refer to it as "Baltimore's secret garden" and "the place to enjoy everything from bingo to Bach." Indeed, there's absolutely nothing retiring about Roland Park Place, where residents 60 years of age and older can continue to take advantage

of in-town living, while enjoying the security and peace of mind that comes with a full array of services, along with health care for life.

A not-for-profit continuing care retirement community, Roland Park Place provides a homelike environment for senior adults who are active and independent, or who need minimal assistance with daily chores. Now owned and operated by Roland Park Place, Inc., it was formed in 1980 by a not-for-profit coalition of the First English Evangelical Lutheran Church, the Lutheran Hospital

of Maryland, and the Lutheran Home and Hospital Association. The community formally opened in 1984, and is fully accredited by the Continuing Care Accreditation Commission for meeting the industry's highest standards of quality.

"From its inception, Roland Park Place was designed to provide seniors the opportunity to live independently," says Greg Lannon, executive director. "This community appeals to retired individuals who are attracted by our commitment to ensuring their quality of life, by our comprehensive activities

program, our lovely facility, and unequaled location."

A Neighborhood Landmark

Located on eight lush acres adjoining the Baltimore neighborhoods of Roland Park and Hampden, the community consists of 235 one- and two-bedroom apartment-style homes—some of which have been designated for assisted living—in a serene country-in-the-city setting. The main building is a luxurious eight-story mid-rise that rests elegantly next door to the property's historic Greenway Cottages. The three Greenway structures, built in the 1860s, are considered the finest local examples of High Victorian Gothic cottage architecture, and were intended by Edward Greenway to serve as summer residences for his family. Today, they provide additional apartments for Roland Park Place residents and a place for overnight guests to stay while visiting the community.

The community's reverence for art and culture extends beyond its own boundaries. Its prestigious North Baltimore location—in close proximity to universities such as Johns Hopkins and to outstanding theaters and world-renowned museums—enables residents, both individually and in groups, to continue exploring the interests of a lifetime.

Emphasizing an Independent Lifestyle

Roland Park Place offers an innovative, independent lifestyle for older adults. In this continuing care retirement community, individuals can live as privately or remain as social as they desire. Residents enter into a long-term contract that provides housing, a full spectrum of services, and nursing care—all in one location. As a result, the lifestyle emphasizes critical elements of retirement living: physical and financial security, in-

ROLAND PARK PLACE OFFERS IN-TOWN LIVING IN A SERENE COUNTRY-IN-THE-CITY SETTING FOR THOSE WISHING TO EXPERIENCE A REWARDING AND FULFILLING RETIREMENT LIFESTYLE.

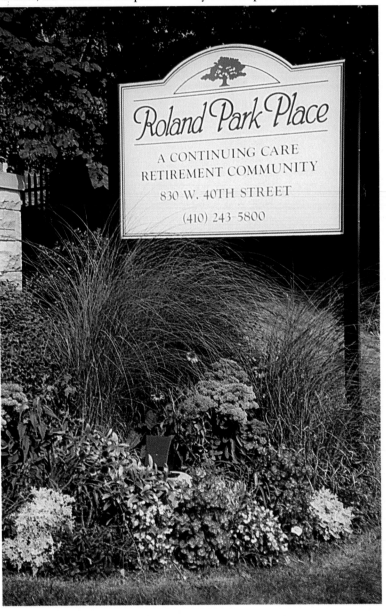

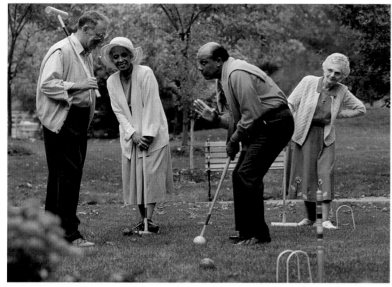

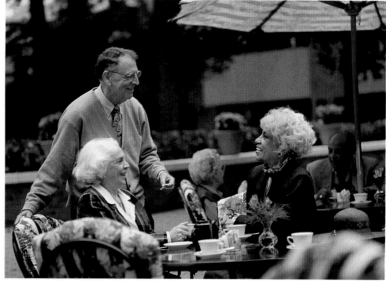

dependence and access to health care, companionship of friends and neighbors, and the right amount of privacy.

Overall, services at Roland Park Place include housekeeping, laundry, 24-hour maintenance and security, valets, and transportation to off-site medical appointments or to group events. Residents are offered a choice of meal plans, and as an added option, meals may be catered in their apartments. Other amenities include an arts and crafts studio, exercise and fitness area, room for social gatherings, 6,000-volume library, beauty salon, convenience store, and full-service bank. If they choose to do so, residents may participate in the educational, religious, and cultural programs and activities offered on the premises, or the varied and exciting planned group outings off-site. Future expansion plans include a wellness center with indoor swimming pool, a greenhouse, additional classroom space

for continuing education courses, and in the Health Care Center, private suites for assisted living.

Access to high-quality medical care is available through the on-site Health Care Center at Roland Park Place. This state-of-the-art facility includes 71 beds licensed for both skilled and comprehensive nursing care. An Ambulatory Care Center also is available. The Health Care Center is staffed with licensed nurses, RNs, LPNs, and certified nursing assistants (CNAs) around the clock. Other associates include a full-time social worker, a certified registered nurse practitioner, a registered dietician, and an activities coordinator. The center's three multipurpose rooms, beautifully appointed dining room, and outdoor patios—along with its professional, dedicated team—are all part of the lifetime health services available to every resident.

To further facilitate the ability of residents to live independently

for as long as possible, Roland Park Place has created the unique Program for Assitance in Living, known as PAL. Through PAL, residents can receive personalized assistance with daily tasks, such as bathing and dressing.

A Community with Value

Since Roland Park Place first opened, the community has remained committed to satisfying the lifestyle needs of its residents. This dedication has never wavered, thanks to a staff that focuses on making a difference in residents' lives. It's a philosophy that is often referred to as the Value of Life at Roland Park Place. It's clear this philosophy leads to a retirement lifestyle with tremendous value. In turn, it's clearly another reason why, in addition to services, activities, and location, Roland Park Place is considered the ideal continuing care retirement community by residents and their families alike.

CLOCKWISE FROM TOP LEFT: THERE'S ABSOLUTELY NOTHING RETIRING ABOUT THE RESIDENTS OF ROLAND PARK PLACE.

DINING WITH FRIENDS IS AN ENJOYABLE EVENT, WHETHER IN ROLAND PARK'S INTERIOR DINING ROOM OR OUTDOORS ON ITS COOL, COURTYARD PATIO.

THE MAIN BUILDING IS A LUXURIOUS EIGHT-STORY MID-RISE THAT RESTS ELEGANTLY NEXT DOOR TO ROLAND PARK PLACE'S HISTORIC GREENWAY COTTAGES.

THE PICTURESQUE COURTYARD PROVIDES A LOVELY SETTING FOR A QUIET STROLL, BIRD WATCHING, LISTENING TO A JAZZ CONCERT, OR JUST ENJOYING A PICNIC WITH FAMILY MEMBERS.

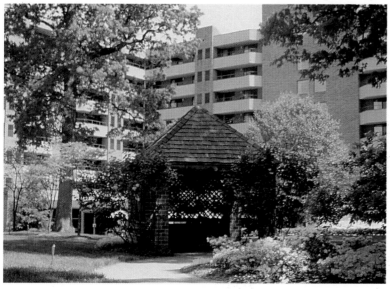

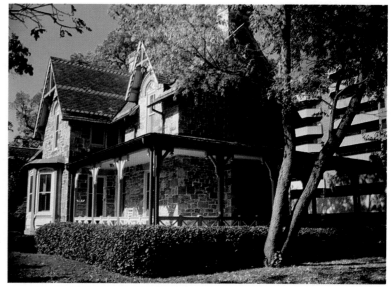

Baltimore Marriott Inner Harbor

THE BALTIMORE MARRIOTT INNER HARBOR, A BASEBALL'S THROW FROM Oriole Park at Camden Yards, offers the best of both worlds to Baltimore visitors. Its leisure guests appreciate the Marriott's location, which is within a short stroll of the Ravens' new stadium and the Inner Harbor, featuring attractions such as Harborplace, the National Aquarium,

and the Maryland Science Center. For corporate travelers, Baltimore's downtown business district is within easy walking distance, the Baltimore Convention Center is directly across the street, and the hotel is just a few minutes from Interstate 95 and a short, 12-minute drive to Baltimore-Washington International Airport.

The Baltimore Marriott, opened in 1985, is the city's preeminent hotel for business functions, featuring more than 14,000 square feet of meeting and banquet space that includes everything from boardrooms to exhibit areas, ballrooms to breakout rooms. Its capacity ranges from a board meeting for 10 to a conference or gala event for 500. The Marriott's exceptional status, in fact, was recently recognized by *Sales & Marketing Management* magazine, which honored the hotel with the prestigious 1996 Executive Choice Award in recognition of its outstanding service, facilities, and support in the planning and execution of executive meetings and conferences. "The award," says General Manager Patrick F. Fragale, "speaks well for the commitment of our employees, the quality of service we provide, and the strength of the relationships we've established with our customers."

Excellent Facilities, Abundant Amenities, and Fine Dining

All of the Marriott's 525 oversized guest rooms and suites are equipped with individual climate control, color TV with cable service, in-room pay movies, AM/FM radios, and other amenities guests have come to expect. The hotel also has 34 suites, some with wet bars, refrigerators, and adjoining sleeping rooms. Its Concierge Level features keyed elevator access, turndown service, free continental breakfast, an honor bar with complimentary hors d'oeuvres, and other unique amenities. Other special features include an indoor

pool, 24-hour room service, and the White Cap Tavern.

The heart of the Marriott can be found in its convention services department, where a full-time crew of talented meeting staffers provide the area's most comprehensive assistance on function planning. The Marriott has earned its reputation as the leader in meeting services. Key elements include a wide range of room configurations to ensure a comfortable and productive meeting environment. Flexibility being a hallmark, staffers can easily adapt rooms to suit changing

needs as the function progresses. The hotel has a vast array of resources to support meetings, ranging from state-of-the-art audiovisual equipment to design assistance. A full-service on-site business center also provides faxing, typing, photocopying, and other important functions.

Fragale sums up the hotel's commitment to helping its clients plan and execute superlative functions, saying, "At Marriott, we bring something extra to every meeting we help plan—a tradition of care, concern, and service, and the com-

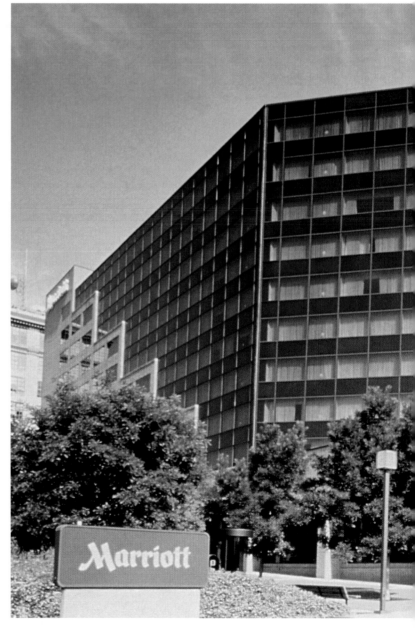

mitment to assuring your meeting the success it deserves."

Since food is an important partner in any business affair, the Marriott chefs take special pride in preparing creative coffee breaks and luncheon menus that refresh the mind and energize meetings.

Of course, the Marriott's capabilities go far beyond meeting planning. In a city known for seafood and ethnic specialties, Promenade, the hotel's restaurant, offers the finest contemporary American cuisine. Newly unveiled is White Cap Tavern, a sleek, casual meeting and greeting place, which in the mornings offers an alternative to traditional breakfast dining with gourmet coffees, espresso, cappuccino, and homemade pastries. From lunchtime until late evening, White Cap Tavern is a wonderful retreat for deliciously prepared light fare com-plemented by the region's finest selection of microbrews on tap, as well as quality Scotches and wines.

Spirit of Hospitality

The Marriott's commitment to providing all guests—whether on a visit for business or pleasure—with the finest personal service originates from its Spirit of Hospitality program. This ongoing effort emphasizes intense training in guest service for all hotel employees. Each week, staff associates are presented with new lessons and exercises aimed at enhancing each guest's experience. These range from emphasizing the importance of greetings to teaching the staff to recognize verbal and nonverbal signs of stress. "The purpose of our exercises is to empower our staff to go the extra mile in serving the guest," Fragale says. "Service is the most important amenity a hotel can offer. Expectations are higher in first-class hotels, and we intend to meet—and exceed—those expectations."

Managed by Prime Hospitality Corporation (NYSE:PDQ), the hotel is part of Marriott International, Inc., the world's leading lodging company. The Marriott Hotels line of upscale, full-service properties encompasses more than 300 hotels throughout the United States and 30 countries and territories. Prime Hospitality Corporation, a leading hotel management company, owns or manages 120 hotels throughout the United States.

Marriott's commitment to quality guest service for leisure and business travelers ensures that the Baltimore Marriott Inner Harbor will continue to serve as an important anchor hotel in the city's ongoing renaissance.

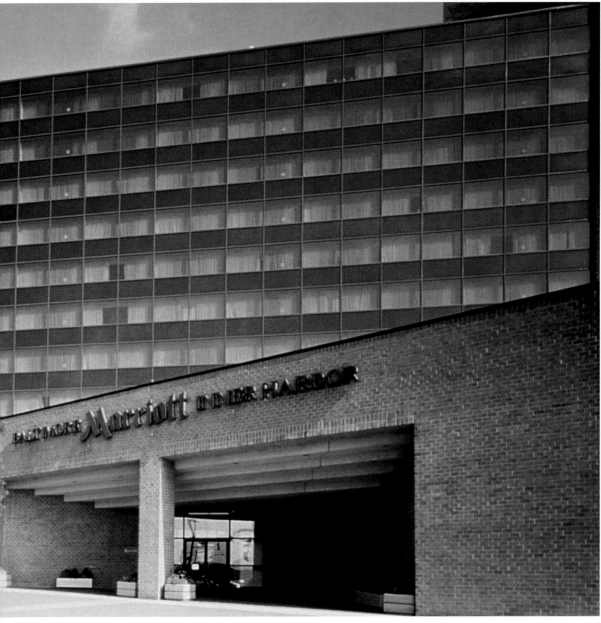

THE BALTIMORE MARRIOTT INNER HARBOR OFFERS THE BEST OF BOTH WORLDS TO BALTIMORE VISITORS. LEISURE GUESTS ARE WITHIN A SHORT STROLL OF ORIOLE PARK, THE RAVENS' NEW STADIUM, AND THE INNER HARBOR, AND CORPORATE TRAVELERS ARE WITHIN EASY WALKING DISTANCE OF THE DOWNTOWN BUSINESS DISTRICT.

Kaiser Permanente

IN ITS FIRST 50 YEARS, KAISER PERMANENTE PIONEERED A NEW WAY OF delivering health care—the innovative, prepaid, group practice approach. In the years following the Great Depression, the organization that would become Kaiser Permanente began by providing construction workers treatment when they were sick or injured, as well as advice on how to stay

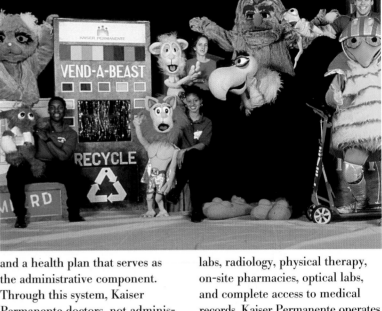

Professor Bodywise IS AN EDUCATIONAL PLAY, PRODUCED BY KAISER PERMANENTE, THAT TEACHES CHILDREN HEALTH AND SAFETY HABITS.

well, all for a payroll deduction of five cents a day. With their doctors and hospitals within easy reach, the new approach to health care worked so well for members and their employers that Kaiser Permanente agreed to cover their families, too.

Kaiser Permanente's membership has since grown, and the company is still pioneering innovations that give its members the quality health care choices they want and deserve. Today, Kaiser Permanente is the oldest and largest not-for-profit health maintenance organization (HMO) in the nation, with 8.6 million members in 18 states and the District of Columbia. The company has led the way through 50 years of change in health care by making quality medical care affordable and accessible.

Serving more than 530,000 members, Kaiser Permanente of the Mid-Atlantic states operates 22 medical centers in the Washington, D.C., and Baltimore areas. Awarded the highest possible level of accreditation by the National Committee for Quality Assurance (NCQA), it consistently receives high ratings in independent member satisfaction surveys.

A Health Plan Like No Other

Kaiser Permanente has two separate arms—a medical group consisting of doctors, and a health plan that serves as the administrative component. Through this system, Kaiser Permanente doctors, not administrators, make all medical decisions. It is this fundamental structure—the partnership between medicine and management—that has led to success and member satisfaction. The medical group has more than 550 physicians—more than 96 percent of whom are board certified—who represent an even mix of primary and specialty care.

Kaiser Permanente's Baltimore-area medical centers are located in Charles Plaza, Severna Park, Towson, White Marsh, and Woodlawn. In addition to primary and specialty care, services include ambulatory surgery, labs, radiology, physical therapy, on-site pharmacies, optical labs, and complete access to medical records. Kaiser Permanente operates two mental health centers and an imaging center in the Washington metro area. Members also can take advantage of the plan's partnerships with area hospitals such as St. Agnes and the Greater Baltimore Medical Center.

Investing in What Counts

As a not-for-profit organization, Kaiser Permanente invests in outreach programs for each community it serves, offering free education and materials about health issues to children and teenagers. In addition, the plan serves its members by reinvesting its income in the latest technology; the best health care regimens; and programs that promote safe, healthy, and more fulfilling lives for those it serves.

And the company is still getting by on five cents: Out of every health care dollar collected, Kaiser Permanente spends only five cents on administration and related costs. All the rest goes directly to patient care, research, medical equipment, and meeting the needs of its members.

KAISER PERMANENTE BELIEVES IN PROVIDING ITS MEMBERS WITH CONVENIENCE. THE WHITE MARSH MEDICAL CENTER, LOCATED IN BALTIMORE, OFFERS MANY SERVICES UNDER ONE ROOF, INCLUDING PRIMARY AND SPECIALTY CARE, LAB, RADIOLOGY, VISION SERVICES, AND PHARMACY.

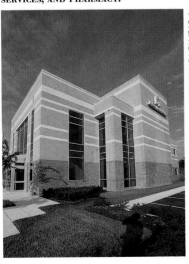

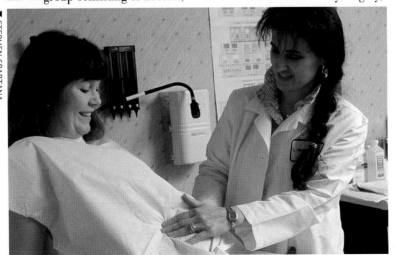

STEPHEN SPARTANA

Snelling Staffing Network

FOR MORE THAN A DECADE, NETWORK RECRUITERS, INC., DOING BUSINESS as Snelling Staffing Network, has provided Baltimore-area employers with staffing solutions. In 1996, the franchise, which is locally owned by a diverse group, placed some 1,700 individuals in temporary and direct-placement employment opportunities in four areas: administrative and

secretarial; accounting and finance; laboratory and scientific; and creative design and marketing. Skills range from entry level office clerks to PhD scientists. Snelling has offices in Annapolis, Columbia, Timonium, Bel Air, and Baltimore.

Network Recruiters, Inc., was founded in 1986 by Robert E. Greene, the company's chairman; Linda S. Kaestner, company president; and a group of local investors. Snelling has a distinctive philosophy. "We are the only staffing service to recognize that the employment process can't begin until a plan is in place," Kaestner says. "By facilitating the transition from school to work—and from one career or one job to a new one—Snelling offers solutions to important workforce needs."

Snelling Staffing Network is preparing for the next century through an approach known as Challenge 2000, a strategic plan that strengthens Snelling's foundation while also preparing for the years ahead. "As we enter the 21st century," Kaestner says, "we will expand our capabilities in job creation, work development, employment, and career development for individuals and organizations. We have already adapted our approach to a technology- and knowledge-driven economy."

Challenge 2000 targets a number of different areas. The company's goal, both now and for tomorrow, is to provide its associates with not only a job, but also a unique opportunity to enjoy a more rewarding employment experience. At the same time, Snelling's plan emphasizes continued strategic alliances, partnerships, active engagement with area colleges and universities, community leadership, and civic involvement.

"We are committed, professional staffing and employment consultants dedicated to individual and organizational success," Kaestner says.

An Array of Services

Snelling Staffing Network offers six types of employment opportunities, including temporary, temp-to-hire, freelance, contract, direct hire, and student interships. Through its Career Development Services, people and organizations can utilize key employment related assistance such as skill and aptitude testing, software and basic office skills training, and professional development products and services. Other offerings include career evaluations, professional employment consulting, and Professional Employer Organization (PEO) Services.

While providing its business clients with administrative and accounting employees is the backbone of Snelling's operation, the company has successfully carved out a niche in more unusual industries. Its creative group handles talented professionals in the areas of graphic design, event planning, animation, Internet/Web solutions, photography, desktop publishing, and dimensional design. Snelling's Laboratory and Technical group matches lab technicians to scientists with employers; these include industry specialists in chemistry, microbiology, research and development, manufacturing, pharmaceutical, quality control, regulatory affairs, and biotechnology.

Even as Snelling continues to expand into new industry niches, while maintaining existing ones, the company is committed to growing the central Maryland economy in numerous ways, from training to partnership development. This commitment, coupled with the company's commitment to its clients, will serve Snelling Staffing Network well into the future.

"We will continue to evolve as a company that is not only innovative and profitable, but also a company that is ethical and socially responsible," Greene concludes.

FROM LEFT:
NETWORK RECRUITERS, INC. CHAIRMAN AND CEO ROBERT E. GREENE

NETWORK RECRUITERS, INC. PRESIDENT AND COO LINDA S. KAESTNER

NETWORK RECRUITERS, INC. TREASURER AND CFO BRUCE H. WEBSTER

NETWORK RECRUITERS, INC. VICE PRESIDENT HAROLD I. MASTER

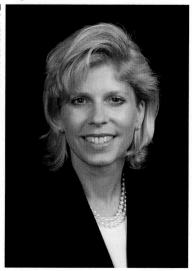
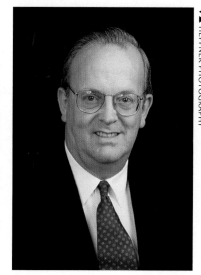
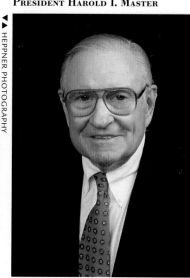

Trigen Energy Baltimore

TRIGEN IS ABOUT RECYCLING ENERGY. IN FOLLOWING ITS MISSION TO PROVIDE energy with half the fuel and half the pollutants of conventional generation, Trigen provides heating, cooling, and, where applicable, electricity to medium to large consumers, including commercial office buildings; hospitals; universities; hotels; city, state, and federal office

buildings; industrial and manufacturing facilities; public housing; convention halls; and stadiums.

The trend in business today is to outsource energy requirements to companies that specialize in the efficient and environmentally responsible production of energy. Fuel prices are rising, environmental issues are taking on greater significance, and replacement and maintenance of equipment is expensive. Finding effective ways to impact the cost of doing business is growing increasingly complex. Trigen Energy Baltimore is one of the leading companies in the energy industry, offering customers a choice for their energy needs.

Trigen Energy Baltimore is a wholly owned, regional-operating subsidiary of Trigen Energy Corporation. A publicly traded company on the New York Stock Exchange, Trigen is the nation's leading commercial developer, owner, and operator of district energy systems.

One example of Trigen's innovativeness is the powerful process of "trigeneration," a patented trigeneration machine sequentially generating heat, electricity, and chilled water from a single fuel source. This process increases efficiency and minimizes pollutants by converting the reject heat that is generated by burning fuel in a thermal energy process or in power production into other forms of end-use energy. The result: clean, efficient energy, in some cases exceeding 90 percent efficiency versus the typical utility power plant efficiency of 33 percent. With Trigen, customers not only save precious capital, time, and energy, but they significantly reduce pollutants.

An Industry Leader

In February 1985, Trigen (then known as the Baltimore Steam Company) was selected by the City of Baltimore, the Public Service Commission of Maryland, and the Baltimore Gas and Electric Company to purchase, operate, and manage the district steam system serving the central business district of Baltimore. The company immediately started making district heating a viable energy alternative for Baltimore through innovative management and operation techniques.

From the start, Trigen negotiated its own purchases of gas at the wellhead and made its oil purchases in bulk. An additional program involved the negotiation of a 20-year contract to purchase steam from the BRESCO waste-to-energy plant. This proactive fuel management lowered the cost of steam service for all customers and earned the Baltimore Steam Company the Department of Energy's Award for Energy Innovation.

Over the next few years, the company served the community under the name of Baltimore Thermal Energy Corporation. In December 1993, the company's name was changed to Trigen-Baltimore Energy Corporation to reflect its association with Trigen Energy Corporation, a nationally recognized leader in district heating and cooling systems. Today, the company name is simply Trigen Energy Baltimore. The

SINCE OCCUPYING ITS FIRST BUILDING IN DOWNTOWN BALTIMORE, TRIGEN HAS BEEN THE UTILITY AGENT FOR ALL ENERGY SERVICES, INCLUDING ELECTRICITY (LEFT).

PCS, BASED IN HANOVER, IS A PARTNER IN TRIGEN'S NEW, PATENTED FOAMING TECHNOLOGY (RIGHT).

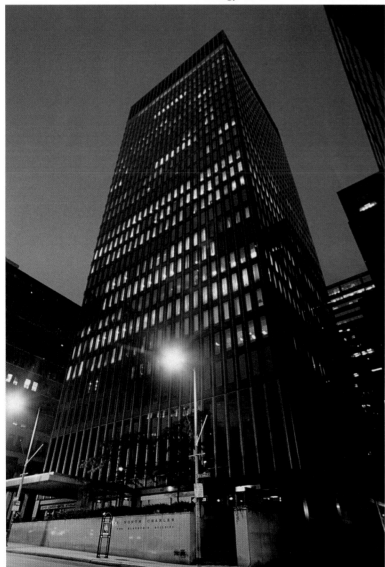

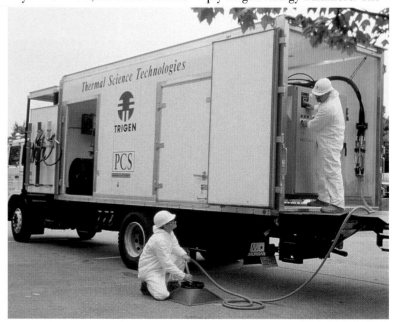

corporation provides Trigen Energy Baltimore with a resource of financial and operational professionals to assist in the implementation of technological advances and aggressive marketing programs.

Advancements in Technology

The heating and cooling of buildings historically has been an added responsibility of property managers, most of whom do not have experience in the energy industry. Trigen's only focus is on the efficient and environmentally responsible heating and cooling, and—where applicable—electricity, of large complexes.

In order to maintain a leadership position in the industry, Trigen invests heavily in research and development. This investment has led to the development of new equipment and systems. New patented insulation techniques have been instituted for pipe already in the ground, adding greater efficiency and reducing vapor; new, state-of-the-art computer control systems have been installed in many of the company plants, improving efficiency, reliability, and safety; and new metering instruments and telemetry improve accuracy and response time. The company was awarded a U.S. patent in March 1995 for its energy-efficient trigeneration machine, used primarily in district chilled water applications, and the company holds several other patents with several pending.

Trigen Energy Baltimore continues to search for ways to stay abreast of developing technologies. Trigen Energy Baltimore's system includes more than 1.5 million pounds per hour of boiler capacity and 17 miles of distribution piping, serving 350 customers. The system delivers 2 billion pounds of steam annually.

Since 1985, the company has invested more than $65 million in system improvements and expansion. This investment, coupled with the dedicated efforts of its employees, has allowed Trigen Energy Baltimore to experience more than 60 percent increase in unit growth over the past five years. Trigen Energy Baltimore today owns and operates four plants in Baltimore, located in East Baltimore near Dunbar High School, South Baltimore near the Baltimore RESCO trash energy plant, Saratoga Street near GSA's Metro West building, and the recently awarded Cherry Hill power plant.

Serving a Community

Trigen Energy Baltimore now serves most of the commercial buildings in the downtown business district, including many of the city's newest signature buildings.

As a company, Trigen is committed to making Baltimore a better place to live and work. To that end, Trigen contributes a great deal of financial and human resources to community projects. Whether it's removing snow after harsh winter storms, clearing and planting grass on empty city lots in disrepair, or donating heating oil to city public schools in need, Trigen is dedicated to Baltimore.

In 1996, Trigen Energy Baltimore was awarded the very first Diversity Award of the Chesapeake Human Resources Association for its outstanding minority hiring and contracting record.

Additionally, the company successfully runs a student co-op program—combined with a scholarship that is linked to student performance and designed to provide business experience to high school students. The company also sponsored an art contest in commemoration of Baltimore's Bicentennial Celebration. Three students were awarded scholarships directly as a result of this contest.

Trigen Energy Baltimore is at the forefront of the revival and growth of Baltimore. A significant goal of the company—and its dedicated personnel—is to be an active participant in the overall economic development of the Baltimore community.

STATE-OF-THE-ART COMPUTERIZED CONTROL TECHNOLOGY IS THE NORM FOR ALL TRIGEN POWER PLANTS (LEFT).

TRIGEN ENERGY BALTIMORE MANAGEMENT TEAM INCLUDES (FROM LEFT) WAYNE LUOMA, PAT DUDLEY, JERRY GLAZER, JIM ABROMITIS, FRED McCATHORINE, AND JOE CRANSTON (RIGHT).

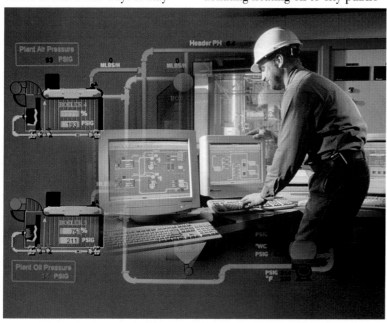

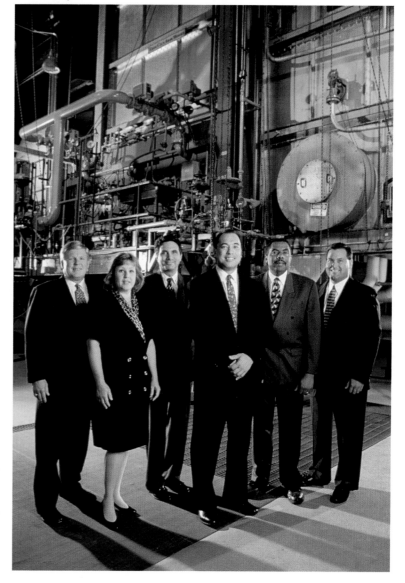

Harbor Court Hotel

FOR MORE THAN A DECADE, BALTIMORE'S HARBOR COURT HOTEL HAS exemplified elegance and grace. The European-style hotel, which opened in 1986, offers an unprecedented combination of luxury and refinement with virtually every modern convenience. ❧ "The Harbor Court is the best of two worlds," says Werner Kunz, managing director of the hotel. "Our

surroundings are serene, harking back to a more gracious era, when service was impeccable, restaurants offered the finest cuisine, and guests were pampered. And yet, the hotel is also designed for the sophisticated guest with 21st-century needs, such as computer capabilities, meeting rooms, 24-hour catering, a fitness center with indoor pool, and other modern amenities."

A Charming Hotel

Owned by David Murdock, the Harbor Court Hotel enjoys a scenic location on Baltimore's Inner Harbor and commands a sweeping view of the heart of the city. Within a five-

minute walk of the hotel are the National Aquarium; Oriole Park at Camden Yards; the Maryland Science Center; the downtown business district and the Baltimore Convention Center; and Harborplace, Baltimore's festival marketplace. Yet the Harbor Court remains an elegant retreat, where guests can relax after having savored the city's many charms.

Among these charms is the hotel itself. In addition to its exotic and warmly comfortable gathering areas, including a library stocked with volumes from all over the world, the Harbor Court boasts 203 luxuriously appointed guest rooms and suites.

Every guest room deftly combines elegance and comfort, providing a minibar, bathrobes, hair dryers, bathroom televisions, and dual-line telephones. Each of the hotel's 25 specialty suites is equipped with a four-poster bed, an oversized marble bathroom, a six-foot bathtub, and three dual-line telephones. The distinctive Harbor Court Suite features two bedrooms, a marble wet bar, a working fireplace, a dining room that seats 12 people, three bathrooms, and a baby grand piano. Many of the guest rooms, and all of the suites, enjoy tremen-

dous views of the Inner Harbor.

A New Standard for Gourmet Cuisine

None other than Cesar Ritz said, "For if the success of a hotel is dependent upon its kitchens and its table—as it is—the kitchens and restaurant in their turn are dependent upon the management. What is good food if not finely served?"

The Harbor Court strives to live up to the standard set by the great hotelier in its two unique restaurants with a team of professionals that includes Galen Sampson, executive chef of the Harbor Court Hotel; Michael Delcambre, chef at Hampton's; and James Zambito, head chef at Brighton's. Each chef believes that atmosphere, service, and cuisine are integrally related elements of equal value.

The most touted of the Harbor Court's restaurants is Hampton's. "At Hampton's, our philosophy has always been to create a sense of timelessness, of an older, more gracious world that combines elegance and pampering—for all the senses," says Kunz.

Seductive elegance, gracious service, and daringly prepared, seasonal cuisine are hallmarks

OPENED IN 1986, THE HARBOR COURT HOTEL HARKS BACK TO A MORE GRACIOUS ERA, WHEN SERVICE WAS IMPECCABLE, RESTAURANTS OFFERED THE FINEST CUISINE, AND GUESTS WERE PAMPERED (LEFT).

THE LIBRARY AT THE HARBOR COURT IS STOCKED WITH VOLUMES FROM ALL OVER THE WORLD (RIGHT).

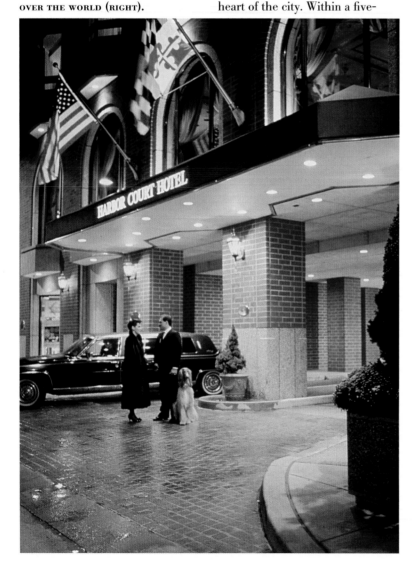

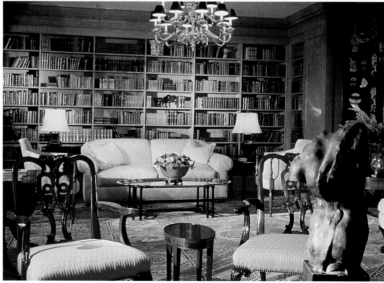

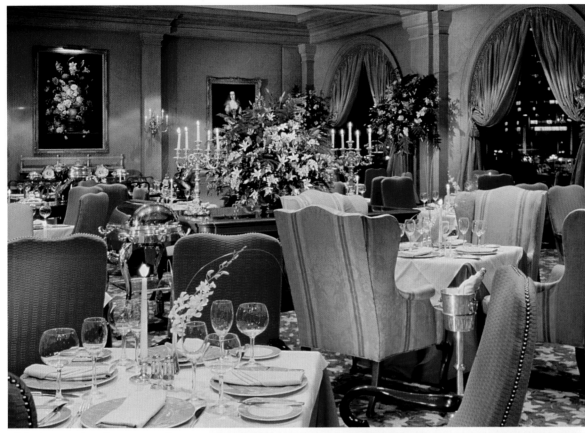

of the internationally renowned
restaurant. For atmosphere alone,
Hampton's is considered to be one
of the grandest dining rooms in
America. Decorated with fruit-
wood molding and walls that are
covered with salmon moiré, the
high-ceilinged, spacious room over-
looks Baltimore's glittering Inner
Harbor. Antique mahogany break-
fronts, Chinese lacquered screens,
lightly scented gardenias floating
in glass bowls, and overstuffed
wing chairs imbue the restaurant
with a sense of grandeur and of
intimacy, enhanced by the generous spacing of the tables to ensure
privacy.

Hampton's may well be considered the centerpiece of the Harbor
Court's culinary universe, but it is
by no means the hotel's only source
of well-prepared, high-quality cuisine. Serving breakfast, lunch, afternoon tea, and dinner, Brighton's
retains the elegant decor of Hampton's, but features traditionally prepared dishes in an informal, light,
and airy café. With its lemon yellow and verdant green schemes,
the restaurant resembles a garden
atelier.

At the exotic Explorer's
Lounge, the city's finest selections

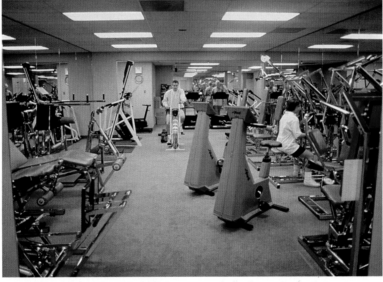

of single malt Scotch, rare cognac,
fine cigars, and wines by the glass
mingle with cool jazz every night
of the week. The lounge also features hand-painted safari scenes
and intriguing objets d'art.

Expresso, Etc., located beside
the hotel's lobby, is a wonderful
gourmet-to-go delicatessen, offering everything from fresh pastries
and sandwiches to gourmet coffees
and newspapers.

The hotel's extensive catering operation receives the same
attention to quality and detail.
In addition to its comprehensive

facilities for business meetings
and dining functions, the Harbor
Court is the city's most prestigious
location for weddings and social
affairs.

Serving Business Is Good Business

The Harbor Court offers unparalleled business services.
"Serving business is good
business," Kunz says, "and we
offer traditional facilities for
business-oriented travelers, as
well as custom-arranged services."
For example, the hotel has created

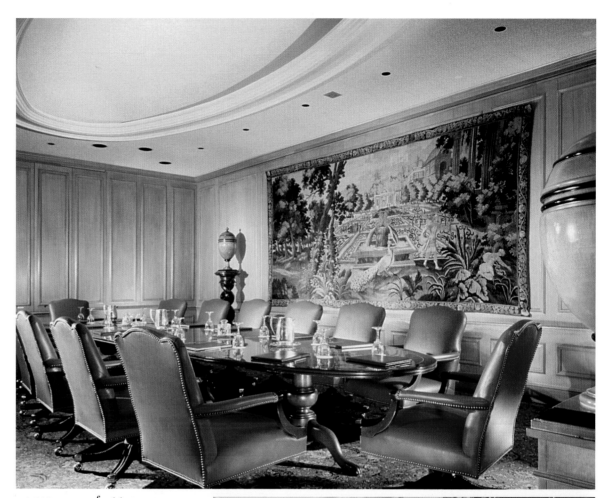

a 3,500-square-foot temporary office—complete with a 25-person conference room, three private offices, a secretary's station, a kitchen, and private rest rooms—for long-term business needs in Baltimore.

Corporate facilities of the more traditional variety include more than 10,000 square feet of meeting space with 11 meeting rooms to accommodate a diversity of functions. The corporate meeting rooms can be arranged in various patterns, including theater, classroom-style, U-shaped, conference, reception, and banquet.

Among the hotel's function rooms are three dedicated boardrooms and meeting rooms that can accommodate groups ranging from 24 to 150 people. In addition, the Harbor Court offers the 320-capacity Whitehall Ballroom. A graceful, elegant space appointed with several antiques, it is Baltimore's only ballroom with a harbor view.

The Harbor Court also offers an array of services that will help facilitate any business function. These include convention coordination, simultaneous translation

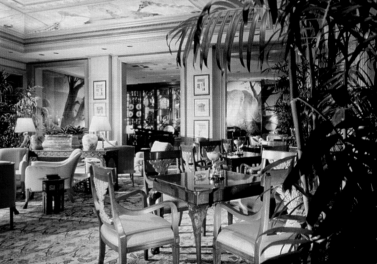

services, and state-of-the-art audio-visual equipment.

The hotel operates the full-service Executive Business Center, which offers guests such support services as photocopying, faxing, shipping, and graphic design. The center is equipped with computer terminals featuring a selection of software. Secretarial services are available, and all guest rooms are equipped with modem-capable, dual-line telephones.

An Award-Winning Hotel

The Harbor Court's overall excellence has been duly rewarded. To date, the hotel has won more lodging and dining awards than any other in Baltimore history. A member of the prestigious Preferred Hotels & Resorts Worldwide, which includes such internationally acclaimed properties as the Ritz in Paris, the Mansion on Turtle Creek in Dallas, and the Peninsula in Hong Kong, the Harbor Court

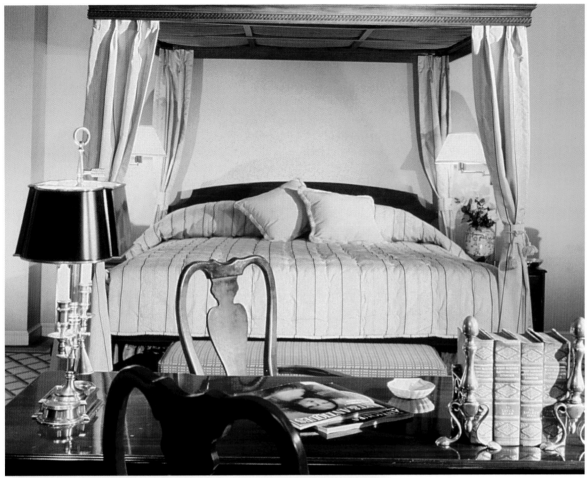

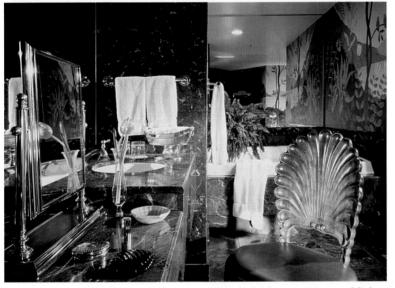

recently was named Preferred Hotel of the Year. "This award," Kunz says, "makes an important statement about our hotel's preeminent record of quality and service."

Other distinguished awards include AAA's four-diamond award and *Mobil Travel Guide*'s four-star distinction. The Harbor Court received the Gold Key Award from *Meetings and Conventions* magazine and The Pinnacle Award from *Successful Meetings* magazine,

both of which recognize establishments boasting superior meeting staffs, meeting rooms, guest rooms, food and beverage services, reservations handling, and recreational facilities. The hotel was the sole Maryland establishment to be so honored.

The Harbor Court was also ranked 11th on the prestigious *Condé Nast Traveler* Readers' Poll of the best hotels nationwide and was included on the magazine's Gold List of best places to stay. In addition,

Zagat has rated the Harbor Court as the best in Baltimore.

On a local level, the hotel has made a promise to be a responsible member of the community. As Baltimore undergoes a second renaissance, spurred by Oriole Park at Camden Yards, the expansion of the new convention center, and other additions, the Harbor Court remains committed to playing an important role—one that attracts travelers of distinction—in the growth of the city.

For Kunz, the Harbor Court occupies a special niche in Baltimore's growing lodgings marketplace. "Exceptional is just one way to express what our guests, who include international critics, business travelers, Hollywood stars, heads of state, kings and princes, weekend tourists, honeymooners, and local patrons, are saying about our hotel," Kunz says. "We're proud that in our first decade, we've contributed to Baltimore's first and second renaissances. We look forward to participating in ongoing rebirths as this unique, historic city continues to adapt and transform itself for the future."

Integrated Health Services, Inc.

INTEGRATED HEALTH SERVICES, INC. (IHS), HEADQUARTERED IN OWINGS Mills, is a highly diversified health care provider, offering a wide spectrum of post-acute medical and rehabilitative services. These include subacute care, home health care, inpatient and outpatient rehabilitation, respiratory therapy, skilled nursing, hospice care, and diagnostic services. ∾ IHS offers a

continuum of medical services that benefit both patients and payers. For patients, the company's services provide a single source of care from hospital to home. For payers, IHS offers the benefit of dealing with one health care supplier; the efficient delivery of integrated services reduces costs while improving clinical outcomes.

Founded in Baltimore in 1986, IHS has grown from its initial niche of operating private, high-quality nursing homes, to becoming a pioneer and industry leader in subacute care, to today's industry-leading position as a developer and operator of full-service post-acute care networks. From its beginnings, says Robert N. Elkins, founder and

chairman of IHS, the company has been an innovator in the health care industry. "Our industry is in the midst of a national passion for change, which is fine with us, because we are the change," Elkins explains. "We're at the very forefront of reform and proud to be part of the solution. Hospital stays, as we have known them, will never be the same again."

Building the Post-Acute Care Network

The IHS post-acute care network is a bold, new way to treat medically stable patients. It is an approach that is reshaping the way Americans view the period of care that follows serious illness

or hospitalization. More than mere alternatives to any one traditional medical model, full-service IHS networks support patients from hospital discharge through recovery. Upon release from an acute care hospital setting, patients usually are discharged either to their homes or to subacute medical units.

Currently, IHS is one of the country's largest home care providers, offering services at more than 500 sites across the nation. Due to advances in technology, patient preferences, and the demographics of an aging adult population, home-based care is increasingly popular, fostering independence and comfort while also providing quality medical services. When integrated within a post-acute network, home health care enhances the continuity of a patient's well-being, lowers overall treatment costs, and serves as a virtually seamless referral source for other IHS specialty medical services.

The company's subacute and nursing/rehabilitation centers, which number more than 600 in 40 states, operate literally as mini-hospitals, where patients receive the equivalent of traditional hospital care at a much lower cost. Treatment specialties include pulmonary care, rehabilitation, wound and infectious disease management, orthopedics, neurology, oncology, cardiovascular care, and nutritional support.

IHS also is successfully targeting health maintenance organizations (HMOs) with a one-stop shopping approach that enables insurers to contract with a single full-service provider, rather than with separate, unaligned services. To date, IHS has more than 425 contracts with HMOs and other managed care organizations—one

FOR PATIENTS, INTEGRATED HEALTH SERVICES, INC. PROVIDES A SINGLE SOURCE OF CARE FROM HOSPITAL TO HOME.

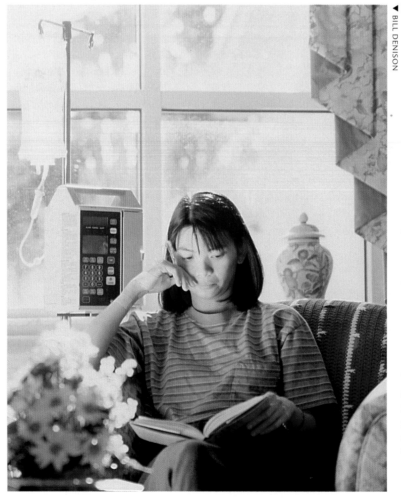

BILL DENISON

of the largest utilization rates in the industry.

IHS presents benefits administrators with an opportunity to control costs while maximizing the benefits of quality care. As America's health care climate continues to change rapidly, IHS emphasizes further growth and expansion. It is adding new medical services for patients and offering expanded efficiencies in cost management for payers. "With cost containment as the primary force behind the industry's metamorphosis," Elkins says, "IHS is committed to offering efficient, high-quality alternatives to the rising costs of prolonged hospitalization."

Dynamic Growth and Innovation

Building from this base, IHS's strategic blueprint for the years ahead follows the managed care model for controlling costs and ensuring positive, predictable clinical outcomes. IHS seeks long-term value for its investors through a strategy of continually assessing shifts in the volatile national health care environment and realigning its resources. This is reflected today in an aggressive move toward shared, at-risk partnering, and capitated rate arrangements with HMOs and other managed care payers.

IHS strives to build its networks through acquisitions and partnerships that strengthen its geographic base and the variety of services it offers. Recent purchases include the acquisition of five home care companies, making IHS one of the largest providers of home health services in the country.

The Future

Since 1986, Integrated Health Services has added a new dimension to America's health care continuum. Today, due to its national post-acute care networks, IHS has become a single source of care, from medical treatment to rehabilitation and home recovery. By incorporating a full range of services within one system, IHS is able to provide efficient health care delivery, predict and control costs, and monitor outcomes. The result? "Our approach gets high marks from patients, case managers, physicians, and payers," Elkins says. "Outcome data and quality measurements show that our care is among the best anywhere."

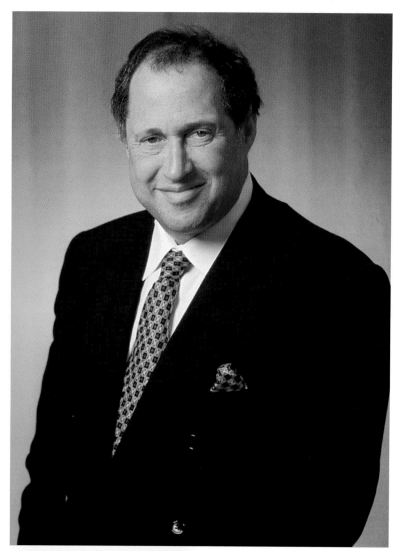

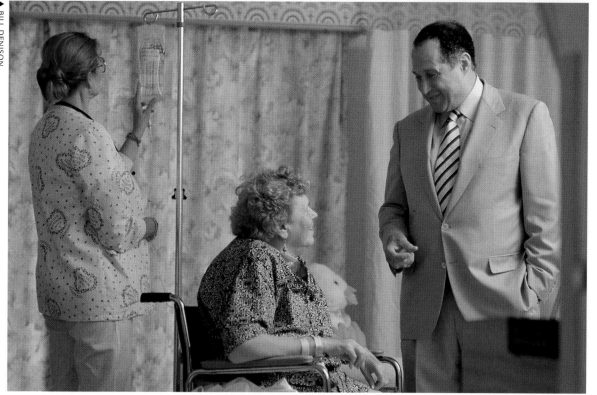

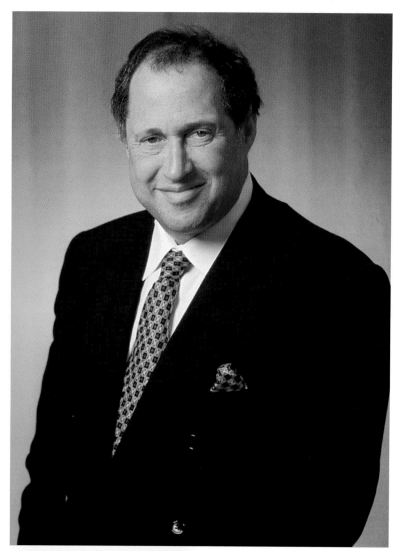

ROBERT N. ELKINS, FOUNDER AND CHAIRMAN OF IHS, SAYS, "OUR INDUSTRY IS IN THE MIDST OF A NATIONAL PASSION FOR CHANGE, WHICH IS FINE WITH US, BECAUSE WE ARE THE CHANGE" (TOP).

DUE TO ADVANCES IN TECHNOLOGY, PATIENT PREFERENCES, AND THE DEMOGRAPHICS OF AN AGING ADULT POPULATION, HOME-BASED CARE IS INCREASINGLY POPULAR, FOSTERING INDEPENDENCE AND COMFORT WHILE ALSO PROVIDING QUALITY MEDICAL SERVICES (BOTTOM).

Helix Health

THE WAY HEALTH CARE IS DELIVERED IS VERY DIFFERENT TODAY. WHILE a variety of forces have reshaped how people get care, the central question remains—how can health care organizations responsibly, conveniently, and economically meet their patients' needs for quality care? To answer that question, Helix Health is changing the face of health care.

Helix Health's mission is to do more than just react to the constantly changing health care environment. Instead, its philosophy is to listen to those it serves and to respond in sensitive, sensible, and imaginative ways to deliver health care that is helpful, personal, cost-effective, and caring—health care with humanity, health care that greets patients with a smile.

Going into the Neighborhoods

Helix Health's challenge and commitment is to bring a full range of quality health care services closer to the community—making them comfortable, personal, easy to get to, and easy to use. Helix is comprised of community hospitals, over 50 doctors' offices, and five urgent care centers on campuses located throughout Baltimore neighborhoods. From Dundalk to Bel Air, White Marsh to Lutherville, Towson to Glen Burnie, and Cross Keys to Catonsville, Helix has programs and doctors to serve its patients.

One of the most effective ways that Helix contains costs, maintains quality, and provides convenient services is by offering the right level of care in the right setting. For example, patients who may have once had long and costly stays in critical care beds can now safely be moved to an intermediate care location for recovery and rehabilitation services. In addition, after a patient has been discharged from critical care, Helix offers short-term, intermediate care in both its hospital and nursing home facilities.

Helix is also broadening the spectrum of services it offers outside of the traditional hospital setting. Helix recognizes that no one wants to go to or stay in a hospital if they don't have to. The simple solution is close-by, easy-to-use health care facilities that allow patients to be as independent as possible while also providing quality care.

That's why, at Helix, primary care, intermediate care, and home care are high priorities. With more than 200,000 home health and hospice visits a year, its commitment continues to grow. Helix is dedicated to being a good neighbor: never losing sight of the people it serves and always being there when it's needed—right around the corner or right down the street.

World-Renowned Specialists

Patients whose problems require sophisticated diagnostic capabilities and specialized care can count on Helix Health to provide a wealth of the right resources and medical professionals. Helix continues to build upon its stellar reputation by recruiting nationally renowned specialists in the fields of cardiology, neonatology,

CLOCKWISE FROM TOP:
HELIX HEALTH'S HIGH-TECH OBSTETRIC SERVICES INCLUDE NEONATAL INTENSIVE CARE UNITS, GENETIC COUNSELING, AND IN VITRO FERTILIZATION PROGRAMS.

HELIX'S PHILOSOPHY IS TO LISTEN TO THOSE IT SERVES AND TO RESPOND WITH HEALTH CARE THAT IS HELPFUL, PERSONAL, COST-EFFECTIVE, AND CARING.

HELIX PATIENTS WHOSE PROBLEMS REQUIRE SOPHISTICATED DIAGNOSTIC CAPABILITIES AND SPECIALIZED CARE CAN COUNT ON THE RIGHT RESOURCES AND MEDICAL PROFESSIONALS.

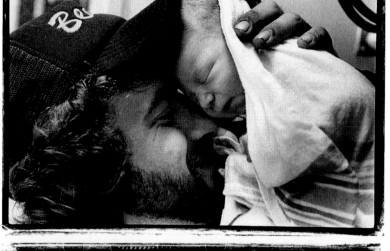

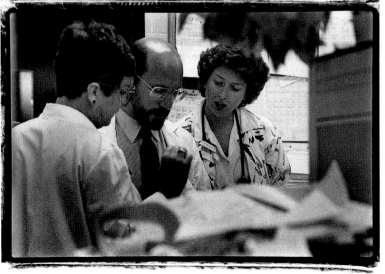

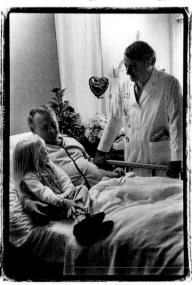

orthopedic and hand surgery, rehabilitation, oncology, and mental health.

In cardiology, for example, Helix Heart Care offers a full scope of services, which are expertly provided by one of the top physician groups in the country. From chest pain management programs to state-of-the-art cardiac catheterization laboratories, Helix Health's cardiovascular program is now one of the largest and most highly acclaimed in the region.

Helix's obstetric/gynecology services are equally notable. Its doctors care for more pregnant women than any other health care organization in the area. Helix's high-tech obstetric services include neonatal intensive care units, genetic counseling, in-womb surgery, and in vitro fertilization programs.

The Helix orthopedic program also offers a wide array of services—from rheumatology to surgery—which are available in satellite offices throughout the region. The Helix rehabilitation program also deserves special mention, as it includes the oldest and largest hospital-based comprehensive patient care program in the state.

Other Helix specialties include oncology, endocrinology, pulmonary services, geriatric medicine, urology, plastic surgery, vascular surgery, and oral surgery.

Being in Two Places at Once

Helix is expanding the boundaries of its community, not to be big, but to be responsive to the way people live and work in Baltimore, Washington, D.C., and everywhere in between. Now, more than a highway connects the two metropolitan areas. The largest health care delivery systems in both Baltimore and Washington— Helix Health and Medlantic Healthcare Group—have formed a partnership to serve the corridor that is rapidly becoming one big region rather than two isolated cities.

The new partnership, called BWHealth, is headquartered in Columbia, Maryland. The idea behind BWHealth is to provide opportunities for information and technology sharing between the two systems, so that each system achieves greater efficiency and

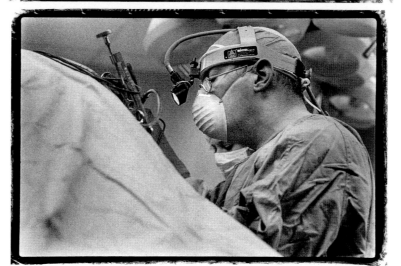

economy. Instead of competing with each other, they complement one another.

Through Medlantic, residents of the Baltimore-Washington community have increased access to Washington Hospital Center and its major centers of excellence, which include Washington Heart, Washington Cancer Institute, and MedSTAR Shock-Trauma Center. Likewise, Medlantic patients have

access to Helix services.

So Helix is not only in two places at once, but in dozens of places—growing, expanding, keeping pace with the region, and making health care healthier. Helix Health is always monitoring the pulse of the community to learn what works, what doesn't, and what's needed so everyone can enjoy good health and a sense of well-being.

PATIENTS OF ALL AGES BENEFIT FROM THE RESPONSIBLE, CONVENIENT CARE OFFERED BY HELIX HEALTH.

HELIX CONTINUES TO BUILD UPON ITS STELLAR REPUTATION BY RECRUITING NATIONALLY RENOWNED SPECIALISTS IN THE FIELDS OF CARDIOLOGY, NEONATOLOGY, ORTHOPEDIC AND HAND SURGERY, REHABILITATION, ONCOLOGY, AND MENTAL HEALTH.

HS Processing L.P.

TUCKED INTO A SHADED ENCLAVE NEAR SPARROWS POINT, THE GIGANTIC warehouses that comprise HS Processing L.P.'s facility tell the story of a region—and an industry—that is prospering again. ∿ During Baltimore's romantic shipbuilding era, steel played a paramount role in the economics of the city and surrounding counties. Centered on

Bethlehem Steel, which in turn spawned a number of industrial manufacturers that supported the trade, Baltimore's eastern communities boomed, employment levels were high, and wages were fair.

Modern times saw a drastic reduction in the demand for steel; therefore, Baltimore's economic focus shifted to other industries. The outlook for steel processing was gloomy.

State-of-the-Art Facilities

HS Processing L.P. looked at the positive side and in September 1988, opened the first of two state-of-the-art Baltimore-area facilities. Located in Dundalk, the plant's primary function, both then and today, is to "slit" and "edge" cold rolled steel. In April 1990, HS Processing L.P. opened its second site—this one in Sparrows Point—designed to "pickle" and "oil" hot rolled coils. Together, the two facilities provide such clients as Bethlehem Steel, U.S. Steel, and other domestic and foreign offshore mills with hot and cold rolled processing—an integral component in manufacturing materials that eventually find their way to numerous and diverse parts of steel products.

In HS Processing's industrial warehouse, which is the length of three football fields, nearly half a million tons of steel are annually buffed—or pickled—with a hydro-

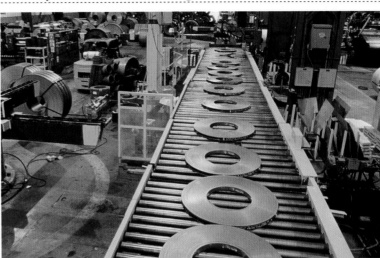

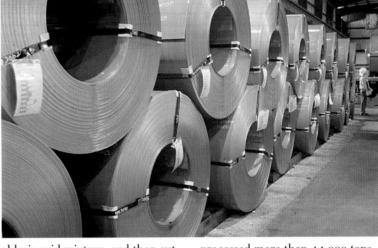

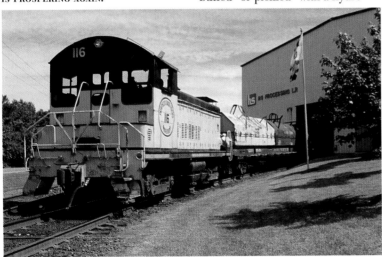

CLOCKWISE FROM TOP:
HS PROCESSING'S FORT HOLABIRD PARK SLITTING FACILITY WAS OPENED IN 1988.

IN THE COMPANY'S INDUSTRIAL WAREHOUSE, WHICH IS THE LENGTH OF THREE FOOTBALL FIELDS, NEARLY HALF A MILLION TONS OF STEEL ARE ANNUALLY BUFFED—OR PICKLED—WITH A HYDROCHLORIC ACID MIXTURE, AND THEN CUT AND SLIT TO SIZE.

TUCKED INTO A SHADED ENCLAVE NEAR SPARROWS POINT, THE GIGANTIC WAREHOUSES THAT COMPRISE HS PROCESSING'S FACILITY TELL THE STORY OF A REGION—AND AN INDUSTRY—THAT IS PROSPERING AGAIN.

chloric acid mixture, and then cut and slit to size. The process involves removing the scale, discoloration, and dirt that mars the look of raw steel, and turning it into a sleek, polished product. The giant coils of this processed steel, which are stored in the Sparrows Point facility, measure from 800 feet to nearly a mile in length. Each can weigh up to 60,000 pounds.

Solid Growth

Since the opening of the Dundalk and Sparrows Point plants, HS Processing has carved out a firm niche for itself. Since 1990, quality, on-time production and delivery have transformed the Sparrows Point plant from a one-shift operation to a seven-day, 24-hour operation for the past three years. In August 1996, the plant

processed more than 44,000 tons of steel.

"In coming to Baltimore, we felt that HS Processing could provide an important support service to customers like Bethlehem Steel," says Al Kunaniec, Sparrows Point plant manager, who recently announced plans for the construction of a 60,000-square-foot building to handle additional storage and processing. "We're just as pleased, however, in seeing Baltimore's manufacturing base grow once again. It's important not to forget that this is a staple of Baltimore's economic engine."

It is all part of HS Processing's philosophy of providing the areas it serves with a multitude of quality services and products, ensuring that the company and Baltimore will continue to grow together.

Pro Staff

IN A BUSINESS WHERE PEOPLE COUNT FOR EVERYTHING, PRO STAFF has emerged as a leader by providing a service very different from traditional staffing services. As companies have become increasingly concerned about maximizing productivity, matching resources to demand, and controlling staffing costs, Pro Staff has responded by developing flexible, cost-effective staffing solutions tailored to clients' specific needs.

In one case, that might mean recruiting hundreds of production personnel who can assemble medical devices to a zero-defect standard. In another, it's 15 highly specialized information technology engineers for the major launch of a new asynchronous transfer mode at a telecommunications and data exchange provider. In yet another, it's providing up to 250 people of various disciplines to staff a corporate headquarters for relocation—or simply finding that one superstar, all-around employee. Pro Staff's people prove themselves willing and able to tackle virtually any staffing and recruitment assignment, calling on the core competencies that make them the best at what they do. A complete explanation of services is available through Pro Staff's toll-free number, 800-938-WORK.

A People Business

Understanding that people make the difference in providing the quality staffing that clients expect, Pro Staff acts as an ongoing resource to provide skilled temporary and flexible employees who are committed to outstanding performance. Pro Staff recruits and retains the best people by offering exceptional benefits, training, advancement opportunities, incentives, and awards.

Personal attention is equally integral. "One of the things our people most often mention is they feel we know them better as individuals than any other service," says Doug Dobbs, executive vice president of Pro Staff.

Founded in 1982 in Minneapolis by Pro Staff President Jeff Dobbs, the company offers its staffing expertise in the Maryland market in an expansive array of skills and disciplines, including office and administrative, accounting and finance, medical administrative, and information technology (IT) consulting. Building on its 15-year-

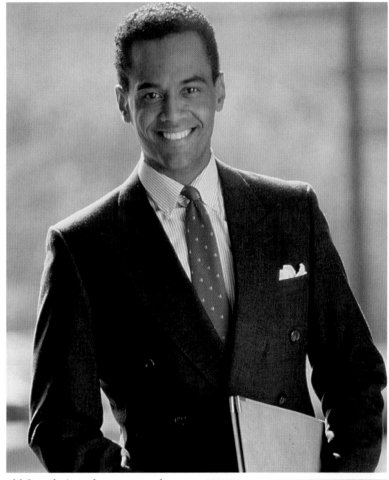

old foundation, the company has grown to more than 195 offices nationwide.

As Jeff Dobbs shares, much of Pro Staff's growth comes from word-of-mouth referrals. "Many of our clients are sent to us by other clients," Dobbs says. "And, many of our employees are referred to us by other employees."

Pro Staff opened in Maryland in 1989 and has grown rapidly to include seven Baltimore-area offices. Gail Smith, general manager for Pro Staff in Maryland, is a staffing industry veteran who knows very well why Pro Staff is unique. Says Smith, "We do things differently here at Pro Staff. We are working for authentic 'win-win' success for our clients and our employees. And our decisions are made here at the local level."

And that's right in line with Pro Staff's major objective: to be

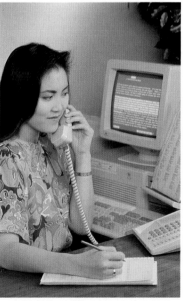

not only recognized as the premier provider of staffing services, but also as the most innovative and reliable supplier of quality staffing, creating a more productive and cost-effective workforce.

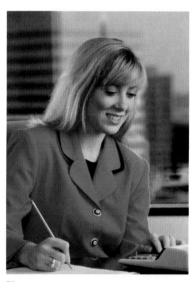

UNDERSTANDING THAT PEOPLE MAKE THE DIFFERENCE IN PROVIDING THE QUALITY STAFFING THAT CLIENTS EXPECT, PRO STAFF ACTS AS AN ONGOING RESOURCE TO PROVIDE TEMPORARY AND FLEXIBLE EMPLOYEES WHO ARE COMMITTED TO OUTSTANDING PERFORMANCE.

RE/MAX Advantage Realty

FOR REALTORS AT RE/MAX ADVANTAGE REALTY, THE BUYING AND SELLING of residential properties is more than a job; it's a mission. "We are not truly in the real estate business," says Alex Karavasilis, co-owner. "We're in the people business. We don't buy and sell properties; we facilitate transactions." ❧ What purchase could be more emotional than buying a home? "A house is much more than bricks and sticks," Karavasilis explains. "It's shelter, safety, security, family, comfort, and personal expression." With that understanding, the approach of RE/MAX Advantage Realty associates is one that combines high-quality customer service and industry professionalism toward everyone from buyers and sellers to a first-time condominium purchaser to a major corporate relocation prospect.

THE ASSOCIATES OF RE/MAX AD-VANTAGE REALTY HAVE MADE JOHNS HOPKINS HOSPITAL'S CHILDREN'S MIRACLE NETWORK A CORPORATE— AS WELL AS PERSONAL—FOCUS ON THE LOCAL LEVEL (TOP).

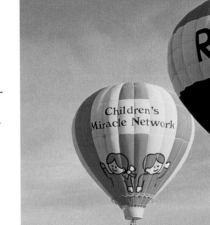

Modern History

RE/MAX Advantage Realty, part of an international real estate sales organization, was founded in Columbia, Maryland, in 1988. In 1992, Karavasilis and Leslie Rock, who are both certified real estate brokers, acquired the firm, bringing to it vast experience and expertise in local real estate. They now oversee a 75-agent base that covers a large part of the Baltimore metropolitan area, including Baltimore City and the counties of Anne Arundel, Baltimore,

RE/MAX ADVANTAGE REALTY, PART OF AN INTERNATIONAL REAL ESTATE SALES ORGANIZATION, WAS FOUNDED IN COLUMBIA, MARYLAND, IN 1988.

Carroll, Frederick, Howard, Harford, Montgomery, and Prince Georges. RE/MAX Advantage Realty is head-quartered in Columbia, with an additional office in Eldersburg.

Over the years, building on the strengths of its regional, national, and international presence, the RE/MAX organization has enjoyed consistent growth. In 1996 alone, market share in Howard County, for example, rose to 34.3 percent. RE/MAX Advantage Realty offices generated more than $160 million in volume and recorded one of the highest sales volume per associate in Greater Baltimore, selling one home every seven hours.

Karavasilis credits this success to the bright and talented professionals of the firm and intensive and ongoing training his associates experience. "Our industry has its own continuing education programs, which are valuable, but in addition to those, we have RE/MAX Advantage Realty grad school. People come here to get their 'master's' and 'doctorates.'"

To that end, in-house training does not rely merely on technical issues, such as the latest sales techniques, marketing tips, and product and service information. What is just as important is good inter-personal skills and an understanding of buyer and seller psychology. The RE/MAX Advantage Realty approach is not just about providing excellent service, but in em-pathizing with its clients. "If our agents really focus on the needs of their client," Karavasilis says, "the financial rewards will always follow."

A Revolutionary Approach

RE/MAX stands for "real estate maximums." The organization, a leader in innovation and service around the world, was launched in Denver

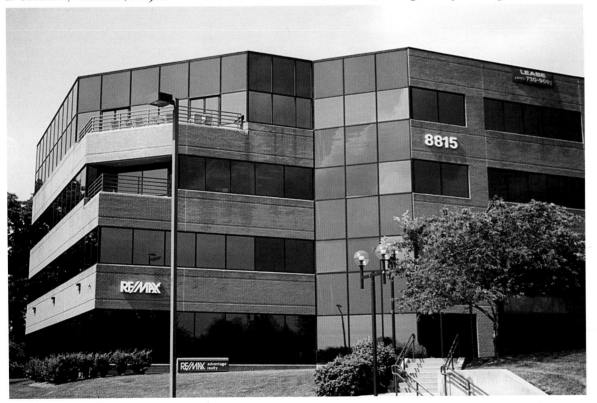

in 1973 by Dave and Gail Liniger. The RE/MAX network includes more than 46,000 members in more than 2,800 offices in the United States, Canada, Australia, the Caribbean, Europe, Israel, Mexico, and South Africa. Under the RE/MAX franchise name, these independently owned and operated offices provide real estate services in residential, commercial, referral, relocation, and asset management. Since its inception in 1973, the RE/MAX organization has experienced 24 consecutive years of growth, attracting sales associates who lead the industry in professional designations, experience, and production.

The RE/MAX difference is evidenced by the company's structure. In exchange for sharing equally in office overhead and management fees, RE/MAX sales associates receive 100 percent commission. Unlike traditional residential real estate companies, which require that experienced professionals often subsidize newcomers to the field, RE/MAX associates pay their fair share and reap the optimum return. Among agents, the system is designed to promote cooperation rather than competition.

As a result, RE/MAX attracts full-time top producers who enjoy full ownership of their business. The average RE/MAX agent has a seasoned knowledge of the industry and more than a decade of experience. "The idea," Karavasilis says, "is to be in business for yourself, not by yourself." That is why, with its progressive office environment, RE/MAX Advantage Realty is styled more like a law firm than a realty company. There is a vast range of support services for agents, ranging from marketing and promotional services to case processing and bulk mailing. Business and financial planning is available as well. And for customers, the RE/MAX Advantage Realty one-stop-shop approach, which offers assistance with lenders, title companies, and other related services, as well as professional real estate representation, ensures that RE/MAX Advantage Realty associates provide the ultimate in customer service and satisfaction.

An additional advantage is the strength of the international

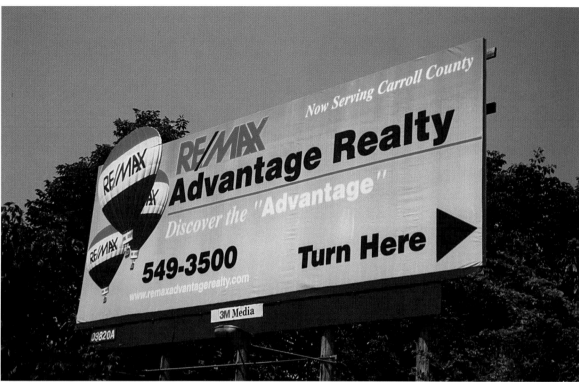

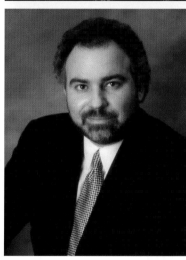 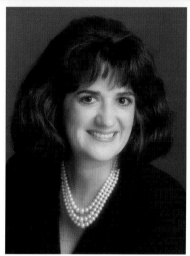

ALEXANDER K. KARAVASILIS (LEFT) AND LESLIE H. ROCK (RIGHT), BOTH CERTIFIED REAL ESTATE BROKERS, ACQUIRED RE/MAX ADVANTAGE REALTY IN 1992, BRINGING TO IT VAST EXPERIENCE AND EXPERTISE IN LOCAL REAL ESTATE.

organization. A worldwide referral network simplifies communication between agents for maximum results.

Community Contributions

While the RE/MAX Advantage Realty ownership team is amply focused on business, both Karavasilis and Rock—along with their agents—are committed to contributing to the local communities. Interested in supporting economic development, Rock, a mayoral appointee for the Baltimore City Commission for Women, has helped develop the nation's first Women's Business Center. She also was involved in the renovation of the Disabled American Veterans' facility. Karavasilis has made Johns Hopkins Hospital's Children's Miracle Network

a corporate—as well as personal—focus on the local level. Members of the firm itself, through an annual charity golf tournament, have donated thousands of dollars to the organization over the past few years.

The unique entrepreneurial environment created by RE/MAX Advantage Realty is integral to the company's success, fostering flexibility and service orientation. It also focuses on the needs of the client, believing that providing the very best possible service to all clients will result naturally in financial reward. It is a revolutionary approach that has propelled RE/MAX Advantage Realty and its associates into industry leadership, and has given the associates, clients, and personnel of the firm a real advantage.

International Youth Foundation

ARMED WITH A $67 MILLION GRANT FROM THE W.K. KELLOGG Foundation, Rick Little had a plan to link socially aware corporations with youth programs worldwide. The result? An independent, international, nongovernmental organization known as the International Youth Foundation (IYF). Dedicated to improving the conditions and prospects for children and youth, IYF was established after some two years of consultation with more than 300 leaders in business, philanthropy, government, and social services in more than 30 countries.

From the outset, the need for an organization that would focus solely on children and youth was overwhelming. Nearly 1 billion children will be born during the 1990s with 97 percent of those births occurring in poor countries. By 2000, young people under the age of 20 will, for the first time in modern history, make up nearly half the world's population—a demographic shift that has profound implications for the world economy.

The International Youth Foundation acts as a channel between worthy programs and corporations seeking to make financial contributions. "More than ever, the success of business is directly related to the success of societies, families, and communities in preparing a competent workforce," says Arnold Langbo, chairman of the Kellogg Company in Battle Creek, Michigan. "We consider it good business to view corporate philanthropy not only as charity, but as wise and strategic investments in our future."

CLOCKWISE FROM TOP:

THE INTERNATIONAL YOUTH FOUNDATION (IYF) BELIEVES EVERY CHILD SHOULD HAVE ACCESS TO FUNDAMENTAL RESOURCES, SUCH AS A SAFE PLACE, A CARING ADULT, A HEALTHY START, MARKETABLE SKILLS, AND AN OPPORTUNITY TO SERVE. IN THE PHILIPPINES, IYF HAS WORKED TO EXPAND THE AVAILABILITY OF THESE RESOURCES TO MORE YOUNG PEOPLE. WHILE VISITING A YOUTH PROGRAM IN MANILA, IYF FOUNDER AND CEO RICK LITTLE TALKS WITH TWO BOYS WHO ONCE LIVED AND WORKED ON THE STREET.

IYF WAS FOUNDED IN 1990 TO BRING WORLDWIDE SUPPORT TO THE MANY EXCEPTIONAL LOCAL EFFORTS THAT ARE CHANGING YOUNG LIVES IN EVERY CORNER OF THE GLOBE.

HOPE FOR ALL CHILDREN IS THE UNIVERSAL MESSAGE BEING PUT FORTH BY THESE STREET AND WORKING CHILDREN IN THE PHILIPPINES DURING A MARCH IN SUPPORT OF THEIR RIGHTS.

Focused on the Future

Since its founding, the International Youth Foundation, which in 1996 relocated its worldwide headquarters from Battle Creek to Baltimore, has remained true to its original philosophy: to identify, strengthen, and expand effective programs that promote positive youth development and to encourage greater understanding and application of knowledge about what works for young people.

Today, the organization works in partnership with national and regional foundations, which make donations to existing programs that have already proved effective in meeting the needs of young people.

Such programs are preventive in nature and promote the confidence, character, competence, and connectedness of young people to their family, peers, and community. The programs provide a range of support and services in such areas as vocational training, health education, recreation, cultural tolerance, environmental awareness, and the development of skills in leadership, conflict resolution, and decision making.

Other efforts include increasing global awareness of children and youth issues, strengthening the organizational abilities of youth program leaders, and increasing international philanthropy in support of children and youth. Funds

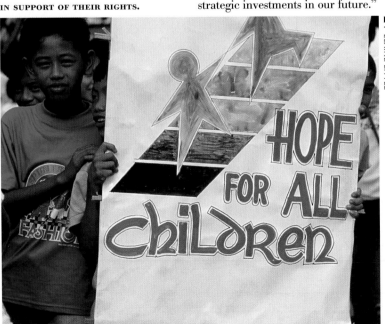

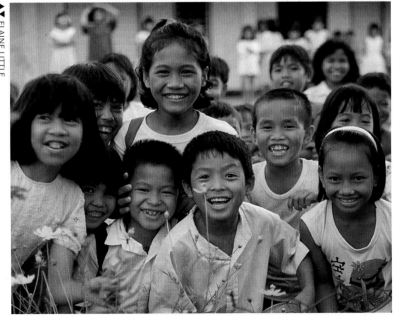

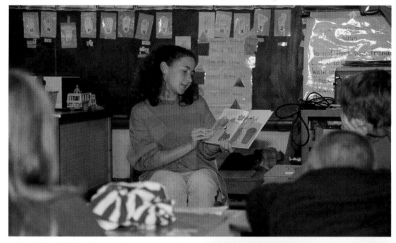

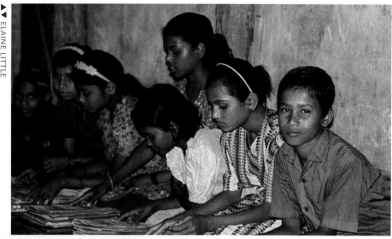

ELAINE LITTLE

raised by IYF are used on a matching basis to create challenges and incentives for donors to support its activities.

Effective Corporate Giving for Youth

IYF's original mission was to provide national and international corporate communities with links to exceptional programs in need of funding. The challenge facing IYF was this: Corporations have long had a history of aiding communities in countries in which they are based, yet they are often discouraged by the difficulty of making charitable investments outside their home countries.

Thanks to IYF, such potential donors can now make wise and strategic investments in proven youth initiatives beyond their national borders. In addition, IYF combines its funds with those of other donors to increase impact and ensure effective use. By removing these obstacles to international grant making, IYF enables donors to make a real difference.

Most of the problems that threaten young people today—poverty, illiteracy, substance abuse, unemployment, crime, and sexually transmitted diseases—respect no national boundaries. The International Youth Foundation serves as a catalyst to identify and expand efforts aimed at solving these serious concerns, as well as to create partnerships with philanthropic-minded businesses to aid in this mission.

In the United States, for instance, the Coca-Cola Valued Youth Program seeks to prevent students from dropping out of school by training them as tutors of elemen-

tary school children. The program, which operates in 40 schools across the country, successfully shows that students can be encouraged to excel if they have proper role models and support to increase self-worth.

In Brazil, a multifaceted program coordinates the activities of more than 40 organizations reaching out to 900,000 street-based children nationwide. It offers these youth services providers valuable training and education, while advocating more effective policies aimed at protecting the rights of Brazilian youth.

The Don Bosco Industrial Skills Training Program in the Philippines provides poor urban youth with vocational skills training and job placement opportunities; to date, the program has successfully placed 90 percent of its graduates each year.

And in the United Kingdom, the Prince's Youth Business Trust teaches entrepreneurial skills to young people all over Britain by combining expert advice from corporate executives with grants and investment capi-

tal. Since it began, the trust has assisted more than 33,000 young people and helped to create 60,000 jobs.

New Partnership Networks

In addition to working closely with the business community, IYF also has created a network of national foundations throughout the world. In this effort, the organization helps leaders in many countries create self-sustaining foundations that in turn identify and support the most effective local efforts. In addition, IYF provides these national foundations with matching grants to complement locally based funding. Currently, the organization has partnerships with foundations in Australia, Ecuador, Germany, Ireland, the Philippines, Poland, Slovakia, South Africa, Thailand, and the state of Oaxaca, Mexico.

Effective giving for youth is the goal: With IYF, there is now a foundation for it.

CLOCKWISE FROM TOP LEFT: A HIGH SCHOOL STUDENT IN SOUTH CAROLINA READS TO CHILDREN WITH SPECIAL LEARNING NEEDS AS A PART OF A SERVICE LEARNING CURRICULUM DESIGNED BY QUEST INTERNATIONAL, AN IYF-SUPPORTED PROGRAM. FOUNDED IN 1975, QUEST PROGRAMS IMPACT MORE THAN 1.5 MILLION YOUNG PEOPLE ANNUALLY IN 30 COUNTIES.

YOUNG PEOPLE IN RURAL BANGLADESH LEARN TO READ AND WRITE AS A RESULT OF A NONFORMAL, PRIMARY EDUCATION PROGRAM OFFERED BY THE BANGLADESH RURAL ADVANCEMENT COMMITTEE (BRAC). BRAC IS ONE OF NEARLY 150 SUCCESSFUL PROGRAMS OPERATING IN MORE THAN 30 COUNTRIES THAT HAVE BEEN IDENTIFIED BY IYF AND ITS PARTNER FOUNDATIONS AS EXAMPLES OF BEST PRACTICE.

IN POLAND, WHERE FEW RECREATIONAL AND CULTURAL OPPORTUNITIES ARE AVAILABLE TO YOUTH, NONGOVERNMENTAL ORGANIZATIONS HAVE EMERGED TO FILL THE VOID. SINCE BEING ESTABLISHED WITH SEED FUNDING FROM IYF IN 1992, THE POLISH CHILDREN AND YOUTH FOUNDATION HAS MADE MORE THAN 300 GRANTS TO NONPROFIT ORGANIZATIONS BENEFITTING OVER 800,000 YOUNG PEOPLE THROUGHOUT THE COUNTRY. ADDITIONAL INFORMATION ABOUT IYF'S WORK IS AVAILABLE ON ITS WEBSITE AT HTTP://WWW.IYFNET.ORG.

Inphomation Communications Corporation

A HIGHLY ACCLAIMED DIRECT RESPONSE MARKETER, INPHOMATION Communications Corporation brings to bear unparalleled in-house resources to create high-impact consumer campaigns that involve television infomercials, short-form television spots, national retail distribution, direct mail, space advertising, media management,

credit card syndication, back-end sales, and aftermarket distribution.

Based in Baltimore, the company is responsible for the country's most successful infomercials, including *Making Love Work* with Barbara De Angelis and *Psychic Friends Network* hosted by Dionne Warwick, which has generated more than 10 million calls since its inception in 1990. Headed by Michael Warren Lasky, a visionary in the area of direct marketing and mass retailing, Inphomation Communications stands at the forefront of electronic and mass retailing.

A highly regarded Brooklyn-born entrepreneur, Lasky began Inphomation Communications

Corporation in 1981 as a print and direct-mail organization. Based on his successful experience in direct marketing, he viewed the emerging infomercial industry as the next logical business step.

Today, Inphomation ranks among the largest and most profitable direct marketing organizations in the world, employing a staff of more than 60 in the areas of creative marketing, production, media management, product fulfillment, client relations, and administration. In addition to its Baltimore headquarters, Inphomation maintains its own fully equipped Los Angeles production operation, featuring an in-house creative team that

develops, creates, and produces many of the company's successful projects.

An Award-Winning Lineup

As the country's preeminent infomercial producer, Inphomation Communications is the only company in industry history with a 100 percent success record; the only company to simultaneously place three blockbuster hits at the top of the infomercial charts; and the only company with the longest-running, most successful infomercial ever, *Psychic Friends Network*. In addition, Inphomation Communications' *Making Love*

SHIPPING TERMINAL CONTAINER OPERATIONS AT THE PORT OF BALTIMORE

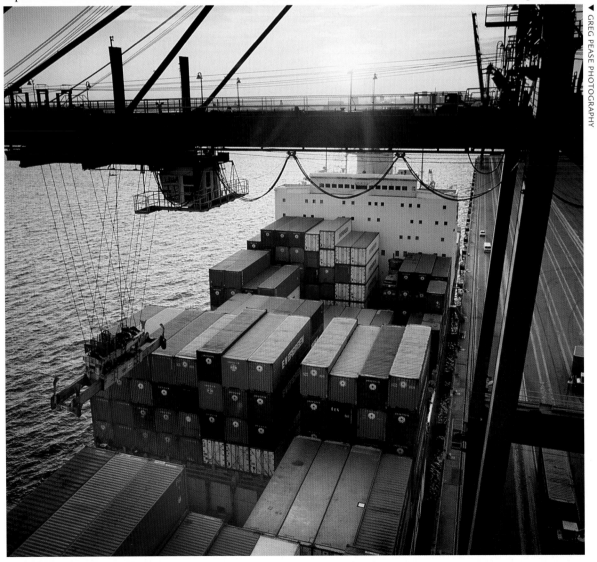

Work infomercial with Barbara De Angelis received NIMA International's 1994 Infomercial of the Year award and generated in excess of 300,000 sales. A follow-up *Making Love Work* infomercial is currently airing across the nation.

Inphomation also joined forces with angler Roland Martin for the infomercial *The Helicopter Lure*, which was launched with massive success on television and in retail. The infomercial promotes the most remarkable tackle box innovation since the invention of the hook—essential for both serious fishermen and beginners alike.

Based on the unprecedented success of *The Helicopter Lure*, Inphomation Communications launched a new infomercial television series, *The American Sportsmaster*. The new series of half-hour television infomercial programs presents Martin as host for a wide range of innovative, new products for today's fishing enthusiasts. Produced on location, Inphomation's new series will also feature such popular cohosts as country artists Mel Tillis and Jerry Clower.

Improving Baltimore's Quality of Life

Lasky's vision has not been confined, however, to his infomercial successes. In 1995, he created the Lasky Family Foundation, which has quickly established itself as a substantive contributor to its neighbors in need in the Baltimore metropolitan area. With its commitment to "improving the quality of life in the Greater Baltimore community by partnering with organizations and agencies whose goal is to serve and save our children," the foundation has worked diligently to make a difference in the future of prominent Baltimore institutions such as the Johns Hopkins Pediatric Oncology Department, Babe Ruth Museum, Baltimore Zoo, and Maryland Special Olympics.

Lasky, a father of three and grandfather of one, is deeply committed to helping lift the burdens of disease and strife from those least able to fend for themselves—the community's children. That is why the Lasky Family Foundation's

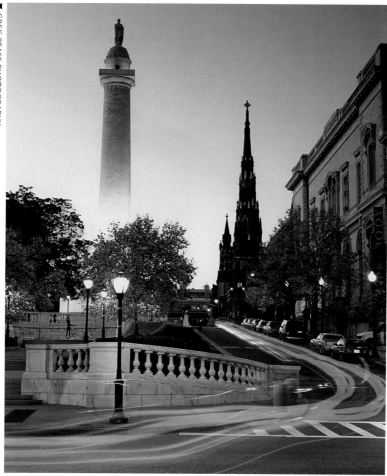

BALTIMORE'S WASHINGTON MONUMENT

largesse will continue to expand in the months and years ahead.

Pioneering the Next Century in Consumer Marketing

From direct response marketing to the world of retail distribution, Inphomation Communications has risen to become an important new supplier of products to all areas of retail distribution, representing its own products as well as those from client manufacturers.

To introduce products to retail, Inphomation Communications recently established a Short Form division to launch products for maximum consumer impact prior to the products' retail rollout. The newly formed division has already yielded the successful introduction of such products as the Magic Brush, a patented new styling tool, as well as a range of exciting new products currently in development.

Recently, Inphomation also moved into the broadcast syndication arena with the production of the television series *The Love Psychic*. Merrill Heatter, the four-time Emmy-award-winning producer

responsible for more than 25 game show series, including *Hollywood Squares*, has joined forces with Inphomation to produce the first-run weekly half-hour relationship game show that stars popular psychic Linda Georgian.

After achieving tremendous success in the domestic marketplace as a leader in the burgeoning infomercial industry, Inphomation has entered the international television arena as a producer and packager of infomercial programming. Inphomation began its international foray by adapting its infomercial blockbuster *Psychic Friends Network* for broadcast in Canada and major European markets. The company is applying its extensive direct marketing experience and resources to territories throughout the world, introducing direct marketing systems across Europe.

A recognized leader in all areas of television and print direct response, and a trendsetter in all areas of mass retail, Inphomation Communications is helping to pave the way for the next century in consumer marketing.

CIENA Corporation

HUNDREDS OF JOBS HAVE OPENED UP IN THE BALTIMORE AREA AS THE result of the growth of CIENA Corporation. CIENA has developed a unique technology that can expand the capabilities of the global information superhighway. ❧ CIENA first came to market in 1996 with a product called the MultiWave™ 1600, which allows

telephone companies to transmit 16 times the amount of information that they previously had been able to send over one optical fiber by using a process known as dense wavelength division multiplexing (DWDM). The system got the attention of major carriers Sprint and WorldCom, which now are aggressively installing it into their networks.

CIENA also got Wall Street's attention in a major way. In 1997, CIENA completed an initial public offering that achieved a $3.44 billion valuation overnight, making it the largest stock sale by a start-up company in history, and zooming CIENA up the ladder of corporations to be taken seriously in the Baltimore area.

Not one to rest on its laurels, CIENA also has gained important recognition throughout the world. The company already is selling its products to major telecommunications carriers in Japan, Teleway Japan Corp. and Japan Telecom, and to Cable & Wireless in the United Kingdom.

Because of its early start and the superior capabilities of its system, CIENA has become the worldwide leader in the field deployment of open architecture DWDM systems. These systems are becoming an integral part of the global information superhighway.

The Baltimore connection is well in place. CIENA has corporate headquarters in Linthicum and manufacturing facilities in both Linthicum and Savage. It has brought a strong telecommunications presence to the region's high-tech corridor.

Meeting the Challenge

CIENA was founded in 1992. Its goal was to provide products and systems that would help people better communicate as the demand for capacity along telephone lines expanded. Increased demand largely has been the result of people becoming more

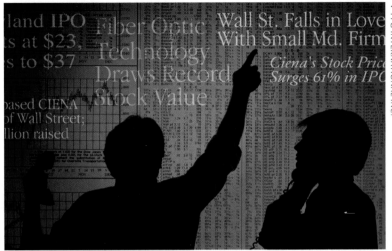

▼ FPG INTERNATIONAL INC.

CIENA CORPORATION RAISED $115 MILLION AS PART OF ITS INITIAL PUBLIC OFFERING ON FEBRUARY 7, 1997, GIVING THE COMPANY A TOTAL VALUATION OF $3.4 BILLION AND LAUNCHING IT INTO THE FORTUNE 500.

PRESIDENT AND CEO PATRICK NETTLES SHOWS OFF A GIFT PRESENTED TO THE COMPANY AS IT FORMALLY OPENED NEW CORPORATE AND MANUFACTURING OFFICES IN LINTHICUM ON JUNE 25, 1997.

productive and learning how to effectively communicate, using such tools as the Internet, fax machines, and videoconferencing.

CIENA's challenge was to create a technology to provide a path for this information growth, using existing telephone lines and, thereby, avoiding the vastly more expensive approach of laying additional lines. In the past, increased capacity had simply involved making the lasers pulse at faster speeds to send more information. However, this method was limited, and researchers were encountering problems with the lasers at higher speeds and with the older fiber that had to carry the increased number of pulses the lasers were producing.

Enter CIENA and DWDM.

The *Wall Street Journal* describes DWDM this way: "The technique is roughly equivalent to using a bundle of flashlights, each with a different colored light, in place of a single flashlight, to transmit data through fiber-optic networks. Each color can carry a stream of information that does not interfere with the streams of other colors."

Each of these streams of light represents tens of thousands of bits of information that then are decoded back into telephone conversations, data, or video. A fiber pair can accommodate 32,000 telephone conversations simultaneously with a standard system. With CIENA's product, more than 768,000 telephone calls can

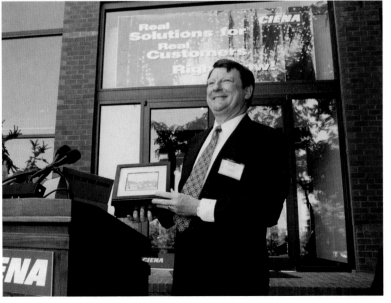

run at the same time on a fiber pair.

These solutions enable carriers to expand fiber bandwidth, improve network reliability, and significantly reduce the cost of providing new broadband services. Working with existing networks of new fiber installations, CIENA's system enables the flexible provisioning of additional bandwidth, without requiring an upgrade of existing network transmission equipment.

CIENA's early success came from a mixture of talents. David Huber provided much of the vision; Patrick Nettles supplied the business experience; John Bayless, as head of venture capital company Sevin Rosen Funds, provided the venture capital; Steve Chaddick headed up product engineering; and Lawrence Huang cemented the first critical customer accounts. Of those principals, Nettles remains as president and CEO; Bayless continues as chairman; Chaddick is senior vice president for products and technologies; and Huang is senior vice president for sales and marketing.

Global Presence

From the time of its founding, CIENA has successfully established a global leadership position for its family of fiber-optic bandwidth solutions. The primary product has been the MultiWave 1600 DWDM system, which increases capacity up to 40 billion bits per second and only requires signal boosts every 120 kilometers. This product already is in its second

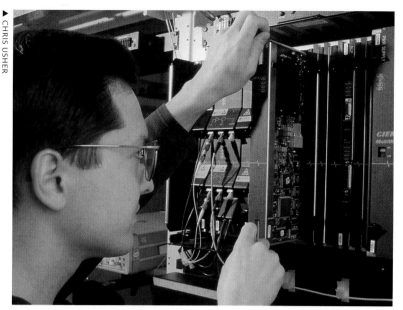

generation, with introduction of the improved MultiWave Sentry™ system.

CIENA's first and largest customer is Sprint, the global telecommunications carrier that has been using the advantages of fiber optics for more than a decade. Sprint is at the forefront in integrating long-distance local and wireless communications services.

Cable & Wireless Communications expects to use CIENA's system to send and receive messages along its U.K. terminus to a transatlantic fiber-optic route.

In its efforts to broaden company product lines, CIENA is introducing three additions to its Multi-Wave 1600 innovation. These include a 40-channel terminal, which will have the effect of hooking 40 lasers up to the same fiber; an optical add-drop multiplexer, which allows customers to terminate individual

signals at various locations; and a network manager system.

Local Commitment

While CIENA is focused on strengthening its role as a worldwide leader in the telecommunications industry, it also is committed to its presence in Baltimore. In a very short period of time, CIENA has become one of the fastest-growing employers in the state of Maryland, increasing its work base by an amazing 600 percent in the last year.

CIENA develops systems to unlock fiber bandwidth, improve network reliability, and significantly reduce the cost of providing new broadband services. It is providing real-life solutions to combat the emerging bandwidth and capacity needs telephone companies are facing now, and will continue to be challenged by in the future.

CLOCKWISE FROM TOP:
THOMAS SATO, A CIENA CORPORATION FIELD DEPLOYMENT TECHNICIAN, CHECKS OUT A MULTIWAVE DENSE WAVELENGTH DIVISION MULTIPLEXING SYSTEM PRIOR TO SHIPMENT.

ONE ELEMENT OF CIENA'S MANUFACTURING OPERATIONS INCLUDES CIRCUIT BOARD ASSEMBLY. A MANUFACTURING EMPLOYEE SOLDERS A COMPONENT ONTO ONE OF THESE BOARDS.

ERICA JONES IS A FIBER-OPTIC ASSEMBLER IN CIENA'S GROWING MANUFACTURING OPERATIONS. THE COMPANY CURRENTLY HAS MANUFACTURING OPERATIONS IN BOTH LINTHICUM AND SAVAGE.

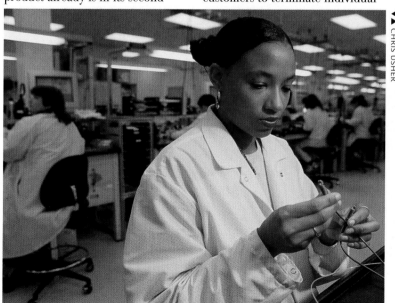

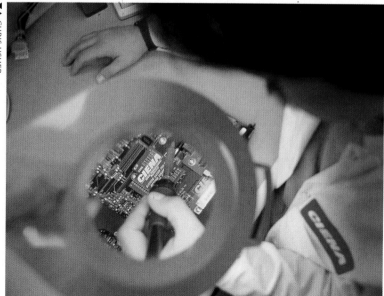

NationsBank Corporation

NATIONSBANK IS KNOWN FOR ITS COMMITMENT TO DOING BUSINESS IN all sectors of the communities it serves. In Baltimore, the bank's customers enjoy the most extensive selection of banking centers, ATM locations, PC banking, and telephone banking choices. "Our customers tell us that convenience and value are their top priorities,"

says NationsBank President Bill Couper. "We realize that customers want to bank in ways that make sense for their lifestyles. Everyone—parents, students, business owners—is trying to make the best use of their time."

Financial Partner

To serve customers better, NationsBank organized itself into three major customer groups: the General Bank, the Institutional Group, and Financial Services. The General Bank is a franchise of more than 3,000 banking centers and commercial banking offices in 16 states and the District of Columbia. The Institutional Group acts as a leading provider of credit, investment banking, capital markets, and specialized financial services to larger domestic and international corporations and institutions. And the Financial Services group specializes in corporate finance, commercial real estate, project finance, capital assets, business inventory financing, and consumer credit. Through its affiliates, NationsBank customers gain access to a wide range of investment products designed to meet their needs.

Neighbor

Many customers first get to know NationsBank by visiting a banking center, talking to friends about their bank, or viewing the bank's Web site at www.nationsbank.com. Then they notice the convenient locations. At major professional sporting and cultural events, they see that NationsBank invests in and advertises locally at games, exhibits, civic festivals, and affordable housing programs. They realize that one of the largest financial services companies in the United States can offer them a great many options.

Naturally, the bank's most valuable resource is its people. Helpful associates, experienced lenders, and skillful managers welcome the opportunity to provide solutions and tools to make dreams attainable.

Associates are equally committed to their families, friends, and

THROUGH VOLUNTEERING, NATIONSBANK ASSOCIATES BUILD PLAYGROUNDS, CREATE AFFORDABLE HOMES, AND STRENGTHEN HEALTH AND HUMAN SERVICES PROGRAMS.

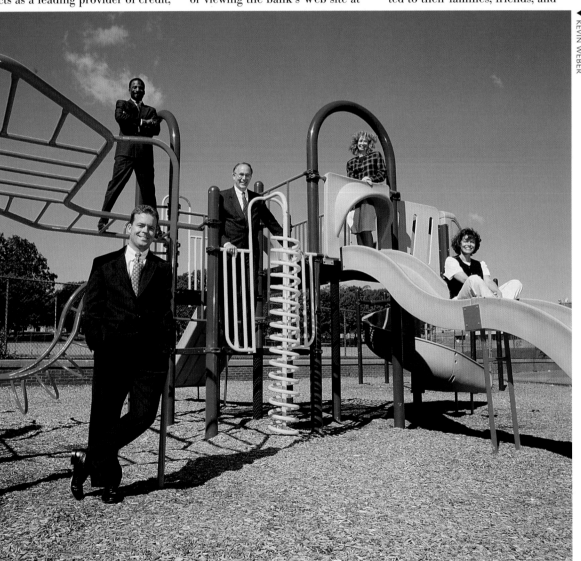

◀ KEVIN WEBER

neighbors. They volunteer their time and talents at more than 100 nonprofit or civic organizations in Greater Baltimore, including Habitat for Humanity. They create playgrounds, raise funds for medical research, coordinate the NationsBank Volunteer Council, and lead the community's United Way campaign. They are lending their hands to make the future brighter for people from all walks of life.

Connector

Entrepreneurs looking for ways to launch or expand their businesses discover that NationsBank has a whole division dedicated to helping small-business owners. And because the bank is a Small Business Administration Preferred Lender, results with SBA loans are just what busy people need: shorter loan applications, competitive rates, lower down payments, and longer repayment terms.

As a cosponsor of the Small Business Resource Center in down-town Baltimore, NationsBank helps people from all over Maryland gain access to free business information. Retired executives from public and private companies are happy to consult just once—or many times—with goal-oriented entrepreneurs.

"We believe the most critical and lasting contribution we can make is to enable the region to grow economically," says Couper. "This means not only attracting employers and helping to create jobs, but also contributing to organizations that enhance the infrastructure and quality of life in the Baltimore region."

NationsBank actively invests in institutions of higher education and education-related programs, and it supports key health and human services organizations in the area. In addition to investing in the region's significant cultural institutions and landmarks, the bank sponsors major sports franchises in its marketplace.

Another way to help the region grow is by investing in affordable housing developments, small businesses, and specialized financial institutions. Through these neighborhood development initiatives, NationsBank revitalizes low- and moderate-income neighborhoods.

Through affordable mortgage programs and special mortgage products, NationsBank provides home mortgage and home improvement lending to qualified applicants of all income levels and races.

Employer

NationsBank is one of America's best companies for working parents, as determined by *Working Mother* magazine. For the fifth consecutive year, NationsBank has been named to the publication's list of Top 10 Companies for Working Mothers. The list spotlights outstanding work environments for women and tracks workplace trends relating to families.

BALTIMORE'S SMALL BUSINESS RESOURCE CENTER OFFERS A WEALTH OF FREE INFORMATION, AND IS CO-SPONSORED BY NATIONSBANK, THE U.S. DEPARTMENT OF COMMERCE, THE SMALL BUSINESS ADMINISTRATION, AND BELL ATLANTIC.

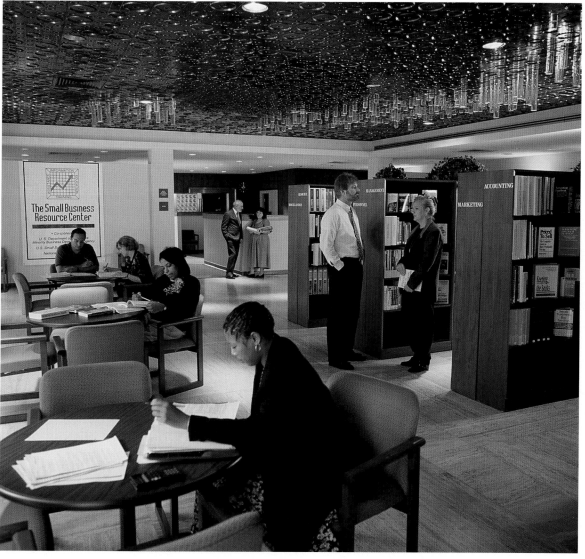

Guilford Pharmaceuticals Inc.

GUILFORD PHARMACEUTICALS INC. IS A BIOPHARMACEUTICAL COMPANY engaged in the development of novel products in two principal areas: targeted and controlled polymer-based drug delivery products for the treatment of cancer and other diseases, and novel therapeutic and diagnostic products for neurological disorders. ❧ Guilford's mission is to become a world leader in the discovery and development of novel pharmaceutical products for the purpose of improving human health and enhancing quality of life. A publicly traded company (NASDAQ: GLFD), Guilford Pharmaceuticals pursues innovation, fosters creativity, and vigorously supports research to better understand human biology; disease pathogenesis; and the pharmacology, safety, and effectiveness of its products.

CRAIG R. SMITH, CHAIRMAN, PRESIDENT, AND CEO, FOUNDED GUILFORD PHARMACEUTICALS INC. IN 1993 (RIGHT).

THE GLIADEL® WAFER, DEVELOPED BY GUILFORD, IS THE FIRST NEW TREATMENT FOR BRAIN CANCER IN 20 YEARS AND DELIVERS HIGH CONCENTRATIONS OF A CANCER CHEMOTHERAPEUTIC AGENT DIRECTLY TO THE TUMOR SITE FOLLOWING THE SURGICAL REMOVAL OF THE TUMOR (BELOW).

Innovative Research and Drug Discovery

Craig R. Smith, chairman, president, and CEO, founded Guilford Pharmaceuticals Inc. in 1993. The company now occupies 83,000 square feet of office and laboratory space, accommodating more than 180 highly skilled employees.

In its relatively short existence, Guilford has already made several medical breakthroughs. GLIADEL®, the company's treatment for brain cancer, is the first new treatment for this disease in 20 years. GLIADEL is a small, white polymer wafer that is implanted in the cavity created when a neurosurgeon removes a cancerous tumor from the brain. The wafer gradually degrades, much like a bar of soap, and delivers BCNU, a cancer chemotherapeutic agent, directly to the tumor site in high concentrations for an extended period of time without exposing the rest of the body to toxic side effects. GLIADEL is marketed throughout the United States by Rhône-Poulenc Rorer Inc.

The targeted treatment of cancer with polymer-based products may be important for cancers other than brain cancer as a treatment for tumor recurrence after surgical resection. Guilford plans to develop its polymer technology with a variety of chemotherapeutic agents for possible applications in the targeted treatment of cancers such as ovarian, breast, head and neck, lung, esophageal, hepatic, pancreatic, and colon, among others. Preliminary research and development work is proceeding with taxoid compounds, including paclitaxel.

DOPASCAN® is a diagnostic test under development by Guilford to treat Parkinson's disease, one of the most common and debilitating neurodegenerative conditions. It is estimated that about 800,000 people in the United States suffer from Parkinson's disease, a disorder resulting from the loss of dopamine neurons in the area of the brain that controls muscle tone and movement.

An intravenous injection of DOPASCAN is followed 12 to 24 hours later by the acquisition of images by brain scanning equipment. If degeneration of neurons has occurred, the uptake of DOPASCAN is reduced.

Clinical trials of the drug have demonstrated that DOPASCAN can differentiate patients with Parkinson's disease from those without the disease, thus enabling more appropriate decisions regarding drug therapy—particularly earlier initiation of therapy with neuroprotective agents in confirmed cases of Parkinson's. It could also help avoid unnecessary drug therapy in non-Parkinson's cases, thereby avoiding the costs and side effects of inappropriate drug use. DOPASCAN has been licensed to—and is being developed by—Daiichi Radioisotope Laboratories for Japan, Korea, and Taiwan.

Neurotrophic Drugs

Guilford Pharmaceuticals is developing novel drugs to promote nerve regeneration and repair, called neuroimmunophilin ligands, for the treatment of neurodegenerative disorders. The degeneration of nerve cells in the brain resulting from certain diseases and conditions can cause a loss of either central nervous system function (as in

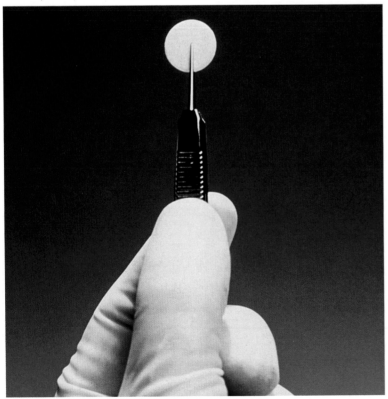

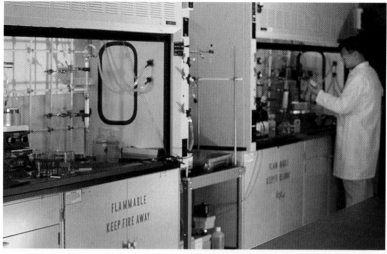

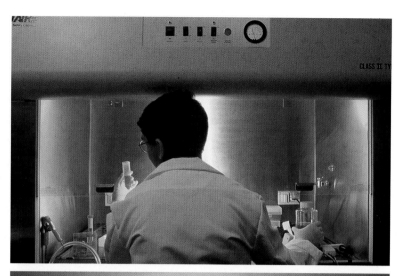

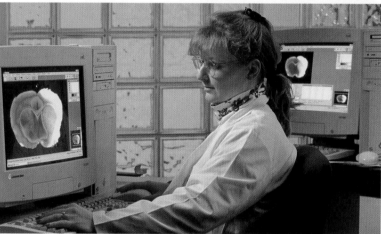

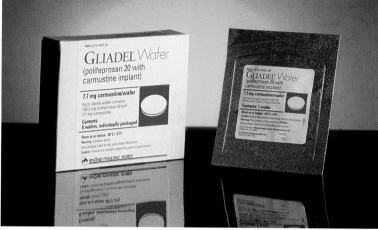

Alzheimer's or Parkinson's disease) or peripheral nerve function (such as in peripheral neuropathies). Under normal circumstances, damaged nerves have a very limited ability to regrow, which poses a major obstacle for the treatment of these conditions.

On August 21, 1997, Guilford and Amgen announced that they have entered into an agreement granting Amgen worldwide rights for Guilford's FKBP-neuroimmunophilin ligands for all human therapeutic and diagnostic applications. Amgen will conduct and pay for all clinical development and manufacturing of products, and will market the products worldwide.

Neuroprotective Drugs

Guilford also is developing novel compounds to protect brain cells against damage from two types of ischemia. Focal ischemia is the temporary loss of blood flow to a localized region of the brain that usually occurs during a stroke, and global ischemia is temporary loss of blood flow to the entire brain that occurs during cardiac arrest.

Guilford is developing neuroprotective compounds in three programs: compounds that prevent the presynaptic release of glutamate (NAALADase inhibitors); compounds that inhibit PARP, an intracellular enzyme that is increased during stroke; and compounds that inhibit NOS, another intracellular enzyme that is elevated during stroke.

Guilford scientists have discovered a new mechanism of action that can modulate presynaptic glutamate release, based on inhibition of the enzyme NAALADase. Guilford has synthesized and filed a number of patent applications on proprietary compounds and uses of this novel method of intervention. In experimental animal models of stroke, the prototype NAALADase inhibitor compound GPI-5000 has demonstrated an 80 percent neuroprotective effect. Preventing glutamate release presynaptically is distinguished from other approaches of blocking glutamate uptake postsynaptically, and may be a more effective or safer means of achieving a neuroprotective effect in stroke and other neurodegenerative disorders.

NAALADase inhibitors are also being investigated for potential utility in other disorders believed to be mediated by excessive release of glutamate, including amyotrophic lateral sclerosis (ALS)—commonly known as Lou Gherig's Disease—epilepsy, Parkinson's Disease, Huntington's Disease, traumatic head and spinal cord injuries, peripheral neuropathies (such as diabetic neuropathy), and schizophrenia. Animal studies conducted in a number of these disorders have demonstrated positive and encouraging results to date.

Guilford is also developing therapeutics for cocaine addiction and other addictive behavior. The goal of the venture is to identify and develop selective cocaine antagonists that can be used in the treatment of cocaine addiction.

Faced with the challenges of serious diseases with no current effective treatments, Guilford has carved a niche in discovering and commercializing improved therapeutics and diagnostics for cancers and serious neurological diseases.

GUILFORD PHARMACEUTICALS OCCUPIES 83,000 SQUARE FEET OF OFFICE AND LABORATORY SPACE, ACCOMMODATING MORE THAN 180 HIGHLY SKILLED EMPLOYEES.

Systems Alliance Inc.

SYSTEMS ALLIANCE INC., HEADQUARTERED IN HUNT VALLEY, WAS FOUNDED IN 1993 as a high-profile information systems services company, providing professional service and integrated solutions to organizations and companies throughout the Mid-Atlantic region. ❧ Khosrow Golshan and Michael Jakubik formed the company to primarily address the

consulting needs of clients using traditional mainframe technology.

But Systems Alliance has evolved and expanded. Working with its clients to successfully manage their transitions to advanced network computing platforms, Systems Alliance develops sound migration strategies, designing and implementing effective solutions, and providing efficient follow-up and technical support.

Delivering Comprehensive Solutions

Systems Alliance provides quality services in four distinct areas. Through its application development division, skilled personnel offer client/server services in areas of project management, system design, graphical user interface development, HTML, and intranet/Internet, among others. In addition, consultants also handle a range of mainframe services, including project management, year 2000 support, system design, and application development.

Networking services, currently in great demand, include network infrastructure design and support, network management, Internet, intranet, installation, service contracts, and mainframe system integration. A third division, help desk services, provides customers with technical support on matters ranging from the simple to the complex.

A fourth division, one that Systems Alliance is expanding, is training and education, which includes year 2000 support, system design, client/server concepts, application development, Web page design, databases, and operating systems. In addition, this division organizes and oversees on-site training programs for clients who wish to become more familiar with technology.

"With our technical expertise, our positioning has always been

to serve clients as an extension of their organization," Golshan says. "This helps them maintain a technical edge in today's competitive business environment. We are able to develop, support, and manage mainframe systems, network infrastructure, and business applications, as well as provide hands-on education and training."

Marrying Service and Expertise

Systems Alliance holds high levels of authorization for Novell and Microsoft, the two major network operating system vendors in the marketplace. Within these two systems, company experts are adept at solving complex integration problems across a variety of software and hardware platforms, operating systems, and equipment, including Windows NT & Back Office, OS/2, LAN Manager, Netware, UNIX, VMS, TCP/IP, and high-speed disk design.

For many Systems Alliance clients, these unfamiliar phrases seem like an incomprehensible foreign language. That's why high-quality customer service is an integral component for Systems Alliance.

"Our strength has always been in the quality of our people," Jakubik

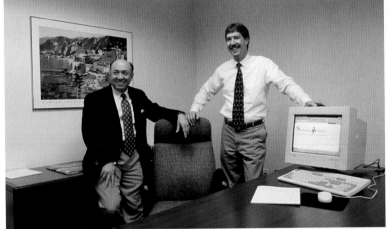

ROGER MILLER

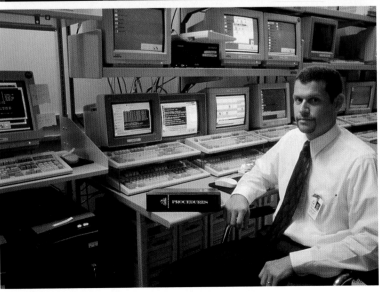

ROGER MILLER

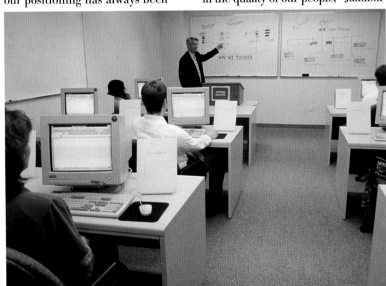

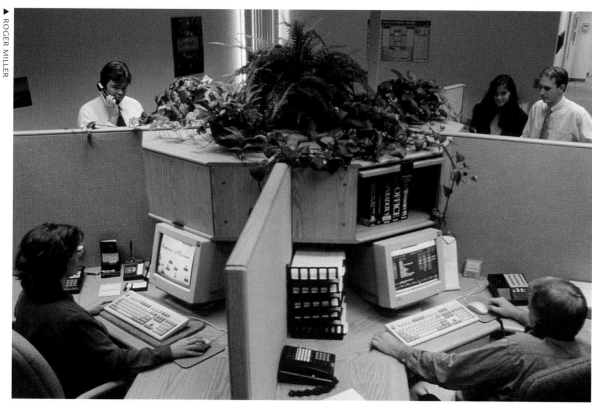

THE HELP DESK FACILITIES FOR SWEETHEART CUP AND NIRO INC. ARE LOCATED AT SYSTEMS ALLIANCE.

says. "We regard our mission as one that focuses both on leading-edge expertise and a stimulating and rewarding one-on-one business relationship with our clients. That commitment to service transforms us from a mere service provider to a strategic business partner."

Systems Alliance's training mission is as important as any other service it offers. Explains Golshan, "Many organizations are now realizing the critical importance of education as they make the transition to the client/server environment. What we provide is a skills framework for client/server technology with a series of challenging, product-independent courses for both network platforms and client/server applications."

The company's training programs fall into two categories: technical workshops, which are aimed at certified netware engineers and Microsoft certified systems engineers, and fundamental skills training, which is designed to maximize the benefits and minimize the risks of client/server migration.

Specialized workshops focus specifically on employees in the fields of business management, technical management, and technical staff. For instance, business

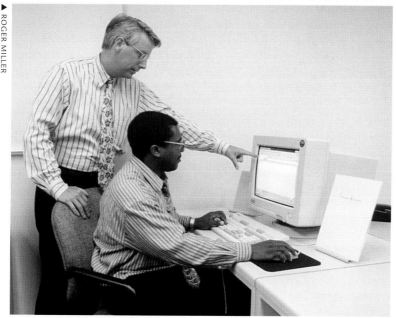

manager training involves executive-level seminars that illustrate the importance of information technology, as well as providing more practical lessons on client/server fundamentals and business process reengineering. For technical managers, training focuses on business aspects of networking projects that give participants an overall perspective on the work they do. And because the nuts and bolts of most information technology projects remain with the technical staff, this group receives a sound foundation in specific prod-

ucts that will be used in system implementation—along with course offerings in advance network programming and development methodologies.

In 1996, in response to a growing number of clients in the Baltimore/Washington, D.C., high-tech corridor, Systems Alliance opened a second office in Rockville, Maryland. Today, with more than 60 employees, Systems Alliance looks forward to continued success in developing and marketing its expertise in the ever changing computer systems industry.

VICE PRESIDENT OF OPERATIONS SCOTT BELT (LEFT) INSTRUCTS A STUDENT AT SYSTEMS ALLIANCE'S IN-HOUSE TRAINING FACILITY.

The Annie E. Casey Foundation

A PRIVATE, CHARITABLE ORGANIZATION, THE ANNIE E. CASEY FOUNDATION has a treasured history of helping to build better futures for disadvantaged children in the United States. In 1994, the foundation selected Baltimore as its national headquarters, honoring the city by making it a part of the foundation's mission. ᕲ "In relocating our

corporate headquarters," says Douglas W. Nelson, president of the Casey Foundation, "we were looking for an affordable place to do business, a range of housing and community choices for our staff, and an environment that was relevant to the urban focus of much of our work."

Already, the foundation has granted more than $20.7 million in support to the city and state in areas ranging from an initiative to help Maryland reform its child welfare system to supporting a Johns Hopkins University study of a model childhood immunization project. Through its Direct Services Grants Program, the foundation has awarded grants to more than 69 community-based organizations that directly serve children and families in Baltimore. In addition, the foundation's New England-based direct services arm, Casey Family Services, which provides a comprehensive range of services to disadvantaged children, has just opened its eighth division in Baltimore.

"Baltimore is more than an investment site for Casey," Nelson says. "It is our home. Being good corporate citizens means encouraging this city to flourish and grow."

A Philosophy for Modern Times

The mission of the Casey Foundation is to foster public policies, human service reforms, and community efforts that more effectively meet the needs of today's children and families. The foundation makes grants that help states, cities, and communities fashion innovative, cost-effective responses to these needs. The foundation currently supports one or more projects in each of the 50 states and the District of Columbia.

The Casey Foundation was established in 1948 by Jim Casey, one of the founders of United Parcel Service, and his siblings, George, Harry, and Marguerite. They named the organization in honor of their mother.

Today, the Casey Foundation has more than 60 employees and annual grant budgets that exceed $93 million. Major initiatives include KIDS COUNT—the organization's flagship program—a national and state-by-state effort to track the economic, social, and physical well-being of children in the United States. The annual *KIDS COUNT Data Book* provides policy makers and citizens with benchmarks to measure the welfare of children.

It also is used to enrich local, state, and national discussions concerning the condition of youngsters.

Other important programs include Assessing the New Federalism, an Urban Institute project that tracks changing social policies; Family to Family: Reconstructing Foster Care, which supports the efforts of states to redesign systems of foster care; and Plain Talk, a neighborhood-based initiative aimed at helping adults, parents, and community leaders communicate more effectively with sexually active young people to protect them from pregnancy and sexually transmitted diseases.

The foundation also is involved in mental health initiatives, education reform, programs for juvenile offenders, projects to rebuild communities and link disadvantaged young adults with good jobs, and system reform efforts at the state and local levels.

Over the coming years, the Casey Foundation will devote increasing resources to demonstrating that distressed neighborhoods can become family-enhancing communities. With youth as its priority, the organization will continue to strengthen America's very foundation.

AMONG THE COMMUNITY-BASED ORGANIZATIONS THAT HAVE RECEIVED GRANTS FROM THE ANNIE E. CASEY FOUNDATION ARE THE BABE RUTH BIRTHPLACE FOUNDATION (LEFT), WHICH ENABLES YOUTH TO PLAY LITTLE LEAGUE BASEBALL WHILE DEVELOPING LEADERSHIP AND OTHER SKILLS, AND THE NEW SONG COMMUNITY LEARNING CENTER (RIGHT), WHICH PARTNERS WITH PARENTS TO DEVELOP THE LITERACY SKILLS OF THEIR PRESCHOOL CHILDREN.

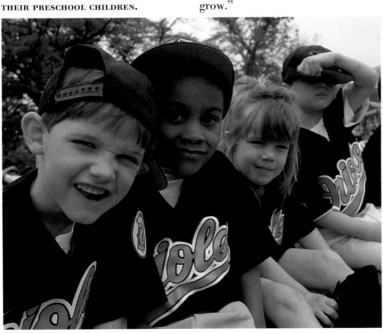

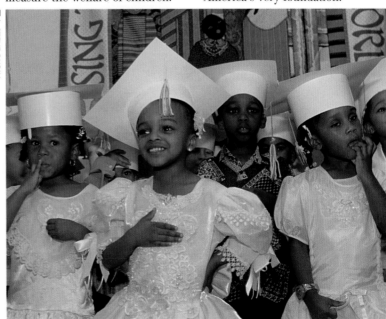

▲ STEVE RUBIN

Avesta Sheffield East Inc.

AVESTA SHEFFIELD HAS BEEN MAKING STAINLESS STEEL SINCE IT WAS invented for the production of fine cutlery in Sheffield, England, and since it was first mass-produced in Avesta, Sweden. Even today, Avesta Sheffield is one of the world's leading suppliers of stainless steel, with an extensive range of products and a well-developed marketing and distribution network.

In March 1995, Avesta Sheffield acquired Eastern Stainless Corp., a stainless steel plate producer in Baltimore, from Armco Inc. of Pittsburgh. The Baltimore facility—which has been producing steel for various companies since 1919—now gives Avesta's North American Division a melting shop and facilities for the production of CPP (continuously produced plate).

The melting shop, which consists of a 50-ton electric arc furnace, a 50-ton AOD, and a continuous caster, has an annual capacity of 150,000 tons. A new CPP line, adopted at the beginning of 1996, allows the facility to process coil weighing up to 25 tons into CPP material measuring up to 2,000 millimeters in width and 15.8 millimeters in thickness.

A Commitment to Baltimore

At the time of the Baltimore acquisition, Avesta Sheffield promised the state of Maryland it would implement extensive measures for improving the environment in and around the facility. These measures, which include flue, gas, and water purification, among other things, were implemented during 1996 at a cost of around $14 million.

According to Michael Rinker, president of the North American Division, "The acquisition of Baltimore was confirmation of Avesta Sheffield's commitment to North America as its third home market. We wanted to continue to grow our business here. That would be accomplished primarily through further investment in local production. We will continue to import products, but we want to be thought of as a local producer, and we'll continue to invest heavily in the facilities that we have in North America."

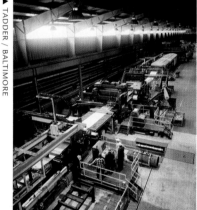

▶ TADDER / BALTIMORE

Besides its Baltimore facility, Avesta Sheffield operates a stainless plate mill in New Castle, Indiana; a stainless pipe and tube mill in Wildwood, Florida; and a stainless bar joint production venture with Teledyne Allvac in Richburg, South Carolina.

Long-Term Growth

Stainless steel is a material with considerable potential for development. During the past few decades, demand has grown at a rate of 4 to 5 percent annually—much higher than the growth rate for carbon steel. This trend is expected to continue as new applications for stainless steel are developed in fields such as environmental protection, hygiene, and construction. New markets and applications provide new opportunities for the profitable sale of Avesta Sheffield stainless steel as the company continues to intensify its focus on products with a high degree of added value and profitability. The company's financial and broad geographical strengths give Avesta Sheffield a sound foundation from which to achieve its goal of becoming the world's leading supplier of stainless steel.

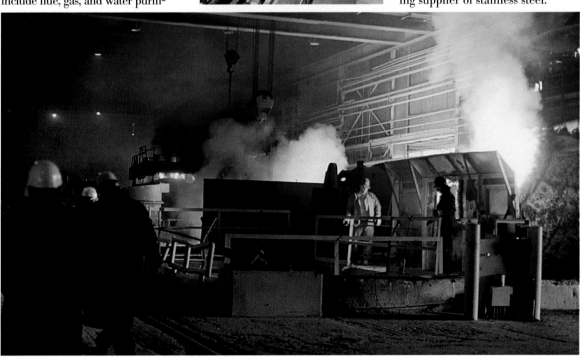

▶ TADDER / BALTIMORE

AVESTA SHEFFIELD'S NEW CCP LINE ALLOWS THE FACILITY TO PROCESS COIL WEIGHING UP TO 25 TONS INTO CCP MATERIAL MEASURING UP TO 2,000 MILLIMETERS IN WIDTH AND 15.8 MILLIMETERS IN THICKNESS (TOP).

THE MELTING SHOP, WHICH CONSISTS OF A 50-TON ELECTRIC ARC FURNACE, A 50-TON AOD, AND A CONTINUOUS CASTER, HAS AN ANNUAL CAPACITY OF 150,000 TONS (BOTTOM).

Treasure Chest Advertising

AS THE NATION'S LEADING PRODUCER OF ADVERTISING INSERT PROGRAMS and circulation-building newspaper supplements such as Sunday comics, Sunday magazines, television listing guides, and special supplements, Treasure Chest Advertising (TC Advertising) is committed to one basic principle: helping customers achieve success. "We under-stand that today's intensely competitive marketplace requires our customers to continually explore innovations that enhance business, increase profits, and contribute to growth," says Donald E. Roland, president and chief executive officer. "Helping our customers succeed is our definition of customer service."

TC Advertising provides compelling, cost-efficient products and high-impact advertising solutions to 300 of the largest-circulation newspapers in the United States and nearly 700 leading regional and national retailers. The company produces more than 22 billion advertising inserts annually for retail customers, and it is America's largest producer of Sunday comics and television magazines.

In addition to providing printing services for major retailers and newspapers, the company has expanded to offer consumer and media research, targeted direct mail services, electronic prepress, transportation, and Internet solutions.

The Rise to the Top

Founded in California in 1967 by Robert and Paul Milhous, Treasure Chest Advertising began as a small, weekly shopper called the *Treasure Chest of Values*. Bob Milhous, a onetime ad salesperson for yellow pages telephone directories, was an ardent believer in the power of print advertising. In an effort to expand his company, he purchased his own printing press and began selling ad circulars. Committed to providing solutions to its retail customers, TC Advertising was a pioneer in the advertising insert industry.

In 1993, R. Theodore Ammon founded Big Flower Press with a vision to develop a company that could provide advertising solutions for its customers. The first acquisition made by Big Flower Press was TC Advertising in August 1993. In the years since, TC Advertising, which now has 4,500 employees, has experienced dramatic growth. As a subsidiary of Big Flower, a $1.4 billion company, TC Advertising has benefited from synergies with affiliated companies Webcraft Technologies and Laser Tech Color. Webcraft Technologies is America's market leader in highly targeted, personalized direct mail. Laser Tech Color is the industry leader in outsourced digital prepress, content management, and Web site services. The coordination between the companies, coupled with TC Advertising's customer knowledge, leads to successful advertising solutions.

A Wide Scope of Capabilities

TC Advertising has long understood the importance of insert advertising. "It's a medium," Roland explains, "that attracts the eye of three-quarters of newspaper readers and helps 50 percent of those readers make specific purchase decisions." Until recently, images for advertising inserts were provided by conventional cameras, but with the advent of digital imaging, TC Advertising can provide digital photography for its clients that can be used in weekly advertising inserts, as well

CLOCKWISE FROM BOTTOM RIGHT: WITH A WORKFORCE OF MORE THAN 4,500, TC ADVERTISING'S INDUSTRY EXPERTS WORK IN PARTNERSHIP WITH CUSTOMERS FROM CONCEPTION TO COMPLETION—DEVELOPING, PRODUCING, AND DISTRIBUTING THE MOST INNOVATIVE, COMPELLING, AND COST EFFECTIVE ADVERTISING PROGRAMS.

TC ADVERTISING IS THE LEADING PRODUCER OF NEWSPAPER COLOR COMICS, PRINTING 48 PERCENT OF THE NATION'S SUNDAY COMICS.

TC ADVERTISING'S CORPORATE HEADQUARTERS, LOCATED IN BALTIMORE'S INNER HARBOR SINCE 1995, OFFER EASY ACCESSIBILITY TO ITS CUSTOMERS AND PRODUCTION FACILITIES.

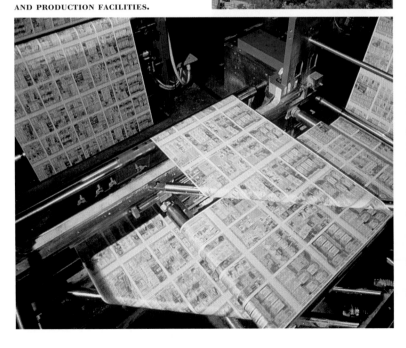

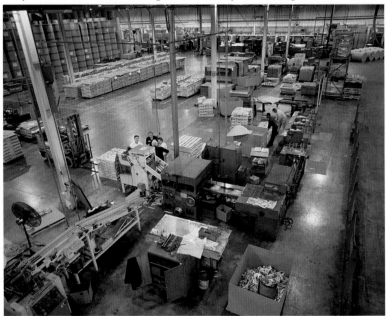

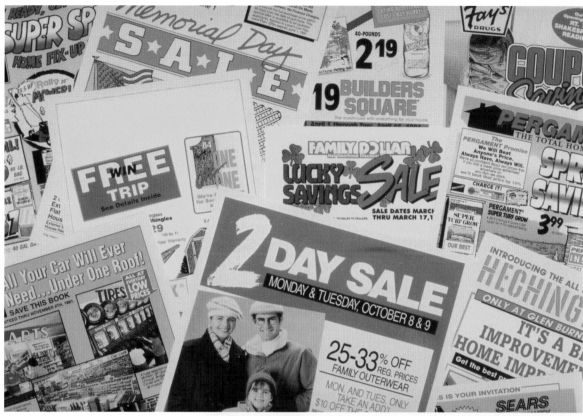

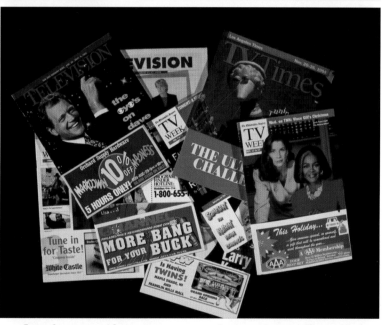

as for daily newspaper ads, direct mail, catalogs, signage, and Web pages. This new capability maximizes content management efficiency while offering enhanced flexibility.

New advances in technology also have expanded target marketing capabilities. "Today, you can do so much more with an advertising image," Roland says. "You can produce numerous versions of inserts, customer-focused direct mail, and Internet Web pages." These new possibilities allow the advertiser's message to be spread to a wider variety of consumers. For example, TC Advertising helped a major supermarket chain—with stores in ethnically diverse metropolitan areas—create ad inserts for a broad-based population, as well as for specific Hispanic and Vietnamese communities.

New Facilities, New Services

TC Advertising recognizes that fulfilling customer needs requires more than technology; it requires attention to such details as convenience and efficiency. The company's corporate headquarters, located in Baltimore's Inner Harbor since 1995, was selected with convenience in mind. The Mid-Atlantic region offers easy accessibility to TC Advertising's customers and to production facilities.

In order to provide customers with even greater convenience, TC Advertising operates a national network of production facilities. As a result, 94 percent of the U.S. population resides within a 250-mile radius of one of TC Advertising's facilities, guaranteeing quicker delivery and unparalleled convenience.

This national scope allows TC Advertising to produce ads that are targeted to specific regions of the country. For example, an advertising insert for a national retailer can be printed in several facilities across the United States in as many as 30 different versions—with each

version targeting specific merchandise for that region.

With its ongoing efforts to provide customers with a full range of advertising services, TC Advertising has made strategic acquisitions, and is developing innovative services such as Target Reach, a revolutionary software system that enables customers to target inserts to specific demographic audiences.

Through more than three decades of expansion and transformation, TC Advertising remains committed to helping its customers grow their businesses through quality, efficiency, and innovation.

Sylvan Learning Systems, Inc.

When Sylvan Learning Systems, Inc., one of the world's largest private providers of educational services, relocated its worldwide corporate headquarters in 1996 to Baltimore's Empowerment Zone, it was the first major public corporation to do so in two decades. Sylvan's relocation also was significant because it was the first step toward establishing Baltimore as an international hub for companies in the rapidly expanding for-profit educational services industry.

"I envision Baltimore as a kind of Silicon Valley for corporations in the education business," says Douglas Becker, co-CEO. "As Silicon Valley became the place to be if you were in the computer business, we believe Baltimore will be the place to be for those in education."

Sylvan Learning Systems has built its strong reputation in the field of supplementary educational programs through a commitment to high standards and rigorous attention to quality. The company's reputation for obtaining results in its Sylvan Learning Centers—both in retail locations and in schools—continues to fuel consistent growth. Through partnerships with educational institutions and organizations, such as Johns Hopkins University and the National Geographic Society, the company continues to explore new avenues for growth and new ways to provide supplementary education to students at all points on the academic spectrum.

Sylvan's goal is to become the world's leading "lifelong learning" company, able to seamlessly deliver educational and testing services to learners of all ages. Its services range from supplemental instruction for pre-K through 12th grade to pre- and postgraduate courses to professional development in the workplace. Combining the technologies of the information age—satellite technology, intranets, and the Internet—with a network of site-based learning centers, Sylvan is establishing worldwide distribution capabilities.

Success Begets Success

Sylvan's success rests on performance. Through its ability to achieve outstanding results in its Sylvan Learning Centers and school-based programs, the company first established a strong reputation in the field of supplemental education. That success fueled growth, enabling Sylvan to expand into the field of adult education and computer-based testing.

Sylvan's performance has earned it an outstanding reputation and prestigious partnerships in every area of its business, including major corporations, organizations, educational institutions, and associations. The synergy among the supplemental education programs, adult education divisions, and computer-testing arena is the cornerstone for the company's success.

As it continues to build market share and expand internationally, the company's ability to sustain its reputation for excellence will depend on one thing alone: Sylvan's ability to achieve results for each of its customers—for the schools, families, organizations, corporations, and individuals who use its services.

Creating New Markets

The company got its start in 1991, when Becker and R. Christopher Hoehn-Saric, co-CEO, purchased Sylvan Learning Centers, a then-struggling educational services firm, from Kinder-Care, Inc. Since then, Sylvan has expanded to more than 700 centers. Much more than a tutoring service, these individualized programs use a diagnostic and prescriptive approach to pinpointing students' academic strengths and weaknesses.

Currently, the Sylvan Learning Centers network is composed of hundreds of franchisees who are participating members of the communities in which they live and work, as well as dozens of company-owned centers. The network is expanding as existing franchisees open additional centers in their own territories and new franchisees join the network. Additionally,

SYLVAN'S INDIVIDUALIZED PROGRAMS USE A DIAGNOSTIC AND PRESCRIPTIVE APPROACH TO PINPOINTING STUDENTS' ACADEMIC STRENGTHS AND WEAKNESSES.

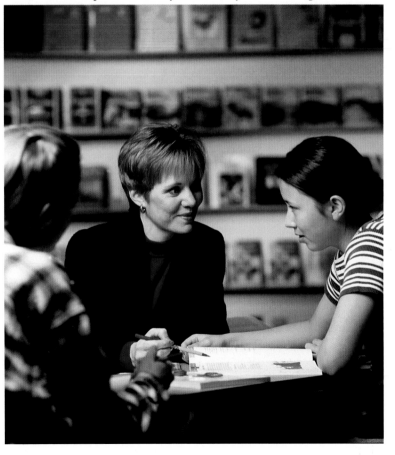

Sylvan is entering new regions outside of the United States, and franchise territories are now being created in Hong Kong, South Korea, China, Israel, and other areas. The company-owned Sylvan Learning Centers serve as "hubs of excellence" to demonstrate successful practices to franchisees.

Success through Partnership

Since its inception, Sylvan's strategy for growth has been to forge partnerships with the education establishment. The company has achieved tremendous success in finding ways to be a good partner to well-regarded, highly credible organizations.

In 1993, Sylvan forged its first partnership with a public school district when it was retained by Baltimore City Public Schools to provide supplemental education services to struggling students within five public elementary schools. Since then, the company's services to school districts have expanded to serve students in kindergarten through 12th grade in hundreds of public, private, and parochial schools across the United States. Sylvan supports the school curricula by focusing on the needs of struggling students, working with them individually to accelerate their learning and help them reenter the learning mainstream.

Through its partnerships with academic organizations, professional associations, and licensing bodies, Sylvan has grown into the leading global provider of computer-based testing services. The company has an exclusive relationship with Educational Testing Service (ETS) to deliver all ETS standardized tests that are computerized, including the Graduate Record Examination, the Graduate Management Admissions Test, the Test of English as a Foreign Language, professional tests for nurses and teachers, and many more. In addition, through its worldwide network of testing centers, Sylvan delivers computer-based tests to license and certify such professionals as doctors, architects, stockbrokers, insurance agents, airplane pilots, and more than 100 others. This experience in testing adults has paved the company's way toward educating and training

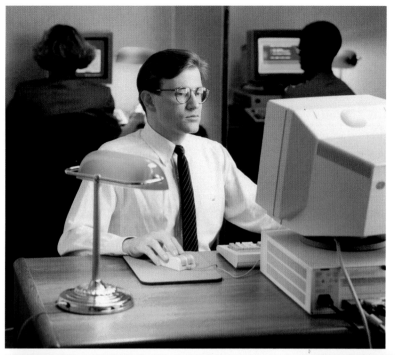

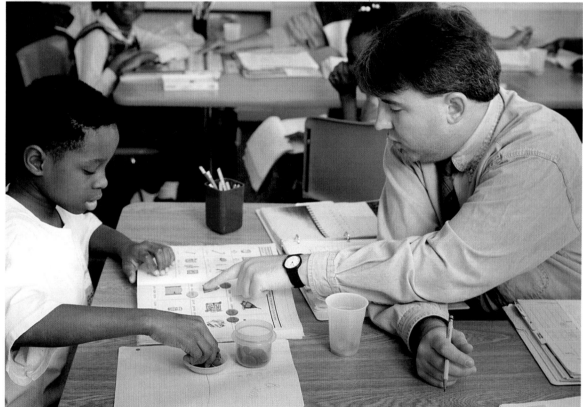

adults. In 1996, in a joint venture with MCI Communications Corporation, Sylvan established the world's first international distribution network for adult professional education and training—Caliber Learning Network, Inc.

Another important partnership has allowed the company to launch a first-of-its-kind education experience for students in grades three through eight. Together with the National Geographic Society, Sylvan offers MindSurf, an after-school program in which students participate in fun and educational activities at many elementary and middle schools throughout the Baltimore area and across the country.

Although it has set its sights on global industry leadership, Sylvan has not forgotten its roots. Recently, the company established the Sylvan Learning Foundation, which will award grants to support education projects throughout the United States. The foundation initially will focus on organizations located in its hometown of Baltimore.

SYLVAN SUPPORTS THE SCHOOL CURRICULA BY FOCUSING ON THE NEEDS OF STRUGGLING STUDENTS, WORKING WITH THEM INDIVIDUALLY TO ACCELERATE THEIR LEARNING AND HELP THEM REENTER THE LEARNING MAINSTREAM.

Baltimore Ravens

IN THEIR INAUGURAL SEASON OF 1996, THE BALTIMORE RAVENS HAD 10 SELLOUTS in 10 games and sold more than 54,000 season tickets. Indeed, the Ravens filled a tremendous void when NFL football was brought back to Charm City after a 13-year absence. ⌁ Ravens Head Coach Ted Marchibroda, one of the most popular coaches in the game of professional football, enjoys a historical

presence in Baltimore, holding a similar position with the Baltimore Colts from 1975 to 1979. His 1996 appointment as the head coach for the Ravens came 21 years to the day after his first head coaching position with the "old Colts."

Record-Breaking Support

The team name became official on March 29, 1996, when more than 33,748 callers to *The Baltimore Sun* voted to name the club the Ravens. It was a record-breaking response to *Sundial*, a popular interactive feature of the newspaper.

On June 5, the team announced its colors—black, purple, and metallic gold. A crowd of 4,000 fans joined members of the team and watched a fashion show with models dressed

in Ravens' colors at The Gallery at the Inner Harbor. To open the inaugural season's festivities in August, a football was passed through city neighborhoods and eventually delivered by Ravens' owner Art Modell into the hands of Mayor Kurt Schmoke at a massive gathering of fans at the Inner Harbor. A standing-room-only crowd of 3,700 came to a downtown hotel for the 1997 draft.

In response to this overwhelming support from the community, Modell established the Ravens Foundation for Families last year. Its mission is to contribute to charities and nonprofit organizations, thereby enhancing the quality of life of the numerous families, neighbors, and friends who have welcomed the team to Baltimore.

The Cream of the Crop

The Ravens' first NFL draft was viewed as a successful one, with the emergence of Jonathan Ogden, a Washingtonian and UCLA offensive lineman, who was named all-rookie in his first year. Ogden moved from left guard to his natural position at left tackle during the 1997 season. Linebacker Ray Lewis, the Ravens' second first-round selection in 1996, led the team's defense with 142 tackles. Quality new players like linebackers Peter Boulware and Jamie Sharper were drafted in 1997.

Quarterback Vinny Testaverde marked his first appearance in a Pro Bowl as a Baltimore Raven, following the 1996 season. Testaverde won the Baltimore Quarterback Club's Most Valuable Player award, finished second in the NFL in passing yards (4,177), and threw for 33 touchdowns (second in the NFL). His 88.7 quarterback rating was second in the American Football Conference and third in the NFL.

During the 1996-1997 season, the Ravens dedicated their final home game to Memorial Stadium as a tribute to the facility and to the American veterans the stadium honors. The team opens its 1998 season at the new stadium at Camden Yards.

DURING THE 1996 SEASON, THE RAVENS SOLD OUT ALL 10 OF THEIR HOME GAMES AND SOLD MORE THAN 54,000 SEASON TICKETS (TOP).

LED BY QUARTERBACK VINNY TESTAVERDE, WHO FINISHED SECOND IN THE 1996 NFL SEASON IN PASSING YARDS AND TOUCHDOWNS, THE RAVENS BROUGHT PROFESSIONAL FOOTBALL BACK TO BALTIMORE TO AN OVERWHELMING COMMUNITY RESPONSE. CONSTRUCTION IS NOW COMPLETE ON THE NEW STADIUM AT CAMDEN YARDS, WHERE THE TEAM OPENED ITS 1998 SEASON (BOTTOM RIGHT).

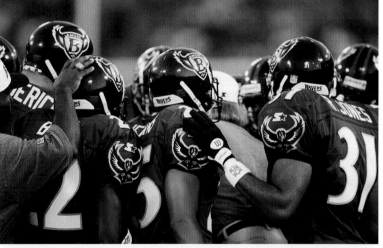

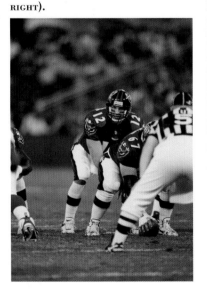

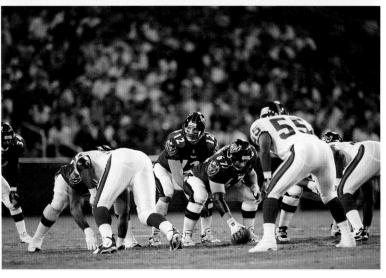

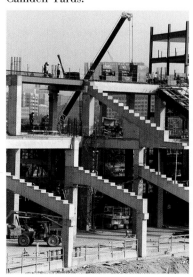

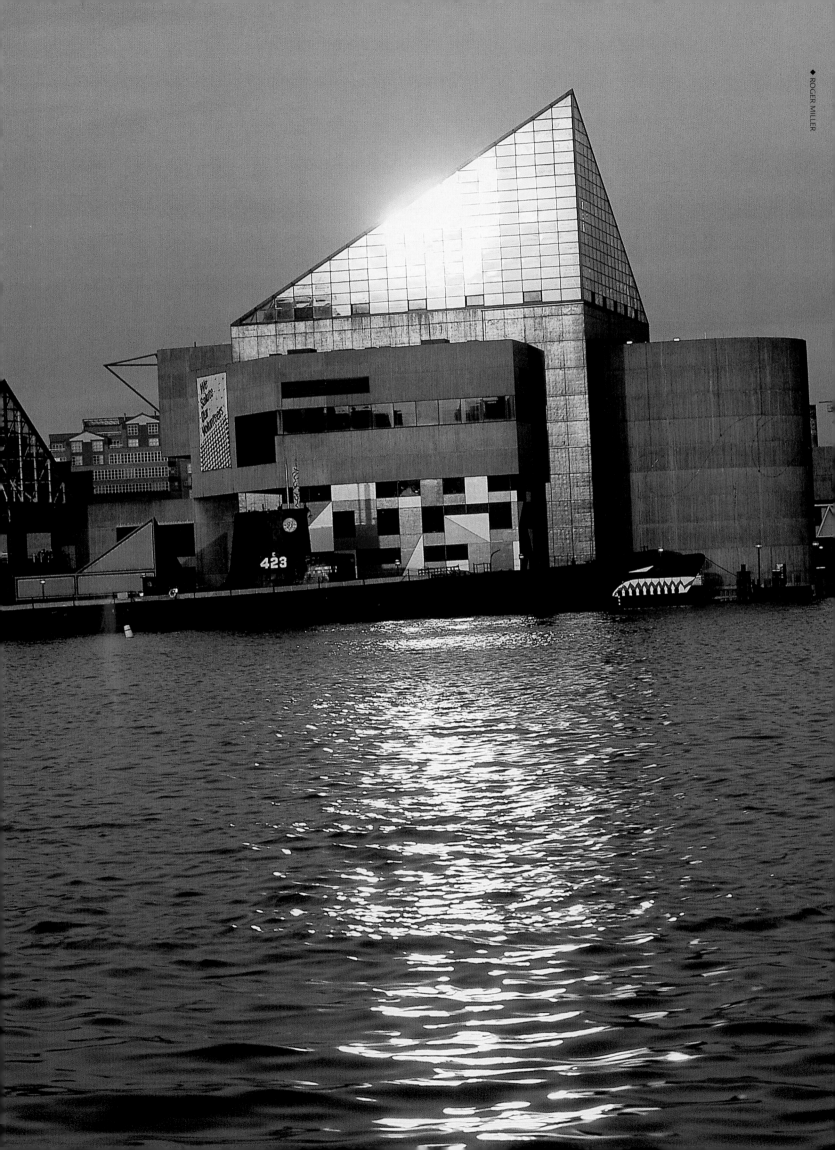

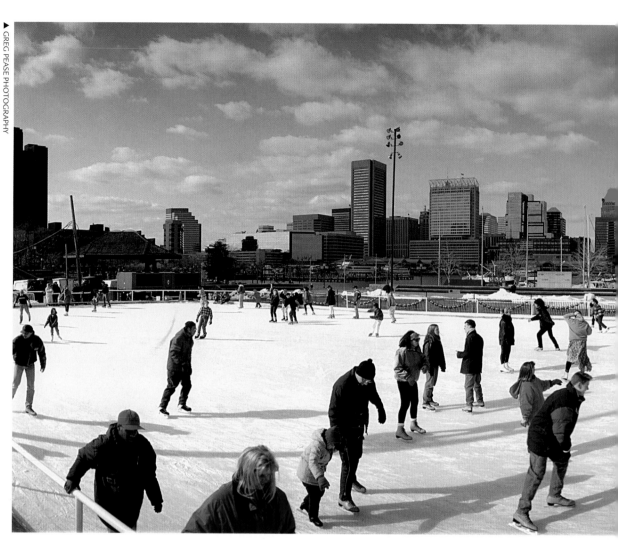

Photographers

STEVE BAKER is an internationally published photographer who has contributed to more than 100 publications. With a degree in journalism from Indiana University, he is the proprietor of Highlight Photography, specializing in assignments for such clients as Eastman Kodak, Nike, Budweiser, the U.S. Olympic Committee, and Mobil Oil, which has commissioned seven exhibitions of his work since 1994. Baker is author/photographer of *Racing Is Everything*, and he has contributed to two other Towery publications, *Indianapolis: Crossroads of the American Dream* and *Nashville: City of Note*. Currently, Baker resides in Indianapolis.

DAVE BOARMAN JR. was born in Baltimore and now lives just outside the city in Catonsville. Although he studied chemistry and physics at St. Mary's College of Maryland, he has decided to pursue a career in photography. Currently, Boarman does freelance work, and is employed by Roger Miller Photo, Ltd. He enjoys all areas of photography, but his strengths are in landscape and natural scenes. Boarman loves the outdoors, especially mountain biking and kayaking.

A. AUBREY BODINE was a Maryland institution for nearly 50 years until his death in 1970. A photographer for the *Baltimore Sunday Sun*, he was the subject of Johns Hopkins University Press' *A. Aubrey Bodine, Baltimore Pictorialist*. Some 10,000 of Bodine's images are featured in the Peale Museum alone.

NIKI BROWN, a native of Baltimore, recently graduated from the University of Maryland, Baltimore County where she studied photography for four years. Photographing architecture and people is Brown's main interest, but she also loves to capture abstract images on film. Currently, Brown is a manager at Festival Photo, and some of her recent projects have included taking pictures of local musicians and shooting portraits.

JIM BURGER, originally from Uniontown, Pennsylvania, has lived in Baltimore since 1978. He graduated cum laude from the Maryland Institute-College of Art

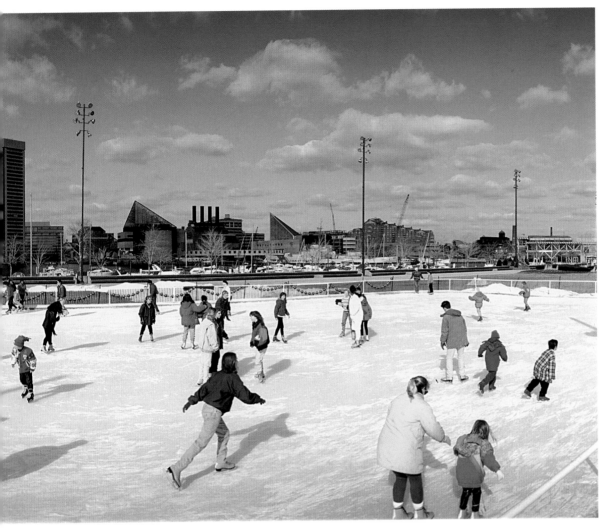

with a bachelor of fine arts. For several years, Burger served as a contributing photographer to *Baltimore City Paper* and ART-SCAPE. Presently, he works for *The Baltimore Sun*. In 1982, Burger received a Baltimore's Best Award for his work.

KELLY CONNELLY, a native of Baltimore, specializes in images of bands and musicians. She works for *Music Monthly* magazine and was voted Best Photographer in that publication's 1996 reader poll. Connelly graduated from New York University with a bachelor's degree in fine arts.

HOWARD DAVIS, a lifelong Baltimorean, is president of Davis Studios Inc., a full-service com-mercial advertising studio special-izing in photographs of people, products, and food. His clients include Black & Decker, Blue Cross/Blue Shield of Maryland, Amtrak, Maserati, Ramada Inns, and Westinghouse. Davis has received many awards for his work and is listed in *Who's Who in Advertising*.

MIDDLETON EVANS has dedicated his photography career to recording Maryland's diverse scenery, includ-ing everything from fishermen lobstering off the Ocean City coast to Amish farmers gathering maple sap in the state's Appalachian highlands. Recently, he released *Maryland's Great Outdoors*, a photojournal documenting the state's natural heritage, dramatic landscape, outdoor recreation, and vast array of wildlife. Evans is currently working on pictorial books on Baltimore and Maryland, as well as a natural heritage sample of the Mid-Atlantic region.

HENNY GARFUNKEL is a self-taught photographer who specializes in streetlife and people photography. Her work has been featured in *Entertainment Weekly*, *Newsweek*, *In Style*, *Interview*, *Harper's Bazaar*, and the *Village Voice*, among other publications. Origin-ally from Providence, Garfunkel graduated from the University of Rhode Island with a bachelor's degree in child psychology, and moved to New York City in the 1970s. ☛

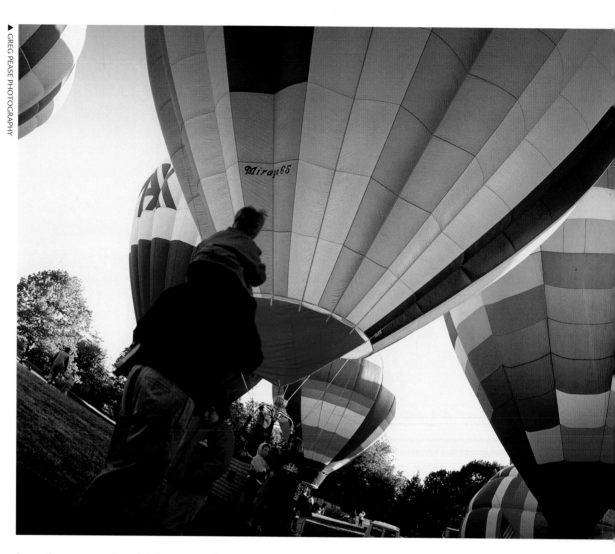

JULIE GREEN, a native of Tulsa, specializes in equine sports journalism and environmental investigations. Drawing on her education at the University of Missouri School of Journalism, as well as her studies under master photojournalist Alex Webb, Green has been published in 42 U.S. and 35 foreign newspapers; 12 books on equines; and *Guitar Player, Orion, Life*, and *Horse Illustrated* magazines.

BILL McALLEN is a freelance photographer and a lifelong resident of Baltimore. Between assignments, he enjoys exploring his hometown from behind the lens of a camera, seeking out the people who add vitality to the city—those who believe old buildings are worth saving and parks are essential. McAllen lives in Baltimore with his wife, Ellen, as well as two cats and four very rare South Baltimore terriers.

MIKE McGOVERN lives in Baltimore where he operates McGovern Photography. He specializes in portraits and institutional photo illustration, and his clients include *Baltimore Magazine*, the *Washington Post, Newsweek*, and several other magazines. A graduate of the Rhode Island School of Design, McGovern enjoys mountain biking.

NICHOLAS McINTOSH has been an amateur photographer since the late 1980s and has recently decided to make it his career. He works as a first assistant at Greg Pease & Associates, and his main photographic interests center around his first love, rock and roll. Currently, McIntosh plays drums in one band and bass in another. His photography has appeared in numerous fanzines and on several album covers.

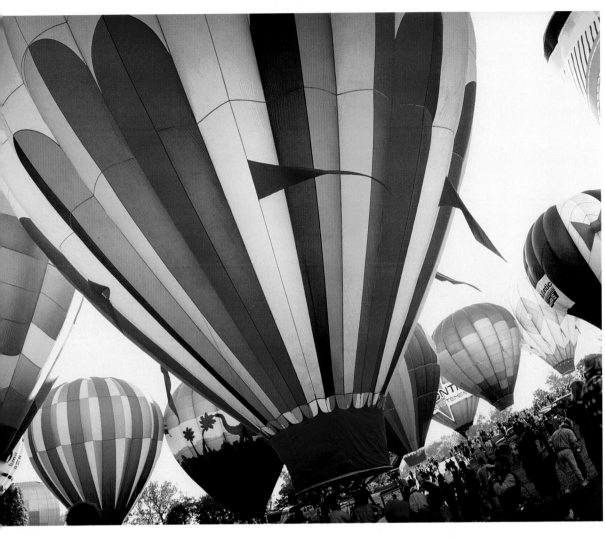

GREG PEASE is a Baltimore-based photographer specializing in corporate and industrial photography. Since beginning his career as a commercial photographer in 1974, he has won numerous awards, and his images have been published in books, magazines, and advertisements worldwide. Best known for his regional landscape and maritime photographs, Pease is coprincipal of Greg Pease & Associates with his wife, Kelly.

BOB SCHATZ, who lives and works in Nashville, specializes in corporate, advertising, and stock photography for such clients as DuPont, IBM, NationsBank, UPS,

and Service Merchandise. His images have been published in numerous magazines, including *Travel & Leisure*, *Business Week*, *Fortune*, and *Time*, as well as in Towery Publishing's *Memphis: New Visions, New Horizons* and *Nashville: City of Note*. Schatz is the recipient of numerous Addy awards, and has completed a monthlong assignment in Syria, Jordan, Israel, Greece, and Turkey.

JAMES D. SCHERLIS, a lifelong Baltimorean, studied at the University of Maryland and the University of Baltimore School of Law. The owner of James Scherlis Photography, he specializes in

editorial/feature, performing arts, and stock photography, as well as teaching and mentoring budding photographers. An internationally recognized cameraman, he is the official photographer for the National Symphony, Peabody Conservatory of Music, and Library of Congress Music Division.

Other photographers and organizations that contributed to *Baltimore: Charm City* include the Maryland Historical Society, Maryland State Archives, and Peter Owen.

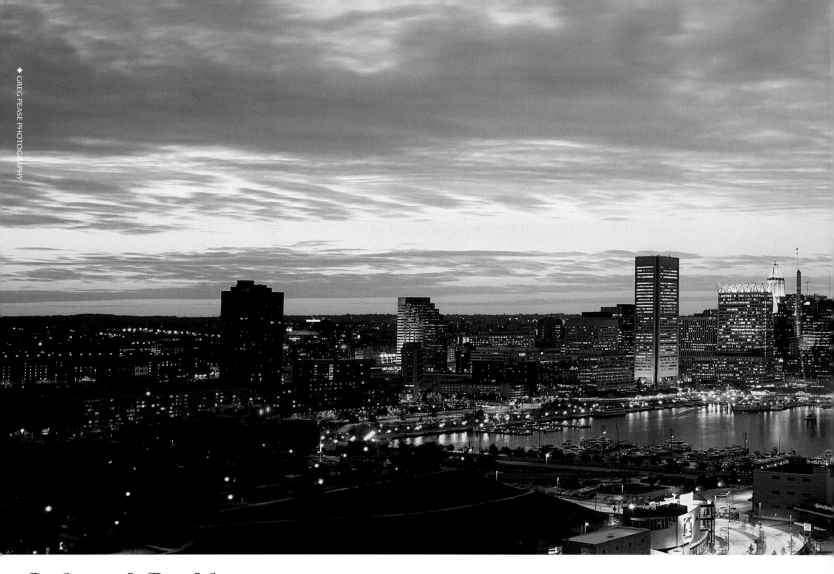

Index of Profiles

The Afro-American Company of Baltimore City, Inc. 278

Alban Tractor Co. Inc. 298

Annie E. Casey Foundation 386

Avesta Sheffield East Inc. 387

Baltimore Business Journal 346

Baltimore Life Insurance Co. 272

Baltimore Marriott Inner Harbor 356

The Baltimore Museum of Art 286

Baltimore Opera Company 294

Baltimore Ravens 392

Baltimore Spice, Inc. 312

The Baltimore Sun 260

Baltimore Symphony Orchestra 279

The Baltimore Zoo 268

Broadmead, Inc. 330

Cellular One 348

CIENA Corporation 378

Colliers Pinkard 292

ECS Technologies, Inc. 334

Edenwald/General German Aged People's Home, Inc. 269

Eisner Communications 310

Fila U.S.A., Inc. 350

Great Blacks In Wax Museum, Inc. 347

Guilford Pharmaceuticals Inc. 382

H&S Bakery 313

Harbor Court Hotel 362

Helix Health 368

HS Processing 370

Inphomation Communications, Inc. 376

Integrated Health Services, Inc. 366

International Youth Foundation 374

Johns Hopkins 270

Kaiser Permanente 358

Legg Mason, Inc. 282

Lever Brothers Company 289

Loyola College in Maryland 263

Management Recruiters of Baltimore/Timonium 332

Maryland Historical Society 262

Maryland Office Relocators 352

Maryland Science Center 329

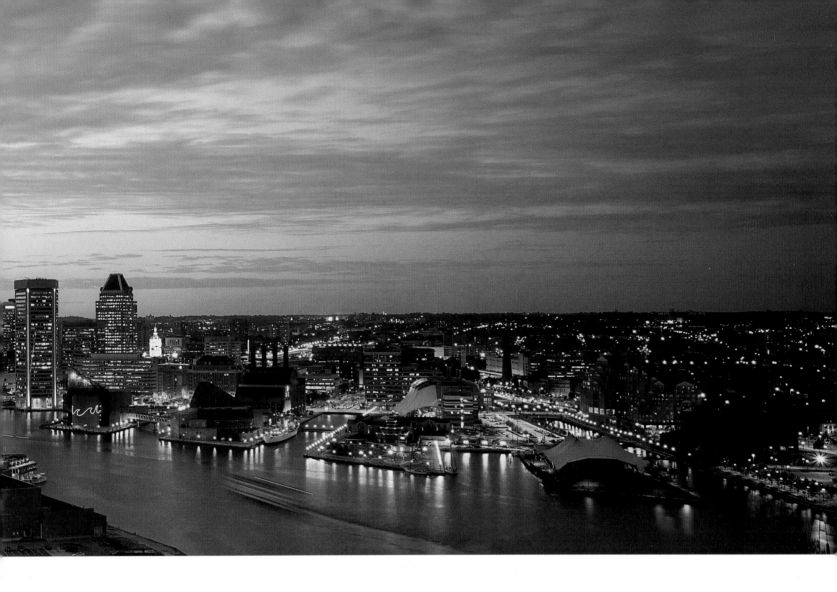

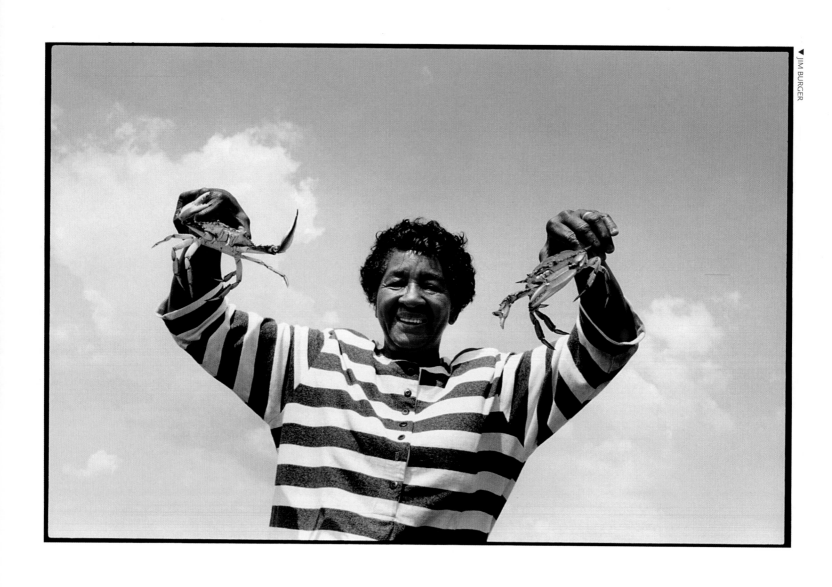